CONTRIBUTORS

ELLEN E. ANDERSON, M.D.

Instructor of Surgery, The Medical College of Pennsylvania, Philadelphia, Pennsylvania

Abdominal Procedures

JAY MORRIS ARENA, M.D.

Professor of Pediatrics and Director of the Poison Control Center, Duke Medical Center, Durham, North Carolina

Poisonings

SUBHASH C. BANSAL, M.D.

Associate Professor of Surgery and Director of Surgical Research, The Medical College of Pennsylvania, Philadelphia, Pennsylvania

Immunologic Alterations in Acute Illness and Injury

BÉLA BENCZE, M.D.

General Director, Hungarian National Emergency and Ambulance Service, Budapest, Hungary

EMS in Hungary

GARRETT E. BERGMAN, M.D.

Assistant Professor of Pediatrics, The Medical College of Pennsylvania, Philadelphia. Pennsylvania

Pediatric Emergencies

ROBERT E. BINDA, JR., M.D.

Assistant Professor, Department of Anesthesiology, University of Pittsburgh School of Medicine; Staff Anesthesiologist, Children's Hospital, Pittsburgh, Pennsylvania

Renal Failure and Fluid-Electrolyte Imbalance

WILLIAM FRANCIS BOUZARTH, M.D.

Clinical Professor of Neurological Surgery, The Medical College of Pennsylvania; Deputy Director, Department of Neurosurgery, Episcopal Hospital, Philadelphia, Pennsylvania

Neurosurgical Procedures; Head and Spinal Injuries; Disaster Preparedness

EDWARD L. BRADLEY, III, M.D.

Associate Professor of Surgery, Emory University School of Medicine; Attending Surgeon, Emory University Hospital; Attending Surgeon, Grady Memorial Hospital; Consultant, Atlanta Veterans Administration Hospital, Atlanta, Georgia

Alimentary Tract Obstruction

GARRY L. BRIESE

Executive Director, Florida Chapter, American College of Emergency Physicians, Jacksonville, Florida

EMS Transportation

RICHARD A. BROSE, Ph.D.

Associate Professor of Medicine, University of Missouri–Kansas City School of Medicine; Director, Emergency Medical Services Training and Research Center, University of Missouri–Kansas City School of Medicine, Kansas City, Missouri

Categorization of Emergency Facilities

JOHN BULETTE, M.D.

Assistant Professor, Department of Psychiatry, The Medical College of Pennsylvania, Philadelphia, Pennsylvania

Evaluation of the Potentially Suicidal Patient

FRANK M. CALIA, M.D.

Professor of Medicine, University of Maryland School of Medicine; Chief, Medical Service, Veterans Administration Hospital, Baltimore, Maryland

Infectious Diseases

GEORGE J. CARANASOS, M.D.

Associate Professor of Medicine, University of Florida, College of Medicine; Chief, Division of General Medicine, Shands Teaching Hospital, Gainesville, Florida

Drug Reactions

RICHARD WAYNE CARLSON, M.D., Ph.D.

Assistant Professor of Medicine and Assistant Director, Shock Research Unit and the Center for the Critically Ill, University of Southern California School of Medicine, Los Angeles County/USC Medical Center and the Hollywood Presbyterian Medical Center, Los Angeles, California

Cardiovascular System Failure

NANCY L. CAROLINE, M.D.

Medical Director, Magen David Adom, Tel Aviv, Israel

Acute Respiratory Insufficiency; Respiratory Care Techniques and Strategies

ELSIE R. CARRINGTON, M.D.

Professor and Chairman, Department of Obstetrics and Gynecology, The Medical College of Pennsylvania and Hospital of The Medical College of Pennsylvania, Philadelphia, Pennsylvania

Obstetric and Gynecologic Procedures

C. GENE CAYTEN, M.D., M.P.H.

Assistant Professor of Surgery, University of Pennsylvania School of Medicine; Director, Center for the Study of Emergency Health Services; Attending Surgeon, Hospital of the University of Pennsylvania, and Veterans Administration Hospital, Philadelphia, Pennsylvania

Traumatology; EMS Planning and Evaluation

YOGINDER K. CHITKARA, M.D.

Research Associate, Alma D. Morani Laboratory of Surgical Immunobiology, The Medical College of Pennsylvania, Philadelphia, Pennsylvania

Immunologic Alterations in Acute Illness and Injury

STEPHEN D. CLEMENTS, JR., M.D.

Assistant Professor of Medicine, Emory University School of Medicine; Attending Physician, Emory University Hospital, Atlanta, Georgia

Disorders Caused by Coronary Atherosclerotic Heart Disease; Effect of Electrolyte Abnormalities on the Electrocardiogram

LEONARD A. COBB, M.D.

Professor of Medicine, University of Washington; Director, Division of Cardiology, Harborview Medical Center, Seattle, Washington

Sudden Death

ERRIKOS CONSTANT, D.D.S., M.D., F.A.C.S.

Assistant Clinical Professor of Surgery, Michigan State University College of Human Medicine, East Lansing; Staff Surgeon (Plastic Surgery), Michigan State University Olin Health Center, East Lansing; Staff Surgeon (Plastic Surgery), Sparrow Hospital, St. Lawrence Hospital, Ingham Medical Center, Lansing, Michigan

Facial Trauma

MILTON CORN, M.D.

Professor of Internal Medicine, Georgetown University School of Medicine; Director, Emergency Department, Georgetown University Hospital, Washington, D.C.

Bleeding Disorders

R ADAMS COWLEY, M.D.

Professor of Thoracic and Cardiovascular Surgery, University of Maryland School of Medicine; Director, Maryland Institute for Emergency Medical Services, Baltimore, Maryland

Specialized Patient Care Units; Operating Rooms

ROBERT H. DAILEY, M.D.

Clinical Associate Professor of Medicine and Community and Ambulatory Medicine (Emergency Medicine), University of California at San Francisco; Chief, Department of Emergency Medicine, Valley Medical Center, Fresno, California

Difficulty in Breathing

JOHN K. DAVIDSON, M.D., Ph.D.

Professor of Medicine, Emory University School of Medicine; Director of Diabetes Unit, Grady Memorial Hospital, Atlanta, Georgia

Diabetic Ketoacidosis; Hyperglycemic States

WILLIAM E. DeMUTH, JR., M.D.

Professor of Surgery, The Pennsylvania State University College of Medicine, Philadelphia; General Surgeon, The Milton S. Hershey Medical Center, Hershey, Pennsylvania

Neck Trauma

ROBERT L. DONALD, M.D.

Clinical Assistant Professor of Medicine, University of Texas Medical School, Houston, Texas; former Chairman, Committee on Emergency Medical Services, American Medical Association, Texas Medical Association, and Harris County Medical Society; former Delegate from the AMA to the Commission on Emergency Medical Services; charter member of the American College of Emergency Physicians

EMS Transportation

MICHAEL E. ERVIN, M.D.

Assistant Clinical Professor, Wright State University School of Medicine; Director of Emergency Services, Miami Valley Hospital; Medical Director of Western Ohio Emergency Medical Services, Dayton, Ohio

Minor Surgical Procedures

RICHARD L. FABIAN, M.D.

Instructor in Otolaryngology, Harvard Medical School, Boston; Chief of Plastic Service and active staff member, Massachusetts Eye and Ear Infirmary, Boston; Chief of Surgery, E. K. Shriner Center for Mental Retardation, Waltham; Active Staff, N. E. Deaconess Hospital, Boston; Consultant in Otolaryngology, Veterans Administration Hospital, W. Roxbury, Massachusetts

Otolaryngologic Procedures

ALAN O. FEINGOLD, M.D.

Assistant Professor of Clinical Medicine, Emory University Medical School, Atlanta; Staff Physician, Dekalb General Hospital and Grady Memorial Hospital, Decatur, Georgia

Disorders of the Red Blood Cells; Splenomegaly

ROBERT DAVID FINK, M.D.

Clinical Associate Professor, Department of Psychiatry, University of Tennessee, Center for the Health Sciences; Superintendent, Memphis Mental Health Institute; Consulting Psychiatrist, Alcohol and Drug Dependence Clinic, Memphis Mental Health Institute, Memphis, Tennessee

Intoxication and the Alcohol Abstinence Syndrome

GERALD F. FLETCHER, M.D.

Professor of Internal Medicine (Cardiology), Emory University School of Medicine; Director of Internal Medicine, Georgia Baptist Hospital, Atlanta, Georgia

Insertion of a Temporary Transvenous Pacemaker

URI FREUND, M.D.

Hadassah Medical Center, Jerusalem, Israel

Cardiovascular System Failure

ARNOLD P. FRIEDMAN, M.D., F.A.C.P.

Professor of Neurology, University of Arizona Medical School; Attending Neurologist, Tucson Medical Center and St. Joseph's Hospital, Tucson, Arizona

Headache

AURÉL A. GÁBOR, M.D. (deceased)

Hungarian National Emergency and Ambulance Service, Budapest, Hungary

EMS in Hungary

JOHN T. GALAMBOS, M.D.

Professor of Medicine, Emory University School of Medicine; Chief of Gastroenterology, Grady Memorial Hospital; Associate Physician, Gastroenterology, Emory University Hospital, Atlanta, Georgia

Hepatic Disease

DONALD S. GANN, M.D.

Professor of Emergency Medicine, The Johns Hopkins University School of Medicine; Director, Division of Emergency Medicine, and Surgeon, The Johns Hopkins Hospital, Baltimore, Maryland

General Body Response to Trauma

JAMES G. GARRICK, M.D.

Head, Division of Sports Medicine, and Associate Professor, Department of Orthopedics, University of Washington, Seattle, Washington

Emergencies in Sports

JAMES E. GEORGE, M.D., J.D.

Emergency Physician, Underwood Memorial Hospital, Woodbury, New Jersey;
Board Member, American College of Emergency Physicians

Medicolegal Problems

JAMES E. GERACE, M.D., Maj., M.C.

Chief, Pulmonary Disease Service, Tripler Army Medical Center; Associate Clinical
Professor of Medicine, University of Hawaii; Visiting Pulmonologist, University of
Hawaii and Queens Medical Center, Honolulu, Hawaii

Near-Drowning

GEOFFREY GIBSON, Ph.D.

Associate Professor, The Johns Hopkins University School of Medicine and The
Johns Hopkins University School of Hygiene and Public Health, Baltimore, Maryland

Utilization of EMS

RAY W. GIFFORD, JR., M.D.

Head, Department of Hypertension and Nephrology, The Cleveland Clinic Foundation, Cleveland, Ohio

Hypertensive Crises

LEON GOLDMAN, M.D.

Professor and Chairman, Department of Dermatology; Director, Laser Laboratory,
University of Cincinnati Medical Center; Director, Dermatology, Cincinnati General
Hospital and Children's Hospital Medical Center, Cincinnati, Ohio

Laser and Microwave Injuries

ROBERTA BECKMAN GONZALEZ, M.D.

Clinical Associate in Medicine, University of Pennsylvania Medical School, Presbyterian University of Pennsylvania Hospital, and Graduate Hospital, Philadelphia,
Pennsylvania

Endocrinologic Problems

GARY J. GRAD, M.D.

Clinical Assistant Professor, Downstate Medical Center; Acting Director, Child and
Adolescent Outpatient Department, Kings County Hospital Center, Brooklyn, New
York

Psychiatric Emergencies

BARBARA HARTLEY GREENE, M.D.

Assistant Professor of Medicine, Emory University School of Medicine; Staff Physician, Grady Memorial Hospital, Atlanta, Georgia

Porphyrias; Pheochromocytoma

ARTHUR H. GRIFFITHS

Communications Specialist, Division of Emergency Medical Services, Public Health
Service, U.S. Department of Health, Education, and Welfare, Washington, D.C.

EMS Communications

WILLIAM F. HAMILTON, Ph.D.

Associate Professor of Decision Sciences and Management, Wharton School, University of Pennsylvania; Associate Director, Leonard Davis Institute of Health and Economics, University of Pennsylvania, Philadelphia, Pennsylvania

Financing the EMS

LINTON C. HOPKINS, M.D.

Assistant Professor of Neurology, Emory University School of Medicine; Attending Neurologist, Emory University Hospital and Grady Memorial Hospital, Atlanta, Georgia

Neuromuscular Diseases

J. WILLIS HURST, M.D.

Professor and Chairman, Department of Medicine, Emory University School of Medicine, Atlanta, Georgia

Chest Pain

LOREN A. JOHNSON, M.D.

Instructor in Emergency Medical Technology, Orange Coast College, Costa Mesa; Emergency Physician, Saint Francis Hospital, Lynwood, California

Trauma Due to Cold; Toxic Bites and Stings

E. JEFF JUSTIS, JR., M.D.

Clinical Assistant Professor of Orthopaedic Surgery, University of Tennessee College of Medicine; Consultant in Hand Surgery to Tennessee and Mississippi Crippled Children Services; Active Staff, The Campbell Clinic, Baptist Memorial Hospital, City of Memphis Hospital; Consulting Staff, LeBonheur Hospital and Arlington Hospital, Memphis, Tennessee

Trauma to the Hand

ALAN S. KAPLAN, M.D., M.P.H.

Director, Professional Programs, Office of the Assistant Commissioner for Professional and Consumer Programs, Food and Drug Administration, Rockville, Maryland

Legislative Aspects of Emergency Care

LESTER KARAFIN, M.D., F.A.C.S.

Professor of Urology, The Medical College of Pennsylvania; Clinical Professor of Urology, Temple University Medical Center; Chief, Section of Urology, Hospital of The Medical College of Pennsylvania; Attending Urologist, Temple University Hospital and St. Christopher's Hospital for Children, Philadelphia, Pennsylvania

Genitourinary Injuries

DOROTHY KARANDANIS, M.D.

Assistant Professor of Medicine, Emory University School of Medicine, Atlanta, Georgia

Diseases of Veins

JAMES W. KELLER, M.D.

Assistant Professor of Medicine, Emory University School of Medicine; Attending Hematologist and Medical Oncologist, Emory University Hospital and Grady Memorial Hospital, Atlanta, Georgia

Disorders of Leukocytes

ROBERT R. KELLY, M.D.

Emergency Physician, Salem Memorial Hospital, Salem, Oregon

Pericarditis

A. RICHARD KENDALL, M.D.

Professor and Chairman, Department of Urology, Temple University School of Medicine; Clinical Professor of Urology and Attending Urologist, The Medical College of Pennsylvania; Attending Urologist, St. Christopher's Hospital for Children, Philadelphia, Pennsylvania

Genitourinary Injuries

THOMAS C. KENNEDY, M.C.P.

Staff Associate, Center for the Study of Emergency Health Services, University of Pennsylvania, Philadelphia, Pennsylvania

Accident Prevention, Consumer Education and Community Involvement in EMS

YEHEZKIEL KISHON, M.D.

Lecturer in Internal Medicine, University of Tel-Aviv Medical School; Associate Director, Heart Institute, Sheba Medical Center, Tel-Hashomer, Israel

EMS in Tel-Aviv

NATHAN S. KLINE, M.D., F.A.C.P., F.R.C.Psych.

Director, Rockland Research Institute, Orangeburg; Clinical Professor of Psychiatry, College of Physicians and Surgeons, Columbia University, New York; Attending Physician, Lenox Hill Hospital, New York, New York

Psychiatric Emergencies

DAVID HOWARD KNOTT, M.D., Ph.D.

Clinical Associate Professor, Department of Psychiatry, University of Tennessee Center for the Health Sciences; Medical Director, Alcohol and Drug Dependence Clinic, Memphis Mental Health Institute; Assistant Superintendent, Research and Training, Memphis Mental Health Institute, Memphis, Tennessee

Intoxication and the Alcohol Abstinence Syndrome

WILLIAM G. LAVELLE, M.D.

Instructor in Otolaryngology, Harvard Medical School, Boston; Chief of Otolaryngology, Whidden Memorial Hospital, Everett; Active Staff, Massachusetts Eye and Ear Infirmary and Children's Hospital Medical Center, Boston, Massachusetts

Otolaryngologic Procedures

JEFFREY A. LEONARD, M.D.

Clinical Associate Professor, Department of Psychiatry, University of Pennsylvania, Attending Psychiatrist, Institute of Pennsylvania Hospital, Philadelphia, Pennsylvania

Headache

ROBERT L. LEOPOLD, M.D.

Professor of Psychiatry, School of Medicine; Professor of Health Care Systems, Wharton School; University of Pennsylvania, Attending Psychiatrist, Hospital of the University of Pennsylvania; Associate Neurologist, Psychiatrist, Graduate Hospital of the University of Pennsylvania; Attending Psychiatrist, Institute of Pennsylvania Hospital, Philadelphia, Pennsylvania

Crisis Intervention Services

DAVID G. LEVINE, M.D.

Assistant Clinical Professor of Psychiatry, School of Medicine, University of California, San Francisco; Mental Health Director and Program Chief, Community Mental Health Services, Marin County, California

Alcohol and Drug Abuse

JEAN-PIERRE LINDENMAYER, M.D.

Assistant Professor of Psychiatry, State University of New York; Acting Director, Psychiatric Inpatient Service, University Hospital, Downstate Medical Center, Brooklyn, New York

Psychiatric Emergencies

JOSEPH LINDSAY, JR., M.D.

Professor of Medicine, Division of Cardiology, The George Washington University School of Medicine; Director of Coronary Care Unit, George Washington University Hospital, Washington, D.C.

Aorta and Peripheral Arteries

GEORGE I. LITMAN, M.D.

Chairman, Sub-council of Cardiology, Northeastern Ohio Universities College of Medicine; Chief, Cardiology Service, Akron General Medical Center, Akron, Ohio

Use of Flow-Directed Balloon Tipped Catheter

GERALD L. LOONEY, M.D., M.P.H.

Assistant Professor, Department of Emergency Medicine, University of Southern California School of Medicine; Attending Staff, LAC-USC Medical Center; Director of Emergency Department, Glendale Adventist Medical Center, Glendale, California

EMS Manpower and Training; Education in the Emergency Department

MILTON N. LURIA, M.D.

Professor of Medicine and Health Services, University of Rochester School of Medicine and Dentistry; Physician, Strong Memorial Hospital, Rochester, New York

Syncope

WILLIAM R. MacAUSLAND, JR., M.D.

Associate Clinical Professor in Orthopaedic Surgery, Harvard Medical School; Assistant Clinical Professor in Orthopaedic Surgery, Tufts University Medical School, Boston, Massachusetts

Orthopedic Procedures; Trauma to Extremities and Soft Tissues

JAMES ROBERTSON MACKENZIE, M.D., F.R.C.S.(C.), F.A.C.S.

Assistant Clinical Professor of Surgery, McMaster University; Active Staff, Hamilton General Hospital; Chief of Emergency Department and active staff member, Chedoke General Hospital; Associate Staff Member, McMaster University Medical Center, Hamilton, Ontario, Canada

Abdominal Trauma

KARL G. MANGOLD, M.D.

Clinical Instructor, University of California, San Francisco; Vice President, American College of Emergency Physicians; Director, Department of Emergency Medicine, Vesper Memorial Hospital, San Leandro, California

Financing the Emergency Department

BENEDICT S. MANISCALCO, M.D.

Assistant Professor of Medicine (Cardiology), University of South Florida College of Medicine, Tampa, Florida

Cardiogenic Shock

JOHN P. MARIANO, B.S.

Emergency Medical Services Coordinator, Philadelphia Department of Public Health, Philadelphia, Pennsylvania

Disaster Preparedness

FRANK I. MARLOWE, M.D.

Associate Professor of Otolaryngology, The Medical College of Pennsylvania; Staff, Hospital of The Medical College of Pennsylvania; Staff, Presbyterian–University of Pennsylvania Medical Center; Consultant, Naval Regional Medical Center, Philadelphia, Pennsylvania

Vertigo

KENNETH L. MATTOX, M.D.

Assistant Professor of Surgery, Cora and Webb Mading Department of Surgery, Baylor College of Medicine; Deputy Surgeon-in-Chief and Director of Emergency Surgical Services, Ben Taub General Hospital, Houston, Texas

Hemoptysis

LEON MENZER, M.D.

Instructor in Neurology, Harvard Medical School; Instructor in Neurology, Tufts University Medical School; Assisting Physician in Neurology, Boston City Hospital, Boston, Massachusetts

Convulsions

SYLVIA H. MICIK, M.D.

Associate Professor, Clinical Pediatrics and Community Medicine, University of California School of Medicine, La Jolla; Director of Emergency Medical Services, San Diego; Attending Physician, University of California Medical Center, San Diego, California

Poison Control Centers

JAMES DEWITT MILLS, JR., M.D.

Clinical Instructor in Medicine, Georgetown University, Washington, D.C.; Chairman, Emergency Department, Mt. Vernon Hospital, and Emergency Department, Alexandria Hospital, Alexandria, Virginia

Organization and Staffing of the Emergency Department

JOHN A. MONCRIEF, M.D.

Professor of Surgery, Medical University of South Carolina, Charleston, South Carolina

Burns

WILLIAM W. MONTGOMERY, M.D.

Professor of Otolaryngology, Harvard Medical School; Senior Surgeon in Otolaryngology, Massachusetts Eye and Ear Infirmary; Chief, Head and Neck Tumor Clinic, Massachusetts General Hospital and Massachusetts Eye and Ear Infirmary; Consultant in Otolaryngology, Children's Hospital Medical Center, Boston, Massachusetts

Otolaryngologic Procedures

JACK COLBERT MORGAN, M.D.

Clinical Instructor, Department of Psychiatry, University of Tennessee Center for the Health Sciences, Memphis, Tennessee

Intoxication and the Alcohol Abstinence Syndrome

GARY G. NICHOLAS, M.D.

Assistant Professor of Surgery, The Pennsylvania State University College of Medicine, Philadelphia; General Surgeon, The Milton S. Hershey Medical Center, Hershey, Pennsylvania

Trauma to the Neck

EDDY D. PALMER, M.D.

Clinical Professor of Medicine, Rutgers Medical School, Piscataway; Attending Physician, Hackettstown Community Hospital, Hackettstown, New Jersey

Hematemesis and Melena

LEONARD F. PELTIER, M.D., Ph.D.

Professor of Surgery, University of Arizona College of Medicine; Chief, Orthopedics, Arizona Medical Center, Veterans Administration Hospital, Tucson, Arizona

Fat Embolism

THOMAS N. PERLOFF, M.Sc.

Associate Director, Urban Health Services Center, University of Pennsylvania, Philadelphia, Pennsylvania

The Health Maintenance Organization; National Health Insurance

ROBERT PAUL PROULX, M.D.

Associate Professor, Los Angeles County/USC Medical Center; Emergency Department Physician, St. Joseph Medical Center, Burbank, California

Heart Distress

JOHN JOSEPH PURCELL, JR., M.D.

Assistant Clinical Professor of Ophthalmology and Director of Cornea Service, Saint Louis University School of Medicine; Director of Cornea and External Disease Service, Saint Louis University Hospitals and Saint Mary's Hospital, Saint Louis, Missouri

Examination of the Eye and Its Adnexa; Ocular Trauma

JONATHAN E. RHOADS, JR., M.D.

Assistant Professor of Surgery and Attending Surgeon, The Medical College of Pennsylvania; Chief of Surgery, Philadelphia Veterans Administration Hospital, Philadelphia, Pennsylvania

Vascular Procedures

ARTHUR E. RIKLI, M.D., M.P.H.

Professor, Department of Community Health and Medical Practice, University of Missouri, Columbia, Missouri

Tokyo EMS

JAMES R. ROBERTS, M.D.

Instructor of Emergency Medicine, The Medical College of Pennsylvania; Attending Physician, Department of Emergency Medicine, Frankfort Hospital, Philadelphia, Pennsylvania

Snakebites

PETER ROSEN, M.D.

Director, Division of Emergency Medicine, Department of Health and Hospitals, Arizona Medical Center, Veterans Administration Hospital, Tucson, Arizona

Hypovolemic Shock

CONSTANTINE C. ROUSSI, M.D.

Chairman, Department of Emergency Medicine, Akron General Medical Center, Akron, Ohio

Diarrhea

ROBERT BARRY RUTHERFORD, M.D.

Associate Professor of Surgery, University of Colorado Medical School; Associate Professor of Surgery, Colorado General Hospital, Denver, Colorado

Trauma to the Peripheral Vascular System

G. ANTHONY RYAN, M.D., B.S., M.P.H.

Senior Lecturer, Department of Social and Preventive Medicine, Monash University, Melbourne, Australia

EMS in Australia

THOMAS D. SABIN, M.D.

Associate Professor of Neurology, Boston University; Director, Neurologic Unit, Boston City Hospital, Boston, Massachusetts

Coma; Confusion; Convulsions; Neurologic Emergencies

ALFRED M. SADLER, JR., M.D.

Clinical fellow in medicine at Harvard Medical School, Department of Internal Medicine; Resident Physician, Department of Medicine, Massachusetts General Hospital, Boston, Massachusetts

Emergency Medical Services in Perspective

BLAIR L. SADLER, J.D.

Vice President, Scripps Clinic and Research Foundation; Director, Green Hospital of Scripps Clinic, California

Emergency Medical Services in Perspective

ARTHUR P. SAFRAN, M.D.

Assistant Professor of Medicine, Instructor in Neurology, Boston University; Instructor in Neurology, Tufts University; Lecturer on Neurology, Harvard University, Boston; Staff, The Framingham Union Hospital, Framingham; Staff, Neurological Unit, Boston City Hospital, Boston, Massachusetts

Confusion

ATEF A. SALAM, M.D.

Associate Professor of Surgery, Emory University School of Medicine; Director of Vascular Surgery Service, Grady Memorial Hospital, Atlanta, Georgia

Upper Gastrointestinal Bleeding

HERBERT STANLEY SHUBIN, M.D. (deceased)

Associate Professor of Medicine and Associate Director, Shock Research Unit and the Center for the Critically Ill, University of Southern California School of Medicine, Los Angeles County/USC Medical Center and the Hollywood Presbyterian Medical Center, Los Angeles, California

Cardiovascular System Failure

HARVEY M. SILVERMAN, M.D.

Emergency Physician, Springfield Hospital, Springfield, Vermont

Smoke Inhalation

MARK E. SILVERMAN, M.D.

Associate Professor of Medicine (Cardiology), Emory University School of Medicine; Attending Cardiologist, Grady Memorial Hospital and Piedmont Hospital, Atlanta, Georgia

Arrhythmias

DAVID P. SIMMONS, M.D.

Clinical Instructor in Orthopaedic Surgery, Harvard Medical School, Boston, Massachusetts

Orthopedic Procedures; Trauma to Extremities and Soft Tissues

HOWARD M. SIMONS, M.D.

Assistant Dermatologist, University of Pennsylvania School of Medicine, Philadelphia; Physician-in-Chief, Dermatology Department, Abington Memorial Hospital, Abington; Attending Dermatologist, Doylestown Hospital, Doylestown, and Warminster General Hospital, Warminster, Pennsylvania

Pruritus; Dermatologic Emergencies

ALVIN J. SLOVIN, M.D.

Assistant Professor of Surgery, The George Washington University School of Medicine, Washington, D.C.

Vascular Emergencies

GEORGE L. SPAETH, M.D.

Professor of Ophthalmology, Jefferson Medical College; Director of Glaucoma Service and Attending Surgeon, Wills Eye Hospital; Associate Ophthalmologist, Graduate Hospital, Philadelphia, Pennsylvania

Examination of the Eye and Its Adnexa; Ocular Trauma

H. HARLAN STONE, M.D.

Professor of Surgery, Emory University School of Medicine; Chief of Trauma, Burn, and Pediatric Surgical Services at Grady Memorial Hospital; Attending Surgeon, Emory University Hospital, Atlanta, Georgia

Gastrointestinal Emergencies; Gastrointestinal Inflammations

CHARLES HERBERT STUART-HARRIS, M.D., D.Sc., F.R.C.P.

Professor and Postgraduate Dean of Medicine, The University of Sheffield, Sheffield, England

Atmospheric Pollution

PANAGIOTIS N. SYMBAS, M.D.

Professor of Surgery, Thoracic and Cardiovascular Surgery Division, Emory University School of Medicine; Director, Thoracic and Cardiovascular Surgery Department, Grady Memorial Hospital; Attending Surgeon, Emory University and Veterans Administration Hospital, Atlanta, Georgia

Chest and Heart Injuries

J. WILLIAM THOMAS, M.B.A.

Lecturer, Wharton School, and Associate Director, Center for the Study of Emergency Health Services, University of Pennsylvania, Philadelphia, Pennsylvania

EMS Planning and Evaluation

THORSTEN THOR

Managing Director, SPRI (The Swedish Planning and Rationalization Institute), Stockholm, Sweden

Stockholm EMS

JAMES R. UNGAR, M.D.

Attending Physician, Department of Family Practice, Los Alamitos General Hospital, Los Alamitos, California

Respiratory Emergencies

GEORGE L. VOELZ, M.D.

Health Division Leader, University of California, Los Alamos Scientific Laboratory, Los Alamos, New Mexico

Radiation Injury

JULIAN A. WALLER, M.D., M.P.H.

Professor and Chairman, Department of Epidemiology and Environmental Health, University of Vermont College of Medicine; Consultant in Injury Control and Emergency Medical Services, Vermont Health Department, Burlington, Vermont

Epidemiologic Factors

STEPHEN G. WAXMAN, M.D., Ph.D.

Assistant Professor of Neurology, Harvard Medical School, and Visiting Assistant Professor of Experimental Neurology (Biology), Massachusetts Institute of Technology, Cambridge; Assistant Neurologist, Beth Israel Hospital, Boston, Massachusetts

Coma

SAMUEL B. WEBB, JR., Ph.D.

Associate Professor of Public Health and Director of the Program in Hospital Administration, Department of Epidemiology and Public Health, Yale University School of Medicine, New Haven, Connecticut

Emergency Medical Services in Perspective

MAX HARRY WEIL, M.D., Ph.D.

Clinical Professor of Medicine and Biomedical Engineering and Director of the Shock Research Unit and the Center for the Critically Ill, University of Southern California School of Medicine, Los Angeles County/USC Medical Center and the Hollywood Presbyterian Medical Center, Los Angeles, California

Cardiovascular System Failure

NANETTE K. WENGER, M.D.

Professor of Medicine (Cardiology), Emory University School of Medicine; Director, Cardiac Clinics, Grady Memorial Hospital, Atlanta, Georgia

Pulmonary Embolism

ROBERT L. WHIPPLE, III, M.D.

Clinical Assistant Professor of Medicine (Cardiology), Emory University School of Medicine, Atlanta, Georgia

Cardiogenic Shock

C. H. WILSON, JR., M.D.

Professor of Medicine and Director, Division of Rheumatology–Immunology, Emory University School of Medicine; Attending Physician and Chief of Rheumatology, Grady Memorial Hospital and Emory University Hospital, Consultant and Chief of Rheumatology, Atlanta Veterans Administration Hospital, Atlanta, Georgia

Acute Arthritis

JACLYNE M. WITTE, B.A.

Research Assistant, Massachusetts Eye and Ear Infirmary, Boston, Massachusetts

Otolaryngologic Procedures

ROBERT J. WOLFSON, M.D.

Professor and Head, Division of Otolaryngology, The Medical College of Pennsylvania, Associate in Otolaryngology, Presbyterian Hospital, University of Pennsylvania Medical Center, Philadelphia, Pennsylvania

Vertigo

THEODORE E. WOODWARD, M.D.

Professor and Head, Department of Medicine, University of Maryland School of Medicine, Baltimore, Maryland

Infectious Disease

MOHAMMED T. YOUNIS, M.D., M.S. (surgery)

Assistant Professor of Surgery, The Medical College of Pennsylvania; Attending Surgeon and Director of the Surgical Intensive Care Unit, Hospital of The Medical College of Pennsylvania; Consultant, Veterans Administration Hospital, Philadelphia, Pennsylvania

Evaluation of Acute Abdominal Pain

PREFACE

Before the book there is the Preface. But before either book or Preface, there is the idea of the book. Dr. George Schwartz, himself an emergency physician and teacher, recognized in the early 1970s that there was a need for a comprehensive textbook of emergency medicine. The literature of this burgeoning discipline had, up to that point, consisted largely of manuals, handbooks, and periodicals. What was needed was far different: a book that would of necessity be large; a book that would begin with pathophysiology and end with the patient; a book that would address itself to the entire spectrum of care in the emergency department: minor and major, undifferentiated and clear-cut, medical and surgical. Epidemiologic, administrative, and legal aspects would also be covered. In short, it was to be a book that would help codify this rapidly growing field.

The editorial staff first met almost five years ago to plan in detail the contents of such a book. In view of the diversity of subject matter, it seemed wise to engage the efforts of diverse editors, all intimately involved in emergency medicine, each with his special area of expertise: an emergency physician, an anesthesiologist/critical care physician, who established the first physician fellowship program in critical care medicine, an internist/cardiologist, an internist with special knowledge of emergency medical care systems, and a surgeon who had established one of the first emergency medicine residencies in the United States. Each editor then took responsibility for selection of contributors from across the country.

The overall outline of the text deserves mention. Part I analyzes mechanisms of vital organ failure and death. It addresses the pathophysiology of such problems and the therapeutic methods for reversal. Part II is devoted to the fundamental procedures and techniques needed for effective care of the seriously threatened patient. Part III is divided into three sections: the first considers some common patient presentations, chosen because of their frequency and importance in everyday practice; the second section is concerned with management of the traumatized patient and special problems of trauma; the third describes the management of the patient who becomes suddenly and seriously ill for reasons other than trauma. Part IV describes the organizational aspects of providing appropriate emergency care: the out-of-hospital services, the epidemiology, information flow, communications, transportation, and the systems development needed to "take the health services system to the patient." Also addressed in this section is the organization of the acute care capacity of the hospital itself; in addition there is a brief description of foreign models of emergency medical service. The book concludes with a consideration of the legal and legislative issues in emergency medicine and with a broad view of the psycho-socio-economic aspects of the field.

Although the book is written for physicians with varied training and experience working in emergency departments, some concepts conveyed apply also to the short-term management of patients with acutely life-threatening conditions in prehospital settings. Some procedures which, for safe performance, require skills beyond those taught in emergency medicine are not covered.

In one sense, a Preface is a misnomer: though it is placed before the rest of the book, it is always written after the book is ready. Nevertheless, what we wanted to say before, we are quite happy to be able to say afterward.

THE EDITORS

ACKNOWLEDGMENTS

To the Contributors go our special thanks for many things. Their individual aims were on target and came out of many physician years of concern with the problems of the patient in the emergency department. Many of the contributors are deeply involved in the education of residents in emergency medicine. Others are no less committed, by way of the traditional disciplines, to improving the care of the patients in the emergency department.

Appreciation is certainly due Brian Decker, Medical Editor at W. B. Saunders Company, for his sensitive guidance and trust during the development of this book. John Dyson of Saunders copyedited the manuscripts and his experienced hand aided greatly. In addition, thanks are due Andrew J. Piernock, Jr., and the Saunders production crew, whose skill can be seen on every page.

Many persons were involved in the joyful labor of bringing forth this textbook. In acknowledgment of some of the people who helped and without whom this book would not have been possible, Dr. George Schwartz thanks his secretaries, Valerie McDaniels, Kathleen McNamee, and particularly Pat Fredericks; his family — Loretta, Ruth, and Rebecca; Dr. Waldo Nelson and Dr. Howard Kirz for their inspiration; and in the final stages Patricia Parkinson. Dr. Peter Safar is grateful to Eva, Philip, and Paul. Dr. John Stone thanks his secretary, Mae Nelson, and his family: Lu, Johnny, and Jim, who understood. The section on emergency medical systems, together with the organizational, legislative, and legal aspects of emergency care, could not have been done without the inspired help of Dr. Joseph A. Fortuna, who knew where everybody was and what they were doing. The complexity of managing the entire transaction with the multiple contributors to this section was resolved through the organizing capability of Nancy J. Wink, M.S.N. Also, Dr. David Wagner gratefully acknowledges the residents — wherein the future begins.

CONTENTS

VOLUME 1

PART III CLINICAL EMERGENCY MEDICINE

SECTION 1 – EVALUATION OF SELECTED COMMON PRESENTATIONS

SECTION 2 — TRAUMATIC EMERGENCIES

VOLUME 2

SECTION 3 – NONTRAUMATIC MEDICAL AND SURGICAL EMERGENCIES

Chapter 40
RESPIRATORY EMERGENCIES.. 855
James R. Ungar

Chapter 41
CARDIAC EMERGENCIES 890

Section 3

Chapter 40

RESPIRATORY EMERGENCIES

James R. Ungar

AIRWAY OBSTRUCTION

For practical purposes airway obstruction may be considered as arising from blockage of normal airflow at any point in the respiratory tract. It represents one of the gravest emergencies encountered by physicians and paramedical personnel alike.

The emergent nature of the obstruction in the airway is a function of several factors, including the location and degree of compromise of the airway at that particular location, the premorbid cardiopulmonary status of the patient, and the rapidity with which the obstruction develops.

Recognition

Regardless of the predisposing factors, the greatest therapeutic gift that the victim of airway obstruction can receive is to have his rescuers recognize that an obstructed airway exists in the first place. In keeping with this train of thought, it is interesting that the first line of defense in airway obstruction management usually is not the emergency physician but the lay individual, since most airway obstructions do not originate in the Emergency Department. Whereas temporizing emergency measures frequently are adequate to sustain patients who have suffered obstructions distal to the carina, the paramount importance of on-the-scene emergency maneuvers to open and maintain patency of a completely obstructed upper airway cannot be overemphasized. In the latter instance, the alternative to successful resuscitative efforts invariably leads to frantic transport of an asphyxiating patient, who more often than not is either dead on arrival at the emergency care center or so badly brain-damaged from anoxia that even the most heroic resuscitative efforts are fruitless. It stands clear that the general public must be made more cognizant of the emergency maneuvers for establishing and clearing the obstructed airway before we can hope to improve the mortality and morbidity associated with this catastrophic event. The responsibility for educating both paramedical and lay individuals rests in the hands of the emergency physician as an extension of his role.

Airway obstructions can be divided into two major categories: (1) obstructions superior to the carina which, by their anatomic location, embarrass influx of inspired air to the point where expedient emergency measures are required for the victim's survival; and (2) airway obstructions distal to the carina which compromise airflow in the bronchi or smaller airways, and as such usually are not so immediately life-threatening.

UPPER AIRWAY OBSTRUCTION

Upper airway obstruction in the strict sense involves blockage of airflow superior to the larynx, but we shall stretch the definition somewhat so that it encompasses all the airways proximal to the tracheal bifurcation.

Causes

By far the most common cause of upper airway obstruction is anatomic blockage of the posterior pharynx by the tongue during states of unconsciousness. In this state the tongue relaxes and falls backward against the throat, while at the same time the head falls forward on the chest and adds to the obstructive element. Other common causes of upper airway obstruction include disease states such as severe tonsillitis: swelling of the soft tissues (especially laryngeal) as occurs in angioneurotic edema; material such as vomitus, mucus, blood, teeth, or dentures in the upper airway; and extrinsic elements such as food, trinkets, and toys. Diphtheria, although rare, can be a very serious cause of obstruction.

Recognition

At times a partially obstructed airway can be recognized by labored breathing or excessive respiratory efforts, often involving the accessory muscles of respiration, and by soft tissue retractions of the intercostal, supraclavicular, and suprasternal spaces. In complete, or nearly complete, upper airway obstruction (more often than not due to a foreign body) there is tremendous inspiratory effort on the part of the patient, who may have his head thrown backward. The patient frequently is cyanotic and exhibits signs of choking such as distention of the eyes, bulging of the lips, and salivation. He may attempt to cough, but usually does not do so. The accessory respiratory muscles are extremely active, and paradoxical breathing also may be noted in which the chest sinks on inspiration while the abdomen rises (with the reverse sequence occurring on expiration). Despite these efforts, no air is moved. After a peridod of time that varies with the pre-incidental arterial oxygen content, respiratory effort ceases. After a further period of time, cardiac arrhythmias develop that eventually progress to a fatal ventricular arrhythmia. Death caused by a foreign body obstructing the upper airway is at times extremely rapid; it implies that hypoxemia is not the only lethal factor, but that vasovagal

responses from afferent vagal stimulation can cause cardiac arrest (which, of course, must still be contended with even if the offending foreign body is removed expeditiously).

The "Café Coronary"

A mechanism for sudden demise by upper airway obstruction entails the inhalation of large boluses of food. Traditionally, this has been reported as occurring in the middle-aged denture-wearer who, while attending a luncheon or dinner, has too many drinks and then attempts to swallow too large a piece of food. This becomes lodged in his upper airway, causing a total obstruction. Because of either hypoxia or the above-mentioned vagal-induced cardiac arrest mechanism, the patient collapses and is thought by those around to have sustained a "coronary." In fact this type of airway obstruction secondary to food inhalation has been called the "café coronary." There should be an extremely high index of suspicion of asphyxiation as being the cause of sudden collapse in a restaurant or at the dinner table, and the most important predisposing factor appears not to be age, dentures, or type of food, but the patient's state of sobriety. If manual removal is not possible and no instruments are available, the Heimlich maneuver has been successful.*

Resuscitation of Patients with Upper Airway Obstructions

The most important factor for successful resuscitation is immediate opening of the airway. This is accomplished by hyperextending the head, and sometimes this simple maneuver is all that is required to relieve upper airway obstruction (i.e., the tongue). To perform the head tilt, it is necessary to have the victim on his back. The rescuer places one hand under the patient's neck and his other hand on the forehead; while lifting up on the neck, pressure is exerted upon the forehead in the opposite direction. By hyperextending the head and neck, the tongue is drawn anteriorly from the posterior

*See pages 187 and 857.

pharynx, and this component of anatomic obstruction is relieved. The head tilt method is satisfactory for relieving the great majority of anatomic upper airway obstructions. If, however, the air-passage still is not opened adequately, additional forward displacement of the mandible may be required, using the "triple-airway maneuver." This entails the rescuer placing his fingers behind the victim's mandibles, and (1) forcefully displacing the mandible anteriorly, while (2) tilting the head backward, and (3) using his thumbs to retract the lower lip, allowing rescue breathing to be performed through the mouth as well as through the nose.* If, after the airway is sufficiently open, the patient remains apneic, artificial ventilation must be started immediately.

There are some modifications for opening the airway in small children and infants. The most important difference lies in the anatomic variance of the child's neck and trachea. The neck of a small child or infant is so pliable that it can easily be overextended; at the same time, the cartilaginous support of the trachea is significantly less than in older children, aldolescents, and adults. Thus, airways can be compressed readily by exaggerating the head tilt, and instead of relieving the anatomic obstruction, an iatrogenic one can be created in its place.

It is imperative that caution be exercised to avoid extension of the neck in cases in which there is a likelihood of cervical spine fracture. In this circumstance, the airway is opened using a modification of the jaw-thrust maneuver, in which the rescuer places his hands on either side of the patient's head and maintains it there in a fixed neutral position. The mandible is displaced anteriorly, using the index fingers. If intubation is necessary, nasotracheal intubation is preferred.

Unless there is an extremely high index of suspicion, the rescuer should not waste time looking for foreign bodies in the upper airway. The presence of upper airway obstruction caused by a foreign body will become more than evident upon initial attempts at ventilating the patient. If (1) the airway has been opened properly, (2) the victim is not breathing spontaneously, and (3) the rescuer is unable to inflate the lungs

by rescue breathing, an immediate attempt should be made to clear the airway with the fingers. The patient is rolled onto his side away from the rescuer, whose knee is placed under the victim's shoulders for support. The patient's mouth is opened, using the thumb and index finger working in opposing directions for leverage, while the rescuer's other hand is free to finger-sweep the mouth and pharynx of the victim in an attempt to clear the obstructing mass. Repeated attempts may be required. This technique is all well and good, provided the rescuer's fingers are long enough to reach the occluding object. Many restaurants and places of public dining have been stimulated to acquire large plastic forceps, called appropriately enough "choke-savers." Essentially they function to extend the useful range of the fingers for extricating foreign bodies that have lodged in the upper airway, but are too deep for digital removal. The forceps is introduced into the mouth and as deeply as possible into the posterior pharynx; the ends then are brought into apposition, and the forceps removed in one continuous motion. There has been significant vocal objection from members of the medical profession regarding the use of this instrument by lay individuals because of potential trauma. However, a laceration of the pharynx, tonsillar pillar, or soft palate is a fair trade for the patient's life. In the Emergency Department, one can replace the "choke-saver" with a long curved Kelly clamp or Magill forceps.

If these maneuvers are unsuccessful in clearing the airway, the victim should be rolled on his side toward the rescuer, who then delivers sharp blows to the interscapular region with the heel of his hand. After each blow, and before artificial ventilation is attempted, the patient's mouth should be probed to detect any foreign body that may have been dislodged in the process. The procedure is that of Henry J. Heimlich, who advocates the use of sudden increases in intrathoracic pressure to produce forceful expulsion of endotracheal foreign bodies. His technique essentially entails sharp upward elevation of the diaphragm, frequently inducible by sharp, sudden, and forceful abdominal compression. In the adult this can be performed by placing the arms around the patient's abdomen from behind, interlocking the hands, and applying the force in the epigastrium (similar to a short yet forceful

*See also Procedure, page 188.

"bear-hug"). A somewhat safer procedure is to perform the maneuver with the arms around the midchest. In the infant, similar results may be obtained by sharp, inward squeezing of the lower thoracic cage, or a sharp blow to the midback. The working hypothesis of the technique lies in the suggestion that most inhaled foreign bodies lodge at a point in the slightly downward-tapering larynx at a point too narrow for further passage of the bolus. Impaction occurs only in the "inspirational" direction, resulting in early asphyxia, since the body lodges in the larynx after exhalation and during early inspiration. The net result leaves the victim with very little in the way of effective tidal volume to expel or cough up the occluding object. There is, however, enough residual volume of air in the lungs adequately to dislodge the foreign body if the chest or abdomen is forcefully and rapidly compressed. Although still somewhat controversial, the Heimlich procedure at least makes sense in theory—certainly it is better than letting a patient choke to death through fear of breaking ribs, lacerating a liver, or trying a procedure that has yet to become deeply entrenched into the folklore of medical "recipes." Many successful foreign body expulsions have been reported as a result of the Heimlich maneuver, and in life-threatening obstruction the procedure should be attempted.

Tracheostomy and Cricothyreotomy

If all the foregoing efforts are unsuccessful, the remaining courses of action are tracheostomy or cricothyreotomy. The latter is the more easily performed procedure for the lay person. Here, the cricothyroid space is palpated between the laryngeal prominence and the cricoid cartilage.* A knife or other sharp instrument suitable for making an incision is employed. The sharp tip of the instrument at hand is placed transversely, exactly in the midline, and pressed firmly through the skin and membrane to a depth of about 2 cm. Even if the knife is introduced too deeply it most likely will come to rest harmlessly against the posterior aspect of the cricoid cartilage, missing the esopha-

---

*See also Procedure, page 420.

gus below and the vocal cords above. The stoma then is dilated and, if necessary, may be enlarged by extending both ends of the incision tranversely. A cannula or suitable substitute then is inserted into the airway and fastened to the neck as required. If dictated by circumstances, rescue breathing may be performed directly over the wound.

AIRWAY OBSTRUCTIONS DISTAL TO THE CARINA

Most endobronchial foreign bodies occur in children who suddenly inspire while they have foreign bodies in their mouths. Common examples of aspirated foreign bodies include vegetable fragments such as beans, peanuts, carrots, or corn; additional items may be nails, pins, screws, thumbtacks, and other small metallic objects. Although sensory afferents produce an expulsive cough when the surface of the upper airway is stimulated, these particular nerve endings do not extend below the carina, so that relatively large foreign bodies can lodge below this level and give no sign of their presence. Usually, however, characteristic symptoms of an endobronchial foreign body do occur, and essentially consist of (1) recurrent spasmodic cough, with periods of quiescence between spasms; (2) an audible wheeze, usually heard during both inspiration and expiration; and (3) increasing dyspnea.

Often, the characteristic wheeze can be heard without a stethoscope by placing the ear on the patient's chest or close to his open lips.

If the time is taken to elicit a careful history, almost all instances of aspiration will be found to have been preceded by an episode of sudden coughing and choking that marked the moment of occurrence. After such an episode there usually is a delay of anytime from several hours to days before the classic triad of symptoms becomes manifest. In certain instances, when a relatively inert small nonmetallic foreign body is aspirated, the only finding is that of asymptomatic atelectasis, found on routine roentgenogram or in the evaluation of mild recurrent cough. It should be noted that the aluminum "flip-tops" on cans visualize poorly on x-ray.

Additional valuable information can be

obtained by careful auscultation and percussion of the chest. The chest findings vary according to the type of bronchial obstruction present. If the foreign body has produced complete bronchial obstruction, the concomitant is atelectasis, which results in decreased or absent breath sounds and dullness to percussion over the involved lung field. If the atelectasis involves a large amount of lung tissue (lobar involvement or greater), there will be a mediastinal shift toward the obstructed side. In many instances of partial bronchial obstruction, air is permitted access to the alveoli, but is prevented from passing out proximal to the obstruction because of a ball-valve obstructing mechanism. This results in obstructive emphysema of the involved lung segment. Breath sounds are distant to absent; percussion reveals hyper-resonance on the affected side, and chest x-ray shows a mediastinal shift to the opposite side (DeWeese and Saunders, 1973*). A ball-valve obstruction in a major bronchus produces early signs of dyspnea, and may require prompt intervention to prevent death from asphyxia. The involved lung becomes emphysematous, and the mediastinal shift to the opposite side may compress the uninvolved lung sufficiently to cause respiratory insufficiency.

Opaque foreign bodies usually are visible on chest x-rays. When atelectasis is present, the cardinal sign on chest roentgenogram is clouding of the atelectatic segment. In the instance where an entire lung is atelectatic, there will also be narrowing of the intercostal spaces and elevation of the ipsilateral hemidiaphragm. The mediastinum shifts to the involved side. When obstructive emphysema is present, the involved lung is overaerated and the mediastinum is shifted to the opposite side. Regardless of the direction of the mediastinal shift, it frequently is easier to see under fluoroscopy than in a single roentgenogram. It is best to obtain both inspiratory and expiratory films (plain) of the chest when an endobronchial foreign body is suspected. In atelectasis, the mediastinal shift is seen in the inspiratory view when the uninvolved lung is full of air; in obstructive emphysema, the shift to the opposite side is noted during expiration when the lung is partially empty.

*Figure 15, p. 165.

Foreign bodies of the bronchi are best removed through a bronchoscope. In infants and small children, bronchoscopy is best performed without general anesthesia, especially if significant respiratory difficulty has already developed. Oxygen must always be delivered through the bronchoscope, since the instrumentation involved further compromises the caliber of the airway. On occasion, it is necessary to discontinue attempts at removal of a foreign body if the procedure is prolonged. A later attempt, after the child has been given a period of rest with supplemental oxygen, may insure a safer procedure.

On occasion, sharp metallic foreign bodies that have gone undetected for months or years can erode the bronchus in which they have lodged and enter the pulmonary parenchyma to produce a lung abscess. When this occurs, the abscess must be drained and the foreign body removed by a transthoracic approach.

Use of Postural Drainage

A recently revived technique for the initial management of foreign bodies in the bronchi is that of postural drainage. Coupled with chest physiotherapy for the first 24 hours after the aspiration has been detected, this has been employed successfully when the patient is not in respiratory distress. The rationale here is that gravitational assistance occasionally can move a foreign body to a point in the respiratory tract where it can be either spontaneously expectorated or made more accessible to endoscopic removal. During the 24-hour period, bronchodilators are inhaled hourly for five minutes at a time, and antibiotics are given if indicated. At the end of that period, endoscopic removal is performed if the foreign body has not dislodged spontaneously.

It is important not to overestimate the ease with which foreign bodes can be retrieved by bronchoscopy. In small infants, in particular, it can be quite hazardous. Most smaller hospitals do not stock the 3-mm. bronchoscope needed for a child less than 1 year old. Furthermore, good forceps to pass through these bronchoscopes are a fairly recent development. Even if the procedure is successful, the attendant complications of pneumonia, cardiac arrest, pneumomediastinum, and atelectasis should always be anticipated. In some instances, thoracotomy is the only way to remove the offending object.

DECOMPENSATED CHRONIC OBSTRUCTIVE PULMONARY DISEASE

Chronic obstructive pulmonary disease, usually the result of repeated chronic and acute bronchitis with eventual tissue damage, scarring, and alveolar hyperinflation, may result in chronic hypoxia and retention of carbon dioxide.

With hypercapnia the respiratory center may lose the sensitivity to the normal CO_2 drive to respiration, leaving the hypoxic drive as dominant. Giving high levels of oxygen may abolish this drive to respiration sufficiently to produce a period of apnea. Thus, carefully monitored oxygen delivery is essential. Care must be taken with the use of morphine and similar drugs that reduce the sensitivity of the medullary respiratory center to CO_2.

Other problems in such patients include secondary polycythemia and increased blood viscosity. Pulmonary hypertension may develop due to increased pulmonary vascular resistance, with eventual cor pulmonale. Bleb formation may occur on the lung surface, and with rupture a pneumothorax occurs; if this is a tension pneumothorax, it can be rapidly lethal.

Emergency Treatment of Pulmonary Emphysema

Most patients with COPD in fact have both chronic bronchitis and emphysema. The differentiation between these two conditions is of academic interest but of little clinical importance. Prognosis is a function of degree of airway obstruction and severity of the clinical condition, not one of classification. In addition, the treatment of COPD is symptomatic at any stage, and management is based on the presenting symptoms, regardless of clinical diagnosis. Therefore, for practical purposes, the treatment of a severe bronchitic is identical to that of a patient with obstructive emphysema.

Treatment of Acute Respiratory Failure in COPD

Acute respiratory failure in COPD is directly correlated with an inability to maintain an adequate alveolar ventilation. Many of the general features of treatment of this complication have been discussed in the section on acute respiratory failure.*

The decision to employ mechanical ventilation in COPD is not an easy one to make, and must be based on an over-all clinical appraisal of the patient's status, including signs of breathlessness, airway obstruction, and accumulation of tracheobronchial secretions. The most important factor in deciding on a specific aid to ventilation is the patient's sensorium. Conservative measures are much preferred in the alert patient, regardless of the disturbances in arterial blood gases. On the other hand, intubation and mechanical ventilation are indicated in a case of acute respiratory acidosis in a patient with a depressed sensorium that renders him unable to cooperate.

Treatment Without Intubation

The preferred first step in a patient with reasonably intact sensorium is that of low flow oxygen, either by nasal cannula at 1 to 2 liters per minute, or by Venturi mask, usually at 24 to 28 per cent ambient oxygen. The aim of therapy is to restore the PaO_2 to around 60 to 70 mm. Hg without causing undue respiratory suppression and attendant hypercapnia. If the $PaCO_2$ begins to rise under this management, it can be relieved to some degree by IPPB treatments administered for 15 to 30 minutes at a time and repeated every three to six hours as necessary. Contained within the IPPB treatments should be sympathomimetics nebulized by the respirator; a cardiac monitor is necessary to detect any arrhythmia. It is advantageous to deliver large tidal volumes during IPPB treatment, since improvement of alveolar ventilation is one of the prime objectives of IPPB therapy in acute respiratory failure.

---

*See Chapter 3.

Pneumothorax is an absolute contraindication to IPPB therapy, unless a chest tube is in place. Severe bullous emphysema presents a relative contraindication.

Parenteral xanthine derivatives and corticosteroids are given by continuous I.V. infusion. A suggested dosage is 500 mg. hydrocortisone and 1000 mg. aminophylline added to 1000 ml. of 5 per cent dextrose in water and run in over a 24-hour period. An initial I.V. loading dose of 100 to 200 mg. of hydrocortisone will induce a more rapid reversal of severe bronchospasm.

Effective tracheobronchial toilet is of utmost importance. Chest physiotherapy should be instituted as soon as possible. Nasotracheal suction is indicated in the patient who is unable to clear his tracheobronchial secretions. Postural drainage may produce copious amounts of sputum.

Antibiotics are indicated in the patient who presents with evident infection of an acute nature in the bronchopulmonary system. If pneumonia is present, and the causative agent cannot be identified from an expectorated sputum sample, transtracheal aspiration can be done, or bronchoscopy with selective collection of lower airway secretions should be performed for culture and sensitivity. However, if bronchospasm is present, such procedures may worsen the condition and should be deferred. Until such cultures are done, an initial choice of antibiotic should be broad spectrum, such as cephalothin or ampicillin.

Congestive heart failure should be treated promptly and vigorously with diuretics and digitalis, even if there is only a suspicion that this process is occurring, since the normal radiographic findings in congestive heart failure might be absent in the patient with COPD. Cor pulmonale is difficult to treat effectively, although some clinical response certainly will occur with this regimen.

Management of the patient with acute respiratory failure requires close monitoring of cardiac rhythm, vital signs, arterial blood gases, and mental status in order effectively to follow the progress of the therapeutic regimen and to recognize the indications for endotracheal intubation. An important sign of deterioration in the patient's condition is alteration of mental status. Although the restless, agitated, combative, and sometimes paranoid patient is difficult to control, it may be vital to determine whether such a state is resulting from hypoxia.

Treatment Requiring Endotracheal Intubation

The purpose of endotracheal intubation is to provide: (1) the conduit for a respirator to supply optimal alveolar ventilation; and (2) improved tracheobronchial toilet.

The patient remains intubated until he is able to achieve effective ventilation spontaneously.

The major indications for endotracheal intubation are deterioration of the patient's mental status, and inability effectively to clear retained tracheobronchial secretions. A cuffed endotracheal tube is inserted, either by nasal or oral routes, and is attached to a volume-limited respirator. The lowest inspired oxygen concentration that can maintain the PaO_2 between 55 and 75 mm. Hg is employed, to minimize the dangers of oxygen toxicity. Resistive efforts to mechanical ventilation on the part of the patient should be counteracted by the use of sedatives or opiates, and the respiratory rate and tidal volume delivered to the patient should be adjusted to prevent too rapid a fall in $PaCO_2$. These patients quite frequently are predisposed to concomitant hypokalemic, hypochloremic metabolic alkalosis, and as such require administration of acidifying agents such as ammonium chloride, potassium chloride, and acetazolamide. Too rapid lowering of the $PaCO_2$, without first correcting the metabolic alkalosis, can precipitate fatal alkalotic encephalopathy.

The goal of therapy should be to restore a normal pH, rather than a normal PCO_2. Frequent blood gas determinations are mandatory, especially in patients on assisted ventilation. The results should be available within minutes so that appropriate changes can be rapidly instituted. Immediately after intubation, a chest roentgenogram should be obtained to insure correct positioning of the endotracheal tube. The cuff of the tube should be deflated for 20 to 30 seconds every four hours to minimize tracheal damage as much as possible. As a rule, tracheostomy should be performed after three days if extubation cannot be expected in the first four to five days.

RESPIRATORY EMERGENCIES ASSOCIATED WITH ASTHMA AND THE CHRONIC OBSTRUCTIVE PULMONARY DISEASES

Bronchial Asthma

Asthma is a *symptom complex* of varied etiology characterized by exaggerated responsiveness of the trachea and bronchi to various stimuli, and is manifested by difficulty in breathing caused by generalized narrowing of the airways associated with bronchospasm, mucosal edema, and retained secretions. Some authorities consider the element of reversibility to be important.

A number of factors, working alone or in combination with one another, are known to contribute to the development and precipitation of the asthmatic process. These include hereditary factors, histopathologic associations (IgE), and physiologic abnormalities of the airways that cause them to over-react to a number of stimuli totally harmless to a non-asthmatic Infectious process of the upper airway, emotional and endocrine factors, exposure to allergens or nonspecific irritants, air pollution, and even exercise are known to precipitate bronchospasm and wheezing. The two main categories, *intrinsic* (inciting cause within a person's own body) and *extrinsic* (reactive to external inducer), have been used frequently to help to classify the condition. The differentiation, of course, relates not so much to treatment of the acute episode as to prevention, which may be quite difficult, particularly when emotional upsets trigger attacks. At present, there is little one can do to control the autonomic nervous system reaction, although biofeedback techniques may offer future progress in therapy.

Regardless of the inciting factor (intrinsic or extrinsic), the final common pathway often reveals a similar clinical picture of acute attack in each patient, despite differences in the primary cause.

Asthma, then, is a symptom complex of varied etiology characterized by exaggerated responsiveness of the bronchi to various stimuli, which results in obstruction of the lower airways and dyspnea.

PATHOPHYSIOLOGY OF THE ACUTE ASTHMATIC ATTACK

Airway obstruction is the hallmark of the acute asthmatic episode, and is due primarily to three major factors: *edema; bronchospasm;* and *retained secretions*. The contribution of these factors to the attack may differ, with resultant variation of response to therapy. For example, if the major component is bronchospastic, relief of the spasm will rapidly relieve the symptoms. On the other hand, if there has been prolonged mucosal edema and tenacious mucus, relief of bronchospasm may offer comparatively little physiologic relief, and therapy must focus on reducing edema and freeing secretions.

The net effect of the asthma attack is that of increased resistance to airflow, which results in decreased pulmonary compliance and subsequent diminution of the effective forces of expiration to a point necessitating the use of accessory respiratory muscles. The additional expiratory forces result in a marked increase in transpulmonary pressure. Excessive small airway closure supervenes, which increases the obstructive component. Hyperinflation of the lungs consequently occurs, producing increased residual volume and increased alveolar dead-space, with a marked diminution in alveolar ventilation. Airway obstruction results in alteration of ventilation/perfusion relationships.

Hypoxemia develops early, and the patient initially compensates by hyperventilation, resulting in a decreased $PaCO_2$. If airway obstruction progresses, or as respiratory muscles fatigue, alveolar hypoventilation becomes generalized, with concomitant CO_2 retention and respiratory acidosis. Hypoxemia is worsened by the increased amount of oxygen consumed as a result of the increased work of breathing. The finding of a rising PCO_2 is indicative of respiratory fatigue , and a picture of acute respiratory failure may develop.

As the situation becomes critical, the derangements in blood gases and acid-base balance produce profound upsets in metabolism and in the function of multiple organ systems. Cardiac arrhythmias and even arrest may be precipitated by the severe hypoxemia, hypercapnia, and acidosis—particularly in a patient whose heart has been sensitized previously by inhalants such as isoproterenol.

The hypoxemia and acidosis produce pulmonary vasoconstriction leading to right ventricular overload and right heart failure, which further accentuates the ventilation/perfusion mismatching through alveolar hypoperfusion. The marked hypercapnia causes cerebral cortical depression, cerebral vasodilatation, and increased intracranial pressure.

MANAGEMENT OF THE ACUTE ASTHMATIC ATTACK

Effective asthmatic therapy is aimed at:
(1) reversing bronchospasm;
(2) improving alveolar ventilation;
(3) liquefying intrabronchial secretions and decreasing mucosal edema; and
(4) minimizing anxiety.

Oxygen is basic therapy in almost all cases, but unless it is humidified, undesirable drying of secretions will occur. Acidbase disturbances usually are corrected with improvement of ventilation, but at times correction of pH with bicarbonate is necessary.

TREATMENT

Therapy must be individualized, owing to the variability in the contribution of the derangements (bronchospasm, edema, secretions) to the episode from patient to patient, as well as variability in patient response. A recording spirometer may be used to evaluate objective response to therapy.

A patient may feel better without a substantial change in ventilatory mechanics, and certainly disappearance of wheezing is a potentially unreliable sign, since this reflects phenomena of larger airways. In more severe cases, objective evidence of response can be obtained through serial arterial blood gas measurements.

PHARMACOLOGIC AGENTS EMPLOYED

Epinephrine. This usually is the most effective agent in reducing the symptoms of an acute attack. Its action is primarily upon the bronchospastic component. It also seems to counteract fatiguing respiratory muscles. Epinephrine, however, is associated with side-effects, and must be used with caution

in the elderly. The presence of heart disease or hypertension also limits its use. For adults without heart disease, 0.3 to 0.5 cc. of a 1/1000 aqueous epinephrine solution generally can be given subcutaneously with safety. The dose can be repeated in 20 to 30 minutes if response has been inadequate. Ethylnorepinephrine hydrochloride (Bronkephrine) is a synthetic sympathomimetic amine with bronchodilating properties similar to epinephrine, but with reduced pressor effects. Therefore, it offers greater safety in the hypertensive patient. Since it has less central nervous system excitatory effects, it has been suggested for use with children. Adult dosage is 0.5 to 1.0 cc. (approximately double that of aqueous epinephrine), and children's dosages must be modified according to age and weight.

Long-acting preparations of epinephrine in oil (usually 0.2 to 0.5 cc. of 1/500 solution) will exert effects for up to 12 hours, but uptake may be variable. These preparations generally are used once a satisfactory response to aqueous epinephrine has been obtained. Epinephrine is the mainstay of most asthma treatment, but patients in status asthmaticus may become refractory to it.

Isoproterenol. This agent also primarily relieves bronchospasm and is given usually in nebulized form (for an average-sized adult, 0.5 cc. of 1/200 isoproterenol is mixed with 2 cc. of normal saline).

The dangers include stimulation of cardiac arrhythmias and an occasional increase in intrapulmonary shunting. In some patients, persistent use of isoproterenol will increase symptoms.

Methylxanthines (e.g., Theophylline, Aminophylline). These drugs are effective bronchodilators and also act to reduce mucosal edema. The most effective way to administer aminophylline is to give an intravenous loading dose of 5 mg./kg. of weight—the rate not to exceed 25 mg. per minute—followed by an intravenous infusion of approximately 0.9 mg./kg. per hour.

Dangers include precipitation of cardiac arrhythmias and the very frequent side-effect of vomiting. Rectal administration may be used in milder cases. The vomiting and reflex vagal action also may induce arrhythmias.

Cholinergic Blocking Agents (e.g., Atropine, Scopolamine). Such agents have theoretic advantages, since cholinergic agents produce bronchospasm in asthmatic individuals (the basis of the "methacholine test" in which inhaled methacholine produces bronchospasm in asthmatics at a dose which does not cause any significant changes in nonasthmatics). However, from a practical standpoint, these agents cause further drying of secretions and tend to depress ciliary activity. Scopolamine has the added disadvantage of producing severe confusion in some patients.

Atropine has its greatest therapeutic use if the inciting cause of asthma is an ingested or inhaled cholinergic substance.

Corticosteroids. These can be given in a single bolus of hydrocortisone, 100 to 300 mg. I.V., or prednisone, 40 to 60 mg. orally. Their use should be reserved for an asthmatic attack that is not responding to the usual measures or for when the patient has been taking an oral cortisone preparation and has discontinued it before the attack. The mechanism of action seems to be to reduce mucosal edema and to decrease the sensitivity of the bronchial smooth muscle to the inciting factors. If the asthmatic reaction is part of an over-all anaphylactic reaction, corticosteroids should be used immediately.

Secretion Moistening and Loosening Agents. Normal saline is useful in a nebulizer, and a high humidity environment is similarly helpful. Agents such as acetylcysteine (mucolytic agents) can be useful at a usual dosage of 3 to 5 cc. of 5 per cent or 10 per cent N-acetylcysteine in a nebulizer, but caution must be exercised since bronchospasm may be increased in sensitive individuals. Expectorants are useful adjuncts. In this regard, adequate hydration is essential.

Anxiety-reducing Agents. Since anxiety is present in asthma attacks and may even be the precipitating factor, sedation often is helpful. Barbiturates have been used, but because of their duration of action, respiratory depressant effects, and enzyme-inducing properties, other sedatives (e.g., diazepam, chlordiazepoxide, etc.) are being used more frequently.

TREATMENT OF INCITING FACTORS

(1) *Infections.* Broad-spectrum antibiotics (tetracycline, ampicillin) are used to treat respiratory infections that are a frequent stimulating factor for asthma. In children, erythromycin or ampicillin is preferable.

(2) Treatment of allergic conditions early in their course may prevent progression to asthma.

MECHANICALLY ASSISTED BREATHING

The patient who can cooperate has been found to benefit greatly from intermittent positive pressure breathing (IPPB) combined with aerosol bronchodilator therapy.

TREATMENT OF RESPIRATORY INSUFFICIENCY

Early recognition is the mainstay of effective therapy of respiratory insufficiency. *Progressive bronchospasm over a 12-hour period in the face of adequate bronchodilator therapy is an absolute indication for hospitalization.* Arterial blood gases are the most effective indicators of deterioration with the findings of hypoxemia and progressive hypercapnia.

Once hospitalized, the patient requires vigorous hydration by both the oral and intravenous routes. For I.V. fluid therapy, a hypotonic polyionic solution is employed, the amount depending on the degree of dehydration determined by urine output and daily weights. In addition, an ultrasonic nebulizer may aid in the rehydration process.

Intravenous corticosteroid therapy, using hydrocortisone or one of its soluble analogues, has been found to be of benefit in the treatment of respiratory insufficiency associated with status asthmaticus. A large initial bolus of hydrocortisone is injected I.V. Total eosinophil count is a guide to assessing steroid dosage. Optimum dose of steroids is considered to be that quantity that produces a 50 per cent or greater eosinopenic response. Initially, 100 to 200 mg. of hydrocortisone can be given, and repeated hourly. Clinical response can be taken as a guide instead of the eosinopenic response, which has had diminishing use.

Intravenous bronchodilator medication, usually in the form of aminophylline in a dosage not to exceed 3 gm. in a 24-hour period, is indicated early in the course of therapy. In sensitive individuals cardiac arrhythmias may occur, necessitating reduction in dosage and limiting its usefulness. The synergistic action of isoproterenol and theophylline should be exploited by administering the former by IPPB at regular intervals, if the patient can tolerate the procedure.

Hypoxia is a constant feature of even mild asthmatic attacks, and frequently approaches critical levels during respiratory insufficiency. It must be treated promptly by administration of continuous low-flow humidified oxygen, beginning at 2 liters/min. by nasal cannula. If required, the percentage of ambient oxygen may be regulated by the use of Venturi masks.

If the patient's condition continues to deteriorate under this management protocol, as manifested by physical signs, symptoms, and laboratory data after 12 hours of vigorous therapy, his condition must be considered critical.

Ominous signs occurring in asthmatic respiratory insufficiency include: *fatigue; hypotension; hypoventilation; somnolence; asterixis; coma;* and *pulsus paradoxus.* The latter is detected by any change in the systolic blood pressure between inspiration and expiration that is in excess of 10 mm. Hg. This finding is a manifestation of extremely elevated intrapulmonary pressures associated with pulmonary overdistention. At this point, it is imperative to monitor arterial blood gases closely, to determine if and when a ventilator is needed.

Once the diagnosis of respiratory insufficiency or respiratory failure is confirmed the major concern is immediate improvement of the alveolar ventilation. This requires endotracheal intubation and the use of a volume-controlled respirator.

Accompanying acidosis should be treated by intravenous administration of sodium bicarbonate, according to the following suggested dosage:

Adults: mEq. HCO_3^- = (25 mEq./liter − observed HCO_3^-) × 0.5 body weight in kg.

Children: mEq. HCO_3^- = Base deficit (mEq./liter) × 0.3 body weight in kg.

Using dynamic ventilatory measurements coupled with arterial blood gas determinations, various pathophysiologic stages of the asthmatic patient may be identified:

	MILD (%)	MODERATE (%)	SEVERE (%)	RESPIRATORY INSUFFICIENCY (%)
$FEV_1/FVC^{\times 100}$	70–75	50–70	50	15
$FEF_{25\text{-}75}$	70–80	40–70	40	– – –
PEF	70–80	40–70	40	15
MVV	65–80	40–65	40	– – –
SBO	2–3	3–6	6	– – –
Blood Gases	PaO_2 70–80 (room air) $PaCO_2$ < 40			PaO_2 60 (with supplemental 40% oxygen blood given) $PaCO_2$ 60 pH 7.3

Where: FEV$_1$ = Forced expiratory volume in one second.
FEF$_{25\text{-}75}$ = Forced expiratory flow between 25 and 75% of the FVC.
FVC = Forced vital capacity.
PEF = Peak expiratory flow.
MVV = Maximal voluntary ventilation.
SBO = Single breath oxygen test.

CHILDHOOD STATUS ASTHMATICUS

The treatment of status asthmaticus in the pediatric age-group is worthy of special attention. A useful time-tested procedure in the management of this problem is that of S.M. Robbins at Philadelphia's Children's Hospital. Asthmatic children presenting to the Emergency Department are given the following: (1) intravenous fluids; (2) up to three injections of 1/1000 epinephrine (0.01 cc./kg. at half-hour intervals); (3) chloral hy-

drate (30 mg./kg.); and (4) intravenous aminophylline (5 mg./kg.) by rapid infusion over a 20-minute period, unless the patient has been medicated with oral theophylline within four hours or is vomiting profusely.

If the child returns within 24 hours, or if he has been receiving steroids within six months of the attack, he is given hydrocortisone (4 mg./kg.) intravenously. When a patient shows no sustained response to such aggressive outpatient therapy, he is admitted with a diagnosis of status asthmaticus.

To aid in the evaluation of disease se-

	0	1	2
PO_2	70–100 in air	70 in air	−70 in 40% oxygen
Cyanosis	None	In air	In 40% oxygen
Inspiratory breath sounds	Normal	Unequal	Decreased to absent
Accessory muscles used	None	Moderate	Maximal
Expiratory wheezing	None	Moderate	Marked
Cerebral function	Normal	Depressed	Coma

verity, a clinical scoring system has been devised according to the above format. Scoring is done by totaling the numbers in each column. A score of 5 or more is indicative of impending respiratory failure.

MANAGEMENT OF STATUS ASTHMATICUS IN CHILDREN

The patient is put at bed-rest in a tent, and humidified oxygen is administered in an initial concentration of 40 per cent, with the F_1O_2 being adjusted in an effort to maintain the PaO_2 at 70 mm. Hg or greater.

Intravenous fluids are administered to counteract dehydration and provide maintenance requirements. These, in addition to their hydrating function, act as an expectorant by preventing inspissation of airway secretions. *Intravenous steroids* should be given early in the course of therapy; it has been shown that these achieve maximal improvement in vital capacity within the first three hours of administration.

CORRECTION OF ACIDOSIS

Acidosis in asthmatics is a product of CO_2 retention or ketosis from lactic acid production, associated with increased work of breathing. Upon drawing arterial blood gases, the base deficit is determined and the metabolic acidosis corrected by administration of sodium bicarbonate, as seen by the formula:

$NaHCO_3$ (mEq.) = body weight (kg.) × 0.30 × base deficit in mEq./liter.

In cases where the base deficit has not been determined, the dosage of sodium bicarbonate is empirically 2 mEq./kg. One-half of the designated dosage is given by slow I.V. push, and the remaining half is placed in the intravenous infusion and given over a four-hour period.

The great majority of children with status asthmaticus are either apprehensive or agitated. Sedation has been found to be extremely beneficial in allaying apprehension. Chloral hydrate is relatively safe and generally well-tolerated by children. It is given orally or rectally in dosage of 30 mg./kg., with repeat dosages at 20-minute intervals if the first dose does not achieve the desired sedative effect. However, the drug should not be administered more than three times in the initial attempts to calm the child.

Intravenous bronchodilator therapy, usually in the form of aminophylline, is given in the dosage previously recommended over a 20-minute period while cardiovascular response is monitored closely. One should look for toxic side-effects, including tremors or convulsions (CNS toxicity), tachycardia and arrhythmias (cardiovascular toxicity), and vomiting and hematemesis (gastrointestinal toxicity).

IPPB in conjunction with nebulized isoproterenol has been advocated by some to break acute asthmatic attacks. This benefit is well-documented; however, children with acute asthmatic attacks frequently are quite reluctant to place anything over their faces because of profound air hunger, and often resist the attempts at IPPB administration. This compounds their anxiety and can predispose them to unnecessary fatigue. It is for this reason that subcutaneous epinephrine coupled with intravenous aminophylline is perferred to IPPB, since its efficacy is the same and it generally is better tolerated by children.

When the work of breathing is progressive to the point of exhaustion in the child with status asthmaticus, inadequate alevolar ventilation develops and $PaCO_2$ begins to rise. The diminished alveolar ventilation, coupled with $\dot{V}/\dot{Q}^*$ mismatching, further compromises an already decreased PaO_2. When the PaO_2 falls below 70 mm. Hg, with

---

*$\dot{V}/\dot{Q}$ = ventilation/perfusion.

an F_1O_2 of 40 per cent or greater, it is highly suggestive of the onset of respiratory failure. Additional criteria for this diagnosis in childhood status asthmaticus include: (1) severe inspiratory retractions; (2) absence of inspiratory breath sounds; (3) generalized muscular weakness; (4) decreased sensorium; (5) cyanosis in 40 per cent ambient oxygen; or (6) a PO_2 of 40 mm. Hg. When any three of these signs, plus a $PaCO_2$ of 65 mm. Hg or greater, are present, the patient's condition is critical and urgent measures are required to save his life.

There are two general schools of thought on the method of therapy in the highly critical situation. The first is that of pulmonary bronchoscopy and bronchial lavage, followed by nasotracheal intubation and mechanical ventilation. The disadvantage of this procedure is the significantly high incidence of attendant bronchospasm in children with status asthmaticus.

The second mode of therapy seems safer, although great care must still be taken. It consists of a carefully monitored infusion of isoproterenol with an infusion pump. The medication is given in an initial dosage of 0.1 μg./kg./min., with 15-minute increments of 0.1 μg./kg./min. until the pulse rate approaches 200 beats per minute, or the clinical condition as manifested by $PaCO_2$ and PaO_2 begin to improve. If this is unsuccessful, nasotracheal intubation and mechanical ventilation are necessary for survival.

RESPIRATORY INFECTIONS

The natural defense mechanisms of the lung are extremely efficient in preventing the contamination of the alveoli from particulate matter and bacteria. On the other hand, the upper respiratory tract contains an abundance of infectious micro-organisms that would produce serious disease if allowed access to the alveoli. Despite the remarkable efficacy of the respiratory tree in preventing parenchymal infection, the defense mechanisms are not impregnable, as evidenced by the high incidence of pulmonary infections in causing significant morbidity and mortality in infectious disease processes.

Clinical infection of the respiratory tract is mostly localized to the trachea and bronchi. Ordinarily, the mucous lining of the trachea and the bronchi is constantly being propelled upward to eliminate particulate matter deposited on it during ventilation. When the foreign matter is irritating to the larger airways, the cough mechanism aids in more rapid expulsion of the entrapped particles in the mucous sheet. However, as is true of defense mechanisms in general, the respiratory cleansing action can be inhibited by a number of processes that (depending on such factors as the virulence of the organisms inhaled, the dosage of the infectious material, and the patient's resistance to the infectious process) may or may not result in clinically significant parenchymal disease. Most conditions mentioned here are covered in more detail in other chapters. However, particular conditions warrant mention here in order to alert the emergency physician to the greatest dangers of such diseases, and to emphasize particular highlights of relevance in the emergency situation.

Epiglottitis

The disease is characterized by the abrupt onset of fever and extreme sore throat, which may proceed to complete respiratory obstruction within hours. The obstruction is the cause of death, and early tracheostomy may be essential in progressive cases. The course may be fulminant.

The mechanism of the upper airway obstruction begins with inflammation in the epiglottis which then curls posteroinferiorly, resting immediately superior to the glottic orifice, and thereby occluding the laryngeal inlet. Complete obstruction may occur by further enlargement of the epiglottis, or by obstruction of the already narrowed glottic orifice by a bolus of tenacious mucus.

PRESENTATION

Clinically, the presenting symptom usually is extreme throat pain associated with dysphagia and anorexia. There generally is retention of secretions with copious and visible puddling of pharyngeal mucus, resulting in drooling as an external sign. Irritability and marked restlessness, caused by air hunger and hypoxia, appear fairly early in the course of the disease. Owing to progressive airway obstruction, dyspnea invariably presents in the first eight hours of the syndrome. Constant features are edema and a striking fiery-red appearance, so that a "cherry-red" epiglottis is seen on depression of the tongue and examination of the pharynx. Examination of the chest is unremarkable except for diminished breath sounds, indicating poor air exchange.

The rapidity with which respiratory obstruction occurs in epiglottitis has made tracheotomy the cornerstone of conservative management. Only in the extremely stable patient, who, after a significant period of intensive observation by medical personnel, shows no evidence of either cyanosis or progressive respiratory distress, is treatment without tracheotomy justified.

Croup

The basic croup syndrome can be caused by infectious, mechanical, or allergic factors. In addition, there is another distinct category known as "spasmodic croup." Initially, this form of croup was thought to be due to allergy or immaturity of the larynx, frequently seen in the "nervous child." Typically, this form of croup develops suddenly at night, tends to be recurrent, and usually is associated with a minor upper respiratory tract infection. The major portion of laryngeal obstruction in this form of croup is due to spasm, with a lesser degree of actual subglottic edema. Such young patients frequently awaken with frightening dyspnea and stridor, which often clears before arrival in the Emergency Department.

Regardless of the specific etiology, there are a number of important factors that predispose to the croup state.

Age is an important factor: the majority of patients with croup are between the ages of 3 months and 3 years. This is in contradistinction to the patients with bacterial croup (*Hemophilus influenzae* and diphtheritic), whose peak age incidence is 3 to 7 years.

In all cases of croup, throat examination must be performed, but this procedure can-

not be taken lightly. Although the child often is feverish, semiconscious, and unresponsive to verbal commands, he is also apprehensive and extremely sensitive to any disturbances. No matter how gentle the examining physician may be in performing the throat examination, in doing so he can initate laryngospasm leading to complete respiratory obstruction. Therefore, before undertaking the examination, one must be ready to perform endotracheal intubation and tracheotomy or cricothyroid puncture.

If spasm of the larynx is the predominant feature rather than edema, administration of syrup of ipecac may produce prompt relief of symptoms. It is assumed that ipecac acts to relax the larynx by working through a vagal reflex. Although it usually is given in subemetic doses (one drop for each month of age up to 2 years, with older children receiving 2 to 5 ml.), the full therapeutic effect of the medication sometimes is not realized until vomiting has occurred. Thus, any child who has been given ipecac must be closely observed in the hour after administration to prevent aspiration. If symptoms subside, one can assume the disease is largely due to spasm. Valuable information can be obtained thus, without resorting to laryngoscopy. Spasmodic croup also has been shown to respond favorably to bronchodilators such as aminophylline.

The use of tracheotomy in croup has been decreasing and is becoming rare, partly owing to the introduction of newer treatments, such as racemic epinephrine.

Mortality from croup is reported in some studies to be as high as 2.7 per cent. There is evidence to suggest that mortality, if not the over-all incidence of tracheotomy, can be decreased by the use of racemic epinephrine delivered by positive pressure ventilator. Most children with infectious croup show dramatic and almost immediate relief when given racemic epinephrine nebulized by compressor through a face mask. However, in many instances the relief is only temporary, and repeat treatment in three to four hours is needed.

STEROIDS IN CROUP

Although these are widely used, the evidence of benefit is still uncertain. Their use may be more justified if laryngospasm is a prominent feature.

Pneumonia

Pneumonia is well discussed in other sections, but several points deserve emphasis here because of their practical significance in the Emergency Department.

(1) Bacteremia is common in the early stages of pneumococcal pneumonia, and can result in metastatic abscesses. A buffy coat examination (stained) may allow rapid diagnosis.

(2) When irritation of the diaphragmatic pleura occurs, pain may be referred to the abdomen and can mimic acute abdominal conditions. In addition, there may be shoulder and neck pain. Pleuritis or pleuritic-type symptoms, on the other hand, usually are located at the site of the pain.

(3) A fulminant form of pneumoni still occurs occasionally, with rapid hypoxemia and death from cardiac arrhythmias.

(4) Sputum gram stain is a useful Emergency Department technique that can make possible more accurate antibiotic therapy.

(5) Staphylococcal pneumonias should be treated with an antibiotic that is effective against penicillinase-producing organisms, owing to the virulence of the pneumonia-causing tissue necrosis and multiple lung abscesses.

(6) *Hemophilus influenzae* pneumonia is rare in adults, but more common in children under the age of 6. Metastatic spread to meninges and joints is a serious possible sequela.

(7) *Klebsiella* pneumonia is rare except in alcoholics and the aged-debilitated. Lung abscess frequently is seen.

(8) Mycoplasma pneumonias are common and respond to erythromycin or tetracycline; an elevated "cold agglutinin" titer in excess of 1:256 suggests the diagnosis.

ACUTE
RESPIRATORY FAILURE

Although the recognition of acute respiratory failure has been simplified by an arbitrary definition based on blood gas test abnormalities (PaO_2 less than 50 mm. Hg; $PaCO_2$ greater than 50 mm. Hg), there is no universal agreement on the definition of acute respiratory failure (ARF). The problem is complex, in that acute respiratory failure may be the primary condition and other organ changes are secondary—or a critically ill patient may develop lethal respiratory complications.

The hallmarks of ARF are a reduction in functional residual capacity, decreased pulmonary compliance, and mismatching of alveolar ventilation/capillary blood flow. These changes are secondary to (1) an abnormal pattern of gas distribution, with closure of alveoli or airways or both; and (2) an increase in pulmonary extravascular water with interstitial edema, either because of an increased pulmonary capillary hydrostatic pressure associated with congestion of the pulmonary vasculature, and or an increased pulmonary capillary endothelial permeability with exudation of plasma into the interstitial spaces. A large variety of nondescript pathologic processes, which in reality may be distinct clinical entities, are all capable of producing the changes associated with ARF.

It is not so important to categorize a patient as having "wet-lung," "post-transfusion lung," "shock lung," or "oxygen-toxicity" lung as it is to recognize and treat the pulmonary derangements that each of these syndromes more or less to the same degree produce. Even CNS hypoxia results in autonomic nervous system changes, with increased pulmonary vascular resistance and development of a similar pulmonary picture.

Accumulation of water in the lungs is a universal finding in ARF, even in patients without primary cardiac disease. On the microscopic level, the endothelium has been incriminated as a particular target of damage that leads to deposition of fluid first into the interstitial space. With more severe damage the "leaky cells" allow passage of red cells, plasma, and other formed elements of the blood. The end-result seen at autopsy is heavy hemorrhagic lungs resembling the liver in consistency.

From a pathophysiologic standpoint, the initiating stimulus for fluid accumulation in the lung varies with the inciting factor of ARF. The clinical manifestations tend to be remarkably constant, however. The chest x-ray changes vary from localized fluffy densities to diffuse opacification, with progressive impairment in mechanics of ventilation and gas exchange. The etiology usually is related to chronic lung disease, but any condition leading to weakness of the respiratory muscles, injury to pulmonary endothelium, depression of the respiratory center, or severely impaired ventilation/perfusion relationships may result in ARF.

The pulmonary capillary endothelium is far more permeable to lipid-insoluble substances (water) than is the alveolar epithelium, and consequently fluid first begins to collect in the interstitial spaces, rather than in the alveoli. In fact, fluid will not accumulate in the alveoli until the interstitium is well filled. Once the alveoli are filled with fluid, they become nonfunctional from a ventilatory point of view, and contribute to "true physiologic shunting" even in the absence of airway collapse. Alveolar filling with fluid represents the most important physiologic stage of pulmonary edema, since it marks the time when significant interference with oxygen diffusion across the pulmonary membrane occurs. Prior to alveolar filling, there is little derangement of oxygenation.

Assessment of respiratory function is vital for the provision of adequate respiratory care at all stages of treatment in ARF.* The patient who is on a respirator should have monitoring of rate, tidal volume, minute volume, and end-tidal PCO_2. These airway measurements supplement the evidence from arterial blood gases and allow sometimes essential minute-to-minute decisions to be made. Fiberoptic bronchoscopy also can be useful in detecting lesions that can account for clinical changes.

More sophisticated equipment (unavailable in most hospitals) allows direct values of compliance and resistance to be derived from the pressure and volume data by a computer. The following discussion deals with information that can be calculated as described, but which in advanced centers can be indicated by computer read-out.

Tests of Oxygenation

Efficiency of oxygen uptake in the lungs is expressed by the alveolar-arterial oxygen difference, and the right-to-left shunt as a fraction of the cardiac output ($\dot{Q}_S/\dot{Q}_T$), and is the most sensitive index of pulmonary complications leading to acute respiratory fail-

---

*See Chapter 3.

ure. Under normal conditions $\dot{Q}_S/\dot{Q}_T$ varies from 2 to 5 per cent of the cardiac output. In ARF values as high as 50 per cent have been recorded, and survival can be expected only with mechanical ventilation with inspired oxygen concentrations of 80 to 100 per cent. Even when breathing 100 per cent oxygen, a patient with a 50 per cent shunt would have a PaO_2 of only 40 mm. Hg.

Under conditions in which complete hemoglobin saturation can be assured (PaO_2 150 mm. Hg or greater), the shunt equation can be simplified to:

$$\frac{\dot{Q}_S}{\dot{Q}_T} = \frac{P(A-a)O_2 \times 0.0031}{P(A-a)O_2 \times 0.0031 + C(a-\bar{v})O_2}$$

where 0.0031 is the factor required to convert partial pressure of oxygen into oxygen content at 37° C., and $C(a-\bar{v})O_2$ is the arterial-mixed venous oxygen content difference. Precise calculation of the shunt equation thus requires measurement of mixed-venous oxygen content in a pulmonary artery sample. The Swan-Ganz balloon catheter allows the pulmonary artery to be catheterized without fluoroscopy, and provides the additional advantage of monitoring both pulmonary artery and capillary wedge pressures.

The magnitude of the $P(A-a)O_2$ is most obviously influenced by the inspired oxygen tension. When it is high, a small fall in the arterial oxygen tension due to anatomic shunting will result in a large $P(A-a)O_2$. If the F_IO_2 is low, the same change in arterial oxygen content is associated with a smaller $P(A-a)O_2$, since the PaO_2 is not high enough to produce full saturation (the implication being that the $P(A-a)O_2$ will be smaller during air-breathing than during oxygen breathing).

ARF of nonobstructive origin presents primarily as true physiologic shunting arising from perfused areas of the lung that are totally unventilated. By placing the patient on 100 per cent oxygen for a 20-minute period, and then drawing an arterial blood sample, the PaO_2 can be determined; the $P(A-a)O_2$ and $\dot{Q}_S/\dot{Q}_T$ can subsequently be calculated, and their magnitude and changes serve to guide the therapeutic scheme. In contrast, chronic obstructive pulmonary disease is associated with large ventilation/perfusion mismatch. The $P(A-a)O_2$ is characteristically low in these patients during oxygen breathing, and consequently is not a useful index of changes in the pulmonary status.

Treatment of Acute Respiratory Failure

Since patients with acute respiratory failure are highly susceptible to development of pulmonary edema, great care must be taken to avoid circulatory overload. Administration of diuretic agents frequently is indicated, and usually, once a diuretic is needed, a potent agent such as furosemide (Lasix) is needed parenterally. The monitoring of intake, output, hourly urine outputs, and body weight changes allows titration of diuresis. Airspace closure, retention of bronchial secretion, and regional pulmonary edema can be greatly minimized by frequent changes in body position.

Once pulmonary edema becomes associated with hypoxemia, the inspired oxygen concentration must be increased. If a ventilator is necessary, an appropriate ventilatory pattern must be established (e.g., by changes in salt and tidal volume). Care must be taken, however, if chronic CO_2 retention has led to decreased sensitivity of the CO_2 respiratory drive. High O_2 flow can abolish the hypoxic drive to respiration in such cases and lead to apnea. If the ventilator is triggered by the patient, adjustment must be made to allow for automatic control.

Use of Salt-Poor Albumin

The simultaneous administration of salt-poor albumin with diuretic agents is open to debate in the treatment of pulmonary edema associated with acute respiratory failure. Proponents of the use of albumin in conjunction with diuretics state that this practice will uniformly decrease an elevated $P(A-a)O_2$, and this has been shown to be true. Those who oppose the routine use of albumin argue that this practice increases intravascular volume, and they further add that there is no conclusive evidence that albumin will mobilize water from the lung. It also stands to reason that, if ARF is associated with pulmonary capillary damage, any albumin added will be quickly lost in the extravascular space. The growing consensus to date is that colloid should be administered only in the face of hypoalbuminemia, or if there is circulatory evidence that hypoalbuminemia accompanies vigorous diuresis.

Unreliability of Central Venous Pressure As Guide

It has been common medical practice to monitor central venous pressure (CVP) as an adjunct to fluid therapy in patients susceptible to overload and subsequent pulmonary edema. Right atrial pressure, however, is an unreliable index of blood volume in many patients (e.g., those with hemorrhagic or septic shock, or with drug intoxication), since left-sided heart failure may be present in spite of low CVP. If whole blood, albumin, or salt solutions are infused in an attempt to raise the CVP to normal levels, interstitial pulmonary edema with a rising $P(A-a)O_2$ are almost certain sequelae. The situation can be facilitated by the use of a Swan-Ganz catheter to measure pulmonary wedge (left atrial) pressure, an estimation of left ventricular performance. In the absence of wedge pressure determinations, fluid replacement should be based upon establishment of a satisfactory urinary output despite subnormal central venous pressures.

Pulmonary complications usually develop insidiously over a period ranging from several hours to several days before they become clinically apparent. Once morphologic changes have become so apparent on the chest x-ray, they are indicative of advanced disease accompanied by drastic reduction in ventilatory reserve. The final stages tend to evolve rapidly into full-blown acute respiratory failure. Once advanced, the pulmonary changes of ARF are at best only slowly reversible; treatment in itself tends to add to the insult, owing to the need for high inspired oxygen concentrations — which in itself tends to produce shunting and abnormalities in the ventilation/perfusion ratio, with need for large tidal volumes and high airway pressures without which adequate gas exchange could not occur.

Under normal circumstances, the work of breathing accounts for 2 to 3 per cent of the total oxygen consumption; in the face of ARF, the work of breathing may increase several-fold over normal values particularly since obstruction to expiration frequently develops. The latter results from inability to synchronize the motion of the diaphragm with the muscles of the chest wall, and in so doing significantly increases the work of breathing. Despite the increased oxygen cost of ventilatory efforts, only a small fraction of the total oxygen consumption is involved. Fever, shivering, and restlessness also contribute to the increased oxygen consumption, and must be minimized when conservation of oxygen consumption is critical to survival. When muscle fatigue supervenes, rapid decompensation occurs and ventilator support is essential.

Artificial Ventilation*

One of the most useful means of minimizing excessive oxygen consumption in patients with ARF is that of artificial ventilation. Also, introduction of PEEP (positive end-expiratory pressure) can improve the P_{O_2}.

Artificial ventilation was first applied in patients with primary ventilatory failure: poliomyelitis; infectious polyneuritis; tetanus; myasthenia gravis; chest wall trauma with chest wall instability; and massive obesity, with or without impairment of the central regulation of breathing. The inherent problem in such cases lies in the nervous, muscular, or skeletal apparatus of breathing, with morphologic changes in the lung occurring

---

*See Chapter 3 for use of ventilators.

secondarily if treatment is delayed or inadequate. Deterioration of pulmonary function is heralded by a decrease in vital capacity, a widened $P(A-a)_{O_2}$, and tachypnea. With reduction in the vital capacity, there follows a diminution of the cough and sigh mechanisms, with subsequent retention of pulmonary secretions, atelectasis, and pneumonia. Advanced respiratory failure results in hypercapnia and respiratory acidosis. Guidelines have been developed to aid the clinician in determining the need for endotracheal intubation and mechanical ventilation (Table 1). Some specific patient problems follow, but certain general principles of ventilator therapy are set out below.

(1) In patients with normal lungs, the P_{CO_2} usually is corrected to a near-normal value through alterations in mechanical dead-space.

(2) In the "stiff lung" with decreased compliance, treatment usually is directed at correcting the cause of the low functional residual capacity. PEEP may find its greatest use in supporting oxygenation in such cases, although the circulatory changes that can be produced may limit its value. The pressure should not exceed 15 cm. of H_2O (and should preferably be less). The need for PEEP may be reduced through supportive means, e.g., removal of secretions, use of bronchodilators, use of diuretics, and treatment of infection.

(3) In those patients with chronic lung disease with very little obstructive component, mechanical ventilation should be avoided if at all possible. The principal thrust of therapy should be to maintain adequate oxygenation.

Deeply comatose patients should have a

TABLE 1   Guidelines for Ventilatory Support in Adults with ARF

MEASUREMENTS	NORMAL RANGE	TRACHEAL INTUBATION AND VENTILATORY SUPPORT INDICATED
Mechanics		
Respiratory rate	12–20	above 35
Vital capacity (ml./kg.)	65–75	less than 15
FEV_1 (ml./kg.)	50–60	less than 10
Inspiratory force (cm. water)	75–100	less than 25
Oxygenation		
Pa_{O_2} (mm. Hg)	75–100 (air)	less than 70 on mask oxygen
$P(A-a)_{O_2}$ (mm. Hg)		
after 10 minutes of 100% oxygen	25–65	greater than 450
Ventilation		
Pa_{CO_2} (mm. Hg)	34–45	greater than 55 except in COPD
V_D/V_T	0.25–0.40	greater than 0.60

cuffed endotracheal tube placed to prevent aspiration of saliva, vomitus, and blood, and to facilitate removal of secretions. Mechanical ventilation should be initiated as dictated by diminishing ventilatory drive or increasing abnormality of arterial blood gas determinations. The combination of hypercapnia and hypoxemia is extremely deleterious to patients with acute brain injuries.

Mechanical Ventilation in ARF Secondary to Acute Pulmonary Disease Such as Pneumonitis

Acute pulmonary disease early in its course shows reflex hyperventilation and respiratory alkalosis. The ventilatory system usually is intact, although diminished inspiratory force is prevalent, secondary to weakness and fatigue directly related to the increased work of breathing. There also are seen, early in the course of the disease, increases in both the $P(A-a)O_2$ and the ratio of dead-space to tidal volume (V_DV_T). Eventually, if progressive and untreated, pulmonary compliance markedly decreases and there is a major reduction in vital capacity, with respiratory failure. Indications for intubation are listed in Table 1.

Mechanical Ventilation for ARF Secondary to Chronic Obstructive Pulmonary Disease

The indications for intubation and artificial ventilation are more stringent in this group of patients, for many reasons. First, these patients are more or less acclimatized to chronic hypoxemia, and as such are capable of withstanding low arterial oxygen tensions. Also, ARF tends to be a recurrent problem in the patient with chronic lung disease. Next, artificial ventilation is no easy chore in the patient with chronic obstructive pulmonary disease, and is associated with an increased risk of complications such as tension pneumothorax and acute circulatory collapse. Once placed on artificial ventilation, these patients frequently manifest rapid and significant reductions in $PaCO_2$ to the point where cardiac arrhythmias, hypotension, or

fatal cerebral complications supervene. Finally, patients with advanced chronic obstructive disease show decreased elastic recoil of the lungs, with less tendency for alveolar collapse. Marked reductions in vital capacity are not necessarily followed by atelectasis. Thus, artificial ventilation in this group of patients is indicated only as a last resort, and certainly not until vigorous attempts have been made to reverse hypoxia without producing excessive hypercapnia. These measures include: (1) antibiotics for treatment of superimposed infection; (2) adequate chest physiotherapy and postural drainage; and (3) relief of associated bronchospasm and bronchial edema. In severe exacerbations of their disease processes, some of these patients will develop profound hyoxemia (PaO_2 less than 40 torr = mm Hg), which responds surprisingly well to low-flow (3 liters/min.) oxygen. Thus, a substantial rise in arterial oxygen content is attainable with a small increment of PaO_2, because the oxyhemoglobin dissociation curve is steep in this PaO_2 range. Relief of hypoxemia without concomitant suppression of chemoreceptor drive or excessive hypocapnia is the hallmark and goal of "controlled oxygen therapy."

Assisted Ventilation in Bronchial Asthma

Patients with bronchial asthma differ from those with emphysema in having an unimpaired response to carbon dioxide. Even in severe asthma the $PaCO_2$ is characteristically low, with a rise to normal or hypercapnic levels reflecting critical decompensation. Hypoxemia, in contrast, is present even in mild attacks, and worsens as the attack progresses. Close observation is the cornerstone of decision to use a ventilator, inasmuch as progressive hypercapnia associated with exhaustion, in face of vigorous therapy with high humidity oxygen, intravenous fluids, bronchodilator drugs, and corticosteroids, is a definite indication for endotracheal intubation and assisted ventilation. Heavy sedation, usually intravenous morphine, and (occasionally) complete paralysis using d-tubocurarine, are required to allay apprehension and prevent patient resistance to the respirator.

Positive End-expiratory Pressure in ARF

Application of continuous positive airway pressure of 2 to 5 cm. water by face mask during spontaneous breathing (continuous positive pressure breathing, CPPB, or positive end-expiratory pressure (PEEP) was used initially as an effective supplement to oxygen therapy in patients with acute pulmonary edema secondary to left ventricular failure or inhalation of noxious gases. The rationale behind this mode of therapy was that CPPB decreased venous return to the right side of the heart and exerted pressure on the pulmonary capillaries to prevent egress of fluid. CPPB also has been advocated as a means of maintaining airway patency during expiration in patients with obstructive pulmonary disease. The value of PEEP in treating patients with severe hypoxemia is now well established, and it has caused renewed interest in the use of CPPB in ARF on patients who are spontaneously breathing. Experience is now accumulating that, in selected intubated patients with at least severe ARF CPPB pressures up to 10 cm., water may reduce severe hypoxemia and obviate the need for total mechanical ventilation.

Treatment-related Complications in ARF

Continuous exposure to oxygen at one atmosphere pressure (100 per cent) causes pulmonary injury. One of the first deleterious effects on pulmonary function is a fall in vital capacity, which becomes more rapidly progressive after 60 hours of exposure to one atmosphere. Hyperbaric oxygen exposure at two atmospheres pressure causes a reduction in vital capacity and pulmonary compliance after an average of only eight hours. In the light of this information, it would seem that the patient with severe respiratory failure who requires high concentrations of oxygen in the inspired gas for relatively long periods of time would be a perfect candidate for the detrimental effects of this otherwise life-sustaining gas. However, the evidence is not so clear-cut.

Morphologic postmortem examination of lungs of patients after long exposure to high oxygen concentrations revealed them to be heavy, "beefy," and edematous. Microscopically there was congestion, intra-alveolar hemorrhage, and edema. Fibrin exudate with prominent hyaline membrane formation was prevalent without associated inflammatory response. This is typical of the early exudative phase. A later proliferative phase has been recognized in patients receiving mechanical ventilation with inspired oxygen concentrations of 80 to 100 per cent after a seven- to ten-day period. This phase is characterized by pronounced alveolar and inter-alveolar septal edema, with fibroblastic proliferation and prominent hyperpalsia of the alveolar lining cells. However, a cause-and-effect relation between the morphologic changes and oxygen therapy has yet to be documented. Interstitial and intra-alveolar edema, hemorrhage, and hyaline membranes are nonspecific responses to a number of injuries. Oxygen is only one of these, and the occurrence of nonspecific morphologic changes cannot be taken as evidence of a specific oxygen effect. Withholding oxygen in a patient who is extremely hypoxemic, for fear of inducing oxygen damage to the lungs, would kill the patient long before the first signs of oxygen toxicity ever entered into the clinical picture. The current rationale for oxygen therapy in ARF is based upon the assumption that an F_IO_2 of 50 per cent or higher is likely to produce serious changes when used for more than two days. The higher the F_IO_2, the more rapid will be the onset of damage. Except in patients with chronic hypoxemia, an F_IO_2 (inspired oxygen percentage) should be selected that will result in a PaO_2 in the normal range. If an F_IO_2 above 50 per cent is necessary to maintain a normal PaO_2, it may be desirable to settle for a PaO_2 in the slightly hypoxemic range. In making this decision, one must assess the patient's cardiovascular status and his ability to increase oxygen transport by increasing cardiac output. His tolerance to hypoxemia also must be borne in mind.

Circulatory Responses to Intermittent Positive Pressure Ventilation

The systemic circulatory response to IPPV and PEEP is somewhat unpredictable. A transient reduction in cardiac output may be expected when mechanical ventilation is first initiated, and a rise when it is terminated. Once circulatory adjustment to artificial ventilation has occurred, variations in ventilatory pattern, even with large changes in mean airway pressure, generally are well tolerated, except by patients with advanced emphysema, hypovolemia, or impaired adrenergic activity.

Adverse Effects of Prolonged Endotracheal Intubation and Tracheostomy

Ulceration of the larynx is the primary lesion associated with prolonged endotracheal intubation. If intubation is of short duration, the lesion tends to be superficial, although deeper ulceration may occur. In prolonged intubations, severe damage to the larynx presents as hoarseness, dysphagia, impaired laryngeal activity, and varying degrees of respiratory obstruction. The laryngeal damage is primarily a function of pressure necrosis. Avoidance of such damage can be facilitated with fiberoptic bronchoscopy to detect early changes.

Another hazard of prolonged intubation is that of sudden occlusion of the tubal lumina by plugging. Kinking is a major hazard; obstruction of the tube by secretions is not always preventable. To obviate any potentially disastrous consequences, facilities for prompt replacement of endotracheal tubes should be kept at the bedside.

A clinical syndrome has been described that is associated with prolonged mechanical ventilation through a tracheostomy tube with attached cuff; it consists essentially of upper airway obstruction of varying degree. Symptoms usually develop within six weeks of extubation, but occasionally can be delayed until up to 18 months later. The most common symptoms are diminished effort tolerance, dyspnea, hacking cough, and a sensation of not being able to clear the throat. Auscultation over the trachea may aid in the diagnosis and localization of this process, which is known as tracheal stenosis. Stridor is a late feature of the illness. Precise information concerning the lesion is best obtained by an air tracheogram.

When tracheomalacia is present, intermittent narrowing of a tracheal segment may be observed with fluoroscopy and cineradiography. Bronchoscopy provides the most definitive diagnostic information; however, it often results in increased secretions and edema, which may aggravate the already compromised tracheal lumen, worsen the obstruction, and force urgent surgical intervention. Thus, bronchoscopy is best deferred until the time of definitive surgical intervention.

Trauma to the trachea from tracheostomy tubes can occur at the tip of the tube, at the level of the stoma, or opposite the inflatable cuff. Among patients receiving artificial ventilation, the maximal damage and deformity typically develops at the level of the inflatable cuff. Tracheoesophageal fistulas or major arterial hemorrhages from erosion can occur, but fortunately are rare complications. The usual end-result is healing, with subsequent scarring and fibrosis. Narrowing is minimal and clinically insignificant.

Respiratory obstruction may be caused either by polypoid granulation tissue at the stoma (these usually are small and seldom pose major therapeutic problems), or the far more serious deformities of the trachea that follow more extensive tissue destruction. These typically develop at the stoma and opposite the inflatable cuff; they are often extensive, and far more difficult to treat.

ASPIRATIONS AND INHALATIONS

Aspirations

Aspiration is the process of inhaling either solid or liquid material into the respiratory tract. It generally occurs when there is depression of the patient's level of consciousness, although this is not universally true. Thus, it is most apt to occur in the debilitated, in the stroke victim, in the patient with brain tumor or other intracranial mass lesion, or as a consequence of drug or alcoholic intoxication and anesthetic administration. Each of these states or conditions is associated with depression or elimination of the normal protective mechanism of reflex glottic closure associated with the acts of swallowing or vomiting. Oil aspiration is somewhat different in that it may seep into the trachea while eliciting little in the way of a gag reflex.

Aspiration of large solid material has been discussed under the section dealing with airway obstructions; aspiration of smaller solid particles is perhaps best covered under the discussion of inhalations; water aspirations are related to drowning and are covered elsewhere in the text.*

From the standpoint of this discussion, we shall focus our attention on the various forms of aspiration pneumonia and its attendant complications.

LIPOID PNEUMONIA

Lipoid pneumonia is an acute pneumonitis elicited by the aspiration of certain oils, particularly vitamin and mineral oils, into the lungs. Access to the airway is through the use of oily nose-drops, defective swallowing mechanisms, forceful administration of oily preparations to crying infants and children, or the aspiration of oily laxatives taken at bedtime. If accidental ingestion has occurred, oil aspiration may occur with induced or spontaneous vomiting.

The lesion produced is an organizing bronchopneumonia, with an abundance of macrophages and desquamated alveolar lining cells. With time it may progress to pulmonary fibrosis with obliteration of the pulmonary vasculature and contraction of the pulmonary parenchymal tissues, consequent bronchial distortion, and in some cases bronchiectasis.

The aspirated oil is partly eliminated by the lymphatic route after ingestion by macrophages and by the sputum. The latter is a combined effect of ciliary propulsive forces and expectoration. When the oil is contained in the sputum, the etiology of the pneumonitis may be determined by cytologic and histochemical studies of 24-hour sputum specimens.

ASPIRATION PNEUMONIA

Aspiration pneumonia results from the introduction of oral bacterial flora into the lower respiratory tract. They usually are mixed infections caused by anaerobic and aerobic streptococci, bacteroides, or fusibacteria. These bacteria are normal inhabitants of the oral cavity and upper airways, and usually are not associated with disease in their native locations; however, if they are introduced into the alveoli, pneumonia invariably results.

The predisposing factors for the development of aspiration pneumonia are those of aspirations in general. Patients usually are mildly-to-moderately ill, but can become quite toxic under certain circumstances.

Aspiration pneumonia need not be limited to that caused by normal flora, but on occasion is invoked by gram-negative bacilli, especially in hospitalized patients and ambulatory patients receiving antibiotics. Under these circumstances the normal oral flora may become altered, so that there is an overgrowth by gram-negative forms that, upon being aspirated, elicit gram-negative bacillary penumonia. Sputum gram-stain is a valuable diagnostic tool in differentiating the causative organism and in deciding upon specific antimicrobial measures. Transtracheal aspiration has more hazards, but offers the advantage of an increased likelihood of isolating the causative organism.

The most virulent form of aspiration pneumonia results from the aspiration of acidic gastric juice. When the pH of the aspirate is less than 2.5 and the volume is sufficiently large, the mortality is high — exceeding 70 per cent in some series. The pathologic manifestations vary from an acute inflammatory reaction with epithelial destruction, hemorrhage, and edema, to nearly-complete parenchymal destruction. Initially the process invokes an intense bronchospasm, followed by a brief period of apnea which becomes a shallow tachypnea pattern. There is a prompt rise in pulmonary artery pressure, while the systemic pressure falls to hypotensive levels. In general the pressures return to normal levels in about an hour, but may fall again later, especially in massive aspirations. The patient characteristically shows evidence of pulmonary hemorrhage and edema in the form of bloody sputum, which has a frothy character. The outpouring of proteinaceous edema fluid exceeds the amount of red cells lost from hemorrhage, and the net result is hemoconcentration, as manifested by a rising hematocrit with a fall in plasma volume. There is a fall in blood pH and evidence of significant right-to-left pulmonary shunting. The derangements in arterial blood gas determinations vary with the degree of insult: minimal injury invokes the blood gas changes of hyperventilation, with an increased pH and a fall in the $PaCO_2$; with severe injury there is a fall in the arterial blood pH, hypoxia, and a rise in the arte-

*See page 792.

rial tension of carbon dioxide. If the patient survives, the sequelae usually are those of interstitial pulmonary fibrosis.

Another form of aspiration pneumonia that may be encountered by the emergency physician arises from the aspiration of fluid contents of the obstructed intestine. This form of aspiration is associated with a particularly virulent, and often fatal, pneumonia. Following aspiration there is a gradual respiratory depression characterized by hypoxia, hypercapnia, tachypnea, and tachycardia. Gross changes early after aspiration show the trachea and bronchi to be filled with thin, frothy secretions, and the lungs exhibit scattered areas of hemorrhage and atelectasis. Microscopic examination reveals areas of pulmonary parenchymal destruction surrounded by zones of hemorrhage, edema, and acute inflammatory reaction. Later autopsy findings (about 20 hours post-aspiration) show the trachea and bronchi to be filled with thick, mucoid material, with complete obstruction of the smaller bronchi and associated areas of distal atelectasis. Histologic examination reveals atelectasis with early pneumonitis. Initially, the fatal outcome of aspiration pneumonia secondary to obstructed intestinal contents was thought to be due to production and systemic absorption of endotoxins. However, more recent experimental evidence seems to indicate that death is due to progressive respiratory failure caused by mechanical obstruction of distal bronchi. This may account for the frequent clinical observation in these patients of progressive and persistent hypoxia and hypercapnia, which is refractory to even the most aggressive measures, suggesting a mechanical obstruction that shows no signs of clearing. Administration of systemic antibiotics has not improved the survival rate. Pathogens usually cannot be recovered from the blood, and the characteristic changes in portal or systemic blood pressure associated with endotoxic shock are conspicuously absent, strengthening the hypothesis that mortality is related to obstructive phenomena rather than bacteria.

The outcome of aspiration pneumonias in general depends on the amount and type of material aspirated. In addition to the general supportive therapy common to pneumonias, specific measures will be dictated by the clinical circumstances. In aspiration pneumonia secondary to normal flora, penicillin is the antimicrobial choice, a seven day course of therapy usually being sufficient. Gram-negative bacillary aspiration pneumonia is treated empirically with gentamicin until definitive culture reports are obtained. If acid gastric contents are aspirated as well, a short course of corticosteroids (24 to 48 hours) may be useful to attenuate the associated chemical pneumonitis, provided therapy can be initiated within a few hours of the aspiration. The treatment of obstructed intestinal content aspiration remains supportive in nature unless evidence of infection occurs. Postural drainage is important in assisting drainage of the irritating aspirated fluid.

Complications of Aspiration Pneumonia. Although all pulmonary abscesses are not sequels to aspiration of infectious material, this process is by and large the most common cause of lung abscess. Abscesses also may arise from hematogenous spread of organisms in septicemias and in septic pulmonary infarcts. Even aseptic infarcts, by devitalizing parenchymal tissue, may precipitate abscess formation. Necrotizing pneumonitis caused by Friedländer's bacillus, staphylococci, and streptococci also may induce lung abscess. In the vast majority of cases of lung abscess, resolution can be obtained by bronchoscopy, antibiotics, and postural drainage. The abscess wall collapses, fibrosis occurs, and healing results through scarring. Recognition of an abscess is the key role of the emergency physician, since the routine treatment for pneumonitis may be ineffective if abscess formation has occurred.

Pulmonary parenchymal disease with infection, along with prolonged bronchial obstruction, are the two principal predisposing factors in the pathogenesis of bronchiectasis. Both of these are characterized by some reduction in the volume of effective lung tissue and concomitant traction on bronchial walls. This traction, combined with weakening of the bronchial walls by infection, results in bronchial dilatation or bronchiectasis. When the parenchymal infection is of short duration, the bronchiectasis is reversible, as seen in atelectasis and pneumonia. Prolonged bronchial obstruction in the face of infection results in nonreversible bronchiectasis. Distal to the bronchiectatic segment, the alveoli are relatively unaerated, and the current of air generated during coughing is inadequate to expel bronchial secretions, which stagnate and become secondarily infected. In longstanding disease, the accumulated secretions destroy much of the bronchial wall, including cilia and muscle. Large anastomotic connections develop between the bronchial and pulmonary vessels, and may produce hemoptysis. Since the segments of bronchiectatic lung frequently are functionless in terms of gas exchange, they may account for a significant amount of pulmonary shunting. Any pulmonary condition tends to be exaggerated, therefore, if bronchiectasis is present.

Inhalations

The surface area of the pulmonary gas exchange surface has been estimated to cover 140 square m. This is comparable to the gastrointestinal surface area, and is some 50 times greater than the adult skin surface area. Thus, the pulmonary portal of entry represents a significant surface area of exchange of gases, vapors, and even particulates. The significance of inhalation of toxic chemicals via the pulmonary route takes on added significance when one considers that undegraded noxious materials can be delivered directly to the brain and other vital organs without first passing through the liver, where deactivation and detoxification might otherwise occur.

The degree of absorption of the inhaled chemical is dependent in large measure on the physical state of the material in question. Fumes, vapors, and gases are molecular in size or in the submicron range, and as such are absorbed into the pulmonary capillaries in accordance with established physicochemical laws. The site of action of these materials is a function of their solubility and the dosage presented to the respiratory tract.

Highly soluble vapors (such as ammonia) usually are trapped in the aqueous mucus lining of the turbinates and pharynx, so that little if any of the vapor reaches the lower respiratory tract unless the inhaled dosage is quite high. This would then overwhelm effectively the trapping mechanism of the upper airways, and allow sufficient quantities of the noxious material to reach the lower respiratory tract and alveoli and produce a chemical burn of the lungs, with subsequent development of pulmonary edema. In contrast, gases of relatively low aqueous solubility will produce relatively little upper respiratory tract irritation, although they readily reach the lower respiratory tree where they initiate inflammatory reactions of varying degree. For example, phosgene gas is relatively insoluble in water. Even if inhaled in small doses, it readily reaches the alveoli, where it slowly hydrolyzes to hydrochloric acid and results in delayed pulmonary edema. Thus, in general, gases or vapors of lower water solubility are more capable of inducing significant reactions in the lower respiratory tract than are those of higher water solubility.

The rate at which a gas or vapor diffuses is dependent on the partial pressure gradient between the alveolar air and the pulmonary capillary. The partial pressure in the blood is primarily a function of the solubility of the gas or vapor in what is, for all practical purposes, an aqueous medium. Nonpolar (slightly soluble) gases or vapors saturate the blood at a rate directly proportional to pulmonary blood flow. Because of the diminished solubility of nonpolar compounds in the blood, there is limitation of uptake, and they rapidly reach equilibrium with the vascular compartment. The net effect of establishing this equilibrium is to diminish the pressure gradient for diffusion between the alveoli and the capillaries, and to reduce the effective driving force for absorption between the ambient air and the body tissues. For soluble gases or vapors, the rate of blood saturation is directly proportional to alveolar partial pressure, since the rate of uptake is not hindered by solubility considerations.

The rate of absorption of gases or vapors in general can be altered by physical activity and disease states. The rate of absorption can be greatly increased by increasing capillary blood flow in the lungs, as this tends to increase the volume of blood presented to the alveoli per unit time and allows more rapid uptake of the gas in question. In patients with impaired hepatic or renal function, a more rapid accumulation of toxicants occurs than in a normal individual.

INHALATION OF PARTICULATE MATTER

The large bulk of inhaled particulate matter is cleared and removed in the upper airway. The bronchi and bronchioles also play an important role in the removal of particulate matter. As repeated branchings take place with only a slight increase in cross-sectional area, the surface area of the walls is greatly increased. Owing to the increased surface area, particles are more likely to impinge on the mucous coat than on the upper air passages. This "bronchiolar filter" has inherent ciliary action that causes particles lodged on the mucous film to be swept to the oropharynx. Many of the smaller particles reach the alveoli, where removal by ciliary action is not possible. Here, removal is accomplished by alveolar phagocytes, termed "dust cells" after the particulate matter they contain. Following phagocytosis of the particles on the alveolar walls, the debris is deposited in the pulmonary connective tissue or the lymphatics.

The ability of particulate matter to produce a local or systemic effect via the pulmonary portal of entry is largely dependent on the physical nature of the material. The chemical nature is of secondary importance, since particles too large to reach the lower airways and alveoli have less pathologic potential, regardless of their chemical composition. It is particle size, density, and surface area that determine biologic activity.

Particles larger than 5 μ in diameter usually are not important factors in eliciting pulmonary inflammatory reactions, or in permitting absorption. Mass normally is a function of size. Large particles, once set in motion, have more inertia than smaller particles. Because of the numerous changes of airflow direction in the respiratory tree, particles with high kinetic energy and inertia are most likely to impinge on the upper airway, since they are relatively incapable of changing directions, and follow the branches of the respiratory tract. Depth of pulmonary penetration also is a function of particle density: the greater the density, the less the probability of deep penetration. Another important factor that inhibits larger particles from deeply penetrating the respiratory tract is their tendency to stay suspended in air for relatively short periods of time in comparison to smaller and lighter particles.

Once impingement occurs in the upper air-conduction passages, the particulates are removed as described above. The chemical properties of the particulate become important in determining the nature of the bio-logic response in those particles that have deeply penetrated the lung.

SPECIFIC INHALATIONS

In our modern industrialized age, a growing concern for the emergency physician lies in the early detection, management, and awareness of complications associated with the inhalation of pollutant gases and a wide variety of noxious industrial compounds.

Frequently encountered pollutant gases such as carbon monoxide, nitrogen dioxide, sulfur dioxide, and ozone are all capable of inducing hypoxemia and increasing the susceptibility to infection by diminishing ciliary activity, and by a direct action on alveolar macrophages to interfere with their phagocytic properties and their subsequent lytic action. In addition, all these compounds are able, through oxidant-induced cellular and biochemical changes, to induce emphysematous changes in the lung.

One of the major toxic reactions associated with inhalation of toxic gases or fumes is that of acute pulmonary edema. The overall incidence of chemically-induced pulmonary edema is relatively small, but the frequency is not at all negligible. The early recognition of this problem is important, since therapy and prognosis differ in many respects from that of pulmonary edema from heart failure observed in usual clinical practice.

"Lag-phase" from Time of Exposure to Development of Pulmonary Edema. Frequently, a "lag-phase" is encountered after inhalations; this represents an appreciable time interval of as long as 10 to 12 hours between exposure and development of pulmonary edema. The emergency physician must be acutely aware of this possibility, since close observation is indicated in all cases of exposure to industrial intoxicants capable of eliciting this phenomenon. Among the industrial agents known to produce delayed pulmonary edema are phosgene, phosphorus compounds, methyl bromide, cadmium fumes, oxides of nitrogen, ozone, and dimethyl sulfate.

The mechanisms responsible for the development of acute pulmonary edema following exposure to these compounds have not been fully elucidated. In general, there is the working hypothesis that toxic agents produce direct toxic injury upon the alveolar-capillary membranes, increase endothelial permeability, and induce the transudation of fluid from the capillary into the interstitial spaces and alveoli.

The mechanism of injury following exposure to nitrogen dioxide and dimethyl sulfate is believed to arise from conversion of these agents into more chemically irritating substances at the cellular level; thus, nitrogen dioxide is converted to nitric acid, and dimethyl sulfate becomes sulfuric acid upon inhalation.

Certain other agents such as hydrogen fluoride, hydrogen sulfide, chlorine, ozone, and phosgene also produce irritation of the bronchial tree and result in an acute chemical bronchitis.

In addition, delayed hypoxemia as a result of pulmonary edema has been shown to be a frequent concomitant of smoke inhalation, suggesting that all patients with a history of severe smoke inhalation should be monitored with serial arterial blood gas determinations even in the absence of clinical radiologic evidence of pulmonary edema, and should be treated with controlled oxygen guided by the blood gas determinations. The details of smoke inhalation will be covered in a separate section.*

Treatment of Pulmonary Edema Secondary to Toxic Inhalations. The most effective therapy of chemically-induced pulmonary edema calls for oxygen to be administered under controlled positive pressure, with judicious use of nebulized bronchodilators for the correction of attendant bronchospasm. Intravenous corticosteroids, followed by oral steroid supplementation for several days, have been found to be beneficial in more severe cases. Nebulized nonirritant fluids will help prevent secondary bacterial pneumonia. If superimposed bacterial pneumonitis is suspected, broad-spectrum antibiotic coverage is indicated pending definitive culture reports. In certain circumstances, tracheostomy is required either for respiratory failure or to aid in the clearing of secretions. Morphine is contraindicated in certain intoxications, such as those arising from ozone and hydrogen sulfide, since both of these intoxicants act as CNS depressants, and profound respiratory depression can occur when morphine is used in conjunction with them.

CARBON MONOXIDE

The ubiquitous nature of carbon monoxide makes it of great concern to the emergency physician, since it can be lethal if the inspired air contains as little as 0.1 vol. per cent. Carbon monoxide is tasteless, odorless, and nonirritating to the mucous membranes, so that it can be inhaled without the victim's awareness. It is present in automobile exhaust, in coal gas, in water gas, in exhaust from heat stoves and furnaces with inadequate ventilation, in smoke from burning buildings, and in coal mine fires.

In 1895, Haldane demonstrated that the detrimental effect of carbon monoxide in the inhaled air is a function of anoxia, and that carbon monoxide in itself is not toxic. Carbon monoxide has an affinity some 210 times that of oxygen for hemoglobin, forming a relatively stable compound, carboxyhemoglobin, that does not dissociate significantly during a passage through the lung or tissue capillaries. Therefore, the fraction of the blood hemoglobin bound to carbon monoxide is functionally ineffective. In addition, the remaining hemoglobin available for transport of oxygen develops an increased oxygen affinity, tending to reduce tissue capillary PO_2 and hamper oxygen unloading to the tissues.

Symptoms of Carbon Monoxide Poisoning. The earliest symptoms of carbon monoxide poisoning are slight headache with muscular weakness, palpitations, dizziness, and mental confusion. Excitement and bizarre behavior may follow. These symptoms progress to coma when the carboxyhemoglobin level exceeds 40 per cent. Carboxyhemoglobin has a cherry-red color, which accounts for the frequency with which the lips of a carbon monoxide-poisoned individual are reported to be of this color. Levels of 10 per cent may be found in smokers and in tunnel workers, and mild symptoms can occur at this level. Carboxyhemoglobin level determination is the best guide as to how therapy should proceed.

Treatment. The goal of therapy is to drive the carbon monoxide off the hemoglobin molecule, while at the same time maintaining adequate oxygenation to the tissues. This usually requires the administration of 100 per cent oxygen, and sometimes even

---

*See page 837.

hyperbaric oxygen administration in the most severe cases. Treatment with oxygen will reduce the concentration of carboxyhemoglobin by 50 per cent within 40 minutes of initiation of therapy; without the use of oxygen, a similar drop in carboxyhemoglobin would require four hours.

PULMONARY BURNS

With recent improvements in the management of shock and sepsis due to burns, the problem of respiratory tract damage, with its associated derangements in pulmonary function, now accounts for an increasing proportion of the major complications and for many eventual deaths in patients who have sustained thermal injuries. The exact cause of the various disturbances in respiratory function is uncertain; in fact, respiratory problems develop in some individuals who have sustained only minimal body surface burns. The inhalation of noxious substances certainly plays an important role in respiratory tract dysfunction, especially when one considers that substances rich in nitrogen — such as mattresses and padded materials — whether filled with wool or polyurethane, release hydrogen cyanide during combustion; polyvinyl chlorides produce hydrochloric acid fumes when burning; and some plastics evolve toluene di-isocyanate which, even in minute amounts, causes intense respiratory tract irritation. In addition, the lethal effects of carbon monoxide are all too well known to the fire-fighter.

The inhalation of hot gases alone can damage the lungs, and the greater the specific heat directly reaching the lung parenchyma, the more devastating the injury becomes. An even greater number of calories are liberated when partial combustion of an inflammable vapor is completely oxidized in the deeper recesses of the tracheobronchial tree.

It is most likely that a combination of these various factors, working in whole or in part, is responsible for the clinical condition now referred to as the "pulmonary burn."

The degree and severity of the resultant disease process varies with the nature and extent of the injury, and no pathognomonic features as such are demonstrable in the lungs at autopsy. Depending on the time lapse between the incurring of the "pulmonary burn" and the institution of intervening therapy, a spectrum of pathologic findings may be observed, ranging from pulmonary congestion, edema, and alveolar thickening to parenchymal hemorrhage, bronchial and bronchiolar epithelial desquamation, and alveolar disruption, and on to bronchopneumonia, lung abscess, and even extensive pulmonary necrosis.

A method has yet to be discovered to diagnose accurately and consistently a pulmonary burn in the antemortem state. Only gross and microscopic examination of the smaller bronchioles and pulmonary parenchyma is capable of revealing the changes that characterize the acute phase of this type of inhalation injury. However, there are certain *external* signs highly suggestive of the diagnosis:

(1) flame burns about the neck and face;

(2) singed nasal vibrissae or mucosal burns of the nose, lips, mouth, and throat;

(3) external flame burns that were incurred in a closed space where heated air or noxious gases, or both, might have been inhaled.

With the exception of severe respiratory distress associated with bronchospastic wheezes in the first few hours following injury, the three criteria described above represent the only means of arriving at a correct early diagnosis. Other physical signs generally are delayed in their appearance and reflect the expected late complications of pneumonia, pulmonary edema, or both.

A raspy cough associated with soot in the sputum is certainly suggestive of the diagnosis, but is seldom found without the presence of the three basic criteria as well. Positive changes on the chest x-ray parallel the morphologic changes in the chest, but appear anytime from 24 to 48 hours after some form of respiratory distress has developed. Bronchoscopy may be of value in selected cases, but seldom offers any more information than the three major criteria in combination with simple examination of an expectorated sputum sample.

Pulmonary function studies usually are of limited value, since the patient generally is hypoxemic to begin with and is unable to cooperate to the full extent required by the tests. Apart from careful observation of ventilatory effort, cyanosis, signs of cerebral hypoxia, labial and lingual edema, and respiratory rate, there are few guidelines to follow during the course of therapy. Objective data can be obtained from the use of arterial blood gas analysis on a serial basis. This allows an over-all assessment of the status of the patient's lungs during treatment, and gives valuable information concerning improvement or deterioration.

A wide range of clinical features are associated with the cause and extent of pulmonary burns. Patients with the most severe pulmonary damage manifest a specific progression through three separate clinical stages, whereas those with lesser degree of insult will show one, or at most two, of these stages. If treatment is to be successful, specific measures must be taken for each problem as it arises in the given clinical stage. There is no such thing as a "routine" or "prophylactic" measure in the handling of a pulmonary burn; each and every therapeutic measure must have a specific indication.

The three clinical stages of pulmonary burns are: (1) *respiratory distress;* (2) *pulmonary edema;* and (3) *bronchopneumonia.*

Stage I: Respiratory Distress. This initial phase is noted only in those individuals who have sustained a major pulmonary burn. It becomes apparent anytime from a few minutes to as long as 24 hours after the injury. Manifestations include rapid and labored respirations in association with cyanosis, lethargy, and often erratic behavior secondary to cerebral hypoxia. Auscultation of the chest reveals distant breath sounds, wheezes secondary to bronchospasm, and "croupy" cough. The chest x-ray almost always is normal at this stage, and even bronchoscopy or laryngoscopy performed at this time will reveal only mild mucosal edema. Arterial blood gases, on the other hand, reveal a severe derangement reflecting acidosis, hypoxemia (PO_2 usually less than 50 mm. Hg), and possibly hypercapnia (PCO_2 in the 50 to 80 mm. Hg range).

Although the clinical picture is one of upper airway obstruction, rarely if ever does tracheostomy produce any lasting relief, and in fact the direct tracheostomy-related late complications of fulminating pneumonia and pulmonary edema constitute a relative contraindication to this procedure as a first line of treatment. When it is performed during this stage there usually is no improvement, and in some cases profuse pulmonary edema may be induced by sudden removal of the glottic barrier, necessitating the use of positive pressure ventilation to save the patient's life. Therefore, in this first stage at least, we should consider tracheostomy as a procedure of last resort.

TREATMENT OF RESPIRATORY DISTRESS STAGE. Over 50 per cent of the patients who manifest respiratory distress do so because of reflex bronchospasm induced by trauma to the bronchial mucosa. These patients usually are aided by being placed in a croup tent or by putting their heads in a child-size croupette with high flow oxygen and maximum humidity setting. Checks of the oxygen concentration within the croup tent or croupette should be made frequently, using an oxygen meter. If improvement by these techniques is not forthcoming, as determined by continuing respiratory distress and a PO_2 below 70 mm. Hg, bronchospasm should be relieved through the use of bronchodilators. Unfortunately, the usual pharmacologic agents used for this purpose (e.g., aminophyllin) are seldom effective, and about the only means that achieves any measure of lasting success is the use of intravenous corticosteroids given in a single and large dose (1500 to 3000 mg. hydrocortisone sodium succinate) over a period of one to five minutes. If necessary the dose can be repeated in eight to 12 hours.

A few individuals with severe respiratory distress fail to respond to humidity, oxygen, and steroids. This is either due to the fact that the lungs have been destroyed by the mechanism of injury, or (rarely) because the upper airway has been obstructed by laryngeal edema, crusting, or inspissated mucus. Tracheotomy must be performed at this time, bearing in mind that only in the exceptional instance does survival occur when associated with true laryngeal obstruction and when the other conservative measures have failed.

Stage 2: Pulmonary Edema. The second stage typically appears some eight to 36 hours after burn injury, although it may appear earlier if induced by such factors as injudicious administration of fluids, congestive heart failure, or the performance of early tracheotomy. Its onset may be sudden or insidious. During the acute phase the chest x-ray may be normal, but classical radiologic signs will appear within four to 12 hours.

TREATMENT OF PULMONARY EDEMA FROM PULMONARY BURNS. As previously suggested, the causes of pulmonary edema may be single or multiple. The pulmonary injury may be the major inciting factor, but it need not be the only one. Heart failure and fluid overload are complications that can be either avoided or dealt with before they overwhelm the clinical picture. Intravenous fluid therapy should contain some element of colloid, and should be adjusted to produce a urinary output of between 40 to 50 cc. per hour. Introduction of a CVP line, or better still a Swan-Ganz catheter, will forewarn against impending heart failure and/or circulatory overload. Continuation or initiation of a digitalis compound also may be indicated, particularly in the elderly. *The most important preventive measure to avoid precipitation of pulmonary edema is delay in performing tracheostomy.* Removal of the glottic barrier results in an increase in intraalveolar pressure, even so minimal an amount as to push the patient into a more fulminant form of pulmonary edema.

For the great majority of patients whose pulmonary edema is on the basis of fluid overload, congestive failure, or the respiratory injury itself, simple measures usually are effective in therapy. Fluid restriction, intravenous diuretics, and rapid digitalization are instituted. If the external burn surface is large, diuretics usually are not required, as the patient tends to lose any excess fluid accumulated in the lungs through the burn area in an hour or two. During the acute phase, fluid mobilization may be accomplished by positive pressure ventilation with oxygen through a face mask.

In a few patients, especially those in whom the pulmonary edema is secondary to the pulmonary burn itself, or to the performance of premature tracheostomy, the more routine measures for combating the process are unsuccessful. Under these circumstances, the effective means of sustaining life and reversing the process is to use a positive pressure ventilator. If a tracheostomy has already been performed, a volume-limited ventilator is fitted onto a cuffed tracheostomy tube. In all other circumstances, the patient requires endotracheal intubation with a cuffed endotracheal tube, followed by ventilatory assistance.

Stage 3: Pneumonia. All patients who survive the first 72 to 96 hours of pulmonary burn develop pneumonia to some varying degree. When onset is early, especially in the face of using a contaminated positive pressure ventilator or if steroids have been administered more than once, the bronchopneumonia may become extensively necrotizing and may progress rapidly to a multitude of small, confluent parenchymal abscesses. These patients show an ever-deteriorating picture of respiratory failure and sepsis, as manifested by positive blood cultures for *Staphylococcus aureus* or *Pseudomonas aeruginosa,* or both. Once sepsis supervenes on top of respiratory insufficiency, death soon follows.

Fortunately, most patients develop only a mild-to-moderate bronchopneumonia, with increased volume of purulent tracheobronchial secretions; blood cultures usually are negative, but the sputum contains a variety of pathogens that invariably become predominantly *Ps. aeruginosa* in the course of a few weeks. Ventilatory problems, and especially respiratory failure, are rare.

Treatment is primarily directed at providing an adequate tracheobronchial toilet: vigorous coughing; expectorants; occasional nasotracheal suctioning; and humidification, using a croupette. Systemic antibiotics are indicated *only* in the face of severe pulmonary sepsis. Even so, frequent sputum cultures should be obtained to derive information about the bacterial content in the respiratory tract in case the pneumonia should worsen. Prophylactic antibiotics neither prevent nor lessen the severity of pneumonia associated with the pulmonary burn. IPPB may be helpful in loosening any retained secretions; however, secretions occasionally may become so voluminous or obstructive in nature as to warrant repeated bronchoscopies or even tracheostomy for successful removal.

Indications for Endotracheal Intubation in Pulmonary Burns.
(1) Severe burns of the face, mouth, and nares, with rapidly increasing edema in these areas.

(2) Increasing stridor and a decreasing PaO_2.

(3) Increasing edema and immobility of the vocal cords on repeated laryngoscopy.

(4) To prevent aspiration of food and secretions.

(5) Profuse tracheobronchial secretions not responsive to suctioning.

(6) Management requires positive pressure ventilation.

OTHER RESPIRATORY DISORDERS

Acute Mountain Sickness

Acute mountain sickness and high altitude pulmonary edema are likely clinical variants of the same disorder. A given patient may suffer from either condition or both; there is a definite time lag between arrival at high altitude and onset of illness, and victims of either disorder become oliguric during the time lag and respond well to induced diuresis.

Before actually looking at these disorders in closer detail, let us review the physiology involved in high altitude environments.

The transportation of an individual to a higher altitude reduces the inspired oxygen tension, leading to a decreased PaO_2 and stimulation of the aortic and carotid bodies to increase minute ventilation, which in turn lowers $PaCO_2$ and increases arterial pH, which tends to reduce minute ventilation acting through the medullary respiratory center. In a matter of minutes to hours the decreased $PaCO_2$ leads to a decreased cerebrospinal fluid PCO_2, which raises the pH of the CSF. This tends to diminish minute ventilation through the chemosensitive regions on the medullary surface. If the individual remains at high altitude, a series of compensatory changes take place. First, the concentration of bicarbonate in the CSF decreases through active transport into the blood, and results in a drop in the pH of the CSF, which increases the minute ventilation. Next, erythrocyte, 2,3-diphosphoglycerate (2,3-DPG) increases, shifting the HbO_2 curve to the right, and increases the delivery of oxygen to the tissues. The decreased PaO_2 stimulates erythropoietin production in the kidney and leads to an increase in the formation of RBCs. The kidney also compensates for the increased arterial pH by excreting an alkaline urine and Na^+, to reduce plasma concentration of HCO_3^-. The decreased arterial PO_2 tends to increase pulmonary vascular resistance. Even healthy individuals occasionally develop acute pulmonary edema in the absence of left ventricular failure.

Acute pulmonary edema on ascending to high altitudes is a condition that has been observed in nonacclimatized individuals from lower altitudes when they are introduced rapidly to great altitudes. The same problem also is encountered when acclimatized persons return to their native high altitude environment after having spent a short period of time at or about sea level conditions.

The mechanism for the development of pulmonary edema is not at all clear. Left ventricular failure is not the cause, since there is absence of hypertension at the pulmonary capillary level. The possibility of increased pulmonary capillary endothelial permeability remains to be thoroughly investigated. It is known that the rapid rise in pulmonary artery pressure upon arrival at high altitude can produce pulmonary edema without a concomitant elevation of pulmonary wedge pressure. The reasons for this phenomenon remain unclear.

Patients who develop high altitude pulmonary edema experience a greater degree of hypoxemia than those who do not. This is apparently related to a special susceptibility. This hypoxemia can be greatly accentuated by exercise or heavy physical exertion, and may explain the many instances in which pulmonary edema develops in persons who perform unusual or prolonged physical activity upon returning to high altitude.

Sleep is another factor contributing to hypoxemia at high altitude in susceptible patients, and may account for the fact that high altitude pulmonary edema frequently develops during sleep.

ONSET

Acute mountain sickness occurs several hours after arrival at high altitude, and does not respond readily to oxygen therapy. The time lag between arrival at high altitude and onset of symptoms excludes any direct relationship between hypoxia and acute mountain sickness; by contrast, a notable feature in those developing mountain sickness during this lag period is the onset of antidiuresis, against which therapy prevents as well as relieves the illness.

Diuresis, a usual phenomenon developing in mild hypoxia, apparently is due to decreased circulating levels of ADH. This occurs as a consequence of inhibitory impulses originating from deformation receptors in the left atrium when it becomes distended by a large volume of blood, as occurs in hypoxemic-induced hyperventilation. Oliguria associated with severe anoxia seems to be due to a sudden discharge of ADH from hypoxic stress secondary to pulmonary congestion and Cheyne-Stokes respiration. In severe illness with pulmonary congestion, antidiuresis is further promoted by increasing hypoxia, reduced splanchnic flow, and sodium retention. Neurogenic vasoconstriction of renal vessels occurs when arterial oxygen saturation is less than 50 per cent. The splanchnic blood flow may also be compromised by pulmonary vascular congestion, which by virtue of its low pressure and distensible characteristics may hold a considerable quantity of blood.

RECOGNITION

The most common presenting complaint encountered in acute mountain sickness is headache. This is followed shortly by anorexia, nausea, and dyspnea. Patients frequently complain of insomnia, muscular weakness, and chest pains. Although visual disturbances, papilledema, convulsions, and coma have occurred in more severe cases, the only consistently demonstrable abnormality is a slight-to-moderate elevation of CSF pressure. In fatal cases, the predominant postmortem findings are cerebral and pulmonary edema.

TREATMENT

The mainstay of therapy is diuresis. Furosemide is the drug of choice and has been found to be most effective in relieving symptoms. Given in a dosage of 80 mg. every 12 hours for two days, beginning immediately after arrival at high altitude, it significantly reduces the incidence and severity of the acute mountain sickness and high altitude pulmonary edema in fresh entrants, as well as in former residents. The prevention is complete in high altitude pulmonary edema, and nearly so in acute mountain sickness. In severe mountain sickness associated with pulmonary edema, diuresis may be enhanced by administering morphine intravenously for one dose at the same time that the first dose of furosemide is administered. The beneficial effect of morphine is apparently related to a redistribution of blood to the periphery, lowering pulmonary blood volume, relieving pulmonary edema, and reducing pulmonary hypertension. Of additional merit is the ability of morphine to augment furosemide diuresis when oliguria

is associated with severe anoxic stress. This is related to the power of morphine to stimulate release of ACTH, as long as it does not cause respiratory depression and sensory impulses are intact. In patients with neurologic manifestations, betamethasone is used in conjunction with furosemide. Betamethasone promotes diuresis and relieves cerebral edema associated with acute mountain sickness.

In order for diuresis to be successful in either prevention or treatment of acute mountain sickness, more than 900 cc. of urine must be produced in adults in the first 24 hours.

Myasthenia Gravis

Myasthenia gravis is a motor-end-plate disease associated with a breakdown of neuromuscular transmission, and manifested by rapid fatigue of voluntary muscles and delayed recovery following exercise. The diagnosis should be considered in patients with a history of easy fatigue and weakness within voluntary muscles without an associated diminution in muscle mass.

RECOGNITION

The more common presenting symptoms include diplopia, a reflection of weakness within the extraocular muscles, ptosis, and proximal muscle weakness. The disease invariably is progressive, with eventual involvement of limb muscles, muscles of speech, mastication, and deglutition. In the more advanced stages respiratory muscles become afflicted, with resultant inhibition of ventilatory effort. It usually is not until the disease is fairly well advanced that muscle atrophy becomes evident.

VENTILATORY FAILURE IN MYASTHENIA GRAVIS

The incidence of ventilatory failure associated with myasthenia gravis is estimated to be about 10 per cent. This complication usually is not seen early in the course of the disease, since the respiratory muscles do not become afflicted until the disease is fairly well advanced. By the time ventilatory failure occurs, the patient has been taking medication for quite some time; thus, it is essential to have a careful history and documentation of the manner of taking and the response to medication. In a significant proportion of patients, it is possible to distinguish on an historical basis alone whether a serious deterioration in condition is on the basis of cholinergic or myasthenic crisis. In addition, it is important to question the patient about possible use of additional medications that might adversely affect his myasthenic state. A good example is quinine, or consumption of food or beverages containing it, since quinine will exacerbate myasthenia gravis.

MYASTHENIA CRISIS

As related to myasthenia gravis, myasthenia crisis is a condition of severe respiratory failure due to weakness of the respiratory muscles, with frequent concomitant weakness of the bulbar musculature. Ventilatory efforts are extremely weak, coughing is qualitatively and quantitatively poor, and deglutition is compromised, resulting in hypoxia, retention of secretions, and frequently pneumonitis. This is due to the basic disease state, and can be treated with anticholinesterase medications. It must be differentiated from the "cholinergic crisis."

CHOLINERGIC CRISIS

Cholinergic crisis results from overmedication with anticholinesterase drugs (e.g., neostigmine). It is characterized by two kinds of effects.

(1) *Muscarinic effects.* Abdominal cramps, nausea, diarrhea, excessive sweating, hyperhydrosis, salivation, lacrimation, visual blurring, miosis, and excessive bronchial secretions secondary to parasympathetic over-response.

(2) *Nicotinic effects.* Weakness, muscle fasciculations, slurred speech, muscle cramps, and dysphagia. These effects are a reflection of overdepolarization at the neuromuscular junction.

Resistance. This may be defined as insensitivity of the neuromuscular junction to anticholinesterase medication, manifested by decreasing responsiveness to progressively increasing dosages of medication, and eventual development of cholinergic effects. A cholinergic crisis frequently develops without improvement in muscular function. Resistance frequently is seen with infections, menses, pregnancy, emotional stress, or thyrotoxicosis. Resistance is especially common with pneumonia, or even simple upper respiratory tract infections.

Tensilon Test. The differentiation of cholinergic from myasthenic crisis is at times extremely difficult. The two types of crisis can be distinguished by a simple but extremely informative maneuver known as the Tensilon Test. The test is based upon objective muscular changes in response to intravenous administration of the parasympathomimetic, edrophonium (Tensilon). The clinical response is observed carefully and timed with serial observations of the strength of eyelid, eye, face, tongue, and extremity muscles. Following the rapid intravenous administration of Tensilon, 2 mg., the patient is closely observed for signs of improvement in muscular strength as in the myasthenic crisis, or worsening of the symptoms of too much cholinergic medication as manifested by increasing weakness, facial or deltoid fasciculations, or twitches or spasms of the eyelids. The response to Tensilon is typically most evident 30 seconds to two minutes after injection. The Tensilon effect lasts for a very short time, so that worsening of symptoms, when it occurs, is not progressive.

Treatment Considerations in Myasthenia Crisis. In the treatment of myasthenic crisis, drugs must assume a subordinate role to the establishment and maintenance of an adequate airway and the assurance of adequate pulmonary function.

In severe crisis, time should not be wasted initially in distinguishing between the disease or the medication as the cause. If the patient is gravely ill, with deteriorating ventilatory function and hypoxia, endotracheal intubation and mechanical ventilation are indicated. The airway must be kept clear of secretions, for which frequent suctioning will be required. Pneumonia should be excluded as either a concomitant or precipitating factor. All anticholinesterase medication should be withdrawn, and the patient observed closely. If he is in cholinergic crisis, the effects should resolve within 12 to 24 hours; if he has shown significant improvement during this time, he may be given a trial of anticholinesterase medication in the form of a Tensilon test. If the response of the test indicates that cholinergic function has returned, the patient may be restarted on medication at this time. If he is in myasthenic crisis due to a lack of medication, anticholinesterase responsiveness will be present early.

Frequently, patients show crisis because of drug resistance, and increasing dosages of medication fail to improve their condition. The effect can either be myasthenic or cholinergic crisis, but in either case the neuromuscular junction is insensitive to anticholinesterases, and further exposure to these drugs will only exacerbate the crisis. These patients should be intubated and placed on a volume-limited ventilator for a minimum of 72 hours. After the initiation of mechanical ventilation, all anticholinesterase medication should be withdrawn. At the end of the first 72 hours, and for each day thereafter as indicated, the patient should be tested with Tensilon for anticholinesterase responsiveness. Occasionally, a period of drug withdrawal is all that is required to resensitize the neuromuscular junction to the anticholinesterase medication.

Spontaneous Pneumothorax

Spontaneous pneumothorax refers to a collapse of the lung as a result of rupture of the visceral pleura. The more common causes include rupture of emphysematous blebs or bullae, or rupture of subpleural tuberculous foci through the visceral pleura. Trauma may be involved as a possible inciting factor in some cases, but usually the pneumothorax occurs in the absence of straining or physical exertion. In some instances, a spontaneous pneumothorax may occur in the presence of a pulmonary or mediastinal tumor.

Until recent years, the presence of a spontaneous pneumothorax was thought to be indicative of the presence of pulmonary tuberculosis. It is now well established that, in the apparently healthy individual, it usually is due to nontuberculous defects in the pleural and subpleural tissues. When a pneumothorax occurs spontaneously in the face of pulmonary tuberculosis, there generally is ample radiologic evidence of the tuberculous infestation.

RECOGNITION

The usual presenting symptoms are those of sudden pleuritic chest pain and shortness of breath in varying degrees. In some cases, the symptoms may be so mild as to be overlooked entirely by the patient, and the pneumothorax is detected as an incidental finding on chest roentgenogram. At the other extreme is the life-threatening complication of tension pneumothorax, with its associated profound dyspnea and circulatory collapse. Since emphysematous blebs or bullae frequently are bilateral, an occasional patient will develop bilateral spontaneous pneumothorax.

The degree of pneumothorax produced by rupture of a bleb or bulla may vary widely. The size and character of the visceral pleural defect, and the nature and location of pre-existing visceroparietal pleural adhesions, may be factors in determining the size and chronicity of the pneumothorax.

Tension Pneumothorax

A potentially life-threatening emergency develops from a specific complication of pneumothorax referred to as tension pneumothorax. This condition develops because of the progressive increment of positive pressure in the pleural space by a ball-valve action of the air leak in the visceral pleura. During inspiration, air is introduced into the pleural space. At end-inspiration the pleural leak seals, preventing access of intrapleural air, and hence expulsion through the respiratory tree. The situation is worsened by deep, gasping respirations, which are common in the anxious and dyspneic victims of tension pneumothorax. These deep inspirations serve to introduce large volumes of air into the pleural space. Eventually, intrapleural pressure increases to the point where the mediastinal structures are shifted to the side opposite the pneumothorax, and when the intrapleural pressure becomes sufficiently great, venous return to the heart is compromised and the patient quickly expires from acute circulatory collapse.

RECOGNITION

The victim of a tension pneumothorax is extremely dyspneic, and cyanosis is common. There is pronounced jugular venous distention and arterial hypotension, which progresses rapidly to shock. The trachea is shifted to the contralateral side—an external manifestation of the mediastinal shift.

In general, the diagnosis of simple spontaneous pneumothorax is made readily by chest x-rays. In equivocal cases, expiratory films will aid in establishing the diagnosis by sharpening the contrast between the lung and the pleural air.

Treatment depends on the size of the collapse and whether or not the pneumothorax is under tension. If there is only slight retraction of the lung from the chest wall and minimal symptoms, observation alone is all that is indicated. Reabsorption of the pneumothorax occurs at a rate of about 1 per cent per day. The pneumothorax will reabsorb, since the sum of the partial pressures of the dissolved gases in venous blood is less than atmospheric pressure. Arterial blood is approximately equilibrated with alveolar gas, and therefore the sum of the gas partial pressures in it approaches atmospheric pressure. For example, in mixed venous blood, the P_{O_2} has fallen 55 mm. Hg, while the P_{CO_2} has risen only 5 mm. Hg, leaving a deficit of 50 mm. Hg. In a pneumothorax, the pressure inside the pleural space will approximate atmospheric. This pressure will be about 40 mm. Hg greater than the sum of gas pressure in venous blood, and results in a gradient for reabsorption into the venous compartment. IPPB therapy is contraindicated if tube thoracostomy is not performed. On the other hand, some physicians advocate chest tubes in all instances of pneumothorax, believing this to be the safest course.

If more than 20 per cent of the lung has collapsed, a rubber catheter for closed thoracostomy drainage, with or without suction, may be employed for several days. In most instances, a water-type seal of drainage is sufficient. Suction should be employed if the air leakage is considerable, or if the patient is threatened by respiratory insufficiency. The 20 per cent figure refers to volume, and therefore what is considered a small pneumothorax (nonprogressive, and observable without insertion of chest tubes) involves only a slightly discernible movement of the visceral pleura away from the chest wall.

TREATMENT OF TENSION PNEUMOTHORAX

Treatment of tension pneumothorax constitutes a medical emergency of the highest priority. A needle should be inserted immediately into the pleural space. If the pressure is positive throughout the respiratory cycle, as indicated by the plunger on the syringe being pushed back, the plunger should be removed until atmospheric pressure is attained. The needle then may be attached to a thoracic pump or an underwater trap. Once the tension pneumothorax is under control, chest tubes may be inserted for continued drainage of residual air.

References

Adair, J. C., et al.: Ten-year experience with IPPB in the treatment of acute laryngotracheobronchitis. Anesth. Analg. 50:649, 1971.
Ahlquist, R. P.: A study of the adrenotropic receptors. Am. J. Physiol. 153:586, 1948.
Bates, D. V.: Chronic bronchitis and emphysema. N. Engl. J. Med. 278:546, 600, 1968.
Bates, D. V., Macklem, P. T., and Christie, R. V.: Respiratory Function in Disease. 2d ed. Philadelphia, W. B. Saunders Co., 1971.
Berenberg, W., and Kevy, S.: Acute epiglottitis in childhood. A serious emergency, readily recognized at the bedside. N. Engl. J. Med. 258:18, 870, 1958.
Bernstein, I. L.: Allergic Diseases of the Respiratory Tract. In Baum, G. L. (ed.): Textbook of Pulmonary Diseases. Boston, Little, Brown & Co., 1965.
Cameron, J. L., Anderson, R. P., and Zuidema, G. D.: Aspiration pneumonia, a clinical and experimental review. J. Surg. Res. 7:44, 1967.
Casarett, L. J.: Toxicology: the respiratory tract. Annu. Rev. Pharmacol. 11:425, 1971.
Christensen, J. B., and Telford, I. R.: Synopsis of Gross Anatomy. New York, Harper & Row Publishing Co., 1966.
Collins, J. T., Palmer, A. S., and Head, L. R.: A graphic method for bedside estimation of pulmonary arteriovenous shunting. Surg. Gynecol. Obstet. 136:129, 1973.
Comroe, J. H., Jr.: Physiology of Respiration. Chicago, Year Book Medical Publishers, Inc., 1962.
Comroe, J. H., Jr., et al.: The Lung, Clinical Physiology and Pulmonary Function Tests. 2d ed. Chicago, Year Book Medical Publishers, Inc., 1962.
Copenhaver, W. M.: Bailey's Textbook of Histology. Baltimore, Williams & Wilkins Co., 1964.
Cramblett, H. G.: Croup—Present day concept; American Academy of Pediatrics Proceedings. Pediatrics 25:6, 1071, 1960.
Cudkowicz, L., and Armstrong, J. B.: The bronchial arteries in pulmonary emphysema. Thorax 8:46, 1953.
Davenport, H. W.: The ABC of Acid-Base Chemistry. 5th ed. Chicago, University of Chicago Press, 1969.
DeWeese, D. D., and Saunders, W. H.: Textbook of Otolaryngology. St. Louis, C. V. Mosby Co., 1973.
Donnellan, W. L., Poticha, S. M., and Holinger, P. H.: Management and complications of severe pulmonary burns. J.A.M.A. 194:1323, 1965.
Dunbar, J. S.: Upper respiratory tract obstruction in infants and children. Caldwell lecture, 1969. Roentgenology 109:227, 1970.
Eden, A. N., Kaufman, A., and Renato, Y.: Corticosteroids and croup. J.A.M.A. 200:5, 1967.

Eller, W. C., and Haugen, R. K.: Food asphyxiation—restaurant rescue. N. Engl. J. Med. 289:81, 1973.

Emmanuel, G. E., Smith, W. M., and Briscoe, W. A.: The effect of intermittent positive pressure breathing and voluntary hyperventilation upon the distribution of ventilation and pulmonary blood flow to the lung in COPD. J. Clin. Invest. 45:1221, 1966.

Gardner, H. G., et al.: The evaluation of racemic epinephrine in the treatment of infectious croup. Pediatrics 52:1, 52, 1973.

Garzon, A. A., et al.: Respiratory mechanics in patients with inhalation burns. J. Trauma 10:57, 1970.

Heckscher, T., Bass, H., and Oriol, A.: Regional lung function in patients with bronchial asthma. J. Clin. Invest. 47:1063, 1968.

Hirsch, E. F., et al.: Discontinuance of respiratory assistance after pulmonary insufficiency. Am. J. Surg. 125:645, 1973.

Ishizaka, K., and Ishizaka, T.: Biological function of E antibodies and mechanisms of reaginic hypersensitivity. Clin. Exp. Immunol. 6:24, 1970.

Johansson, S. G. O., Bennich, H., and Berg, T.: The clinical significance of IgE. Progr. Clin. Immunol. 1:157, 1972.

Jordan, W. S., Graves, C. L., and Elwyn, R. A.: New therapy for post-intubation laryngeal edema and tracheitis in children. J.A.M.A. 212:585, 1970.

Kleinfeld, M.: Acute pulmonary edema of chemical origin. Arch. Environ. Health 10:942, 1965.

Lecks, H. I., Wood, D. W., and Kravis, L. P.: Childhood status asthmaticus: recent clinical and laboratory observations and their application in treatment. Clin. Pediatr. (Phila.) 5:209, 1966.

Leeson, C. R., and Leeson, T. S.: Histology. Philadelphia, W. B. Saunders Co., 1967.

Levine, G., et al: Gas exchange abnormalities in mild bronchitis and asymptomatic asthma. N. Engl. J. Med. 282:1277, 1970.

Lichtenstein, L. M., and DeBernardo, R.: The immediate allergic response: in vito action of cyclic AMP active and other drugs on the two stages of histamine release. J. Immunol. 107:899, 1971.

Lloyd, T. C., Jr., and Wright, G. W.: Evaluation of methods used in detecting changes of airway resistance in man. Am. Rev. Resp. Dis. 87:529, 1963.

Margolis, C. Z., Ingram, D. C., and Meyer, J. H.: Routine tracheotomy in Hemophilus influenzae type B epiglottitis. J. Pediatr. 81:1150, 1972.

Mays, E. E.: An arterial blood gas diagram for clinical use. Chest 63:793, 1973.

McFadden, E. R., Jr., and Lyons, H. A.: Airway resistance and uneven ventilation in bronchial asthma. J. Appl. Physiol. 25:365, 1968.

McLaughlin, R. F., and Tueller, E. E.: Anatomic and histologic changes in early emphysema. Chest 59:592, 1971.

Miller, W. F.: Intermittent positive pressure breathing. Minn. Med. 47:272, 1964.

Mittman, C., et al.: Smoking and chronic obstructive lung disease in alpha-1-antitrypsin deficiency. Chest 60:214, 1971.

Morse, H. R.: Unusual cases of tracheobronchial obstruction. Ann. Otol. Rhinol. Laryngol. 18:812, 1972.

Orr, T. S. C.: Mast cells and allergic asthma. Br. J. Dis. Chest 67:1, 1973.

Pattle, R. E.: Surface Tension and the Lining of the Lung Alveoli. In Caro, C. G. (ed.): Advances in Respiratory Physiology. Baltimore, Williams & Wilkins Co., 1966.

Polk, H. C., and Stone, H. H.: Contemporary Burn Management. Boston, Little, Brown and Co., 1971.

Pontopiddan, H., et al.: Acute respiratory failure in the adult. N. Engl. J. Med. 287:743, 1972.

Pontopiddan, H., et al.: Acute respiratory failure in the adult. N. Engl. J. Med. 287:799, 1972.

Pontopiddan, H., Geffin, B., and Lowenstein, E.: Acute respiratory failure in the adult. N. Engl. J. Med. 287:690, 1972.

Preston, F. W., and Beal, J. M.: Basic Surgical Physiology. Chicago, Year Book Medical Publishers, Inc., 1969.

Rapkin, R. H.: Tracheotomy in epiglottitis. Pediatrics 52:426, 1973.

Reed, C. E., and Siegel, S. C.: Asthma. New York, Medcom Press, Inc., 1974.

Robe, E. F.: Infectious croup. III. Hemophilus influenzae type B croup. Pediatrics 2:559, 1968.

Schottelius, B. A., and Schottelius, D. D.: Textbook of physiology. St. Louis, C. V. Mosby Co., 1973.

Selkurt, E. E.: Physiology. Boston, Little, Brown & Co., 1966.

Senaloza, D., and Sime, F.: Circulatory dynamics during high altitude pulmonary edema. Am. J. Cardiol. 23:369, 1969.

Singh, I., et al.: Acute mountain sickness. N. Engl. J. Med. 280:4, 175, 1969.

Sladen, A., Zanxa, P., and Hadnott, W. H.: Aspiration pneumonitis—the sequelae. Chest 59:448, 1971.

Smith, G., et al.: Treatment of coal-gas poisoning with oxygen at 2 atmospheres pressure. Lancet 1:816, 1962.

Snider, G. L.: Interpretation of the arterial oxygen and carbon dioxide partial pressure—a simplified approach for bedside use. Chest 63:801, 1973.

Sodeman, W. A., and Sodeman, W. A.: Pathologic Physiology: Mechanisms of Disease. Philadelphia, W. B. Saunders Co., 1974.

Stone, H. H., and Martin, J. D., Jr.: Pulmonary injury associated with thermal burns. Surg. Gynecol. Obstet. 129:1242, 1969.

Sussman, S., et al.: Dexamethasone in obstructive respiratory tract infections in children. Pediatrics 34:851, 1964.

Thorn, G. W.: Clinical considerations in the use of corticosteroids. N. Engl. J. Med. 264:775, 1966.

Vilinskas, J., Schweizer, R. T., and Foster, J. H.: Experimental studies on aspiration of contents of obstructed intestine. Surg. Gynecol., Obst. 135:568, 1972.

West, J. B.: Distribution of gas and blood in the normal lungs. Br. Med. Bull. 19:53, 1963.

Wood, D. W., Downs, J. J., and Lecks, H. I.: The management of respiratory failure in childhood status asthmaticus. Experience with 30 episodes and evolution of a technique. J. Allergy Clin. Immunol. 42:261, 1968.

Young, J. A., and Crocker, D.: Principles and Practice of Inhalation Therapy. Chicago, Year Book Medical Publishers, Inc., 1973.

Zarem, H. A., Rattenborg, C. C., and Harmel, H. H.: Carbon monoxide toxicity in human fire victims. Arch. Surg. 107:851, 1973.

Chapter 41   CARDIAC EMERGENCIES

A. Recognition and Treatment of Arrhythmias
B. Emergency Evaluation and Treatment of Disorders Resulting from Coronary Atherosclerotic Heart Disease
C. Cardiogenic Shock
D. Pulmonary Edema
E. Hypertensive Crises
F. Pericarditis
G. Recognition and Treatment of Pulmonary Embolism
H. Infective Endocarditis
I. Effect of Electrolyte Abnormalities on the Electrocardiogram

A. RECOGNITION AND TREATMENT OF ARRHYTHMIAS

Mark E. Silverman

Arrhythmias and their side-effects are alarming, and therfore a common reason to seek emergency advice. The patient may be aware that he has had a disturbance of rhythm, which he may describe as a palpitation, skipping, fluttering, jumping in the chest, or runaway heart, or he may experience only a secondary effect such as dizziness, syncope, seizures, chest discomfort, or dyspnea. Because of the diversity of presentations and the frequent disappearance of the arrhythmia prior to reaching the emergency room, the diagnosis may be difficult to make unless the physician questions the patient very closely.

The following information should be obtained when an arrhythmia is suspected.

(1) *Current attack:*

When did it start?

Where were you and what were you doing?

Did it begin abruptly or gradually?

Did it end abruptly or gradually?

How long did it last?

Were you able to count the pulse rate?

Was the rhythm regular or irregular?

Can you mimic the rate and rhythm by patting your fingers on top of the other hand?

Were there associated symptoms such as chest discomfort, weakness, dizziness, fainting, visual blurring, sweating?

What medications do you take?

What is your consumption of cigarettes, coffee, tea, alcohol, or diet pills?

(2) *Prior attacks:*

Have you had similar attacks in the past? (If so, obtain above information.)

If so, how frequently do they occur, and have you been examined or had an electrocardiogram recorded during an attack?

Have you found any positions, maneuvers or medications that have halted or prevented attacks?

Have you ever been told that you have "W-P-W"?

Do you have recurrent chest pain or discomfort?

(3) *Review of medical history*

Is there a history of heart disease, heart attack, enlarged heart, or heart murmur?

Is there a history of lung disease, blood clots to the lung, or medications for the lung?

Is there a history of chronic anxiety or recent emotional distress?

Is there a history of high blood pressure? Thyroid disease? Thyroid medication?

The extent of questioning and examination will of course depend on the clinical status of the patient. The physician must always be alert to the possibility of a serious underlying cardiac problem, such as a myocardial infarction or pulmonary embolus, that will require immediate disposition to an intensive care area.

TIPS IN UNRAVELING ARRHYTHMIAS

If you are fortunate enough to capture the arrhythmia on paper, the next step is to analyze the type of rhythm disturbance.

(A) Do not rely on a single lead.

P waves, like beautiful women, may not be fully appreciated from a single view. Too frequently, a diagnosis is made from a single monitor lead that is misleading. Simultaneous leads, a 12-lead electrocardiogram, an esophageal lead, and sometimes an intraatrial recording may be necessary.

(B) Look for the P waves.

In tachyrhythmias, P waves often are obscured by the closely preceding QRS–ST–T waves. These should be scrutinized for notches, small peaks, or negative deflections that could represent hidden P waves. By careful comparison with previous cycles, P waves may become apparent as a suddenly peaked T wave or a bump in the ST segment. Sometimes the P wave will be exposed by increasing the paper speed to 50 mm./second or doubling the standardization.

(C) Try to find a common P–P interval.

The atrial rate is determined by using

TABLE 1

TYPE OF ARRHYTHMIA	ATRIAL RATE	VENTRICULAR RESPONSE	P WAVE	P-R INTERVAL	QRS DURATION	CAROTID MASSAGE
Sinus Tachycardia	100–200	1:1	sinus	normal	normal°°	transient slowing
Atrial Fibrillation	–	irregular 50–250	fibrillatory base line	absent	normal°°	transient slowing
Atrial Flutter	180–400°	2:1 3:1 etc.	sawtooth base line	constant or variable	normal°°	transient increase in A–V block
Atrial Tachycardia	130–250°	1:1	normal or small	normal or short	normal°°	abolishes or no effect
PAT with block	130–250°	1:1 2:1 etc.	normal or small	prolonged	normal°°	no effect
Junctional Tachycardia	100–250°	1:1	inverted II, III, aVf, hidden, or behind QRS	short, hidden, retrograde	normal°°	abolishes or no effect
Ventricular Tachycardia	variable	independent of atrium 100–250°	sinus	A–V dissociation	prolonged	no effect

°Range is approximate.
°°Unless bundle branch block or aberration is present.

calipers or drawing marks on a card. Two promising deflections on the EKG are selected as the potential P–P interval. The card or caliper is then matched to this interval, and stepped progressively up or down the EKG to see if it fits other possible P wave deflections. If the settings do not coincide with the deflections, a different set of deflections is measured and the procedure repeated. Of course, the P wave may not be discernible at all if it is simultaneous with the QRS, or amidst the T wave.

(D) Is there a relationship between the P wave and the QRS?

Once P waves are identified, a relationship between the P wave and QRS must be sought. Which P wave conducts which QRS? Do any of the P waves conduct? The P to QRS intervals are measured to find a repetitive P–R interval, or a sequence that might suggest the underlying structure of the arrhythmia. Sometimes it is helpful to place the EKG on blank paper and draw a vertical line for each P wave and a vertical line for each QRS. Various possible combinations then are attempted by measuring intervals and

connecting the P waves to a QRS until a reasonable sequence is established.

(E) Analyze the QRS.

Arrhythmias are conventionally divided into "supraventricular" and "ventricular" in origin. A supraventricular origin implies that the focus is located above the division of the bundle branches to the ventricles, and includes the sinus node, atria, A–V node, and surrounding junctional tissue, and the bundle of His. Since the impulse can conduct through the normal ventricular conducting system (unless aberration or bundle branch block is present), the QRS duration is normal (less than 0.12 sec.). Ventricular arrhythmias originate below the division of the bundle branches, and therefore do not have ready access to normal conducting pathways. For this reason, the QRS is prolonged (greater than 0.11 sec.) and the morphology is often bizarre.

(F) Compare the electrocardiogram with previous tracings.

Prior tracings may easily solve an electrocardiographic mystery. Previous evidence of ectopic beats, atrial or ventricular, may be used as evidence of the origin of the current arrhythmia. The shape of the P wave and P–R interval may be compared to the tachyrhythmia in question. A question of aberration may be resolved if a previous tracing demonstrates that bundle branch block is present. The finding of Wolff-Parkinson-White syndrome on a previous EKG may provide the reason for a bizarre arrhythmia.

(G) Utilize evidence from physical examination.

Analysis of neck veins for the presence or absence of A waves, cannon waves, or flutter waves is useful in sorting out the atrial arrhythmias. Variation in heart sound intensity and abnormal splitting of the second heart sound may help to identify certain arrhythmias.

(H) Consider using carotid sinus massage and edrophonium chloride (Tensilon).

The effect of vagal stimulation on the heart should be taken advantage of to slow A–V conduction, decrease the ventricular rate, and expose the presence or absence of P waves and their rate and configuration. An arrhythmia that is slowed or converted by these maneuvers is almost always supraventricular, since the ventricle scarcely is affected by these maneuvers.

Carotid sinus massage is performed with the patient in a supine position, and the head slightly hyperextended and turned about 20° to the left to expose the area of the carotid sinus. The EKG is monitored and recorded continuously while the area of the carotid sinus is lightly massaged for three to five seconds, with the fingertips moving in a direction parallel to the course of the artery. If this is unsuccessful, more vigorous pressure can be tried. If the right side is not effective, the left carotid sinus can be approached, or the patient can be asked to perform a Valsalva maneuver during the massage. Both carotids should never be stroked simultaneously, and great care must be taken in the elderly, and in patients with a carotid artery bruit or a history of stroke. Occasionally, profound bradycardia or suppression of all pacemakers, resulting in asystole, can occur. Fortunately, this almost always is temporary; however, atropine should be available, as well as equipment for initiating cardiopulmonary resuscitation. Rarely, the offending arrhythmia may be enhanced by carotid sinus massage, or ventricular fibrillation may be precipitated.

Tensilon potentiates the effect of vagal stimulation by interfering with acetylcholinesterase, the enzyme that breaks down the mediator of vagal influence, acetylcholine. The effects are similar to carotid sinus massage. Tensilon is preferable to other parasympathomimetic drugs like Prostigmin, because its onset and duration of action is brief (1 to 3 minutes). The drug is given as a 5 to 10 mg. bolus quickly injected intravenously, while the EKG is monitored. Occasional side-effects include abdominal cramps, salivation, tachypnea, perspiration, and muscle fasciculations.

I) Check the medicines the patient is taking.

Digitalis, thyroid, quinidine, procainamide, amphetamines, and bronchodilators are all potent contributors to arrhythmias. Certain arrhythmias are more likely to be drug-induced than others—for example, atrial fibrillation is rarely digitalis-induced, whereas junctional tachycardia is common in patients taking this drug.

(J) Check the electrolytes and blood gases.

Although there may be other reasons for an arrhythmia, the underlying cause may be spurred into action by hypoxia, electrolyte imbalance, or an acid-base problem.

(K) Is there a response to medication?

Observation of the response to medications may provide some information. For example, a tachyrhythmia subdued by lidocaine is more likely to be ventricular than atrial.

DISTURBANCES OF SINUS DISCHARGE

Sinus Tachycardia

RECOGNITION

In sinus tachycardia (Fig. 1), the pacemaker is located in the sinoatrial node and discharges at a rate exceeding 100 beats/min. Depending on the cause of the sinus tachycardia, the age of the patient, and the capabilities of the conducting system, rates as high as 180 to 200/minute may be attained. A slight variation in the rate is common. There is conduction of each impulse through the atria to the ventricle; therefore, a P wave is associated with each QRS com-

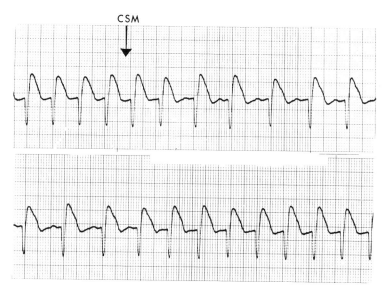

Figure 1. Sinus tachycardia. The sinus P wave is obscured within the descending limb of the T wave. Carotid sinus massage (CSM) transiently slows the sinus rate and exposes the P wave. The rate then increases. The strips are continuous.

plex, and the P–R interval is constant. Unless bundle branch block or ventricular aberration occurs, the QRS interval is narrow. Carotid massage usually produces a slowing of the heart rate, with a gradual return to the original rate as the vagal effects decrease.

THERAPY

Sinus tachycardia usually is a normal response of the heart to an external stress, or it can be an important clue to underlying cardiovascular pathology. Treatment is directed to discovery of the underlying abnormality. Among the more common stresses to be excluded are anxiety, fever, pain, exhaustion, excitement, exercise, and the use of drugs such as epinephrine, isoproterenol, and atropine. Sometimes patients are unaware that they are taking drugs containing epinephrine, thyroid, and amphetamine derivatives (hormone pills, diet pills, bronchodilators). Hyperthyroidism, anemia, pulmonary emboli, A–V fistula, myocarditis, congestive heart failure, and pheochromocytoma may have sinus tachycardia as a prominent finding.

Sinus Bradycardia

RECOGNITION

Sinus bradycardia is present when the sinus node discharges at a rate of 60 beats or less each minute. If the sinus rate falls significantly below 60, the A–V junction may "escape" temporarily and provide a "default" mechanism that maintains the heart rate. In the absence of A–V block or bundle branch block, each P wave is conducted with a normal P–R interval and a narrow QRS interval.

THERAPY

Sinus bradycardia often is a normal finding, particularly in people with excellent physical conditioning. It may occur because of high vagal tone resulting from nausea, inferior myocardial infarction, or occasionally fright. The sinus node discharge also can be slow because of sinoatrial disease (see below). No therapy is usually necessary if the rate is above 50 beats/minute, the blood pressure is normal, and the patient asymptomatic. If acute treatment is indicated, atropine, 0.3 to 1.0 mg., is given subcutaneously or intravenously.

Sinus Arrhythmia

RECOGNITION

A variation in the rate of sinus node discharge is termed "sinus arrhythmia." This is quite common in children, and may be related to respiration.

THERAPY

No therapy is necessary.

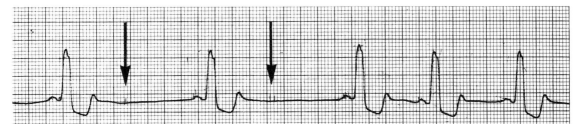

Figure 2. Sinus arrest. The arrows point to the anticipated location of the sinus P wave. The last three P waves document the rate of the sinus discharge. The P–P interval of the first three P waves is double the succeeding P–P intervals, indicating a transient 2:1 sinus block.

The "Sick Sinus" Syndrome

RECOGNITION (Fig. 2)

The ability of the sinus node to discharge regularly may be seriously impaired by a variety of diseases. This is found most commonly in the elderly, and is referred to as a "sick sinus node" or chronic sinoatrial disease. The sinus rate is usually slow, and may fail to discharge for one or more cycles. This is recognized on the EKG by the absence of the expected P wave (sinus pause or arrest), resulting in a lengthy pause until the next P wave occurs or the junction or ventricle escapes. The prolonged P–P interval may be a multiple (2:1, 3:1, etc.) of the usual sinus rate. Occasionally, a Wenckebach periodicity of the sinus rate can be plotted. The junctional tissue may also be diseased and may fail to escape after an appropriate interval. Dizziness, syncope, or cardiac arrest may then occur. Patients often present because of unexplained dizzy spells or syncope, and the only witness to the unreliable sinus node is the persistent sinus bradycardia. Monitoring studies may reveal the underlying mechanism of the symptoms. Patients with the sick sinus syndrome also are subject to recurring supraventricular tachyrhythmias. These include premature atrial beats, atrial fibrillation, atrial tachycardia, and atrial flutter. The "brady-tachy" syndrome aptly describes the clinical problem.

THERAPY

If the patient is asymptomatic, no therapy is necessary. A permanent pacemaker is required if dizziness or syncope are related to a sick sinus. Patients with the "brady-tachy" syndrome are often managed with a combination of a permanent ventricular pacemaker and antiarrhythmic drug, such as quinidine or procainamide. An atrial pacemaker can be used if the A–V junction is not diseased.

ECTOPIC SUPRAVENTRICULAR BEATS

RECOGNITON

Supraventricular beats (Fig. 3) originate either in the atria (premature atrial contractions/PACs) or junctional tissues (premature junctional or nodal contractions/PJCs or PNCs). They are considered premature when they occur prior to the expected sinus impulse. They may arise from a single ectopic impulse, or occasionally may be multifocal in origin. The ectopic impulse may be conducted through the A–V node to the ventricle and produce a QRS, or may be "blocked" by refractory tissue that has not recovered from the preceding impulse.

A PAC is recognized by a premature P wave differing in configuration from the sinus-originated P wave. Frequently, the PAC is so premature that it is partially or completely obscured by the preceding ST or T wave. If the P wave cannot conduct to the ventricle, noncompensatory pauses will result. Indeed, "unexplained" pauses frequently are due to blocked PACs. If the premature impulse can conduct to the ventricle, the P–R interval is usually normal.

Impulses arising from the low atrial area, A–V node, and His bundle are referred to as junctional or low atrial in origin. The spread of the impulse is almost the reverse of the sinus wave, and results in inversion of the P wave in leads II, III, and aVf. Depending on its exact origin and the rate of conduction to the ventricles, the P wave may be in front of, in the middle of, or behind the

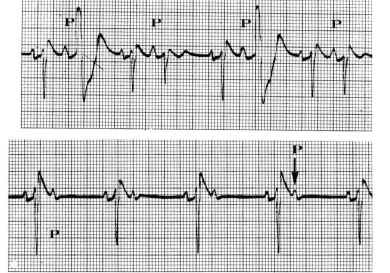

Figure 3. Premature atrial contractions. The upper strip illustrates premature atrial impulses (P) that are conducted. There is aberrant conduction of alternate premature atrial contractions. The bottom strip reveals premature P waves that are not conducted (blocked PACs).

QRS. A short P–R interval is usually, but not always, present when the P wave leads the QRS.

THERAPY

Premature supraventricular beats are common and may be an incidental finding in an otherwise normal heart. Sometimes they occur because of anxiety, exhaustion, hypoxia, drugs, pulmonary emboli, hyperthyroidism, or underlying heart disease. Treatment is not necessary unless they produce troublesome palpitations, or lead to bursts of atrial flutter, atrial fibrillation, or junctional tachycardia. If indicated, quinidine, procainamide, or propranolol may be tried.

ECTOPIC VENTRICULAR BEATS

RECOGNITON

Ventricular ectopic beats (PVCs or VPBs) originate below the division of the bundle branches in the septum or walls of the ventricles. They usually are premature and may follow the preceding sinus beat by a constant interval (fixed coupling). If a PVC follows each sinus beat, the rhythm is often referred to as ventricular bigeminy. The PVC may arise from a single focus or may be multifocal in origin. The PVC is recognized because of the altered, prolonged QRS, which is not preceded by a P wave. Occa-

sionally, there will be retrograde conduction to the atria from a PVC, producing a P wave that is inverted in leads II, III, and aVf following the QRS. The PVC often depolarizes the A–V node and blocks the conduction of the next sinus P wave, resulting in a "compensatory pause." If the PVC is very early, the A–V tissue may recover in time for the next sinus beat to be conducted without interruption. The PVC in this case is said to be "interpolated."

THERAPY

PVCs may occur in people who have no evidence of heart disease, or may be a sign of underlying heart disease, drug toxicity, hypoxia, electrolyte imbalance, stimulants (coffee, tea, tobacco, anxiety, etc.). Treatment is not necessary for the asymptomatic person without heart disease. If dizziness or uncomfortable palpitations occur, quinidine, procainamide, or propranolol can be tried. PVCs can be very difficult to eradicate, and side-effects and toxicity caused by overzealous treatment should be an important concern. PVCs are not necessarily treated in patients with heart disease. Underlying causes should be considered and eliminated if possible. Treatment usually is indicated if PVCs are early in the cycle (landing on or near the preceding T wave—"R on T"), multifocal, in chains of two or more, or are contributing to heart failure, angina, or dizzy spells. Treatment with intravenous lidocaine, procaina-

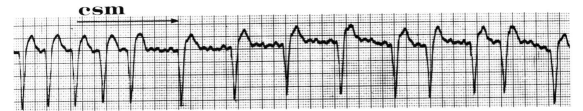

Figure 4. Atrial fibrillation. Carotid sinus massage (CSM) transiently slows the ventricular response, revealing the fibrillatory baseline. The ventricular rate than accelerates.

mide, or propranolol may be necessary in patients who are acutely ill, particularly in the setting of an acute myocardial infarction. Oral quinidine, procainamide, and propranolol are the choices in a stable patient.

ATRIAL FIBRILLATION

RECOGNITION

In atrial fibrillation (Fig. 4), there is an uncoordinated, random firing of atrial muscle fibers. There is no dominant pacemaker. When enough atrial fibers depolarize simultaneously, A–V conduction of the impulse may occur, discharging the ventricular conduction system. Because of the random nature of the atrial discharge and the corresponding variability in impulses traversing the A–V node, the ventricular rate is grossly irregular: it may vary from as slow as 40 to as rapid as 250/minute, but usually is between 80 and 150. There are no discernible P waves, and the electrocardiographic base line is finely or coarsely tremulous. Occasionally, oscillations resembling P waves may be present; however, they are not repetitive and no P–P interval can be plotted. The QRS is narrow unless bundle branch block or aberration is present. Carotid sinus massage may produce no response, or may slow the ventricular rate and lead to an irregular return to the previous rate.

THERAPY

Initial therapy depends on the rapidity of the ventricular response, the status of the patient, the etiology of the atrial fibrillation, and the medications the patient is taking. In an emergency, cardioversion may be required. This is not ordinarily necessary unless the tachycardia is extreme, and hypotension occurs. Usually, however, the prime objective is to slow conduction through the A–V node, and thereby decrease the ventricular rate. The drug of choice is digitalis, although propranolol is also highly effective if the patient is not in severe heart failure. Frequently, there will be a reversion to sinus rhythm following digitalis. If this does not occur, but the ventricular rate is slowed, correction of the atrial fibrillation may proceed at a more leisurely pace. Underlying disorders, particularly pulmonary emboli, hyperthyroidism, and mitral stenosis, should be corrected if possible. Atrial fibrillation related to myocardial infarction is often transient, and responds to treatment with digitalis and treatment of the accompanying congestive heart failure. If reversion of the atrial fibrillation has not yet occurred and is still deemed necessary, the patient should be started on quinidine or procainamide. Cardioversion can then be administered if necessary. This rhythm is only rarely digitalis-induced. When the physician is faced with the dilemma of a patient with atrial fibrillation and possible digitalis intoxication, two choices are possible. If the patient is not symptomatic, digitalis should be stopped and the rate and rhythm carefully observed. When the rhythm is poorly tolerated, digitalis can be given in cautious increments and the response noted. It is wise to remember that digitalis almost always is indicated in rapid atrial fibrillation with an irregular ventricular rate, and only rarely should be withheld. When the ventricular response is regular, digitalis intoxication resulting in A–V block, and consequent need for a junctional pacemaker, must be considered.

ATRIAL FLUTTER

RECOGNITION (Fig. 5)

In atrial flutter, the pacemaker is located ectopically in the atria outside the sinus node. The rate of discharge of this focus can

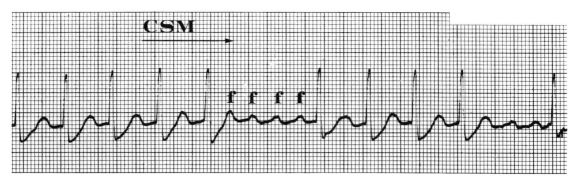

Figure 5. Atrial flutter. Carotid sinus massage (CSM) transiently increases the A–V block from 2:1 to 4:1 conduction, revealing flutter waves (f).

vary from 180 to 400/minute, but characteristically is around 250 to 300/minute. Atrial flutter is identified by the sawtooth morphology of the "flutter waves," usually seen to best advantage in lead II or V_1. The sawtooth expression is produced by the positive and negative deflection of each flutter wave. Since the A–V conducting system is not capable of transmitting atrial impulses at this rate of bombardment, there is usually a physiologic block of 2:1 or greater. A Wenckebach conduction pattern is also frequent, resulting in grouping of ventricular beats. The most common pattern of A–V conduction is 2:1. If the atrial rate is 280, a ventricular rate of 140 results. At this rate, the flutter waves may be obscured within the QRS–T complexes and atrial flutter may be overlooked. A ventricular rate of 140 or 150 should always be eyed suspiciously for evidence of atrial flutter. Atrial tachycardia can be difficult, if not impossible, to differentiate from atrial flutter. Generally, the atrial rate is slower (150 to 200) in atrial tachycardia; however, in the range of 200 to 250, the two rhythms may seem identical. The QRS is narrow unless there is an associated bundle branch block or aberration. The QRS is related to the P wave, although it is often difficult to decide which P wave is producing which QRS, particularly if there is varying A–V block. Carotid sinus massage rarely reverts the rhythm. There may be no response, or the degree of block may be increased transiently with a jerky return to normal as the block decreases from 4 to 1, to 3 to 1, to 2 to 1.

THERAPY

Digitalis is usually the initial therapy. However, some cardiologists feel that the initial treatment should be cardioversion, beginning at low energy and raising until the rhythm reverts to normal. One can begin with 10 watts/second (10 joules) and increase by 10-joule increments. Cardioversion is more dangerous in the digitalized patient than in the untreated patient.

Many cases of atrial flutter may spontaneously revert to sinus rhythm once digitalis has slowed the ventricular rate and improved myocardial performance. Occasionally, inordinately high dosages of digitalis may be required before atrial flutter is brought under control. Cardioversion is extremely successful in reverting the flutter rhythm. If both digitalis and cardioversion are unsuccessful, quinidine, procainamide, or propranolol may be useful adjuncts for further management. Quinidine and procainamide can enhance conduction through the A–V node and occasionally can increase the ventricular rate to alarming levels by changing the block from 3:1 to 2:1, or from 2:1 to 1:1. For this reason, digitalis or propranolol is always given before quinidine or procainamide is started. Cardioversion may be tried again after these agents have been started. Atrial pacing at very high rates (150 to 800/min.) also has been effective in converting atrial flutter to sinus rhythm.

PAROXYSMAL ATRIAL TACHYCARDIA (PAT)

RECOGNITION

In atrial tachycardia (Fig. 6) the pacemaker is "ectopic," located somewhere in the atria outside of the sinus node. The rate of discharge of this pacemaker may be as slow as 130 or as rapid as 250. Typically, the

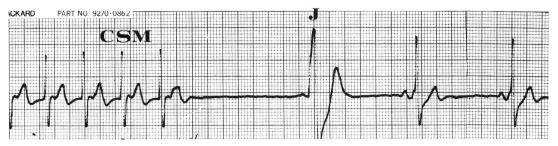

Figure 6. Paroxysmal atrial tachycardia. Carotid sinus massage (CSM) abolishes the arrhythmia and results in a period of sinus suppression with a junctional (J) escape beat.

rate is between 150 and 180, and often, though not invariably, rigidly regular, with no variation from one minute to the next. P waves are present, but are difficult to see because they are often of low amplitude and obscured within the closely preceding T wave. Each impulse is conducted to the ventricle (1:1 conduction) unless atrioventricular block results in conduction of two or more (2:1, 3:1, etc.) atrial impulses for each ventricular depolarization. This is referred to as "PAT with block," and is often a sign of digitalis intoxication. The QRS is narrow unless bundle branch block or ventricular aberration occurs. Classically, carotid sinus massage either has no effect or is followed by an abrupt return to a regular sinus rhythm (except in the case of "PAT with block").

THERAPY

Vagal-mediated parasympathetic stimulation by carotid massage is the initial form of therapy, which frequently will revert the rhythm to sinus rhythm. Tensilon may prolong or augment the parasympathetic blockade of the A–V node, and is sometimes effective even when carotid massage fails. When carotid sinus massage (either side) and Tensilon (5 to 10 mg. I.V.) are ineffec-

tive, other vagal stimulating maneuvers can be tried, but these are rarely successful. They include Valsalva maneuver, gagging, and standing the patient on his head. Ocular pressure is hazardous and should not be used. If the systolic blood pressure is below 120 mm./Hg, elevating the blood pressure may convert the arrhythmia. This is accomplished by using a peripheral vasoconstrictor such as phenylephrine. A dosage of 0.25 to 0.5 mg. can be given straight intravenously, or 10 to 20 mg. can be added to 250 cc. 5 per cent dextrose in water. This is dripped in at a rate sufficient to elevate the systolic blood pressure from 120 to 150 mm. Hg. If the arrhythmia does not convert spontaneously, carotid sinus massage should be tried again. If these efforts prove unsuccessful, digitalis or cardioversion is necessary. The severity of the symptoms dictates the rate of digitalis administration. The effects of digitalis, and the improvement of myocardial efficiency with a slower heart rate, may eradicate the atrial tachycardia. If control of the ventricular rate is difficult, or if the atrial tachycardia persists despite ventricular slowing, cardioversion usually will abolish the atrial arrhythmia. When this is not available, quinidine, procainamide, or propranolol may be employed. Rapid atrial pacing has also been

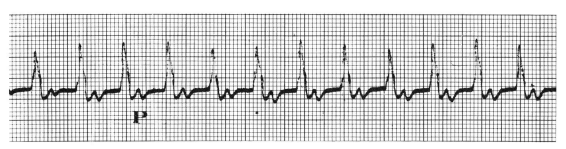

Figure 7. Junctional tachycardia. A retrograde P wave (P) follows each QRS and distorts the ST segment.

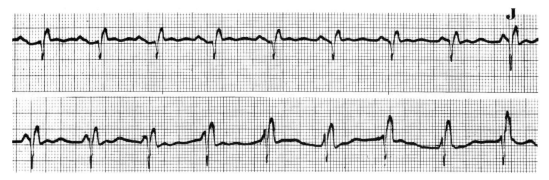

Figure 8. A–V dissociation. A mildly accelerated junctional rhythm (J) usurps control of the ventricles from the sinus node. The strips are continuous.

utilized effectively in converting atrial tachycardia.

JUNCTIONAL (NODAL) TACHYCARDIA

RECOGNITION

Junctional or nodal tachycardia (Figs. 7, 8) indicates that the ectopic focus is located within the area between the low atrium and the ventricular conducting system. Because the A–V node itself has not been shown capable of spontaneously initiating impulses, the term "junctional" is used. This term also recognizes that a wider anatomic area can be responsible for this rhythm. The rate of a junctional tachycardia can be anywhere between 100 and 250/min. A rate of 140 to 150/min. is most common. Because the electrical impulse is initiated near the origin of the ventricular conducting system, the P wave is conducted retrogradely, and therefore is usually inverted in leads II, III, and aVf. Since the impulse is conducted to the ventricle as quickly as to the atria, the P wave is intimately attached to the QRS, either preceding it by an interval less than 0.10 second, simultaneous with it and not seen, or tagging just behind. The terms high, mid, and low nodal, depending on whether the P wave is in front of, within, or behind the QRS, are no longer appropriate to use. This is because the rate of retrograde conduction, rather than its anatomic origin, determines the position of the P wave relative to the QRS. There is usually 1:1 conduction of each junctional impulse, and the QRS is narrow unless there is bundle branch block or ventricular aberration. Carotid sinus massage either has no effect, or is followed by an abrupt return to a regular sinus rhythm.

THERAPY

Although junctional tachycardia may occur in apparently normal hearts, it is frequently induced by digitalis intoxication, or may occur following a myocardial infarction or cardiac surgery. Junctional tachycardia is treated exactly like atrial tachycardia, using carotid massage, Tensilon, other vagal maneuvers, or vasoconstrictors, followed by digitalis or cardioversion if necessary. If the patient is taking digitalis, digitalis intoxication is assumed and the drug is discontinued. This arrhythmia should be suspected particularly when the ventricular rate becomes faster and regular in the patient with atrial fibrillation who is receiving digitalis. Junctional tachycardia associated with a myocardial infarction, cardiac surgery, or myocarditis is often transient, and may not require therapy. If the ventricular rate is rapid or congestive heart failure is present, digitalis is given. If the arrhythmia persists, antiarrhythmic agents such as propranolol, procainamide, or quinidine may be used. Cardioversion is effective and may be used if other measures fail.

GENERAL CONCEPTS IN THE MANAGEMENT OF ATRIAL AND JUNCTIONAL TACHYRHYTHMIAS

The major initial concern in the treatment of the atrial and junctional tachyrhythmias is the ventricular rate of response to the onslaught of atrial impulses. The physiologic consequences of the rapid ventricular rate include shortening of the diastolic filling period, abbreviation of the time for coronary flow, increased ventricular work and oxygen consumption, and a variable cardiac output. This may aggravate congestive heart failure, precipitate angina pectoris or myocardial infarction, initiate life-threatening ventricular arrhythmias, or produce syncope. In addition, the rapidly or irregularly contracting ventricle may alarm the patient greatly. Treatment of all arrhythmias depends on diagnosing the type and the underlying etiology, if possible. Several possible therapeutic approaches may be used.

(1) *Removing or treating the offending basis of rhythm disturbance.*

The causes include drug effects (particularly digitalis but also thyroid, amphetamines, catecholamines, and nicotine), electrolyte imbalance, myocardial damage, pericarditis, pulmonary embolus, myocarditis, hyperthyroidism, rheumatic fever, and hypoxia.

(2) *Slowing or abolishing the excessive atrial rate.*

This may be accomplished by carotid massage, Tensilon, antiarrhythmic drugs (including quinidine, procainamide, Dilantin, lidocaine, and propranolol), and by cardioversion.

(3) *Reducing the number of atrial impulses reaching the ventricles by prolonging the refractory period of the A–V node.*

Digitalis is usually the drug of choice, although in selected cases propranolol may be preferred. In addition to its effects on the A–V node, digitalis improves myocardial efficiency by increasing the force of myocardial contraction. This results in an increase in cardiac output and coronary flow that may play an important role in eradicating the arrhythmia.

Occasionally, the exact rhythm cannot be diagnosed with assurance. If digitalis toxicity can be excluded, digitalis can be given. Because quinidine and procainamide may enhance conduction through the A–V junction, these drugs should *not* be given prior to adequate digitalis. Cardioversion usually is effective in all atrial tachyrhythmias and may be used if available. If the rhythm disturbance is related to digitalis, cardioversion may result in more serious arrhythmias, and is contraindicated.

THE WOLFF-PARKINSON-WHITE SYNDROME

RECOGNITION

The Wolff-Parkinson-White syndrome (Fig. 9) is considered separately, since the bizarre nature of this arrhythmia can easily mislead the unsuspecting diagnostician. Patients with this syndrome are subject to paroxysmal tachyrhythmias that are almost always supraventricular in origin. Atrial tachycardia is the most frequently associated arrhythmia, but atrial fibrillation and atrial flutter are also common. The mechanism may vary from one time to the next in the same patient. Because of the presence of an anomalous pathway, the supraventricular impulse has two available routes to the ventricle. If the A–V node is the chosen pathway, the QRS is narrow. If the supraventricular impulse reaches the ventricle via the anomalous pathway, a bizarre QRS with an initial delta wave is transcribed. The usual

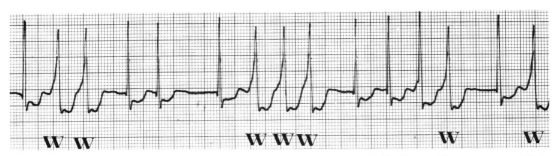

Figure 9. Wolff-Parkinson-White syndrome. The basic rhythm is atrial fibrillation. The complexes with the narrow QRS are conducted via normal conducting pathways. The complexes marked as W begin with a marked delta wave due to early ventricular excitation through a bypass tract. The grossly irregular rhythm is the clue that the rhythm is atrial fibrillation and not runs of ventricular tachycardia.

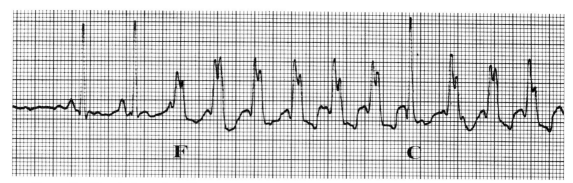

Figure 10. Ventricular tachycardia. Two sinus beats are followed by a fusion beat (F) leading off a run of ventricular beats. A capture beat (C) transiently interrupts the ventricular rhythm. Cardiac arrest occurred in this patient seconds after this EKG was recorded.

physiologic delay in the A–V node is circumvented, and the ventricular rate is often extremely rapid. Ventricular rates exceeding 200 and approaching 300/min. may occur. The prolonged QRS and alarming heart rate simulate ventricular tachycardia; however, closer inspection usually will reveal a grossly irregular ventricular rate, delta waves, and a concordant QRS pattern across the precordial leads. In addition, there is often a mixture of narrow and wide QRS intervals.

THERAPY

Treatment is highly individualized for the patient with the W-P-W syndrome. Frequently, the best therapy is discovered by trial and error. In general, atrial tachycardia is treated exactly like the garden variety PAT. There is some concern that digitalis is potentially dangerous in the treatment of atrial fibrillation and atrial flutter in W-P-W. Digitalis, because of its effect in increasing the atrial rate and delaying impulses in the A–V node, actually may facilitate conduction through the pathway and accelerate the ven-

tricular rate greatly. Nevertheless, digitalis is still usually effective in treating these arrhythmias. Propranolol, in a dose of 0.25 to 0.5 mg./min. I.V. to a total dose of 5 mg., has proved effective. Lidocaine, quinidine, and procainamide also are useful, singly or in combination with digitalis or propranolol. Cardioversion almost always is successful, and should be performed immediately if the patient is acutely ill.

VENTRICULAR TACHYCARDIA

RECOGNITION

Three ventricular beats in a row constitute ventricular tachycardia (Figs. 10, 11). The rate of the ectopic ventricular focus may be regular or irregular and from 100 to 250 beats/min., the rate of 150 to 200 beats/min. being most common. The rhythm is often initiated by a ventricular premature beat striking on the upstroke of the T wave (R on T).

The rapid depolarization of the ventricle is conducted retrogradely, depolarizing the

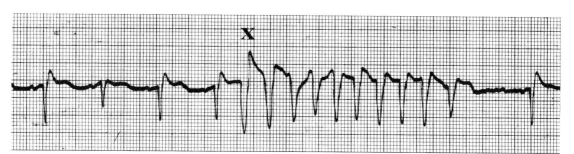

Figure 11. Ventricular tachycardia. A premature ventricular beat (X) strikes on the T wave, initiating a transient burst of ventricular tachycardia.

junctional tissue. The P wave, therefore, usually arrives at the A–V node, finds it already depolarized, and is unable to conduct. Occasionally a sinus P wave arrives between ventricular beats and is able partially or completely to conduct through to the ventricle. When the ventricle is depolarized solely by the P wave, the ventricle is said to be "captured," and the beat is called a "capture beat." This is recognized by the narrow QRS identical to a normally conducted sinus beat. If the ventricle is depolarized by partial conduction of the P wave and simultaneous conduction of an ectopic ventricular beat, the resultant QRS may reflect the contribution of both impulses, and is termed a "fusion beat." The finding of capture or fusion beats is very suggestive, although not absolutely diagnostic, that the arrhythmia is ventricular in origin. Since the atrial rate is independent of the ventricular rate, the P waves are not related to the QRS, and the atria and ventricles are "dissociated." The rapid ventricular rate usually obscures the P waves so that they are seen only intermittently. The ventricular beats originate outside the conducting tissue spreading through myocardium, and therefore the QRS is wide and often splintered in configuration. Carotid sinus massage has no effect on ventricular tachycardia.

Differentiation of Ventricular Tachycardia and Supraventricular Tachycardia with Aberration (Fig. 12)

Supraventricular tachycardia with aberration of conduction may simulate ventricular tachycardia and be difficult or even impossible to distinguish from it. The term "aberration" applies when an impulse originating above the ventricles (supraventricular) is conducted in a circuitous path through the ventricles, rather than by the normal ventricular conducting pathways. A QRS wider than normal results. This usually is because of incomplete recovery of one or more of the bundle branches at the time that the impulse reaches the ventricles. For this reason, aberration is more likely to occur with rapid rates or with premature beats. Because the right bundle branch is usually the last portion of the bundle branches to recover, the aberrant beats most often have a right bundle branch block configuration (rSr' in lead V_1). Aberration is favored by a long-short sequence, i.e., a long preceding R–R interval and a short coupling interval to the beat in question. The following criteria have been proposed to help distinguish aberrant beats from ventricular ectopic beats.

FACTORS FAVORING VENTRICULAR TACHYCARDIA

(1) Presence of fusion beats or capture beats.

(2) Tachyrhythmia begins with premature beat striking on T wave.

(3) qS or rS morphology in lead V_6.

(4) All QRS complexes are one direction (all positive or all negative) in V leads (excluding Wolff-Parkinson-White syndrome).

(5) Previous isolated beats that were felt to be ventricular in origin.

(6) Retrograde QRS to P interval (R to P) greater than 0.10 second.

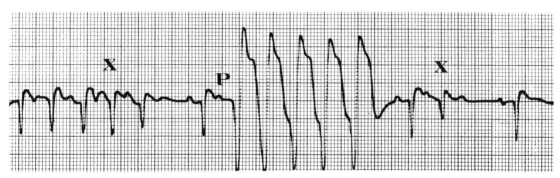

Figure 12. Supraventricular tachycardia with aberration. Frequent premature atrial beats (X) are noted. After a long cycle a premature atrial contraction (P) results in a brief run of aberrant beats. The long-short sequence and obvious premature P wave suggest that the tachyrhythmia is supraventricular with aberration.

FACTORS FAVORING ABERRATION

(1) P waves precede and are related to the QRS.

(2) The initial direction of QRS is identical with sinus-conducted QRS in lead V_1.

(3) rSr' in V_1 and qRS in V_6 morphology.

(4) Configuration of QRS similar to QRS of previously known supraventricular beats.

(5) Retrograde QRS to P (R to P) interval less than 0.10 second.

(6) Rhythm is slowed or terminated by carotid sinus massage.

THERAPY

Ventricular tachycardia is usually a grave arrhythmia requiring rapid therapy. The patient and monitor leads should always be checked, since artifacts from scratching, loose leads, etc., commonly masquerade as ventricular arrhythmias. A precordial blow is sometimes all that is necessary to revert the arrhythmia. Since supraventricular tachycardia with aberration or bundle branch block closely simulates ventricular tachycardia, carotid sinus massage may be tried. A bolus of 50 to 100 mg. of lidocaine, followed by an intravenous concentration of 2 to 4 mg./min., is the next choice. A second bolus can be given to raise the serum level; however, a total dose of 750 mg./hour should not be exceeded. If this does not work, intravenous propranolol, procainamide, or Dilantin may be tried. If drugs are ineffective, bedside cardioversion is required. Intravenous Valium, 5 to 20 mg., usually produces enough sedation to permit the electroshock. If this fails, hypoxia, drug toxicity, or electrolyte abnormalities are a possibility and should be checked. Restoration of the blood pressure and coronary perfusion with vasopressors may also be beneficial. A ventricular pacemaker may be used to "overdrive" the ventricular tachycardia. After the pacemaker has wrested control of the ventricle from the ectopic focus, the rate can be cautiously decreased. This mode of therapy is very effective in patients with recurrent bursts of ventricular beats, particularly if there is an underlying slow sinus rhythm. Occasionally, the ventricle has to be paced at a rate of 110 to 120 to suppress the ventricular tachycardia. The most important therapy of ventricular tachycardia is its prevention before it can occur. Drug intoxication (particularly digitalis, but also procainamide, quinidine, epi-

nephrine, isoproterenol, and Aramine), anoxia, and electrolyte disturbances must be considered suspect.

Frequent premature ventricular contractions, complete heart block with a slow ventricular rate, rapid atrial tachycardias, or very slow sinus rhythms may predispose to ventricular tachycardia, especially in the setting of a myocardial infarction. Prompt recognition and treatment of these arrhythmias, including intracardiac pacing if necessary, can prevent the development of the more dangerous arrhythmia of ventricular tachycardia.

ACCELERATED IDIOVENTRICULAR RHYTHM

RECOGNITION

An accelerated idioventricular rhythm (Fig. 13) (slow ventricular tachycardia) is a frequent guest in acute myocardial infarction. It is an escape rhythm and differs from the usual form of ventricular tachycardia by its slow rate (60 to 130/min.), the usual presence of sinus bradycardia, multiple fusion beats, and the lack of clinical symptoms. The ventricular beats occur late in the cycle, and for that reason often intermingle or "fuse" with the sinus beat that already has partially depolarized the ventricle. The rhythm appears to play with the sinus rhythm, weaving in and out, depending on the sinus rate. The ectopic beats are not preceded by a P wave (unless they occur simultaneously with the sinus-conducted beat), and are ventricular in appearance with a wide QRS.

THERAPY

It is important to recognize this arrhythmia, for it often does not require treatment. The impulse of the inexperienced physician is to give lidocaine, which can be harmful by suppressing the sinus node and the ectopic rhythm, resulting in a profound bradycardia or even asystole. The correct therapy is to watch carefully or to use atropine to accelerate the sinus rate. If the ventricular rate exceeds 110, lidocaine may be necessary.

VENTRICULAR FIBRILLATION AND STANDSTILL

The terminal rhythm disturbance may be either ventricular fibrillation or ventricu-

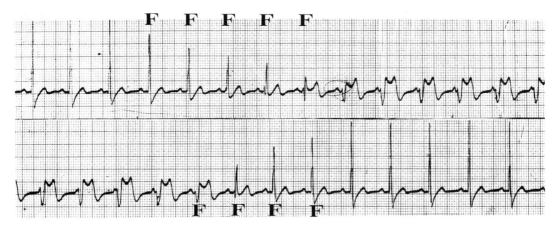

Figure 13. Accelerated ventricular rhythm. The strips are continuous. The ventricular and sinus rates are very similar, producing a series of fusion beats (F) at the beginning and end of the arrhythmia.

lar standstill. Although both of these rhythms may be spontaneously self-reverting and may be attested to only by transient dizziness or a syncopal (Stokes-Adams) episode, they usually require immediate and concerted attention. The two rhythms cannot be differentiated by bedside diagnosis, and distinction is possible only by an electrocardiogram. The term "cardiac arrest" applies to both of these rhythms, and usually announces itself by signs of central nervous system anoxia—a sudden loss of consciousness, or a seizure.

RECOGNITION OF VENTRICULAR FIBRILLATION

Ventricular fibrillation (Fig. 14) is immediately recognized by the completely chaotic oscillations of the isoelectric line, without any discernible QRS. The oscillations may be of relatively low amplitude, or very coarse and uneven in appearance. Occasionally, there is some difficulty in distinguishing where ventricular tachycardia ends

and ventricular fibrillation begins. There is no clinical problem in diagnosis, for no pulse is palpable and the patient rapidly becomes unconscious.

THERAPY

A precordial blow is occasionally enough of a stimulus to convert the ventricular fibrillation to a more desirable rhythm. If this is ineffective, the cardiac output must be maintained by external massage together with adequate ventilation. Neither can succeed without the prompt institution of the other. This requires a firm surface on which to place the patient, suctioning of any material that may be blocking the airway, positioning of the head, and establishing an airway by any means available, including mouth-to-mouth breathing if necessary. The inevitable acidosis is neutralized by several ampules of $NaHCO_3$. Inability to revert these arrhythmias can usually be ascribed to failure to correct anoxia and acidosis, or delay in treatment. Success is directly related to

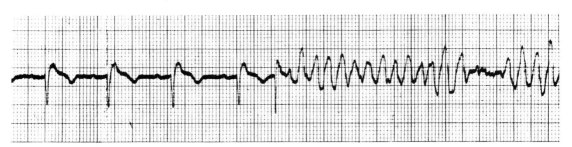

Figure 14. Ventricular fibrillation. A premature beat of uncertain origin initiates a period of ventricular fibrillation.

the time lapse between arrest and therapy. For this reason, if there is any delay in obtaining electrocardiographic documentation, electroshock ("blind defibrillation") should be administered immediately, on the assumption that ventricular standstill will not be affected adversely and that ventricular fibrillation will be reverted.

A defibrillator should be made ready as quickly as possible, and conducting jelly or saline pads applied to the paddles. These may then be placed either in the anterior-posterior position, or at the apex and upper right sternal border. Two hundred to 400 watt-seconds of electrical energy are discharged through the paddles. External massage is reinstituted immediately, and the success of the maneuver is determined by feeling for pulses and observing for spontaneous movement or respirations. If unsuccessful, the acidosis should again be corrected and a higher current delivered. In the meantime, an EKG should be positioned and the exact rhythm disturbance delineated. Further therapy will be dictated by the type of rhythm.

RECOGNITION OF STANDSTILL (ASYSTOLE)

Ventricular standstill is apparent because of the unwavering, thin, isoelectric line, disturbed only by an occasional P wave or a rare QRS. This is often preceded by a very irregular, slow ventricular rhythm.

THERAPY

The immediate maintenance of the circulation, ventilation, and correction of acidosis is identical to the treatment for ventricular fibrillation. Pacemaker activity must be established. A precordial blow with the fist, or needling the myocardium, may stimulate electric depolarization. Intracardiac or intravenous injection of epinephrine (5 cc. of a 1:10,000 solution) or Isuprel (0.2 mg.), with or without calcium gluconate (10 cc.), followed by cardiac massage to circulate the drug, may initiate pacemaker excitement. If a good CVP line is present, intracardiac injection is unnecessary. Isuprel may be given by continuous I.V. drip (1 mg. in 500 cc. 5DW). External pacing may be tried, but this rarely is effective. If available, a pacemaker wire can be inserted through a needle into the heart by percutaneous left ventricular puncture, or preferably transvenously into the right ventricle.

The prevention of ventricular fibrillation or ventricular standstill constitutes a most important point of therapy. These rhythms are frequently preceded by other rhythm disturbances, especially frequent premature ventricular contractions, ventricular tachycardia, and third-degree heart block. Treatment directed at correcting these rhythms may prevent cardiac arrest. Careful attention to the electrolytes, particularly the potassium, may be very helpful in prevention.

The patient most likely to arrest is the one who has just arrested. For this reason, preparations must be made on the assumption that he will again arrest in the next few minutes. If the physician cannot be present continually, it is imperative that he fully educate the nurse so that she is aware of the warning signs of impending ventricular arrhythmias. A review of the events leading up to the cardiac arrest, the drugs that the patient is taking, and the electrolyte, pulmonary, and renal status before and after the arrest, may yield clinical information that could prevent a future arrest. A repeat physical examination and complete EKG should be undertaken to establish new base lines.

ATRIOVENTRICULAR BLOCK

Normal Electrophysiology

The electrical impulse originating from the sinoatrial (S–A) node is transmitted through conducting pathways within the atrial wall to the atrioventricular (A–V) node. The A–V node is located in the lower portion of the right atrium above the tricuspid valve. After a transient delay in the A–V node, the impulse continues from the A–V node through the bundle of His to the bundle branches and ventricular conducting system. The P–R interval on the EKG measures the time interval between the sinus node discharge and ventricular depolarization (onset of QRS). The normal P–R interval generally ranges from 0.12 to 0.20 second.

Atrioventricular Block

The term "heart block" refers to a delay in conduction, or a failure of the impulse to

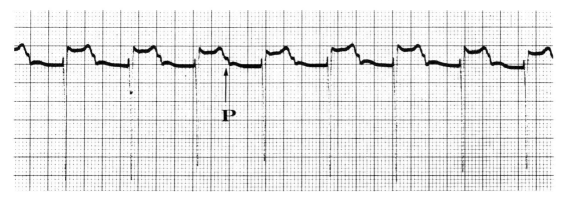

Figure 15. First degree heart block. The P–R interval is prolonged to 0.40 second. The P wave (P) is hidden in the descending limb of the T wave.

reach the ventricular conducting system. This could occur in the atrium, at the level of the A–V node, in the His bundle, or in the bundle branches to the ventricle.

Heart block is further classified as to the degree of conduction disturbance.

RECOGNITION OF FIRST-DEGREE HEART BLOCK (Fig. 15)

The P–R interval is 0.20 second or greater, and all P waves are conducted to the ventricle. Intervals as long as one second between the P wave and the QRS are possible. First-degree heart block can be produced by a conduction impairment at any level from the atrium through the bundle branches.

RECOGNITION OF SECOND-DEGREE HEART BLOCK

One or more P waves fail to conduct to the ventricle (dropped beats). There are two types of second-degree heart block.

Mobitz Type I–"*Wenckebach Phenomenon*" (Fig. 16). There is progressive prolongation of A–V conduction, until conduction is completely interrupted and a ventricular beat is dropped. This is seen on the EKG as an increasing P–R interval, until a P wave is not conducted to the ventricle. The resultant pause allows time for the A–V conducting tissue to recover, and the P wave can again be conducted at a shorter P–R interval. The progressive lengthening of the P–R interval then repeats itself until the next pause. The space produced by the dropped beat separates the Wenckebach cycles and gives the appearance of "group-beating"—often a clue to the underlying Wenckebach periods. The length of the Wenckebach period is described by counting the number of P waves and QRS complexes that group together, i.e., 3:2, 5:4, etc. There are two other characteristics that help to unmask a Wenckebach rhythm—the first R–R cycle of the Wenckebach period shortens more than the following R–R cycles, and the R–R cycle containing the dropped P wave is less than twice the preceding R–R cycle.

The presence of A–V Wenckebach periods usually implies involvement of the area of the A–V node. Since this area is located on the inferior (diaphragmatic) surface of the heart, A–V Wenckebach commonly accompanies an inferior myocardial infarction. Digitalis intoxication is another

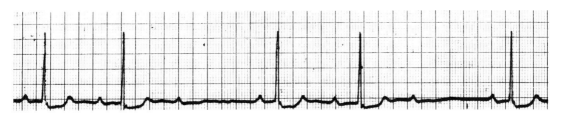

Figure 16. Second degree A–V (Wenckebach) block. A 3:2 A–V Wenckebach is illustrated.

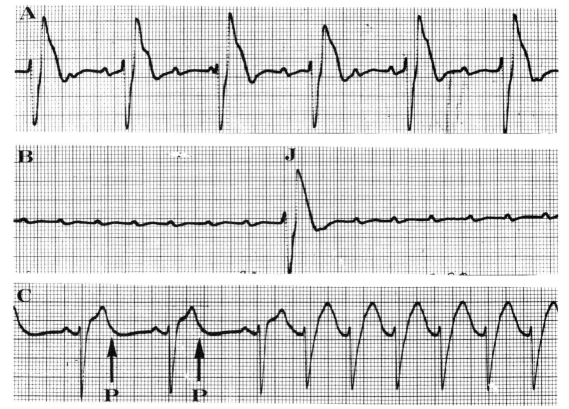

Figure 17. Second degree A–V (Mobitz II) block. The strips are not continuous but are taken from the same patient. Strip A shows complete A–V block with a junctional escape rhythm. Strip B shows a prolonged period of systole due to complete A–V block with a single escape junctional beat (J). Strip C shows 2:1 A–V block with the nonconducted P wave hidden in the T wave (arrows). The 2:1 conduction abruptly returns to 1:1 in the middle of the strip.

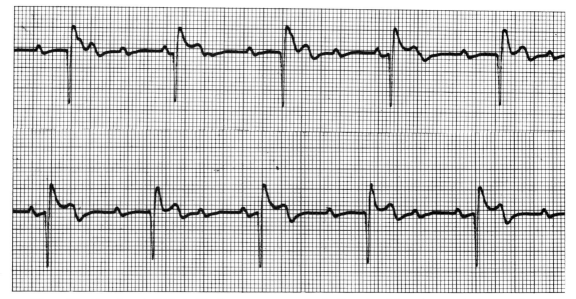

Figure 18. Complete A–V block. The P waves are completely dissociated from the ventricular complexes because of complete A–V block. A junctional rhythm is responsible for the ventricular depolarization.

cause of a Wenckebach conduction disturbance.

Mobitz Type II (Fig. 17). In this type of second-degree heart block, the P–R interval remains constant, with intermittent failure of P waves to conduct—that is, a P wave occurs but is not followed by a QRS. Mobitz Type II block is less common than Wenckebach, and is a sign of severe permanent impairment of the conducting system, usually distal to the A–V node. The most common setting is an anterior myocardial infarction. Because a Mobitz Type II block often is produced by extensive damage to the ventricular conducting system, the QRS usually is wide.

Recognition of Third-Degree Heart Block (Fig. 18). In third-degree (complete) A–V block, none of the atrial impulses succeeds in conducting through to the ventricle. Therefore, the atrium and ventricle beat independently of each other—the P waves and the QRS complexes are not related. Third-degree heart block may be intermittent, occurring transiently between long periods of apparently normal conduction, or permanent. The area of the complete block may be located anywhere from the atrial connections to the A–V node to the bundle branches.

If the patient is to survive, there must be a pacemaker below the level of the block. Usually, a junctional pacemaker at a rate of 40 to 60 beats/min. comes to the rescue. The resulting QRS is usually narrow. If the junctional tissue does not rise to the occasion, a ventricular pacemaker will often supply a rate of 20 to 40 beats/min. The QRS is then broad.

GENERAL CONCEPTS IN THE MANAGEMENT OF HEART BLOCK

The effective ventricular rate, not the degree of atrioventricular block, is the primary concern in the management of heart block. Many patients have no difficulty with a heart rate in the 40s or 50s, and do not require electrical or drug therapy. Other patients cannot tolerate these rates without problems such as syncope, angina pectoris, congestive heart failure, hypotension, or the emergence of dangerous arrhythmias.

On the coronary care unit, two different types of heart block are delineated, each with its own prognosis and treatment.

Heart Block with Inferior Myocardial Infarction

Heart block is very common in inferior myocardial infarction, because the area containing both the A–V node and the inferior (diaphragmatic) portion of the heart is usually supplied by the same (right) coronary artery. Heart block is transient, rarely lasting longer than a week, and appears in a predictable, progressive fashion. Initially, the P–R interval lengthens to greater than 0.20 second (first-degree heart block). This is succeeded by Wenckebach periods (second-degree heart block) of variable length. The patient then may, or may not, develop complete (third-degree heart block) atrioventricular block.

With inferior myocardial infarction there is usually a reliable, relatively speedy junctional pacemaker below the level of the block that stimulates the ventricle 50 to 60 times a minute. If the ventricular rate is enough to prevent symptoms or complications, no therapy is required, although intermittent use of atropine (0.3 to 1.5 mg. subcutaneously or I.V.) is justified in an attempt to diminish the excessive vagal effects that often occur in inferior infarction and increase the heart block. If the junctional pacemaker is not dependable, or if the slow rate allows ectopic ventricular arrhythmias to surface, a transvenous ventricular pacemaker is necessary. Isoproterenol can be used to increase the rate, but it is difficult to control and may precipitate more dangerous arrhythmias. A pacemaker may also be necessary in the patient with A–V block and heart failure. In this case, control of the ventricular rate allows digitalis to be used safely.

Heart Block with Anterior Myocardial Infarction

When heart block occurs with anterior myocardial infarction, there is invariably extensive myocardial damage, either from the new infarction alone or from a new infarction superimposed on previous infarctions. Heart block in this new situation is often highly capricious, developing without warning and possibly producing sudden death. Since the damage is often widespread, and the area of the block distal to the A–V node, ventricular, rather than junctional, pacemakers must be relied upon. Their inherent

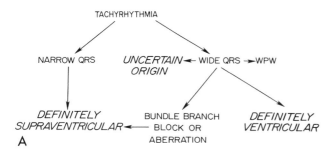

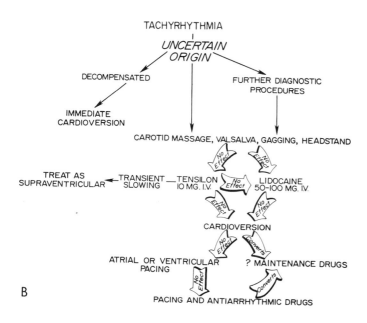

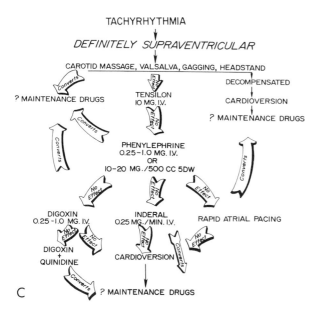

Figure 19. Algorithms for analyzing and treating tachyrhythmias.

A, The analysis of a tachyrhythmia.

B, An algorithm for the therapy of a tachyrhythmia of uncertain origin.

C, An algorithm for the therapy of a supraventricular tachyrhythmia.

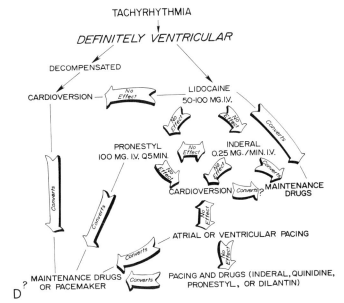

Figure 19. Continued. D, An algorithm for the therapy of a ventricular tachyrhythmia.

rate of discharge is slower (20 to 30/min.), and often undependable or tardy in firing. For these reasons, asystole or ventricular arrhythmias are common. Certain electrocardiographic patterns may forewarn of the development of complete heart block. These include a leftward or superior mean QRS axis with a RBBB configuration in the V leads, a Q in lead V_1 with a RBBB pattern, and a Mobitz Type II heart block. A prophylactic transvenous ventricular pacemaker usually is inserted in these situations, since there may not be time when block suddenly develops. The mortality is very high in anterior infarction with heart block, because of the extensive injury, and there is some doubt whether the patient will survive even with a pacemaker. Nevertheless, a pacemaker is warranted, even though the eventual salvage may not be great.

References

Abildskov, J. A., Millar, K., and Burgess, M. J.: Atrial fibrillation. Am. J. Cardiol. 28:263, 1971.

Bellet, S.: Clinical Disorders of the Heart Beat. Philadelphia, Lea & Febiger, 1971.

Cheng, T. O.: Atrial pacing: its diagnostic and therapeutic applications. Progr. Cardiovasc. Dis. 14:230, 1972.

Chokshi, D. S., Mascarenhas, E., Samet, P., et al.: Treatment of sinoatrial rhythm disturbances with permanent cardiac pacing. Am. J. Cardiol. 32:215, 1973.

Chung, E. K.: Appraisal of multifocal atrial tachycardia. Br. Heart J. 33:500, 1971.

Chung, E. K.: Principles of Cardiac Arrhythmias. Baltimore, Williams & Wilkins Co., 1971.

Cohn, L. J., Donoso, E., and Friedberg, C. K.: Ventricular tachycardia. Progr. Cardiovasc. Dis. 9:29, 1966.

Collinsworth, K. A., Kalman, S. A., and Harrison, D. C.: The clinical pharmacology of lidocaine as an antiarrhythmic drug. Circulation 50:1217, 1974.

Cranefield, P. F.: Ventricular fibrillation. N. Engl. J. Med. 289:732, 1973.

Cranefield, P. F., Wit, A. L., and Hoffman, B. F.: Genesis of cardiac arrhythmias. Circulation 47:190, 1973.

Dighton, D. H.: Sinus bradycardia. Autonomic influences and clinical assessment. Br. Heart J. 36:791, 1974.

Dreifus, L. S., and Watanabe, Y.: Current status of diphenylhydantoin. Am. Heart J. 80:709, 1970.

Fisch, C., and Knoebel, S. B.: Recognition and therapy of digitalis toxicity. Progr. Cardiovasc. Dis. 12:71, 1970.

Hoffman, B. F., Rosen, M. R., and Wit, A. L.: Electrophysiology and pharmacology of cardiac arrhythmias. III. The causes and treatment of cardiac arrhythmias. Part A. Am. Heart J. 89:115, 1975.

Jelinek, M. V., Lohrbauer, L., and Lown, B.: Antiarrhythmic drug therapy for sporadic ventricular ectopic arrhythmias. Circulation 49:659, 1974.

Josephson, M. E., Caracta, A. R., Ricciutti, M. A., et al.: Electrophysiologic properties of procainamide in man. Am. J. Cardiol. 33:596, 1974.

Kistin, A. D.: Problems in the differentiation of ventricular arrhythmias from supraventricular arrhythmia with abnormal QRS. Progr. Cardiovasc. Dis. 9:1, 1966.

Lichstein, E., et al.: Incidence and description of accelerated ventricular rhythm complicating acute myocardial infarction. Am. J. Med. 58:192, 1975.

Lindsay, J., Jr.: Quinidine and countershock: a reappraisal. Am. Heart. J. 85:141, 1973.

Lown, B., Temte, J. V., and Arter, W. J.: Ventricular Tachyarrhythmias: clinical aspects. Circulation 47:1364, 1973.

Marriott, H. J. L.: Practical Electrocardiography. Baltimore, Williams & Wilkins Co., 1972.

Marriott, H. J. L., and Sandler, I. A.: Criteria, old and new, for differentiating between ectopic ventricular beats and aberrant ventricular conduction in the presence of atrial fibrillation. Progr. Cardiovasc. Dis. 9:18, 1966.

Mason, D. T.: Digitalis pharmacology and therapeutics: Recent advances. Ann. Intern. Med. 80:520, 1974.

Moss, A. J., and Davis, R. J.: Brady-tachy syndrome. Progr. Cardiovasc. Dis. 16:439, 1974.

Narula, O. S.: Wolff-Parkinson-White syndrome. a review. Circulation 47:872, 1973.

Pick, A., and Langendorf, R.: Recent advances in the differential diagnosis of A-V junctional arrhythmias. Am. Heart. J. 76:553, 1968.

Resnekov, L.: Present status of electroversion in management of cardiac dysrhythmias. Circulation 47:1356, 1973.

Rosen, K. M.: Cardiac arrhythmias (part 3). Junctional tachycardia: mechanisms, diagnosis, differential diagnosis, and management. Circulation 47:654, 1973.

Samet, P.: Cardiac arrhythmias (part 2). Hemodynamic sequelae of cardiac arrhythmias. Circulation 47:399, 1973.

Sandler, I. A., and Marriott, H. J. L.: The differential morphology of anomalous ventricular complexes of RBBB-type in lead V_1: ventricular ectopy versus aberration. Circulation 31:551, 1965.

Schlant, R. C., and Hurst, J. W.: Advances in Electrocardiography. New York, Grune & Stratton, Inc., 1972.

Smith, T. W.: Drug therapy: digitalis glycosides (2nd of two parts). N. Engl. J. Med. 288:942, 1973.

B. EMERGENCY EVALUATION AND TREATMENT OF DISORDERS RESULTING FROM CORONARY ATHEROSCLEROTIC HEART DISEASE

Stephen D. Clements, Jr.

In the early and mid-1960s, it was noted that constant monitoring of patients with myocardial infarction led to early recognition and treatment of life-threatening arrhythmias. Mortality statistics improved in groups of patients with myocardial infarctions. Further attempts to improve treatment of these patients facilitated prompter recognition of critical symptoms and signs and speedy entrance into coronary care monitoring units.

The Emergency Department at present has become an important area for receiving patients with clinical manifestations of coronary atherosclerosis. Furthermore, we now know that over one-half of fatalities from coronary atherosclerotic heart disease involve sudden death outside the hospital (Spiekerman et al., 1962; Kuller et al., 1966). In many individuals who experience sudden death, prodromal warning clues can be identified, such as a changing pattern of angina or episodes of prolonged pain (Soloman et al., 1969).

This knowledge has resulted in an extension of the facilities of the Emergency Department to mobile units for early monitor care, and patient and physician education so that early entrance into health care systems can be accomplished.

Regardless of coronary care units and better physician and patient education, some 600,000 individuals die each year in this country of coronary atherosclerotic heart disease. (Feinleib and Davidson, 1972). Early and correct identification of the coronary syndrome is important for appropriate therapy. Important early decisions commonly are made in Emergency Department settings.

There has been increasing awareness that angina pectoris and myocardial infarction are parts of a *continuum* of clinical manifestations of coronary atherosclerotic heart disease. The following sections will outline these manifestations and offer suggestions for initial management. Basic clinical taxonomy follows the outline set forth in the recent edition of *The Heart* (Hurst et al., 1974) (Fig. 1).

Heberden's description of angina in the late 1700s has stood the test of time in that those classic subjective complaints are encountered today in individuals suffering from angina pectoris (Heberden, 1772). The latter is commonly a short-lived discomfort rather than a pain. Patients relate that it is a sensation of tightness, slight burning, "indigestion-like" heaviness, or heavy pressure in the chest. Some have a sensation of impending doom and others have a vague, not necessarily unpleasant, discomfort often misinterpreted as originating from some other organ system. The discomfort often is so mild that it is ignored for a long time before its source is identified correctly. Frequently, it is localized to the substernal area, but it may involve the epigastrium, neck, elbows, interscapular areas, or mandible.

Most commonly, angina pectoris is precipitated by a measurable amount of exercise and relieved by rest. Some patients will tell of walking up a flight of stairs and devel-

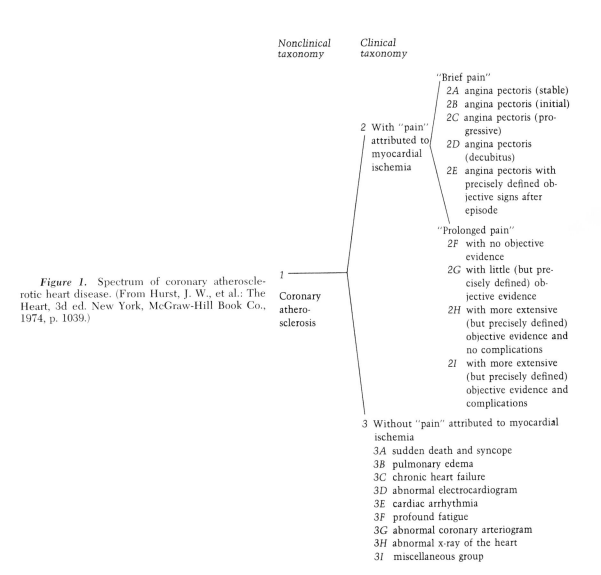

Figure 1. Spectrum of coronary atherosclerotic heart disease. (From Hurst, J. W., et al.: The Heart, 3d ed. New York, McGraw-Hill Book Co., 1974, p. 1039.)

Nonclinical taxonomy

Clinical taxonomy

2 With "pain" attributed to myocardial ischemia

"Brief pain"
2A angina pectoris (stable)
2B angina pectoris (initial)
2C angina pectoris (progressive)
2D angina pectoris (decubitus)
2E angina pectoris with precisely defined objective signs after episode

"Prolonged pain"
2F with no objective evidence
2G with little (but precisely defined) objective evidence
2H with more extensive (but precisely defined) objective evidence and no complications
2I with more extensive (but precisely defined) objective evidence and complications

1 Coronary atherosclerosis

3 Without "pain" attributed to myocardial ischemia
3A sudden death and syncope
3B pulmonary edema
3C chronic heart failure
3D abnormal electrocardiogram
3E cardiac arrhythmia
3F profound fatigue
3G abnormal coronary arteriogram
3H abnormal x-ray of the heart
3I miscellaneous group

oping substernal discomfort, or mowing a round of grass, or shoveling a certain amount of snow. In addition to exercise, emotional stress notoriously induces angina pectoris. A disturbing pattern is that which occurs at rest, while either supine or sitting. This commonly is referred to as *angina decubitus*. This carries a more grave prognosis, usually signaling severe obstructive disease. *Nocturnal angina pectoris* is part of this spectrum, and may be associated with early left ventricular dysfunction that occurs shortly after assuming the recumbent position and is due to increased venous return. Digitalis may help this type. Another variety is that associated with rapid eye movement sleep and dreaming (Nowlin et al., 1965). This occurs later at night after sleep has begun, and may awaken the patient; it probably will not be helped significantly by digitalis.

Angina pectoris characteristically is relieved by sublingual nitroglycerin, starting to take effect one-and-one-half to two minutes after administration and being complete in about five minutes. Sometimes a second and third nitroglycerin tablet may be required, but this usually represents a break in the usual pattern and is a danger signal.

Patients not uncommonly experience discomfort on first arising, during such activities as shaving or taking a shower; then, as the day goes by, they tolerate more activity without developing angina pectoris. A similar phenomenon occurs on the golf course when the discomfort starts while the patient walks the first hole; passes away with rest or nitroglycerin; and is absent during the remainder of the round. Another interesting observation is the so-called "walk-through" phenomenon (MacAlpin and Kattus, 1966). Some individuals can continue walking after the development of discomfort, which disappears after a brief period. The mechanisms of early morning angina pectoris and the "walk-through" phenomenon are not entirely clear, but some think it is related to the opening up of collateral channels.

From the clinical standpoint, then, coronary atherosclerotic heart disease should be viewed as a spectrum (Fig. 1). Certainly *painful* syndromes represent a large part of the spectrum, although at other times the patient may manifest coronary atherosclerotic heart disease *in the absence of pain*. For example, cardiac arrhythmias, syncope, or sudden death may be first manifestations of cor-

onary atherosclerotic heart disease. Hurst and Logue have offered a useful taxonomy that represents clear definitions of the elements of this spectrum, and it is to be hoped that this will promote better understanding of modes of treatment and better recognition of syndromes requiring specific treatment (Hurst et al., 1974).

BRIEF PAIN

By definition, *angina pectoris* is a discomfort of brief duration, usually lasting three to five minutes, occasionally five to 15 minutes, but never 30 minutes to two hours. In an Emergency Department or other initial encounter area, a patient whose subjective complaints suggest angina pectoris caused by coronary atherosclerosis must be evaluated carefully in order to define the syndrome. Correct definition results in appropriate therapy.

Angina Pectoris, Stable

This is brief discomfort that occurs at a relatively fixed frequency, has predictable precipitating characteristics, and is relieved promptly by rest and nitroglycerin. By definition, no change has taken place in this pattern in one month.

The objective data that can be collected as one formulates the problem of angina pectoris are important. If an attack is witnessed, blood pressure may be noted to be elevated, sometimes going up before the patient experiences discomfort; arrhythmias may develop and signs of left ventricular dysfunction may appear. Occasionally one may palpate an ectopic impulse that appears and disappears with an attack; an atrial or ventricular gallop or transient reversed (paradoxic) splitting of second sound, or even a murmur of mitral regurgitation from papillary muscle dysfunction, may develop. Some patients experience breathlessness during an attack, occasionally as a chief complaint and certainly indicating transient pulmonary congestion.

In patients with stable angina, the *resting* EKG frequently is normal. The EKG *during an attack* may be normal or may show characteristic ST segment depression in certain leads. If angina occurs under observation, an EKG should be made to discover any ischemic changes. Occasionally, the EKG will show ST segment elevation in leads that correspond to the compromised area of the myocardium (Prinzmetal et al., 1959; Prinzmetal et al., 1960). In the office setting under stable conditions it is helpful to quantitate exercise tolerance while monitoring the EKG. Characteristic electrocardiographic changes of myocardial ischemia give positive objective data to the diagnosis. If this is in question, electrocardiographically monitored treadmill stress testing may be helpful for diagnostic purposes.

The treatment of angina pectoris, stable, consists of nitroglycerin, propranolol, and other general measures such as weight reduction in the obese patient, discontinuing smoking, and the avoidance of situations that repeatedly precipitate discomfort. Planning should include long term follow-up, preferably by the same physician. Emergency physicians can identify and appropriately treat this syndrome, educate the patient, and thus get him off to a good start.

Angina Pectoris, Initial

This is defined as a first episode of *brief* pain caused by myocardial ischemia. Angina may be stable for months, followed by a pain-free interval of several weeks; a recurrence of angina at this point is of the same significance as the very first episode.

This variety should be treated as if a small infarction had occurred; that is, hospitalization is indicated if the patient contacts the physician soon after the discomfort. If a few days have passed, management probably can be carried out safely at home. After a few days rest, activity can be increased gradually over the next few weeks.

The patient should be educated about coronary atherosclerosis and given nitroglycerin to be used as needed. Propranolol should be considered if episodes of pain or discomfort recur in the future.

Angina Pectoris, Progressive

This implies a change in the usual pattern or an accelerating frequency of discomfort. Some episodes may occur at rest.

Treatment usually consists of hospitalization and the use of nitroglycerin, Isordil, and propranolol. If the cycle is not interrupted by rest and this therapy, some patients should be considered for coronary arteriography and coronary bypass surgery.

Angina Pectoris, Decubitus

In this type, patients experience discomfort at rest while either sitting or lying down. This is a bothersome symptom, and along with progressive angina pectoris is considered to represent a "preinfarction syndrome."

Treatment usually consists of hospitalization and treatment with nitroglycerin, Isordil, and propranolol. Persistent symptoms signal the need to consider coronary arteriography and coronary bypass surgery.

Sometimes, patients have brief pain and yet have associated electrocardiographic changes or enzyme changes. Of course, these patients have small or moderate-sized infarctions and require management as such.

PROLONGED PAIN

Patients who experience prolonged chest pain, i.e., 30 minutes or more, usually require serial observations in the coronary care unit over the next few days. One of the problems encountered when dealing with coronary atherosclerotic heart disease is the tendency to consider myocardial infarction as a single entity. This causes special difficulty at the time of initial contact with the patient. *If positive objective evidence is required, such as dead zones and ST and T wave changes, grave errors can be made. The EKG has been particularly misleading in this setting, especially since it may well be normal when the patient is first seen.*

In the Emergency Department setting, it is important to realize that the evaluation of patients with chest pain does not necessarily produce a definitive answer, but it does allow the choice of the appropriate observation unit so that more definitive data can be collected. Certainly, when a patient with typical pain pattern and classic electrocardiographic changes enters the Emergency Department, and myocardial infarction is clearly present, the course of action is clear. On the other hand, a patient with 30 minutes or more of chest pain with normal EKG and physical findings should be sent to coronary care for observation without delay.

Subjectively, patients may complain of "heavy pressure," burning sensations, or hard pain in the substernal area. The discomfort commonly radiates to the left arm, neck, jaw, interscapular region, or sometimes the right arm, and sometimes may be several hours in duration. Persistent pain incompletely relieved by opiates is a troublesome complaint.

Objective findings on first encounter are quite variable. Commonly there are no abnormal findings. Blood pressure, however, may be at one extreme or the other. Hypertensive responses are frequent. Hypotensive shock states are dreaded and are associated with poor prognosis. When left ventricular dysfunction is present, neck veins may be distended. Rales may be present at the lung bases when frank pulmonary congestion is present. Ectopic impulses may be noted at the precordial area. Aortic closure may be delayed owing to poor left ventricular function, and reversed splitting of second heart sound can result. Atrial and ventricular gallop sounds at apex are common. The mid-to-late systolic murmur of papillary muscle dysfunction sometimes occurs. Rarely, a holosystolic murmur at left sternal border, associated with a thrill and a state of vascular collapse, signals ruptured ventricular septum. Pulmonary edema and an apical holosystolic murmur suggests ruptured papillary muscle. Arrhythmias may be apparent at the bedside.

The EKG may show one of several abnormalities: ST changes, T wave changes, or Q waves plus ST-T wave changes. The so-called "hyperacute" T changes of infarction are not uncommon. These rapidly evolve to Q waves, ST elevation, and peaked waves,

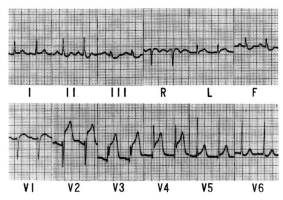

Figure 2. Admission tracing recorded during the initial phase of anterior myocardial infarction demonstrating "peaked" T waves and marked ST segment elevation in leads V2 to V4. Both mean T vector and ST vector are pointing toward the acutely injured area. (Reprinted from Hurst, J. W., and Wenger, N. K. (eds.): Cardiology for Nurses. New York, MEDCOM, 1978, p. 51; in press.)

followed by T-inversion (Figs. 2 and 3). Arrhythmias will be discussed later.

Chest x-ray may be normal or may show distention of upper lobe veins on a six-foot upright posterior-anterior x-ray. Alveolar edema is a discouraging finding, indicating severe left ventricular dysfunction.

POINTS IN DIFFERENTIAL DIAGNOSIS

Proper early assessment leads to appropriate treatment. In deciding upon the correct diagnosis, several differential points often cause confusion.

(1) Sometimes the discomfort of acute cholecystitis presents with a midline lower

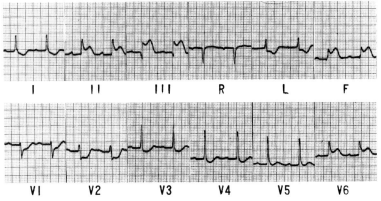

Figure 3. Admission tracing demonstrating initial changes of acute inferior myocardial infarction. Initial forces are horizontal with small Q waves in lead II, F and prominent Q wave in lead III. ST segment vector points inferiorly, to the right, and posteriorly toward the injured area. During the initial phase the T vector points inferiorly toward the infarcted and injured area. (Reprinted from Hurst, J. W., and Wenger, N. K., (eds.): Cardiology for Nurses. New York, MEDCOM, 1978, p. 51; in press.)

substernal component, and may be mistaken for the discomfort of myocardial ischemia. As the process develops, more localization occurs and correct assessment of the problem is more obvious.

(2) Acute viral pericarditis at times poses a difficult problem. The pain frequently is severe, and has substernal and often left supraclavicular or left interscapular components, aggravated by inspiration and relieved by sitting up. Opiates commonly do not give complete relief, yet corticosteroids intravenously may be of dramatic diagnostic as well as therapeutic value. Of course, pericarditis may be secondary to recent or remote myocardial infarction, or may accompany aortic dissection or trauma. Serial observations frequently are required to separate these entities.

(3) Dissecting aneurysm of the aorta may cause severe sudden onset of chest pain, usually with radiation to the back, and of a "tearing" quality. Associated pericarditis may indicate aortic "sweating" into the pericardium or pericardial bleeding. Involvement of the coronary arteries can result in myocardial infarction. Alteration in peripheral pulses, hypertension, and sternoclavicular pulsations together with widened mediastinum on x-ray afford clues to the underlying problem.

(4) Pulmonary embolism may cause substernal pain of acute onset, and results in EKG changes that mimic inferior myocardial infarction or both inferior and anterior infarct. Hypotension, supraventricular arrhythmias, and pulmonary edema may accompany embolism. Clues to the correct diagnosis are a high index of suspicion in certain settings, such as immobilized states, postoperative states, peripheral venous disease, and the use of oral contraceptive drugs. If one requires pleuritic pain, wedge-shaped infiltrates, and hemoptysis for the diagnosis, many instances of pulmonary embolism will be overlooked.

(5) Hyperventilation with associated sharp anterior chest pain commonly is mistaken for myocardial ischemia, and can be separated out if the symptoms are reproduced by overbreathing the patient.

(6) Peptic ulcer disease usually results in burning pain in the epigastric area, but sometimes the lower substernal location of the pain causes concern about possible cardiac origin. Rupture of the esophagus, associated with prolonged vomiting and retch-

ing, usually has associated left pleural fluid of gastric origin or mediastinitis.

(7) Pancreatitis may be confused with myocardial ischemia but, of course, has associated elevated amylase and a component of back pain. The clinical setting offers a clue: usually alcohol has been ingested to excess. Interesting and imperfectly understood EKG changes sometimes accompany pancreatitis. These changes may mimic inferior myocardial infarction.

CLINICAL SYNDROMES IN MYOCARDIAL INFARCTION

In patients with clinical manifestations of coronary atherosclerotic heart disease, certain syndromes may be present on initial contact that require prompt action.

Pulmonary Edema

The patient complains of shortness of breath and may have elevated venous pressure and systemic arterial pressure in addition to rales and wheezes over the lung fields. Sometimes heart sounds are difficult to hear because of restlessness and pulmonary noise, but ventricular gallop sounds are common. Treatment consists of getting the patient into a sitting position or elevating the head of the bed, oxygen by mask, morphine, and Lasix and digoxin intravenously. Sometimes positive pressure oxygen helps. The hypertensive response sometimes seen in this setting usually responds to the above treatment. There has been interest lately, however, in altering afterload with vasodilators, such as nitroprusside, phentolamine, and even intravenous nitroglycerin, while monitoring the pulmonary capillary wedge pressure with a Swan-Ganz catheter (Fanciosa et al., 1972; Chatterjee, et al., 1973; Kelly, et al., 1973; Flaherty, et al., 1975). This maneuver, when done, should be instituted after the patient is under surveillance in the C.C.U.

Severe Pain

Relief of pain is important, since increased catecholamine levels may aggravate arrhythmias. Hypertensive responses to pain cause myocardial oxygen consumption to increase, and may enlarge infarct size. Morphine sulfate, intravenously in increments of a few milligrams, may be titrated for relief of pain. If bradycardia or nausea occur as a result of morphine, 0.6 mg. of atropine should be given I.V. Demerol, 50 to 100 mg. I.V., is preferred by some (because of its "atropine-like" effect) in face of inferior infarction, since vagotonia and A-V block sometimes are early complications in such patients.

Shock

When patients present with hypotension and evidence of underperfusion of organ systems—such as the central nervous system, kidney, skin, and extremities—serious problems are ahead. Blood pressure may be in the 70 to 80 range. The neck veins may indicate elevated or low venous pressure. Heart sounds may be faint. Once this syndrome is identified in the Emergency Department, a good intravenous line should be obtained. If hypovolemia is present, intravenous fluids should be given. If bradycardia accompanies hypotension, atropine should be administered to increase the heart rate. If measurement of left atrial pressure can be made later, the finding of a low LA pressure suggests that more volume is needed. If the heart simply has low output in the face of satisfactory filling pressure, measures to increase the stroke volume have to be considered. Dopamine, Isuprel, and norepinephrine are possible treatments, each having some disadvantages. Under special circumstances, the intra-aortic balloon pump may be useful (Dunkman, et al., 1972).*

Ruptured Ventricular Septum

A state of shock usually accompanies this condition. Occasionally, the patient may have reasonably good cardiac function. The problem is recognizable by a loud holosystolic murmur at the left sternal border, frequently associated with a thrill. If cardiac output is low, the murmur may not be so loud. Significant left-to-right shunts usually

are associated with high venous pressure. Early surgical correction of these defects is associated with high mortality; however, an apparent improvement in surgical mortality may, in fact, indicate that some deaths have occurred during the waiting period, and those who eventually undergo surgery are those with lesser risk (Graham et al., 1973; Jones et al., 1975). Certainly, if the patient is hemodynamically stable, the longer surgical intervention can be postponed, the better the chance of survival.

Papillary Muscle Dysfunction and Rupture

Patients with myocardial ischemia or infarction may develop mid- to late-systolic crescendo-decrescendo murmurs at the apex, due to failure of the papillary muscles to contract properly. These murmurs may not require specific action, but recognition is important, since mitral regurgitation may aggravate the borderline left ventricular function. The papillary muscles may rupture and produce massive mitral regurgitation with gross pulmonary edema. If this syndrome is recognized, valve replacement is necessary. The mortality in this situation is high, with or without surgery.

Cardiac Rupture

Occasionally, a patient with infarcted myocardium may present with tamponade caused by a rupturing heart. A rare patient has had pericardiocentesis and prompt surgery with success (Cobbs et al., 1973). Rarely, murmurs of blood gushing through a small hole from the heart to the pericardium have been noted (Logue and Bishop, 1950).

Electromechanical Dissociation

When electric activity persists on EKG, although no cardiac output can be detected, prognosis is poor. One should ensure that tamponade is not present and that hypovolemia has been corrected. High potassium states can cause this—in addition to infarction with vascular collapse. If beta-adrenergic agents such as isoproterenol, dopamine, epinephrine, and calcium have been tried, little else can be done.

---

*See Cardiogenic Shock, page 922.

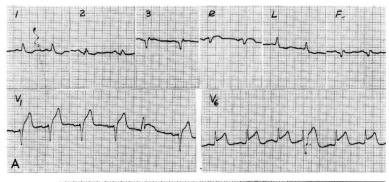

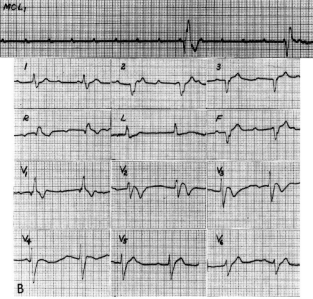

Figure 4. A, Admission tracing that shows an old inferior infarction and peaked T waves plus ST segment elevation in leads V_1 and V_6 (present also in leads V_2 through V_5), indicating "hyperacute" changes of anterior infarction.

B, The top MCL_1 rhythm strip, taken about 24 hours after admission, demonstrates high-grade A–V block that abruptly developed, resulting in a state of disorientation and combativeness. Atropine and isoproterenol, in addition to external massage, increased the ventricular rate, and a transvenous pacemaker was inserted. Note the right bundle branch block pattern and the left axis deviation not present on admission tracing.

Bradycardia and Asystole

Occasionally, patients present with a "cholinergic storm" state with bradycardia and hypotension. Slow heart rates, especially less than 50 beats per minute, associated with hypotension or arrhythmia, should be treated with atropine, 0.6 to 1.0 mg. I.V. Increasing the heart rate often will "overdrive" ventricular arrhythmias that are occurring at heart rates in the 50 to 60 range. If patients with inferior infarction have A-V block, and yet heart rate is greater than 50 and blood pressure is adequate for organ perfusion, a pacemaker may not be needed. If *symptomatic* bradycardia is present, secondary to A-V block and unresponsive to atropine, a transvenous pacemaker is necessary. In the setting of anterior infarction, left axis deviation, and right bundle branch block, a pacemaker is needed if and when A-V block occurs. The development of new left

axis deviation and right bundle branch block, under observation, should call for a pacing catheter in place in the right ventricle, or certainly one ready for use at the bedside (Fig. 4). Regardless of pacing, many patients with left axis deviation and right bundle branch block do not survive because of pump failure (Waters and Mizgala, 1974; Godman et al., 1970; Atkins et al., 1973). Asystole is associated with a poor prognosis and is commonly a terminal state, resulting from the patient's going through a sequence of more treatable arrhythmias — such as ventricular tachycardia and ventricular fibrillation.

Ventricular Premature Beats and Ventricular Tachycardia

If ventricular premature beats or ventricular tachycardia is present on initial contact, prompt treatment with lidocaine, 50 to 100 mg. I.V., followed by a drip at 2 to 5 mg. per minute, usually will abolish the arrhythmia. Some use Pronestyl, 100 mg. I.V., followed by a 1-mg./cc. concentration drip used at up to 1 gm. per hour to control the arrhythmia. Prompt DC cardioversion is indicated if ventricular tachycardia is present and the hemodynamic situation is in jeopardy. Antiarrhythmic drugs should follow this cardioversion.

Ventricular Fibrillation

Prompt defibrillation, followed by ventilation if needed, is important. If a patient suspected of having infarction suddenly becomes pulseless, ventricular fibrillation should be suspected and prompt "blind" defibrillation should be accomplished. Some Emergency Departments have defibrillators with built-in electrodes on the paddles that allow instantaneous rhythm identification. One must remember that the predisposing factors are still present after defibrillation, and measures should be started to prevent recurrence of the arrhythmia. Lidocaine or pronestyl should be started I.V., followed by a drip.

Supraventricular Arrhythmia

Atrial tachycardias identified on initial contact sometimes require prompt treatment, especially if associated with hypotension. Carotid sinus massage or Valsalva maneuver frequently convert these. Small doses of digoxin intravenously, followed by repeat carotid sinus massage or Valsalva maneuver, often are helpful. One to 2 mg. of propranolol, I.V., has been very useful in this setting.

Atrial fibrillation requires that the ventricular response be controlled with digoxin, unless hypotension is present and the atrial kick of sinus rhythm is desperately needed. In this latter instance, DC cardioversion is indicated.

Atrial flutter (usually with 2:1 block) can aggravate cardiac function considerably, and some physicians believe that low watt second cardioversion should be used promptly, followed by digoxin. An alternate approach is digoxin, usually at rather high doses at four-hour intervals, which may revert this rhythm to atrial fibrillation and then to normal sinus rhythm.

OTHER CLINICAL SYNDROMES

These deserve special attention, since coronary arteriography and surgical help may be needed at an early date.

Pain of Myocardial Ischemia Associated with Marked, yet Reversible, EKG Changes

(a) Sometimes patients show dramatic ST depression of several millimeters during pain, reverting to normal after pain has subsided. This evidence, commonly gathered in the Emergency Department, may be a clue to a main left coronary artery lesion or other "critical lesion" that requires intensive, prompt medical or surgical treatment.

(b) Occasionally, a patient may be observed to have ST segment elevation during pain that reverts to normal as pain subsides (Fig. 5). This is the so-called "Prinzmetal angina" (Prinzmetal et al., 1959; Prinzmetal et al., 1960), and represents a spectrum of anatomic defects. At one end of the spectrum are normal vessels with spasm, and at the other end may be a high grade lesion in the left anterior descending before the first septal perforating vessel. If this evidence is present on EKG, many believe that a prompt coronary arteriogram should be performed. One should not confuse this with the hyperacute stages of infarction that rapidly evolve over a few hours and are not reversible.

The importance of prompt monitoring of patients having attacks of myocardial ischemia cannot be overemphasized. If the patient presents to the Emergency Department with chest pain, subjective data (history alone) will suggest that the discomfort either is or is not of cardiac origin, or there may be doubt about the origin. If the discomfort suggests myocardial ischemia or infarction, a survey should be made for complications. Initial treatment of these can be begun, and prompt portage to the coronary care unit made. If the origin of the discomfort is in doubt—regardless of EKG or x-ray findings—the patient must be monitored. Long

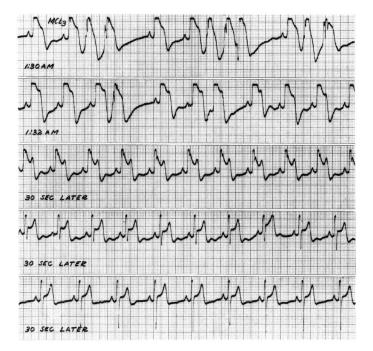

Figure 5. Prinzmetal angina: MCL₃ rhythm strips that were taken over a 3.5-minute period during a brief episode of chest discomfort. Note the marked ST segment elevation, increased R wave with loss of S wave, and the arrhythmia. Over this brief period the ST segments returned to baseline, and discomfort subsided.

periods of deliberation may result in sudden unrecognized changes in the patients condition and delayed therapy.

References

Atkins, J. M., et al.: Ventricular conduction blocks and sudden death in acute myocardial infarction. Potential indications for pacing. N. Engl. J. Med. 288:281, 1973.

Chatterjee, K., et al.: Hemodynamic and metabolic responses to vasodilator therapy in acute myocardial infarction. Circulation 48:1183, 1973.

Cobbs, B. W., Hatcher, C. R., and Robinson, P. H.: Cardiac rupture: three operations with two long-term survivals. J.A.M.A. 223:532, 1973.

Dunkman, W. B., et al.: Clinical and hemodynamic results of intra-aortic balloon pumping and surgery for cardiogenic shock. Circulation 46:465, 1972.

Fanciosa, J. A., et al.: Improved left ventricular function during nitroprusside infusion in acute myocardial infarction. Lancet 1:650, 1972.

Feinleib, M., and Davidson, M. J.: Coronary heart disease mortality: a community perspective. J.A.M.A. 222:1129, 1972.

Flaherty, J. T., et al.: Intravenous nitroglycerin in acute myocardial infarction. Circulation 51:132, 1975.

Godman, J. J., Lassers, B. W., and Julian, D. G.: Complete bundle branch block complicating acute myocardial infarction. N. Engl. J. Med. 282:237, 1970.

Graham, A. F., et al.: Ventricular septal defect after myocardial infarction. Early operative treatment. J.A.M.A. 225:708, 1973.

Heberden, W.: Some account of a disorder of the breast. Med. Trans. R. Coll. Physicians Lond. 2:59, 1772.

Hurst, J. W., et al.: The Heart, 3rd ed. New York, McGraw-Hill Book Co., 1974.

Jones, E. L., et al.: Myocardial revascularization combined with intracoronary infusion of hyperosmolar solution in early management of postinfarction ventricular septal defect. Circulation 52:170, 1975.

Kelly, D. T., et al.: Use of phentolamine in acute MI associated with hypertension and left ventricular failure. Circulation 47:729, 1973.

Kuller, L., Lilienfeld, A., and Fisher, R.: Epidemiological study of sudden death due to atherosclerotic heart disease. Circulation 35:1056, 1966.

Logue, R. B., and Bishop, L. J.: Rupture of the heart causing a systolic murmur and thrill. J.A.M.A. 144:757, 1950.

MacAlpin, R. N., and Kattus, A. A.: Adaptation to exercise in angina pectoris. Circulation 33:183, 1966.

Nowlin, J. B., et al.: The association of nocturnal angina pectoris with dreaming. Ann. Intern. Med. 63:1040, 1965.

Prinzmetal, M., et al.: Angina pectoris. 1. A variant form of angina pectoris. Preliminary report. Am. J. Med. 27:375, 1959.

Prinzmetal, M., et al.: Variant form of angina pectoris, previously undelineated syndrome. J.A.M.A. 174:102, 1960.

Soloman, H. A., Edwards, A. L., and Killip, T.: Prodromata in acute myocardial infarctoin. Circulation 40:463, 1969.

Spiekerman, R. E., et al.: The spectrum of coronary heart disease in a community of 30,000: clinicopathologic study. Circulation 25:57, 1962.

Waters, D. D., and Mizgala, H. F.: Long-term prognosis of patients with incomplete bilateral bundle branch block complicating acute myocardial infarction. Role of pacing. Am. J. Cardiol. 35:1, 1974.

C. CARDIOGENIC SHOCK

Benedict S. Maniscalco,
and Robert L. Whipple, III

Cardiogenic shock is a major complication of acute myocardial infarction that may be responsible for more than 15 per cent of deaths among all patients with myocardial infarction. Despite the modern therapeutic and technologic advances in modern coronary care units, the mortality rate from cardiogenic shock remains in excess of 75 per cent. The more stringent the criteria used to define this syndrome, the higher the mortality rate.

Cardiogenic shock may be defined as a syndrome in which there is a drastic reduction in regional blood flow leading to progressive deterioration of tissue perfusion and organ function as a direct result of myocardial dysfunction, i.e., inadequate cardiac output. It is characterized by hypotension, with a systolic arterial pressure of less than 90 mm. Hg or a drop more than 60 mm. Hg in previously hypertensive patients. In addition, there are signs of inadequate perfusion in regional vascular beds: (1) the skin is cool and clammy, which reflects increased sympathoadrenal discharge with vasoconstriction of cutaneous and visceral vascular beds; (2) central nervous system effects as the result of decreased cerebral blood flow are agitation, confusion, and obtundation; (3) urinary output is below 20 cc./hr. and urinary sodium content is decreased, reflecting inadequate renal blood flow. The peripheral pulses usually are weak and thready, and may be absent, an additional sign of intense peripheral vasoconstriction. Cardiac symptoms consist of recurrent or persistent chest pain.

Metabolic acidosis and lactic acidosis may be precipitated because of tissue hypoxia. Hypoxemia occurs in all patients with shock, and hyperventilation may be present to compensate for the abnormal hydrogen ion accumulation. Therefore, hypocapnia may be present as an early sign (see Table 1).

All therapeutic modalities, whether pharmacologic, mechanical, or surgical, seek to restore the circulation to normal by increasing cardiac output, decreasing peripheral vascular resistance, and improving regional blood flow.

This definition of cardiogenic shock implies that inadequate left ventricular function is the sole etiologic factor for the presence of the shock syndrome. Other causes, therefore, must be excluded (see Table 2).

PATHOLOGY

Cardiogenic shock may occur in many forms of heart disease. Therefore, this discussion is limited to cardiogenic shock as a result of myocardial infarction and coronary atherosclerotic heart disease.

TABLE 1 Clinical Diagnosis of Shock

1. Hypotension
   - (a) Systolic BP < 90 mm. Hg
   - (b) Drop ≧ 60 mm. Hg in systolic BP in patient with prior hypertension
2. Reduction in Regional Blood Flow
   - (a) Skin—cool, clammy, cyanotic, mottled
   - (b) CNS—agitation, confusion, somnolence, obtundation
   - (c) Kidney—urinary flow < 20 cc./hr.
   - (d) Pulses—weak, thready, absent
   - (e) Heart—recurrent or persistent chest pain

TABLE 2 Other Causes of Shock in Myocardial Infarction

1. Drugs
   - (a) Narcotics
   - (b) Tranquilizers
   - (c) Diuretics
   - (d) Cardiac depressants—quinidine, lidocaine, Dilantin
   - (e) Antihypertensives
2. Cardiopulmonary
   - (a) Arrhythmia—bradycardia, tachycardia, A-V dissociation
   - (b) Dissecting aortic aneurysm
   - (c) Cardiac tamponade
   - (d) Pulmonary embolus
3. Systemic
   - (a) Gastrointestinal hemorrhage
   - (b) Ruptured viscus
   - (c) Acute pancreatitis
   - (d) Septicemia
   - (e) Primary metabolic acidosis, i.e., diabetic ketoacidosis, lactic acidosis

Pathologic reports vary in their findings with respect to the location of infarcts, the number of primary branches of coronary arteries obstructed, and the incidence of occlusion in secondary branches. However, attempts to quantitate the amount of mycardium involved uniformly report that at least 40 per cent of the left ventricular myocardium is affected (Page, et al., 1971). Thus, a loss of 40 per cent of available contractile elements, either recently or in the past, is the major pathologic determinant of cardiogenic shock.

Histologically, the zone of infarction contains myocardial cells that are: (1) frankly necrotic; (2) ischemic, but still viable; and (3) normal. The fate of the latter two cellular types is determined by the balance between oxygen supply and oxygen demand. Obviously, judicious therapy is indicated in order to salvage as much myocardium as possible, since it appears that the degree and severity of left ventricular dysfunction correlates with the ultimate *size* of any particular myocardial infarction or the sum of all areas of infarction.

It is not clear whether the extent of necrosis seen at postmortem is purely the result of the duration of shock, or also is related to the therapy instituted. Data have accumulated indicating that the latter factor may be of equal importance to the former. The balance between O_2 supply and O_2 demand is delicate, and both may be affected by therapy.

The major determinants of myocardial oxygen consumption (MVO_2) are set out below.

(1) Preload, i.e., the end-diastolic myocardial fiber length that is determined primarily by left ventricular end-diastolic pressure.

(2) After-load, i.e., aortic impedance and peripheral vascular resistance.

(3) Contractile state of the myocardium, which is greatly affected by catecholamines.

(4) Heart rate.

Recent studies have elucidated the effect of various forms of therapy on MVO_2 in acute myocardial infarction, and their role in increasing or limiting the ultimate size of the infarction. Such information may be of great practical importance in the judicious selection of therapy for patients with myocardial infarction and shock. These facts will be discussed below.

PATHOPHYSIOLOGY

The decrease in contractile mass of the left ventricle as a result of myocardial infarction leads to a depressed ejection fraction with an *obligatory rise* in left ventricular end-diastolic pressure (LVEDP).

The classic Starling Curve equates ↑ LVEDP with ↑ left ventricular end-diastolic volume (LVEDV) and an increase in end-diastolic fiber length that theoretically would result in increased contractility. However, this classic Starling relationship does not necessarily obtain in acute myocardial infarction, because of concomitant changes in ventricular compliance (Diamond, 1972).*

Changes in ventricular compliance help to explain the presence of a normal heart size in acute myocardial infarction, despite large elevations of LVEDP. A decrease in compliance often presents in these patients, preventing a large rise in left ventricular end-diastolic volume (LVEDV) and thus maintaining a shorter left ventricular radius. By the Laplace relationship, MVO_2 would be lower with a small left ventricular radius, and this may serve as a protective mechanism.

A rise in LVEDP appears mandatory to maintain cardiac output in the face of decreasing left ventricular compliance, and thus may not represent "heart failure" in the traditional sense. Left ventricular failure, therefore, should be defined in terms of *reduced cardiac work* that interrelates pressure generation of the left ventricle and cardiac output, rather than isolated elevation of LVEDP.

Experimental studies have shown the presence of a myocardial depressant factor (MDF) in shock states. Its role in acute myocardial infarction is still unknown. Elaborated from the pancreas, MDF causes a breakdown of lysosomal membranes with elaboration of cellular enzymes. In experimental studies, its action may be reversed by the administration of steroids and calcium. MDF may play an active role in the late

---

*Ventricular compliance is defined as a change in left ventricular volume per unit change in left ventricular diastolic pressure ($\Delta V/\Delta P$). Thus, if a greater pressure change were required to deliver the same volume of blood from the left atrium to the left ventricle, ventricular compliance would be decreased.

stages of shock after prolonged tissue hypoxia.

Other factors may affect left ventricular function adversely. They include: (1) hypoxemia; (2) hypovolemia; (3) arrhythmias (especially severe bradycardia, tachycardia, or A-V dissociation); and (4) acute mitral regurgitation; ventricular septal rupture.

Hypoxemia, invariably present in shock, aggravates myocardial ischemia, leading to further extension of the zone of necrosis and decreased cardiac output. Metabolic or lactic acidosis leads to decreased contractility, owing to the negative inotropic effect of the hydrogen ion (acidity).

Hypovolemia limits venous return, and generally is related to increased losses of extracellular fluid from vomiting and sweating and to "third space" losses. The infarcted ventricle may *require* a larger end-diastolic pressure and volume to support stroke volume because of the decreased ejection fraction. Thus, hypovolemia must be corrected.

Arrhythmias, either bradycardia or tachycardia, may contribute significantly to decreased left ventricular output. Bradycardia will reduce cardiac output, since stroke volume may be limited by intrinsic myocardial dysfunction. Atropine usually will correct the slow heart rate. Tachyrhythmias limit cardiac output by decreasing diastolic filling time, and may aggravate myocardial dysfunction by increasing myocardial oxygen consumption. Sinus tachycardia is compensatory and not to be treated primarily. Correction of other factors contributing to left ventricular dysfunction generally will slow the heart rate to physiologic levels.

Atrial infarction, atrial fibrillation, or atrioventricular dissociation, with their loss of atrial contribution to LV filling, may cause abrupt and severe hemodynamic consequences. If possible, normal sinus rhythm should be restored, since cardiac output may fall by as much as 25 per cent or more when the atrial "kick" is lost.

Acute mitral regurgitation secondary to ischemic papillary muscle dysfunction or rupture and ruptured interventricular septum seriously compromise cardiac output by further decreasing effective forward stroke volume.

THERAPY OF CARDIOGENIC SHOCK

The major components of therapy include the following.

(1) Monitor clinical parameters.
(2) Pharmacologic therapy:
    (*a*) vasopressors;
    (*b*) vasodilators;
    (*c*) digitalis.
(3) Mechanical circulatory assistance.

Monitor Clinical Parameters

The patient should be located in an intensive care unit where frequent clinical observations may be recorded. These include continuous electrocardiographic monitoring, frequent monitoring of vital signs, and measurement of arterial blood gases and hemodynamic parameters.

Urinary flow should be recorded on an hourly basis by use of an indwelling catheter in the bladder; flow rates of < 20 cc./hr. usually are seen in cardiogenic shock. Measurement of urinary output also is helpful in calculating fluid balance and therapy. Twice-daily weighings usually involve too much movement of the patient.

When proper equipment is available for hemodynamic monitoring in the intensive care area, right-sided pressures and arterial pressures should be monitored continuously.

The Swan-Ganz flow-directed balloon catheter allows right heart catheterization at the bedside. It is introduced into a median basilic vein and directed from the arm to the pulmonary artery and pulmonary capillary wedge (PCW) position without fluoroscopic control in the vast majority of cases by simple observation of the pressure wave forms.[*]

The pulmonary artery end-diastolic pressure (PAEDP) and pulmonary capillary wedge pressure usually, but not always, reflect left ventricular end-diastolic pressure, and thus may be of great clinical value. Once the PCW pressure is obtained, the balloon is deflated and withdrawn to the pulmonary artery and left in this position. Once PAEDP is measured, if it correlates closely with the PCW pressure, succeeding measurements are taken in this position. Between measurements, the balloon should remain deflated in order to avoid serious potential complications.

Additional advantages for the Swan-Ganz catheter are the ability to (1) obtain

---

[*]See Procedures Section, page 332.

blood samples for determination of cardiac output; (2) detect shunts in the case of rupture of the ventricular septum; and (3) note from the PCW wave form whether mitral regurgitation is present.

Arterial pressure is monitored by insertion of a small percutaneous cannula in the brachial or radial artery.* †

After measurement of left ventricular end-diastolic pressure, arterial pressure, and cardiac output, other parameters of cardiac performance may be calculated. These include stroke volume, stroke work and their indices, peripheral resistance, and so on. The method for these calculations may be found elsewhere.

Thus, initial hemodynamic measurements allow accurate characterization of the shock and observation of the effects of therapeutic interventions.

Patients in cardiogenic shock fall into class IV of Killip's classification for left ventricular dysfunction in acute myocardial infarction (Wolk, et al., 1972). Left ventricular end-diastolic pressure generally is greater than 25 mm. Hg (normal 8 to 12). However, approximately 5 per cent of patients initially put into this class will be found to have normal or low LVEDP secondary to previously discussed alternative etiologies. It is important to identify this group because they will respond to volume expansion. Cardiac output and index are markedly depressed, and stroke-work index (SWI) almost always is less than 25 g-m/m². SWI of <20 is associated with a mortality greater than 80 per cent.‡

---

*If pressure monitoring equipment is not available, central venous pressure should be monitored. Great caution must be exercised in the interpretation of such measurements, since CVP reflects events only on the right side of the heart. Since the vast majority of myocardial infarctions occur in the left ventricle, there is no consistent relationship between LVEDP and CVP measurements (Russell and Rackley, 1974).

†See Procedures Section, page 355.

‡Stroke work index is calculated in g-m/m² from the formula:

$$SWI = \frac{(MSP - PAEDP \text{ or } LVEDP) \times SI \times 1.36}{100}$$

Where:
MSP = mean systolic pressure
PAEDP = pulmonary artery end-diastolic pressure
LVEDP = left ventricular end-diastolic pressure
SI = stroke volume corrected for body surface area

Pharmacologic Therapy

VASOPRESSORS

The great paradox of drug therapy for cardiogenic shock is that available vasopressors such as norepinephrine, metaraminol, etc., that increase cardiac output and raise blood pressure do so *at the expense of increasing myocardial oxygen consumption* (MVO₂). This in turn is likely to increase the extent of tissue necrosis and infarct size.

An ideal agent for power failure might: (1) have a positive inotropic effect (↑ contractility); (2) increase cardiac output; (3) decrease LVEDP; (4) decrease peripheral vascular resistance; (5) dilate selected vascular beds; (6) have little or no chronotropic (↑ heart rate) effects; and (7) produce only little or no increase in MVO₂ (myocardial oxygen consumption).

Of the currently available agents, dopamine appears to the authors to be the vasopressor of choice. With careful titration of the infusion rate needed for each individual patient, in doses of 1 to 17 mg./kg./min., the following effects of dopamine are noted.

(1) Increased myocardial contractility through direct β-receptor stimulation and indirect stimulation of the release of norepinephrine.

(2) Increased adrenergic activity leading to vasoconstriction of both arterial and venous vascular beds.

(3) Selective dilatation of renal and mesenteric vascular beds.

(4) A mixed chronotropic effect that has a proportionately smaller effect on contractility than either isoproterenol or norepinephrine.

(5) In higher doses, vasoconstrictor effects are greater than vasodilatory effects.

In patients with cardiogenic shock, dopamine will have the following effects.

(1) It will increase cardiac output and improve all indices of left ventricular function.

(2) If peripheral vascular resistance is low, it will return mean arterial pressure toward normal.

(3) Total peripheral vascular resistance decreases in response to the positive inotropic effects of dopamine in patients who initially manifest intense peripheral vasoconstriction.

(4) It will increase renal and splanchnic blood flow.

(5) It will increase cardiac output to a greater extent than norepinephrine but a lesser than isoproterenol; however, it causes less rise in MVO_2 than either.

In short, dopamine compares favorably with the ideal vasopressor and is recommended as the initial inotropic drug of choice.

VASODILATORS

Recently, investigators have reported the efficacy of carefully monitored therapy with vasodilating drugs such as nitroprusside and/or phentolamine in both low output states and frank cardiogenic shock (Franciosa, et al., 1972; Walinsky, et al., 1974). Hemodynamic improvement usually occurs within five to ten minutes after beginning an infusion. Left ventricular end-diastolic pressure is reduced, systemic and pulmonary vascular resistances decrease, and there is a slight decrease in mean arterial pressure. The result is an increase in cardiac output, cardiac index, and stroke work index.

These changes are effected by careful control of the infusion rate and without a significant increase in heart rate or precipitate drop in arterial pressure in most cases. Thus, normotensive and even hypotensive patients may benefit from such therapy. Care must be taken to insure a diastolic intra-aortic pressure of 60 to 65 mm. Hg or greater. Diastolic pressures below this level would seriously compromise coronary blood flow.

The over-all result of vasodilator therapy should be improved hemodynamics, which should restore a more equitable balance between myocardial oxygen supply and demand, limit infarct size, and salvage ischemic myocardium. Although only limited clinical experience has been reported to date, vasodilator therapy may play a more prominent role in the future in the treatment of cardiogenic shock.

Although pharmacologic doses of corticosteroids do exert a vasodilating effect, their experimental use is predicated on possible benefits at the cellular and subcellular level. Controlled experimentation will determine whether they have any future place in therapy.

DIGITALIS

The inotropic effects of digitalis are well recognized, and its role in the treatment of left ventricular failure is universally ac-

cepted. However, its role in the therapy of cardiogenic shock is not clear, since the increase in myocardial contractility of noninfarcted myocardial muscle segments causes an obligatory rise in myocardial oxygen consumption. Our recommendation is to administer digitalis to patients in cardiogenic shock with left ventricular failure and dilatation. By the Laplace relationship, left ventricular dilatation leads to increased myocardial oxygen consumption on the basis of increased ventricular radius and wall tension. The beneficial effects of digitalis in decreasing ventricular radius (thereby decreasing MVO_2) are felt to outweigh the theoretical deleterious effects secondary to increased contractility (with the obligatory rise in MVO_2).

Thus, we would endorse the use of digitalis in cardiogenic shock with left ventricular enlargement. Caution must be taken to avoid digitalis intoxication, in view of the increased sensitivity to this drug in patients with hypoxemia and decreased renal blood flow. Doses, therefore, should be reduced to avoid this complication. Frequent monitoring of arterial blood gases and serum electrolytes (especially K^+) is essential.

Other agents that have been used without discernible benefit include glucagon, calcium, and adenosine phosphate compounds.

Mechanical Circulatory Assistance

The hemodynamic effects of intra-aortic balloon pumping are: (1) a reduction in peak left ventricular pressure; (2) a reduction of LVEDP: (3) an increase in mean aortic diastolic pressure; (4) an increase in cardiac output; and (5) an augmentation of diastolic coronary blood flow.

The net results are: (1) a reduction in left ventricular preload and afterload; (2) reduced myocardial oxygen consumption; (3) decreased infarct size; (4) increased perfusion at the periphery of the infarct.

This is accomplished by positioning the balloon catheter tip just distal to the left subclavian artery after introducing it from the femoral artery. Synchronization is required with the QRS complex of the standard EKG or arterial pressure wave form. Inflation occurs on the T wave, utilizing CO_2 or helium. Proper sensing can occur with heart rates of up to 180 beats per minute. When the balloon is inflated, intra-aortic pressure is increased and diastolic coronary blood flow is augmented. The balloon is deflated with the onset of ventricular systole, and intra-aortic pressure (afterload) falls, allowing an increased left ventricular stroke volume.

The balloon pumping device has been used extensively in clinical trials in cardiogenic shock, and has proved of great benefit in a large number of cases. When it is used in combination with the vasodilator agents, synergistic beneficial effects are reported.

Potential complications and contraindications for the use of balloon pumping are reviewed in "Suggestions for Further Reading" at the end of this chapter.

Balloon pumping is of particular value for temporary support of the circulation when further diagnostic studies (e.g., cardiac catheterization) are needed in anticipation of emergency cardiac surgery.

SUMMARY

Cardiogenic shock is a life-threatening complication of acute myocardial infarction. Emergency measures must be taken to support the circulation and to restore adequate blood flow to local vascular beds.

Cardiogenic shock is associated with at least a 40 per cent loss of contractile elements of left ventricular myocardium. Stroke volume and cardiac output are reduced markedly (but not always), and left ventricular end-diastolic pressure is elevated with resulting pulmonary congestion.

While hypotension persists, continued extension of the infarction occurs. Therapy is directed at salvaging ischemic myocardium and limiting infarct size by correcting hemodynamic abnormalities. Initial evaluation must include a search for other possible causes of the shock state, which must receive immediate or concomitant correction if found.

Correction of hypovolemia or arrhythmia may relieve the hemodynamic problems in a small percentage of patients. The roles of vasopressors, vasodilators, digitalis, and balloon pumping are reviewed.

References

Diamond, G., and Forrester, J. S.: Effect of coronary disease and acute myocardial infarction on left ventricular compliance in man. Circulation 45:11, 1972.

Franciosa, J. A., et al.: Improved left ventricular function during nitroprusside infusion in acute myocardial infarction. Lancet 1:650, 1972.

Page, D. L., et al.: Myocardial changes associated with cardiogenic shock. N. Engl. J. Med. 285:133, 1971.

Walinsky, P., et al.: Enhanced left ventricular performance with phentolamine in acute myocardial infarction. Am. J. Cardiol. 33:37, 1974.

Wolk, M. K., Scheidt, S., and Killip, T.: Heart failure complicating acute myocardial infarction. Circulation 45:1125, 1972.

Suggestions for Further Reading

Braunwald, E., and Maroko, P. R.: The reduction of infarct size: an idea whose time (for testing) has come. Circulation 50:206, 1974.

Chatterjee, K., and Swan, H. J. C.: Vasodilator therapy in acute myocardial infarction. Mod. Concepts Cardiovasc. Dis. 63:119, 1974.

Chatterjee, K., et al.: Hemodynamic and metabolic responses to vasodilator therapy in acute myocardial infarction. Circulation 48:1183, 1973.

Epstein, S. E., et al.: The early phase of acute myocardial infarction: pharmacologic aspects of therapy. Ann. Intern. Med. 78:918, 1973.

Gunnar, R. M., Loeb, H. S., and Rahimtoola, S. H.: Shock in Myocardial Infarction. New York and London, Grune & Stratton, 1974.

Kones, R. J.: Cardiogenic Shock. Mount Kisco, N.Y., Futura Publishing Company, 1974.

Lefer, A. M.: Role of a myocardial depressant factor in shock states. Mod. Concepts Cardiovasc. Dis. 62:59, 1973.

Maroko, P. R., et al.: Factors influencing infarct size following experimental coronary artery occlusions. Circulation, 43:67, 1971.

Parmley, W. W., et al.: Hemodynamic effects of non-invasive systolic unloading (nitroprusside) and diastolic augmentation (external counterpulsation) in patients with acute myocardial infarction. Am. J. Cardiol. 33:818, 1974.

Resnekov, L.: Mechanical assistance for the failing ventricle. Mod. Concepts Cardiovas. Dis. 63:81, 1974.

Russell, R. O., and Rackley, C. E.: Hemodynamic Monitoring in a Coronary Intensive Care Unit. Mount Kisco, N.Y., Futura Publishing Company, 1974.

Willerson, J. T., et al.: Intra-aortic balloon counterpulsation in patients in cardiogenic shock, medically refractory left ventricular failure and/or recurrent ventricular tachycardia. Am. J. Med. 58:184, 1975.

D. PULMONARY EDEMA

John H. Stone

Pulmonary edema is a clinical syndrome of air-hunger and breathlessness that may result from many diverse causes (Table 1). In the Emergency Department the clinical picture of pulmonary edema may not indicate the specific etiology because of the similar ultimate pathophysiologic changes: accumulation of fluid within the alveolar or interstitial spaces of the lung, resulting in *hypoxemia* and *abnormal pulmonary function* (the latter characterized by decreased lung compliance, increased work of breathing, abnormal ventilation-perfusion relationships, decreased vital capacity, and impaired gas exchange across the alveolocapillary membrane).

ETIOLOGY OF PULMONARY EDEMA

Many clinical settings, both cardiac and noncardiac, may be associated with clinical and radiologic evidence of pulmonary edema. Recognizing that in some instances our knowledge of etiology remains incomplete, it is nevertheless helpful to think of pulmonary edema as a *continuum of disease* in terms of its pathogenesis (Fishman, 1972). On the one hand, there are instances caused by rather pure *hemodynamic* or *physical forces* (classic examples are mitral stenosis and left ventricular failure); at the other end of the continuum are the situations in which *altered permeability* of *the alveolocapillary interface* plays a major role (e.g., pulmonary edema which follows inhalation of toxic gases). A given entity that results in the clinical picture of pulmonary edema can then be placed along this continuum and its place modified as our knowledge of etiology is extended. For example, in the pulmonary edema associated with *uremia*, both *hemodynamic factors* (left ventricular failure, hypertension, hypervolemia, high cardiac output associated with anemia) and *permeability factors* can usually be implicated. In the pulmonary edema of *influenzal viral pneumonia*, the pathogenesis seems to be largely an *alteration of permeability* of the alveolar epithelial or pulmonary capillary beds.

The following discussion is directed toward recognition and treatment of *cardiogenic pulmonary edema*, primarily that which is secondary to *left ventricular failure*, statistically the most common cause of the syndrome. The reader is referred elsewhere in this book to a discussion of the discrete clinical entities that may be associated with pulmonary edema. In addition, an excellent discussion emphasizing the noncardiogenic forms of pulmonary edema is recommended (Robin et al., 1973).

CARDIOGENIC PULMONARY EDEMA

RECOGNITION

In its fully developed form, cardiogenic pulmonary edema is not difficult to recognize. The initial presentation of the patient in the Emergency Department, however, may be confused with other causes of breathlessness (pulmonary emboli, bronchial asthma, pneumothorax) from which it must be differentiated.

Subjective findings include dyspnea, orthopnea, paroxysmal nocturnal dyspnea, and cough. The patient is usually terrified and may later relate having had *angor animi* (a sense of impending doom). Alterations of mental status, ranging from agitation and confusion to stupor, may occur as a result of decreased cerebral blood flow and hypoxemia. The patient with myocardial infarction may also complain of chest discomfort.

Objective findings include any or all of the following: (1) tachypnea; (2) wheezing; (3) rales at the lung bases; (4) elevated jugular venous pressure; (5) atrial and/or ventricular gallop sounds on cardiac auscultation; (6) pulsus paradoxus (because of the marked respiratory excursions); (7) rapid "thready" pulse and/or pulsus alternans; and (8) abnormalities of precordial palpation (displaced cardiac apex, abnormal systolic bulges).

In advanced pulmonary edema, cyanosis may be present. Some patients may produce the typical frothy pink sputum. Diaphoresis is common because of the work of breathing. The patient will spontaneously assume an upright posture unless he is obtunded.

TABLE 1   Major Etiologic Factors in the Pulmonary Edema Syndrome

1. HEMODYNAMIC FACTORS
   Left ventricular failure
   Mitral valve obstruction (mitral stenosis, left atrial myxoma)
   Volume overload (e.g., overtransfusion)
   Cardiac arrhythmias

2. ALTERED PERMEABILITY
   Inhaled toxic gases; smoke inhalation
   Infections (viral, bacterial) of the lung
   Endotoxemia
   Drowning
   Aspiration pneumonia
   Anaphylaxis; adverse drug reactions
   Adult respiratory distress syndrome

3. DECREASED PLASMA ONCOTIC PRESSURE
   Hypoalbuminemia of nephrosis, hepatic disease

4. EXCESS NEGATIVE INTRAPLEURAL PRESSURE
   Re-expansion of pneumothorax

5. MISCELLANEOUS: MIXED/UNKNOWN ETIOLOGIC FACTORS
   Neurogenic (after head trauma; postictal)
   Heroin overdose
   High altitude pulmonary edema
   Pulmonary embolism

Edema of the extremities or sacrum may of course be present in the patient with an acute exacerbation of chronic heart failure.

The chest x-ray is a valuable adjunct in recognition of pulmonary edema (Hublitz and Shapiro, 1974). In cardiogenic pulmonary edema, the heart is usually enlarged. Two major exceptions to this are (1) acute myocardial infarction before the heart has had time to dilate and (2) mitral stenosis with atrial fibrillation and rapid ventricular response. In noncardiogenic forms of pulmonary edema, the heart is usually normal in size, unless influenced by coexisting cardiac disease.

The x-ray may detect abnormalities in heart size, individual cardiac chamber enlargement, pleural (and subpulmonary) effusions, fluid in the interlobar fissures, and a redistribution of blood flow in the lungs away from the bases and to the upper lobes (resulting in prominent upper lobe vessels).

The chest x-ray has been used to divide pulmonary edema into two major stages—an "earlier" form known as interstitial pulmonary edema and the more florid alveolar pulmonary edema. In the *interstitial* form, the edema is localized to the interface between alveoli and pulmonary capillaries. Its radiologic appearance is characterized by (*a*) the septal "B" (and "A") lines of Kerley, (*b*) a diffuse reticular pattern to the lung fields, and (*c*) perivascular and peribronchial "cuffing" (or blurring of the usually distinct margins of these structures). In *alveolar* pulmonary edema, there is transudation of fluid into the alveoli, resulting in a characteristic x-ray picture showing, in the most advanced form, homogeneous radiopacities radiating symmetrically from the perihilar areas, the so-called "butterfly" appearance.

Pulmonary edema may at times be *localized* or *unilateral*. Several factors may be involved in such instances, including (1) the patient's posture (lying on one side only, for example) and the attendant effects of gravity and (2) *prior* pulmonary problems (chronic obstructive pulmonary disease, pneumonia, pulmonary emboli), which may have modified the pulmonary vascular bed, including its lymphatic drainage. Unilateral pulmonary edema has also been reported after rapid re-expansion of pneumothorax (Humphreys and Berne, 1970), a finding probably related partly to the negative intrapleural pressure of the chest tube.

The clinician should be aware that considerable dissociation may occur between the patient's signs and symptoms and the chest film. A patient with an acute myocardial infarction, for example, may clinically appear quite ill with overt dyspnea, whereas his chest x-ray may, at least initially, show a normal heart size and rather subtle early signs of interstitial pulmonary edema, such as pulmonary venous engorgement and Kerley "B" lines. On the other hand, even after left-sided cardiac pressures have returned to normal, there may be a temporal "lag" in the radiologic appearance with respect to clinical improvement because of relatively slow removal of intra-alveolar fluid.

Arterial blood gases are useful in confirming the presence and severity of hypoxemia. In addition to hypoxemia, derangements in P_{CO_2} and pH are common and have been described *classically* as showing (1) a reduced P_{CO_2} (hypocapnia) and (2) normal to somewhat alkaline pH, reflecting a respiratory alkalosis.

Recent evidence, however (Aberman and Fulop, 1972), indicates that either respiratory acidosis (hypercapnia) or metabolic (lactic) acidosis may be present in many patients with pulmonary edema. The reasons for these aberrations are not entirely clear (they may at times be a reflection of the stage at which the patient is first seen in the course of the disease). Blood-gas findings are emphasized here because they have implications for therapy (see below) and because they underscore the need for objective verification of the patient's respiratory-metabolic status in this clinically precarious situation.

The electrocardiogram in pulmonary edema is most useful for the assessment of dysrhythmias, which may require specific treatment themselves. In the patient with acute myocardial infarction, the EKG is helpful in diagnosis only when it is positive.

TREATMENT

The treatment of pulmonary edema secondary to left ventricular failure consists of (1) general measures (some of which may be useful in both cardiac and noncardiac forms) and (2) attempts to improve the cardiac performance (either by "unloading" the left ventricle or by improving cardiac contractility). The major therapeutic measures available are summarized below; overlap will be noted between the above two broad categories.

General Measures

A *calm medical team* is an absolute necessity that may be more difficult to achieve than is ordinarily thought; nevertheless, it is critical to allaying the patient's anxiety and fright.

The patient will spontaneously *sit upright* unless he is obtunded, and he should be assisted in maintaining this posture.

Oxygen by nasal cannula or a plastic mask should be given. The patient is usually so air-hungry at first that he may not tolerate a tight-fitting mask. Administration of oxygen can be monitored by arterial Po_2; if, with other therapy, the Po_2 does not rise above 50 mm. Hg, mechanical ventilation in the form of positive pressure breathing may be necessary. Either intermittent positive pressure breathing (IPPB) or positive end-expiratory pressure breathing (PEEP) may be employed. The advantages of improved oxygenation and reduction of further transudation into the alveoli obtained with IPPB or PEEP must be weighed in the individual clinical situation against the known potential of these techniques for seriously impeding venous return and precipitously reducing the cardiac output (especially in the hypovolemic or already hypotensive patient). They may also lead to rupture of pulmonary blebs with pneumothorax and pneumomediastinum.

Equipment for *suctioning* of tracheal secretions should be readily available.

Rotating tourniquets are important and especially helpful because their effects are immediate and rapidly reversible. Blood pressure cuffs set above venous pressure, but below arterial pressure, are the most comfortable tourniquets and should be rotated among three extremities at a time.

Aminophylline may be helpful because of its effects in (1) reducing pulmonary venous pressure, (2) improving renal blood flow (promoting diuresis), (3) increasing myocardial contractility, and (4) dilating the bronchial tree. The drug should be given *slowly* intravenously in an initial dose of 250 to 500 mg. Its side effects include nausea and vomiting, hypotension, and increased ventricular irritability.

Diuretics such as furosemide (40 mg. IV) may be quite helpful in promoting a reduction in blood volume. A rapid onset of action (5 to 15 minutes) follows intravenous administration. There is also evidence that furosemide causes an *immediate* decrease in venous tone ("medical phlebotomy"), which is independent of its diuretic effects and which is also desirable (Dikshit et al., 1973). Care must be taken that excessive diuresis does not result in hypotension, which may worsen the clinical situation. This is especially true in patients with previously normal blood volume, such as those with fresh myocardial infarction, acute left ventricular failure and *translocation* of fluid to the lungs (as opposed to those with more chronic left ventricular failure and hypervolemia).

Sodium bicarbonate is *rarely* indicated, even with metabolic acidosis, and its use may well be harmful (increased hyperosmolarity, rapid shift in arterial pH, and decreased oxygen unloading because of a shift to the left of the oxyhemoglobin dissociation curve) (Grossman and Aberman, 1976).

Measures to Improve Cardiac Performance

Morphine is the single most important drug in the treatment of pulmonary edema secondary to left ventricular failure. It should be given slowly, intravenously, in doses of 3 to 5 mg., titrating the dose according to the respiratory rate (a most valuable clinical sign in this situation) and the clinical condition of the patient. Judicious use of morphine is *not* contraindicated even in those patients with CO_2 retention (Aberman and Fulop, 1972); its use, together with other conventional treatment, may in fact prevent the need for endotracheal intubation and mechanical ventilation. In the patient with CO_2 retention, of course, monitoring of blood gases is even more important than in the patient with a normal or low PCO_2.

Morphine has several actions that are of benefit to the patient with pulmonary edema secondary to left ventricular failure. They include (1) "pharmacologic phlebotomy" or pooling of blood in the capacitance vessels, (2) reduction of central respiratory drive and respiratory rate, (3) a decrease in systemic arterial resistance with resultant decrease in cardiac work, and (4) very important, relief of the patient's anxiety—he may still be short of breath but is less concerned about it. An increase in cardiac contractility following the use of morphine has been noted, but this takes 15 to 30 minutes to become manifest.

Phlebotomy of 250 to 500 cc. may be indicated at times and may be especially helpful when inadvertent overtransfusion or overhydration results in pulmonary congestion. The best technique for phlebotomy includes withdrawal of blood into a blood bank bag so that it can be retransfused should untoward effects result.

Digitalis may be given to patients not already receiving the drug. Digoxin in a dose of 0.5 mg I.V. is the usual choice. Its ability to *increase cardiac contractility*, while taking some 15 to 30 minutes to manifest itself, may be useful in preventing recurrence of pulmonary edema once it is controlled. Its other major effect, *slowing of AV conduction*, makes it especially useful in the treatment of patients with atrial fibrillation and a rapid ventricular response. Patients with fresh myocardial infarction and those with hypokalemia are more sensitive to digitalis, which may be reflected in ventricular arrhythmias.

Cardioversion may be life-saving in certain cardiac rhythm disturbances, three dramatic examples being (1) ventricular tachycardia, (2) atrial fibrillation with uncontrolled ventricular response in the patient with mitral stenosis, and (3) atrial arrhythmias in patients with hypertrophied left ventricles (such as aortic stenosis, idiopathic hypertrophic subaortic stenosis, and hypertensive cardiovascular disease) in whom the onset of the arrhythmia (and loss of the "atrial kick" of sinus rhythm) may be devastating.

Other agents to improve cardiac contractility, such as *dopamine*, may be useful in selected patients, particularly those with hypotension secondary to decreased cardiac contractility.

The need to lower blood pressure with appropriate antihypertensive agents in the patient with a hypertensive crisis and pulmonary edema is obviously an important part of the treatment.

Recently, *nitroprusside* has been used for its ability to immediately reduce cardiac afterload. It has been found useful in patients with acute mitral regurgitation as well as in patients with cardiomyopathies in whom temporary potentiation of "forward flow" may be beneficial (Chatterjee, 1975). Its use may, however, be accompanied by precipitous lowering of blood pressure and concomitant reduction in coronary artery perfusion. The drug is therefore, appropriately utilized *only* in situations in which continuous hemodynamic monitoring is available.

References

Aberman, A., and Fulop, M.: The metabolic and respiratory acidosis of acute pulmonary edema. Ann. Intern. Med. 76(2):173, 1972.

Chatterjee, K.: Vasodilator therapy for heart failure (editorial). Ann. Intern. Med. 83:421, 1975.

Dikshit, K., Vyden, J. K., and Forrester, J. S.: Renal and extrarenal hemodynamic effects of furosemide in congestive heart failure after acute myocardial infarction. N. Engl. J. Med. 288:1087, 1973.

Fishman, A. P.: Pulmonary edema, the water-exchanging function of the lung. Circulation 46:390, 1972.

Grossman, R. F., and Aberman, A.: Emergency management of acute pulmonary edema (editorial). Ann. Intern Med. 844:488, 1976.

Hublitz, U. F., and Shapiro, J. H.: The radiology of pulmonary edema. CRC Crit. Rev. Clin. Radiol. Nuclear Med. p. 389, June 1974.

Humphreys, R. L., and Berne, A. S.: Rapid re-expansion of pneumothorax — a cause of unilateral pulmonary edema. Radiology 96:509, 1970.

Robin, D., Cross, C. E., and Zelis, R.: Pulmonary edema. N. Engl. J. Med. 288(5 and 6):239 and 292, 1973 (two-part article).

E. HYPERTENSIVE CRISES

Ray W. Gifford, Jr.

RECOGNITION

Recognition of a hypertensive crisis depends not so much on the absolute level of blood pressure as on the clinical status of the patient. For example, a blood pressure of 180/100 mm. Hg in a patient with evidence of aortic dissection or acute left ventricular failure should be treated promptly with appropriate parenteral antihypertensive agents, whereas a blood pressure of 240/140 mm. Hg found on routine examination of an aysmptomatic patient without evidence of target organ disease may require no emergent therapy or even hospitalization, if provision is made for prompt evaluation and management on an ambulatory basis.

History

Hypertensive encephalopathy is the prototype of the hypertensive crisis, because it occurs only in association with hypertension, and acute reduction of blood pressure will reverse the signs and symptoms within a few hours. The patient with hypertensive encephalopathy usually presents with severe generalized headache, blurring of vision, vomiting, and confusion. If the patient is coherent enough to give a history, the physician will learn that these symptoms evolved gradually over a period of several hours, sometimes a day or two. If the patient has had occasion to have his blood pressure measured there is almost invariably a history of hypertension, often of long standing, which has been treated inadequately, if at all, or the patient may have stopped taking his medications a week or more before onset of symptoms.

Sometimes, by the time the patient comes under medical surveillance, he is obtunded or even comatose, so that the history must be obtained from a family member. When no observer is present to relate the details of onset of symptoms, the physician is faced with the differential diagnosis of coma in a hypertensive patient; this includes acute cerebral infarction (usually the brain stem), intracerebral hematoma, subarach-

noid hemorrhage, head injury, uremia, and diabetic coma, to mention the most common conditions (Table 1).

DIFFERENTIATION OF INTRACRANIAL BLEEDING FROM HYPERTENSIVE ENCEPHALOPATHY

Unlike hypertensive encephalopathy, intracranial bleeding, whether it be subarachnoid or intracerebral, usually leads to loss of consciousness within an hour to two, but often within minutes, after abrupt onset of severe headache, and the resulting coma is deeper than that observed in hypertensive encephalopathy. Most patients with acute cerebral infarction or "stroke in progress" do not have headache as a prominent part of their symptomatology, and most do not lose consciousness unless the infarction is in the brain stem (vertebral-basilar distribution). When this occurs, the coma usually is preceded by a constellation of symptoms that can be similar to those of hypertensive encephalopathy, including dysarthria, dysphagia, diplopia, confusion, and paresis of one side of the face and the opposite extremities. The onset of coma in brain stem stroke may be delayed for several hours after onset of symptoms, but it is unusual for the prodromal symptoms to last 24 to 48 hours as is characteristic of hypertensive encephalopathy. Focal neurologic symptoms usually wax and wane in hypertensive encephalopathy, whereas they become progressively worse in acute cerebral infarction.

Physical Examination

Patients with hypertensive encephalopathy usually have blood pressure in excess of 250/150 mm. Hg unless hypertension is of recent onset (e.g., acute glomerulonephritis in children and eclampsia), in which case hypertensive encephalopathy may occur when blood pressure is no higher than 180/110 mm. Hg. Patients with acute head injury and intracranial hematoma may have blood pressure in excess of 250/150 mm. Hg, but most of those with acute cerebral infarction and subarachnoid hemorrhage do not have hypertension of this magnitude.

Evidence should be sought of trauma to the head, such as lacerations, contusions, hematomas, dried blood in the scalp, and bleeding from the ears and nose.

The presence of malignant (group IV) hypertensive retinopathy with severe arteriolar constriction, exudates, hemorrhages, and papilledema is strong evidence for hypertensive encephalopathy, but the absence of these findings does not rule it out. Furthermore, there is always the possibility that patients with cerebral hemorrhage or infarction can have retinopathy of malignant hypertension. Most patients with hypertensive encephalopathy do have severe retinal arteriolar constriction, both focal and generalized, even if they do not have exudates, hemorrhages, and papilledema, and the diagnosis of hypertensive encephalopathy should be questioned if arteriolar spasm is absent or minimal. However, any patient with significant hypertension is likely to have retinal arteriolar constriction. Unilateral papilledema, without retinal hemorrhages and exudates, suggests an intracranial space-occupying lesion such as tumor or hematoma. Subhyaloid hemorrhages may occur with subarachnoid hemorrhage, and this finding on funduscopy will confirm the diagnosis.

Nuchal rigidity is strong evidence favoring subarachnoid hemorrhage, either primary or from an intracerebral hematoma that has penetrated into the ventricular system and permitted blood to get into the subarachnoid space. It usually does not occur until several hours after the hemorrhage. Hypertensive encephalopathy does not produce nuchal rigidity (Table 1).

Neurologic examination is important and helpful. In contrast to cerebral hematoma or infarction, the neurologic signs produced by hypertensive encephalopathy are migratory, transitory, and often subtle, and cannot be explained by a focal cerebral lesion (Table 1). Frequently, there are no neurologic abnormalities other than alteration in consciousness, as described above, with or without hyperirritability as manifested by generalized muscular twitching. Coma usually is more profound in patients with cerebral hemorrhage or brain stem stroke than in those with hypertensive encephalopathy. Focal or generalized convulsive seizures can occur with hypertensive encephalopathy, intracerebral hematoma, or subarachnoid hemorrhage.

Abnormalities in respiration, such as Cheyne-Stokes or Biot breathing and cardiac arrhythmias, are associated more frequently with cerebral or subarachnoid hemorrhage or brain stem infarction than with hypertensive encephalopathy.

Laboratory Findings

When the history and physical findings are suggestive of hypertensive encephalopathy, antihypertensive therapy should be started without waiting for the results of laboratory examinations. Therapy can be appropriately modified subsequently if results of laboratory examinations indicate that the diagnosis is in error or reveal the presence of unsuspected complications (e.g., renal failure).

When there is little doubt about the diagnosis, the initial stat laboratory evaluation should include a hemogram, urinalysis, serum electrolytes and creatinine (or BUN), and electrocardiogram. Further studies should be postponed until the crisis is controlled.

When the patient is comatose or too obtunded to give a reliable history, and no witnesses are present to describe the onset of his illness, a more extensive stat investigation is warranted, although this should be carried out as expeditiously as possible so that appropriate antihypertensive treatment can be started without undue delay. This usually means a trip to the Radiology Department for roentgenograms of skull and chest. If the situation demands it, there is no reason why this cannot be done after the patient has received an injection of diazoxide, or while an infusion of sodium nitroprusside is running.° Other studies should include a standard SMA 12, a "coma profile" (barbiturate level, blood acetone, and ammonia), and a kidney profile (sodium, potassium, chloride, CO_2, BUN, and serum creatinine). *Examination of cerebrospinal fluid is sometimes indicated but must be done*

°See section on treatment.

TABLE 1   Important Clinical Features In Differential Diagnosis of Hypertensive Encephalopathy

DISORDER	RAPIDITY OF ONSET OF SIGNS AND SYMPTOMS	CHARACTER OF HEADACHE	LEVEL OF CONSCIOUSNESS	SIGNS	CHARACTERISTIC PROGRESSION
Hypertensive Encephalopathy	Rapid onset over 12-48 hours on background of abrupt increase in BP	Severe and generalized —recent onset	Restless, clouding of consciousness, to frank coma	Vomiting, visual disturbance, transient migratory and focal signs, focal and generalized seizures	Progressive unless treated
Cerebral Infarction	Rapid—minutes to hours. Occasionally stuttering onset	Often no headache or mild. Rarely severe	Inattentive or mildly lethargic. Coma rare except with brain stem infarction	Focal deficits usually fixed after abrupt or stuttering onset	Improve gradually and progressively over days to weeks
Cerebral Embolus	Usually very sudden onset, often with fixed deficit immediately	Headache usually not a major component	Same as cerebral infarction	Same as cerebral infarction	May show somewhat more rapid initial improvement than in atherothrombotic infarction
Subdural Hematoma (a) acute	(a) Onset in hours to days of progressive deterioration on background of trauma	(a) Almost invariably severe headache	(a) Varying but generally progressive deterioration → coma	(a) Mental irritability, confusion, hemiparesis. Aphasia, hemianopia not common	(a) Progressive deterioration until surgical intervention
(b) chronic	(b) Subacute onset over weeks or longer, with or without obvious history of trauma	(b) Varying and intermittent dull headache in 80-90%	(b) Often waxing and waning levels of consciousness, or progressive deterioration	(b) Same as acute, with more gradual progression	(b) Usually irregular deterioration → dementia or coma until surgery

TABLE 1 Important Clinical Features In Differential Diagnosis of Hypertensive Encephalopathy—Continued.

DISORDER	RAPIDITY OF ONSET OF SIGNS AND SYMPTOMS	CHARACTER OF HEADACHE	LEVEL OF CONSCIOUSNESS	SIGNS	CHARACTERISTIC PROGRESSION
Brain Tumor	Days, weeks, or even months	Recurrent headache in person previously free of them	Normal or mildly impaired until advanced stages or until changed by catastrophic event	Dependent upon localization of tumor and degree of edema	Slow progression
Hypertensive Parenchymal Hemorrhage (a) "capsular"* (b) pontine (c) cerebellar	(a), (b), (c) Usually very rapid over minutes to an hour with nausea, vomiting, rapid development of focal signs	(a) Sudden, severe headache (b), (c) Sudden severe headache with occipital localization	Often rapid deterioration to deep coma	(a), (b) Severe, *dense,* focal deficit in motor system (c) Diplopia, cerebellar signs, brain stem compression	(a) Either stabilizes or progresses to death rapidly (b) Sudden deep coma, often with early death (c) Surgical emergency that often ends in death without rapid intervention
Subarachnoid Hemorrhage	Very rapid onset. Seizure may occur with onset or soon after.	Very rapid onset of severe headache, often localized, and becoming generalized	Normal to deep coma depending on secondary involvement	Cranial nerve deficit, particularly III & VI. Fever, vomiting, stiff neck. Aphasia, hemiparesis, and other focal signs due to secondary effects	Variable—spontaneous recovery or death from rebleeding, infarction, parenchymal destruction

*Refers to effects of thalamic or putaminal hemorrhage.
Source: reprinted with permission of Grune & Stratton from Gifford, R. W., Jr., and Westbrook, E.: Hypertensive encephalopathy; mechanisms, clinical features and treatment. Progr. Cardiovasc. Dis. 17:115, 1974.

TABLE 2   Laboratory Examinations That May Be Helpful in Differential Diagnosis of Hypertensive Encephalopathy

| | CSF EXAMINATION | | | | |
DISORDER	PRESSURE	PROTEIN	CELLS	BRAIN SCAN	ELECTRO-ENCEPHALOGRAM
Hypertensive Encephalopathy	nl or ↑	nl or ↑	Clear, few cells	Normal	Diffuse theta or delta
Cerebral Infarction	nl, may ↑ after 2-3 days with swelling	normal to <100 mg.%	Nl with mild reaction after 2-3 days	Uptake in involved area after 4-7 days	Focal theta and delta
Cerebral Embolus	nl, may ↑ after 2-3 days with swelling	normal to <100 mg.%	Normal or ↑ RBC. May develop xantho-chromia	Uptake in involved area after 4-7 days	Focal theta and delta
Subdural Hematoma	nl or ↑	nl or ↑	Normal or ↑ in RBC. May be xanthochromic	Normal early. Abnormal with time. Crescent defect	Normal or unilateral voltage decrease with slowing
Brain Tumor	nl or ↑	nl or ↑	Normal or few unless seeding or necrosis of tumor	Often focally posi-tive initially, and remains so	Supratentorial – focal slow Infratentorial – bilateral or asynchronous bursts of slow
Hypertensive Parenchymal Hemorrhage	↑	nl or ↑	Frequently bloody	Becomes positive in involved area after several days	Focal slow, then may become diffusely abnormal
Subarachnoid Hemorrhage	Usually ↑	↑	Frankly bloody	May become positive after several days in areas of paren-chymal damage	Diffusely abnormal, perhaps lateralizing in time

(Reprinted with permission of Grune & Stratton from Gifford, R. W., Jr., and Westbrook, E.: Hypertensive encephalopathy: mechanisms, clinical features and treatment. Prog. Cardiovasc. Dis. *17*:115, 1974.)

with extreme caution, especially if there is a suspicion of increased intracranial pressure. Patients with hypertensive encephalopathy may have increased CSF pressure (although this is not always the case even when papilledema is present), but the fluid is clear. Bloody fluid not due to a traumatic tap rules out hypertensive encephalopathy and confirms the diagnosis of subarachnoid hemorrhage, which may be due to spontaneous bleeding, rupture of a congenital A-V malformation or "berry" aneurysm, or extension of a cerebral hematoma into the subarachnoid space (Table 2). Xanthochromic fluid can occur with extensive hemorrhagic infarcts or subdural hematomas in addition to old subarachnoid bleeding, but never occurs with hypertensive encephalopathy.

If indicated, a stat electroencephalogram may be made with a portable instrument while the patient is receiving parenteral hypotensive therapy. In hypertensive encephalopathy, the EEG may show transient focal disturbances, or bilaterally synchronous sharp and slow waves, or both; however, it is nonspecific and nonlocalizing,

whereas it can be lateralizing in cerebral and subdural hematoma and some hemispheric infarctions (Table 2). The brain scan usually is normal in the acute phase of cerebral infarction or hemorrhage, and in subarachnoid hemorrhage. It is normal and remains so in hypertensive encephalopathy, whereas in the other conditions an abnormal focus may develop after a few days. The EMI scan is more helpful than the isotope scan in identifying hematomas early, but shows no abnormality in hypertensive encephalopathy.

OTHER HYPERTENSIVE CRISES

There are other hypertensive emergencies, but most are discussed elsewhere in this book and this chapter. Some are so self-evident that detailed discussion of their differential diagnosis is unnecessary. They include: acute left ventricular failure; acute coronary insufficiency; eclampsia; dissecting aneurysm of the aorta; pheochromocytoma;

drug interactions; acute glomerulonephritis; acute hypertension in the postoperative period; severe body burns; and malignant hypertension.

Acute Left Ventricular Failure

When hypertension, regardless of its severity, coexists with acute left ventricular failure, reduction of blood pressure with parenteral agents is almost always indicated, especially when the failure is due to hypertensive heart disease. Reducing the work load on the left ventricle usually restores cardiac compensation dramatically, sometimes without the need for digitalis.

Acute Coronary Insufficiency

Acute coronary insufficiency, with or without acute myocardial infarction, sometimes can cause an abrupt and alarming increase in blood pressure, perhaps through a reflex mechanism (Horwitz and Sjoerdsma, 1964). The blood pressure may reach levels in excess of 250/150 mm. Hg. The accompanying chest pain is the diagnostic tip-off, and the EKG usually shows changes of acute ischemia or infarction.

Eclampsia

Eclampsia should be viewed as hypertensive encephalopathy occurring in a pregnant woman, usually in the last trimester. Differential diagnosis usually presents no difficulties if one keeps in mind that pregnant women also are predisposed to rupture of congenital aneurysms of the circle of Willis. Convulsions are more likely to occur in women with eclampsia and children with acute glomerulonephritis (see below) than in other patients with hypertensive encephalopathy. Furthermore, symptoms of hypertensive encephalopathy appear at lower levels of blood pressure in eclampsia and acute glomerulonephritis than in other patients with hypertensive encephalopathy.

Acute Glomerulonephritis

Patients with acute glomerulonephritis, especially children, are susceptible to hypertensive encephalopathy with convulsions. The diagnosis usually is easy because there aren't many conditions in childhood that are associated with acute onset of hypertension, proteinuria, hematuria, and cylindruria with or without azotemia.

Dissecting Aneurysm

This condition is discussed elsewhere in this book. Hypotensive therapy has become the treatment of choice for most patients.

Pheochromocytoma

Pheochromocytoma should be suspected in any patient with severe hypertension, especially if the blood pressure is unusually labile and the patient has excessive sweating, paroxysmal headache, palpitations (with or without tachycardia), and a variety of arrhythmias. Sometimes, patients with pheochromocytoma present with hypertensive encephalopathy. Diagnosis depends on finding increased concentrations of free catecholamines in the blood or urine, or increased concentrations of VMA and/or metanephrines in the urine. Although almost every patient with hypertensive crisis of any type should be screened for pheochromocytoma, one should not wait for the results of tests to be reported before initiating hypotensive therapy.*

Drug Interactions

Very similar to the hypertension of pheochromocytoma is the acute hypertensive crisis precipitated by the interaction between monoamine oxidase inhibitors (MAOI) and drugs (ephedrine, tyramine, amphetamines) or foods and beverages containing tyramine (Chianti wine, cheddar cheese, naturally fermented beers, chicken livers, pickled herring) that release tissue catecholamines. The presenting complaint usually is severe headache, coming on abruptly after ingestion of the offending drug or food. Other features suggesting pheochromocytoma, such as sweating, tachycardia, and tremor, may or may not be present. The blood pressure usually is in excess of

---

*See next section.

220/130 mm. Hg, and may be much higher. Appropriate treatment should be instituted promptly before waiting for results of determinations of urinary catecholamines, VMA, and metanephrines, which usually take several days. Fatal cerebral hemorrhages have been reported as a result of this type of drug interaction. In this situation of intense adrenergic stimulation, an alpha blocking agent (such as phentolamine) is a better choice on physiologic grounds, although a vasodilating agent (nitroprusside) can be effective,* and is easier to use.

Postoperative Hypertension

Occasionally, hypertension occurring in the immediate postoperative period requires parenteral treatment, if for no other reason than that the patient still is taking nothing by mouth. Sometimes it is a true emergency, either because the blood pressure is extremely high, or because even moderate hypertension is a threat to recently placed vascular suture lines.

Body Burns

For reasons that have never been elucidated, extensive body burns sometimes are accompanied by severe hypertension. Most patients die, not from the hypertension but from the extensive burns.

Malignant Hypertension

Retinal hemorrhages, exudates, and papilledema signify the presence of malignant hypertension with necrosis of small arteries and arterioles. Even in the absence of symptoms or evidence of target organ disease, this represents a quasi-emergency requiring reduction of blood pressure within 48 hours.

TREATMENT

Hypotensive Drugs (Tables 3 and 4)

DIURETICS

Since all the antihypertensive agents listed in Table 3 have the propensity for

causing retention of fluid and sodium, a rapidly acting diuretic (e.g., furosemide, 80 to 120 mg., or ethacrynic acid, 50 to 150 mg.) usually should be given intravenously at the onset and repeated as often as necessary to prevent fluid retention, normally one to three times daily as long as parenteral medication is necessary. Larger doses than those suggested may be necessary for patients with renal insufficiency. If the patient is obviously dehydrated and volume-depleted at onset, the diuretic may be omitted for the first 24 to 48 hours, but it usually becomes necessary eventually to counteract overexpansion of plasma and extracellular fluid volumes. Judicious use of a diuretic enhances the effectiveness of all the agents in Table 3, and prolongs the action of all except sodium nitroprusside, phentolamine, and trimethaphan, which have very short durations of action and hence must be given by continous infusion.

VASODILATORS

Sodium Nitroprusside. Sodium nitroprusside is the most potent and most consistently effective agent available for management of hypertensive crises of any description. The only contraindication to its use is inability to monitor the patient closely in an intensive care unit, because its onset of action is almost instantaneous but its duration is so evanescent that close surveillance is mandatory to keep the blood pressure within the desired range. An infusion pump is helpful, but this does not obviate the need for frequent (usually $\bar{q}$ three to five minutes at least initially) measurements of blood pressure. An intra-arterial line for measuring blood pressure continuously is useful but not absolutely necessary.

Sodium nitroprusside is a versatile drug, because one can lower the blood pressure as rapidly or as slowly as desired and can maintain it at any level by appropriate adjustment of the infusion rate; accidental hypotension is corrected automatically and promptly by slowing the rate of infusion or temporarily stopping it. Consequently, it is safe to use when the diagnosis is questionable and the physician has lingering doubts about the advisability of reducing blood pressure rapidly with agents that have a prolonged effect.

Sodium nitroprusside has a very favorable effect on left ventricular function in the failing heart, because it reduces both after-

---

*See section on treatment.

load and preload (Cohn, 1973). Moreover, it is the only antihypertensive agent listed in Table 3, except for phentolamine, that is effective in managing hypertension associated with pheochromocytoma or MAOI drug interactions.

Sodium nitroprusside is converted to thiocyanate, which can cause acute toxic psychosis and delirium if the blood level exceeds 10 to 12 mg./100 ml. This rarely occurs except in patients with advanced renal failure, and then only after several days. As a precautionary measure, it is advisable to determine blood thiocyanate concentrations every 48 hours during infusions of sodium nitroprusside. If toxic levels are obtained, the drug must be withdrawn.

Diazoxide. Diazoxide also is a potent and rapidly acting hypotensive agent that must be given by bolus injection to be effective because it is rapidly bound to plasma protein (Sellers and Koch-Weser, 1973). Its advantage is convenience, because once the maximal hypotensive effect is realized, usually within three to five minutes after the bolus injection, the blood pressure remains at rather stable levels for up to 12 hours, thus obviating the need for the meticulous monitoring required when sodium nitroprusside is used. However, by the same token, one is committed to whatever hypotensive response may occur and if the diagnosis was in error or the hypotensive response too great, one is faced with the administration of a pressor agent to counteract the effect of the diazoxide.

Some clinicians have suggested giving bolus I.V. injections of 100 mg. of diazoxide every 15 to 20 minutes until the blood pressure is at the desired level. This is a cumber-

TABLE 3 *Antihypertensive Drugs for Parenteral Administration in Managing Hypertensive Crises*

DRUGS°	ROUTE OF ADMINISTRATION AND DOSAGE (MG.) I.M.	ROUTE OF ADMINISTRATION AND DOSAGE (MG.) I.V.	ONSET OF ACTION (MIN.)	DURATION OF ACTION	IMPORTANT SIDE-EFFECTS
Vasodilators Sodium nitroprusside (Nipride)		50–200/liter by infusion	Instantaneous	2-3 min.	Retching, vomiting, agitation, cutis anserina, flushing, tachycardia, thiocyanate intoxication
Diazoxide (Hyperstat)		200–300 by bolus injection (within 30 sec.)	3-5	4-12 hrs.	Nausea, vomiting, flushing, tachycardia, headache, angina, hyperglycemia
Hydralazine (Apresoline)	10–50	200/liter by infusion	20-30	3-6 hrs.	Headache, tachycardia, palpitation, angina, flushing
Sympathetic Depressants Reserpine (Serpasil)	1–5	1–5 from syringe in 3-5 min.	120-180	4-8 hrs.	Somnolence, stupor, unpredictable hypotension, activation of peptic ulcer
Methyldopa (Aldomet Ester)		300–600 in 100 ml. over 30-60 min.	120-180	4-8 hrs.	Somnolence
Pentolinium (Ansolysen)	2–10		20-30	4-6 hrs.	Atony of bowel and bladder; paralysis of accommodation
Trimethaphan Camsylate (Arfonad)		1000/liter by infusion	5-10	5-10 min.	
Phentolamine (Regitine)	5–10	5–10 by bolus inj. or 200/liter by inf.	Instantaneous	5-20 min.	Tachycardia, palpitations, headache, flushing

°In most cases a rapidly acting diuretic (furosemide or ethacrynic acid) should be given intravenously at the beginning and at appropriate intervals throughout treatment with these agents (see text).

TABLE 4 *Hypotensive Drugs of Choice for Parenteral Administration in Managing Some Hypertensive Crises*

CRISIS	DRUG(S) OF CHOICE	SATISFACTORY ALTERNATIVE DRUGS	RELATIVELY CONTRAINDICATED DRUGS
Hypertensive encephalopathy	Sodium nitroprusside Diazoxide	Hydralazine Trimethaphan Pentolinium	Reserpine Methyldopa
Acute intracranial hemorrhage	Sodium nitroprusside	Trimethaphan	Reserpine Methyldopa Diazoxide
Acute cerebral infarction	Sodium nitroprusside	Trimethaphan Hydralazine	Reserpine Methyldopa Diazoxide
Head injury	Sodium nitroprusside	Trimethaphan Hydralazine	Reserpine Methyldopa Diazoxide
Acute left ventricular failure	Sodium nitroprusside	Trimethaphan Pentolinium Diazoxide	Hydralazine
Acute coronary insufficiency	Sodium nitroprusside	Reserpine Methyldopa	Hydralazine Diazoxide
Eclampsia	Sodium nitroprusside Diazoxide	Hydralazine	Pentolinium Trimethaphan
Acute glomerulo-nephritis	Sodium nitroprusside Diazoxide	Hydralazine	
Dissecting aneurysm	Reserpine + Trimethaphan + Guanethidine, p.o. + Propranolol, p.o.	Sodium nitroprusside + Propranolol, I.V.	Diazoxide Hydralazine
Pheochromocytoma and MAOI drug interactions	Sodium nitroprusside	Phentolamine	All others
Postoperative hypertension	Sodium nitroprusside Diazoxide	Reserpine Methyldopa Hydralazine	Pentolinium Trimethaphan
Extensive body burns	Sodium nitroprusside Diazoxide	Reserpine Methyldopa Hydralazine	
Malignant hypertension	Diazoxide Reserpine	Methyldopa Sodium nitroprusside Hydralazine	

some alternative if the patient cannot be placed in an intensive care unit for monitoring an infusion of sodium nitroprusside.

Diazoxide can cause severe hyperglycemia in some patients. This is infrequent, but it is advisable to determine blood glucose concentrations daily for patients receiving this agent.

Hydralazine. In the past, hydralazine was used either intravenously or intramuscularly (see Table 3 and 4) for management of acute hypertensive crises associated with acute glomerulonephritis or toxemia of pregnancy. It causes a reflex tachycardia and increases the cardiac output, and hence should not be used in patients with pre-existing heart disease. Now that sodium nitroprusside and diazoxide are available it is used less frequently.

SYMPATHETIC DEPRESSANT DRUGS

Reserpine. Except for dissecting aneurysm and acute hypertension associated with coronary insufficiency, there is little indication for the use of reserpine in managing hypertensive crisis. Its maximal hypotensive effect is not realized for two to three hours after intravenous or intramuscular administration, and this is too long to wait for most emergencies. Moreover, it causes somnolence bordering on stupor in some patients, and therefore interferes with clinical evaluation of patients with head injuries, hypertensive encephalopathy, and stroke. Its unpredictable effect sometimes leads to severe and prolonged hypotension.

Methyldopa. Methyldopa shares the same disadvantages as reserpine, except that its soporific effect is somewhat less and undesirable hypotension does not occur as often.

Ganglion Blocking Agents. Pentolinium and trimethaphan are effective and prompt-acting hypotensive agents that do not cause somnolence or stupor. Because they block the autonomic ganglia, they also depress the parasympathetic system and thereby cause atony of the bowel and bladder, which is particularly undesirable in the immediate postoperative state. Trimethaphan has a short duration of action and, like sodium nitroprusside, it must be given by continuous intravenous infusion under close surveillance in an intensive care unit. Tachyphylaxis frequently develops to the hypo-

tensive action of trimethaphan. Except for the management of hypertension associated with acute dissecting aneurysm, it is not used much any more; it has all the disadvantages of sodium nitroprusside, but is less effective and causes more side-effects.

Phentolamine. This is an alpha adrenergic blocking agent with a short duration of action that is specifically effective in managing hypertension associated with pheochromocytoma or drug interactions with MAOI. It usually is not effective in managing crises from other causes, and for this reason it has been used as a diagnostic test for pheochromocytoma. However, it does produce a depressor effect in enough patients with severe hypertension from any cause to minimize its value as a diagnostic procedure. Bolus injections have such a short duration of action that it is cumbersome to treat patients in this manner. Consequently, continuous infusions of the drug are preferable when indicated to treat hypertension secondary to excess circulating catecholamines. Sodium nitroprusside is equally effective and has become the agent of choice for management of this type of hypertension.

Management of Certain Crises

Table 4 summarizes the agents of choice for the various types of hypertensive crises. Only those which are controversial are discussed in detail here.

HYPERTENSIVE ENCEPHALOPATHY

All authorities agree that prompt reduction of blood pressure to normal or near-normal levels is indicated for patients with hypertensive encephalopathy as soon as the diagnosis is made or even strongly suspected. However, the diagnosis is not always easy, and the differential includes conditions on which there is not uniform agreement about the desirability of lowering blood pressure precipitously (see p. 942). In any case, most patients should be in an intensive care unit if they are comatose or semicomatose, because patency of the airway must be assured and precautions must be taken in case convulsions occur. Therefore, monitoring a sodium nitroprusside infusion presents no additional problem, and this is the drug of choice. Diazoxide is a satisfactory alternative if close observation is impossible and if the diagnosis is not in doubt.

CEREBRAL HEMORRHAGE

There is an unresolved controversy about the advisability of reducing blood pressure for patients with subarachnoid or intracerebral hemorrhage. Preliminary results of a cooperative study have shown that hypotensive therapy is less effective than antifibrinolytic therapy in patients with acute subarachnoid hemorrhage (Nibbelink and Sahs, 1972). Some physicians actually advocate keeping blood pressure at low normotensive or even hypotensive levels for patients with intracranial bleeding. Angiographic demonstration of severe arterial spasm adjacent to bleeding sites has aroused the fears of others that reduction of blood pressure will cause more ischemia in these areas. Gradual reduction of blood pressure with sodium nitroprusside seems warranted. If the neurologic deficit seems to worsen as blood pressure declines, the rate of infusion can be slowed or stopped, and the original blood pressure is quickly restored. Diazoxide is relatively contraindicated because one has so little control over its effect.

CEREBRAL INFARCTION

There is even more controversy over the advisability and benefit of reducing blood pressure for patients with acute cerebral infarction. Until blood pressure exceeds 190/110 mm. Hg it is probably wise to do nothing to control it, unless the patient is also in congestive heart failure. If it exceeds these arbitrary limits, an infusion of sodium nitroprusside may be administered cautiously to keep the blood pressure between 160/90 and 190/110 mm. Hg, provided the neurologic deficit does not worsen.

ECLAMPSIA

The management of hypertension associated with eclampsia is another controversial area. Many obstetricians prefer to control the convulsions with magnesium sulfate, empty the uterus, and not treat the blood pressure per se, because they fear that this would reduce placental perfusion even more and jeopardize the fetus. There are no stud-

ies to confirm or contradict this contention. Most internists and some obstetricians treat eclampsia as they would hypertensive encephalopathy in other settings, with intravenous furosemide and either sodium nitroprusside or diazoxide. There is agreement that the uterus should be emptied as soon as possible. Diazoxide, being a generalized smooth muscle relaxant, usually stops or slows active labor, but this can be restored with oxytocic agents.

CORONARY INSUFFICIENCY

When severe hypertension (e.g., >220/130 mm. Hg) accompanies coronary insufficiency or acute myocardial infarction, it seems reasonable to relieve the ischemic left ventricle of the additional work-load imposed by the hypertension. On the other hand, a precipitate drop in blood pressure might be equally hazardous. Drugs of choice include sodium nitroprusside infusion or intramuscular reserpine (no more than 1 mg.), the objective being to maintain blood pressure at levels of 150/90 to 170/110 mm. Hg.

Plans

Regardless of the cause of the hypertensive crisis, the objective should be to control the blood pressure with oral medications as soon as practicable so that the nuisance of parenteral treatment can be eliminated. Whenever patients are conscious and able to take medications, appropriate oral treatment should begin simultaneously with the parenteral treatment.

Radiologic and laboratory investigations that have been delayed until the crisis has been controlled may be undertaken while the patient is still on parenteral therapy if they seem important to the immediate management of the patient. Unless there are compelling reasons to the contrary, however, control of blood pressure should be maintained even if it means following the patient into the operating room or the angiographic laboratory with a sodium nitroprusside drip while he has cerebral angiograms, coronary angiograms, or aortograms.

COMPLICATIONS

Potential complications include: (1) those inherent in the disease with which the hypertension is associated, and they are as numerous and diverse as the diseases themselves; (2) the nonspecific effect of rapid reduction of blood pressure (e.g., cerebral or myocardial ischemia or infarction or renal failure); and (3) specific side-effects of the individual drugs (e.g., hyperglycemia from diazoxide, or thiocyanate intoxication from sodium nitroprusside).

Patients with hypertensive crises are seriously ill, and many are doomed to die or have major residual disability regardless of how expertly they are managed. Nevertheless, *judicious* reduction of blood pressure (which is not necessarily synonymous with *cautious* reduction of blood pressure), using agents appropriate for the condition being treated, is much more often helpful than harmful.

The alert clinician can anticipate untoward effects of rapidly lowering the blood pressure and guard against them by using agents that have a short duration of action, permitting prompt restoration of original levels of blood pressure if necessary. In this regard, it should be emphasized that even advanced renal failure is not a contraindication to the parenteral use of potent hypotensive agents. One can always resort to dialysis to replace kidney function, but one has no replacement for brain or cardiac function. Lastly, the physician who is well informed regarding the pharmacology and side-effects of the drugs he uses can detect untoward reactions early, before they become major problems.

References

Cohn, J. N.: Vasodilator therapy for heart failure; the influence of impedance on left ventricular performance (editorial). Circulation 48:5, 1973.

Gifford, R. W., Jr., and Westbrook, E.: Hypertensive encephalopathy: mechanisms, clinical features and treatment. Progr. Cardiovasc. Dis. 17:115, 1974.

Horwitz, D., and Sjoerdsma, A.: Some interrelations between elevation of blood pressure and angina pectoris. Hypertension. Proc. Council for High Blood Pressure Research, Am. Heart Assoc. 13:39, 1964.

Nibbelink, D. W., and Sahs, A. L.: Antifibrinolytic therapy and drug-induced hypotension in treatment of ruptured intracranial aneurysms. Trans. Am. Neurol. Assoc. 97:145, 1972.

Sellers, E. M., and Koch-Weser, J.: Influence of intravenous injection rate on protein binding and vascular activity of diazoxide. Ann. N.Y. Acad. Sci. 226:319, 1973.

Suggested Reading

A.M.A. Committee on Hypertension: The treatment of malignant hypertension and hypertensive emergencies. J.A.M.A. 228:1673, 1974.

Koch-Weser, J.: Current concepts: hypertensive emergencies. N. Engl. J. Med. 290:211, 1974.

Palmer, R. F., and Lasseter, K. C.: Sodium nitroprusside. N. Engl. J. Med. 292:297, 1975.

Toole, J. F., and Patel, A. N.: Cerebral Vascular Disorders, 2d ed. New York, McGraw-Hill Book Co., 1974, p. 412.

F. PERICARDITIS

Robert R. Kelly and John H. Stone

Pericarditis is defined as an inflammation of the fibroserous sac surrounding the heart. In addition, the process usually involves the epicardium to some degree. It may be acute and self-limited, recurrent, or chronic. A multitude of etiologic agents are responsible and may be grouped for the sake of simplicity under three major categories: infectious, noninfectious, and autoimmune-hypersensitivity states (see Table 1). The majority of cases fortunately are acute and self-limited, resulting either from a viral infection or, by exclusion, from some ill-defined idiopathic cause.

SYMPTOMS

The patient often relates having recently suffered with symptoms of either a viral-like upper respiratory infection or gastroenteritis. This may then be followed by nonspecific complaints of malaise, fever, arthralgias, dyspnea, or dysphagia in conjunction with the sudden onset of sharp parasternal or epigastric pain.

The *character of the pain* may be nonspecific, but frequently it is distinctive and worthy of careful evaluation. It has been shown that only the inferior portion of the

TABLE 1 *Major Causes of Acute Pericarditis*

1. Infectious
   a. Viral
   b. Bacterial
   c. Tuberculous
   d. Fungal
   e. Parasitic

2. Noninfectious
   a. Metabolic
      (1) Uremia
      (2) Myxedema
   b. Neoplastic
   c. Dissecting aneurysm of aorta
   d. Acute myocardial infarction
   e. Radiation injury
   f. Traumatic

3. Presumed hypersensitivity-autoimmune etiology
   a. Collagen vascular disease
   b. Acute rheumatic fever
   c. Following pericardial injury
      (1) After myocardial infarction (Dressler's)
      (2) After trauma (blunt or penetrating)
   d. Serum sickness
   e. Drug-induced (e.g., procainamide, hydralazine)

4. Idiopathic

external parietal pericardium is pain-sensitive, and it is anatomically adjacent to the diaphragmatic pleura. It is postulated, then, that pericardial innervation traverses the left phrenic nerve, taking origin from cervical nerve roots (Fowler, 1974). This may explain why pericardial pain usually is *pleuritic*, occasionally associated with hiccups, and commonly referred to the neck, trapezius ridge, shoulder, or upper arm. The pain may be aggravated by swallowing, twisting or turning of the trunk and by reclining; partial relief is often obtained by leaning forward in the upright position. Sometimes the pain may be *constant*, simulating that of myocardial infarction, or *absent*, especially in the chronic forms secondary to tuberculosis, uremia, or neoplasia.

The differential diagnosis that arises with pericardial pain includes myocardial infarction, pneumonia, pulmonary emboli or infarction, pneumothorax, dissecting aneurysm, pleurisy, or intercostal neuralgia. In addition, an occasional patient may complain of palpitations secondary to atrial arrhythmias or of dyspnea, orthopnea, lightheadedness and syncope due to cardiac tamponade. In contrast, patients with chronic pericarditis are often asymptomatic.

CLINICAL FINDINGS

Physical Examination. The *pericardial friction rub* is pathognomonic of pericarditis. It is a mono-, bi-, or triphasic "scratchy, grating" sound, seemingly close to the ear, and is heard best along the left midsternal edge. It is best appreciated with the patient leaning forward in held expiration or in a crawling position. The triphasic rub occurs most commonly and is secondary to pericardial-epicardial or pleural contact during ventricular systole, diastole, and atrial systole. The latter component may be superimposed on the ventricular diastolic sound in tachycardic states and obviously is lost in the presence of atrial fibrillation.

The intensity of pericardial rubs varies greatly with respiration and position; their fleeting, transitory nature may require frequent repeated auscultation. For this reason, *the absence of a rub in the emergency room in no way excludes the diagnosis of pericarditis.*

Rubs may at times be confused with murmurs. Spodick (1971) cites (1) the unusual location of maximal intensity (mid-left sternal edge) along with (2) failure to radiate in patterns expected for murmurs as helpful in distinguishing the two. The intensity of the friction rub is not indicative of the degree of pericardial effusion.

Pericardial effusion is invariably present as part of the inflammatory process, regardless of the etiology; its hemodynamic significance is primarily related to the *rapidity of accumulation* and only secondarily to the *amount.* Traumatic injuries may produce cardiac tamponade with as little as 150 to 200 cc., whereas a liter or more of fluid may be present in slowly accumulating uremic effusions. Pericardial effusion alone is not indicative of pericardial inflammation, since it may accompany the anasarca of cardiac failure, nephrosis, or hepatic failure.

Cardiac tamponade may be defined as impaired diastolic filling of the heart because of increased intrapericardial pressure, resulting in a critical reduction of cardiac output. Classically, the triad of increased venous pressure, arterial hypotension, and a small quiet heart has been described as indicating tamponade. Traumatic injuries may indeed produce this classical triad, but other causes often result in an enlarged cardiac silhouette without reduction in heart sounds or apical

TABLE 2   Common Causes of Cardiac Tamponade

1. Trauma
   a. Penetrating
   b. Blunt
   c. Iatrogenic (pericardiocentesis, transvenous cardiac pacing)
2. Neoplasm
3. Infection
4. Rupture of heart, aorta
5. Anticoagulant therapy in pericarditis

impulse. Patients with tamponade usually present as either pale or cyanotic, sitting upright, extremely anxious and dyspneic, or in shock with coma. Inspection of the neck veins reveals an elevated jugular venous pressure, a positive hepatojugular reflux, and *Kussmaul's sign* (an abnormal elevation instead of the normal fall in jugular venous pressure with inspiration). The *paradoxic pulse* (inspiratory decline of greater than 10 mm. Hg in the systolic blood pressure) should be looked for with the aid of a blood pressure cuff; if the blood pressure is inaudible, palpation of the femoral artery may show a decreased pulse amplitude with inspiration. Neither Kussmaul's sign nor the paradoxic pulse is pathognomonic for tamponade, since they may be present in the patient with

asthma and chronic obstructive pulmonary disease (because of the wide swings in intrathoracic pressure). A detailed discussion of the pathophysiology of the paradoxic pulse and Kussmaul's sign is available elsewhere (Goldman, 1975). Table 2 lists the common causes of cardiac tamponade. Cardiogenic shock secondary to myocardial infarction may mimic tamponade but should be differentiated from it by the history as well as prominent gallop rhythm, significant pulmonary congestion, and characteristic EKG changes.

Laboratory. Laboratory aids in the diagnosis of pericarditis with effusion or tamponade include (1) chest x-ray and/or fluoroscopy, (2) electrocardiogram, (3) echocardiogram, (4) pericardiocentesis, and (5) surgical biopsy. The *chest x-ray* may show a diffusely enlarged cardiac silhouette with a loss of chamber definition often referred to as the "flask" or "water-bottle" heart; if serial roentgenograms are available, an increase in the cardiac silhouette without pulmonary congestion may suggest the diagnosis. Traumatic injuries may produce hemopericardium and tamponade without a significant increase in over-all cardiac size. *Fluoroscopy* may show decreased pulsations; an epicardial fat line may be seen as a radiolucent strip well within the cardiac margins on fluoroscopy (or at times on the lateral chest film).

The *electrocardiogram* is abnormal in

R.E. 17508

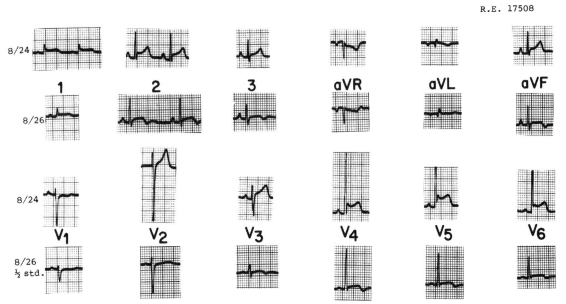

Figure 1. Evolution of EKG changes in a young man with presumed viral pericarditis: initial ST segment elevation (8/24) followed by diffuse T inversion (8/26).

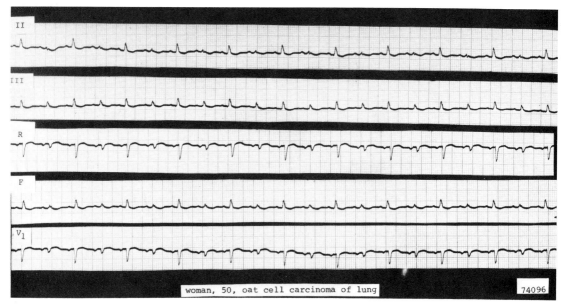

Figure 2. Electrical alternans, with alternating height of the QRS complexes, in a patient with malignant pericardial effusion.

90 per cent of patients with acute pericarditis, but the "typical" evolutionary changes described below occur much less frequently. The electrocardiogram changes are due not to pericarditis *per se* but to the concomitant epicarditis; they consist of diffuse concave *ST-segment elevation* in the limb and precordial leads except for ST depression in aVR and V₁. After a few days to weeks, the ST segments become isoelectric with concomitant T-wave inversion (Fig. 1). This persists for weeks or months and then usually returns to normal. With large effusions, low voltage or electrical alternans of the QRS complex may be found (Fig. 2). Total electrical alternans of the P waves and QRS complexes frequently indicates effusion, often malignant in origin.

According to Spodick (1971), sinus tachycardia is the rule in pericarditis except in uremic pericarditis and in cases of inferior infarction with bradycardia. Atrial arrhythmias, atrial flutter and fibrillation, are not uncommon due to the proximity of the sinoatrial node to the inflamed epicardial surface. Spodick warns, however, that atrial arrhythmias in acute pericarditis often point to underlying heart disease.

Echocardiography is a relatively new but accurate, noninvasive method for demonstrating pericardial effusion. It has obviated, except in a minority of cases, the need for angiography.

Pericardiocentesis for diagnostic purposes should not be performed in the emergency room, but only as part of a therapeutic maneuver in life-threatening cardiac tamponade. Pericardial fluid analysis (sugar, protein, cell count, cytology, cultures) and/or surgical biopsy are inpatient procedures indicated when clinical deterioration is present and diagnosis is uncertain. The technique for performing pericardiocentesis is described in detail in the Procedures Section of this text.

VARIETIES OF PERICARDITIS

In *viral pericarditis*, identified viral agents include Coxsackie A and B, influenza, echo, mumps, herpes simplex, varicella, and adenovirus. Approximately 28 per cent of cases (Fowler, 1974) give a history of preceding upper respiratory tract or enteric illness occurring two to three weeks before the abrupt onset of chest pain. Arthralgias, myalgias, and fever, usually low grade but occasionally to 104°F, accompany the illness. In addition, some cases may show transient pulmonary infiltrates and pleural effusions. The process usually resolves within a few days or within three to six weeks; recurrence of symptoms is noted approximately 23 per cent of the time (Fowler, 1974). Serious complications such as tamponade or myocarditis (the latter heralded by conduction disturbances, transient Q waves, and high myocardial enzyme elevations) are rare.

Idiopathic pericarditis is diagnosed by excluding known causes; a viral or autoimmune etiology is suspected but not proved. The symptoms, associated findings, and course are identical to those of viral pericarditis, except for the absence of myocarditis.

Purulent pericarditis is usually a complication of other disease processes and primarily results from extension of mediastinal or pulmonary infections into the pericardium by surgical entry or traumatic penetration. Hematogenous metastases from skin, soft tissues, and bone are less common. The primary process or its treatment with antimicrobial agents may mask the pericardial infection. A friction rub and classic electrocardiogram pattern are absent in more than half of these patients, but cardiomegaly secondary to large effusion is common. Etiologic agents include both gram-positive and gram-negative bacteria and mycotic organisms. Pericardial fluid analysis and culture are necessary for correct diagnosis and treatment. Surgical removal of the pericardium may be necessary.

Tuberculous pericarditis occurs in 5 to 10 per cent of tuberculous patients, but it may be difficult to demonstrate tuberculous infection elsewhere. Spread from infected mediastinal nodes (Fowler, 1974) appears to be the most common portal of entry into the pericardium. There is a 10 to 12 times greater incidence in blacks than in whites. The onset is usually insidious, with persistent low-grade fever, weight loss, and progressive cardiac enlargement, often leading to a presentation with either cardiac tamponade or constrictive pericarditis (see below). The tuberculin skin test is usually positive with rare exception. Culture of the sanguineous effusion has a low yield and should be supplemented by pericardial biopsy in patients in whom the clinical situation requires bacteriologic confirmation.

Pericarditis of acute myocardial infarction: 1 in 5 cases of acute myocardial infarction is complicated by the development of clinical pericarditis, usually within two to four days after onset but sometimes as late as 10 days after infarction. Its development signifies epicardial injury. Large effusions are rare and suggest either bleeding from anticoagulant use or, terminally, myocardial rupture.

The *postpericardial injury syndrome* includes the postpericardiotomy (surgical), postmyocardial infarction (Dressler's), and post-traumatic injury (penetrating and nonpenetrating) syndromes. All three syndromes are identical in clinical manifestations, occurring within three days to several months after injury. Chest pain and fever up to 104°F, are the prominent features along with pulmonary infiltrates, effusions, arthralgias, and leukocytosis. The course is usually benign unless complicated by anticoagulant therapy and is self-limited to one or two weeks' duration, although recurrences may occur up to two years after injury. The clinical manifestations seem to result from a hypersensitivity reaction produced through the formation of antiheart antibodies after the initial injury to the pericardium and/or myocardium (Engle et al., 1975; Lessof, 1976).

Autoimmune diseases: Pericarditis may be present in up to 40 per cent of the cases of systemic lupus erythematosus (SLE) and often precedes other manifestations of the disease; in contrast, in rheumatoid arthritis, pericarditis usually follows a well-documented peripheral arthritis. In SLE, positive serum and pericardial fluid LE cell "preps," and antinuclear antibodies facilitate the diagnosis, whereas rheumatoid patients demonstrate characteristically low pleural or pericardial fluid glucose. In both entities, the process is usually benign, responding to treatment of the systemic disease, and is of little prognostic significance. Certain drugs, notably procainamide and hydralazine, may induce a lupus-like syndrome which usually remits with discontinuation of the drug.

Previously considered a terminal event in the patient with chronic renal failure, *uremic pericarditis* now occurs in 10 to 15 per cent of patients on chronic hemodialysis; the pericarditis may develop despite amelioration of the uremic syndrome by dialysis. These patients have significant chest pain, loud friction rubs, and large (often hemorrhagic) pericardial effusions. Typical electrocardiographic changes are infrequent in uremic pericarditis. Pericarditis in uremia is often found in conjunction with heart failure and pulmonary congestion. Cardiac tamponade frequently occurs in such patients, probably as a result of the increased bleeding tendency and platelet function abnormalities of chronic uremia, as well as the anticoagulation required for hemodialysis. In addition, clinically significant tamponade may be *unmasked after dialysis* because of the attendant reduction in plasma volume and filling pressure of the heart.

Neoplastic pericarditis: Benign as well as malignant tumors may involve the pericardium. Of the malignant processes, lung and breast carcinoma, mesothelioma, sarcoma, lymphoma, and leukemic infiltration are the most common. Malignant effusions frequently produce complete electrical alternans of the electrocardiogram and often lead to cardiac tamponade. The use of irradiation in the treatment of neoplasms may lead to a postirradiation pericarditis.

Penetrating wounds of the heart (gunshot, stab, cardiac resuscitation, CVP line, pacemaker implantation) and blunt trauma have produced *traumatic pericarditis.* Associated cardiac injuries may occur including rupture of the heart, papillary muscle dysfunction, interventricular or atrial septal defects, and myocardial contusion.

DISPOSITION AND TREATMENT

With rare exception, the patient presenting with pericarditis should be admitted to the hospital for accurate diagnosis and monitoring. The routine hospital ward will suffice in most instances, except for patients with associated atrial arrhythmias and signs of incipient or actual tamponade or in those cases secondary to trauma, myocardial infarction, or dissecting aneurysm in which intensive care monitoring is required.

Treatment, of course, must be directed toward the underlying etiology. For patients with acute viral or idiopathic pericarditis and the postpericardial injury syndromes, reassurance, bed rest, and analgesia with either aspirin or indomethacin is adequate in most situations. The indiscriminate use of corticosteroids, although very effective in alleviating pain and symptoms, is to be discouraged. First of all, their use in undiagnosed bacterial or tuberculous disease could be catastrophic. Second, observers have noted a "steroid dependency"—on attempting to taper or discontinue the drug, a recurrence of the clinical manifestations often occurs, prompting long-term use with its greater potential for side effects. On the other hand, in serious clinical situations, such as pericarditis secondary to acute myocardial infarction, short-term steroid use is justified and may reduce the requirements for narcotics.

Dialysis patients with uncomplicated uremic pericarditis frequently obtain relief from indomethacin and may be referred back to their dialysis center for increased frequency or duration of dialysis.

Pericardiocentesis is essential therapy when life-threatening cardiac tamponade presents in the emergency room, especially in patients with chest trauma who do not respond to the usual volume replacement and chest tube insertion for hemopneumothorax or tension pneumothorax. If purulent pericardial fluid is obtained during a *therapeutic tap,* initial antimicrobial therapy should be based on Gram stain or acid-fast stain.

Constrictive Pericarditis

This condition results when the healing of an acute fibrinous, serofibrinous, or especially hemorrhagic pericarditis results in the formation of a nondistensible scar obliterating the pericardial cavity, encasing the heart, and limiting diastolic filling.

SYMPTOMS

Patients with this disorder complain of exertional dyspnea and fatigue, mild orthopnea, and swelling of the abdomen and, less commonly, the ankles. Epigastric discomfort secondary to ascites and hepatosplenomegaly may also be noted. Fluid retention is usually very gradual, taking place over months to years (occasional patients have developed symptoms in a few weeks). A past history of acute pericarditis may be elicited. A *mistaken* diagnosis of nephrotic syndrome or hepatic cirrhosis may have been made in the past because of anasarca.

CLINICAL FEATURES

The prominent feature of this disease is *elevated systemic venous pressure,* reflected in distended neck veins, hepatic and splenic engorgement, ascites, and less commonly, pedal edema. The neck veins often demonstrate Kussmaul's sign and other highly suggestive wave forms. The liver may be firm because of cardiac cirrhosis, but the hepatosplenomegaly and ascites should not be misdiagnosed as cirrhosis of the liver if attention is paid to the distended neck veins. The paradoxic pulse is seldom present, and the blood pressure is normal to low. The lung fields are usually clear except in hypoalbuminemic patients, in whom pleural effusions may be present. The cardiac examination often reveals a "small quiet heart" without a palpable apical impulse, but heart sounds of normal intensity and even modest cardiomegaly may be found. Heart murmurs and a pericardial friction rub are unusual, but a *pericardial knock*, resembling a premature third sound, is often heard.

Laboratory studies pertinent to the diagnosis include a characteristic but not diagnostic *EKG* demonstrating (1) *low-voltage QRS complexes*, primarily in the limb leads, with (2) *generalized flattening or inversion of the T waves* and (3) *notched, broad P waves*. *Atrial arrhythmias*, especially atrial fibrillation, occur in *25 to 30 per cent of the patients*. *Roentgenographic studies* usually show clear lung fields, occasionally pleural effusions, with a normal to slightly enlarged cardiac silhouette. *Pericardial calcification* is present in approximately 50 per cent of the cases, although it may also be seen in chronic pericarditis without constriction. *Fluoroscopy* and *echocardiography* may well be helpful.

DISPOSITION AND TREATMENT

Once signs and symptoms of constrictive pericarditis become present, surgical decortication is indicated.

References

Engle, M. A., Zabriskie, J. B., Senterfit, L. B., and Ebert, P.A.: Postpericardiotomy syndrome. Mod. Concepts Cardiovasc. Dis. 44:59, 1975.

Fowler, N. O.: Pericardial disease. *In* Hurst, J. W., et al. (Eds.): The Heart, 3rd ed. New York, McGraw-Hill Book Co., 1974, p. 1387.

Goldman, M. J.: Pericarditis. Presented at the Medical Staff Conference, University of California San Francisco. West. J. Med. 123:467, 1975.

Lessof, M. H.: Postcardiotomy syndrome: pathogenesis and management. Hosp. Practice Sept. 1976, p. 81.

Spodick, D. H.: Differential diagnosis of acute pericarditis. Progr. Cardiovasc. Dis. 14:192, Sept. 1971.

Suggestions for Further Reading

Braunwald, E.: Pericardial disease. *In* Wintrobe, M. M., et al. (Eds.): Harrison's Principles of Internal Medicine, 7th ed., New York, McGraw-Hill Book Co., 1974, p. 1210.

Hogan, P. J.: Pericarditis. *In* Beeson, P. B., and McDermott, W. M. (Eds.): Textbook of Medicine, 14th ed. Philadelphia, W. B. Saunders Co., 1975, p. 1044.

Symbas, P. N.: Traumatic Injuries of the Heart and Great Vessels. Springfield, Ill., Charles C Thomas, Publisher, 1972.

Spodick, D. H.: Acute cardiac tamponade. Progr. Cardiovasc. Dis. 10:64, 1967.

Wood, P.: Chronic constrictive pericarditis. Am. J. Cardiol. 7:48, 1961.

G. RECOGNITION AND TREATMENT OF PULMONARY EMBOLISM

Nanette K. Wenger

Pulmonary embolism is both the most common pulmonary disease and the most common cause of death in most general hospitals; because its manifestations are deceptively nonspecific, a high index of suspicion is necessary to enable the institution of appropriate diagnostic measures and the requisite sequential plan of management.

Patients at high risk for the development of pulmonary embolism include those with thrombophlebitis; patients requiring prolonged bed rest or immobilization; postoperative or postpartum patients; those with cardiac arrhythmias or congestive heart failure; those with extensive trauma; excessively obese patients; those with malignant neoplasms or debilitating diseases; women receiving oral contraceptive agents; and those with varied abnormalities of the blood clotting mechanism.

CLINICAL HISTORY

Sudden unexplained dyspnea, in a predisposed patient, is the most frequent clinical presentation; at times, this may be associated with cough or with nonspecific chest discomfort. The classic triad of hemoptysis, pleuritic chest pain, and dyspnea is rarely encountered. Syncope and clinical evidence of an acute cardiovascular episode are uncommon; characteristically, this presentation with hypotension, tachycardia, chest pain, and congestive heart failure (often mimicking acute myocardial infarction) indicates massive life-threatening pulmonary embolism.

PHYSICAL EXAMINATION

The physical findings also are often nonspecific in patients with small-to-moderate pulmonary embolism. Tachypnea and tachycardia are common; there may be an increased intensity of the pulmonic component of the second heart sound, but fixed splitting of the second heart sound is uncommon. A third or fourth heart sound may be heard. Lung rales may be present, but pleural and pericardial friction rubs are unusual, as is cyanosis. Evidence of thrombophlebitis—disparity of the leg diameter, redness, tenderness, warmth, and a Homan's sign—is an important diagnostic feature when present; unfortunately, it occurs in less than one-half of patients with documented pulmonary embolism. However, not infrequently, clinical evidence of thrombophlebitis appears after the diagnosis of pulmonary embolism has been made.

As stated, the patient with massive, life-threatening pulmonary embolism may have hypotension, tachycardia, congestive heart failure, and evidence of acute cor pulmonale; cyanosis may be detected in this small subgroup of patients.

ROUTINE LABORATORY STUDIES

There is no specific diagnostic laboratory test for pulmonary embolism.

The most frequent electrocardiographic changes are nonspecific alterations of the ST segment and T wave. The $S_1Q_3T_3$ pattern occurs uncommonly, as does evidence of right ventricular "strain." The electrocardiographic abnormalities may mimic those of acute myocardial infarction or anterior ischemia.

The chest x-ray may be normal in one-quarter to one-third of patients. The abnormalities, when encountered, most often include an infiltrate and elevation of the hemidiaphragm on the side of the embolus. A classic Hampton's hump is unusual.

The oft-cited triad of an elevated bilirubin and LDH in the presence of a normal SGOT has not proved of value; usually, all three parameters—bilirubin, LDH, and SGOT—are within the normal range. The white blood cell count is not unduly elevated in pulmonary embolism and, indeed, may be normal. Suspicion of pneumonia, rather than pulmonary embolism, as the etiology of a symptomatic pulmonary infiltrate should be raised when the white blood cell count is greater than 15,000/cc.

An arterial blood Po_2 of greater than 90 mm. Hg, prior to the administration of oxygen, virtually excludes significant pulmonary embolism, as most patients with this problem have some degree of hypoxemia. Marked hypoxemia is usual with massive pulmonary embolism accompanied by hypotension and/or congestive heart failure.

FURTHER DIAGNOSTIC PROCEDURES

The diagnostic procedure indicated is radioisotopic pulmonary perfusion scanning, a simple noninvasive test that can identify areas of malperfusion in the pulmonary vascular bed. If the diagnosis of pulmonary embolism is seriously entertained, 5000 to 7500 units of heparin I.V. should be administered prior to diagnostic studies to patients for whom anticoagulant therapy is not contraindicated; if the lung scan results are negative, the heparin can be discontinued.

A technically adequate, negative pulmonary scan virtually excludes significant pulmonary embolism. However, many pulmonary scans provide equivocal information. This is particularly so when an infiltrate in the lung field on the plain chest film corresponds to the area of malperfusion on the lung scan. In this instance, identification of venous thrombi in the legs (by phlebography, by impedance plethysmography, or by ^{125}I fibrinogen scanning) may provide additional information.

Although a definitive diagnosis of pulmonary embolism is made at pulmonary angiography, this procedure is not needed or indicated in the majority of patients with pulmonary embolism; pulmonary angiography should be performed only on those for whom surgical intervention may be contemplated. This group includes patients for whom anticoagulant therapy is contraindicated, or those with massive pulmonary embolism, unresponsive to medical therapy, for whom pulmonary embolectomy may be recommended.

PLAN OF CARE

Medical Management

PULMONARY EMBOLISM WITHOUT LIFE-THREATENING CARDIOVASCULAR DYSFUNCTION

The patient should be at bed rest, and symptomatic therapy should be given for the thrombophlebitis, if present—local heat, elevation, etc. Acetaminophen, 325 to 650 mg. orally every four to six hours, is recommended for the patient with minimal or mild chest pain, as it will not interfere with subsequent oral anticoagulant therapy. For patients with severe chest pain, particularly of the pleuritic variety, morphine sulfate can both control the pain and markedly decrease apprehension; 1 mg. of morphine should be given slowly, intravenously, as needed, up to a dose of 5 to 10 mg.

Heparin anticoagulation is the management of choice because of its rapid and predictable action; it should be administered to all patients without a specific contraindication to anticoagulant therapy. Heparin dosage should be designed to maintain the Lee White clotting time at 25 to 30 minutes one hour before the administration of the next dose. In general, a dosage of 10 units of heparin per pound of body weight per hour can attain this degree of anticoagulation. There is good evidence that patients whose Lee White clotting time is in excess of 60 minutes (one hour before the next heparin dose) have a significantly increased incidence of bleeding complications, whereas patients with a Lee White clotting time below 20 minutes have an increased incidence of recurrent pulmonary embolism.

Ideally, heparin should be administered by continuous intravenous infusion, i.e., maintaining a constant intravenous flow rate designed to achieve a Lee White clotting time of 25 to 30 minutes. Where this is impractical, intermittent intravenous heparin, using a heparin lock to avoid repeated venipuncture, is recommended, using the above dosage guidelines. The disadvantage of this mode of administration is that, after each dose of heparin, the clotting time is, for a few hours, essentially "infinite," increasing the risk of bleeding complications. Intramuscular or subcutaneous heparin should not be administered to patients with acute pulmonary embolism, as the absorption may be unpredictable with variations in systemic blood pressure and tissue perfusion.

MASSIVE PULMONARY EMBOLISM WITH LIFE-THREATENING CARDIOVASCULAR DYSFUNCTION

The management of these patients involves primarily the support of the circulation. Isoproterenol is the drug of choice, administered as 1 to 2 mg. per 500 cc. 5 per cent dextrose and water, as, in addition to its positive inotropic effect, it acts as a pulmonary vasodilator to decrease pulmonary artery pressure. If isoproterenol is ineffective in restoring the blood pressure, or if it results in undue tachycardia or arrhythmia, 1 to 2 ml. of a 2 per cent solution of l–norepinephrine in 500 cc. of 5 per cent dextrose and water should be used. If hypovolemia is indicated by a low or normal pulmonary artery pressure (as determined by Swan-Ganz catheter measurement), intravascular volume expansion should be attempted.

Additional therapy should include digitalis, diuretic agents, and antiarrhythmic drugs as required to control right ventricular failure and the occasional associated arrhythmias.

Higher than usual doses of heparin (7,500 to 15,000 units I.V. every four hours for at least the first 24 hours) are recommended for patients with massive pulmonary embolism, as this has been reported to decrease mortality.

Should the above regimen prove ineffective in maintaining adequate blood pressure levels and an adequate urine output, pulmonary angiography should be considered as a preparation for surgical intervention.

Surgical Management

Surgical management is necessary for patients with contraindications to anticoagulant therapy, such as actively bleeding gastrointestinal or genitourinary lesions; significant abnormality of coagulation or platelet function; recent cerebrovascular accident or intracranial, spinal cord, or retinal surgical procedure; cerebral neoplasm; severe renal or hepatic disease; extensive trauma or burns; uncontrolled hypertension with severe retinopathy; and so on. Surgical management also is indicated for patients in whom pulmonary embolism recurs on adequate anticoagulant therapy.

The surgical procedure indicated is interruption of the inferior vena cava; this is designed to prevent recurrent pulmonary embolism. This procedure is also indicated in patients with documented massive pulmonary embolism (including those undergoing pulmonary embolectomy), who are thought not able to tolerate a recurrent episode of pulmonary vascular obstruction.

Inferior vena caval interruption may be accomplished transvenously, using local anesthesia, by the placement of a Mobin-Uddin umbrella filter or any of the newer modifications of this device. Alternate surgical approaches, requiring general anesthesia, include ligation, plication, or clipping of the inferior vena cava.

The major risks of the "umbrella" filter include penetration or perforation of adjacent structures, migration of the filter, and re-embolization; however, the morbidity and mortality are far less than those encountered with surgical interruption of the inferior vena cava.

Vena cava ligation is more effective in preventing recurrent pulmonary emboli than is vena caval clipping or plication, but is associated with a higher incidence of disabling leg sequelae. For the patient with severe cor pulmonale, partial interruption of the inferior vena cava appears to afford greater safety; sudden reduction of venous return to the heart, as occurs with total inferior vena cava ligation, has been associated with increased mortality.

For patients with massive pulmonary embolism, unresponsive to the medical regimen outlined above (e.g., those patients in whom the hypotension, hypoxemia, or cardiac failure remains refractory or those sustaining a cardiac arrest), consideration of emergency pulmonary embolectomy is warranted. This requires prior angiographic confirmation of pulmonary embolization, because of the excessively high mortality associated with surgery in a patient with an incorrect diagnosis. The institution of cardiopulmonary by-pass is recommended prior to the performance of the diagnostic procedure, with by-pass being continued during the pulmonary embolectomy and the subsequent inferior vena caval interruption.

References

Bryant, L. R., et al.: Massive pulmonary embolism: a plan of medical management. South. Med. J. 67:825, 1974.

Eberlein, T. J., and Carey, L. C.: Comparison of surgical managements for pulmonary emboli. Ann. Surg. 179:836, 1974.

Reul, G. J., and Beall, A. C.: Emergency pulmonary embolectomy for massive pulmonary embolism. Circulation 50:236, 1974. (Suppl. II.)

Sasahara, A. A.: Therapy for pulmonary embolism. J.A.M.A. 229:1795, 1974.

Sasahara, A. A., et al.: The urokinase pulmonary embolism trial: a national cooperative study. Circulation 47: 1973. (Suppl. II)

Webster, J. R., and Marquardt, J. F.: Pulmonary embolism: silent killer of the elderly. Geriatrics 29:46, 1974.

Wenger, N. K., Stein, P. D., and Willis, P. W., III: Massive acute pulmonary embolism: the deceivingly nonspecific manifestations. J.A.M.A. 220:843, 1972.

H. INFECTIVE ENDOCARDITIS

John H. Stone

The cardiac valves and endocardium may be primarily involved by a wide variety of organisms: bacteria, fungi, and even Rickettsia. It appears that almost any structure that projects into the cardiac stream may be involved by endocarditis. In view of the likelihood that transient bacteremia is a very common phenomenon, it is often unclear why some patients develop endocarditis and others do not. Hearts altered by prior rheumatic, congenital, or syphilitic disease are most commonly involved; but infection apparently also may be superimposed on previously normal valves. Intracardiac prostheses (valves, patches) may become infected; endocarditis has also been reported in association with heart diseases of unclear etiology, such as idiopathic hypertrophic subaortic stenosis (IHSS) and the click-murmur syndrome (Barlow's). At times more subtle is the endovascular infection that may be set up in distant reaches of the circulatory system on such entities as A–V fistulae, aortic aneurysms, or normal blood vessels (mycotic aneurysms, peripheral emboli). Right-sided endocarditis (tricuspid valve) is a problem that occurs particularly in the intravenous drug user and may present primarily as a metastatic pneumonia. This is especially true in infections caused by *Staphylococcus aureus*.

Because of its widely variable clinical presentations, infective endocarditis is one of the great medical mimics and may be notoriously difficult to diagnose early. Early recognition and treatment can occur only when the emergency physician maintains a high index of suspicion. The emphasis of this discussion, therefore, will be on *Recognition*.

RECOGNITION

Infective endocarditis is one of the oldest examples of that group of diseases (including the collagen vascular diseases) which may present with evidence of multisystem involvement. Apparently disparate clinical findings often become disturbingly understandable in retrospect when considered within the unifying diagnosis of endocarditis. Endocarditis clearly should be entertained in the differential diagnosis of fever in any patient with cardiac murmurs or abnormalities. Even here, however, problems arise because the clinical distinction between "functional" and "organic" heart murmurs may be difficult—*and* patients with proven endocarditis may be afebrile when seen. Night sweats may be a helpful clue when present—but constitutional symptoms such as anorexia, fatigue, and malaise are nonspecific enough to be easily attributable to processes other than endocarditis. The most common cause of splinter hemorrhages in the nails is not endocarditis, but local trauma. Signs traditionally considered "classic," such as petechiae, splenomegaly, evidence of embolization and clubbing of the fingers, should be expected in a *minority* of patients when the diagnosis is first made: in this light, although such findings should be searched for, they might well be considered "late signs" of the disease process (Vogler, et al., 1962). Infective endocarditis is best analyzed as a number of interrelated sets of signs and symptoms—or *syndromes of clinical presentation*. Here again, some of these can be considered only "late" findings, unfortunately.

CARDIAC SYNDROMES

The sudden onset of congestive heart failure in patients with previously well compensated disease should suggest the possibility of endocarditis. The finding of a *new* heart murmur (especially a regurgitant murmur) may be an important clue. Myocarditis as well as localized suppuration (e.g., paravalvular abscess) may occur and result in conduction defects and arrhythmias. Since endocarditis is the most frequent cause of *coronary artery emboli* (Wenger and Bauer, 1958), a patient with fresh myocardial infarction in the proper clinical context (fever, murmur) is a prime candidate for this diagnosis. *Pericarditis* can, of course, occur as a sequel to this embolic type of infarction, just as it may following infarction of more usual etiology. Purulent pericarditis frequently is a concomitant of staphylococcal endocarditis.

THROMBOEMBOLIC EPISODES

Arterial emboli are the second most frequent complication (after congestive heart failure) of infective endocarditis; the clinical incidence ranges from 15 to 35 per cent (Weinstein and Schlesinger, 1974). Many neurologic syndromes may be mimicked: *hemiplegia; seizures; meningitis; subarachnoid hemorrhage.* Such complications have been reported in almost one-third of patients with endocarditis at some point during the disease. Unexplained onset of *peripheral gangrene* may be the first clue to the proper diagnosis. Occlusion of a large peripheral vessel should suggest fungal endocarditis, which is characterized by large, friable vegetations. In this regard, patients with acute arterial obstruction should always have the surgically retrieved clot cultured and stained for bacteria and fungi, since this may be the only site from which the diagnosis can be made. (A left atrial myxoma, which may closely simulate endocarditis, may also present in this embolic fashion, and the diagnosis may be made by examination of the embolized tissue.)

Splenic, renal, and *bone* infarctions may occur and may pose difficult differential diagnostic problems at first. *Septic arthritis* has been described. Many patients will complain of migratory arthritis early in the course of the disease and an erroneous diagnosis of rheumatic disease may be suspected. It seems likely that some arthralgias as well as other manifestations previously thought to be *embolic*—such as *Roth spots* (oval pale retinal lesions surrounded by hemorrhage) and *Osler nodes* (firm, tender, red/purple lesions on the pads of the fingers and toes)— are in fact signs of an acute allergic *vasculitis* (Weinstein and Schlesinger, 1974). There is some disagreement about *Janeway lesions* (macular, non-tender hemorrhagic areas on the palms and soles) for which both embolic and vasculitic etiologies have been proposed (bacteria have been cultured from them in a few cases).

CENTRAL NERVOUS SYSTEM SYNDROMES

As noted above, major emboli to the central nervous system are frequent in patients with endocarditis. The onset of *neurologic deficit* (e.g., hemiplegia) in the context of fever and cardiac murmur should raise this possibility, especially in the younger patient in whom the more usual possibilities may not be expected.

In addition to embolic phenomena, *metastatic infections* to the brain and mycotic aneurysms may occur. Purulent and sterile forms of *meningitis* may occur. A triad of disease including meningitis, pneumonia, and endocarditis (*"Osler's triad"*) has been emphasized in clinical lore, with the admonition that when two of the three entities are present, the third should be looked for also.

As emphasized by Weinstein and Schlesinger (1974), however, in the patient with endocarditis, "headache, nuchal rigidity, and mild cerebrospinal fluid pleocytosis do not necessarily represent pyogenic meningi-

tis; they may result from cerebral emboli that involve relatively silent areas of the cortex and produce, few, if any, localizing neurologic manifestations."

Multiple *cerebral abscesses* may develop. *Brain abscess* of a more localized form is more common in patients with cyanotic congenital heart disease because of the obligatory right-to-left shunt.

Mycotic aneuryms may occur widely throughout the body on such vessels as the coronary arteries, abdominal aorta, superior mesenteric and splenic arteries. Within the central nervous system, rupture of these aneurysms may produce findings of subarachnoid or intracerebral hemorrhage.

Psychiatric syndromes, including frank psychosis, also have been described in patients with endocarditis.

RENAL SYNDROMES

In addition to embolic involvement which may cause renal infarction, pyelonephritis may be simulated. A type of diffuse or focal glomerulonephritis (with proteinuria, abnormal urinary sediment, and hematuria), presumably on an immunologic basis, may occur. Frank renal insufficiency has been described in a small percentage of patients, and this group of uremic patients may run a relatively afebrile course. (Conversely, patients on chronic hemodialysis with A-V shunts in place are at increased risk for the development of endocarditis.)

UNEXPLAINED PROBLEMS AFTER SURGICAL PROCEDURES

Persistent fever and constitutional symptoms following surgical procedures should suggest the need for blood cultures. These include cardiac surgery, dental surgery, genitourinary tract instrumentation, and gynecologic–obstetric procedures, including childbirth.

"RIGHT-SIDED" ENDOCARDITIS

Recent work has better defined this entity, which is seen in increased incidence in addicts who use drugs intravenously. Murmurs may well be *absent* in this group of patients (tricuspid valve regurgitation should be looked for as systolic pulsations of the deep jugular venous pulse). Atrial and/or ventricular gallops may be present. Pleuritic chest pain, pulmonary emboli, and recurrent pulmonary infections in the patient with a history of drug abuse should strongly suggest this diagnosis. Blood cultures usually are positive, the most common organism being the *Staphylococcus aureus*, but fungal and gram-negative organisms also have been seen. Involvement of the *left* cardiac valves in this clinical situation is not uncommon with Staphylococcal organisms and is especially frequent with gram-negative and fungal infections.

ENDOCARDITIS IN DEBILITATED PATIENTS

Patients, especially those in the older age groups, with certain debilitating illnesses (such as cancer, cirrhosis, and diabetes) and those on immunosuppressive agents, including steroids, may develop infective endocarditis which, at least initially, is obscured by extracardiac manifestations of their underlying disease, resulting in delayed diagnosis.

A *nonbacterial* or *marantic* endocarditis with *sterile* vegetations on the cardiac valves has been described in association with a wide spectrum of diseases, most frequently near-terminal carcinoma. Petechiae, fever, murmurs, and emboli may combine to make the clinical picture in this form of endocarditis indistinguishable from that found in the infective variety.

LABORATORY FINDINGS

Fastidious attention to collection and proper incubation of *blood* for *cultures* (aerobic, anaerobic, and fungal) is critical in the diagnosis of endocarditis. Four to six venous blood cultures are almost always adequate. Cultures should be held for *three weeks* or until positive. Penicillinase should be added to the cultures of those patients recently on penicillin; if the clinical situation is not acute, such patients should not be treated immediately but should be re-cultured after being off antibiotics for 24 to 48 hours. (In this connection, much subsequent clinical confusion may be obviated by obtaining blood cultures *before* administration of antibiotics for seemingly trivial fevers in patients with known cardiac valvular disease.)

Although the most frequent causative agent is the *Streptococcus viridans* (depending in part on the patient population being reported and whether or not the author differentiates "subacute" from "acute" endocarditis), the bacteriologic spectrum of endocarditis seen is very wide and includes staphylococci, enterococci, fungi, some gram-negative organisms, and many others. Staphylococcal infection is especially likely to be seen in postoperative cardiac patients and drug addicts and may result in a particularly virulent form of the disease sometimes categorized as "acute" endocarditis.

It should be kept in mind that an uncertain percentage of patients, from 5 per cent to as high as 15 per cent in some series, will have negative blood cultures in spite of clinical/pathologic evidence of endocarditis.

Other laboratory data may not be specific enough to be helpful. Although a normochromic-normocytic anemia and elevated sedimentation rate are common, they may not be of significant value to the clinician except as supporting data. The white blood cell count may be normal, elevated, or low. Urine sediment findings may be helpful in the total clinical context. A high titer of rheumatoid factor may serve as supporting data in patients suspected of having endocarditis and should fall with appropriate therapy. In a patient with neurologic involvement, cerebrospinal fluid pleocytosis is common and should not be confused with viral meningitis.

INITIAL THERAPY

Since treatment of endocarditis involves close attention to detail (serum dilutions, in vitro testing) over several *weeks*, only the *Initial Plans* for therapy will be outlined here. Duration of therapy, special problems such as drug sensitivity, and therapy for unusual organisms are beyond the scope of this discussion, and the reader is referred to *Suggestions for Further Reading* for these and other aspects of treatment.

Following appropriate blood cultures (at least *four* via separate venipunctures, over several hours):

A. *If organism is unknown* and *immediate treatment is deemed necessary* prior to results of blood cultures (e.g., clinical diagnosis appears certain, or the patient is critically ill): Ampicillin, 12 gm./day I.V. (divided doses) *or* penicillin G, 24 million units/day I.V. (divided doses).

Plus

Gentamicin 1 to 1.7 mg./kg. I.M. every eight hours.

UNLESS

1. Staph. aureus is suspected (e.g., I.V. drug user): Nafcillin, 12 gm./day I.V. (divided doses) *in addition to* above schedule using ampicillin and gentamicin.

2. Patient is sensitive to penicillin: vancomycin, 2 gm./day I.V. (divided doses) *and* gentamicin, 1 to 1.7 mg./kg. every eight hours. (*Note:* the combination of vancomycin and gentamicin is *nephrotoxic;* rapid desensitization to penicillin in the patient with a history of "penicillin reaction," though also involving some risk to the patient, may be a reasonable alternative for consideration—the above regimen using penicillin/ampicillin plus gentamicin may then be followed (Green, et al., 1967).

B. *If organism is known:*

Streptococcus viridans: Penicillin G, 10–20 million units/day I.V. (divided doses) *plus* streptomycin, 0.5 gm. I.M. every 12 hours.

Enterococcus: Penicillin G, 20 million units/day I.V. (divided doses) *plus* streptomycin, 0.5 to 1 gm. I.M. every 12 hours.

Staphylococcus: Nafcillin, 12 gm./day I.V. (divided doses).

(N.B.: These regimens are suggested *initial* therapies only and must be reassessed in the light of subsequent data, blood cultures, sensitivity studies, renal function tests, and the like.)

PREVENTION OF BACTERIAL ENDOCARDITIS

Patients with heart disease of diverse etiologies (rheumatic, congenital, other), as noted above, are at increased risk of developing endocarditis when undergoing dental/surgical procedures that may be associated with bacteremia. Although controlled data to validate the following recommendations are not available, they may serve as guidelines designed to prevent endocarditis in such patients. The recommendations are part of a statement prepared by the Committee of Rheumatic Fever and Bacterial Endocarditis of the Council on Cardiovascular Disease in the Young of the American Heart Association. The full statement is available

from the American Heart Association, with whose permission it is reprinted (Kaplan et al., 1977).

For Dental Procedures and Surgery of the Upper Respiratory Tract

Prophylaxis for Dental Procedures and Surgical Procedures of the Upper Respiratory Tract

	Most congenital heart disease;[3] rheumatic or other acquired valvular heart disease; idiopathic hypertrophic subaortic stenosis; mitral valve[4] prolapse syndrome with mitral insufficiency	Prosthetic heart valves[5]
All dental procedures that are likely to result in gingival bleeding[1, 2]	Regimen A or B	Regimen B
Surgery or instrumentation of the respiratory tract[6]	Regimen A or B	Regimen B

[1]Does not include shedding of deciduous teeth.
[2]Does not include simple adjustment of orthodontic appliances.
[3]E.g., ventricular septal defect, tetralogy of Fallot, aortic stenosis, pulmonic stenosis, complex cyanotic heart disease, patent ductus arteriosus or systemic to pulmonary artery shunts. Does not include uncomplicated secundum atrial septal defect.
[4]Although cases of infective endocarditis in patients with mitral valve prolapse syndrome have been documented, the incidence appears to be relatively low and the necessity for prophylaxis in all of these patients has not yet been established.
[5]Some patients with a prosthetic heart valve in whom a high level of oral health is being maintained may be offered oral antibiotic prophylaxis for routine dental procedures except the following: parenteral antibiotics are recommended for patients with prosthetic valves who require extensive dental procedures, especially extractions, or oral or gingival surgical procedures.
[6]E.g., tonsillectomy, adenoidectomy, bronchoscopy, and other surgical procedures of the upper respiratory tract involving disruption of the respiratory mucosa.

REGIMEN A—PENICILLIN

1. Parenteral-oral combined:

Adults: Aqueous crystalline penicillin G (1,000,000 units intramuscularly) **mixed with** *procaine penicillin G* (600,000 units intramuscularly). Give 30 minutes to 1 hour prior to procedure and then give penicillin

V (formerly called phenoxymethyl penicillin) 500 mg. orally every 6 hours for 8 doses.*

Children:† Aqueous crystalline penicillin G (30,000 units/kg. intramuscularly) **mixed with** *procaine penicillin G* (600,000 units intramuscularly). Timing of doses for children is the same as for adults. For children less than 60 lb. the dose of penicillin V is 250 mg. orally every 6 hours for 8 doses.*

2. *Oral:***

Adults: Penicillin *V* (2.0 gm. orally 30 minutes to 1 hour prior to the procedure and then 500 mg. orally every 6 hours for 8 doses.)*

Children:† Penicillin *V* (2.0 gm. orally 30 minutes to 1 hour prior to procedure and then 500 mg. orally every 6 hours for 8 doses.* For children less than 60 lb. use 1.0 gm. orally 30 minutes to 1 hour prior to the procedure and then 250 mg. orally every 6 hours for 8 doses.)*

For Patients Allergic to Penicillin
Use *either Vancomycin* (see Regimen B)

or use

Adults: Erythromycin (1.0 gm. orally 1½ to 2 hours prior to the procedure and then 500 mg. orally every 6 hours for 8 doses.)*

Children: Erythromycin (20 mg./kg. orally 1½ to 2 hours prior to the procedure and then 10 mg./kg. every 6 hours for 8 doses.)*

REGIMEN B – PENICILLIN PLUS STREPTOMYCIN

Adults: Aqueous crystalline penicillin G (1,000,000 units intramuscularly) **mixed with** *procaine penicillin G* (600,000 units

intramuscularly) *plus Streptomycin* (1 gm. intramuscularly). Give 30 minutes to 1 hour prior to the procedure; then penicillin V 500 mg. orally every 6 hours for 8 doses.*

Children:† Aqueous crystalline penicillin G (30,000 units/kg. intramuscularly) **mixed with** *procaine penicillin G* (600,000 units intramuscularly) *plus streptomycin* (20 mg./kg. intramuscularly). Timing of doses for children is the same as for adults. For children less than 60 lb. the recommended oral dose of penicillin V is 250 mg every 6 hours for 8 doses.*

For Patients Allergic to Penicillin
Adults: Vancomycin (1 gm. intravenously over 30 minutes to 1 hour). Start initial vancomycin infusion ½ to 1 hour prior to procedure; then *erythromycin* 500 mg. orally every 6 hours for 8 doses *

Children:† Vancomycin (20 mg./kg. intravenously over 30 minutes to 1 hour).‡ Timing of doses for children is the same as for adults. *Erythromycin* dose is 10 mg./kg. every 6 hours for 8 doses.*

Genitourinary Tract and Gastrointestinal Tract Surgery or Instrumentation

Bacteremia may be caused by surgery or instrumentation of the genitourinary tract (especially urethral or prostatic manipulations, including urethral catheterization whether the urine is infected or not). It may also accompany surgery and instrumentation of the lower gastrointestinal tract and of the gallbladder, and may be associated with obstetric infections such as septic abortion or peripartum infection. Documented cases of bacterial endocarditis have been recorded following these procedures, and antibiotic prophylaxis to prevent this infection should be employed.

Endocarditis following uncomplicated vaginal delivery is extremely rare; the necessity for antibiotic prophylaxis has not been firmly established. Likewise, upper gastrointestinal endoscopy (without biopsy), percutaneous liver biopsy, proctoscopy, sigmoidoscopy, barium enema, pelvic examination, dilatation and curettage of the uterus, and uncomplicated insertion or removal of intrauterine devices (IUD's)—although occasionally associated with bacteremia—have only very rarely, if ever, been associated with development of infective endocarditis.

---

*In unusual circumstances or in the case of delayed healing, it may be prudent to provide additional doses of antibiotics even though available data suggest that bacteremia rarely persists longer than 15 minutes after the procedure. The physician or dentist may also choose to use the parenteral route of administration for all of the doses in selected situations.

†Doses for children should not exceed recommendations for adults for a single dose or for a 24-hour period.

For those **patients receiving continuous oral penicillin for secondary prevention of rheumatic fever, alpha hemolytic streptococci which are relatively resistant to penicillin are occasionally found in the oral cavity. While it is likely that the doses of penicillin recommended in Regimen A are sufficient to control these organisms, the physician or dentist may choose one of the suggestions in Regimen B or may choose oral erythromycin.

‡For vancomycin the total dose for children should not exceed 44 mg./kg./24 hours.

Based upon currently available evidence, they do not require antibiotic prophylaxis in most patients with underlying heart disease. However, since the patient with a prosthetic valve appears to be at especially high risk, it may be wise to administer antibiotic prophylaxis with these procedures. This empiric recommendation is based more upon concern than definitive data.

Enterococci (e.g., *Streptococcus fecalis*) are frequently responsible for endocarditis following genitourinary tract and gastrointestinal tract surgery or instrumentation. Although bacteremia and even sepsis with gram-negative bacteria may follow instrumentation of the genitourinary tract or gastrointestinal tract, these organisms only rarely cause bacterial endocarditis. Thus, antibiotic prophylaxis to prevent endocarditis following these procedures should be directed primarily against enterococci. Because these procedures are usually performed in a hospital or clinic, parenteral antibiotics are recommended.

Suggested antibiotic regimens for gastrointestinal and genitourinary tract surgery and instrumentation are shown below:

For Gastrointestinal and Genitourinary Tract Surgery and Instrumentation*

Adults: Aqueous crystalline penicillin G (2,000,000 units intramuscularly or intravenously) **or** *ampicillin* (1.0 gm. intramuscularly or intravenously) **plus** *gentamicin* [1.5 mg./kg., (not to exceed 80 mg.) intramuscularly or intravenously] **or** *streptomycin* (1.0 gm. intramuscularly).

Give initial doses 30 minutes to 1 hour prior to procedure. If gentamicin is used, then give a similar dose of gentamicin and penicillin (or ampicillin) every 8 hours for two additional doses.† If streptomycin is used then give a similar dose of streptomycin and penicillin (or ampicillin) every 12 hours for two additional doses.†

Children: Aqueous crystalline penicillin G (30,000 units/kg. intramuscularly or intravenously) **or** *ampicillin* (50 mg./kg. intramuscularly or intravenously) **plus** *gentamicin* (2.0 mg./kg. intramuscularly or intra-

venously) **or** *streptomycin* (20 mg./kg. intramuscularly). Timing of doses for children is the same as for adults.†

For Those Patients Who Are Allergic to Penicillin†

Adults: Vancomycin (1.0 gm. intravenously given over 30 minutes to 1 hour) **plus** *streptomycin* (1.0 gm. intramuscularly). A single dose of these antibiotics begun 30 minutes to 1 hour prior to the procedure is probably sufficient, but the same dose may be repeated in 12 hours.†

*Children:*** Vancomycin‡ (20 mg./kg. given intravenously over 30 minutes to 1 hour) **plus** *streptomycin* (20 mg./kg. intramuscularly). Timing of doses for children is the same as for adults.†

---

*In patients with significantly compromised renal function, it may be necessary to modify the dose of antibiotics used. Some of these doses may exceed manufacturer's recommendations for a 24-hour period. However, since they are only recommended for a 24-hour period in most cases, it is unlikely that toxicity will occur.

†During prolonged procedures, or in the case of delayed healing, it may be necessary to provide additional doses of antibiotics. For brief outpatient procedures such as uncomplicated catheterization of the bladder one dose may be sufficient.

**Doses for children should not exceed recommendations for adults for a single dose or for a 24-hour period.

‡For vancomycin the total dose for children should not exceed 44 mg./kg./24 hours.

References

Green, G. R., Peters, G. A., and Geraci, J. E.: Treatment of bacterial endocarditis in patients with penicillin hypersensitivity. Ann. Intern. Med. 67:235, 1967.

Kaplan, E. L. (Committee Chairman), et al.: Prevention of bacterial endocarditis. Circulation 56:139A, 1977.

Vogler, W. R., Dorney, E. R., and Bridges, H. A.: Bacterial endocarditis, a review of 148 cases. Am. J. Med. 32:910, 1962.

Weinstein, L., and Schlesinger, J. J.: Pathoanatomic, pathophysiologic and clinical correlations in endocarditis. N. Engl. J. Med. 291:832, 1122, 1974.

Wenger, N. K., and Bauer, S.: Coronary embolism: review of the literature and presentation of fifteen cases. Am. J. Med. 25:549, 1958.

Suggestions for Further Reading

Kaye, D. (ed.): Infective Endocarditis. Baltimore, University Park Press, 1976.

I. EFFECT OF ELECTROLYTE ABNORMALITIES ON THE ELECTROCARDIOGRAM

Stephen D. Clements, Jr.

Laboratory determination of serum electrolytes requires more than a few minutes. A preliminary answer to a life-threatening electrolyte question may be obtained from the electrocardiogram. The EKG is a sensitive indicator of certain electrolyte abnormalities; specifically, it reflects ionic concentrations at the level of the cell membrane and the transmembrane potential of all cardiac cells. Changes in ionic concentrations and transmembrane potentials are reflected in the surface EKG (Fig. 1).

Potassium and calcium alterations have predictable and reversible effects on the EKG (Surawicz, 1967). Changes due to hyperkalemia are more prominent in the presence of hypocalcemia and hyponatremia.

POTASSIUM

Hyperkalemia causes the following electrocardiographic changes (Surawicz, 1967; Wenger and Herndon, 1974; Winsor, 1968).

(1) Tall peaked symmetrical T waves.

(2) Increased QRS duration.

(3) Decreased P wave amplitude and increased P wave duration, sinoatrial block, prolonged PR interval, atrial fibrillation, and atrial standstill.

(4) Further QRS prolongation, ectopic ventricular activity, ventricular fibrillation.

The earliest EKG of hyperkalemia usually is a symmetric peaking of the T waves. This may occur in the 5.5 to 6.0 mEq./liter range and is not altogether specific for hyperkalemia (Figs. 1 and 2). Some normal individuals have tall peaked T waves, especially during periods of bradycardia. U waves usually accompany the normal tall peaked T waves, whereas in the presence of hyperkalemia U waves are small to absent.

As potassium rises above 6 mEq./liter, the resting membrane potential is decreased, as is upstroke velocity of the action potential. Decreased rate of ventricular depolarization results in QRS prolongation. As potassium reaches higher levels, the QRS becomes more more prolonged and tends to merge with the T wave (Fig. 1, *D*). At this stage the T wave may lose its peaked appearance, owing perhaps to altered depolarization.

As the QRS becomes even more prolonged, arrhythmias occur, including atrial fibrillation, other supraventricular arrhythmias, and ventricular tachycardia. Absent P waves may indicate continued sinus node rhythm and failure of the atrium to depolarize. Impulses may be conducted to the ventricle through the internodal pathways. Higher levels of potassium result in ventricular fibrillation and arrest in diastole.

The administration of calcium intravenously may reverse the cardiac toxicity of hyperkalemia; calcium should be given cautiously to the patient on digitalis, however, since digitalis toxicity may be enhanced thereby. Sodium bicarbonate and glucose/insulin infusions also cause movement of po-

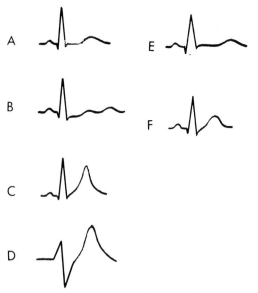

Figure 1. Surface EKG changes indicating potassium and calcium concentrations; normal (A), hypokalemia (B), hyperkalemia (C), severe hyperkalemia (D) hypocalcemia (E), and hypercalcemia (F).

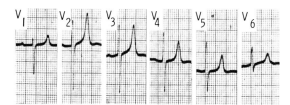

Figure 2. Tall peaked T waves with no alterations of QRS. The changes are relatively mild for the degree of hyperkalemia in this patient (K = 8.3 mEq./liter and Na = 138 mEq./liter).

tassium into the cells, and will ameliorate the electrolyte disturbance until the underlying cause can be identified.

Hypokalemia increases resting membrane potential and prolongs the duration of the action potential. This results in the following electrocardiographic changes (Fig. 3A and B).

(1) Slight peaking of the P wave.

(2) ST segment depression.

(3) Loss of T wave amplitude and increase in U wave amplitude.

(4) An apparent prolongation of the Q-T interval—Q-T interval when measurable may be normal.

Peaked P waves are not commonly noted in the presence of hypokalemia. ST segment depression occurs regularly and may be exaggerated by exercise-induced tachycardia. T waves become low in amplitude. The Q-T interval is difficult to measure since the U wave fuses with the T wave, simulating a long Q-T interval.

Arrhythmias may be multiple, especially in the presence of what ordinarily would be usual doses of digitalis. Supraventricular arrhythmias, ventricular premature beats, ventricular tachycardia, and fibrillation may occur.

Potassium has a variable effect on AV conduction; however, hyperkalemia in general slows AV conduction, as does profound hypokalemia. There is some evidence to suggest that the effect of potassium on AV conduction is related also to the rate of change of the potassium level. Careful attention should be given to potassium in patients with cardiac disease, in particular those with conduction abnormalities and those on digitalis and potent diuretics.

CALCIUM

Hypercalcemia is seen in such malignant diseases as carcinoma of the breast with bone metastases, multiple myeloma, and other disorders such as hyperparathyroidism and hypervitaminosis D. Calcium plays an important role in the contracting myocardium and its excitability.

Elevated levels of calcium are reflected in the EKG as shortening of the Q-T interval and QRS complex. The former sometimes produces an apparent S-T segment elevation because of the early T waves. This, coupled with slight peaking of the T wave, may mimic an early phase of infarction (Fig. 4).

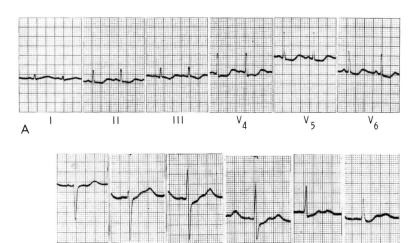

Figure 3. A, Mild changes of hypokalemia showing ST segment depression, low T wave amplitude, and T waves merging with U waves. The Q-T interval appears long for this heart rate. Potassium was 3.3 mEq./liter.

B, More profound changes of hypokalemia with ST segment depression and prominent U waves.

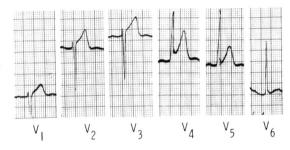

Figure 4. Extreme hypercalcemia (15 mEq./liter) showing short Q–T interval and ST segments so short that they are pulled up by the T waves mimicking injury pattern.

Conduction abnormalities and even ventricular fibrillation may result at very high serum calcium levels.

Emergency measures for hypercalcemia include saline diuresis and furosemide; subsequent therapy is directed at the underlying cause of the disturbance.

Hypocalcemia frequently is seen in advanced renal disease, pancreatitis, hypoparathyroidism, and malabsorption syndromes.

Electrocardiographic changes in hypocalcemia include slight shortening of the P-R interval and QRS duration, and prolongation of the Q-T interval (Fig. 5). The increased Q-T interval actually is due to S-T segment prolongation and little or no T wave alteration. Extreme degrees of hypocalcemia have been associated with T wave changes.

The coexistence of hypocalcemia and hypokalemia results in the T wave merging with the U wave. Hypocalcemia and hyperkalemia, as commonly seen in renal failure, result in a tall peaked T wave following a long S-T segment.

MAGNESIUM

Magensium disturbances are not as

clearly reflected in the EKG as are potassium and calcium. High levels of magnesium in animals result in electrocardiographic changes somewhat similar to those seen in hyperkalemia. Some studies indicate that magnesium administered in hypocalcemic situations will reverse the electrocardiographic effects of hypocalcemia. Magnesium sulfate has long been used as an antiarrhythmic agent, and still may be useful in certain situations.

HYPOTHERMIA

In the Emergency Department setting, patients presenting with accidental hypothermia have characteristic EKGs that have some features common to electrolyte disorders. Bradycardia, atrial fibrillation, muscle tremor artifact, prolonged QRS complexes with "J" point abnormality, T wave changes, and prolonged Q-T interval are seen in hypothermic patients (Fig. 6). The most characteristic feature is the terminal QRS abnormality or "J" wave, seen most prominently in the lateral precordial leads. This abnormality, when easily noticed, signals profound hypothermia and commonly accompanies severe illness (Clements and Hurst, 1972).

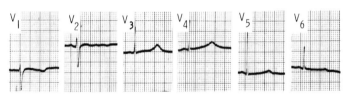

Figure 5. Long Q–T interval in a patient with a calcium level of 5.4 mEq./liter.

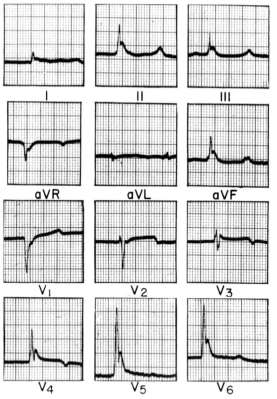

Figure 6. Admission electrocardiogram in a patient with a body temperature of 75° F. Heart rate was 40 beats per minute and Q-T interval is prolonged. Atrial fibrillation present. Prominent QRS terminal force abnormality ("J" wave) most easily identified in lead V₅. (Reprinted with permission from *The American Journal of Cardiology* 29:729, May 1972.)

DRUGS

Certain drugs affect the EKG in ways similar to those of electrolyte abnormalities (Winsor, 1968). Digitalis alone poses few problems, but the combination of digitalis and quinidine produces a pattern indistinguishable from hypokalemia. Quinidine and Pronestyl both cause QRS prolongation at higher doses. The phenothiazines may prolong the Q-T interval and initiate ventricular arrhythmias or A-V conduction disturbances. A wide variety of drugs is known to produce changes in the EKG (Surawicz and Lasseter, 1970). These effects must be taken into account when examining the EKG for evidence of electrolyte disturbances.

References

Clements, S. D., and Hurst, J. W.: Diagnostic value of electrocardiographic abnormalities observed in subjects accidentally exposed to cold. Am. J. Cardiol. 29:729, 1972.

Surawicz, B.: Relationship between electrocardiogram and electrolytes. Am. Heart J. 73:814, 1967.

Surawicz, B., and Lasseter, K. C.: Effect of drugs on the electrocardiogram. Progr. Cardiovasc. Dis. 13:26, 1970.

Wenger, N. K., and Herndon, E. G., Jr.: Endocrine and Metabolic Diseases. In Hurst, J. W., et al. (eds.): The Heart, 3d ed. New York, McGraw-Hill Book Co., 1974, p. 1497.

Winsor, T.: Electrolyte abnormalities and the electrocardiogram. J.A.M.A. 203:109, 1968.

Chapter 42

VASCULAR EMERGENCIES

A. Aorta and Peripheral Arteries
B. Diseases of the Veins

A.   AORTA AND PERIPHERAL ARTERIES

Joseph Lindsay, Jr. and Alvin J. Slovin

AORTIC DISEASE

General Considerations

For clinical purposes, aortic disease may be categorized appropriately in accordance with its structural manifestations without great regard to its etiology. The etiology of a thoracic aneurysm, for example, is often obscure clinically and may remain so after postmortem examination. This discussion, therefore, will focus on the major structural aortic disorders, aneurysm, and medial dissection, but since a knowledge of the disease processes that affect the aorta, and of their characteristic pathophysiologic consequences, is important to allow accurate recognition and intelligent management, we shall first consider these matters.

Etiologic and Pathogenic Considerations

ATHEROSCLEROSIS

Atherosclerosis of the aorta, an almost invariable accompaniment of aging, affects the intima primarily. Raised, grayish, fibrous plaques containing lipid form within that layer. Hemorrhage into these plaques, ulceration, calcification, and formation of overlying thrombus complete the pathologic picture. Importantly, the media of the vessel underlying areas of severe intimal injury is weakened by penetration of the process.

Atherosclerosis tends to be most severe in the abdominal aorta distal to the renal arteries, to involve the arch and proximal descending aorta to a lesser degree, and relatively to spare the ascending aorta except for the immediate area of the aortic valve. As might be expected, aneurysm and occlusion of the abdominal aorta are the most frequent clinical manifestations of aortic atherosclerosis.

MEDIAL DEGENERATION

Noninflammatory degeneration of the aortic media is a far less frequent cause of

overt clinical disease than is atherosclerosis. Imprecisely categorized and probably heterogenous in etiology, weakening of the aortic wall resulting from medial degeneration may result in aneurysm formation or medial dissection.

The lesion is most completely manifest in some patients with the Marfan syndrome in whom fragmentation and degeneration of the elastic fibers of the aortic media are extensive. Clefts resulting from the degenerating fibers are filled with a metachromatic mucoid material. The descriptive term cystic medial necrosis is often applied, even though true necrosis is not present. This process is most severe in the ascending aorta, including the aortic sinuses, but less commonly is found in more distal locations in that vessel and in the other large elastic arteries, including the pulmonary artery.

The most frequent clinical manifestation of this process is aneurysm of the aortic root. Enormous dilatation occurs of the sinuses of Valsalva and the aortic ring. The intima is fissured by the dilatation of the underlying media, and limited areas of medial dissection occur. This aneurysmal dilatation characteristically is limited to the ascending aorta, producing the "Florence Flask" appearance on angiography (Figs. 1 and 2). Severe aortic regurgitation, external rupture into the pericardium, or extensive medial dissection may complicate this process. This aortic lesion is also encountered in patients lacking the skeletal and ocular features of the Marfan syndrome, and has been termed idiopathic cystic medial necrosis.

The vast majority of patients with aortic dissection do not have the Marfan syndrome, and their aortic walls typically manifest a relatively mild degree of cystic medial necrosis or a nonspecific degenerative process. Hypertension appears to be a major factor in the genesis of medial dissection in such instances.

AORTITIS

Syphilitic aortitis is still by far the most common infectious disease of the aorta. The

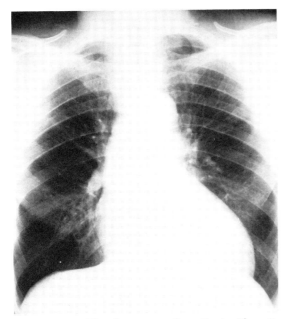

Figure 1. The chest x-ray of a patient with aortic root aneurysm resulting from cystic medial degeneration. Although the aortic lesion is characteristic of that seen in Marfan's syndrome, this patient had none of the skeletal or ocular features of that disorder. The aortogram in this patient is shown as Figure 2. Note that the aneurysm is not visible on the plain film.

spirochetes invade the aortic media by way of the vasovasorum. Thus, the ascending segment and the arch of the aorta, the most richly vascularized segment, are involved with greatest frequency. When examined histologically, the aortic wall is found to be damaged by a patchy mesoaortitis, accompanied by proliferation of the fibrous tissue in the adjacent intima and advantitia. Aneurysm, a frequent clinical manifestation, involving especially the ascending aorta, arch, and proximal descending aorta, is a common complication. Unlike atherosclerotic aneurysms, syphilitic aneurysms are rare distal to the renal arteries. Aortic regurgitation also is a common complication. Occlusion of one or both coronary ostia by the intimal proliferation is less frequent.

Bacterial invasion of the normal aorta is rare, although primary mycotic aneurysms have been reported in infective endocarditis and other septicemias. Secondary infection of a segment with pre-existing disease, notably an abdominal aneurysm, is somewhat more common.

Noninfectious aortitis, uncommon in the U.S., nevertheless has been reported as an

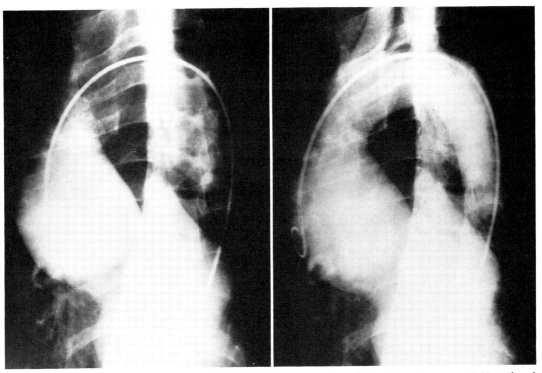

Figure 2. Two frames from the aortogram of the patient whose plain film is shown in Figure 1. Note that the aneurysmal dilatation is limited to the aortic sinuses and proximal aorta. Aortic regurgitation is present.

isolated abnormality, as well as in association with generalized disease processes, such as rheumatic fever, rheumatoid arthritis, scleroderma, and Hodgkin's disease. In the Orient, the occurrence in young women of a nonspecific aortitis is frequent enough to allow investigators to collect substantial series of cases. Occlusion of the orifices of the large branches from the aortic arch is characteristic, but aortic aneurysm also is known. The eponym Takayasu's arteritis, recalls the Japanese ophthalmologist who first described the retinal findings in this disease. A pathologically distinct aortitis of the proximal aorta, found in some patients with ankylosing spondylitis, may result in serious aortic regurgitation. Giant cell arteritis (temporal arteritis, polymyalgia rheumatica) has been reported to involve the aorta and to result in aneurysm and in dissection.

CONGENITAL ANOMALIES

The numerous congenital anomalies of the aortic root and arch vessels are beyond the scope of this discussion. It is noteworthy that aneurysm, dissection, and rupture of the aorta are frequent complications of aortic coarctation.

Aortic Dissection

Medial dissection is said to be the most common life-threatening disease of the aorta. The term "dissecting aneurysm" is often applied, but invites confusion. Pre-existing atherosclerotic or syphilitic aneurysms that are symptomatic from expansion or impending rupture may be considered in a broad sense to be "dissecting." It is important to understand that medial dissection is an entity quite distinct from such lesions in etiology, pathogenesis, and clinical course. Longitudinal cleavage of the medial layer of the aorta by a column of blood is the primary pathologic event. In at least 90 per cent of instances, the cleavage plane communicates with the aortic lumen, frequently, but not invariably, near the proximal limit of the dissection. More than one intimal tear may be found. Those at the more distal portion of the dissection have been termed "re-entry" tears. It is, not clear however, that proximal tears are the sites of "entry," nor that the more distal ones are sites of "re-entry" for the hematoma.

Lethal complications often result from this process. Rupture of the weakened aortic wall is the most devastating of these. Fatal cardiac tamponade due to rupture of the intrapericardial portion of the ascending aorta is the single most common cause of death. When the process is limited to the descending aorta, rupture into the left pleural space is characteristic. Hemorrhage into the mediastinum or the retroperitoneal area is less common. Occlusion of a major aortic branch vessel may ultimately be as lethal as hemorrhage, since life-threatening myocardial, cerebral, renal, or mesenteric ischemia may result. Ischemia of an extremity is common, but somewhat less catastrophic.

It is useful to divide instances of aortic dissection into subgroups based on the anatomic involvement. The nomenclature utilized by DeBakey is widely accepted. The term "type I" aortic dissection is applied when the dissection involves the ascending aorta and extends distally beyond that segment. Many of these extend to the iliac arteries. Characteristically, there is an intimal tear within a few centimeters of the aortic valve. About two-thirds of all instances of aortic dissection are of this variety. Instances in which medial cleavage begins just beyond the left subclavian artery and extends distally are placed in "type III". This variety makes up approximately 30 per cent. DeBakey labeled as "type II" those dissections limited to the ascending aorta. Several of the "type II" cases in the series reported by DeBakey had stigmata of the Marfan syndrome. These cases are so distinct that, in our view, they should not be considered a variety of ordinary aortic dissection. Dissection of the ordinary kind involving the ascending aorta can be managed without regard to the extent of its distal dissection, whereas the lesion seen in the Marfan syndrome presents special problems. Thus, we have not found "type II" a particularly useful subgroup.

RECOGNITION

Pain in the midline of the trunk is the most common presenting symptom of aortic dissection. Typically, it is excruciating, at peak intensity from its inception, and is located in the anterior chest, interscapular area, epigastrium, or lumbar area. The discomfort often is perceived in more than one of these sites, simultaneously or sequentially. Occurrence in sites both above and below the diaphragm is particularly distinctive. For example, the patient who initially appears to have acute myocardial infarction because of severe anterior chest pain should be suspected of aortic dissection if his pain suddenly shifts to the epigastrium or to the lumbar area.

Painless dissection occurs in 10 to 15 per cent of patients in the reported series. Painless dissection seems most frequently to result from an inability of the patient to perceive or to report pain, for example, when a cerebrovascular occlusion has resulted from the dissection. Moreover, syncope is a relatively frequent acute event. Even when preceded by pain, the severe nature of the discomfort often is blunted by the patient's depressed sensorium following the syncopal episode.

Thus, the vast majority of patients with acute aortic dissection will present with severe pain, or as if experiencing an acute neurologic event. Rarely, aortic dissection will be found during a study of a patient with an abnormal aortic silhouette on chest x-ray, with aortic regurgitation, or with loss of an arterial pulsation.

Once the diagnosis of dissection is suspected, a carefully conducted cardiovascular examination will often reveal supporting clues to the diagnosis. The murmur of aortic regurgitation, or the absence or diminution of a major arterial pulse, is detectable in the great majority of patients with type I dissection. These signs, however, are frequently absent in those patients with type III dissection. Less specific findings, such as a systolic murmur, a vascular bruit, or palpable widening of the abdominal aorta, may raise the suspicion of dissection in such cases. Detection of pulsation in either sternoclavicular joint is a particularly helpful finding in those patients who present without more certain physical symptoms.

Since hypertension appears to play a role in the pathogenesis of this disorder, as many as 80 per cent of patients manifest either an elevated blood pressure or evidence of antecedent hypertension. A few patients, particularly those with type III dissection, are severely hypertensive. Arterial pressures exceeding 250/140 mm. of mercury are sometimes found during the acute episode. Acute renal ischemia, due to occlusion by the dissection of a renal artery, has been suspected.

A significant number of patients are hypotensive when initially seen. In the setting of acute dissection, this almost invariably is indicative of hemorrhage or of cardiac tamponade as a consequence of external rupture. It is important to appreciate the significance of hypotension, since certain of these patients will survive long enough to undergo life-saving operative intervention. This is

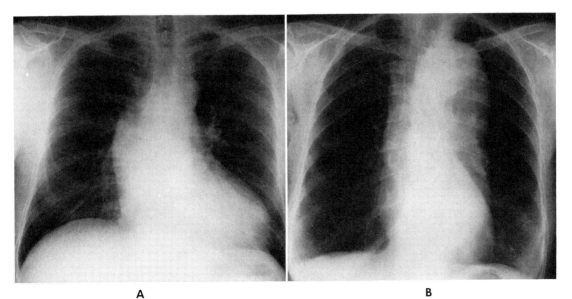

A B

Figure 3. The chest x-rays from two patients showing the characteristic deformities resulting from Type I (*A*) and Type III (*B*) aortic dissection. Chest films of this quality are unusual in the acutely ill patient with this disorder.

evident, since exsanguination temporarily may be prevented by the compression of the hematoma in surrounding tissues, and by the fall in arterial pressure.

Most routine laboratory studies are of little diagnostic significance, but the plain chest radiograph is of considerable value (Fig. 3). The aortic or mediastinal silhouette is almost invariably abnormal. Changes are most specific for aortic dissection when they can be demonstrated to be recent by comparison with previous films. The chest film is likely to be most useful in a negative sense. When the aortic silhouette is convincingly normal on a good quality film, dissection is unlikely. Unfortunately, it is rare for chest x-rays in these very ill patients to be of sufficiently good quality to allow one to feel secure that the aortic silhouette is unequivocally normal.

MANAGEMENT

If the progression of medial dissection can be arrested before external rupture has occurred, and before occlusion of the arterial supply to a vital organ has taken place, the patient should survive. In 1965, Wheat and Palmer reported successful application of potent antihypertensive agents designed to accomplish this purpose. They proposed that simultaneous reduction of both the aortic pressure and the force of myocardial contractility was essential. The same year, DeBakey and his co-workers reported an extensive surgical experience in which mortality from this disorder was favorably altered. After a decade of controversy, there still is not total agreement regarding the precise indications for one or the other of these forms of treatment. Nevertheless, the availability of an effective, readily applicable pharmacologic therapy is of great importance to the emergency physician.

Trimethaphan (Arfonad) is the most widely applied drug for acute management. Intravenous infusion of a solution (1 to 2 mg./ml.) at a rate necessary to reduce systolic arterial pressure to 100 to 120 mm. Hg is recommended. In most patients, this level can be achieved rapidly and maintained by careful adjustment of the infusion rate. The hypotensive effects are quickly dissipated by termination of the infusion. The head of the patient's bed should be elevated to take advantage of the orthostatic effects of the drug. Once a decision has been reached to

manage the patient by pharmacologic rather than operative means during the acute episode, other antihypertensive agents should be begun. Guanethidine, 25 to 50 mg. twice daily by mouth, or methyldopa 250 to 500 mg. three or four times daily intravenously or by mouth, may be used for this purpose. Reserpine, 0.5 to 2.0 mg. intramuscularly, will promptly reduce arterial pressure and the force of ventricular systole, and therefore is useful if the primary medications fail; it is particularly useful when tachyphylaxis to trimethaphan precedes effective control of the blood pressure by long-acting agents. Propranolol, 1.0 mg. every four to six hours intramuscularly, or 80 to 160 mg. or more orally, frequently is added because it reduces the force of ventricular contraction, and thereby the pulsatile force of aortic flow. It may be the principal drug in patients with little or no hypertension. Diuretic therapy is adjunctive and is utilized almost invariably.

Although there appears to be a controversy in the literature regarding specific indications for pharmacologic therapy versus operative intervention, there are, in fact, only a minority of patients in whom this choice is a real issue. Many patients are not candidates for an operation under any circumstances because of advanced age, or chronic cardiac, renal, or pulmonary disease. Another substantial group are not candidates for drug therapy since they have already become hypotensive as a result of hemorrhage or cardiac tamponade. The same is true of those patients who have advanced aortic regurgitation consequent to their dissection. Among those patients in whom the opportunity exists to choose between the two modalities of treatment, most authorities now agree that those with involvement of the ascending aorta should undergo operative treatment at once, whereas those whose dissection is limited to the descending aorta should be managed with drugs. Experience with drug therapy in the former has been unsatisfactory. With these practices in mind, the physician who diagnoses aortic dissection and initiates treatment can reasonably foresee whether or not his patient will undergo an immediate operation, and can plan accordingly.

Antihypertensive therapy should be initiated for all patients who are distinctly hypertensive and who are strongly suspected of aortic dissection. Trimethaphan can conveniently be utilized until aortography is carried out and a decision regarding operative intervention is reached. Dramatic relief of pain often follows reduction of the arterial pressure. The level of blood pressure, the clarity of the diagnosis, and the presence or absence of symptoms must be taken into account in the decision to initiate therapy in mildly hypertensive patients. A decision to interrupt drug therapy and to undertake operative intervention may be triggered by failure of the medications to prevent progression of the dissection, as evidenced by renewed pain, loss of additional pulses, increase in aortic regurgitation, or signs of impending or partial rupture.

Partial or impending rupture of the dissection invariably signaled by hypotension, occurs prior to hospital admission in at least 25 per cent of patients. Drug therapy, of course, is of no benefit in such cases, but heroic surgical therapy may salvage a few.

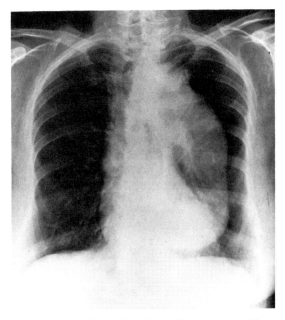

Figure 4. Chest film of an elderly patient with an extensive atherosclerotic aneurysm of the descending aorta. The resulting deformity in this instance could not be distinguished from that produced by medial dissection.

Thoracic Aneurysm

Saccular or fusiform aneurysms of the thoracic aorta are now most commonly due to atherosclerosis and, because of the distribution of that process, characteristically are located in the descending segment. Syphilis, far less common than in years past, is the second most frequent etiologic agent. Involvement of the ascending aorta and arch is usual. Aneurysms of the ascending aorta consequent to medial cystic necrosis, and of the proximal descending segment due to trauma, make up the bulk of the residue. It often is difficult to be certain clinically of the etiology of an aneurysm, and sometimes the question still is unsettled at autopsy.

RECOGNITION

Most thoracic aneurysms are asymptomatic and are first detected on a radiographic examination (Fig. 4). Aneurysms limited to the proximal ascending aorta, particularly those resulting from cystic medial necrosis, may not be clearly visible on a chest radiograph, since much of this aortic segment lies within the aortic silhouette (Fig. 1). Dilatation of the ascending aorta may be suggested by convex distortion of the superior portion of the right cardiac shadow. Patients who have complaints related to their aneurysm most often report deep, diffuse, chest pain, which at times varies with body position and may seem to be related to erosion by the aneurysm of contiguous bony structures. Compression of the tracheobronchial tree, left recurrent laryngeal nerve, or other mediastinal structures may result in dyspnea, hoarseness, dysphagia, or cough. Larger aneurysms and those of the ascending aorta or arch are associated with symptoms more frequently than are those of the descending aorta. As discussed in the next section, symptoms arising from an abdominal aneurysm indicate impending rupture. Although symptoms are reported with "stable" thoracic aneurysms, it is the authors' experience that the abrupt appearance of symptoms or a change in their character is evidence of impending rupture, a matter of great urgency.

Rupture of thoracic aneurysms may produce dramatic clinical syndromes. Erosion into the esophagus or tracheobronchial tree may produce rapid exsanguination or asphyxia from aspiration. Not all rupture is immediately fatal. Erosion into the lung parenchyma may produce recurrent hemoptysis for a period of weeks or months. Rupture into the pulmonary artery produces a continuous murmur indicative of the acute left-to-right shunt.

MANAGEMENT

The emergency physician's principal concern in patients with thoracic aneurysm is the detection of impending rupture, and the immediate referral of such patients to a cardiovascular surgical team. Hypovolemic patients should have their blood volume restored to maintain adequate perfusion, but restoration of the blood pressure to normal may provoke renewed bleeding. In normotensive or hypertensive individuals with impending rupture, the use of agents to reduce intra-aortic pressure, and thereby the hydraulic forces on the aortic wall, is intuitively attractive, but to our knowledge has not been utilized.

Abdominal Aneurysm

Virtually all abdominal aneurysms are atherosclerotic in etiology and, in keeping with the distribution of that process, are located distal to the renal arteries. Detection of asymptomatic aneurysms and recognition of the syndromes produced by rupture or impending rupture of these structures are the proper concerns of the emergency physician.

ASYMPTOMATIC ABDOMINAL ANEURYSM

Forty per cent of the abdominal aneurysms in the series reviewed by Gore and Hirst were asymptomatic. They were discovered incidentally during an investigation of other problems; for example, detection of an enlarged, calcified aorta on lumbar spine x-rays made because of low back pain, or detection of a pulsatile abdominal mass on routine physical examination.

Recognition. Careful evaluation of a pulsatile mass is required, since, to be palpable, an abdominal aneurysm is likely to exceed 4.5 cm. in diameter. A tortuous aorta or, in thin individuals, a prominent aortic pulse may be mistaken for an aneurysm. On the other hand, the thickness of the abdominal wall in obese patients may make an aneurysm appear larger than it really is. Aneurysms involving the iliac arteries characteristically are not found on abdominal palpation, but on rectal or pelvic examination.

Anteroposterior and lateral films of the abdomen logically are the initial step in the evaluation of a suspected or frankly palpable aneurysm. If calcification is present in both walls of the aorta, the diameter of the vessel can be estimated reasonably. If calcification is present in only one wall, tortuosity of the aorta without aneurysm formation cannot be ruled out, and further studies are necessary. A chest film also is useful, since thoracic aneurysm often is associated. If the thoracic aorta appears normal, it is extremely rare for an abdominal aneurysm to extend above the renal arteries.

Abdominal ultrasonography has been found to be most accurate in determining the lumen diameter, wall thickness, and length of the abdominal aneurysm. This technique is particularly valuable in following the size of aneurysms for which operative treatment is not recommended initially.*

Aortography is reserved for final preoperative assessment. Although the value of its routine use is open to debate, many surgeons feel that the information gained from angiographic evaluation of the branch arteries is valuable enough to justify its application.

Management. The danger of rupture of asymptomatic aneurysms greater than 6 cm. in diameter has been estimated to be from 40 to 80 per cent within two to five years from the time of diagnosis. Accordingly, elective aneurysmectomy is recommended for those patients who are considered to be reasonable risks for major abdominal surgery. Although many feel that those with aneurysms less than 6 cm. in size can be followed carefully without operation, the risk of rupture may be as high as 20 per cent in five years. This hazard, and the probability of increasing aneurysm size over the years, causes some surgeons to recommend elective aneurysm resection in such patients under the age of 60 who are good anesthetic risks. Any increase in the size of an asymptomatic aneurysm that is being followed by periodic physical and ultrasound evaluations is an indication for hospitalization and resection.

SYMPTOMATIC ABDOMINAL ANEURYSM

Eighty per cent or more of the patients whose abdominal aneurysms become symp-

---

*See page 376.

tomatic will be dead within one year unless the aneurysms are resected. They are, therefore, of great importance to the emergency physician, whose principal concern will be to suspect the problem, appreciate its urgency, and refer the patient to a vascular surgeon capable of abdominal aneurysmectomy. Five clinical syndromes generally are produced by abdominal aortic aneurysms.

"Expanding" Aneurysms. Expansion may be heralded by the development of lumbar back pain radiating into the left flank or groin, or by abdominal pain in the periumbilical area. The discomfort may be intermittent and mild, or may be continuous with increasing intensity. The aneurysm may be tender to palpation. Epigastric fullness after eating, and nausea and vomiting, may result from impingement by the aneurysm on the third and fourth portions of the duodenum. Whether these signs and symptoms are due to bleeding within the aneurysm walls, or to a leak into the retroperitoneal space, can be determined only at operation. It can be appreciated that these findings are not diagnostic. They are, however, sufficiently characteristic in a patient with a pulsatile abdominal mass to dictate serious consideration of immediate operative therapy.

The diagnosis cannot be discarded in obese patients, particularly those more than 40 years of age, when abdominal palpation does not reveal an aneurysm. Plain films of the abdomen, intravenous pyelogram, or spinal x-rays should be reviewed for the presence of aortic calcification. Abdominal ultrasonography also may be helpful.

Inferior vena caval obstruction presenting as marked edema of the lower extremities has been reported consequent to expansion of an abdominal aortic aneurysm. This is an extremely rare occurrence, as the vena cava usually is displaced to the right by the aneurysm without being compromised.

Ruptured Aneurysms. When an aneurysm ruptures into the retroperitoneal tissues, the patient experiences sudden severe abdominal pain radiating to the back and possibly the groin. Syncope, nausea, and vomiting also may occur. As the retroperitoneal hematoma increases in size and dissects over the musculature, the pain may extend into the hips, flanks, groin, or scrotum. The pain usually is continuous. When first seen by a physician, most of the patients are hypotensive or in outright shock. A tender abdominal mass is usually palpable, consisting of the aneurysm alone or including the retroperitoneal hematoma. Even though shock is present, most patients will stabilize if the parietal peritoneum remains intact. In the majority of cases, sudden death does not occur, and the pain may decrease in intensity. In one recently reported series, the interval from onset of symptoms to arrival at the hospital averaged 9.5 hours. When symptoms are present and the patient's abdomen is too obese to allow recognition of a mass, the diagnosis of a ruptured aneurysm may be made after examination of plain films of the abdomen for evidence of aortic calcification, or for obliteration of the psoas shadows. If the diagnosis still is not confirmed, abdominal paracentesis may be helpful, but need not be positive for blood if the hematoma is confined to the retroperitoneum. An aortogram may be necessary. A fall in hematocrit is observed only after a number of hours have elapsed, and should not be expected early in the course of ruptured aneurysm. Ecchymosis of the flanks or pelvic area also is a late development, usually appearing after the third day.

Once the diagnosis has been made, the patient should be taken to the operating room. Infusions should be started, but large volumes of fluid or blood should be avoided, as elevating the blood pressure may increase the retroperitoneal bleeding and result in intraperitoneal rupture.

The occurrence of gastrointestinal bleeding in the presence of a palpable aortic aneurysm suggests the possibility of an aortoenteric fistula. This aorta usually communicates with the distal duodenum or, less commonly, the jejunum. Death rarely occurs at the first bleeding episode. Episodic bleeding varying in severity can recur over a period of several weeks. An upper gastrointestinal series or an aortogram often will not be diagnostic, and therefore, once the diagnosis is strongly considered, excision of the aneurysm and repair of the intestine should be performed. Although the aortic wall must be considered to be infected, with the use of systemic antibiotics pre- and postoperatively, and at times continuously administered intra-abdominal antibiotics postoperatively, bypass grafts outside of the abdominal cavity (e.g., axillofemoral grafts) have not always been necessary.

Rupture of an arteriosclerotic abdominal

aortic aneurysm into the inferior vena cava is an uncommon event. The size of the communication will determine the severity of the resulting high output congestive failure, edema of the lower extremities, and engorgement of the lower abdominal wall veins. A continuous murmur on abdominal auscultation is characteristic, and aortography will confirm the diagnosis. At the time of surgery, great care must be exercised in handling the aneurysm to prevent entrance of aortic mural thrombus into the vena cava, with resultant pulmonary embolization.

Acute Thrombosis of Abdominal Aortic Aneurysms. Acute thrombosis of an abdominal aortic aneurysm will produce the same symptoms and findings as an aortic saddle embolus, acute thrombosis of the terminal aorta, or bilateral iliofemoral emboli. Severe ischemia of the lower extremities will result in pain, pallor, paresthesias, loss of peripheral pulses, and paralysis. Suspicion that the aortic bifurcation occlusion results from a thrombosed aneurysm arises upon discovery of a palpable abdominal mass.

Surgery should be performed without delay, in order to prevent loss of limb and death. If a thrombosed abdominal aortic aneurysm has been recognized preoperatively, a laparotomy is undertaken, but in the majority of cases the thrombosed aneurysm will not have been recognized, and the distinction between embolic and acute thrombotic occlusion will not be clear. Bilateral incisions exposing the common femoral, profunda femoris, and superficial femoral arteries may be performed under local anesthesia. Restoration of flow can be attempted by retrograde passage of Fogarty embolectomy catheters. If flow cannot be restored, laparotomy should be performed, and it is at this time that the thrombosed aneurysm will be recognized. Intraoperative angiography may be necessary to determine distal patency after clot removal. Postoperatively, the revascularized limbs must be checked for muscle edema, and fasciotomies must be performed if not included in the initial operative procedure. In the series reported by Johnson et al., the operative mortality of patients with acute abdominal aortic aneurysm thrombosis was 53 per cent.

Infected Aneurysms. Although uncommon, infection of an abdominal aortic aneurysm should be considered in any patient with an aneurysm who presents with fever, chills, weight loss, or malaise without an obvious source of sepsis. Moreover, laboratory studies indicative of infection in a patient with an aneurysm who is being considered for surgery should dictate a search for a site of infection prior to elective resection. Blood cultures should be drawn on multiple occasions, since 50 per cent will be positive. Salmonellae, staphylococci, and streptococci are the most common organisms. Once the diagnosis is made, antibiotic therapy should be begun and the patient prepared for operative treatment, since the risk of rupture is great. The duration of antibiotic therapy preoperatively will vary, depending on whether expansion of the aneurysm and impending rupture is suspected. An axillofemoral graft or another type of by-pass outside of the infected tissues should be performed, the aneurysm resected, and both ends of the aorta oversewn. Gram stains and cultures of the aneurysm wall and content should be performed at the time of surgery.

Abdominal Aortic Aneurysms with Peripheral Emboli. Peripheral arterial emboli originating in an aortic or iliac artery aneurysm have been thought to be rare, but the frequency almost certainly has been underestimated, since Lord et al. report a four-year study in which 10 per cent of surgically removed peripheral emboli arose from an aortic aneurysm. It is noteworthy that 29 per cent of the aneurysms resected by them during that period were detected in patients presenting with embolic episodes who were subjected to aortography. Thus, the absence of a palpable mass on physical examination in a patient with a peripheral embolus does not rule out the possibility of its having been thrown off by an aneurysm. Aortography to visualize the abdominal aorta and distal vascular tree should be performed prior to or after embolectomy, unless the embolus is known to be of cardiac origin. In good risk patients, embolectomy should be followed by aneurysm resection.

POSTOPERATIVE COMPLICATIONS OF ANEURYSM RESECTION AND BY-PASS GRAFTING

The diagnosis of an aortoenteric fistula should be considered immediately in any patient presenting with upper or lower gastrointestinal bleeding who has had graft replacement of an aortic aneurysm. Death rarely occurs with the initial episode. Indeed, the patient may have multiple bleeding episodes of varying severity over several weeks. Furthermore, bleeding may appear from months to years after graft insertion. Most fistulous connections are between the proximal graft suture line and the duodenum, but they also may occur between the distal suture line and the ileum if an aortoiliac graft was performed. Direct contact between the bowel and suture line, resulting from inadequate tissue coverage of the graft, appears to be a major source of trouble. Late anastomotic breakdown is attributable to deterioration of silk sutures, or to infection and false aneurysm formation with erosion into the bowel. Fistulas occurring in the early postoperative period usually are the result of infection.

Early surgical exploration is the treatment of choice, since endoscopy, x-ray studies of the G. I. tract, and aortography may fail to demonstrate the source of bleeding. When infection is absent, repair of the bowel and graft suture line may be possible without removal of the graft; however, if infection is encountered at exploration, the treatment consists of total graft excision and revascularization through an uninfected bed employing, for example, an axillofemoral graft.

The second major complication, graft infection, has been reported to occur in 1.3 to 6 per cent of prosthetic reconstructive procedures. At the present time, the rate is probably less than 2 per cent. Controversy still exists over whether this rate can be lowered by the preoperative use of antibiotics, since Szilagyi et al. reported an incidence of graft infection of 1.9 per cent in patients not receiving prophylactic antibiotics. Infection may appear early in the postoperative period, or years later. Gram-negative organisms are the most common invaders after reconstruction of the abdominal aorta and iliac arteries. Staphylococci are more frequent when the infected graft is in the inguinal area.

In addition to an aortoenteric fistula, infection of a retroperitoneal graft may become manifest as graft thrombosis, or as retroperitoneal hemorrhage, or it may result in false aneurysm formation.

Infection of a graft in the femoral area may result in a wound abscess, a sinus tract with purulent drainage or with hemorrhage, an infected false aneurysm, or graft thrombosis. Hemorrhage will almost always occur eventually when an anastomotic site is infected. Infection tends to be localized when a graft remains patent, and to propagate in a thrombosed graft. The femoral limb of an aortofemoral graft must be removed in order to control the infection, and blood flow to the limb must be restored by bypassing the infected site. At the time of surgery, it must be determined whether the abdominal portion of the graft also is infected. If so, total graft excision is required.

The presence of a false aneurysm after aortofemoral grafting does not always imply that infection is present. If signs and symptoms of sepsis are absent, the pulsatile mass may be due to separation of the arterial graft suture line despite the use of synthetic suture material. This problem does not require graft excision, but rather anastomotic repair.

ARTERIAL DISEASE OF THE EXTREMITIES

ARTERIAL THROMBOSIS

Thrombosis may be superimposed on arteriosclerotic arteries, on aortic or peripheral aneurysms, or on arterial by-pass grafts. Resulting symptoms may be chronic or acute.

Thrombosis secondary to atherosclerosis in the superficial femoral artery, the most common site, characteristically results in calf claudication. Distal pulses may or may not be present, depending on the amount of collateral flow. If present, they usually will disappear with exercise.

The signs and symptoms of ischemia are apt to be more severe, and to progress faster the more distal the location of the arteriosclerotic closure: for example, occlusion of the popliteal artery or one or more of the trifurcation vessels. In addition to superficial femoral or popliteal artery occlusion, obstruction at the origin of the deep femoral artery may result in severe and rapidly progressing symptoms of ischemia. Disabling claudication, muscle and skin atrophy, dependent rubor, rest pain, ischemic ulceration, and frank gangrene may occur.

Thrombosis of the distal aorta and iliac vessels, usually superimposed on atherosclerosis, typically results in the progressive development of hip, thigh, and leg claudica-

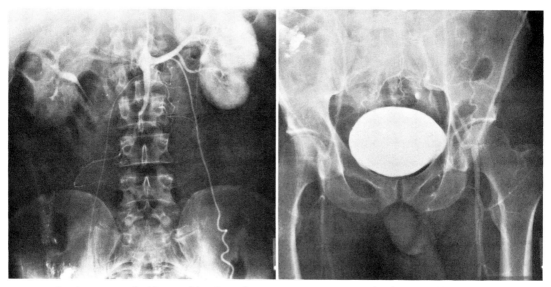

Figure 5. Aortogram of a 43-year-old male with impotence, progressive claudication of both lower extremities, and gangrene of the right third toe. Occlusion of the abdominal aorta below the renal arteries with reconstitution of distal flow is demonstrated. Marked arteriosclerosis of the aorta and iliac arteries was found at surgery. Aortic thrombectomy and aortofemoral by-pass graft resulted in complete relief of symptoms.

tion, as well as impotence. Progression of the occlusive process to involve the femoro-popliteal vessels results in increased ischemic symptoms of the lower extremities (Fig. 5). Propagation of the aortic thrombosis to involve the renal arteries has been docu-mented. Acute thrombosis of an arterio-sclerotic abdominal aorta may occur during sepsis, hypovolemia, or any low cardiac output state (Fig. 6). Arteriography should be followed by Fogarty catheter thromboec-tomy via the femoral arteries. This proce-

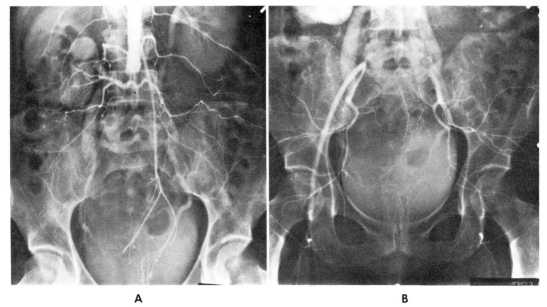

A   B

Figure 6. Aortogram of a 45-year-old female who developed a bile abscess post cholecystectomy. Pain, pares-thesia, loss of pulses, and paralysis of both lower extremities occurred suddenly. Aortography (A, B) revealed occlu-sion of the distal aorta, right common iliac, left common iliac, external iliac, and common femoral arteries. Fogarty thromboembolectomy under local anesthesia resulted in restoration of all pulses following removal of clot and a large rubbery atheroma from the aortic bifurcation. Hydronephrosis is present, but is unrelated.

dure can be performed under local anesthesia, even in a "poor risk" patient.

Thrombosis of an abdominal aortic or peripheral arteriosclerotic aneurysm may give rise to symptoms of acute or chronic ischemia. The diagnosis of thrombosis of a small nonpalpable abdominal aortic or peripheral artery aneurysm may be made only at the time of operation.

ARTERIAL EMBOLISM

Eighty to 90 per cent of arterial emboli originate in the heart chambers. They are most frequent in patients with myocardial infarction, ventricular aneurysm, mitral stenosis, atrial fibrillation, cardiomyopathy, or prosthetic valves. Emboli originating in atrial myxomata are rare, but occasionally may be diagnosed from histologic examination of a peripheral embolus. About 10 per cent of emboli arise from abdominal aortic aneurysms. Peripheral arterial aneurysms, especially of the subclavian and popliteal arteries where movement may play a role in the release of thrombus, may be the source of embolic material, as may the nonaneurysmal arteriosclerotic aorta, in rare cases. In a small percentage of cases, the source of the embolus is unknown (Fig. 7). Emboli tend to lodge at sites of arterial bifurcation, or in areas of arteriosclerotic narrowing. The sudden onset of pain and paresthesia in an affected limb associated with cyanosis, cool skin, and loss of distal pulses is characteristic. Paralysis also will be present when limb viability is threatened. A large embolus that lodges at the aortic bifurcation, a "saddle embolus," may result in ischemia in both lower extremities.

Preoperative arteriography is not regarded by all surgeons as necessary, since in most cases the diagnosis is clear-cut, and embolectomy must be performed within hours of the onset of symptoms; however, the diagnosis may be difficult in individuals with both cardiac disease and peripheral arteriosclerosis who suddenly develop acutely ischemic limbs. Arteriography may show multiple occlusions and severe arteriosclerotic changes (Fig. 8). Information regarding the presence or absence of peripheral pulses prior to the onset of acute ischemia may allow a differentiation between thrombosis and embolism. When this is lacking, the surgeon may attempt to restore flow with the aid of the Fogarty embolectomy catheters, and may employ intraoperative arteriography after removal of the embolus, to determine the patency of the distal tree.

It should be remembered that, in about 2 to 8 per cent of instances of acute embolic or thrombotic occlusion, a syndrome of acute massive ischemic myopathy, myoglobinuria, hyperkalemia, and metabolic acidosis develops. This syndrome, first described by Haimovici in 1960, results in death in 50 to 80 per cent of cases. Thus, following ischemic injury due to vascular occlusion, the patient's urine should be checked for myoglobin and his blood electrolytes and pH should be determined. Renal failure may be prevented. Alkalinization of the urine may

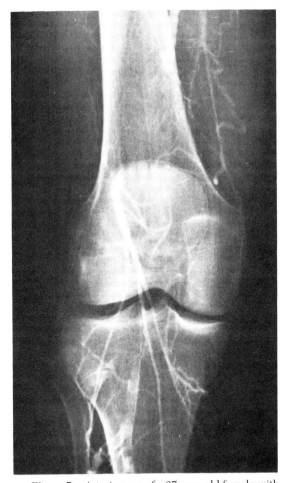

Figure 7. Arteriogram of a 37-year-old female with a history of sudden onset of pain in the right calf and coldness of the lower leg and foot. The aorta and proximal arteries were normal, but the popliteal artery was occluded by clot. Collateral filling of the trifurcation vessels revealed multiple emboli. After successful embolectomy, cardiac catheterization and ventriculography were performed and were normal.

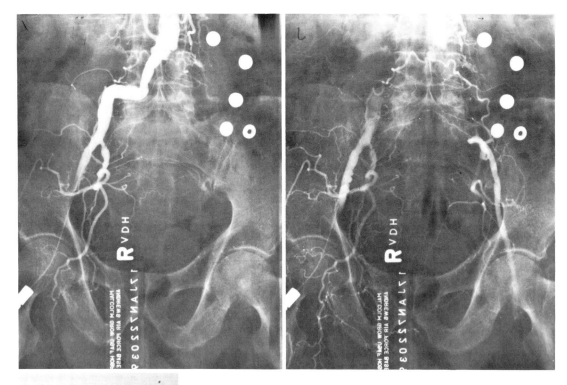

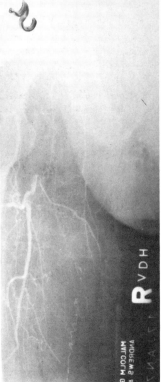

Figure 8. Aortogram of an 85-year-old male admitted for congestive heart failure. He had a history of several old myocardial infarcts, and his rhythm was atrial fibrillation. Pain, paresthesia, and paralysis occurred suddenly in the right leg, accompanied by pain and paresthesia in the left. Of the lower extremity pulses, only a weak right external iliac pulse was present. Both limbs were cold. The right common femoral and superficial femoral arteries were occluded and a clot was present in the profunda femoris. On the left side, the common iliac artery was occluded; the external iliac and common femoral arteries filled by collaterals. All distal pulses had been present prior to the acute episode. Therefore, Fogarty catheter embolectomy under local anesthesia was performed. All pulses were restored.

prevent myoglobin precipitation in the renal tubules. The longer the duration of acute arterial occlusion, the greater the chance of developing this syndrome. Early amputation of an affected limb may be life-saving.

RAYNAUD'S DISEASE AND PHENOMENON

Raynaud's phenomenon, the only common symptomatic vasospastic disorder, is an episodic condition characteristically precipitated by cold or by emotional stress. Classically, there occurs a sequence of three color changes involving one or more fingers, less frequently the toes, and rarely the nose, lips, or ears. At onset, the affected part exhibits marked pallor, often described by the patient as "dead white." Following the pallor, there is a deep cyanosis, which is succeeded in turn by hyperemia (rubor). Pain is not a prominent feature. The total episode seldom lasts longer than 15 minutes. This color sequence is not invariable, and the presence of all components is not necessary for diagnosis. Intense vasospasm of the small cutaneous arteries and arterioles is thought to produce this phenomenon, but the basic mechanism is not known.

The necessity to identify those patients who have an associated disease presents a greater challenge for the physician than recognition of the syndrome. This is an important distinction, since the prognosis is quite benign in the absence of an underlying disease, but the typical Raynaud's phenomenon may be associated with such serious illnesses as systemic scleroderma, rheumatoid arthritis, or systemic lupus erythematosus. The identification of these processes is especially difficult, since the vasospastic phenomena may antedate their other features.

Gifford has suggested the following clues to the existence of an underlying disease.

(1) Abrupt onset; rapid progression to ulceration and gangrene.

(2) Onset after age 50, especially in men.

(3) Unilateral symptoms, especially when confined to one or two digits.

(4) Vasospastic episodes in a warm environment.

(5) Accompanying malaise, fever, weight loss, skin rash.

(6) Prominence of arthralgias, swelling of fingers and hands, and fibrotic symptoms.

(7) Absence of one or more arterial pulsations (except dorsalis pedis).

(8) Abnormal laboratory tests suggesting anemia or protein aberrations.

Apart from the so-called "collagen vascular diseases," numerous other conditions may be associated with Raynaud's phenomenon. Habitual use of vigorously vibrating tools (e.g., pneumatic hammers) has been blamed for its appearance, and the syndrome occasionally appears in pianists or typists.

Raynaud's phenomenon, occurring in the absence of an underlying disease, is termed Raynaud's disease, and is less uncommon than the secondary forms. It is said to be most frequent in young women. Complete assurance as to the benign nature of this complaint cannot be given until several years have elapsed, since, as stated, Raynaud's phenomenon at first may be the sole manifestation of systemic disease.

Acute vasospastic episodes ordinarily do not require therapy because of their transient nature. The emergency physician must be concerned to refer such patients for follow-up diagnosis and therapy. Areas of tissue necrosis are unusual, especially in the primary form, and they are typically small when present.

Prevention of recurrent episodes is of concern for long term management. The affected parts, of course, should be protected from cold exposure. Administration of oral vasodilators such as Dibenzyline or cyclandelate has been suggested. Moreover, reserpine injected into the brachial artery has been reported to reduce the frequency of vasospastic episodes, as has the use of oral reserpine or of methyldopa. Sympathectomy may be of value in the idiopathic variety.

PERIPHERAL ANEURYSMS AND ARTERIOVENOUS FISTULAS

Popliteal aneurysms, the most common peripheral arteriosclerotic aneurysms, are bilateral in about one-quarter to one-third of cases, and may be associated with aneurysms of the abdominal aorta and femoral arteries. Many patients are asymptomatic. Thus, a pulsating mass in the popliteal fossa or the unilateral prominence of a pulse in that area on one side may be detected on routine physical examination; or an asymptomatic popliteal aneurysm may be found during arteriography for other peripheral or abdominal arterial lesions. Gifford and his associates found that symptoms appeared in a majority of 100 patients with popliteal artery aneurysm who were followed for five years.

Although rupture is uncommon, embolization of aneurysmal content or thrombosis of the sac may bring patients with these lesions to the emergency physician. When acute ischemia of the foot, secondary to embolization into the posterior tibial and/or anterial tibial arteries, is the presenting problem, the popliteal artery is patent, and the diagnosis of popliteal aneurysm usually can be made by palpation and confirmed by arteriography. However, when thrombosis of the aneurysm is the cause of acute ischemia of the foot and lower calf, the absence of a pulsatile popliteal mass may lead to the erroneous diagnosis of embolism to the superficial femoral or popliteal artery. In such circumstances, knowledge of the presence of aneurysms elsewhere should increase the examiner's suspicion of this diagnosis. X-ray of the popliteal area for the presence of calcium in the aneurysm may be confirmatory. Arteriography is sometimes helpful, but unfortunately a thrombosed aneurysm may not be detected.

Because of their tendency to be complicated by acute ischemia of the legs, excision of popliteal aneurysms is recommended when the diagnosis is made. Complete arteriography should be performed preoperatively to demonstrate other aneurysms.

As is the case with popliteal aneurysms, arteriosclerotic femoral artery aneurysms are more common in elderly males, approximately one-half of whom are hypertensive. They comprise about one-third of all peripheral aneurysms, frequently are bilateral, and often are associated with other arteriosclerotic aneurysms. Fifty per cent of patients with femoral aneurysms will have one in the abdominal aorta as well.

Almost 50 per cent of the 45 patients with femoral artery aneurysms reported by Cuter and Darling sought care because of thrombosis or acute rupture of the aneurysm. Thrombosis was twice as common as rupture. Expanding or ruptured aneurysms may produce pain, tenderness, femoral nerve irritation, groin ecchymosis, or edema resulting from venous obstruction. Thrombosis of the aneurysm may threaten limb viability or may be followed by intermittent claudication.

Surgical resection is recommended be-cause of the frequency of complications. Preoperative arteriography is essential to detect other aneurysms, and to define the relationship of the aneurysm to the common, deep, and superficial femoral arteries. Emergency surgery is required in patients with ruptured or acutely thrombosed aneurysms.

Arteriosclerotic aneurysms of the subclavian artery are rare, but may be seen in association with arteriosclerotic aneurysms elsewhere. The aneurysm may be an incidental finding on chest x-ray, but may manifest its presence as a mass associated with pain and weakness in the upper extremity attributable to pressure on the brachial plexus. Arteriography will confirm the diagnosis, and treatment consists of excision and graft replacement.

Vascular compression in the thoracic outlet is a far more common cause of subclavian artery aneurysms than is arteriosclerosis. Recurrent distal embolization or acute thrombosis of the aneurysm may occur. Mathes and Salam consider the presence in such patients of ischemic symptoms, unrelated to posture or to position of the upper extremity, to represent recurrent embolization and thus indicate the need for urgent surgical treatment.

TRAUMATIC ANEURYSMS AND ARTERIOVENOUS FISTULAS

Penetrating injuries that cause tangential arterial lacerations may result in the formation of a false aneurysm in which the wall is composed of thrombus and fibrous tissue. False aneurysms may produce symptoms from compression of surrounding structures. They tend progressively to increase in size and eventually to rupture. An arterial injury may not have been suspected at the time of injury. It is wise to carry out arteriography in all cases of penetrating trauma, even if distal pulses are present, whenever it appears from the direction of penetration that the possibility of arterial injury exists.

Penetrating injuries causing simultaneous damage to an artery and adjacent vein may result in arteriovenous fistulas. The diagnosis frequently is delayed, and months or years may pass before the patient returns with symptoms. When the lesion is located in the head and neck area, the patient may complain of a continuous buzzing sound. Arteriovenous fistulas of the lower extremities may result in varicose veins or chronic skin ulcerations. On physical examination, a thrill may be palpable, and a continuous murmur may be audible. If the fistula can be closed by manual compression, the pulse rate may decrease (Branham-Nicaladoni sign). Cardiomegaly and symptoms of congestive heart failure may develop in patients with large shunts.

Arteriovenous fistulas complicate surgical procedures. Iliac artery-to-vein fistulas have resulted from lumbar disk excision or pelvic surgery. Superior mesenteric arteriovenous fistulas have been reported after extensive small bowel resection. Peroneal and posterior tibial arteriovenous fistulas have occurred as a result of the false passage of Fogarty embolectomy catheters.

Early diagnosis, arteriography, and surgical repair are ideal. Conservative management of fistulas that complicate the passage of a Fogarty catheter has been advocated, because of the degree of associated atherosclerotic disease.

References

Brenner, W. I., Richman, H., and Reed, G. E.: Roof patch repair or an aortoduodenal fistula resulting from suture line failure in an aortic prosthesis. Am. J. Surg. 127:762, 1974.

Cooke, P. A., and Ehrenfeld, W. K.: Successful management of mycotic aortic aneurysm: report of a case. Surgery 75:132, 1974.

Cutler, B. S., and Darling, R. C.: Surgical management of arteriosclerotic femoral aneurysms. Surgery 74:764, 1973.

Dardik, H., and Dardik, I.: Popliteal aneurysm thrombosis simulating femoral embolic occlusion: value of intraoperative transfemoral arteriography. Am. Surg. 40:493, 1974.

DeWeese, J. A.: Pedal pulses disappearing with exercise: a test for intermittent claudication. N. Engl. J. Med. 262:1214, 1960.

Dillon, M. L., Young, W. G., and Sealy, W. C.: Aneurysms of the descending thoracic aorta. Ann. Thorac. Surg. 3:430, 1967.

Dolen, J. E., et al.: Dissection of the thoracic aorta—medical or surgical therapy. Am. J. Cardiol. 34:803, 1974.

Gifford, R. W., Jr.: The Arteriospastic Diseases. Cardiovascular Clinics. Vol. III, No. 1. Philadelphia, F. A. Davis Co., 1971, pp. 128–139.

Goldstone, J., and Moore, W. S.: Infection in vascular prosthesis, clinical manifestations and surgical management. Am. J. Surg. 128:225, 1974.

Gore, I., and Hirst, A. E., Jr.: Arteriosclerotic aneurysms of the abdominal aorta: a review. Progr. Cardiovasc. Dis. 16:113, 1973.

Gospard, D. S., and Gaspar, M. R.: Arteriovenous fistula after Fogarty catheter thrombectomy. Arch. Surg. 105:90, 1972.

Hachiya, J.: Current concepts of Takayasu's arteritis. Sem. Roentgenol. 5:245, 1970.

Haimovici, H.: Myopathic-nephrotic-metabolic syndrome and massive acute arterial occlusions. Arch. Surg. 106:628, 1973.

Hardy, J. D., and Timmis, H. H.: Abdominal aortic aneurysms: special problems. Ann. Surg. 173:954, 1971.

Heggtveit, H. A.: Syphilitic aortitis. Circulation 29:346, 1964.

Hirst, A. E., and Gore, I.: Marfan's syndrome: a review. Progr. Cardiovasc. Dis. 16:187, 1973.

Iyengar, S. R. K., Lynn, R. B., and Charrette, E. P.: The use of lateral tomography in patients with abdominal aortic aneurysms. Surg. Gynecol. Obstet. 137:235, 1973.

Johnson, J. M., et al.: Sudden complete thrombosis of aortic and iliac aneurysms. Arch. Surg. 108:792, 1974.

Joyce, J. W., et al.: Aneurysms of the thoracic aorta. Circulation 29:176, 1964.

Lord, J. W., et al.: Unsuspected abdominal aortic aneurysms as the cause of peripheral arterial occlusive disease. Ann. Surg. 177:767, 1973.

Mannick, J. A.: Surgical treatment of aneurysms of the abdominal and thoracic aorta. Progr. Cardiovasc. Dis. 16:69, 1973.

Mathes, S. J., and Salam, A. A.: Subclavian artery aneurysm: Sequela of thoracic outlet syndrome. Surgery 76:506, 1974.

McFarland, J., et al.: The medical treatment of dissecting aortic aneurysms. N. Engl. J. Med. 286:115, 1972.

Murdoch, J. L., et al.: Life expectancy and causes of death in the Marfan syndrome. N. Engl. J. Med. 286:804, 1972.

Paloyan, D., Collins, P. A., and Washburn, F. P.: Superior mesenteric arteriovenous fistula. Am. Surg. 40:481, 1974.

Rainer, W. G., Sodler, T. R., Jr., and Guillen, J.: Ruptured abdominal aortic aneurysm. Logistical and surgical considerations. Am. J. Surg. 126:794, 1973.

Rosen, A. J., Depalma, R. G., and Victor, Y.: Risk factors in peripheral atherosclerosis. Arch. Surg. 107:303, 1973.

Saha, S. P., and Nunn, D. B.: Sudden thrombotic occlusion of abdominal aortic aneurysm. A report of two cases. Am. Surg. 40:246, 1974.

Snider, R. L., Porter, J. M., and Eidemiller, L. R.: Inferior vena caval obstruction caused by expansion of an abdominal aortic aneurysm: report of a case and review of the literature. Surgery 75:613, 1974.

Symas P. N., et al.: Marfan's syndrome with aneurysm of ascending aorta and aortic regurgitation. Am. J. Cardiol. 25:483, 1970.

Tobias, J. A., and Daicoff, G. R.: Aortogastric and aortoileal fistulas repaired by direct suture. Arch. Surg. 107:909, 1973.

Wagner, R. B., and Martin, A. S.: Peripheral atheroembolism: Confirmation of a clinical concept, with a case report and review of the literature. J. Thorac. Cardiovasc. Surg. 73:353, 1973.

Wheat, M. W., Jr., and Palmer, R. F.: Dissecting aneurysm of the aorta. Curr. Probl. Surg. July, 1971.

Willwerth, B. M., and Waldhausen, J. A.: Infection of arterial prosthesis. Surg. Gynecol. Obstet. 139:445, 1974.

B. DISEASES OF THE VEINS

Dorothy Karandanis

THROMBOPHLEBITIS

This disease is characterized by the thrombosis of blood within a vein, with variable inflammatory involvement of the vein wall. The anatomic location of the thrombus and the degree of inflammatory reaction will determine the clinical presentation.

Thrombophlebitis involving the lower extremity is common in the general adult population, and may develop spontaneously in a healthy person. Among hospitalized patients, however, the incidence is incredible; thrombophlebitis develops in 20 to 30 per cent of all surgical patients and in more than 50 per cent of patients undergoing prostatectomy or hip nailing. In many cases, the disease is subclinical, and special techniques are required to document its presence. Postpartum patients and those with chronic disease, terminal cancer, trauma, polycythemia vera, heart failure, or shock also are predisposed to the development of thrombophlebitis. The disease is rare in children and in paraplegics.

Recognition

SUPERFICIAL THROMBOPHLEBITIS

Thrombosis of superficial veins follows local trauma or intravenous therapy, or develops without known antecedent in the varicose veins of the lower extremity. The process is a local one, with heat, redness, swelling, and tenderness confined to the area about the involved vein. A tender thrombosed cord frequently is palpable. The extremity as a whole is not swollen, pallid, or cyanotic. The condition may be confused with bacterial cellulitis or lymphangitis, but the presence of high fever, elevated white blood cell count, tachycardia, or lymphadenopathy helps to differentiate these conditions from superficial thrombophlebitis

Thrombosis of the deep veins of the lower extremity occurs as three distinct clinical types, and is easily distinguished from superficial thrombophlebitis.

PRESENTATIONS OF DEEP VEIN THROMBOSIS

Phlegmasia alba dolens (White, painful inflammation). So-called "milk leg," or extensive deep vein thrombophlebitis, or iliofemoral thrombophlebitis is recognized by swelling of the entire extremity from the toes to the inguinal canal. There is tenderness over the vessels in the groin, and arterial spasm may be present, with decrease in arterial pulsation and pallor or mottling, accounting for the "alba" (white). Onset is sudden, usually developing fully in less than 24 hours. The site of the thrombosis is in the femoral vein above the profunda femoris; many times, the thrombus extends into the external iliac vein up to the common iliac vein. Bed rest and elevation do not cause the swelling to subside, in contrast to localized deep thrombophlebitis. The patient who presents with iliofemoral thrombophlebitis usually has sustained abdominal or pelvic surgery or trauma, or is in the postpartum period.

Phlegmasia cerulea dolens (Blue, painful inflammation). This condition develops when all the veins of the leg are thrombosed (massive deep vein thrombophlebitis), and blood cannot return to the heart. It represents a progression of iliofemoral thrombophlebitis, with extension of the thrombus into the first portion of the vena cava and thrombosis of the whole venous collateral bed of the leg. The leg is swollen, cool, and cyanotic; ischemic tissues covered with blebs may be present, and the toes and foot may be gangrenous.

Localized deep thrombophlebitis. In contrast to the above three presentations of thrombophlebitis, localized deep thrombophlebitis may be clinically inapparent and very difficult to diagnose. The thrombi originate in the deep veins of the calf or the thigh, but clinical symptoms are more prominent when the thrombi are in the calf. There may be very little impairment of function, the thrombus causing either no symptoms or simply a calf heaviness or pain on motion. The involved leg may swell, become slightly cyanotic with use, and clear rapidly with elevation and rest. The swelling may be very slight, and only accurate measurement of calf circumference may bring this out. Swelling above the knee usually is absent. There may be calf or thigh tenderness; pain in the calf or popliteal area on dorsiflexion of the foot with the knee extended (Homans' sign) is a helpful maneuver. More sensitive is the blood pressure cuff test. The cuff is placed about the thigh or the calf and inflated; in the absence of local pathology, patients ordinarily do not complain of pain below 180 mm. Hg. Pain in the 60 to 150 mm. Hg range is considered a positive test. To establish the diagnosis of localized deep thrombophlebitis in doubtful cases, phlebography or scanning after administration of I-125 labeled fibrinogen may be required. Use of a Doppler apparatus by an experienced person may aid diagnosis.

A clinically silent process corresponds pathologically to minimal inflammatory reaction in the wall of the vein, and the terms "phlebothrombosis" or "bland thrombus" are commonly used to connote this. Thrombophlebitis may extend proximally by propagation of a clot tail into the larger veins. In some patients, this clot propagating in the larger veins adheres to the vein wall, causes inflammation, and may ultimately lead to "milk leg"; in others, the clot is bland and simply waves freely in the stream of blood. In this latter situation, pulmonary embolization is more likely to occur, and may be the first manifestation of thrombophlebitis.

Treatment

Thrombosis of superficial veins is usually a self-limited disease. Analgesics, elevation to relieve dependency edema, and elastic stockings are all that is required. Anticoagulation is not indicated.

Treatment of iliofemoral thrombophlebitis should be designed to prevent further acute complications (e.g., the development of phlegmasia cerulea dolens) and to avoid, if possible, the complication of venous insufficiency. Further thrombus formation is effectively halted by anticoagulation and elevation, thus averting any immediate threat to life and limb. Anticoagulation will not lyse existing thrombi; these will become organized, a process that destroys the valves. When recanalization is complete, permitting the flow of blood, the direction of blood flow will not be guided by valves. This postphlebitic limb will be subject to dependent edema with pain and ulceration. To prevent damage to the valves of the deep veins, therefore, it is recommended by some that thrombectomy under local anesthesia be performed as soon as possible, before organization (which is fairly advanced two weeks after the onset of symptoms) results in a clot that is difficult to remove.

The treatment of phlegmasia cerulea dolens includes, in addition to anticoagulation and elevation, vena cava ligation or plication prior to thrombectomy, and amputation of areas of gangrene.

Localized deep thrombophlebitis is treated with anticoagulation and elevation to prevent extension of the thrombus. Thrombectomy usually is not performed, since the small number of involved veins usually does not result in a postphlebitic limb. If a pulmonary embolus occurs in the anticoagulated patient, ligation of the appropriate vessels, if they are known for certain, or interruption of the vena cava, is indicated.

In all forms of thrombophlebitis elevation, calf exercises, early ambulation, and elastic stockings (if tolerated by the patient) help to prevent stasis and further propagation of thrombi. In some instances, so much of the venous return is carried by the superficial veins that elastic stockings compromise the venous return and result in extreme pain. In these cases, external compression should not be used.

Fluid replacement must be adequate to prevent hypotension in patients in whom large amounts of fluid are sequestered in the swollen extremity. Conversely, as the swollen limb improves and the edema clears, congestive heart failure must be guarded against.

Since anticoagulation is immediate with heparin, it is preferred to Coumadin for initiating therapy. Various heparin treatment regimens have been recommended. Heparin may be given by the intermittent intravenous route every four hours in a dose of 5000 to 10,000 units; continuously by intravenous drip (40,000 units in 1000 cc. 5 per cent glucose adjusted to flow about 10 drops per minute); or it may be given subcutaneously, using a very concentrated solution of heparin (20,000 to 40,000 units per ml.) depositing 10,000 units with a No. 25 gauge needle subcutaneously every eight to 12 hours. The Lee-White clotting time is tested just prior to the next injection. The dosage is regulated to keep the clotting time between two and two-and-one-half times normal. In continuous intravenous therapy, the rate of administration is adjusted to keep the clotting time within this level at all times. Good results also have been reported with intermittent intravenous therapy, giving 12,000 units three or four times a day without monitoring clotting time.

Heparin therapy should be continued until the thrombus has become fixed to the endothelial wall and the predisposing factors for thrombosis have been eliminated. Experimentally, a bland peripheral thrombus will become adherent to the vein wall after a period of about eight to ten days. Venous stasis, which is the most important predisposing factor to venous thrombosis, is reduced when the patient is fully ambulatory, or able to perform calf muscle exercises, or when the limb is elevated above heart level. Thus, heparin therapy should be continued for at least eight days, and may be discontinued at that time if the patient is fully ambulatory, or exercising, or is able to have the limb in an elevated position.

Complications

PULMONARY EMBOLISM

It is impossible to state the incidence of pulmonary embolism in thrombophlebitis, since so many cases of the latter remain undiagnosed and resolve without complication. It is certain, however, that a sharp drop in deaths from pulmonary embolism (ten- to twentyfold in some studies) has followed the introduction of heparin for the treatment of suspected and proved thrombophlebitis. Use of low-dose prophylactic heparin in those at high risk of developing thromboembolic disease has been shown in various studies to be both safe and very effective. Aspirin also has been used as a preventive measure owing to its effect on platelets.

VENOUS INSUFFICIENCY

Although unusual following superficial or localized deep thrombophlebitis, venous insufficiency is a frequent sequela to iliofemoral thrombophlebitis, even with administration of adequate heparin. According to some, the only way regularly to prevent venous insufficiency is to remove surgically the iliofemoral clot as soon as possible after the onset of symptoms.

HEMORRHAGIC COMPLICATIONS OF HEPARIN ADMINISTRATION

Significant bleeding during heparin therapy has been infrequent (less than 5 per cent), and only rarely is the cause of significant morbidity or mortality. Among the hemorrhagic manifestations noted are hematemesis following gastric surgery, wound hematoma in postoperative patients, retroperitoneal or bowel wall hematoma, hemarthrosis, microscopic hematuria, and hematoma at venipuncture sites.

Contraindications to the use of heparin include potential or actual gastrointestinal bleeding, blood dyscrasias (especially increased permeability and increased fragility of capillaries), and neurocerebral injury with blood in the spinal fluid. Severe hypertension should be controlled prior to initiation of heparin therapy.

VENOUS INSUFFICIENCY

Failure of the venous valves occurs most commonly in the lower extremity. The valves of the superficial veins, the deep veins, or the valves of the perforating veins that connect the superficial and the deep systems may be involved. Other sites of venous insufficiency (not to be discussed here) include the anal canal, the esophagus in cases of portal hypertension, and the broad ligament.

Clinically significant venous insufficiency usually is the result of a prior episode of thrombophlebitis of the deep veins. Many patients presenting with sequelae of venous insufficiency give a definite history of deep venous thrombosis. Follow-up of large series of patients with extensive deep vein thrombosis shows that 70 per cent develop clinical evidence of venous insufficiency in ten years, and the number increases to 90 per cent if the patients are followed for 15 to 20 years. Other causes of clinically significant venous insufficiency include arterial venous fistulas and congenital absence of valves.

It is estimated that one out of five adult women and one out of 15 adult men have insufficiency of the superficial veins (varicose veins); that 7 million Americans have venous insufficiency severe enough to result in stasis changes in the skin of the legs; and that 20 per cent of these have a venous ulcer.

In the motionless upright position, the venous pressure in the foot (whether or not the valves are competent) approximates that of a column of blood extending from the foot to the heart, about 100 mm. Hg. Venous return from the lower extremity in the upright position, and relief of the high venous pressure in the foot, depend heavily on the activity of the calf muscles. Contraction of these muscles results in a pressure of about 140 mm. Hg in the veins of the calf, and causes them to empty. Blood flow is directed from distal to proximal, and from superficial to deep, by means of valves. As the muscles relax, the venous pressure in the veins of the calf is lowered to about 40 mm. Hg, reflux is prevented by closure of the valve cusps, and more blood enters the "pumping chambers" from the muscles and from the superficial veins by way of the perforating veins. The net result is an increase in blood flow toward the heart and a fall in pressure in the distal superficial veins (even though the superficial veins are not surrounded by a muscle pump). The thigh muscles exert a much lower pressure on exercise, and contribute far less to venous return than the calf muscle with its dense fascia, numerous valves, and its system of perforating veins.

Recognition

VENOUS INSUFFICIENCY CONFINED TO THE SUPERFICIAL VEINS

The superficial veins appear enlarged, elongated, and tortuous. The disease frequently is clinically insignificant. Patients may complain of aching, heaviness, cramping, itching, and burning of the involved extremity, with edema on prolonged standing. There may be occasional spontaneous rupture of a skin venule, or the varicosed vein may become involved in a superficial thrombophlebitis. After many years of involvement, skin changes about the ankle and lower leg, such as telangiectasia, pigmentation, and eczema, may occur. Stasis ulcers are unusual.

VENOUS INSUFFICIENCY OF THE PERFORATING VEINS

Calf muscle contraction causes blood to be directed toward the heart via the deep veins, but, in the presence of incompetent perforating veins, blood is forced into the superficial veins, resulting in venous hypertension of the superficial venous system. This leads to dilatation, elongation, tortuosity, and, finally, incompetence of the superficial system. More important, however, venous hypertension in the perforating veins is reflected in the venules and capillaries of the ankle. If untreated, venous hypertension secondary to incompetent perforating veins leads, inevitably, over a period of years, to the well known sequelae of venular dilatation, edema, pigmentation, induration, and ulceration.

VENOUS INSUFFICIENCY OF THE DEEP VEINS

Most of the venous return from the lower extremity to the heart takes place through the deep veins. During a bout of deep vein thrombophlebitis, superficial veins and other collaterals dilate and accomplish venous return. Phlebography readily demonstrates the newly-opened channels. Recanalization of the thrombosed vein occurs slowly and usually is complete in two years. (In some cases of iliofemoral thrombophlebitis, recanalization never occurs.) The most significant effect of recanalization is that blood will flow without directional control, since the valves in a segment of vein have been destroyed by the thrombophlebitis. In many instances, the vein involved is small or unimportant, and, despite the fact that it is incompetent, there are few or no clinical sequelae. In some instances, however, return of the blood to the heart is compromised, and venous hypertension results, followed by stasis, edema, and so on. In such cases, function actually would be better if the venous return continued through the dilated superficial veins and collaterals whose valves had not been destroyed by thrombophlebitis.

Clinically significant insufficiency of the deep veins frequently is accompanied by, or results in, insufficiency of the perforating veins. Incompetent perforating veins are more numerous, and even more clinically important in the presence of deep venous insufficiency than when occurring alone.

A variety of simple but elegant tourniquet tests have been devised to differentiate accurately the various types and combinations of venous insufficiency. In brief, insufficiency of a superficial system can be demonstrated by elevating the limb to empty the vein, then applying a tourniquet to the superior section of the vein in question, and having the patient arise. Release of the tourniquet results in rapid retrograde filling of the vein if the superficial vein is incompetent. To check the perforating veins, the above is repeated, but the tourniquet is not released. If the perforating veins are incompetent, the vein will fill from below in 20 to 30 seconds. If both deep and perforating veins are incompetent, the superficial veins fill so rapidly from below that one can hardly perform the retrograde filling test. If a superficial vein, engorged following application of a tourniquet, empties on walking with tourniquet in place, the perforators are competent.

In addition to tourniquet tests, phlebography usually is performed to ascertain the state of the entire venous system of the limb, if surgery is to be performed.

Treatment

Venous insufficiency results in a hydrostatic load that leads to interstitial edema. Chronic accumulation of edema is responsible for all the complications. If treatment is successful in controlling edema, an incompetent venous system will not lead to crippling disease. Control of edema requires firm external elastic support and frequent periods of elevation. These simple measures may produce wondrous results and healing. Surgery is required sometimes, however.

Elastic support usually is all that is needed to control the edema and the subjective symptoms that result from insufficiency of the superficial veins. For cosmetic reasons, ligation, division, and extraction of the varicose veins may be performed. Insufficiency of the deep veins and ankle perforators also responds to firm elastic support and periods of elevation. Surgical elimination of incompetent superficial and perforating veins should be carried out when the first signs of venous dilatation at the ankle, and skin irritation or discoloration, appear (between four and five years after a deep vein thrombosis). Despite the associated deep venous insufficiency, there is good response to surgery of the incompetent superficial and perforating veins. Congestion, discoloration, and dermatitis clear, and many patients may not have to wear elastic support.

In cases with persistent iliofemoral vein obstruction, vein by-pass surgery may be indicated, but the results are not dependable. Relief of ankle edema and its consequences still may require surgery of the superficial and perforating veins, but an adequate collateral channel must be demonstrated prior to extirpation of the superficial varicosities. These patients need unremitting elastic support and frequent periods of elevation.

Complications

Hyperpigmentation of the skin and recurrent eczematoid reactions are a consequence of the edema of venous insufficiency. Hyperpigmentation, largely a hemosiderin deposition, results from capillary stasis and hemorrhage. Stasis also results in a lowered oxygen content of the blood, predisposing to necrosis and ulceration. Interstitial fibrosis reduces the blood supply further by compressing the capillaries.

Ulceration is uncommon if only the superficial veins are incompetent. Phlebography shows that patients with swollen ulcerated legs have incompetent perforating veins, and either deep venous incompetence or incompetence of localized calf veins.

Iliofemoral thrombosis without recanalization may be followed by chronic edema of the entire extremity and, occasionally, by lymphedema.

SUPERIOR VENA CAVAL OBSTRUCTION

Obstruction of the superior vena cava produces an easily recognized clinical syndrome. Malignancy (especially bronchogenic carcinoma) accounts for over 75 per cent of all cases. The majority of patients have a carcinoma of the right upper lobe, and roughly 2 per cent of all lung cancers are complicated by superior vena caval obstruction. Less common etiologies include granulomatous or fibrosing mediastinitis secondary to tuberculosis, syphilis, or histoplasmosis. Intrathoracic thyroid, aortic aneurysm, traumatic mediastinal hematoma, irradiation therapy, and infusion of irritating solutions into the superior vena cava also may lead to obstruction. Rarely, obstruction occurs secondary to congestive heart failure, or occurs spontaneously.

There are four main pathways of collateral circulation when the superior vena cava is obstructed: internal mammary, vertebral, azygos, and lateral thoracic. Both the azygos and lateral thoracic veins communicate with the inferior vena cava, and the internal mammary communicates with the vertebral and the azygos. Thus, several routes are available to return blood to the heart. If the azygos orifice into the superior vena cava is obstructed, the flow will be directed to the inferior vena cava. If the azygos anastomosis with the superior vena cava is patent, blood from the head and upper extremity will find its way to the lower unobstructed portion of the superior vena cava by way of the azygos vein, and thence to the heart.

Recognition

Early signs include congestion of the conjunctiva, facial cyanosis, and the appearance of small venules over the chest wall. If the caval obstruction has occurred rapidly, as often is the case in malignancy, in dissecting aneurysm, or when irritating solutions are infused into the superior vena cava, headache, somnolence, respiratory distress, convulsions, periorbital edema, and proptosis may occur because of the sudden rise in the intracranial pressure. There may be edema of the head, neck, arms, and dorsum of the hands and tachycardia with hypotension. As the obstruction becomes more chronic, engorgement and tortuosity of the veins of the head, neck, arms, chest, and abdomen appear. The cyanosis and congestion are confined to the upper half of the body, readily differentiating this condition from constrictive pericarditis and cor pulmonale. All findings are more striking in the recumbent position, and are especially exaggerated when the patient bends over. Venous pressure in the arms is elevated to 200 to 500 mm. H_2O, while the venous pressure in the lower extremities in the supine patient remains a normal 60 to 120 mm. H_2O.

Treatment

If the obstruction develops rapidly, producing cerebral symptoms and deterioration in vital signs, dramatic improvement sometimes may be obtained by decreasing the intravascular volume through the use of diuretics or phlebotomy. Emergency thrombectomy should be considered if the obstruction is due to benign cause, such as infusion of irritating solutions. In most situations, however, the occlusion has occurred more gradually, allowing time for the development of an adequate collateral circulation. In these cases, emergency treatment generally is not required, and eventual treatment will depend on the underlying condition. Most patients tolerate obstruction of the superior vena cava very well, developing adequate collaterals, with a decrease or a disappearance of clinical symptoms over a period of months or years. Thus, if the underlying condition is benign, no specific therapy need be directed at relieving the obstruction if it developed slowly and the patient is comfortable. If the obstruction is due to a rapidly growing malignant lesion, radiation therapy, with or without chemotherapy, is used for palliation; this frequently results in a remission of the symptoms of superior vena caval obstruction. The prognosis is very good in benign disease, but very poor when the disease is malignant.

Complications

Pulmonary emboli are an extremely unusual complication of thrombosis of the superior vena cava. Grafts to by-pass the obstruction usually are not recommended, as these frequently become thrombosed.

References

Abramson, D. I.: Vascular Disorders of the Extremities. 2nd ed. Hagerstown, Maryland, Harper and Rowe, 1974.

Banker, V. P., and Maddeson, F. E.: Superior vena cava syndrome secondary to aortic disease: report of two cases and review of the literature. Dis. Chest. 51:656, 1967.

Bauer, G.: A roentgenological and clinical study of the sequels of thrombosis. Acta Chir. Scand. 86:74, 1942. (Suppl.)

Bauer, G.: Nine years' experience with heparin in acute venous thrombosis. Angiology 1:161, 1950.

Bauer, G.: Clinical experiences of a surgeon in the use of heparin. Am. J. Cardiol. 14:29, 1964.

Brown, R. C., Nelson, C. M. K., and Petronio, T. L.: Angiographic demonstration of collateral circulation in a patient with superior vena caval syndrome. Am. J. Roentgenol. Radium Ther. Nucl. Med. 119:543, 1973.

Cockett, F. B.: The post-phlebitic syndrome. Proc. R. Soc. Med. 63:131, 1970.

Coon, W. W., Park, W. W., and Keller, J. B.: Venous thromboembolism and other venous disease in the Tecumseh Community health study. Circulation 48:839, 1973.

Davis, L. Christopher's Textbook of Surgery. 9th ed. Philadelphia, W. B. Saunders Co., 1968.

Dodd, H., and Cockett, F. B.: The Pathology and Surgery of the Veins of the Lower Limb. Edinburgh, E. S. Livingstone, Ltd., 1956.

Effler, D. B., and Grove, L. K.: Super vena caval obstruction. J. Thorac. Cardiovasc. Surg. 43:574, 1962.

Griffith, G. C., and Boggs, R. P.: The clinical usage of heparin. Am. J. Cardiol. 14:39, 1964.

Haller, J. A., Jr.: Deep thrombophlebitis. Pathophysiology and treatment. Major Probl. Clin. Surg. 6:1, 1967.

Haller, J. A., Jr.: Pathophysiology and management of postphlebitic venous insufficiency. South. Med. J. 63:177, 1970.

Homans, J.: Thrombosis of the deep veins of the lower leg causing pulmonary embolism. N. Engl. J. Med. 211:993, 1934.

Lofgren, K. A.: Treatment of varicose veins. Mod. Treat. 2:1121, 1965.

Lowenberg, R. I.: Early diagnosis of phlebothrombosis with aid of a new clinical test. J.A.M.A. 155:1566, 1954.

Negus, D.: The post-thrombotic syndrome. Ann. R. Coll. Surg. Engl. 47:92, 1970.

Neuschatz, J., and Crosby, W. H.: The prevention of postoperative thrombosis—a simple, safe approach. Arch. Intern. Med. 130:966, 1972.

O'Sullivan, E. F., et al.: Heparin in the treatment of venous thromboembolic disease: administration, control, and results. Med. J. Aust. 2:153, 1968.

Provan, J. L., and Thomson, C.: Natural history of thrombophlebitis and its relationship to pulmonary embolism. Can. J. Surg. 16:284, 1973.

Siderys, H., and Rowe, G. A.: Superior vena caval syndrome caused by intrathoracic goiter. Am. Surg. 36:446, 1970.

Skinner, D. B., Salzman, E. W., and Scannell, J. G.: The challenge of superior vena caval obstruction. J. Thorac. Cardiovasc. Surg. 49:824, 1965.

Smyrnis, S. A., and Kolios, A. S.: Deep vein thrombosis in surgical patients: a phlebographic study. Surgery 73:692, 1973.

Chapter 43

GASTROINTESTINAL EMERGENCIES

A. INTRODUCTION

H. Harlan Stone

With few exceptions, patients suffering from acute disease of an intra-abdominal organ present with pain, bleeding, jaundice, or some combination thereof. Other signs and symptoms may indeed prove to be valuable aids in arriving at the correct diagnosis, or in dictating some more appropriate course of management; yet such additional findings often are merely reflex phenomena, e.g., nausea and vomiting, and may by no means be specifically related to the underlying pathologic process.

(1) *Pain* is probably the most useful of all subjective data. As a general rule, unremitting pain is caused by inflammation. An almost instantaneous onset or the sudden worsening of pain usually indicates an origin from either a vascular accident or rupture of some hollow viscus. Intermittent or so-called "colicky" pain, on the other hand, develops whenever there has been actual anatomic obstruction to the lumen of a peristaltic hollow conduit (e.g., bowel, ureter, cervical os, etc.). Thus, a more precise characterization of pain, that is, whether it is steady or intermittent, easily and relatively accurately differentiates inflammations from nongangrenous mechanical obstructions.

Initially, most pain is visceral in origin and, for conscious appreciation, must be referred to that dermatome served by its specific somatic nerve counterpart. However, with progression and thus extension of the disease process, direct stimulation of parietal nerve endings eventually occurs. This then leads to a significant alteration in the pain pattern because of the almost universal dominance of somatic over visceral afferent impulses. Accordingly, it is this change in the character or location of abdominal discomfort, no matter how slight, that can be so critical a factor in the emergency differential diagnosis of acute abdominal pain.

(2) *Bleeding* into the peritoneal cavity uniformly initiates so mild an inflammatory reaction, that, in the absence of associated conditions such as abdominal wall trauma, either acute anemia or hypovolemic shock becomes the presenting feature. Likewise, hemorrhage into the lumen of the gastrointestinal, urinary, or reproductive tract is usually a relatively painless event that, accordingly, becomes the single most impressive clinical finding.

(3) Lastly, although *jaundice* is not always due to diseases of the liver or biliary duct system, its more frequent association with such diseases makes investigation of these areas absolutely mandatory.

Thus, by using three simple criteria—abdominal pain (be it steady or intermittent), bleeding (into the free peritoneal cavity or into some hollow viscus), and jaundice—the majority of acute abdominal conditions can be sorted easily and rapidly into specific categories that are much more conducive to refinements in diagnosis and initial therapy.

B. INFLAMMATIONS

H. Harlan Stone

PRELIMINARY CONSIDERATIONS

SYMPTOMS

Inflammatory disease within the peritoneal cavity is generally characterized by unremitting abdominal pain or discomfort. Gradual intensification of this pain is associated with the more commonly encountered inflammatory conditions, e.g., penetrating peptic ulcer, acute cholecystitis, pancreatitis, or nongangrenous appendicitis. On the other hand, the rapid worsening of symptoms or a sudden onset of severe abdominal pain at first usually indicates hollow viscus perforation or some vascular catastrophe as a direct complication of the primary disease state.

Splanchnic pain arising as the conscious appreciation of gastrointestinal pathology almost always is referred to its corresponding dermatome, usually is midline, and routinely is nonspecific. Foregut diseases (stomach and duodenum) give symptoms that are epigastric in location; midgut problems (small bowel and right and transverse colons) generally are referred to the periumbilical region; hindgut inflammations (descending and sigmoid colons) have infraumbilical and suprapubic representation.

Since the liver, biliary tract, and pancreas have embryologic origins from the foregut, their initial symptoms accordingly are reflected as epigastric pain. Wider extension of these inflammations eventually leads to irritation of parietal peritoneum in the immediate proximity of the involved organ; thus, overt conscious recognition of the inflammatory locale is of that part of the abdominal topography now receiving maximal stimulation by the resultant suppurative exudate.

Local abdominal tenderness merely confirms the existence of such peritoneal irritation as previously has been furnished by the patient in relating his subjective symptomatology. Since individual reactivity to direct palpation may be confusing, particularly if the patient has a relatively low pain threshold, resort to rebound tenderness generally identifies the site of maximal parietal irritation with much greater accuracy. Rectal examination is just another method of eliciting rebound tenderness, although lateralization to one side or the other and the presence of a discrete pelvic mass are additional items of useful information.

Muscle spasm (or, as it is more commonly called "guarding") is said to be involuntary whenever the inflammatory process is intense, is located directly beneath the area palpated, and is maintained as a continuous muscular contraction. With voluntary guarding, there is, instead, a conscious response on the part of the patient to protect himself against real or anticipated pain consequent to abdominal wall stimulation. A warm hand, left in contact with the abdominal wall for several minutes, usually will permit the examiner to distinguish between these two forms of muscle spasm.

In cases of peritonitis not arising from progression of mechanical intestinal obstruction to bowel gangrene, the onset and severity of nausea, vomiting, and obstipation generally parallel the development and completeness of an adynamic ileus. Audible peristaltic activity similarly reflects the degree of this intestinal paralysis.

With any inflammatory process, presence of a palpable mass suggests induration of a specific abdominal organ, confinement of purulent exudate to a given anatomic region of the abdomen, or even further localization of the infection into a single, well-defined intra-abdominal abscess. Essentially, all such masses are exquisitely tender. Similar findings can be noted on rectal as well as bimanual pelvic examination.

Other remarkable findings that may be associated with peritonitis are: the presence, and especially the tenderness, of an abdominal or groin hernia; fistulous tracts on an acute or chronic basis, with communication to a pre-existing abscess or to some segment of the intestinal tract; and fresh, healing, or mature wounds of the abdominal wall, whether accidentally acquired or produced by operation. Nevertheless, only the combination of a thorough medical history of the present illness, careful inspection of the fully exposed abdomen, and the intelligently executed rectal and/or pelvic examination can insure against the omission of some highly significant item from the emergency data base. This is indeed one time when haste makes waste.

DIAGNOSIS

Routine laboratory tests always should include a complete blood count and urine analysis. Some rapid measurement of red cell mass (hematocrit or hemoglobin) is extremely useful, as it gives evidence of an already established anemia, provides some estimate of the severity of dehydration, or serves as a base line for future reference when hemorrhage is the immediate problem.

The white blood count, with differential, generally reflects the intensity of any inflammatory process. Extreme leukocytosis (greater than 25,000 WBC/cu. mm.) and leukopenia (less than 5000 WBC/cu. mm.) are noted in cases of profound sepsis, or even septic shock. In addition, it is well to rule out the possibility of leukemia, as misdiagnosis can lead to an unnecessary operation and, thus, confrontation with a difficult bleeding diathesis.

Urinalysis is of utmost importance in detecting the presence of urinary tract infection, which may coexist or which may itself alone be responsible for all the patient's symptoms. Pyuria and bacilluria are the prime findings in such cases. Other abnormalities of diagnostic value are the hematuria associated with renal trauma, stone, or tumor; albuminuria of chronic renal disease itself; and isosthenuria of altered tubule function. Equally critical is the recognition of glycosuria in the diabetic (who may present in ketoacidosis with abdominal pain as a prominent symptom); and bile in the urine of patients with liver or biliary tract disease. Other substances occurring abnormally in the urine, such as porphyrins, lead salts, etc., also may warrant attempts at detection under specific circumstances. The gross appearance of the urine (reddened) is an important clue in diagnosing acute intermittent porphyria. In some cases of pancreatitis, the serum amylase may not be elevated, but the two-hour urine amylase will be.

Blood chemistries certainly are valuable in assessing the presence and severity of pre-existing disease states, as well as the magnitude of derangements caused by the acute peritoneal inflammation itself. Serum electrolytes (sodium, potassium, chloride, and carbon dioxide combining power), blood urea nitrogen (BUN), and blood glucose are standards. However, even more useful in arriving at the etiologic basis of the peritonitis are serum concentrations of amylase and bilirubin (both total and direct). Other determinations that often prove useful in the problem case are serum uric acid, calcium, and one or more of the various liver enzymes (especially SGOT).

Even when there is a significantly altered laboratory result, greater reliance almost always must be placed on the patient's history of his present illness and on repeated physical examinations. Laboratory data in general merely provide confirmatory information and guides to more energetic supportive care.

Radiographic study is much more productive in arriving at the correct diagnosis than are any of the standard laboratory tests. Plain films of the supine abdomen will give some idea as to solid organ locations, size, and contour; bowel patterns in relation to displacement, distention, and distribution of intraluminal gas; abnormal masses; free intra-abdominal gas; and the presence as well as approximate quantity of peritoneal fluid.

The upright chest x-ray is almost as important, for it may reveal subdiaphragmatic free gas, pneumonia as the true cause of abdominal symptomatology, sympathetic pleural effusion, and previously unrecognized cardiopulmonary pathology (of major consideration in effecting supportive care, and in both inducing and maintaining anesthesia).

Contrast studies often are required also. Simple air insufflation of the stomach essentially is never contraindicated, since it furnishes information about the size and location of adjacent upper abdominal viscera, and increases the physician's ability to distinguish free intraperitoneal gas in cases of gastroduodenal perforation. On the other hand, barium swallow and upper gastrointestinal series are seldom warranted, except to identify esophageal and esophagogastric pathology and completeness, as well as the probable cause of gastric outlet obstruction. Barium enema is indicated much more frequently, especially to detect the presence of and to determine the level and basis for large bowel obstructions. Only the possibility of a free perforation of the colon contraindicates use of the barium enema, although associated inflammatory processes demand that greater than usual care be taken in introducing the barium suspension.

Intravenous cholangiography (IVC) often is almost diagnostic of cholecystitis and pancreatitis, but nonvisualization of both gallbladder and common bile duct is meaningless. Clinical symptoms and signs usually are more valuable indicators. A much more reliable study is the intravenous pyelogram (IVP), which not only accurately defines upper urinary tract pathology, but also distinguishes most sizeable masses in the retroperitoneal space.

Other diagnostic studies of a more specialized nature indeed may be required, yet such generally are reserved for the patient with either a more perplexing and as yet unresolved problem or with a certain diagnosis that demands better anatomic definition. Accordingly, resorting to sonography or selective arteriography has seldom been necessary on an emergency basis for inflammatory conditions, even though these have proved to be exceedingly valuable diagnostic adjuncts in selected cases; also, the selective arteriography provides a new therapeutic tool — intra-arterial infusion of Pitressin and norepinephrine in GI bleeding.

The abdominal tap, carried out after studies to detect free air, may be of value in detecting free blood in the peritoneal cavity.*

The development of fiberoptic endoscopy has simplified analysis of gastrointestinal problems, particularly bleeding. If endoscopy is to be performed, there should not be massive uncontrolled hemorrhage; moreover, it should take place prior to any barium studies.

SPECIFIC INFLAMMATIONS

Esophagitis

Inflammation of the distal esophagus usually is caused by gastric acid regurgitation, and is by far the most frequent and most significant complication of hiatal hernia. Often there is also a history typical for peptic ulcer disease. Otherwise, symptoms of esophagitis are so prominent that they suppress the conscious appreciation of essentially all other visceral sensations. Finally, one unfortunately all too common cause of esophagitis is the ingestion of some caustic, usually a strong alkali such as lye.

The *pain* of esophagitis is steady and substernal in location (Fig. 1). Inflammation

---

*See page 356.

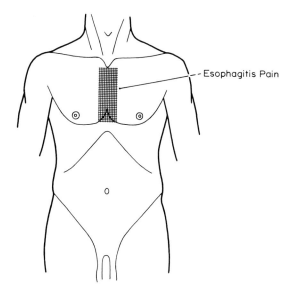

Figure 1. Location of pain of esophagitis.

of the terminal esophagus or esophagogastric junction usually is referred to the mid- or upper sternum, although perixiphoid or epigastric discomfort occasionally may be dominant, particularly if peptic ulcer disease of the stomach or duodenum coexists. Pain is intensified by swallowing, is then accompanied by a fullness in the same areas, and may be relieved dramatically by the eructation of gas or food. However, vomiting can instead worsen or even initiate a similar pain pattern. Such changes in symptoms as induced by vomiting apparently are related to whether that portion of the esophagus proximal to any terminal esophageal obstruction has thereby been decompressed, or whether gastric acid has refluxed up through a segment of esophagus, further irritating an already inflamed mucosa. Because of the close association of chronic symptoms with eating, patients with established esophagitis usually show obvious weight loss. A new development, now being clinically tested, may have future diagnostic use. A mixture of 10–15 cc. of viscous Xylocaine and 20 cc. of antacid is given orally. Initial testing indicates that patients with pain from esophagitis experience marked relief within minutes.

Complications of esophagitis include obstruction, bleeding, and perforation, in decreasing order of frequency. Obstruction can be due to the spasm of acute esophagitis, or to scar contracture developing after only a few months of inflammation. Hemorrhage is rarely massive, but chronic minor bleeding, together with a restricted dietary intake, may account for an otherwise unexplained iron-deficiency anemia. Perforation almost always is the direct result of either endoscopy instrumentation or erosion by an ingested foreign body or caustic agent. Spontaneous esophageal perforation, on the other hand, occurs through a relatively uninflamed esophageal mucosa at the time of forceful vomiting, and bears little relationship to either acute or chronic esophagitis.

Physical findings are quite impressive, that is, except for lip and mouth burns if an acid or alkali has been swallowed, associated malnutrition, the extreme discomfort often produced by an acute episode of pain, or malodorous breath when terminal esophageal obstruction has led to repeated eructations of undigested food from a dilated proximal gullet.

Diagnosis is supported by a barium swallow demonstrating distal esophageal spasm or stenosis, together with an upper gastrointestinal series to identify an associated hiatal hernia or pepetic ulcer. In cases of esophageal obstruction leading to megaesophagus, the esophagus should be aspirated until it is as empty as possible before the patient is sent to be x-rayed. These same radiographic studies are also of aid in differentiating specific causes of esophagitis and, in particular, other reasons for esophageal obstruction, such as tumor or foreign body. Nevertheless, absolute confirmation of the diagnosis of esophagitis can be made only by esophagoscopy, with biopsy of the inflamed mucosa when appropriate. This usually requires hospital admission and several days of postendoscopy observation.

Treatment in the uncomplicated case is directed toward neutralization of the inciting gastric acid. A bland, soft, and possibly even puréed diet and antacids, are therefore prescribed. However. these are only temporary measures, as any associated hiatal hernia or peptic ulcer disease usually requires an operation aimed at correcting any anatomic defect at the esophageal hiatus and/or controlling the acid peptic diathesis.

If obstruction in the terminal esophagus is present, emptying the more proximal esophagus and differentiating the various possible causes of such obstruction definitely are warranted. In addition, the patient will always show evidences of inanition as well as dehydration, for which intravenous fluid therapy is indicated.

Esophagitis caused by an ingested caustic agent should be managed somewhat differently because of its greater propensity for both perforation and later cicatricial occlusion. Following initial evaluation, esophagoscopy usually is performed to confirm the presence of a mucosal injury. Following this, either a soft nasogastric tube is passed, or the patient is asked to swallow a lead bead affixed to the end of a sturdy silk suture. The other end of the tube or suture is then taped to the patient's nose. By this means, an indwelling object prevents complete occlusion of the esophageal lumen when maximal swelling has been reached, and also provides a guide to make subsequent esophageal dilatation a much safer procedure. Antibiotics effective against gram-positive bacteria and anti-inflammatory steroids usually are added to the intravenous fluids given for water and electrolyte maintenance, although the benefit of such drugs has never been proved.

Gastritis

Inflammations of the gastric mucosa can develop on the basis of an ingested irritant, shock, atrophy, bile reflux, or hyperacidity. The process may be acute, subacute, or chronic. Epigastric pain is relatively constant, is characterized by a fullness rather than by any burning sensation, and rarely is relieved by taking food or an oral medication. Nausea, vomiting (occasionally persistent), and even diffuse mucosal bleeding are other symptoms. Mild epigastric tenderness, often associated with voluntary guarding, is generally the only positive physical finding.

The diagnosis of acute gastritis can be confirmed only by gastroscopy, although symptoms usually are sufficient to warrant initiation of therapy, and, if this is met with success, to justify such a diagnostic assumption without further study. Subacute and chronic symptoms always require gastroscopy, as well as upper gastrointestinal series, to identify the specific basis for gastritis, and thereby to dictate definitive therapy directed at correction of the individual cause.

For the acute case, antacids and bland liquids should be prescribed until symptoms have subsided. Nausea seldom, if ever, can be relieved by any medication other than a sedative. If vomiting recurs or persists, hospital admission is required, with gastric decompression by a nasogastric tube until nausea has disappeared. Dehydration is routinely managed by appropriate intravenous fluids. Anticholinergic medications (such as propantheline) can be used to decrease acid secretion. However, to get a good therapeutic response, the dose must be sufficient to cause a marked dry mouth and, usually, blurring of vision. A dose of 30 mg. Pro-Banthine administered every three to four hours normally produces the desired effects.

Peptic Ulcer

SYMPTOMS

Peptic ulcers occur in both the stomach and duodenum. Although hyperacidity, the male sex, and a younger age tend to be associated with ulcerations of the duodenum, any gastric ulcer must always be differentiated from malignant neoplasia. Usually, those patients presenting at the Emergency

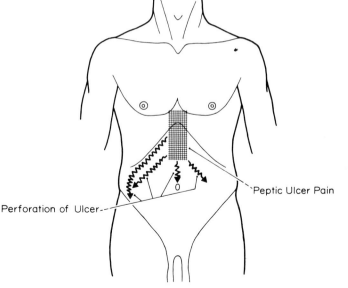

Figure 2. Locations of pain of uncomplicated and perforated peptic ulcer.

Department with ulcer disease have more severe symptoms, and are more likely to have one of the complications, e.g., hemorrhage, obstruction or perforation.

A well-taken patient history is critical to the diagnosis, especially in uncomplicated cases. Everything centers about the characteristic pain pattern. Pain is burning in nature; is located deep in the epigastrium (Fig. 2); develops when the stomach is empty (arising between meals or awakening the patient several hours past midnight, especially following a highly-seasoned dinner, multiple cups of coffee, or alcohol); is relieved by alkali, the ingestion of bland food (milk, crackers, etc.) or vomiting; and recurs periodically, often during phases of metabolic stress or emotional crisis. Symptoms may be acute without a similar prior experience, or may have been present continuously or intermittently for many years. Superimposed upon such a history may be the symptoms of a major complication: (1) upper gastrointestinal bleeding; (2) gastric outlet or duodenal obstruction; and (3) perforation.

Apart from poorly defined upper abdominal tenderness, physical examination of the patient with uncomplicated peptic ulcer disease is seldom remarkable. However, with hemorrhage, blood can be vomited and/or passed per rectum. Obvious bleeding, with or without hypovolemic shock, then becomes the dominant feature. The same is true of gastroduodenal obstructions, in which pain is minimal in the face of per-

sistent vomiting. Nevertheless, local pyloric or duodenal spasm associated with an acute ulcer may indeed mimic the obstruction produced by chronic scar of long term ulcer disease or a gastric tumor.

DIAGNOSIS AND TREATMENT

The diagnosis of an uncomplicated peptic ulcer is made by an x-ray contrast study, i.e., gastroduodenal series, with or without the addition of gastroscopy. Endoscopic biopsy or gastric washings for cytology are indicated only in order to rule out malignancy. Even though all specific studies are reported as negative, a characteristic patient history is sufficient for the diagnosis of active peptic ulcer disease, and therefore for the initiation of therapy.

Between-meal antacids, a multiple feeding bland diet and sedation (e.g., phenobarbital) usually are prescribed. If vomiting is a major factor, immediate hospitalization and nasogastric tube decompression should be instituted. The stomach is kept constantly buffered by antacids, bland food, or acid removal by suctioning. In patients with dehydration or electrolyte disturbances (potassium depletion, with or without resultant alkalosis), intravenous fluids are required, and should contain at least twice the daily requirement of potassium chloride. Close follow-up of all cases, whether hospitalized or not, is mandatory.

With *perforation*, there is the sudden

onset or intensification of epigastric pain, which then radiates almost immediately throughout the abdomen. This pain is usually so intense that the patient breathes in both a rapid and shallow fashion in a vain attempt to splint his abdominal musculature. In fact, he writhes from one position to another in search of some relief from the severe pain. Occasionally, however, the perforation is partially walled off by adhesions, so that gastroduodenal contents leak down the right abdominal gutter and elicit maximal pain in the right lower quadrant, thereby simulating acute appendicitis. For identical reasons, the irritating fluid may instead reach one or both of the diaphragms, and accordingly produce phrenic nerve-mediated supraclavicular pain.

On examination, the abdomen is exquisitely tender, and generally is described as being "boardlike" because of the extreme involuntary spasm of all ventral abdominal muscles. There are no peristaltic sounds, as adynamic ileus is almost instantaneously produced. An upright chest x-ray or lateral decubitus film of the abdomen will reveal free intraperitoneal air in the majority of cases, although its absence by no means rules out a perforation. Resorting to gastroscopy or a formal gastrointestinal series is contraindicated. Patient history and physical examination are more than adequate.

Emergency laparotomy to close the perforation is ideal treatment. Immediate passage of a nasogastric tube and its connection to suction, however, should be the first step taken, as this one measure will reduce considerably the magnitude of subsequent gastroduodenal spill into the peritoneal cavity. Owing to the generalized peritonitis, these patients have sequestered large quantities of extracellular fluid into the peritoneal cavity and accordingly require energetic fluid therapy to replace such losses. Saline or lactated Ringer's solution, occasionally supplemented by plasma, generally is used to resuscitate these patients from their acute dehydration shock. Once a relatively normal central venous pressure and an adequate urine output have been established, operation can be accomplished safely, provided potassium deficiencies have been corrected simultaneously. Antibiotics (e.g., ampicillin or one of the cephalosporins) are added to the intravenous fluids in order to combat any concomitant peritoneal contamination by gram-positive bacteria. Culture and sensitivity tests should be carried out at the time of operation.

In some patients, it is not clear whether ulcer perforation has occurred and has now spontaneously sealed, or whether there merely is a severe and acute nonperforative ulcer diathesis. All such patients should be hospitalized immediately, prepared for surgery, and carefully observed until a firm decision can be made. In either event, nasogastric suctioning and fluid therapy are beneficial.

Enteritis and Colitis

SYMPTOMS AND DIAGNOSIS

Inflammations of the small and large intestines can be due to a wide variety of causes: viral, bacterial, or protozoal infection; ingestion of toxic substances; bowel ischemia; and diseases with as yet undefined etiologies. Autoimmune disease, psychosomatic reactions, and unrecognized infectious agents each have been proposed to explain the latter group.

The onset of enteritis usually is quite sudden. Nevertheless, recurrent episodes and chronicity are not rare, especially in the case of colitis. As a general rule, symptoms include some combination of nausea, vomiting, diarrhea, and abdominal pain. Intensification of abdominal fullness or abdominal cramps often heralds the urge to vomit or defecate, either or both of which may then occur simultaneously or consecutively. Although such symptoms may be relieved somewhat by vomiting or the passage of stool, mucus and/or flatus respite usually is but transient. Vomiting may be projectile, and on occasions may progress to nonproductive retching. Diarrhea generally is watery; may contain blood, pus, or mucus admixed with stool; and may so severely excoriate the anus and perineum as to cause burning pain with each defecation.

Other symptoms are related to the etiology of the enteritis itself, such as sustained high fever, headache, and photophobia in viral enteritis; intermittent chills and spiking fever, with pus or blood in the stool, in bacterial and parasitic infections; manifestations of liver, kidney, and central nervous system toxicity following the ingestion of poisons or even bacterial toxins; and congestive heart failure or other symptoms of the low flow state, with diarrheal stools containing blood and/or sloughed intestinal mucosa in cases of bowel ischemia.

Evidences of dehydration as a result of extracellular fluid and electrolyte loss are the most prominent findings on physical examination, and are proportionate to the severity of vomiting, diarrhea, and fluid sequestration into bowel wall and peritoneal cavity. Hypovolemic shock even may have supervened. Examination of the abdomen usually reveals vague yet diffuse tenderness, no true rebound tenderness, mild voluntary guarding, and hyperactive bowel sounds, often in rushes. Significant electrolyte derangements, complicating peritonitis, or recent belladonna administration should be suspected if the silent abdomen of paralytic ileus is found.

Bowel gangrene or perforation produces typical signs of peritonitis, i.e., diffuse and extreme abdominal tenderness, definitive rebound, involuntary abdominal muscle spasm, hypoactive to absent peristalsis, and near to total cessation of the diarrhea, which may have been bloody.

Occasionally, a tender abdominal mass of indurated bowel, due to inflammation or ischemia, is discovered. Certain chronic diseases, such as regional enteritis or granulomatous colitis, may have required operation previously, and thus surgical scars and complicating fistulas should be noted. Apart from revealing perineal pathology such as fissures and fistulas, rectal examination generally adds little useful information, but almost always inflicts moderate discomfort during any acute episode of diarrhea.

Standard laboratory data are primarily of value as guides to electrolyte therapy, and as base lines for later comparison when the acute phase has subsided. Nevertheless, the degree of leukocytosis does parallel the severity of all inflammation. For example, neutropenia often is noted, not only in salmonellosis (typhoid fever) and viral enteritis, but also in either actual or impending septic shock. Leukocytosis over 20,000 cu./mm. is generally found with bowel gangrene or perforation and its associated peritonitis. In addition, febrile agglutinations should be drawn.

Microscopic examination of a smear of the stool is always indicated. Scraps of sloughed mucosa, amebic trophozoites, chains of staphylococci, and masses of leukocytes can be seen, all of which should considerably influence the diagnosis. Most important of all, however, is the taking of a stool culture. This is critical not only to the correct diagnosis, but also for isolation and subsequent eradication of a responsible focus in those instances of contagious disease.

In cases not suspected of having progressed to perforation and no longer attended by profuse diarrhea, a careful sigmoidoscopic examination should be performed. Search should be made for the diffuse ulceration or pseudopolyps of ulcerative colitis, vertical ulcers with transverse fissures as noted in granulomatous colitis, pus-covered ulcers in amebic colitis, and the dusky bowel mucosa of ischemic colitis.

Plain films of the abdomen and an upright chest x-ray usually reveal the free gas of perforation, bowel loops separated by the exudate of peritonitis, and toxic dilatations of intestinal segments that have progressed to gangrene. However, these are uncommon complications. Instead, most plain radiographs are nondescript. Barium enema is never indicated as an urgent diagnostic procedure, but is of great value at a later date in differentiating the various forms of chronic colitis.

TREATMENT

Treatment is first directed toward fluid and electrolyte repletion in those patients with moderate to severe dehydration. Intravenous fluids, primarily Ringer's lactate, are given fairly rapidly until an adequate urine flow has been established. Acidosis and specific electrolyte deficiencies also are appropriately corrected. Mild dehydration, on the other hand, usually can be managed by clear liquids given orally, once vomiting has ceased. If intravenous therapy is required, however, hospitalization for one or more days of observation is probably wise. Other significant complications—peritonitis, sepsis, and bleeding—automatically warrant emergency hospital admission.

A mixture of belladonna and an antacid is the most common oral medication used to control both vomiting and diarrhea. If diarrhea is the main problem, Kaopectate or, in severe cases, paregoric is prescribed. In any event, nothing except clear, bland liquids should be given by mouth until acute symptoms have subsided.

More specific therapy depends upon the exact etiology. Viral enteritis requires merely the supportive measures already mentioned. Bacterial enterocolitis initially should be treated with parenteral antibiotics, such as ampicillin, until a more definite diagnosis can be made on the basis of culture results.* A confirmed etiology of Salmonella or Shigella may support the initial choice of antibiotic or indicate the need to alter such. Amebic colitis demands specific antimicrobial therapy. Metronidazole (Flagyl), 750 mg. t.i.d., is given orally for ten days, followed by a course of diodohydroxyquin to eradicate remaining cysts. Enteritis due to toxins should be managed according to the type of poison ingested, e.g., heavy metal, organic hydrocarbon, or bacterial toxin.

Patients with contagious infections also should be isolated, and the epidemiology of the process thoroughly investigated in order to detect other victims at an early stage, as well as to eliminate the threat of carriers to the community at large. Reporting such cases to the proper authorities is an absolute public health necessity.

Signs of peritonitis and/or intestinal

------

*See also page 1329.

bleeding indicate the urgent need for fluid therapy with colloid as well as crystalloid, intravenous antibiotics, and possible surgery. Bowel gangrene and perforation—those specific complications responsible for most instances of peritonitis—always demand emergency surgery. These include perforations due to bacterial and amebic enterocolitis, bowel gangrene caused by low flow states and mesenteric embolus or thrombosis, and toxic dilatations of gangrenous bowel due to infection or idiopathic conditions like ulcerative colitis. Perforations are closed, resected, or exteriorized, and all gangrenous bowel is excised with appropriate venting and diverting enterostomies. Nevertheless, those patients with chronic localized peritonitis, which frequently occurs in regional enteritis, probably should be observed and treated with antibiotics and fluid therapy alone. Anti-inflammatory steroids often are indicated in such cases, as well as in fulminating ulcerative colitis, but, if these are administered, the patient always should be hospitalized for closer follow-up.

Appendicitis

Inflammation of the vermiform appendix is primarily due to an obstruction of its lumen. Accordingly, the pain first appreciated may be colicky and referred to the epigastric or periumbilical midline (Fig. 3).

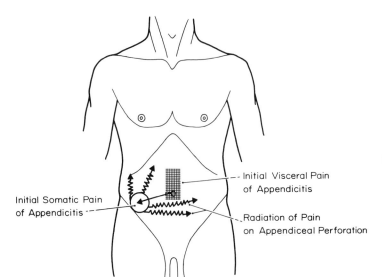

Figure 3. Progression of pain pattern in acute appendicitis.

Initial Visceral Pain of Appendicitis

Initial Somatic Pain of Appendicitis

Radiation of Pain on Appendiceal Perforation

TABLE 1 *Staging Acute Appendicitis*

STAGE	TEMPERATURE	PAIN	NAUSEA, ETC.	TENDERNESS	REBOUND	GUARDING	MASS	PERISTALSIS	LEUKOCYTOSIS
Simple	36–37°C.	Epigastric, or periumbilical; midline	Nausea	Mild, vague to definite RLQ	Mild; to RLQ	Voluntary mild, RLQ	—	Normal	6–8000/cu. mm.
Suppurative	37–38°C.	RLQ usually; occ. to flank (appendiceal location)	Vomiting	Definite RLQ & right flank; right pelvis on rectal exam	Definite; RLQ on abdominal & rectal exam	Voluntary to involuntary; RLQ	—	Hypoactive	10–12,000/cu. mm.
Gangrenous	38–39°C.	Same, with some generalized pain	Vomiting	Same, with some generalized tenderness	Same	Involuntary in RLQ	—	Usually absent	12–15,000/cu. mm.
Perforated	>39°C.	Diffuse abdominal pain	Vomiting	Generalized abdominal tenderness	Diffuse rebound tenderness	Diffuse; involuntary	—	Absent	>15,000/cu. mm.
Abscessed	>38°C.	Pain referred to abscess	Usually both nausea & vomiting	Primarily in vicinity of abscess	Referred to abscess	Involuntary; primarily in vicinity of abscess	Usually in RLQ & pelvis	Hypoactive to absent	>15,000/cu. mm.

With progression of the process, exudate diffuses from the immediate area of the appendix and reaches the adjacent somatic peritoneum, thereby causing pain to radiate to that locale. Gangrene, and then gross perforation, lead to a wider distribution of the irritating bacterial exudate, thus accounting for the signs and symptoms of generalized peritonitis. Finally, with localization of the inflammation into abscess pockets, tender masses can be detected on both abdominal and rectal examination.

This *progression* of appendicitis is reflected by changes in symptoms, signs, and degree of leukocytosis, as altered by the actual anatomic location of the appendix (Table 1). For example, as suppuration occurs, referral of pain to the midline usually is replaced by radiation to the right lower quadrant, although the pain may migrate to the flank if the appendix is retrocecal, or to the low back, hip, or suprapubic region if the appendix extends down into the pelvis. In any event, a careful pelvic examination should be carried out on all females of reproductive age to rule out acute gynecologic inflammatory disease. Similarly, the rectal examination can identify such entities as prostatitis and seminal vesiculitis in the male.

Except for the white blood count, laboratory data are of value only in assisting repletion of fluid and electrolyte losses and in differentiating appendicitis from urinary tract infections, pancreatitis, porphyria, and several other acute conditions. X-rays are of more use, as the presence of an appendiceal fecalith, although a rare finding, almost clinches the diagnosis. In addition, gas patterns of an obstructed small bowel or colon lesion, free intraperitoneal air, and abnormalities on the intravenous pyelogram should be noted, in order to prevent a diagnostic error.

The diagnosis of appendicitis, therefore, also should include an assessment of the anatomic location of the organ, as well as the stage to which the inflammation has progressed. Any question of possibility of appendicitis should warrant just as immediate a hospital admission as if the diagnosis were more certain.

Once this stage has been reached, the patient should be hydrated with Ringer's lactate intravenously in preparation for surgery. The urine concentration and output per hour generally are used as guides for adequacy of fluid therapy. A nasogastric tube also should be inserted. If the clinical diagnosis of appendicitis is definitive, preoperative antibiotics (a cephalosporin or ampicillin) should be begun intravenously in an attempt to control the infection and thereby to avoid perforation as the preparations are made. However, if appendiceal gangrene or perforation is believed to have occurred, an aminoglycoside antibiotic (gentamicin or tobramycin) should be given instead. In general, all supportive efforts are directed toward the delivery of definitive therapy, i.e., appendectomy.

Diverticulitis

Obstruction to the neck of an acquired diverticulum of the colon can produce an inflammatory process similar to appendicitis, though with a more chronic history of intermittency and much less propensity for progression into generalized peritonitis. Almost all patients are above 40 years of age; most are 60 or older.

The onset of symptoms is gradual, with vague midline lower abdominal pain migrating, as suppuration develops, to localize at the site of maximal somatic peritoneal irritation. Usually, the pain, as well as maximal tenderness, is in the left lower quadrant of the abdomen, ocasionally in the left midabdomen or hypogastrium, and, rarely, noted only on rectal examination. Rebound confirms referral to those areas. Peristalsis is normal or hypoactive, and the patient's temperature is relatively low grade (37 to 38° C). The WBC generally ranges between 7000 and 12,000 cu./mm.

After spread of the inflammatory exudate, pain and tenderness are no longer as specifically confined to the left lower quadrant as before. Nausea and vomiting, hypoactive to absent bowel sounds, and fever of 38° C. or greater are then noted. At this time, leukocytosis increases to at least 12,000 cu./mm.

Without localization of the infection, generalized peritonitis with its typical signs and symptoms then develops. At this stage, it may be impossible to delineate the true cause without prior knowledge of the steps in progression.

Sigmoidoscopy probably is contraindicated during the acute inflammation, but plain x-rays are useful in eliminating the possibility of mechanical intestinal obstruction. Whenever the diagnosis is in much doubt, a gentle barium enema can differentiate diverticulitis from other causes of localized peritonitis by demonstrating segmental bowel spasm in the area of inflammation and diverticulosis elsewhere in the colon.

Because of the vomiting and peritoneal exudate consequent to diverticulitis, correction of fluid and electrolyte deficits requires intravenous therapy with solutions such as Ringer's lactate and specific electrolyte supplements. In addition, antibiotics effective against gram-negative rod bacteria should be given intravenously—one of the cephalosporins, ampicillin, or an aminoglycoside. Cleocin or chloramphenicol can be added specifically for their effect on *Bacteroides fragilis*. A nasogastric tube also should be passed, and the patient must not be fed by mouth until all symptoms and signs of acute inflammation have subsided. Accordingly, the diagnosis of diverticulitis always warrants admission to the hospital.

General peritonitis or evidences of severe sepsis may necessitate emergency operation to resect gangrenous or perforated bowel or to divert the fecal stream by installing a proximal colostomy. Preoperative measures are essentially identical to those taken in patients with acute perforated appendicitis.

Perirectal Abscesses

Extensions of infection from the anal canal may go in one of several directions. Laterally and below both the levator and transverse perineal muscles, abscesses present in the perianal region. Extension above the transverse perineal muscles, yet still below the levator, confines the abscess to the ischiorectal space. Inflammation with abscess above the levator and bounded by the rectum medially is referred to as pelvirectal. Differentiation of these is possible only by careful and gentle rectal examination.

Infection in these cases gives symptoms of perineal fullness, pain, and tenderness. The associated sphincter spasm makes defecation quite painful. Systemic signs of sepsis, such as fever and leukocytosis, generally reflect the severity of the process.

The infectious etiology is based upon those bacterial species normally present in stool, i.e., gram-negative rods and various anaerobes. In patients with an impaired resistance to infection (those with diabetes, renal failure, reticuloendothelial diseases, etc.), the infection can be extensive, fulminating, and lethal.

Treatment requires incision and drainage, with débridement of dead tissue if sepsis is profound or the necrosis extensive. Perianal abscesses usually can be drained under local anesthesia, and the patient managed by frequent clinic visits. On the other hand, ischiorectal and pelvirectal abscesses require hospital admission, parenteral antibiotics (ampicillin, cephalosporin, or aminoglycoside), and drainage under general anesthesia. Fluid therapy and control of associated medical conditions likewise must be given due attention.

Cholecystitis and Cholangitis

Acute inflammations of the gallbladder usually, but not always, are associated with gallstones. Onset tends to be relatively sudden, often after a fried meal, and is manifested by nausea, vomiting, and epigastric pain (Fig. 4). With progression, low grade fever (37 to 38° C.) develops; the pain migrates to the right upper quadrant; and both local and rebound tenderness likewise are referred to this area. Advanced cholecystitis is reflected by more exquisite right upper quadrant tenderness, even liver tenderness, and referral of pain to the right supraclavicular and scapular areas; higher fevers, possibly spiking to 39 or 40° C.; and mild jaundice.

Cholecystitis is more common in multiparous and obese females above the age of 40. Repeated and, up to the time of examination, consistently remitting acute bouts are the rule until a more severe and persistent episode occurs. Ductal obstruction and gallbladder dilatation may lead to perforation if surgical intervention is delayed.

Cholangitis, instead, is inflammation within the common duct and its intrahepatic radicals. It may occur intermittently with acute cholecystitis or, as often is noted, as a later postcholecystectomy complication. Symptoms are more severe, and prognosis worse, than is the case with cholecystitis. The liver and entire right upper quadrant are extremely tender. Chills and high spiking fevers (39 to 41° C.) are characteristic, as

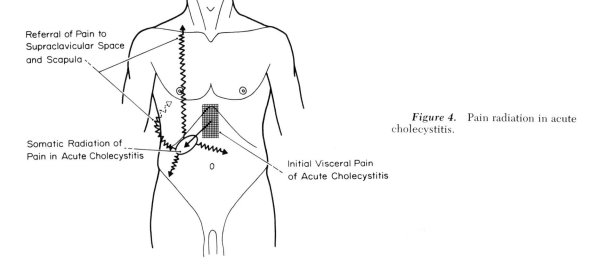

Referral of Pain to
Supraclavicular Space
and Scapula

Somatic Radiation of
Pain in Acute Cholecystitis

Initial Visceral Pain
of Acute Cholecystitis

Figure 4. Pain radiation in acute cholecystitis.

is jaundice, bile in the urine, and WBC in excess of 15,000 cu./mm.

Standard laboratory studies are drawn to determine the degree of leukocytosis, the severity of jaundice, and the general status of liver function after repeated injuries inflicted by biliary tract disease. In addition, electrolytes are useful to direct the required intravenous fluid therapy.

Since less than 15 per cent of gallstones are radiopaque, plain x-rays are of little diagnostic value. However, the intravenous cholangiogram is of considerable assistance in the differential diagnosis from other acute conditions in the upper abdomen, and especially from pancreatitis. Should the common duct visualize and the gallbladder not, a diagnosis of acute cholecystitis is almost assured. On the other hand, an opacified gallbladder, in the absence of identifiable dye in the common duct, strongly suggests pancreatitis. Visualization of both structures rules out acute biliary tract disease; total nonvisualization is meaningless.

All patients with either acute cholecystitis or cholangitis should be hospitalized immediately for observation and possible emergency operation. A nasogastric tube is passed to keep the stomach empty and thereby prevent further stimulation of the gallbladder by gastric acid reaching the duodenum.

Intravenous fluids also are given at rates designed to prepare the patient for prospec-

tive urgent surgery, although improvement in symptoms or a complete remission during such observations makes elective operation after a six-week interval the desired approach. Antibiotics are indicated only for those patients who fail to improve, or who manifest signs of sepsis or cholangitis. Similarly, these same patients probably will require an early operation, within 12 to 36 hours.

Pancreatitis

SYMPTOMS AND DIAGNOSIS

The exact cause of any isolated case of pancreatitis is usually a moot point, although alcoholism, biliary tract disease (especially common duct stones), trauma, hyperparathyroidism, and hypercholesterolemia are common associations. The inflammatory process almost always is sterile, at least initially. There are varying degrees of severity, and it is on this basis that different terms have been coined to describe the disease. The magnitude of physical signs, extent of dehydration, and level of the serum amylase (or rate of urinary excretion of pancreatic amylase) are the parameters commonly used to grade the severity.

Onset usually is gradual over several hours, and is characterized by progressive worsening of relatively steady epigastric pain. Nausea and vomiting then follow. Abdominal examination usually reveals distention, diffuse upper midline tenderness, no masses, and absent to hypoactive peristalsis. The patient's temperature generally is low grade (37 to 38° C.), and the WBC less than 12,000 cu./mm. Dehydration generally is mild at first, but may progress to moderate extremes as vomiting persists and additional fluid is sequestered into the area of inflammation. A scant and concentrated urine output, and significant increases in the hematocrit, reflect the magnitude of extracellular fluid loss. This milder stage customarily is referred to as acute edematous pancreatitis.

More intense inflammation can progress to necrotic and then hemorrhagic forms. In such cases, peritoneal signs are more striking, paralytic ileus is absolute, fever may reach 39 to 40° C., and the WBC usually exceeds 15,000 cu./mm. The serum amylase often is more than five times normal, but instead may be within normal range if the episode of pancreatitis is recurrent in a previously almost destroyed gland, or has produced extensive pancreatic necrosis. Further dehydration, and even retroperitoneal hemorrhage, may be so severe as to have caused moderate to profound hypovolemic shock. Electrolyte derangements are primarily acidosis and, occasionally, a hypocalcemia low enough to cause tetany. Hypoglycemia of a transient, or possibly even permanent, diabetes also is common.

Differentiation of acute pancreatitis from urgent surgical problems such as cholecystitis, cholangitis, perforated peptic ulcer, proximal intestinal obstruction, and mesenteric embolus or thrombosis may be exceedingly difficult in the individual case. It is for this very reason that even mild cases of pancreatitis should be hospitalized and observed on a surgical service. The basic management of pancreatitis is supportive and nonoperative, whereas these other causes of peritonitis almost always require laparotomy. Nevertheless, whenever the exact diagnosis is in doubt, an operation should be carried out to ensure that a correctible surgical lesion has not been overlooked. The amylase determination may be a source of confusion, since it can be elevated in cases of intestinal obstruction and ulcer perforation, as well as in pancreatitis.

Plain x-rays of the abdomen often reveal a proximal loop of jejunum dilated in segmental paralytic ileus—the so-called "sentinel loop." The intravenous cholangiogram, as mentioned before, often will signify pancreatitis by an opacified gallbladder and nonvisualized common bile duct. Free intraperitoneal gas also is absent. However, continued observation is the most reliable means of assuring an accurate differentiation.

TREATMENT

Treatment is based on keeping the intestinal tract at rest, extracellular fluid repletion, and correction of specific electrolyte derangements. A nasogastric tube is passed and connected to continuous suction. Intravenous fluids are then begun, initially in relatively massive quantities, and are administered at rates to maintain the central venous pressure in normal range and the urine output at 50 to 100 ml./hour. Ringer's lactate alone is adequate for mild cases, yet more severe inflammations generally require the addition of large quanitites of colloid—both plasma and blood. Acidosis is corrected by intravenous supplements of sodium bicarbonate, and the hypocalcemia by aliquots of calcium gluconate in a separate intravenous solution. An associated diabetes similarly will require insulin for control until the acute episode has resolved.

Other related problems seldom are noted immediately, but can be life-threatening within several days of hospitalization. These include respiratory failure, delirium tremens, and refractory shock. Late sequelae, on the other hand, may develop after quiescent episodes and present as almost unrelated conditions.

Pseudocysts of the pancreas are sterile abscesses, usually in the lesser peritoneal sac, that have developed as collections of pancreatic juice, inflammatory exudate, and necrotic pancreas. Patients present with either: (1) a tender upper abdominal mass; (2) signs of peritonitis localized to the upper abdomen; or (3) an obstructed duodenum or gastric outlet due to pressure from the pseudocyst. Nausea and vomiting usually are prominent symptoms. Other common, yet not consistent, findings are low grade fever (37 to 38° C), leukocytosis of 12,000 cu./mm. or greater, and significant elevations of the serum amylase.

This diagnosis may be suspected when there is a prior history consistent with pancreatitis, together with the features now presenting. An upper gastrointestinal series reveals displacement of the stomach outline by a retrogastric pancreatic mass, which itself can be demonstrated to be cystic by the sonogram.

Treatment consists of intravenous fluid repletion followed by surgical drainage of the cyst, perferably into the stomach or into a Roux-en-Y segment of jejunum.

C. ALIMENTARY TRACT OBSTRUCTION

Edward L. Bradley, III

GENERAL CONSIDERATIONS

Introduction

Alimentary tract obstruction has become a frequent cause of morbidity and mortality. Although precise data are not available, it has been estimated that one of every five emergency surgical admissions is necessitated by some form of alimentary tract obstruction. It is true that patient response will depend on the cause and nature of the obstruction, but for one specific area, intestinal obstruction, the mortality rate approximates 10 per cent. Since there were approximately 2 million emergency surgical admissions in the U.S. in 1972, it follows that 40,000 people may have died from the effects of alimentary tract obstruction. Needless to say, this mortality is excessive. With widespread and proper application of *presently existing* knowledge, it is likely that this figure could be halved.

Definition and Dangers

Alimentary tract obstruction can best be defined as an intrinsic or extrinsic failure of the normal caudad progression of intraluminal contents.

Such a situation results in several possible complications. Quite apparent is the effect on normal nutrition, which, if permitted to continue, would lead eventually to inanition. Less obvious is the development of dehydration and the threat of alimentary tract perforation with attendant sepsis. These complications are discussed more fully in the section of this chapter dealing with pathophysiology. If abdominal distention is a feature of the obstruction, the resultant expansion in volume of the abdominal contents takes place at the expense of pulmonary volume and expansion. This results

in a decrease in alveolar ventilation and a corresponding increase in unoxygenated blood. Remote effects may result in other organ systems initiated by the fall in arterial oxygenation. Finally, in situations characterized by distention and vomiting, the threat of pulmonary aspiration of regurgitated intestinal contents is ever-present.

Etiology

By far the most common cause of alimentary tract obstruction is the temporary cessation of intestinal activity immediately following abdominal surgery. Fortunately, this process is self-limiting. With regard to causes of persistent obstruction, adhesions account for 40 per cent, carcinoma of the colon 20 per cent, and incarcerated hernia 10 per cent, the remaining 30 per cent being divided among the many causes listed in Table 1. Since the most effective therapy requires a preliminary diagnosis of the cause of any given obstruction, consideration of these should be of therapeutic value. "Common things occur commonly."

Pathophysiology

Although not all sections of the alimentary tract respond to obstruction in an identical manner, certain physiologic truths can be appreciated from a discussion in general terms.

As noted, alimentary tract obstruction exists when intestinal contents fail to progress. Since intraluminal progression of intestinal contents basically is due to an integrated and coordinated contraction of smooth muscle in the intestinal wall (peristalsis), obstruction conceivably could be

TABLE 1   Causes of Alimentary Tract Obstruction

A. MECHANICAL	ESOPHAGUS	STOMACH	DUODENUM	SMALL BOWEL	COLON
1. Congenital	Atresia Stenosis	Pyloric stenosis	Atresia Stenosis Duodenal web Annular pancreas Congenital bands	Atresia Stenosis External hernia	Atresia Stenosis Meconium ileus Imperforate anus Hirschsprung's disease
2. Inflammatory	Stricture	Stricture	Stricture	Adhesions Regional enteritis Abscess Stricture	Granulomatous colitis Ulcerative colitis Diverticulitis Abscess Stricture
3. Neoplastic	Carcinoma Leiomyoma	Carcinoma Lymphoma Sarcoma Polyps	Carcinoma Polyps	Carcinoma Lymphoma Sarcoma Leiomyoma Carcinoid	Carcinoma Sarcoma Lymphoma

4. Miscellaneous	Foreign body
	Achalasia
		Foreign body
		Paraesophageal
		  hernia
		Volvulus
			Foreign body
			Hematoma
			
			Superior mesenteric
			  artery syndrome
				Foreign body
				Hematoma
				Worms
				Gallstone
				Bezoars
				Intussusception
				Hernia
				Volvulus
					Foreign body
					Endometriosis
					Fecal impaction
					Intussusception
					Volvulus

B. PARALYTIC ILEUS
1. Conduction Defects: Na^+ and K^+ abnormalities, as in depletion states and diabetic ketoacidosis
2. Peristaltic Defects: Abnormalities in muscular contraction, as in mesenteric vascular disease and porphyria
3. Neural Irritative States: Overbalanced sympathetic stimulation, as in local or general toxicity and retroperitoneal injuries

produced by either physical obturation to the passage of intestinal contents, or the absence of effective peristalsis. The former condition, referred to as *mechanical* obstruction, and the latter state of functional obstruction, called *paralytic ileus,* arise from two completely different causes, but many similar effects may be produced.

The alimentary tract secretes more than 8000 ml. of fluid into the lumen daily. Since little more than 200 to 400 ml. can be recovered in the feces, the efficiency of the resorption mechanism can easily be appreciated. Increases in intraluminal fluid volume occur in intestinal obstruction. The question whether alimentary tract secretions in obstruction actually are increased, or whether absorption is decreased, has not been resolved. Experimental evidence supporting each theory is available and, in the author's opinion, the two positions are not mutually exclusive. Regardless of the actual mechanism involved, the amount of intestinal fluid residing in the alimentary tract in a given obstruction will be determined by the site of the obstruction. If the site is quite distal, a large amount of fluid will accumulate above the obstruction. With more proximal obstructions, there will be proportionally less intra-luminal fluid, as bowel secretion and absorption take place distal to the obstruction in a normal fashion.

If normal absorption of alimentary tract secretions cannot take place, the extracellular fluid secreted into the lumen is functionally lost to the body. Deficits in extracellular fluid volume can only be replaced by borrowing from the intracellular space. This situation becomes aggravated when repeated episodes of vomiting are a prominent feature of the obstruction. Clearly, the net result is profound dehydration, with the attendant abnormalities in all cellular and subcellular systems dependent on solvent transport. Therefore, in addition to obstruction to the flow of intestinal contents resulting in a loss of nutrition, alimentary tract obstruction invariably produces some degree of dehydration. This development is of great consequence, since the seriousness of the situation has now undergone escalation. It is possible for the human organism to take no external nutrition whatever for periods lasting months, survival being based upon the conversion of stored fat and protein to energy equivalents. In contrast, underlining the importance of fluid homeostasis, is the observation that few would survive two

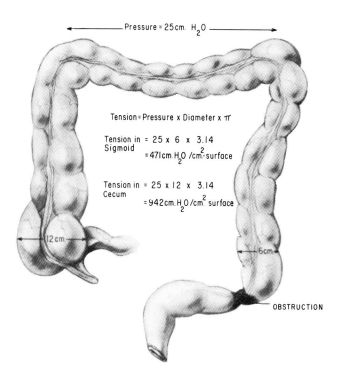

Figure 1. A physical analysis of obstruction relating wall tension to the degree of distention. (From Schwartz, S. I., et al. (eds.): Principles of Surgery. Copyright © 1969 by McGraw-Hill, Inc. Used by permission of the McGraw-Hill Book Co.)

weeks of total fluid deprivation. Persistent extracellular fluid deficits lead to hypotension and shock. Coronary, carotid, and renal thromboses are frequent sequelae of this development in the older age group.

If these were the only problems arising from alimentary tract obstruction, the situation would be sufficiently severe. However, another process occurs which, by itself, places the patient at greatest risk of death: the intestinal tract becomes *distended*. Although simple distention at first may seem innocuous, closer examination reveals the true scope of this complication.

First, distention increases tension in the wall of the alimentary tract simply by an increase in the radius, pressure remaining constant. This relationship for tubular structures is known as Laplace's Law, and is illustrated in Figure 1. As a corollary, one might expect that, since the cecum has the largest radius in the intestinal tract, rupture from the increased pressure would occur most commonly in this location. The general concept of stress and strain in the wall of the alimentary tract as a direct result of distention, leading to tensions exceeding the yield point and subsequently the cohesive forces of the intestinal wall, with resultant rupture, is worthy of our consideration.

Secondly, the immediate antecedent cause of distention is an increase in intraluminal pressure. What is the origin of this excessive pressure? Theoretically, it could have come from increased intraluminal secretion, from gases liberated by the action of bacteria upon stagnant intestinal contents, or from swallowed atmospheric air. Wangensteen and Rea designed a simple experiment to test the hypothesis that intestinal gas was primarily the result of swallowed atmospheric gases (Fig. 2). Not only was this confirmed by the experiment, but, with the absence of intestinal distention in the group with cervical esophagostomies, it was clearly demonstrated that, whatever abnormalities in intestinal fluid secretion and absorption take place in obstruction, they cannot *in and of themselves* produce increased intestinal pressure with subsequent distention. Therefore, the primary cause of intestinal distention is swallowed air.

What are the dangers of increased intraluminal pressure? We have already discussed the increase in wall tension resulting from pressure-induced distention. If we consider for a moment the final distribution of blood supply to the intestine (Fig. 3), it should be clear that intramural blood flow is vulnerable to increases in intraluminal pres-

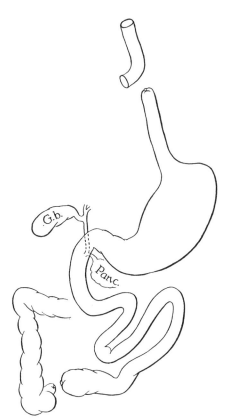

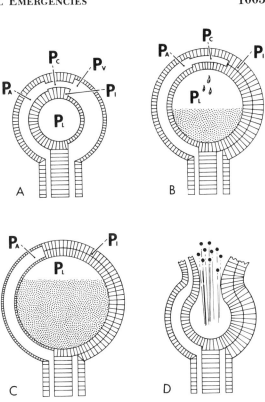

Figure 2. An experimental preparation to investigate the origin of intestinal gas and the mechanism of distention in intestinal obstruction. In dogs subject to ileal obstruction, if an end cervical esophagostomy prevented air swallowing, then little gas, fluid, or distention was present in the obstructed bowel. This work clearly demonstrated that swallowed air was responsible for intestinal distention and that, in the absence of distention, the obstructed gut effectively reabsorbs digestive juices. (From Wangensteen, O. H., and Rea, C. E.: Surgery 5:329, 1939.)

Figure 3. Diagrammatic representation of the effects of increased intraluminal pressure on the intramural blood flow in a cross section of intestinal wall. P_L = intraluminal pressure, P_I = interstitial pressure, P_V = pressure in venule, P_C = capillary pressure, P_A = arteriolar pressure.

A, Normal conditions: $P_L < P_I < P_V < P_C < P_A$.

B, Increased intraluminal pressure secondary to obstruction: $P_L > P_I > P_V$ but $< P_C < P_A$. Since interstitial pressure exceeds venular pressure, venule closes. Shift in Starling equilibrium results in marked outflow of fluid from capillary.

C, Continued increase in intraluminal pressure: $P_L > P_I > P_V > P_C < P_A$. Both venule and capillary now collapsed by surrounding pressure, resulting in a loss of aerobic cellular perfusion and nutrition.

D, Perforation resulting from cellular necrosis when anaerobic metabolism could no longer maintain viability of intestinal wall.

sure. Although the author is unaware of any studies measuring pressures in venules, capillaries, and arterioles in the bowel wall, it is reasonable to assume that values for these vessels are similar to venules, capillaries, and arterioles elsewhere in the body. Under these anatomic circumstances, if intraluminal pressure exceeded venular pressure, we could expect an increase in capillary pressure. Such increases in capillary pressure would result in Starling disequilibrium, to the extent that there would be not only a net increase in extracellular fluid loss from the capillary into the bowel wall, resulting in thickening and edema, but also intraluminal weeping from mucosal capillaries. Since a new capillary exchange equilibrium would then be achieved at a higher pressure, reabsorption at the venular terminal would be diminished. Concurrent with the increase in transcapillary fluid loss into the extravascular spaces, lymphatic flow would increase. Eventually this cycle, if unchecked, would result in reduced arterial inflow, reduced tissue oxygenation, anaerobic cellular metabolism, and tissue acidosis, culminating in the confluent cell death known as necrosis. Such a scenario for perforation of the alimentary tract has been developed solely from distention and an increase in intraluminal pressure exceeding venular pressure. Clearly, any physical factors acting to reduce blood supply in a more abrupt fashion, such as acute vascular occlusion due to thrombosis or volvulus, could promote the preceding change of events in a matter of hours. It is the increase in intraluminal pressure manifested by distention which causes the primary danger in alimentary tract obstruction. When distention can be decompressed by vomiting or other means, as in high jejunal or gastric outlet obstruction, perforation is exceedingly rare.

Do the pressures in the alimentary tract support these concepts? In fact, very little work has been done to support or deny the above suppositions. The bursting strength of the normal human intestine has ranged from 80 to 260 mm. Hg, being in the lower end of this range for colon and higher for small bowel. In the few instances in which intraluminal pressures have been measured proximal to obstructions, small bowel pressures have ranged from 10 to 14 cm. H_2O, and colon pressures from 12 to 52 cm. H_2O. All these pressures increased with either peristalsis or respiration, but in no case have they approached those pressures required to burst the intestine as a result of pressure per se. However, it is necessary to note that, because these were operative data, a Valsalva maneuver, such as might be produced by attempts at defecation, was not performed. It is interesting to speculate that a sudden Valsalva maneuver might increase intraluminal pressure into the region of danger from bursting, particularly with regard to colon distentions.

Since venular pressures are known to be in the range of 10 mm. Hg ($\sim$ 14 cm. H_2O), it can easily be appreciated that intraluminal pressures in mechanical intestinal obstruction may exceed venular pressure, setting in motion the chain of events chronicled above. Sustained intraluminal pressure becomes an important concept in that, if the sustained pressure exceeds the systolic capillary and venular pressure, necrosis must surely follow. However, if the sustained intraluminal pressure is less than systolic pressures in these vessels, cellular nutrition could be interrupted only during periods of peristalsis when intraluminal pressures are temporarily increased. In this set of circumstances, it is unlikely that tissue necrosis could occur. Since the pressure values measured in paralytic ileus are correspondingly lower, intra-

mural vascular obstruction and subsequent necrosis should be less common if considered solely on a basis of pressure. That perforation rarely occurs in paralytic ileus is amply supported by clinical experience.

We might, therefore, view the range of intraluminal pressures in obstruction affecting intramural blood flow as a continuum: i.e., the greater the intraluminal pressure, the less the intramural blood flow and the greater the likelihood of tissue necrosis and perforation. Of course, any factors negatively affecting intramural blood flow, in addition to increased intraluminal pressure, would serve only to hasten necrosis and promote earlier perforation. This situation occurs when the mesenteric blood flow is compromised, resulting in strangulated obstruction. Since the time course preceding perforation is greatly shortened by the addition of extrinsic vascular obstruction to the simple obstruction, the course of therapy also must be accelerated when strangulated obstruction is suspected.

Although the concept of such a continuum is valuable from the standpoint of understanding pathophysiology, in a practical sense the actual measurement of intraluminal pressure is both risky and unnecessary. It is sufficient to recognize that distention is present, since fortunately the degree of distention is a reasonably direct function of the magnitude of intraluminal pressure. Clinically, we may infer that the more distention there is present proximal to an obstruction, the more likely perforation is to occur and, therefore, the more urgent decompression has become.

Another particularly virulent form of intestinal obstruction has been referred to as the "closed-loop"obstruction. This situation exists when neither entrance nor exit of intestinal contents is possible from a segment of bowel. Often such a closed-loop obstruction also is strangulated, as in volvulus or strangulated inguinal hernia, but strangulation is not a prerequisite. An example of a closed-loop obstruction without strangulation would be a distal colon obstruction in the presence of a competent ileocecal valve. The added virulence of this form of obstruction is due primarily to the inherent toxicity of the entrapped intraluminal fluid. Extensive animal experimentation has shown that this intraluminal fluid contains products of bacterial origin that have profound vasodepressive effects. These observations have clear therapeutic implications.

Clinical Manifestations

Signs and symptoms of alimentary tract obstruction depend to a great degree upon the site, the nature, and the duration of the obstruction.

HISTORICAL FEATURES

In the more distal lesions, the most common complaint will be one of distention. This becomes more prominent as the site of obstruction progresses distally from the upper jejunum. In more proximal lesions, clinically evident distention is not a common feature. Its lack can be attributed both to the small volume of bowel proximal to the lesion, and to the ability to decompress very proximal lesions by vomiting. However, with proximal obstruction, protracted and projectile vomiting is quite characteristic. In contrast, as the obstruction progresses distally, vomiting becomes less prominent. However, the nature of the vomitus becomes more characteristic. Regurgitated ileal contents have a distinctly fecal odor, and vomitus of this type is referred to as feculent vomitus.

Another major feature of the history is the presence of irregular bowel function. With complete obstruction, one would not expect continued passage of feces, and this generally is the case. However, it is possible to evacuate bowel contents distal to the obstruction, and thus appear to have a normal bowel movement after complete obstruction has occurred. Clearly then, the only circumstance in which the presence of bowel movements effectively can dismiss the diagnosis of complete obstruction is that of *continued* fecal passage. Obstruction and continued fecal passage can continue to coexist in only one situation, in a high grade incomplete or partial intestinal obstruction. The most common example of this is partial colonic obstruction due to fecal impaction.

A third major determinant found in the history is the existence and nature of associated pain. Quite characteristically, the pain is associated with the major peristaltic wave and therefore is intermittent. Since the major peristaltic wave in the small bowel occurs every two to three minutes, and in the colon occurs at intervals of 15 to 20 minutes, this feature often can be used to localize the site of obstruction. The pain usually is described as dull and cramping, rising slowly in a crescendo pattern, reaching a maximum lasting around 30 seconds, and gradually receding. The etiology of the pain is not known. However, the strong association with peristalsis suggests that forced distention may be an important factor. It is of significant clinical importance to realize that, since *episodic* pain is associated with intestinal peristalsis, it would not be expected to occur in any primary aperistaltic condition.

PHYSICAL FEATURES

Many physical signs are of value in the diagnosis and initial management of alimentary tract obstruction, but two are of paramount importance: the character of the bowel sounds, and the presence or absence of abdominal tenderness.

Although the exact causation of bowel sounds as yet is only suspected, it is well known that they do not occur in the absence of peristalsis. Therefore, a failure to detect bowel sounds after listening for several minutes allows a working diagnosis of paralytic ileus. This in itself does not discriminate among the various causes of paralytic ileus. If bowel sounds *are* present, however, their character is of importance. Bowel sounds in mechanical intestinal obstruction are quite characteristic and frequently pathognomonic in a setting suggesting obstruction. They have been described as high pitched, rushing, and continuous. No amount of verbal description can equal the experience of actually hearing such sounds. In the author's opinion, of equal importance to the character of the bowel sounds is the temporal relationship of the abdominal pain to the peristaltic wave that produces them. Cramping abdominal pain coexisting with the characteristic bowel sounds, and ceasing when the overactive peristaltic activity ceases, is the foundation upon which the diagnosis of mechanical obstruction is made.

Determination of abdominal tenderness is the second major consideration in the physical examination. Uncomplicated alimentary tract obstruction rarely results in other than mild tenderness to palpation. More severe tenderness, particularly in conjunction with rebound tenderness, means parietal peritonitis. This development in a setting of obstruction means either that perforation has already occurred or that gangrenous bowel is present. This is a physical sign of the utmost importance, since the development of bowel necrosis necessarily accelerates the surgical program.

Other physical findings are frequently of value either in assisting in the establishment of the diagnosis, or in helping to define the pathologic stage of the obstruction.

Abdominal distention has been felt to be a sine qua non of obstruction. Although distention is a very common finding in intestinal obstruction, as already mentioned, a high obstruction is not associated with abdominal distention. Therefore, the absence of distention does not obviate the presence of obstruction.

Similar comments may be made with regard to the percussion note. If the bowel is distended with air, the characteristic percussion note may be elicited. An additional consideration is that the bowel may contain more fluid than air, making percussive resonance less likely.

Some have set great store by the presence or absence of feces in the rectum on digital examination. As noted, bowel evacuation may or may not take place distal to a complete obstruction, and therefore, in the author's opinion, this sign is of little prognostic significance.

Since postoperative adhesions are the most common cause of mechanical obstruction, the finding of an abdominal scar in a setting suggesting obstruction is of some help in suggesting the diagnosis and in defining the possible cause of the obstruction. Also, since the second most common cause is incarcerated hernia, an examination of the inguinal and femoral regions should be part of every examination with the possible diagnosis of obstruction. This is particularly true when there have been no previous abdominal surgical procedures.

Diagnosis

In the overwhelming majority of instances, the diagnosis of alimentary tract obstruction will be obvious from the history

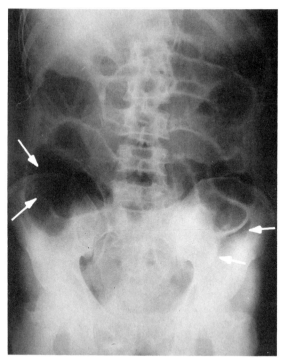

Figure 4. Plain abdominal film of patient with paralytic ileus. Arrows denote the presence of gas in an undistended colon.

and physical examination. Occasionally, further diagnostic studies seem necessary.

No characteristic changes of obstruction are reflected by examination of the patient's blood. Generally, whole blood and serum examinations reveal only some degree of nonspecific dehydration. However, in one specific instance, WBC evaluation may prove to be of benefit. In those instances in which impending or actual necrosis or inflammatory bowel disease is suspected, marked elevations in WBC count are noted quite frequently. In conjunction with fever and moderate abdominal tenderness, the etiology of the alimentary tract obstruction can be strongly suspected. Such suspicions have far-reaching implications for management, as will be discussed below.

By far the most helpful adjunct in diagnosis and management is the abdominal x-ray. Plain films of the abdomen taken with the patient in the recumbent and upright or lateral decubitus positions support the clinical diagnosis, frequently can distinguish between mechanical and paralytic obstruction, and often suggest the anatomic site of the obstruction (Figs. 4 and 5). When the plain film suggests that the obstruction is in the

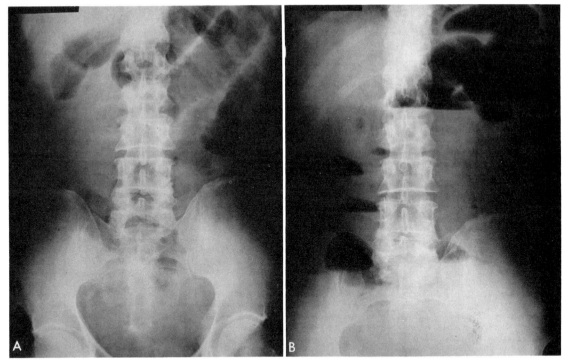

Figure 5. A, Plain abdominal film of a patient with mechanical small intestinal obstruction. Note the absence of colonic gas.

B, Upright abdominal film of the same patient showing air-fluid levels in multiple loops of bowel. By themselves, air-fluid levels are not diagnostic of mechanical obstruction.

colon, many feel that a cautious barium enema for confirmation is in order.

Occasionally, in high mechanical obstruction or in other exceptionally rare instances, an upper gastrointestinal series with small bowel follow-through may be required to confirm a clinical diagnosis.

Management

In our discussion of pathophysiology, we have emphasized the major determinants of morbidity and mortality associated with alimentary tract obstruction: extracellular fluid loss with dehydration, and increases in intraluminal pressure secondary to air swallowing, ultimately leading to necrosis and perforation. It is clear, therefore, in which directions the primary therapeutic efforts initially should be directed.

Before 1930, the surgical mortality rate for acute obstruction was in the range of 30 per cent. At the present time, it is 5 to 10 per cent. Improved anesthesia, the liberal use of antibiotics, and improved techniques in surgery and in patient monitoring all may

have improved over the past 40 years, but the primary reason for the reduction in mortality rate has been an appreciation of the necessity for preoperative rehydration. Since intraluminal fluid sequestration is an almost invariable process accompanying distention, for the reasons discussed (the so-called "third space" type of fluid loss), it follows that all patients with alimentary tract obstruction regardless of etiology are dehydrated, differing only with respect to the degree of dehydration.

A primary effort, therefore, should be directed at rehydration. Since the patient has lost extracellular fluid, the composition of the replacement fluid should closely approximate extracellular fluid. At the present time, this may best be accomplished by the intravenous administration of Ringer's lactate solution in 5 per cent dextrose and water. Potassium supplements should be added as required. Although no precise determinants are available of the total amount of replacement fluid to be given or of the rate of replacement, a few clinical guidelines may be of value. In instances of dehydration, a central venous pressure (CVP) monitoring line is of great assistance. Venous pressure values, particularly when taken in conjunction with hourly urine volumes and pulse and blood pressure information, provide a clinically reliable indication of hydration. As initial goals for the rate and volume of fluid administration, a CVP of >5 and <12 cm. H_2O, hourly urine output exceeding 30 cc./hr., pulse <120, and satisfactory blood pressure should be achieved. Generally, this can be accomplished within five to six hours unless dehydration is particularly severe.

Secondly, as noted, it is of paramount importance to prevent the further intestinal accumulation of swallowed air. Intestinal intubation can effectively prevent continued aerophagic distention, permitting gradual intestinal absorption of gas already present in the intestine. It can serve no useful purpose to debate the efficiency of short versus long intestinal tubes in the absence of reliable quantitative data, and it is sufficient for our purpose to state that nasogastric tube decompression is eminently satisfactory. Appropriate placement and continued patency are clear prerequisites for the proper function of any decompressing tube.

After intestinal intubation and fluid replacement have been started, further studies can be carried out to determine the probable cause of the obstruction. Isolating the probable cause will determine whether future therapy will include surgery.

The basic distinction to be made is whether the obstruction has been produced by mechanical factors requiring surgical correction, or whether the obstruction is a manifestation of primary paralytic ileus and will resolve spontaneously. A most important observation in this regard is the presence of abdominal tenderness. Under this circumstance, in a setting of mechanical obstruction, impending or actual intestinal necrosis has complicated the picture. All therapeutic measures must be accelerated greatly if the patient is to survive. In this specific instance, surgical treatment should be regarded as an emergency.

Uncomplicated mechanical intestinal obstruction, on the other hand, merely represents an urgent surgical situation, to be undertaken when the patient has been rehydrated and is in a more stable condition. Abdominal tenderness in a setting of paralytic ileus usually means that the ileus is secondary to an inflammatory process, such as appendicitis, cholecystitis, etc. Thus, the therapeutic focus should properly be directed to that required by the inflammatory focus itself, since the resultant paralytic ileus is a secondary self-limiting phenomenon. These principles are expressed in the logic flow diagram shown in Figure 6.

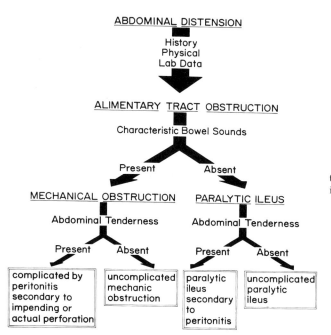

Figure 6. Logic flow diagram emphasizing the clinical importance of abdominal tenderness in alimentary tract obstruction.

SPECIFIC OBSTRUCTIONS

The general principles underlying diagnosis and management of most causes of obstruction have been discussed in the previous section, but certain representative obstructions are either compellingly urgent, sufficiently common, or seemingly divergent from basic principles to warrant individual attention.

Acute Esophageal Obstruction

The diagnosis and management of chronic esophageal obstruction only infrequently confronts the emergency physician. On such rare occasions, the history of dysphagia is sufficiently characteristic to enable proper steps to be taken.

On the other hand, acute esophageal obstruction is a frequent occurrence in emergency practice. Almost all these instances will be a result of foreign body ingestion. An ingestion history usually can be obtained from adults, but the diagnosis in children may be more difficult. One particularly helpful sign in children is excessive drooling. Frequently, the patient will complain of a sensation of the object "sticking" at a certain highly specific level. A history of foreign body ingestion and subsequent substernal pain frequently radiating to the neck should suggest esophageal perforation. In conjunction with cervical subcutaneous emphysema and constitutional reactions, the diagnosis of perforation may be made. More commonly, however, the patient will describe a "feeling" that a foreign body is lodged in the esophagus. If the object is metallic, a chest x-ray will establish whether a foreign body is present, and if so, its exact location. As a *general* rule, any foreign body with no sharp or protruding edges that reaches the stomach will safely traverse the intestinal tract. If the object is not metallic, esophagoscopy may be the only safe diagnostic alternative. In the author's opinion, the low incidence of morbidity of diagnosis and therapy with fiberoptic esophagoscopy is far less significant than the morbidity associated with previous suggestions, such as those advocating the blind forcing of a suspected foreign body down the esophagus and into the stomach by further ingestion or other mechanisms.

One particularly urgent form of acute esophageal obstruction is that produced by a lodgment of food in the esophagus at the level of the larynx, producing esophageal *and* laryngeal obstruction. This condition has properly been called the "café coronary." In the most severe form, the patient may have been calmly eating (usually meat) when he suddenly turned blue and became unconscious. Alcohol intake is a common historical finding. Since this situation is not unlike the sequence of events following an acute myocardial infarction, an initiating esophageal obstruction might not be considered. However, the association with eating should alert the informed physician. An additional helpful feature is that these patients cannot speak. With lesser degrees of laryngeal obstruction, stridor and dyspnea with retractions might substantiate the diagnosis. Urgent removal of the offending plug of material from the esophagus is mandatory. This occasionally can be accomplished by fingers alone, but more commonly by a laryngoscope if one is available and time permits. If attempts at removal of the obstruction fail, tracheostomy should not be delayed.

Acute Gastric Dilatation

Mechanical gastric outlet obstruction producing chronic gastric dilatation can result from a variety of causes. However, acute massive gastric dilatation can occur in the absence of mechanical factors, presumably as a result of paralytic gastric ileus secondary to overactive sympathetic nervous stimulation. Acute gastric dilatation is seen commonly in debilitated patients with nasogastric tubes who are receiving nasal oxygen. Instances of gastric distention leading to bursting have occurred when nasal oxygen has been inadvertently connected to the nasogastric tube. Episodes of acute gastric dilatation also occur frequently in diabetic patients.

Whatever the underlying cause, marked gastric distention occurs, and 4 to 5 liters of extracellular fluid may accumulate. Distention of such a degree may produce interference with pulmonary and cardiac function through elevation of the diaphragm. In addition, such marked and rapid fluid losses may produce dehydration and hypovolemia. Vomiting with massive aspiration is a common sequela. The diagnosis in the described patients may be suspected if there are epigastric distention and tympany, repeated episodes of emesis, frequent singultus, and tachycardia. Untreated acute gastric dilatation may result in fatality. Adequate nasogastric tube drainage and rehydration remain the mainstays of therapy.

External Incarcerated Hernia

Since external incarcerated hernias may be among the most frequent causes of alimentary tract obstruction in emergency practice, and since their management initially may differ from our general therapeutic principles, a brief discussion seems warranted.

By definition, an incarcerated hernia is an irreducible protrusion of abdominal contents beyond the usual confines of the abdominal cavity, without, however, any compromise of the blood supply to the herniated tissue. In contrast, a strangulated hernia exists when the above conditions are met, but blood supply is insufficient to maintain viability. The clinical distinction between incarceration and strangulation is not always as simple as the difference in terms might suggest. Since each strangulated hernia must first pass through a stage of incarceration in its temporal course, at many points in the continuum of development, distinction may be difficult. Generally, the development of necrosis will be heralded by local tenderness, inflammation, fever, and an elevated WBC. It is of the utmost importance to distinguish between these two types of irreducible hernias, since the advent of necrosis will accelerate greatly our mode of therapy.

Three of the most common areas of hernia incarceration are the inguinal, femoral, and umbilical regions. Usually the patient will give a history of noticing the hernia for several years. However, on this occasion the previously reducible hernia cannot be replaced. If none of the signs of actual or impending necrosis are present, manipulative reduction of the hernia may be attempted. Such manipulation, particularly if improperly performed, may result in several complications. If necrosis of the hernial sac con-

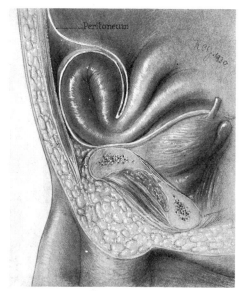

Figure 7. En masse reduction of an inguinal hernia. In this complication, the entire hernia sac and its contents are "reduced" back within the abdomen. However, the intestinal component of the hernia is not reduced from the sac. If sufficient constriction is present at the neck of the hernia sac, necrosis of intestine still confined within the hernia sac can occur. (From Pearse, H. E., Jr.: Strangulated hernia reduced en masse. Surg. Gynecol. Obstet. 53:822, 1931.)

tents is not recognized prior to reduction, generalized peritonitis will result when the necrotic material is returned to the abdominal cavity. Second, it is possible to rupture the incarcerated bowel if undue force is applied in an attempt to reduce the hernia. A third possible complication of incarcerated hernia reduction is that of a reduction en masse, in which the incarcerated mass of tissue is returned to the abdominal cavity but is not released from constriction (Fig. 7). Because of these potential complications, any patient undergoing successful hernia reduction should be followed continuously in a controlled environment until it can be established that none of these potential complications has developed. Surgical repair of the successfully reduced incarcerated hernia should be undertaken at the earliest convenient time to prevent a recurrence.

Failure to reduce the incarceration is an indication for urgent surgical repair in an effort to prevent the development of strangulation and subsequent necrosis. Preparations are similar to those general principles of management previously discussed.

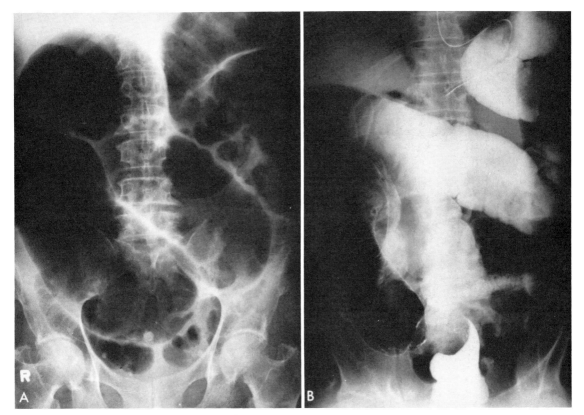

Figure 8.   *A,* Plain abdominal film of a patient with sigmoid volvulus. Note the large gas-filled loop of sigmoid pointing toward the right upper quadrant.

B, Barium enema on this same patient. Some barium has passed the area of twisting into the proximal colon. The tapering sigmoid at the point of twist has been referred to as a "parrot's beak."

Rectosigmoid Obstruction

Obstructions localized to the distal colon and rectum require that the emergency physician be familiar with several specialized forms of management peculiar to this region.

One of the basic dissimilarities in the pathophysiology of mechanical colonic obstruction, when compared to mechanical obstruction at other sites, is whether or not the ileocecal valve is functionally competent. In the 30 per cent of patients in whom this valve is competent, distention is limited exclusively to the colon when a distal obstruction exists. Accumulated gases and subsequent distention cannot be "decompressed" back into the small bowel; a closed-loop obstruction exists. Should the abdominal film suggest a closed-loop obstruction, haste in operative decompression is urgent. If, as is usual, the ileocecal valve is not competent, the abdominal film will suggest a rather generalized dilatation of both small and large bowel. This situation allows more time for rehydration, gastric decompression, and delineation of the obstruction.

The technique of proctosigmoidoscopy is an indispensable aid in the diagnosis and management of rectosigmoid obstructions. Most of the common causes of acute obstruction in this region, fecal impaction, carcinoma, inflammatory colon diseases, volvulus, and foreign bodies, are easily recognizable when seen through the sigmoidoscope. Upon occasion, its use will permit nonoperative decompression of sigmoid volvulus.

The diagnosis of volvulus frequently can be suspected by careful examination of the abdominal films (Fig. 8). A cautious barium enema may reveal the characteristic "parrot's beak." In performing sigmoidoscopy upon such patients, a most valuable piece of equipment is a bronchoscopy shield. If the operator is able to decompress the twisted sigmoid by *gentle* manipulation of the sigmoidoscope, the rapid colonic decompression through the sigmoidoscope will amply justify the use of the shield. If decompression can be obtained with the sigmoidoscope, a large red rubber catheter should be placed in the rectosigmoid area to prevent recurrent intestinal torsion in the post-decompression period. Following nonoperative decompression, strong consideration should be given to elective sigmoid resection in good risk patients, as the recurrence rate is exceptionally high.

It should be clear that no sigmoidoscopic attempt to reduce a sigmoid volvulus should be made if there is any question of the viability of the involved colon. Nonoperative detorsion of necrotic colon will result in death. In general, if sigmoidoscopic detorsion has failed, it is unwise to persist in any further nonoperative attempts, as volvulus represents a classic example of strangulation obstruction.

References

Barnett, W. O., and Hardy, J. D.: Observations concerning the peritoneal fluid in strangulated intestinal obstruction: the effects of removal from the peritoneal cavity. Surgery 43:440, 1958.

Cohn, I., Jr.: Strangulation obstruction: collective review. Surg. Gynecol. Obstet. 103:105, 1956.

Cokkinis, A. J.: The Management of Abdominal Operations. 2nd ed. London, Lewis, 1957.

Drucker, W. R., and Wright, H. K.: Physiology and pathophysiology of gastrointestinal fluids. Curr. Probl. Surg. May, 1964.

Maingot, R.: Abdominal Operations. 5th ed. New York, Appleton-Century-Crofts, Inc., 1969.

Noer, R. J., and Derr, J. W.: Effect of distention on intestinal revascularization. Arch. Surg. 59:542, 1949.

Shields, R.: The absorption and secretion of fluid and electrolytes by the obstructed bowel. Br. J. Surg. 52:774, 1965.

Sperling, L.: Mechanics of simple obstruction: an experimental study. Arch. Surg. 36:778, 1938.

Van Zwalenburg, C. : Strangulation resulting from strangulation of hollow viscera. Ann. Surg. 46:780, 1907.

Wangensteen, O. H.: Intestinal Obstructions. 3rd ed. Springfield, Ill., Charles C Thomas, 1955.

Wangensteen, O. H., and Rea, C. E.: The distention factor in simple intestinal obstruction. An experimental study with exclusion of swallowed air by cervical esophagostomy. Surgery 5:327, 1939.

Welch, C. E.: Intestinal Obstruction. Chicago, Ill., Year Book Medical Publishers, Inc., 1958.

D. UPPER GASTROINTESTINAL BLEEDING: DIFFERENTIAL DIAGNOSIS AND MANAGEMENT

Atef A. Salam

GASTROINTESTINAL BLEEDING

General Considerations

A great variety of lesions may cause bleeding in the gastrointestinal tract. More often than not, this complication manifests itself by hematemesis and passage of blood in the stools. Depending on the extent of blood loss, signs and symptoms of hypovolemia also may be present. "Upper gastrointestinal bleeding" is the term commonly used to describe all cases in which blood is present within the stomach, as evidenced by hematemesis or by the character of the drainage from the nasogastric tube. These features indicate that the source of bleeding is proximal to the ligament of Treitz. Distal to that level, the peristaltic contractions in the intervening loop of bowel normally prevent backflow of blood to the stomach.

Mixing of blood with acid in the stomach leads to the formation of acid hematin, which is the material responsible for the characteristic tarry or melanotic stools that are seen commonly in such cases. This change in the color of stools may be seen with any upper gastrointestinal bleeding in excess of 50 to 100 cc. Because of rapid neutralization of the acid in the duodenum and proximal bowel, no acid hematin can be formed if the bleeding site is in the small or large bowel, with the rare exception of a bleeding peptic ulcer in a Meckel's diverticulum. In most cases, therefore, one can assume that the absence of blood in nasogastric drainage in a patient who is presenting with melena is an indication that the bleeding is no longer active.

Bright red rectal bleeding is characteristic of large bowel lesions, although it may be seen with severe cases of upper gastrointestinal bleeding. The higher the source of bleeding, the more the blood is mixed with the stools. Blood on the surface of the fecal column is characteristic of low rectal or anal bleeding.

DIAGNOSTIC WORK-UP OF UPPER GASTROINTESTINAL BLEEDER

(1) Clinical evaluation.
(2) Endoscopy.
(3) Angiography.
(4) Gastrointestinal series.

Clinical Evaluation

Once the general condition of the patient is stabilized with suitable fluids and blood, as complete a medical history as possible should be obtained. History of heavy drinking is suggestive of esophageal variceal bleeding or erosive gastritis, and bleeding that has been preceded by repeated forceful vomiting is characteristic of Mallory-Weiss syndrome. None of these features, however, is absolutely specific, as evidenced by the fact that the source of bleeding can be identified on the basis of history in only 40 per cent of cases.

Apart from mild epigastric tenderness, abdominal examination usually is negative in patients with bleeding peptic ulcer. In contrast, patients with variceal bleeding usually show some evidence of liver disease such as jaundice, ascites, and enlarged liver or spleen. These signs, however, may be absent in patients with portal vein occlusion, compensated liver cirrhosis, or idiopathic portal hypertension.

Gastroduodenal Endoscopy

Since the advent of fiberoptic gastroscopy, endoscopy has become increasingly popular for the initial evaluation of patients presenting with upper gastrointestinal bleeding. The test does not require general anesthesia and can be done as a bedside procedure. It permits the recognition of the presence of multiple anomalies and, more importantly, the identification of which lesion actually is responsible for the acute hemorrhage.

The diagnostic accuracy and relative ease of performance of gastroduodenoscopy justify consideration of the examination for all patients with acute upper gastrointestinal bleeding. It should be performed as soon as feasible to ensure a high rate of diagnostic accuracy. It should be done before the patient is given any barium, otherwise the field would be obscured. Endoscopy is not recommended in patients with massive bleeding, because of poor visibility and because of the danger of exsanguination or aspiration during the procedure.

Diagnostic Angiography

Celiac, superior mesenteric, and inferior mesenteric angiography has been shown to be very useful in the diagnosis of gastrointestinal bleeding. Selection of the artery to be studied is based on the clinical impression regarding the site of bleeding. In some cases, study may be needed of more than one artery. Bleeding in excess of 0.5 to 1 cc. per minute usually can be detected angiographically as extravasation of contrast medium from the bleeding vessel. Visceral angiography usually is indicated in most cases of gastrointestinal bleeding in which the endoscopic findings have been inconclusive. It is the best method for the demonstration of bleeding sites in the small bowel, such as Meckel's diverticulum or an A-V malformation. Angiographic visualization of the bleeding site is essential in all cases that are being considered for intra-arterial therapeutic infusion. Angiography is most valuable in the work-up of patients with variceal bleeding. The anatomic and physiologic information that is provided by either periarterial or percutaneous splenoportography is essential for the proper selection of operative procedure in each individual case.

Gastrointestinal Barium Study

Gastrointestinal barium study is only of limited value in the diagnostic work-up of upper gastrointestinal bleeding. Manipulation of the patient in the dark room is hindered by the I.V. lines and other equipment used for resuscitation. The patient cannot be examined upright for fear of inducing hypotension. This contributes to the relative inaccuracy of emergency upper gastrointestinal series. Only one-third to one-half of endoscopically proved gastric or duodenal ulcers can be seen on emergency gastrointestinal studies. Since barium contrast study cannot prove a visualized lesion to be the source of bleeding, it should not be used as a primary study if the need for endoscopy or angiography is anticipated, but it should be obtained before the patient is discharged.

BLEEDING PEPTIC ULCER

Peptic ulcer disease usually is responsible for two-thirds of all cases of upper gastrointestinal bleeding. The ratio of duodenal to gastric ulcers in most series is the same as their ratio in the uncomplicated form, indicating that the location of the ulcer does not alter its tendency to bleed. Although granulation tissue at the base of the ulcer is the most likely source, erosion into a blood vessel is seen commonly in patients who require emergency surgical treatment. Hemorrhage from an extragastric major vessel, such as the gastroduodenal or the splenic artery, is often fatal.

Management

Because of the potential danger of exsanguination, all patients with bleeding from peptic ulcer should be hospitalized in an area where they can be observed adequately. Once the blood loss has been replaced and the condition of the patient has been stabilized,* endoscopy should be performed. After the diagnosis of bleeding peptic ulcer has been confirmed, an attempt should be made to treat the patient medically. In most cases, the bleeding stops after a period of bed rest, sedation, and repeated gastric lavage with iced saline. These patients should be put on a strict ulcer diet until the symptoms disappear and until com-

plete healing of the ulcers is confirmed by endoscopic and radiologic examinations. For duodenal ulcer, this medical management may be tried for as long as six months. For gastric ulcer, on the other hand, the absence of any evidence of healing after six weeks of adequate medical management should be considered an indication for surgical treatment. Elective surgical treatment should be considered in all patients who have repeated episodes of bleeding or one episode of life-threatening hemorrhage. Other indications for elective surgical treatment include perforation, obstruction, and, in case of gastric ulcers, malignancy.

The indications for emergency operative control of bleeding from peptic ulcer include threatening exsanguination and an episode of major bleeding subsequent to an initial satisfactory response. Less defined are the criteria for surgical treatment when the bleeding, although not very severe, is persistent despite adequate medical treatment. In such cases, operative treatment should be considered if, after initial restoration of blood volume, the patient continues to require more than one unit per 12 hours to stabilize his vital signs.

Certain technical aspects of the operative management of bleeding peptic ulcer need to be emphasized. Thorough exploration of the entire abdomen should be conducted in order to exclude any other possible source of bleeding. The lesser sac should be opened so that the entire stomach, including the gastroesophageal region, can be examined adequately. The ulcer should be well exposed by opening the stomach or duodenum, and the bleeder should be oversewn by one or more matrix stitches of nonabsorbable suture. Extragastric ligation of the feeding vessel, such as the gastroduodenal artery, also may be needed if the ulcer base is severely inflamed. To protect the patient against further bleeding, a corrective procedure for ulcer diathesis must be performed. This usually consists of vagotomy combined either with pyloroplasty or with antrectomy. Vagotomy and pyloroplasty is the simpler of the two operations, but it has a higher incidence of recurrence of bleeding. It usually is selected for the emergency treatment of bleeding duodenal ulcer in elderly patients with multiple medical problems. Conversely, vagotomy and antrectomy is recommended for young patients with sta-

*See page 541.

ble vital signs, provided that the extent of pathology is compatible with uncomplicated closure of the duodenal stump. Hemigastrectomy, with or without vagotomy, is the procedure most commonly used for the treatment of bleeding gastric ulcer.

Success rates as high as 90 per cent for vagotomy and pyloroplasty, and 95 per cent for vagotomy and antrectomy, have been reported. Operative mortality usually is below 5 per cent in young and otherwise healthy patients, but it may be 20 per cent or higher in elderly patients with complicated medical problems.

BLEEDING ESOPHAGEAL VARICES

Hemorrhage from esophageal varices is a life-threatening complication that is responsible for the death of more than one-third of all patients with liver cirrhosis. Together with erosive gastritis, it accounts for nearly one-third of all cases of upper gastrointestinal bleeding.

In patients with portal hypertension, collateral channels develop between the portal venous bed of the fundus of the stomach and the systemic veins draining the lower third of the esophagus. Circulatory

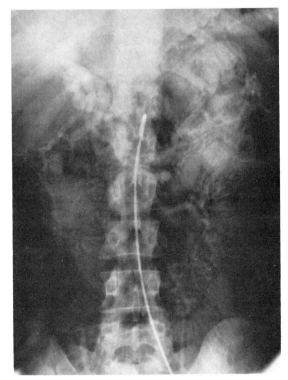

Figure 2. Portal hypertension—prehepatic. Neonatal portal vein thrombosis.

overloading of the submucous venous plexus in this region leads to the formation of gastroesophageal varices. Because of their vulnerable position, these varices frequently rupture, causing serious and sometimes fatal hemorrhage. It is possible that this complication might be triggered in some instances by a sudden rise in venous pressure due to straining, or by repeated mucosal irritation secondary to reflux esophagitis. In most cases, however, no obvious precipitating factor can be found.

According to the site of the circulatory block, portal hypertension may be described as hepatic, prehepatic, or posthepatic. Of the three varieties, hepatic portal hypertension is the most common cause of variceal bleeding (Fig. 1). It usually is due to either alcoholic or postnecrotic cirrhosis, although cases secondary to hepatic fibrosis or schistosomiasis occasionally may be seen. Prehepatic portal hypertension usually is caused by portal venous occlusion as a result of anomalous development of the portal vein or thrombophlebitis secondary to sepsis in the newly-born (Figs. 2 and 3). Although relatively rare, portal vein occlusion is the most

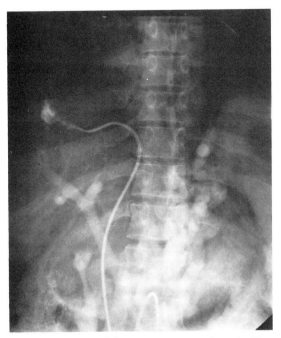

Figure 1. Portal hypertension—intrahepatic. Venous phase of superior mesenteric artery injection showing extensive gastroesophageal varices.

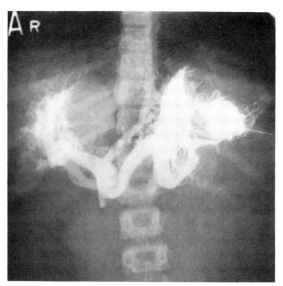

Figure 3. Portal hypertension—prehepatic. Direct splenoportogram showing hilar occlusion of the portal vein.

common cause of upper gastrointestinal bleeding in children. Other causes of portal vein thrombosis occurring later in life include cirrhosis, intra-abdominal sepsis (Fig. 4), or neoplasms. Splenic venous thrombosis is a rare clinical entity that is mostly seen as a complication of alcoholic pancreatitis. In this condition, the venous hypertensive state is

limited to the cardia and other parts of the stomach that normally are drained by the short gastric or gastroepiploic branches of the splenic vein. Since the pressure in the veins along the lesser curvature remains normal, a pressure gradient develops within the stomach wall leading to the formation of gastric, as well as esophageal, varices (Figs. 5 and 6). Posthepatic portal hypertension, commonly known as Budd-Chiari syndrome, is due to hepatic vein thrombosis, with or without inferior venocaval obstruction. In most cases, the cause of venous thrombosis is not clear, although birth control pills have been blamed in some recently reported cases.

Management of Variceal Bleeding

A quick assessment of the general condition of the patient and the severity of bleeding should be made in the Emergency Department. Resuscitative measures should be initiated without delay, and continued while diagnostic procedures are being performed. Unless the bleeding is very severe, an attempt should be made to confirm the diagnosis of esophageal varices versus other causes of upper gastrointestinal bleeding such as gastritis, esophageal tear, or peptic ulceration. Endoscopy is most valuable in this regard, and should be performed as soon as the general condition of the patient allows.

Several techniques have been described for surgical management of variceal bleeding. Mild cases frequently respond to bed rest and repeated gastric lavage with iced saline. For persistent bleeding, an attempt

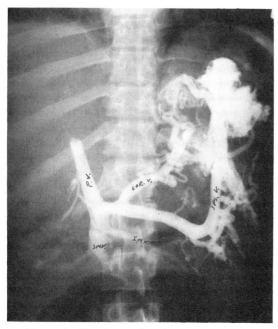

Figure 4. Portal vein thrombosis secondary to abdominal sepsis.

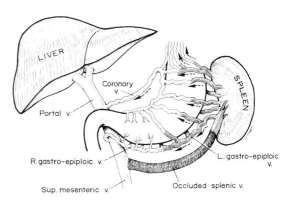

Figure 5. Splenic vein thrombosis. Diagrammatic illustration of collateral circulation.

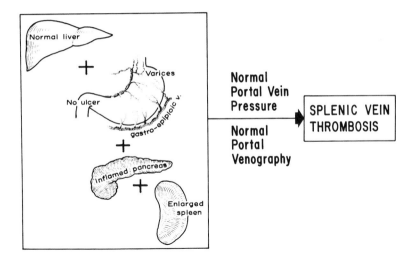

Figure 6. Splenic vein thrombosis: diagnostic features.

should be made to control it either by balloon tamponade (Sengstaken-Blakemore tube) or by intra-arterial vasopressin perfusion. More than two decades of experience with balloon tamponade has established clearly the efficacy of this technique in controlling variceal bleeding. However, because of its high complication rate, an increasing number of clinicians are now advocating the use of intra-arterial vasopressin perfusion initially, reserving balloon tamponade for severe cases in which immediate control of bleeding is mandatory. Further discussion of these two techniques is given at the end of this chapter.

During a bleeding episode, the rate of production of ammonia in the intestine is expected to increase, owing to the action of proteolytic intestinal bacteria on the protein component of the blood within the bowel. Ammonia and other related metabolites play a basic etiologic role in the development of the various mental changes that commonly are associated with variceal bleeding. Certain preventive measures, therefore, should be taken to control the rate of production of these metabolites. An oral nonabsorbable intestinal antibiotic such as neomycin has proved effective in this regard. The usual dose is 2 gm. initially, followed by 1 gm. every six hours. Administration of enema or suppositories to empty the blood in the colon also is recommended in these cases.

Approximately 80 per cent of cases of variceal bleeding can be managed successfully by medical means, at least temporarily. Studies have shown that 60 per cent of such patients rebleed massively within one year at a mortality rate that may reach 50 per cent. On this basis, elective surgical treatment should be considered in all patients who have hemorrhaged once, unless the risk involved is exceptionally high because of severe liver disease or associated medical illness. The superiority of this approach, as compared to medical management, has been confirmed in several well controlled clinical studies. The operation may be delayed for a few weeks until the liver function studies show complete recovery from the worsening effects of the bleeding episode. Remarkable improvement in the condition of the liver often is seen in alcoholic patients who have abstained.

The response to medical management is considered inadequate if the bleeding continues or recurs, as evidenced by the presence of bright red blood in the nasogastric tube and by the continued need for blood transfusion. Further management of these patients should be determined by the extent of their liver disease. Experience has shown that emergency operative treatment usually is well tolerated by patients with good hepatic function and stable liver disease, once vital signs are stabilized. Since the risk involved is not much higher than the risk of elective surgical treatment, emergency operative control of the bleeding should be recommended for these patients early in the course of their treatment if they fail to respond to nonsurgical management.

Conversely, patients with severe liver disease are very poor candidates for emergency operative treatment, on account of the exceedingly high incidence of postoperative liver failure. Continued medical management, therefore, is warranted in such patients as long as the danger of exsanguination is not imminent. The latter approach applies to patients with severe muscle wasting, massive ascites, jaundice (bilirubin more than 2 mg./100), hypoalbuminemia (less than 3 gm. per cent), and marked prolongation of the prothrombin time.

OPERATIVE PROCEDURES FOR THE SURGICAL CONTROL OF VARICEAL BLEEDING

The emergency physician usually will not be the operating surgeon, but it is important to be aware of the surgical procedures that can be employed, and to seek appropriate consultation for selected patients.

(1) *Operations designed to decompress the varices by interrupting the collateral pathways between the portal and systemic venous systems at the gastroesophageal junction.* This category includes transesophageal ligation of varices, gastroesophageal devascularization, and Tanner's operation. Transesophageal ligation of varices is associated with a very high incidence of rebleeding, and should only be used as a temporary procedure in very high risk patients who are not expected to tolerate a more extensive procedure. Splenectomy and gastroesophageal devascularization might succeed initially, but the bleeding is likely to recur within less than two years in more than one-half of the cases. However, this operation may be the only feasible procedure in patients with complete mesosplenoportal venous thrombosis. In order to interrupt the extrinsic, as well as the intrinsic, porta-azygos collaterals, Tanner combines gastric devascularization with transection of the proximal part of the stomach. This operation, however, has not received wide acceptance because of the high incidence of leakage from the devascularized suture line.

(2) *Operations designed to decompress the varices by creating a shunt between the portal and systemic venous systems.* Included in this category are portacaval, conventional splenorenal, and mesocaval shunts (Fig. 7). A well constructed portasystemic shunt almost invariably protects the

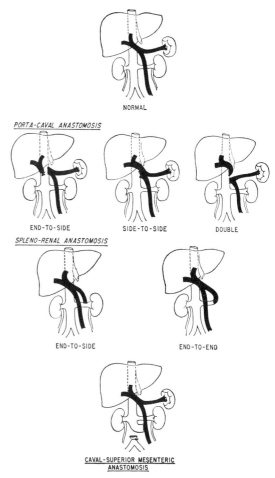

Figure 7. Various forms of portasystemic shunts. (From Schwartz, S. I., et al. (eds.): Principles of Surgery. Copyright © 1969 by McGraw-Hill, Inc. Used by permission of the McGraw-Hill Book Co.)

patient against further variceal bleeding. Recently, however, there has been an increasing awareness of certain negative features of these operations, namely, the high incidence of encephalopathy and delayed hepatic failure. These complications seem to be related to the sudden loss of portal venous blood flow to the liver, which is a constant feature of all types of total portasystemic shunting procedures. In order to avoid these undesirable features, a new procedure, the distal splenorenal shunt, has been described recently. The operation is designed to decompress the variceal bed without interfering with the portal venous blood flow to the liver. In this procedure, the splenic end of the divided splenic vein is anastomosed to the side of the left renal vein, and its central end is oversewn close to its junction with

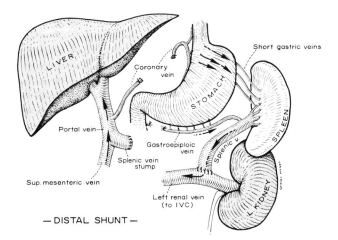

Figure 8. Diagrammatic representation of the distal splenorenal operation.

the superior mesenteric vein. The operation is still in the investigative stage, although encouraging results have been reported recently (Fig. 8).

ACUTE EROSIVE GASTRITIS

The clinical importance of this condition has been appreciated more in recent years since the introduction of the fiberoptic instrumentation made routine diagnostic gastroscopy practically feasible. It is characterized by the development of multiple erosions, ranging from pinpoint size to about 1 cm. in diameter. Microscopically, the pathology is limited to the gastric mucosa, which shows multiple foci of hemorrhage, necrosis, and ulceration. Acute gastritis often is preceded by stress caused by trauma, operation, sepsis, or pulmonary insufficiency. Similar histologic changes often are seen in association with heavy drinking, or prolonged intake of anti-inflammatory drugs such as aspirin or steroids. In some instances, no obvious precipitating factor can be found.

The mechanism of acute gastric mucosal bleeding is not known. A constant pattern of acid hypersecretion has never been demonstrated, but impairment of the gastric mucosal barrier occurs and is physiologically demonstrable by the measured increase in the back-diffusion of hydrogen ions.

Acute erosive gastritis should be considered in the differential diagnosis of upper gastrointestinal bleeding in patients with severe illness secondary to sepsis or multiple injuries. Alcoholic gastritis, another clinical entity, is the most common cause of bleeding in heavy drinkers. *Endoscopic distinction between alcoholic gastritis, variceal bleeding, and Mallory-Weiss syndrome is essential*, since the treatment of these conditions is not the same.

Management

Erosive gastritis is an acute process that may never recur if the patient survives the first episode. Therefore, medical treatment may be continued beyond what is considered as an adequate trial in other conditions such as bleeding peptic ulcer or esophageal varices. Successful control of bleeding from acute gastritis, using intra-arterial vasopressin infusion, has been reported by several investigators in recent years. At the present time, this technique ought to be considered if the bleeding fails to respond to bed rest and gastric lavage, particularly in poor surgical risk patients.

Surgical treatment in this condition remains controversial. Vagotomy and pyloroplasty is a relatively simple operation, but the incidence of rebleeding in various series ranges from 15 to 50 per cent. Total gastrectomy, on the other hand, provides complete protection against bleeding, yet is a rather extensive procedure with considerable morbidity and mortality. Partial gastrectomy and vagotomy generally is considered the operation of choice, being less extensive than total gastrectomy, and more effective than vagotomy and pyloroplasty in controlling the bleeding. Vagotomy and pyloroplasty may be preferred for the treatment of seriously ill patients, but the mortality associated with postoperative recurrence of bleeding in these patients is quite high.

MALLORY-WEISS SYNDROME

The relationship between retching and vomiting, and mucosal or submucosal lacerations at the cardioesophageal junction, was described by Mallory and Weiss in 1929. It has been postulated that the vomiting reflex becomes poorly co-ordinated after repeated episodes of vomiting, and the gastric contents are regurgitated against an unrelaxed esophagus and a contracted diaphragm. In most of the early reports, ingestion of alcohol was stressed as a precipitating factor. More recently, many causes of vomiting other than alcoholism have been reported.

In most instances, the history of retching and vomiting normal gastrointestinal contents before hematemesis permits recog-

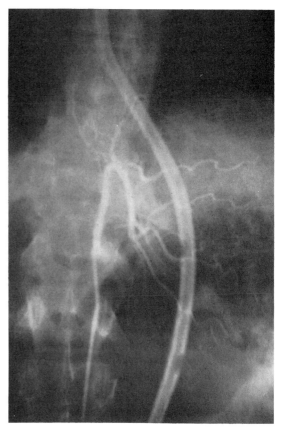

Figure 10. Mallory-Weiss syndrome – after vasopressin infusion.

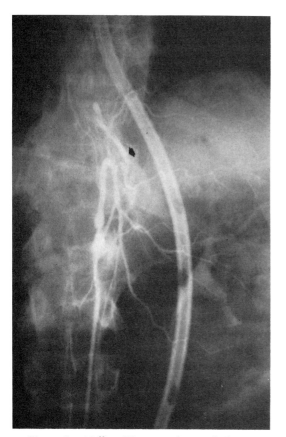

Figure 9. Mallory-Weiss syndrome – before vasopressin infusion.

nition of this condition. The diagnosis can be readily confirmed, if bleeding is active, by selective celiac arteriography (Fig. 9). Endoscopy can be used diagnostically if bleeding has slowed or stopped. Routine use of these diagnostic modalities has shown that this condition occurs more frequently than previously thought.

Management

Medical management, including blood transfusions but without any tubes or surgery, has proved adequate in many patients with Mallory-Weiss syndrome. Some patients have been treated successfully with the balloon tamponade, but the pressure often is insufficient to control the arterial type of bleeding, which fortunately is less common. Intra-arterial vasopressin infusion has been used with increasing frequency in recent years, and the results have been quite encouraging (Fig. 10). Surgical intervention is required when bleeding is massive, recurrent, or unresponsive to intra-arterial infusion. The stomach is opened close to the gastroesophageal junction, and the bleeder is oversewn.

NONSURGICAL TECHNIQUES COMMONLY USED IN TREATMENT OF UPPER GASTROINTESTINAL BLEEDING

Gastric Irrigation with Iced Saline

This is the most widely used technique in the initial management of patients with upper gastrointestinal bleeding. A No. 30 Ewalt nasogastric tube is positioned in the stomach and, using a 60 cc. syringe, the stomach is irrigated with iced saline. The exchange should be rapid enough to achieve maximal cooling of the gastric mucosa. Saline, rather than water, is used to avoid possible water intoxication.

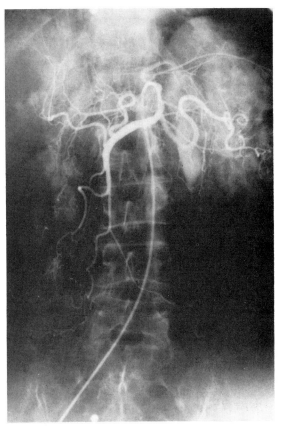

Figure 12. Same patient. Bleeding controlled by vasopressin infusion.

Intra-arterial Vasopressin Perfusion

INDICATIONS

(1) Mucosal lesions, e.g., acute erosive gastritis.
(2) Mallory-Weiss syndrome.
(3) Moderate variceal bleeding in high-risk patients.
(4) Moderate persistent diverticular bleeding.
(5) Bleeding from inoperable tumor of the G.I. tract (Figs. 11 and 12).
(6) A.V. malformation of the GI tract.
(7) Peptic ulcer: I.A.V.P. does not seem to be quite as effective in controlling bleeding from peptic ulcer. Occasionally, however, it may be indicated in patients with severe medical illness such as renal failure or advanced chronic lung disease.

TECHNIQUE

At first the bleeding site is demonstrated by selective variceal angiography. Pitressin,

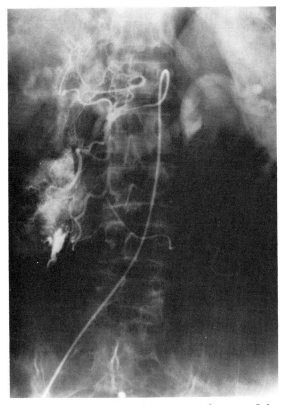

Figure 11. Bleeding from carcinoid tumor of the second part of duodenum.

0.1 to 0.4 unit per minute (depending on the vessel being infused), is administered for 15 minutes. A repeat angiogram is obtained, and the dose of Pitressin infusion is adjusted according to the angiographic findings. Effective vasoconstriction is indicated by significant decrease in the size of the branches of the infused vessels, with good forward flow into the capillary and venous phase without extravasation of contrast (Figs. 11 and 12). During the procedure, continuous EKG and arterial pressure monitoring should be obtained. The infusion is continued for 24 hours, using the same strength as determined by the angiographic response, and then one-half the initial strength for the next 24. This is followed by 24 hours of saline infusion, and, if there are no signs of renewal of bleeding, the catheter is removed. The patient should be kept in an intensive care area during the entire procedure.

FURTHER MANAGEMENT

If the bleeding is controlled, the patient should be worked up and managed medically or surgically, according to the nature of the underlying disease. The criteria of failure of this technique are: (1) recurrence of bleeding after an initial favorable response; or (2) persistence of bleeding as indicated by the continued presence of bright red blood in the nasogastric drainage, and by further need for more than 3 units of blood transfusion during the first 24 hours of infusion therapy. In such cases, it is essential to exclude catheter displacement by repeated angiography before discontinuing the treatment.

COMPLICATIONS

(1) All complications of angiography, such as arterial hematoma, thrombosis, or laceration.

(2) Bowel ischemia.

(3) Liver damage due to inadvertent injection into an anomalous hepatic artery.

(4) Ischemia of the lower limbs due to catheter displacement in the aorta.

(5) Circulatory overload owing to the antidiuretic effect of vasopressin.

Balloon Tamponade for the Treatment of Gastroesophageal Variceal Bleeding

Balloon tamponade usually is done with the Sengstaken-Blakemore tube. This is a rubber tube with three lumens and a gastric and an esophageal balloon. Two of the lumens are used to inflate the balloons, and the third is used for nasogastric suction.

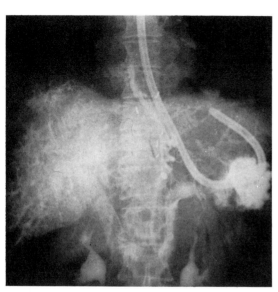

Figure 13. Sengstaken-Blakemore tube before inflation of the balloons. Notice filling of the gastroesophageal varices.

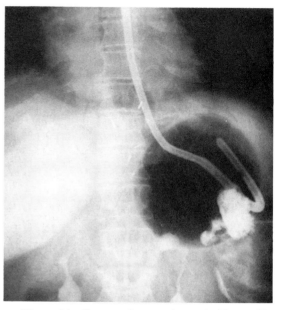

Figure 14. Same patient as shown in Figure 13. Notice nonfilling of esophageal varices with the gastric balloon inflated.

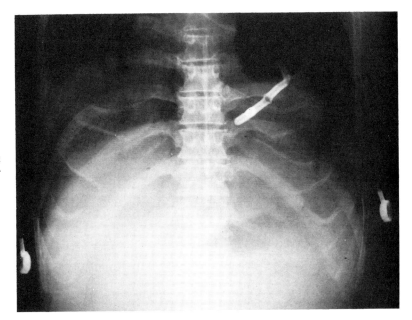

Figure 15. Gastric balloon misplaced in the esophagus inflated by mistake.

INDICATIONS

(1) Severe variceal bleeding.

(2) Moderate or persistent bleeding that requires transfusion of more than 2000 cc. of blood over a period of 24 hours.

TECHNIQUE

Whenever it is feasible, the patient should be placed in an intensive care area where the vital signs can be observed care-fully. Once the tube has been passed into the stomach, 50 cc. of air is injected into the gastric balloon so that its position below the diaphragm can be confirmed radiologically. The gastric balloon then is inflated fully, using a total of 250 to 300 cc. of air (Figs. 13 and 14). In order to tamponade the fundal veins carrying the blood from the gastric veins to the esophageal veins, the tube is put on traction and maintained in this position by fixing it to the mouth-piece of a foot-ball helmet used for this purpose. The posi-

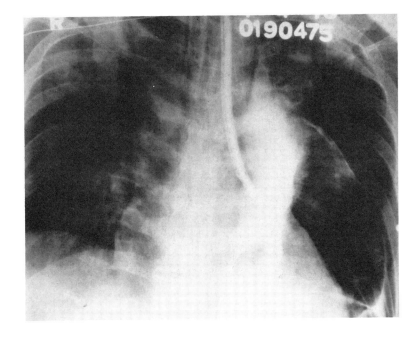

Figure 16. Same patient as shown in Figure 15. Esopha-gogram showing extravasation of contrast in the left pleural space.

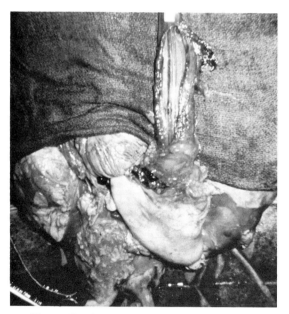

Figure 17. Same patient as in Figure 15, showing laceration of the esophagus at autopsy.

then deflate the balloons, and, if there are no signs of renewed bleeding, remove the tube the next day.

COMPLICATIONS OF THE SENGSTAKEN-BLAKEMORE TUBE

(1) Mucosal necrosis due to excessive or prolonged pressure by the balloon.

(2) Aspiration pneumonitis due to secretions accumulating in the esophagus.

(3) Laceration of the esophagus caused by over-inflation of a misplaced gastric balloon (Figs. 15, 16, and 17).

(4) Airway obstruction due to dislodgement of an under-inflated gastric balloon. If this happens, the tube should be immediately divided and extracted. A pair of scissors should be kept by the bedside for this purpose.

tion of the tube should be adjusted in order to avoid any pressure on the external nose. To prevent aspiration pneumonitis, a separate suction tube is used to evacuate the secretions in the esophagus. In most cases, bleeding can be controlled by the gastric balloon alone, but in some instances direct compression of the bleeding varix by the esophageal balloon also is needed. Because of the danger of esophageal necrosis or laceration, the pressure in the esophageal balloon should not exceed 40 mm. Hg.

FURTHER MANAGEMENT

If the bleeding continues with both balloons inflated, one should first look for correctible causes of failure such as misplacement of the balloons, inadequate tamponade, or misdiagnosis. If none exists, and the liver function tests are satisfactory, emergency operative treatment is indicated. If there are clinical and laboratory signs of liver decompensation, medical management should be continued. Operative treatment in these cases should be used as a last resort.

If the bleeding has been controlled, deflate the balloons intermittently at six-hour intervals to avoid mucosal necrosis. Continue the treatment for 24 to 48 hours,

References

Drapanas, T., et al.: Experiences with surgical management of acute gastric mucosal hemorrhage: a unified concept in the pathophysiology. Ann. Surg. *173*:628, 1971.

Eisenberg, M. M., et al.: Vagotomy and drainage procedure for duodenal ulcer: the results of ten years' experience. Ann. Surg. *170*:317, 1969.

Farris, J. M., and Smith, G. K.: Appraisal of the long-term results of vagotomy and pyloroplasty in 100 patients with bleeding duodenal ulcer. Ann. Surg. *166*:630, 1967.

Hedberg, S. E.: Endoscopy in gastrointestinal bleeding: a systemic approach to diagnosis. Surg. Clin. North Am. *54*:549, 1974.

Herrington, J. L., Sawyers, J. L., and Scott, H. W., Jr.: A 25-year experience with vagotomy-antrectomy. Arch. Surg. *106*:469, 1973.

Nusbaum, M., et al.: Clinical experience with selective intra-arterial infusion of vasopressin in the control of gastrointestinal bleeding from arterial sources. Am. J. Surg. *123*:165, 1972.

Palmer, E. D.: The vigorous diagnostic approach to upper-gastrointestinal tract hemorrhage: a 23-year prospective study of 1,400 patients. J. Am. Med. Assoc. *207*:1477, 1969.

Salam, A. A., et al.: Hemodynamic contrasts between selective and total portal-systemic decompression. Ann. Surg. *173*:827, 1971.

Schwartz, S. I.: Principles of Surgery. New York, Blakiston, McGraw-Hill Book Co., 1969.

Sherlock, S.: Diseases of the Liver and Biliary System. 4th ed. Philadelphia, F. A. Davis Co., 1968.

Warren, W. D., Zeppa, R., and Fomon, J. J.: Selective transplenic decompression of gastroesophageal varices by distal splenorenal shunt. Ann. Surg. *166*:437, 1967.

Wychulis, A. R., and Sasso, A.: Mallory-Weiss syndrome. Arch. Surg. *107*:868, 1973.

E. HEPATIC DISEASE

John T. Galambos

HEPATITIS

Introduction

The most common types of infection of the liver are due to viral agents. These are (occasionally) the E.-B. agent of infectious mononucleosis, or the cytomegalovirus or (rarely) rubella, coxsackie, or ECHO viruses. By far the most common infection of the liver is due to the hepatitis viruses, types A and B (probably also type C). The disease caused by virus A has a short incubation period and used to be called infectious hepatitis. That caused by virus B has a long incubation period and used to be called "serum hepatitis." It is well known that both types of virus can be transmitted by mouth. The fecal-oral route is the dominant mode of transmission for type A hepatitis. The recognized route of infection for type B is parenteral. Other modes of transmission include sexual contact and close person-to-person (possibly droplet but not fecal) transmission.

Recognition

SUBJECTIVE FINDINGS

Viral hepatitis A or B may be asymptomatic. However, patients usually are brought to the Emergency Department because of symptoms, and over 85 per cent have these for less than ten days before the onset of jaundice. The symptoms are: (1) lassitude, loss of appetite, and nausea in over 90 per cent; (2) weakness, fever, vomiting, and headache in 70 to 80 per cent; (3) chilliness, abdominal discomfort, or abdominal pain in two-thirds. It should be noted that abdominal pain can be severe enough to be confused with a surgical abdomen. Surgery should be avoided, since operative mortality rate is very high. Irritability and drowsiness occur in 50 per cent of patients. These symptoms should *not* be confused with the early manifestations of encephalopathy. A flu-like syndrome characterized by sore throat, myalgia, arthralgia, or nasal stuffiness occurs in 20 per cent. Arthralgia is common in hepatitis A; arthritis usually is seen in hepatitis B, probably because of precipitation of antigen–antibody complexes on the synovia. Polyarthritis may be prominent in a few patients, who may or may not become jaundiced subsequently.

Look for dark urine (bilirubinuria) as a clue to hepatitis in symptomatic patients. This finding precedes jaundice by a period of one to four days. Symptomatic but anicteric hepatitis is common among children, but most adults become jaundiced.

OBJECTIVE FINDINGS

The most characteristic observations are dark urine, jaundice, and a tender liver, palpable at, or a few centimeters below, the costal margin. The liver usually is palpable, but is never markedly enlarged. The edge is smooth and rounded and the consistency is firm. It is not as firm and rubbery as a cirrhotic liver, nor is it hard as a liver filled with cancer. Hepatic tenderness may not be easy to elicit because of the patient's unwillingness or inability to permit the physician to palpate the liver. Percussion or brisk pressure in the right hypochondrium or upper right quandrant can elicit pain, however. The spleen is palpable in 15 per cent of patients; some lymph nodes may be enlarged, but generalized lymphadenopathy is not seen in viral hepatitis. Occasionally, small spider angiomata may develop transiently during the acute illness.

The hematocrit and WBC usually are normal; a relative lymphocytosis is common. Atypical lymphocytes (virocytes)up to 10 per cent may be seen. Leukocytosis of 12,000 or over, particularly with a shift to the left, usually indicates a severe, atypical form of hepatitis or another illness. The urine generally is normal, although a mild proteinuria may be seen in addition to bilirubin. Serum bilirubin over 10 mg./dl. usually is not seen in typical viral hepatitis.

The most useful liver (injury) tests (part of multiphasic screening) are the elevation of the SGOT, serum alkaline phosphatase (SAP), prothrombin time (PT), and hepatitis B surface antigen (HBsAg). In about 50 per cent of patients with hepatitis the SGOT is over 500 units. Only an occasional patient with biliary tract disease or alcoholic hepatitis will have SGOT elevations in this range. It must be remembered that the height of the SGOT is not proportional to the severity of liver disease. Patients with asymptomatic or subclinical viral hepatitis may have SGOTs over 2000 units. SAP may be normal or elevated, but it rarely exceeds twice the upper limit of normal. Despite the elevation of SAP, the serum cholesterol is not increased. The serum albumin, although usually decreased somewhat, still remains within normal limits. The gamma globulin usually is under 2 gm./dl. Although typical viral hepatitis may be associated with gamma globulin elevations over 3.5 gm./dl. and albumin below 2.5 gm./dl., these findings generally indicate a chronic hepatitis with or without cirrhosis. The PT is always normal, or becomes normal in 24 hours after vitamin K injection. Prolongation of the PT is the most significant *prognostic* finding: it is evidence of extensive depression of hepatic function, and indicates a fulminant clinical course or a chronic rather than acute illness.

The most definitive diagnostic test of hepatitis B is the HBsAg. The earlier in the course of hepatitis that serum is tested, the greater is the chance to detect this antigen. At or before onset of symptoms of hepatitis B, HBsAg is positive in over 90 per cent of cases. After the onset of jaundice, antigenemia rapidly decreases in frequency. Persistent antigenemia for 13 weeks or longer may indicate the development of chronic hepatitis.

Assessment

When the epidemiologic setting is appropriate, the subjective and objective findings are characteristic, and the diagnosis of acute hepatitis is made without additional procedures. When the diagnosis is uncertain or the course is atypical, a liver biopsy should be performed. A skilled observer can then establish the diagnosis on morphologic grounds.

TREATMENT

Diagnostic Plan

The initial plan is to provide rest, ensure hydration and nutrition, and to establish the diagnosis. Once the disease is suspected, obtain a CBC, HBsAg, bilirubin (fractionation for direct or conjugated and indirect bilirubin is meaningless), SGOT, SAP, albumin, gamma globulins, and PT.

If the diagnosis of typical acute viral hepatitis is uncertain, obtain a liver biopsy. The disease is atypical if the biopsy shows: (1) confluent bridging) necrosis—this form of hepatitis is associated with a 15 per cent mortality rate, 25 per cent risk of chronic active hepatitis, and 30 per cent risk of cirrhosis; or (2) chronic aggressive hepatitis with or without cirrhosis, which may masquerade as acute viral hepatitis. The latter is suspected when the spleen is enlarged and there is a previous history of hepatitis, or when other findings suggest chronic liver disease (ascites, wasting, low albumin and high gamma globulin, LE cells, nuclear or smooth muscle antibodies).

Serum protein electrophoresis is necessary only if the serum albumin is low. The low serum albumin in multiphasic analysis may be a laboratory error in the face of elevated serum bilirubin. Liver scan is unnecessary and expensive.

During typical acute hepatitis, the liver tests need not be repeated more often than at seven- to 14-day intervals. The clearing of jaundice is just as apparent by clinical observation as by laboratory tests. When the patient's clinical illness is severe, the PT should be repeated daily. Persistence of nausea and vomiting, the persistent high plateau of the serum bilirubin concentration, may be manifestations of an atypical form of severe hepatitis.

Liver biopsy also should be considered if the patient had cholestatic hepatitis. In this case, serum bilirubin may rise over 10 mg./dl. and may exceed 25 mg./dl. The serum lipoproteins, SAP, the α_2 and β globulins, and cholesterol are elevated. The SAP is increased to two to three times the upper limits of normal, whereas SGOT usually remains under 300 units.

Therapeutic Plan

There is no specific treatment for viral hepatitis. Treatment can be divided into: (1) the patient; and (2) the contacts.

TREATMENT OF THE PATIENT

BED REST

Hospitalization is necessary only if adequate rest is not possible at home, or if nausea and vomiting preclude adequate oral hydration, let alone nutrition. There is no evidence that enforced bed rest accelerates the rate of healing of typical acute hepatitis, and since prolonged bed rest by itself results in physical debility, it should not be enforced. The clinically ill patient who is nauseated and cannot eat should remain in bed. However, once the appetite and sense of well-being improve, the patient should be allowed to ambulate in his room within the limits of fatigue, regardless of the depth of jaundice, and should be allowed to go to the bathroom. As hepatitis is improving, gradual ambulation can hasten rather than retard the rate of recovery.

The course of illness can be followed by clinical observation of the patient, by examination of the size and tenderness of the liver, and by the following two laboratory tests: bilirubin and SGOT. The prothrombin time should be closely followed only in the acutely ill patient who is at risk of developing fulminant clinical illness. Frequent measurements of bilirubin in the clinically jaundiced patient are a waste of money and effort. However, it is important to follow the trend of serum bilirubin concentrations if clinical illness is severe or prolonged. In typical acute hepatitis, the bilirubin is either rising or decreasing, but usually is not leveling off at a plateau. The SGOT generally falls after the first two weeks of illness. A secondary rise two to three weeks after onset of jaundice is not unusual, however. If there are clinical indications suggesting relapse, examinations twice a week may be required. A secondary rise of the SGOT without clinical symptoms, or secondary rise of the serum bilirubin, need not interfere with progressive ambulation. When the late course of hepatitis is in doubt, a BSP test may be helpful. A normal BSP test in the face of fluctuating or persistently elevated SGOT is a most reassuring observation. If persistent elevation of the SGOT is associated with elevation of bilirubin after three months, it indicates the development of a chronic form of hepatitis.

DIET

For the acutely ill patient, the aim is to provide 16 carbohydrate calories (4 gm. of glucose I.V. or sucrose p.o.) per kilogram of body weight per day. If the patient eats at all, it should be in the morning, as breakfast often provides most of the daily calories. During the recovery phase, forced feeding or high protein or low fat diets serve no useful purpose, and should not be prescribed. Diet should depend on the patient's usual eating habits. One gm. of protein per kilogram, divided into five or six small feedings, usually is well tolerated and is sufficient to promote optimal recovery. During ambulation, excessive alcohol consumption should be discouraged. However, there is no evidence that social drinking is any more harmful after recovery from viral hepatitis than it was before onset. Prolonged abstinence will not benefit these patients. Additional vitamin supplements have no value.

CORTICOSTEROIDS

These should not be used in typical acute viral hepatitis. Corticosteroids do not shorten the clinical illness enough to justify the added risks of: (1) increased rate of relapse; (2) increased rate of chronic hepatitis; and (3) increased rate of gastrointestinal bleeding. The types of patient who may be considered candidates for corticosteroid therapy are: (1) those over 45 years of age whose jaundice is progressively deepened during a three- to six-week period, or in whom anorexia, nausea, and vomiting persist and seriously interfere with hydration and nutrition; and possibly (2) those whose liver biopsy shows confluent (bridging or submassive) necrosis.

ESTROGENS

All forms of estrogens, including birth control pills, should be discontinued during the acute phase of viral hepatitis. Therapy may be reinstituted after recovery.

ANTIEMETICS

If nausea is severe, phenothiazines can be used despite the fact that the patient is jaundiced. Usually, however, nausea and vomiting in typical acute hepatitis subside within a few days without any therapy. Repeated or prolonged administration should be avoided, because the rate of metabolism of these drugs is decreased in hepatitis.

IMMUNE SERUM (GAMMA) GLOBULIN (ISG)

There is good evidence on large-scale studies that this form of therapy is of no value in the treatment of viral hepatitis. Indeed, 45 ml. of commercial ISG had no beneficial effect in patients with clinical hepatitis.

THERAPY OF CONTACTS

If the patient has hepatitis A, ISG should be given to intimate contacts only: i.e., those who could have been exposed to fecal contaminations, through shared bed linen, common use of bathroom, or intimate physical contact. Globulin is indicated for children who are play or household contacts. It is not indicated for school or work contacts, nor for casual visitors. The ISG prophylaxis consists of 2 cc. of commercial globulin for adults, 1 cc. for individuals between 50 and 100 pounds, and 0.5 cc. for children under 50 pounds. In hepatitis B, ISG has no proved value. However, initimates, particularly sexual contacts, may be given 5 ml. of ISG.

COMPLICATIONS

Bone marrow depression, aplastic anemia, or agranulocytosis are rare but well established complications of otherwise typical viral hepatitis.

Fulminant Hepatitis

DEFINITION

This is an acute, fulminant liver disease superimposed on the previously normal liver. The cause may be viral or from drugs (such as halothane, isoniazid, zoxazolamine, oxyphenisatin, ethanol, etc.). The disease is characterized by rapid progression of encephalopathy, coma, and a mortality rate of about 75 per cent in patients under 20 years of age, and over 90 per cent in those over 40 years of age. At autopsy, the liver shows massive necrosis (acute yellow atrophy). In those who survive a clinically identical illness, the liver biopsies within a week of coma may show confluent necrosis, or only minimal-to-moderate changes characteristic of acute viral hepatitis. Massive parenchymal necrosis is not essential for fulminant hepatic failure.

RECOGNITION

SUBJECTIVE FINDINGS

A severe illness may develop either de novo or during the course of an otherwise typical acute hepatitis. The symptoms are those of rapidly progressive anorexia, malaise, irritability, drowsiness, restlessness, and insomnia. These findings must be distinguished from the drowsiness and depression seen in typical acute hepatitis. Look for hyperexcitability, excessive irritability, insomnia at night with somnolence in the daytime, impaired mentation, increasingly severe vomiting. These are followed by the development of obtundation, confusion, and coma. Convulsions may develop, particularly in children.

OBJECTIVE FINDINGS

These are an altered state of consciousness, and the development of incoordination and asterixis (a flapping tremor). The prothrombin time (PT) usually becomes prolonged one or more days before the clinical deterioration, and often is accompanied by decrease of SGOT toward normal. The most ominous objective evidence for fulminant hepatitis is the gradual or rapid decrease of liver size during a severe clinical illness. This clinical course is accompanied by either the development or the return of fever, and by leukocytosis with neutrophilia. Occult gastrointestinal bleeding is common, but significant bleeding also may occur occasionally. Hyperventilation and decreased serum bicarbonate concentration may be the result of encephalopathy.

When rapid deterioration of consciousness suggests fulimant hepatitis, it is imperative that drug therapy be meticulously explored to make sure that the symptoms are not due to excessive sedation. In severe hepatitis, the metabolism of drugs is impaired, and excessive somnolence can be caused by ordinary doses of sedatives or tranquilizers.

TREATMENT

Diagnostic Plan

The patient must be hospitalized under close observation. The diagnosis is documented by demonstrating the characteristic physical and laboratory findings described above; specifically, prolongation of PT, decreasing SGOT, and liver size. Vitamin K therapy is routinely given; it is ineffective and should be stopped in three days. Renal and respiratory failure should be anticipated. Prevent fluid overload, but assure adequate hydration. Insure normal PO_2 by nasal oxygen or by intubation and respirator.

Therapeutic Plan

The only known effective measures for the treatment of fulminant hepatic failure are the maintenance of vital functions, the avoidance of sedation of any type (even in an irritable, restless, unruly patient), prevention of fluid overload or underhydration, and the control of electrolyte imbalance and of lactic acidosis. An unexplained anion gap must be sought by daily determination of serum electrolytes to detect lactic acidosis promptly. An arterial pH is to be obtained when the serum bicarbonate falls below 12 mEq./liter, the electrolytes show an unexplained anion gap, and the urine pH is low. If possible, blood lactate should be measured. However, the initiation of therapy for lactic acidosis should not await the report of blood lactate concentration; it must be treated promptly by infusion of large amounts of bicarbonate and glucose. Hypoglycemia may develop, particularly in children.

In order to avoid overhydration and to provide adequate calories, a nasogastric (NG) tube is placed in the most dependent part of the stomach (document it by x-ray), and 4 gm. of carbohydrate/kg./day is provided. This is done by feeding, via the NG tube, a 25 per cent sucrose solution (one calorie per ml.). For the average adult, 50 cc. is given hourly. This is accompanied by a liquid antacid every two hours, and 1 gm. of neomycin at the beginning of every four-hour cycle. In order to prevent gastric distention in case of decreased gastric emptying, the NG tube is connected to suction for between 210 to 240 minutes in each four-hour cycle.

Corticosteroids have no proved value in the treatment of fulminant hepatitis, and current evidence fails to substantiate any clear-cut beneficial effect. Plasma or blood exchange transfusions have no value. Massive blood exchange, or the so-called "total body wash-out," is an experimental mode of therapy, the worth of which has not yet been established. Ex vivo porcine liver perfusion or charcoal column hemoperfusion also are experimental tools that are not available for general use.

Antibiotics should be used with a great deal of caution, and tetracycline must be avoided. Documented infection must be present before antibiotics are used. They must not be employed as "prophylactic" measures: their metabolism is greatly altered in the face of severe liver disease and anticipated renal failure.

DRUG HEPATITIS

Introduction

Hepatotoxicity due to drugs may be: (1) unpredictable; or (2) predictable. *Unpredictable injury* is a manifestation of hypersensitivity, and is a rare complication of the drug. It is not reproducible in animals and is not dose-dependent. The types of lesion fall into five categories: (*a*) nonspecific hepatitis; (*b*) granulomatous hepatitis; (*c*) simple cholestasis: (*d*) cholestatic hepatitis; and (*e*) (severe) viral hepatitis. The *predictable injury* is due to drugs that have direct toxic effect on the liver; it usually is reproducible in an experimental animal, the injury is dose-dependent, and the lesion is distinctive.

Hypersensitivity Drug Reactions

RECOGNITION

Subjective and objective findings are those described under viral hepatitis or fulminant hepatitis.

A drug history should be obtained. A large number of drugs are associated with well defined types of liver injury. An association is probable if the appropriate type of liver lesion follows therapy with the suspected drug. A list of these drugs and the associated liver lesions is available (Klatskin, 1974). Drug injuries that simulate viral hepatitis usually are severe—for example, halothane hepatitis. This type of injury is rare, but has a 25 to 50 per cent mortality rate when it occurs. It may develop after a single exposure, but it is more common after multiple exposures. It is extremely rare (if it occurs at all) in children.

TREATMENT

Same as for viral hepatitis.

Hepatotoxic Drug Reactions

Hepatotoxic drugs are not prescribed frequently. These are used for cancer chemotherapy—such as mithramycin or urethan or alkylating agents. Methotrexate probably belongs in this group, as it is given for severe psoriasis.

A widely used hepatotoxic drug is ethanol (alcohol). The liver injury is dose-dependent; both the daily dose and the duration of drinking are important. The lesion is distinctive (it was reproduced in the baboon), and the hepatotoxicity is not prevented by a "good" diet.

Alcoholic Hepatitis

RECOGNITION

SUBJECTIVE FINDINGS

Drinking of 160 gm. ethanol/day (pint of 86 proof) or more, or binge drinking, usually is required. Although a few months of drinking may suffice, years of drinking most often precede the development of alcoholic hepatitis. Clinical illness due to this hepatitis is always preceded by recent excessive drinking. The age of the patients ranges from 15 years upward. The peak incidence is in the fifth and sixth decades. The most common symptoms are anorexia (in two-thirds to three-quarters of patients), nausea, vomiting, abdominal pain, and weight loss (in one-half of the patients).

OBJECTIVE FINDINGS

The liver is enlarged in every patient with alcoholic hepatitis, although it may be missed occasionally. Ascites, jaundice, and fever are seen in about one-half of these patients. Splenomegaly is found in one-third, and encephalopathy in 15 per cent of the patients. Cirrhosis may or may not accompany the first clinical manifestation. The exclusion or the documentation of cirrhosis or al-

coholic hepatitis requires liver biopsy. Laboratory abnormalities usually are characteristic, but not pathognomonic. *Note:* Moderately severe alcoholic hepatitis may produce normal liver tests. Anemia is a frequent finding that is present in about three-quarters of patients in the lower socioeconomic groups. Leukocytosis may be marked, but leukopenia also may be seen. A WBC over 10,000 is seen in one-half of the patients. SGOT may be normal; if elevated, it rarely is over 500 units—indeed, it usually is under 300 units. Alkaline phosphatase generally is elevated, but rarely exceeds three times the upper limit of normal. The bilirubin is normal in a one-third to one-half of the patients.

Because of the frequent occurrence of abdominal pain, vomiting, jaundice, fever, and leukocytosis, it is imperative that the patient with alcoholic hepatitis must not be considered to have a surgical abdomen, because his risk of operative mortality is very high.

TREATMENT

DIAGNOSTIC PLAN

Obtain routine blood studies for liver tests and a prothrombin time. Do a liver biopsy to establish the diagnosis. If the prothrombin time is prolonged, the patient's chances of dying with the acute illness are about eight times as high (over 40 per cent) as if the prothrombin time is within four seconds of normal. If the prothrombin time is normal on admission, but becomes prolonged within a week or two, in association with increasing anorexia, the patient is again at increased risk (about 20 per cent) of dying with the acute illness. Patients with symptomatic alcoholic hepatitis should be hospitalized.

THERAPEUTIC PLAN

There is no specific therapy for alcoholic hepatitis. The treatment is similar to that of acute viral hepatitis. Nutritional deficiencies are common, and should be corrected with appropriate diets and vitamins. *Note:* These patients have poor appetites, and a plethora of pills may be harmful. Liquid foods are better accepted than regular diets. Do not prescribe diets that sound good but which the patient does not eat. Corticosteroids have shown no beneficial effect in several controlled clinical trials.

CIRRHOSIS

Introduction

Cirrhosis is the end-stage of various types of chronic hepatitic processes. The microscopic appearance of the cirrhotic liver is not diagnostic of its etiology, but the type of hepatitis associated with the cirrhosis may be diagnostic.

Cirrhosis may be asymptomatic, i.e., it may have no overt clinical manifestations. When it is symptomatic, the findings are due to one or more of the four types of "liver failures" of cirrhosis. These are: (1) parenchymal liver cell failure (chronic hepatitis); (2) renal—lymphatic failure (ascites); (3) CNS failure (encephalopathy; and (4) portal hypertension (GI bleeding). The presence of one type of "failure" need not be accompanied by another. For example, cirrhosis may be mistaken for "hepatitis," "chronic brain syndrome," or "GI bleeding," and thus be easily overlooked.

Recognition

PARENCHYMAL LIVER CELL FAILURE

SUBJECTIVE AND OBJECTIVE FINDINGS

The clinical manifestations of parenchymal liver cell failure in the cirrhotic patient are those of acute or chronic hepatitis. The onset of symptoms generally is insidious, and the laboratory findings are usually but not always characteristic of a chronic disease. Although elevation of gamma globulins is common in cirrhosis, they may be normal; they also may be elevated in chronic active hepatitis without cirrhosis. Signs of nutritional deficiency are late manifestations of the disease, or are associated with alcoholism.

ASSESSMENT

The clinical and laboratory findings of parenchymal liver failure may suggest cirrhosis, but are not diagnostic. Definitive diagnosis requires morphologic examination of the liver.

TREATMENT

Diagnostic Plan. Obtain CBC, liver tests, serum protein electrophoresis, PT, and liver scan. The abnormal hepatic uptake of the radiocolloid (may suggest "filling defects") and increased uptake by the spleen and bone marrow suggest cirrhosis.

The initial plan should include performance of a liver biopsy to prove the diagnosis of cirrhosis, and to identify the activity of the cirrhotic and the chronic hepatitic process.

Therapeutic Plan. A symptomatic patient with cirrhosis who has chronic active hepatitis will benefit from therapy. The recommended treatment is 20 mg. of prednisolone, together with 50 mg. of Imuran, daily. After improvement, the prednisolone is reduced to 20 mg. every other day or 10 mg. daily, and the Imuran is continued. *Note:* Bone marrow depression is very rare on this dose of Imuran. Alcoholic hepatitis with cirrhosis responds to abstinence. Long term corticosteroid therapy for abstaining alcoholic cirrhotics has been associated with a decrease in survival rate.

The diet should provide 1 gm. protein/kilogram of body weight. Nutritional deficiencies should be treated. In the absence of these, additional vitamins are no more helpful than in noncirrhotic patients. The only vitamin supplement that may be of help is vitamin K_1, if the patient's prothrombin time is prolonged. Ten mg. daily for four days will give maximum benefit. Because of the risk of encephalopathy, a high protein diet may be dangerous and is not likely to improve the patient's rate of recovery or chances for longevity. The type of anemia should be identified and the etiology treated as in noncirrhotic patients.

ASCITES

RECOGNITION

Ascites due to cirrhosis must be differentiated from that due to cancer or infection or to a large ovarian cyst.

Subjective Findings. Weight gain and increasing abdominal girth may be accompanied by pedal edema.

Objective Findings. There is no definite pathognomonic test for cirrhotic ascitic fluid. A high protein content in ascitic fluid, together with a low serum albumin concentration, is likely to be due to infection or cancer. However, high protein ascites can be caused by cirrhosis. Chylous ascites may occur in cirrhosis. Bloody ascites suggest hepatoma or tuberculosis. A friction rub over the liver may indicate tumor, but may be due to a fibrinoid exudate of chronic cirrhotic ascites. In women, the differentiation of ascites from a large ovarian cyst may be difficult. One clue is that, in cirrhotic ascites, intestinal gas can be percussed in the middle of the abdomen, whereas an ovarian cyst gives dullness in the midline of the abdomen and the resonance is in the flanks. Finally, make sure that the "fluid wave" in an enlarging abdomen is indeed fluid. Fat may be misdiagnosed for ascites. Fluid is documented by a diagnostic tap.

TREATMENT

Diagnostic Plan. A small needle should be used for a diagnostic paracentesis. Cell count and protein content are measured, and the fluid is cultured because of the high frequency of asymptomatic peritonitis in cirrhotic (alcoholic) patients. The patient should be weighed and the serum electrolytes, BUN and creatinine measured.

Therapeutic Plan. Removal of large amounts of the ascitic fluid is no longer an acceptable mode of therapy of cirrhotic ascites. The first stage of therapy is bed rest and sodium restriction. If the urine sodium/potassium ratio is less than 1, Aldactone (50 mg., three or four times a day) is started and the dose increased to insure a urinary sodium/potassium ratio greater than 1 – preferably greater than 3. The diet should contain no more than 1 gm. of sodium. If the patient has not received diuretic therapy previously, these measures usually are sufficient to induce a satisfactory rate of diuresis. Before diuretic therapy is started, make sure that the patient has an adequate circulating blood volume. This usually is not a problem when the patient has had no prior diuretic therapy, but is a common one in those who have been on diuretics. A decreased effective blood volume should be expanded with plasma until neck veins become visible at 33° elevation, the blood pressure shows no postural drop, and the pulse

pressure is 20 mm. Hg or greater. The rate of diuresis should not exceed 1 lb. a day, preferably no more than 3 to 4 lb a week. Rapid diuresis may be dangerous. If the weight loss is greater than one half pound/day, hematocrit, electrolytes, BUN, and creatinine need to be followed at least two to four times a week. If serum electrolyte concentrations become abnormal, obtain a creatinine clearance. Restriction of fluid intake is not necessary unless the patient's serum sodium concentration is decreasing below 132 mEq./liter. In most patients, fluid restriction is not necessary and is an unwarranted hardship. A serum sodium concentration between 132 and 136 mEq./liter is satisfactory for patients receiving diuretic therapy. After spironolactone (Aldactone) has been given for two days (spot urine Na/K > 1), furosemide (Lasix) is the recommended agent. Chlorothiazides have a much greater propensity to precipitate encephalopathy in cirrhotic patients. Use the minimum amount of furosemide necessary for diuresis. An excessively rapid diuresis is a therapeutic failure.

At all times, remember ascites may be a cosmetic defect or a source of discomfort, but represents no hazard to the patient (unless there is an umbilical hernia). On the other hand, diuretic therapy is hazardous and may lead to a fatal outcome.

Paracentesis should be avoided. On occasion, however, it is necessary because of impending rupture of umbilical hernia or excessive accumulation of fluid in the scrotum, or because tense ascites interferes with respiration. A few liters of ascitic fluid should be removed and the plasma volume expanded with blood or plasma to compensate for reaccumulation of ascites. The latter may be reduced by giving Lasix 40 to 80 mg. I.V. after the plasma infusion.

Removal of large amounts of ascitic fluid can be done if constant intravenous infusion of plasma or sterile reinfusion of ascitic fluid maintains central venous pressure and ensures good urine flow rate. This form of therapy requires close supervision to prevent the rise of hematocrit, BUN, and creatinine by the intravenous infusions of plasma or other protein-containing fluids. This is a very expensive form of therapy that should be resorted to only when a hepato-renal syndrome is impending or when serum osmolarity is falling and is unresponsive to any other measure. The reinfusion of ascitic fluid may be another substitute for the infusion of plasma. This is valuable if the ascitic fluid has high protein and normal electrolyte content and is clear. Again, however, the problem of ascites is not serious enough to warrant extreme measures that are associated with significant risks. The basic problem is functional renal failure.

HEPATIC COMA

Definition

Encephalopathy is the more appropriate term to describe the altered stage of consciousness that usually develops during the course of chronic liver disease. It can be classified in four categories: Stage I, personality changes, inappropriate behavior, euphoria, or hyperexcitability or depression; Stage II, development of asterixis, confusion, disorientation, and later some obtundation; Stage III, stupor, but capable of arousal and responsive to stimuli; Stage IV, coma (may be decerebrate). The abnormal mental and neuromuscular state must be accompanied by liver disease—usually with spontaneous or surgical portosystemic shunt. However, overt parenchymal failure, such as jaundice, need not be present. All stages of encephalopathy are reversible, and recovery is possible.

Encephalopathy of chronic liver disease may be classified as nitrogenous and drug-induced. *Nitrogenous encephalopathy* is associated with elevated blood ammonia and amino acids, and either may be spontaneous or can be precipitated by various events. These include: (1) gastrointestinal hemorrhage; (2) uremia; (3) high protein meals; (4) constipation; (5) diuretics; and (6) probably by infection. *Non-nitrogenous encephalopathy* may be induced by sedatives (including antihistamines), tranquilizers, or narcotics. Nitrogenous encephalopathy is due to a major decrease of the hepatic functional capacity to metabolize nitrogen, the defect occurring in the urea cycle enzymes.

Recognition

SUBJECTIVE FINDINGS

When encephalopathy is superimposed in chronic liver disease, the onset may be the same as described in fulminant hepatitis, but usually is more gradual. Rapid changes from a well-compensated stage to IV + coma can occur within hours or minutes, particularly in patients who have had a portal-systemic shunt operation.

OBJECTIVE FINDINGS

Encephalopathy of chronic liver disease is a clinical diagnosis. It does not require the determination of blood ammonia or electroencephalography. Nitrogenous encephalopathy is associated with elevated blood ammonia, but the height is of no help in diagnosis. The patient may appear normal despite a very high blood ammonia. Drug-induced encephalopathy may not increase blood ammonia. The blood ammonia level may be helpful if it is well within normal limits in the patient who is in coma. This would make nitrogenous encephalopathy unlikely. The characteristic EEG changes are paroxysms of bilaterally synchronous high voltage slow delta waves. However, these are not diagnostic of hepatic encephalopathy, because other metabolic derangements may produce identical findings.

If the patient is under observation, the simplest way to detect the development of encephalopathy is to note the change of handwriting; the inability to draw simple pictures or arrange simple forms with matchsticks; the inability to hold steadily the bulb of blood pressure cuff or to count backward by sixes; and so on. Fetor hepaticus is a characteristic breath odor of encephalopathy, but it is rarely observed now because prompt treatment of encephalopathy with antibiotics abolishes this finding.

Treatment

DIAGNOSTIC PLAN

Identify a precipitating cause and eliminate it. Look for gastrointestinal bleeding; excessively high protein intake for the patient's tolerance; the ingestion of foods of high ammonia content, such as cheeses, salamis, aged processed meats, etc; electrolyte abnormalities, with or without rising blood urea or dehydration. Detect and eliminate sources of infection and correct constipation. Diuretic therapy for ascites is a common precipitating cause. Chlorothiazides are prone to cause coma. When the patient with gastrointestinal bleeding is encephalopathic, transfuse with fresh blood, if possible; stored blood has two to five times the ammonia content of that of fresh blood.

EEG usually is not readily available, and is expensive and unnecessary for the diagnosis of encephalopathy.

Note: During Stage I, the patient often manifests behavioral patterns that under usual circumstances call for sedation. These symptoms are insomnia, restlessness, irritability, and uncontrolled and disturbing behavior. Sedation of any type can push this patient into coma, and therefore must be avoided. The best and most effective therapy for encephalopathy is *prevention.* If at all possible, avoid drugs and surgery—including the portal systemic shunt operation, which is a common initiating cause of recurrent or chronic encephalopathy.

THERAPEUTIC PLAN

During the last decade, no new therapeutic modalities of proved value have been added to the treatment of hepatic encephalopathy. The principles of therapy can be divided into *do* and *do not* categories. In the *do* category, it is important to correct electrolytes and fluid imbalance, and provide adequate carbohydrate calories to prevent endogenous "high protein" breakdown. Promote daily bowel movements. Give 3 to 6 gm. neomycin daily in divided doses; chronic and prolonged use of this drug may produce renal failure. Lactulose therapy is experimental, but offers promise of being as effective as neomycin. Detect and correct infection, but avoid the use of tetracycline. When drugs such as sedatives and phenothiazines are used in patients with chronic liver disease, bear in mind that the metabolic rate is depressed and the half lives prolonged. There are *no* safe sedatives. Colon bypass surgery may be considered as a desperate last measure. Corticosteroids have no value in the treatment of encephalopathy of chronic liver disease. One to 3 gm./day L-dopa may have a beneficial effect, but is still experimental. Its usefulness is not proved, and side-effects may be distressing. In the *do not* category, avoid sedatives (including alcohol), diuretics, ammonia-containing foods, and more protein nitrogen than the patient is able to metabolize without encephalopathy.

References

Galambos, J. T.: Alcoholic Hepatitis. *In* Schaffner, F., Sherlock, S., and Leevy, C. M. (eds.): The Liver and its Diseases. New York, Intercontinental Medical Book Corporation, 1974.

Klatskin, G.: Drug-induced Hepatic Injury. *In* Schaffner, F., Sherlock, S., and Leevy, C. M. (eds.): The Liver and its Diseases. New York, Intercontinental Medical Book Corporation, 1974.

Mosley, J. E., and Galambos, J. T.: Viral Hepatitis. *In* Schiff, L. (ed.): Diseases of the Liver, 4th ed. New York, Intercontinental Medical Book Corporation, 1975.

Popper, H.: Drug-induced Liver Injury. *In* Gall, E. A. (ed.): The Liver. Baltimore, Williams & Wilkins Co., 1973.

Schenker, S., Breen, K. J., and Hoyumpa, A. M.: Hepatic encephalopathy: current status. Gastroenterology 66: 121, 1974.

Chapter 44

OBSTETRIC AND GYNECOLOGIC EMERGENCIES

Elsie R. Carrington

GYNECOLOGIC

Most problems in the spectrum of gynecologic emergencies are associated with genital or abdominal pain with or without fever, menstrual irregularities, abnormal vaginal bleeding, and specific conditions that result in shock. The emergency nature of the problem may be related simply to the intensity of the symptoms for which the patient seeks prompt relief, but many represent threats in terms of morbidity and mortality, much of which can be prevented by early diagnosis and treatment.

Two basic concepts should be emphasized. First, if the woman is in the reproductive years, the possibility of coexisting pregnancy always should be considered; second, if the patient is in the second half of pregnancy and presents with a medical or surgical complication, however mild this may seem, there may be serious consequences. Disorders such as hypertension, urinary tract infection, diabetes, and many others progress rapidly during late pregnancy and may be fatal for the fetus, if not for the mother.

Major Problems in the Emergency Department

PROBLEMS OF PELVIC INFECTION

LOWER GENITAL TRACT

The usual presenting symptoms are discharge, local irritation, and/or intense itching and swelling. *Acute vulvovaginitis* appears in three major forms.

Mycotic Infections (Candidiasis). These are associated with a thin watery discharge, intense itching, and thick, white, cheesy plaques on the vaginal wall. The vulva may be markedly swollen, inflamed, and tender. The high glycogen content of the vulvovaginal tissues is conducive to the possibility of a diabetic state out of control, and this should be considered and urine and blood sugars checked. Definitive diagnosis of the local lesion is made by culture on Nickerson's medium, or by hanging drop to which a few drops of 10 per cent potassium hydroxide have been added.* Local treatment consists of Mycostatin vaginal suppositories, 100,000 units, to be inserted once or twice a day for two weeks, and Mycostatin ointment without hydrocortisone applied externally to the edematous vulva. Hydrocortisone ointment adds little in these cases, but it may be effective in some instances of low grade chronic infections or allergic conditions affecting this area.

Trichomonas Vaginalis. Trichomonas infections are associated with profuse, bubbly, opaque, or yellowish discharge. Punctate red "strawberry spots" frequently are noted on the vaginal mucosa. Intense itching is common, but swelling of the vulvar tissues is unusual unless secondary infection occurs. Definitive diagnosis is made by observing the motile flagellates microscopically in a hanging drop with saline solution. Metronidazole (Flagyl), 250 mg. orally three times a day for 10 to 14 days, is the

---

*See page 460.

most effective treatment. Vinegar douche (2 tablespoons per quart of warm water) may give some relief, but is not curative.

The major problem in treatment of Trichomonas infections is that sexual partners often harbor trichomonads. Recurrent infections in the female require treatment of the consort. Simultaneous treatment of each partner, using the Flagyl regimen described above, is effective. The single dose metronidazine treatment of trichomonal vaginitis has been used in Great Britain during the past two or three years, but only recently has been used in the U.S. The regimen consists of administration of 2 gm. of Flagyl (eight tablets) orally at the same visit. The same dosage is provided for the consort. Side-effects of nausea have been noted in 20 to 25 per cent of cases, but the treatment has been efficacious in a high percentage, and offers the advantage of simplicity and better patient compliance.

Herpetic Vulvovaginitis. Recently a marked increase has been noted in the incidence of lower genital tract infections with herpes virus type II. Lesions are vesicular, sometimes ulcerated, and secondarily infected. The lesions involving the vulva may be excruciatingly painful during the acute stage, which may last for one or two weeks. Treatment is not universally successful. Idoxuridine can be used locally. Better results in relief of pain seem to be achieved with an application of a 1 per cent aqueous solution of neutral red dye to the lesions, followed by photoinactivation using a cool white fluorescent light. A 22-watt bulb should be used and placed about 6 inches from the lesions for 15 minutes.

Chemical Vaginitis. Certain chemicals frequently used as douches can produce deep ulcerations and bleeding, which may be profuse. Potassium permanganate which has not been thoroughly dissolved in the solution is one example. Strong concentrations of creosote is another. If the bleeding is not excessive, it may be controlled by temporary use of a firm 2- or 3-inch wide vaginal pack. Frequently the bleeding is profuse or an arterial spurt may be noted, in which case sutures must be applied.

Bartholinian Abscess. Although abscesses of Bartholin's glands commonly are gonorrheal in origin, other microorganisms often are found, either as the primary cause or as secondary infections. Incision and

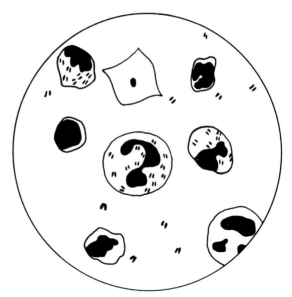

Figure 1. Gram-negative intracellular diplococci in acute gonorrheal infection.

drainage under local anesthesia are easily performed on an emergency basis and bring dramatic relief. Antibiotics are unnecessary unless cellulitis of the surrounding tissue is present. Aspiration of the abscess, with or without instillation of antibiotic, is not curative and should be rejected. The cyst should be marsupialized or excised in about six weeks in order to prevent recurrent infection.

Gonorrhea. Characteristic symptoms of a recently acquired gonorrheal infection include urinary frequency and dysuria and usually a profuse, purulent vaginal discharge. Involvement of paraurethral (Skene's) glands (90 per cent), cervical glands (80 per cent), and Bartholin's glands (20 per cent) becomes evident at varying times after the incubation period of three to five days following exposure. Except for slight dysuria, lower genital tract gonorrhea remains asymptomatic in over 50 per cent of infected women, but in a much lower percentage of infected men. Purulent material obtained from the meatus after stripping of the urethra from above downward, and from the cervical glands, may reveal gram-negative intracellular diplococci on a stained smear (Fig. 1). Definitive diagnosis is made by culture on Thayer-Martin medium.

Treatment at this stage is curative in approximately 95 per cent of cases if adequate amounts of antibiotic agents are given and the level is maintained for an adequate period. A total of 4.8 million units of aqueous procaine penicillin should be divided and administered in two sites at the one visit. Probenecid, 1 gm. orally, should be given 30 minutes before the injection to ensure effective levels by delaying the renal excretion of penicillin. This regimen is likewise effective in aborting incubating syphilis. Long-acting benzathine penicillin should not be used to treat gonorrhea, since bactericidal levels for gonococci are not reached. If the patient is allergic to penicillin, tetracycline, 1.5 gm. orally followed by 0.5 gm. four times a day, should be given for four days up to a total of 9.5 gm. This regimen is contraindicated in pregnant women. Erythromycin, 1.5 gm. orally followed by 0.5 gm. four times a day for four days, up to a total of 9.5 gm., is safe for mother and fetus, but its efficacy appears to be somewhat lower than either of the other drugs. Neither the tetracycline nor the erythromycin regimens can be counted on to treat syphilis, and therefore a blood test for syphilis should be made in such instances.

Untreated or inadequately treated infection spreads by direct extension along the surface of mucous membranes, involves the endometrium for a relatively short period of time, and then extends to the fallopian tubes and other pelvic structures, at which point symptoms of acute infection become evident. This sequence of events commonly, but not invariably, follows a menstrual period.

Therapeutic regimens used for lower genital tract gonorrhea are entirely different from those required for treatment of upper genital tract disease.

UPPER GENITAL TRACT

The most characteristic symptoms are lower abdominal or general abdominal pain and fever.

The terms "pelvic inflammatory disease" (PID) and "tubo-ovarian disease" are used with abandon. This is unfortunate. A more precise diagnosis is often possible at the time of the first examination or after a period of observation. Differentiation of acute salpingitis with or without peritonitis from other entities (abscesses of all sorts, pyosalpinx, tubo-ovarian, pelvic, or ovarian abscess) is important in both planning the

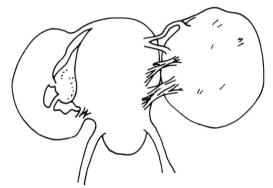

Figure 2. Pelvic inflammatory disease. Pyosalpinx (*left*); tubo-ovarian abscess (*right*).

management and determining the prognosis of the specific problem.

Acute Salpingitis. Purulent material escaping from the fimbriated ends of the tubes causes an acute peritonitis. Not infrequently, the fimbria may seal off after a varying amount of spillage, resulting in a distended inflamed tube filled with pus *(pyosalpinx)* (Fig. 2). In either case, there is marked bilateral tenderness, leukocytosis with a shift to the left, and fever of 101 to 104° F., and peritoneal signs usually are present; the liver also may be tender. At this stage of the disease, no adnexal masses may be palpable unless a pyosalpinx is markedly distended and tense. Surgery is contraindicated in cases of acute salpingitis and in all but the unusual case of pyosalpinx because these conditions generally respond well to high-dosage antibiotic therapy and the peritonitis regimen. Secondary bacterial invaders are common. Ampicillin, 6 gm. per day for a total of seven to ten days, is usually curative. If the infection has been present for several days and is more severe, hospitalization and more aggressive treatment are necessary. Penicillin, 20 to 30 million units per day intravenously, and kanamycin, 0.5 gm. intramuscularly q. 12 hours, should result in marked improvement within a 48-hour period and control of infection within five to seven days. If improvement is not evident within 24 to 48 hours, it is likely that an acute tubo-ovarian or pelvic abscess has developed and that surgical intervention will be necessary after re-evaluation of the pelvic findings.

Tubo-ovarian Abscess (Fig. 2). This condition is characteristically an acute *recur-*

rent pelvic infection. Otherwise the signs and symptoms of pyosalpinx and tubo-ovarian abscess are similar, and the differential diagnosis may be made on the basis of response to therapy within the first 24 to 48 hours of treatment. Failure to respond in this period and continued evidence of peritonitis suggest leakage of tubo-ovarian abscess. Surgical intervention is necessary. Pelvic clean-out, including panhysterectomy with bilateral salpingo-oophorectomy, is the operation of choice because of the extensive destruction and subsequent symptomatology associated with less definitive surgery.

RUPTURED TUBO-OVARIAN ABSCESS. Patients who present with ruptured tubo-ovarian abscess represent acute surgical emergencies. Massive spillage of purulent contents into the abdominal cavity frequently is accompanied by septic shock. Generalized abdominal tenderness, rigidity, and rebound are characteristic. Culdocentesis often reveals free pus, even if the patient is not yet in shock.* Culture of the material obtained usually does not reveal gonococci but, more commonly, coliform or other secondary invaders. Initial steps in management as described for septic shock† must be taken immediately in order that the patient may be transferred to the operating room for definitive surgery as soon as possible. When this is delayed, the mortality rate is well over 50 per cent.

Pelvic Abscess. A pelvic abscess that points into the vagina with bulging of the cul-de-sac is amenable to drainage by posterior colpotomy, breaking up of loculations, and insertion of a mushroom catheter or T-tube for drainage. However, definitive surgery often is necessary several months after the acute process has subsided.

Ovarian Abscess. Isolated ovarian abscesses are not common but are serious, potentially lethal infections. They usually occur as a postoperative complication of vaginal hysterectomy, occasionally after abdominal pelvic surgery. Microorganisms gain access to the substance of the ovaries via perforation of the relatively resistant tunica at needle puncture or resection sites during surgery, or in some cases at a fresh ovulatory stoma. Signs and symptoms are similar to those of tubo-ovarian abscess. Their onset is relatively late in the postoperative period, after the patient has been discharged from the hospital. Pain and fever may develop acutely, and rupture may occur within two or three days. Some progress slowly over the course of three or four weeks before rupture finally occurs. Ovarian abscesses are notoriously inaccessible and unresponsive to antibiotic therapy alone. A palpable tender adnexal mass, found late in the postoperative period in a patient with persistent pain and fever, is a clear indication for reoperation and removal of the infected adnexa. In contrast to tubo-ovarian disease, removal of the remainder of the pelvic organs is not essential to effect a cure.

DIFFERENTIAL DIAGNOSIS

Abdominal pain and fever are common complaints of extragenital conditions. Urinary tract infection or calculi, appendicitis, and diverticulitis always should be considered. In the latter, nausea, vomiting, and a change in bowel habit are more frequent early complaints. Other gynecologic disorders that must be differentiated from pelvic inflammatory processes include the following.

PUERPERAL SEPSIS AND SEPTIC ABORTION

About 20 per cent of all pelvic infections fall into this category. The necrotic decidua is an excellent culture medium for virulent organisms such as coliform, anaerobic streptococci, bacteroides, and clostridia. Vascular and lymphatic changes associated with pregnancy make the surrounding tissue highly vulnerable to spread of infection along these routes (Fig. 3). This is in contrast to the spread of gonorrheal infections along the mucosal surfaces. Pelvic cellulitis is the most common finding. Induration and tenderness of the parametria may be unilateral or bilateral. Further extension results in peritonitis, pelvic abscess, pelvic thrombophlebitis, or septicemia. Pelvic cellulitis commonly is accompanied by spiking fever and chills, tachycardia, and leukocytosis in the range of 30,000. Antibiotic therapy must be started at once without awaiting the report on culture and sensitivity. Gram stain of

---

*See page 462.
†See page 1041.

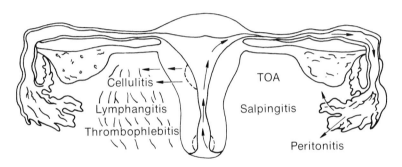

Figure 3. Characteristics of spread of pelvic infection postpartum or post abortion (*left*); gonorrheal infection (*right*).

material, obtained by inserting the swab directly into the uterine cavity, serves as a guide to selection of antibiotic, although in any case the choice should cover a broad spectrum. Penicillin, 10 million units in a liter of fluid I.V., and kanamycin, 0.5 gm. I.M., is an appropriate choice unless evidences of septic shock are present.

SEPTIC SHOCK

The development of hypotension in a patient with pelvic infection calls for immediate action. Mortality rate is high if definitive treatment is delayed. Septic abortion with instrumentation is the most common cause. Other causes include ruptured tubo-ovarian or ovarian abscess, puerperal sepsis, severe pyelonephritis, or amnionitis associated with pregnancy. Lethal effects are related not only to virulence of the infection but also to a marked increase in peripheral vascular resistance, the intense vasoconstriction resulting from the action of endotoxic lipopolysaccharides in the cell wall of gram-negative bacteria. Peripheral blood flow, venous return to the heart, and cardiac output are diminished, and hypotension becomes more profound. The kidneys are the most susceptible target organ, and coronary blood flow may be reduced. The following steps should be taken promptly.

(1) Evaluation should be made of the hemodynamic, cardiopulmonary, CBC, electrolytes, blood gases, and EKG status. A central venous pressure catheter should be inserted. A CVP of less than 5 or 6 cm. of water indicates significant hypovolemia.

(2) The type and source of infection should be ascertained by culture and sensitivity determinations from blood, urine, and material obtained from the uterine cavity, and via cul-de-sac puncture. Gram stain of the smear should be done as an initial screening procedure.

(3) Evaluation of renal function includes

insertion of a Foley catheter and hourly measurement of urinary output. BUN, serum electrolytes, and pH determinations should be obtained.

Effective treatment is dependent on control of infection and correction of the circulatory defect. Fluids should be started immediately. Intravenous infusion, containing 10 million units of penicillin and 1 gm. of chloramphenicol in normal saline solution, will cover the most frequent and serious offenders, including bacteroides. A alternate regimen using clindamycin phosphate, 300 mg. in 100 cc. of normal saline, and given I.V. over a 30-minute period and repeated every eight hours, in addition to kanamycin, 0.5 gm. I.M. q. 12 hours, will cover a similar broad spectrum including bacteroides.

If the blood pressure remains at shock levels for about 30 minutes after the fluids have been running and the antibiotics have been given, hydrocortisone, 1 gm., or its equivalent in other intravenous steroid compounds should be given. The use of corticosteroids in shock remains an equivocal issue. In our experience, their value in dealing with these critical gynecologic problems has been demonstrated repeatedly.

The nidus of infection must be removed as promptly as possible. If the problem is a septic abortion, dilatation and curettage or suction and curettage is performed as soon as the patient is stable. Failure to respond within approximately four hours is indication for hysterectomy, because microabscesses throughout the uterine sinusoids are beyond the reach of curettage. Laparotomy is performed directly without a D&C if the cul-de-sac puncture reveals purulent material. This finding suggests uterine perforation or ruptured postabortal abscess.

PELVIC THROMBOPHLEBITIS

This condition may occur as a complication of any of the upper genital tract infections mentioned above, or may be related to postoperative, postabortal, or puerperal sepsis. The diagnosis is often difficult. Changes within the veins are not readily palpable, although tenderness usually is present. If the process is limited to the pelvic veins, there is no swelling of the legs or other characteristic signs of thrombophlebitis of the lower extremities. The diagnosis should be suspected in a patient with pelvic tenderness who continues to run a septic febrile course despite the use of appropriate antibiotics. These thrombi are inaccessible to antibiotics unless anticoagulation is carried out. Administration of heparin intravenously, and antibiotics including either chloramphenicol or clindamycin to cover bacteroides, is highly effective. Dramatic improvement usually is evident within 24 to 48 hours. Heparin therapy should be continued for approximately ten days.

INTRAUTERINE DEVICE-INDUCED INFECTION

The pregnancy rate in patients wearing these devices is approximately 3 per cent. Pelvic infection may occur in nonpregnant individuals with an IUD in place. However, the occurrence of pregnancy with an IUD in situ is apt to be far more serious and may be associated with septic shock.

If the pregnancy is early and there is no evidence of infection, and if the tail of the device is readily available, the IUD usually may be removed without interrupting the pregnancy, but even in these cases therapeutic interruption should be seriously considered. If the pregnancy is more advanced, the tail of the device disappears into the uterine cavity and the risk of infection is significantly increased. Sepsis may not become apparent until the patient goes into labor, whether early or at term. Therapeutic interruption of the pregnancy clearly is advisable if the gestational age is previable. If intrauterine infection develops, intensive antibiotic therapy, evacuation of the products of conception, and removal of the IUD should be carried out as promptly as possible.

PROBLEMS INVOLVING MENSTRUAL IRREGULARITY, PAIN, AND BLEEDING

The most common cause of a late or missed menstrual period during the repro-

ductive years is pregnancy, and the most common causes for vaginal bleeding in this age-group are related to complications of pregnancy. Although in the final analysis conditions other than pregnancy may prove to be responsible, the potential dangers of obstetric hemorrhage underscore the importance of early diagnosis.

ECTOPIC PREGNANCY

Unruptured. Definitive diagnosis of unruptured extrauterine pregnancy often is exceedingly difficult. The history is of prime importance. Characteristic symptoms include a missed menstrual period; lower quadrant pain (unilateral at first); and vaginal bleeding, which may occur as spotting, dark brownish discharge, or bleeding interpreted by the patient as a menstrual flow. Occasionally, the patient reports no irregularity of the menstrual cycle. Suspicion is raised if there is a history of a chronic inflammatory process, prior abdominal or gynecologic surgery, or a previous condition that would cause adhesions, e.g., a ruptured appendix.

On pelvic examination, softening and cyanosis of the cervix may be noted and the corpus may be slightly enlarged, but rarely beyond a six- to eight-week gestational size. As a rule, marked tenderness is elicited on manipulation of the cervix, but a tender, sausage-shaped adnexal mass may or may not be palpable. It should be emphasized that failure to outline a tubal enlargement does not exclude the diagnosis. The pregnancy test, if positive, may be helpful, but negative tests with unruptured ectopic pregnancies are not uncommon. Culdocentesis is negative in unruptured ectopic pregnancy. Differentiation of this condition from intrauterine pregnancy with corpus luteal cyst often is difficult. However, *the diagnosis of unruptured ectopic pregnancy, if seriously entertained, must be excluded before the patient is discharged.* Laparoscopy, open colpotomy, or, in some cases, laparotomy may be necessary to confirm the diagnosis.

Ruptured. Generalized abdominal pain, shoulder top pain, and syncope are the major complaints. The abdomen is tender, often somewhat doughy, and rebound-positive. The hemoglobin and hematocrit levels and the drop in blood pressure reflect the degree of blood loss. The white blood count may be slightly elevated, but there usually is no shift to the left. Culdocentesis should be carried out promptly. Blood obtained from a cul-de-sac tap usually fails to clot, confirming the diagnosis. Blood should be obtained immediately for typing and cross-matching, and an intravenous infusion of Ringer's lactate solution should be started, using a large bore needle so that the patient can be transferred promptly to the operating room for emergency laparotomy. Hemorrhagic shock can develop rapidly.

Differential Diagnosis. Unruptured ectopic pregnancy, or ectopic pregnancy with mild-to-moderate intra-abdominal bleeding, can mimic so many other conditions that it has been called "the great masquerader." In over 50 per cent of cases, the classic symptoms are not obtained in the history and a discrete adnexal mass is not found on pelvic examination. Common differential problems include the following.

(1) Bleeding into or rupture of corpus luteum cyst.

(2) Threatened or incomplete abortion.

(3) Tubo-ovarian disease. Diagnosis is particularly difficult in patients recently treated with antibiotic (presumably for pelvic inflammatory disease). Fever, leukocytosis, and other signs of infection may be controlled, but not necessarily the pain. About 25 per cent of all tubal pregnancies are associated with pre-existing chronic salpingitis.

(4) Ruptured graafian follicle (mittelschmerz). Episodes of pelvic pain associated with ovulation occur at midcycle without interference of periodic menstrual flow. There may, however, be a small amount of vaginal bleeding due to the relative estrogen withdrawal at midcycle. If there is no blood at the external os, examination of the cervical mucus is particularly helpful. Marked arborization showing sheets of fern patterns in the cervical mucus is characteristic of unopposed estrogen stimulation, which is maximal at the time of ovulation* The presence of pregnancy, whether intrauterine or extrauterine, usually produces enough progesterone to inhibit arborization partially or completely.

(5) Appendicitis. Early and more predominant gastrointestinal symptoms, and leukocytosis with a shift to the left, are the major differential features.

(6) Complications associated with endometriosis, ovarian cysts, and pedunculated fibroids may give rise to signs and symptoms very similar to those of extrauterine pregnancy.

ABORTION

Termination of pregnancy before the end of the 20th week in most states (16th week in Pennsylvania) is considered an *abortion* when the fetal weight is less than 500 gm. Prior to the 28th week of gestation, or in cases of fetal weights between 500 and 999 gm., termination of pregnancy is termed *immature labor*. Premature labor spans the 28th through the 36th week, but the weight range for infants in this category cannot be considered specific, since both low and high birth weight infants for gestational age frequently are found within this group.

Threatened Abortion. Chief complaints of threatened abortion are crampy lower abdominal pain, back ache, and vaginal bleeding, or dark brownish vaginal discharge. The cervix is uneffaced and undilated, and the membranes are intact. At this stage the patient usually can be treated on an out-patient basis, with mild sedation, analgesic, and instruction to return should symptoms progress. Intramuscular injection of a long-acting progestogen is of value only if the condition is due to an inadequate progestational state, one of the less common causes of abortion. Otherwise, the use of these agents may well convert a *threatened* to a *missed* abortion.

If the symptoms become more severe, with the cervix obviously dilated and the membranes clearly visible or ruptured, the patient should be admitted with the diagnosis of *inevitable abortion*. Cramps and bleeding are more severe in connection with *incomplete abortion*, and may be sufficient to produce profound anemia, shock, and even death. An intravenous infusion, to which Pitocin, 10 units, has been added, should be started promptly, using a large-bore needle, and blood should be sent for typing and cross-matching while the patient is transferred to the operating room for D&C or suction curettage. *Septic abortion* is discussed in the section on pelvic infections.

---

*See Figure 3, page 461.

PROBLEMS OF VAGINAL BLEEDING NOT ASSOCIATED WITH PREGNANCY

Vaginal Bleeding in Young Girls. *Trauma* incurred in bicycle, picket fence, and other accidental injuries may result in bleeding, hematoma, and edema of the female genitalia, but they rarely produce any permanent damage. The location of the urethra provides protection against direct injury, but local swelling may cause urinary retention. Bleeding usually can be controlled by external pressure. Deep lacerations should be closed with absorbable suture. Healing with little if any scarring is the rule.

Prolapsed Urethra. Symptoms of prolapse of the urethral mucosa include the appearance of a dark mulberry mass at the vaginal introitus, bleeding, and pain on micturition. The bleeding is never excessive but the appearance of the mass, which occupies the entire area between the labia, is frightening to the parents. Neither the urethra nor the vaginal orifice is visible, but a lubricated catheter inserted in the center of the mass will seek the bladder and confirm the diagnosis. No attempt should be made to reduce the prolapse of this devitalized tissue. The patient should be admitted for surgical correction, a relatively simple operation of excision of the necrotic tissue at the line of demarcation.

Suspected Rape. The medicolegal aspects of rape require careful documentation of the details of the history and physical and laboratory examinations, which subsequently may be made available to law enforcement officers. In some states a physician may not examine a patient until she has been seen by a police surgeon or other specially authorized medical personnel. If the child is less than 16 years of age, some states require that an immediate verbal report be made to designated officials under the "battered child" laws.

The medical problems associated with rape are complex and include immediate care of acute physical or psychic injuries, prevention of venereal disease, and prevention of pregnancy. The following is an abbreviated outline of recommendations distributed widely as a technical bulletin by the American College of Obstetricians and Gynecologists in July 1970. (For a further discussion of rape from the psychiatric viewpoint, see pp. 1194 and 1214–1216.)

(1) Get *consent* — written and witnessed.

(2) Get *history* in the patient's own words.

(3) Record *examination findings* in detail.

(4) Obtain the following *laboratory* specimens:

(a) A *swab from the vaginal pool* and from any suspicious areas around the vulva which can be tested for alkaline phosphatase, blood group antigen of semen, and precipitin test against human sperm and blood;

(b) A *wet mount* of material from the fornix should be examined immediately for motile sperm;

(c) *Smear and culture* for gonococcal infection.

(5) *Protect against disease.* Probenecid, 1 gm., is given orally, and 4.8 million units of penicillin is divided in half and injected into two separate sites. This provides adequate protection against both gonorrhea and incubating syphilis. If the patient is allergic to penicillin, tetracycline, 500 mg. q.i.d., is prescribed for 15 days. Appropriate adjustment of dosage is made for children.

(6) *Protect against pregnancy.* Medroxyprogesterone acetate (Depo-Provera), 100 mg. intramuscularly, or stilbestrol, 25 mg. twice daily by mouth for five days if the patient is in the second half of the menstrual cycle, or stilbestrol, 5 mg. daily for 20 to 25 days beginning prior to midcycle, is protective in a high percentage of cases. If the menstrual period does not begin within a week or ten days after cessation of estrogen, a D&C should be done.

It is important that the following definitions be recognized. *Rape* is coitus without consent of the woman. *Statutory rape* is coitus with a female below the age of consent, usually 16. *Sexual molestation* is noncoital sexual contact without consent. Where there is reasonable doubt, the final opinion recorded should be in terms of alleged or suspected rape.

The emergency physician may be called to testify years after the examination, and the initial record should contain as much description as possible. Photographs can be taken with the patient's consent, and can be extremely useful in the event of legal action. When passing specimens to the laboratory hand, transfers should be the rule, and the name and signature of all those transporting specimens should be written on the chart.

OBSTETRIC EMERGENCIES

EMERGENCY DELIVERY

The potential hazards of emergency delivery include maternal soft tissue damage, retained secundines, and postpartum hemorrhage. The major dangers for the newborn are related to trauma caused by tentorial tears of intracranial hemorrhage, particularly if the delivery is precipitate, and hypoxia or asphyxia if respirations and an airway are not established promptly.

Management. Although the perineal preparation may need to be abbreviated, efforts should be made to obtain the best possible level of asepsis. The delivery should be controlled and steady. No attempt should be made to gain time by locking the patient's lower extremities, or otherwise forcibly holding back the presenting part.

Loops of *cord* about the infant's neck usually can be freed by slipping the cord over the head or over the oncoming shoulder, but if the loops are tight the cord is doubly clamped, cut, and unwound.

The shoulders are rotated into an anteroposterior position, and the anterior shoulder is delivered first by gentle downward traction of the head. At this point, a delay of 30 seconds before delivery of the posterior shoulder allows for uterine muscle contraction. Another 30 seconds between the delivery of the posterior shoulder and the rest of the body allows for further uterine contraction, aimed at decreasing the likelihood of postpartum hemorrhage.

Shoulder dystocia can be a serious problem. Although the head may be fully delivered, impaction of the anterior shoulder above the symphysis imposes greater risk of cord and chest compression, and respiratory efforts are impaired. Direct pressure above the symphysis may bring the anterior shoulder into the pelvis. If this is not suc-cessful, the hand is inserted into the vagina and the posterior shoulder is rotated anteriorly, while a downward and simultaneous corkscrew maneuver is carried out, bringing the posterior shoulder anteriorly under the symphysis.

The third stage carries the greatest risk of the entire labor for the mother. In the Emergency Department setting, *delivery of the placenta* should be conducted in a conservative manner. Spontaneous uterine contractions cause a shearing off or separation of the placenta; the uterus changes from a discoid to a globular shape, and gentle traction on the cord usually is all that is required. Vigorous manipulation or kneading (the Credé method) should be avoided. After the placenta has been delivered, elevation of the uterus out of the lower pelvis and gentle massage promote uterine contractions. *Oxytocics* should be withheld until the placenta has been delivered, in order to avoid "trapping" the placenta and the need for manual extraction under less than ideal conditions. Ergotrate or Methergine, 1 ml. (0.2 mg.), can be given intravenously or intramuscularly after the third stage, unless the patient is hypertensive, in which case an intravenous drip using 10 units of Pitocin dissolved in 1000 ml. of 5 per cent dextrose is advisable.

RESUSCITATION OF THE NEWBORN

Most normal newborns will breathe within the first minutes of life. Gentle bulb suction of the oropharynx, stimulation by gentle towelling, and maintenance of warmth are the essential considerations. *Caution:* Exposing even the normal newborn to cooling should be avoided. Chilling and shivering increase oxygen utilization, and also increase metabolic acidosis and related pulmonary vasoconstriction. Determination of the Apgar score (Table 1) at one and five minutes after birth reflects the newborn's ability to cope with extrauterine life and provides an important guide, not only for the infant's need of resuscitation, but also for the type of resuscitative effort that may be required.

Mechanical Resuscitation. Equipment necessary for resuscitation includes the following.

(1) Rubber suction bulb.

TABLE 1   *The Apgar Scoring System*

SIGN	2	1	0
1. Heart rate	Greater than 100	Less than 100	Absent
2. Respirations	Good, crying	Slow, gasping, irregular	Absent
3. Color	Pink	Extremities cyanotic	Cyanotic
4. Muscle tone	Active motion	Some flexion of extremities	Limp
5. Reflex irritability	Cough, sneeze	Grimace only	No response

(2) Oropharyngeal airways — several sizes.

(3) Infant oxygen mask.

(4) Ambu bag (Hope infant resuscitator).

(5) Suction catheters — No. 8 or 10 French with the DeLee mucus trap attached for oral or wall suction use.

(6) Endotracheal tubes — Cole tubes which are precurved and narrowed at the distal end are preferred. These prevent endobronchial intubation.

(7) Laryngoscope with straight infant blade and blunt tip.

MANAGEMENT

The depressed infant with Apgar score of 5 to 7, heart rate below 100, usually will respond to the following procedures.

(1) Head down position with a 2-inch thickness of towel rolled under the shoulders and head extended.

(2) Stimulation by flicking of the feet. Avoid excessive trauma such as digital rectal stimulation or slapping. These may in themselves induce apnea.

(3) Oxygen by mask.

(4) Pharyngeal fluid that tends to accumulate should be aspirated gently. *Caution:* One of the most common errors in resuscitation of the newborn is the overzealous use of catheter suctioning. Rapid up-and-down manipulation of the catheter deep in the pharynx not only occludes the air passage and prevents the baby from breathing, but the stimulation of the epiglottis involved causes reflex gagging, laryngospasm, apnea, and bradycardia.

The *severely depressed* or comatose infant, Apgar score 0 to 4, heart rate below 100, needs artificial ventilation. If nothing else is available in the emergency situation, mouth-to-mouth resuscitation should be carried out after foreign material has been removed from the oropharynx. The following methods should be available.

(1) Positive pressure oxygen. Initial inflation may require 25 to 45 cm. of water pressure, and subsequent pressure of 10 to 15 cm. of water at a rate of about 30 per minute.

(2) If the chest does not expand with intermittent positive pressure oxygen, laryngoscopic inspection of the airway, suction of obstructing material, and intubation with a Cole tube is indicated.

(3) Oral suction of the trachea with the DeLee mucus trap should be performed before oxygen is blown into the lungs.

(4) Intermittent positive pressure oxygen should be given by mouth to tube, bag and mask, or mechanical resuscitator.

The *asphyxiated infant* frequently will need biochemical resuscitation for correction of metabolic acidosis soon after respirations have been initiated. This should be performed only by those skilled in the technique and in insertion of an umbilical vein catheter. Sodium bicarbonate, 2 to 3 mEq./kg. diluted with an equal volume of 10 per cent glucose, is given slowly over a five-minute period when indicated.

Third Trimester Bleeding and Postpartum Hemorrhage

Vaginal bleeding in late pregnancy always should be considered an emergency until proved otherwise. History of recent occurrence, or the presence of active vaginal bleeding, is ample indication of the need to obtain immediate obstetric consultation and to make preparations for admission to the Maternity Unit.

PLACENTAL SEPARATION

This is the most common cause of late pregnancy bleeding. *Placenta abruptio* is separation of the normally implanted placenta. *Placenta previa* is separation of the

TABLE 2 *Signs of Placental Separation*

PLACENTA PREVIA	PLACENTA ABRUPTIO
1. Painless, bright red bleeding.	1. Pain of varying severity and passage of dark blood.
2. Amount of bleeding and signs of shock are commensurate.	2. Signs of shock often exceed visible blood loss (retroplacental concealed bleeding).
3. Uterus is soft and nontender.	3. Uterus is firm to tetanically contracted and tender.
4. Fetus is palpable; fetal heart tones usually are present.	4. Fetus often is difficult to palpate owing to uterine contraction, which, if tetanic, seriously impairs placental blood flow. Fetal heart tones may be irregular or absent.
5. Blood clotting usually is normal.	5. Blood coagulation defect (hypofibrinogenemia) is associated with severe abruptio.
6. Incidence is not increased in hypertensive disorders.	6. Incidence is significantly increased in hypertensive disorders.

placenta located low in the uterus, near or completely covering the internal os of the cervix. Characteristic signs of these conditions are contrasted as shown in Table 2.

Exsanguinating hemorrhage and profound shock may occur rapidly with either of these complications. On the other hand, the amount of blood visualized can be deceptive, since considerable quantities may be concealed behind the placenta or within the uterus. Recognition of these problems by the emergency physician is important, since certain steps may need to be taken in the Emergency Department without delay. These include the following.

(1) Check maternal vital signs, fetal heart rate, and signs of placental separation as outlined above.

(2) *No vaginal or rectal examinations.* If placenta previa is present, profuse hemorrhage may occur as the placenta is dislodged.

(3) Draw blood for typing and crossmatching, and start intravenous infusion of Ringer's lactate using a large-bore needle for blood transfusion.

(4) Draw an additional 10 ml. of blood, and transfer 5 ml. into each of two separate small test tubes for a clot observation test if there is any suspicion of placenta abruptio.

(5) Transfer to the Maternity Unit as promptly as possible.

POSTPARTUM HEMORRHAGE

Immediate Postpartum Hemorrhage. This condition, which occurs in about 5 per cent of all deliveries, is one of the most sudden and dangerous emergencies in medicine. Hemorrhage is still a leading cause of maternal mortality, and postpartum hemorrhage accounts for approximately 25 per cent of these deaths. Etiologic factors include: uterine atony; retained placental tissues; vaginal, cervical, or uterine lacerations; and coagulation disorders. Coagulation problems that may arise in the immediate postpartum period may have as underlying causes placenta abruptio, amniotic fluid embolism, or intrauterine retention of a dead fetus for a protracted period prior to delivery.

MANAGEMENT. *Avoid delay.*

(1) If the placenta is undelivered and cannot be readily expressed, it should be manually removed, and the uterus should be pushed out of the pelvis and massaged.

(2) If the placenta has been delivered and bleeding persists, inspect the birth canal for lacerations, and explore the uterus for retained secundines or possible rupture.

(3) Draw blood for typing and crossmatching, and start intravenous infusion with Ringer's lactate or physiologic saline to which 10 units of oxytocin should be added. Methergine, 1 ml. (0.2 mg.), may be given I.V. directly.

(4) Bimanual tamponade should be undertaken with one hand in the uterus or against the cervix elevating the uterus out of the pelvis and the other hand on the abdomen so that compression and massage can be more effectively applied.

(5) Packing. Although the use of uterovaginal packing remains controversial, it may prove valuable under these emergency conditions. The uterus and vagina should be methodically and tightly packed, but the uterus should not be overdistended so that it is unable to contract against the pack. Under these conditions, the packing is used as a temporary measure until the patient can be transferred to the operating room.

(6) Failure to respond to these conservative measures requires surgical control by hysterectomy or uterine or hypogastric artery ligation.

Note: An overdistended bladder can be a factor in preventing effective uterine contractions. It is important to make certain that the urinary bladder is emptied by catheterization.

Delayed Postpartum Hemorrhage. Bleeding that occurs after the first 24 hours following delivery most commonly is due to retained *placental fragments.* These increase the risk of continued bleeding, subinvolution, and infection. Attempts to treat this condition with oxytocic prescriptions and by sending the patient home for bed rest are ill-advised. The patient should be admitted for re-examination and uterine curettage under anesthesia.

Placental site bleeding is a less common but potentially dangerous cause of delayed postpartum hemorrhage. This is apparently due to separation or lysis of the fibrin crust over placental site vessels. Bleeding usually begins between the seventh and 12th days postpartum and may be profuse. The patient should be admitted promptly. D&C is usually curative. In a few cases a more agressive surgical procedure will be necessary.

Pre-Eclampsia–Eclampsia

The patient with advancing pre-eclamptic toxemia cannot be treated as an outpatient. Hospitalization is essential. The diagnosis is made on the basis of the cardinal signs — *edema, hypertension,* and *proteinuria* occurring in the second half of pregnancy.

Symptoms do not appear until late in the course of the disease. In fact, the patient who presents in the Emergency Department with headache, visual disturbances (diplopia, blurring of vision, scotomata), or epigastric pain, and who also exhibits the signs of pre-eclampsia, may be in imminent danger of convulsions. The symptoms reflect the effects of the primary vasoconstrictive process, including edema, hypoxia, hemorrhage, and metabolic alterations in tissues, particularly of the brain, retina, liver, kidneys, heart, and the placenta. The patient should be admitted to the Maternity Unit immediately for treatment aimed to achieve the following objectives.

PREVENTION OF CONVULSIONS

Magnesium sulfate is the single most valuable agent in the treatment of severe pre-eclampsia and eclampsia. A total of 10 gm. of a 5 per cent magnesium sulfate solution (5 gm. injected deep I.M. in each buttock), or 2 gm. of a 10 per cent solution is given I.V. *slowly* and 4 gm. in each of the two sites is given I.M.

PROMOTION OF RENAL FUNCTION

An indwelling catheter should be inserted and hourly intake-output record maintained. Osmotic diuretics are seldom needed if magnesium sulfate dosage is adequate. However, if urinary output continues at less than 30 cc. per hour, and fluid shift from the extravascular space back into the vascular space has not been satisfactorily achieved, plasma volume usually is low and the hematocrit elevated. A single I.V. infusion of 700 to 1000 ml. of 5 or 10 per cent dextrose in water over a period of one to two hours improves urinary output, but careful monitoring is necessary to avoid cardiac overload. *Caution:* Thiazide diuretics are contraindicated.

CONTROL OF BLOOD PRESSURE

Antihypertensive agents are not needed unless the blood pressure is inordinately high and fails to respond to the magnesium sulfate. In such cases, an underlying essential hypertension almost certainly is present in addition to a superimposed pre-eclampsia.

DIFFERENTIAL DIAGNOSIS

Pre-eclamptic toxemia must be differentiated from other hypertensive disorders that usually are accentuated by pregnancy — mainly essential hypertension and primary renal disease.

ECLAMPSIA

The occurrence of convulsions and/or coma greatly increases the mortality risk for both mother and fetus. The first steps, which must be taken quickly, are aimed at preventing trauma and hypoxia.

(1) Mouth gag with wrapped tongue blades.

(2) Aspiration of mucus.

(3) Administration of oxygen.

(4) Record vital signs and avoid overtreatment with heavy sedation.

(5) Intravenous magnesium sulfate, 2 to 4 gm. in a 10 or 20 per cent solution administered by *slow* intravenous injection, followed by intramuscular injection of 50 per cent magnesium sulfate in two sites, making a total of 10 gm.

The remainder of the treatment is similar to that prescribed for severe pre-eclamptic toxemia, but as soon as convulsions are controlled the patient should be sent to the Maternity Intensive Care Unit, where stabilization and delivery will be carried out if the gestational age is favorable. Delivery generally is accomplished by induction of labor, since the uterus under these conditions usually is responsive. In a small percentage of cases, cesarean sections will be necessary.

DIFFERENTIAL DIAGNOSIS

Other convulsive disorders may occur late in pregnancy. These include convulsions due to epilepsy, insulin overdose with profound hypoglycemia, trauma, hypertensive encephalopathy, and, occasionally, drug toxicity. These may be distinguished from eclampsia by history if available, by the absence of cardinal signs of severe pre-eclampsia, and by the presence of specific signs of these convulsive disorders.

References

Mattingly, R. F.: High risk gynecology. Clin. Obstet. Gynecol. *16*: June, 1973.

Monif, G. R. G.: Infectious Diseases in Obstetrics and Gynecology. Hagerstown, Md., Harper & Row, 1974.

Osofsky, H. J.: High risk pregnancy with emphasis upon maternal and fetal well being. Clin. Obstet. Gynecol. *16*: March, 1973.

Romney, S. L., et al.: Gynecology and Obstetrics. The Health Care of Women. New York, St. Louis, and San Francisco, McGraw-Hill Book Co., 1975.

Willson, J. R., Beecham, C. T., and Carrington, E. R.: Obstetrics and Gynecology. 5th ed. St. Louis, The C. V. Mosby Co., 1975.

Chapter 45

NONTRAUMATIC OTOLARYNGOLOGIC EMERGENCIES

William W. Montgomery,
Richard L. Fabian,
William G. Lavelle,
and Jaclyne M. Witte

EAR

FROSTBITE

Frostbite is the result of prolonged exposure of the auricle to extremely cold material. It is characterized by hyperemia when mild, or by white ischemia, vesicles, and gangrene when severe.

Treatment. This should include systemic antibiotics, pain medication, heparinization, sterile dressings, and late conservative débridement of gangrenous areas as necessary. Hot or cold applications are *not* recommended.

Complications. These may include secondary bacterial invasions, perichondritis, and autoamputation of the auricle.

BURN

Burns of the auricle can be of thermal, chemical, or radiation origin. Hyperemia is noted when mild injury occurs. Necrosis, blistering, and serum exudation are characteristic of severe burns.

Treatment. This consists of systemic antibiotics, aseptic débridement of exfoliating tissue (especially vesicles), and prevention of crust formation with hydrogen peroxide soaks. Local antisepsis is instituted with Betadine, silver sulfadiazine, or similar agents. Tetanus toxoid booster or Hyper-Tet is given as necessary.

Complications. These include extensive tissue loss and secondary bacterial invasion, particularly with gram-negative organisms.

HEMATOMA

Hematoma can be spontaneous or due to trauma. The upper auricle is the most frequent location. It can be recognized by a well circumscribed blue swelling and dark red transillumination.

Treatment. This begins with aseptic cleansing of the auricle, and incision and drainage of the hematoma before organization occurs. A conforming pressure dressing (Chapter 16) should be applied and systemic antibiotics prescribed.

Complications. These include secondary infection (perichondritis), or organization of clot with subsequent fibrosis and calcification. A "cauliflower ear" deformity results.

PERICHONDRITIS

Perichondritis of the auricle has many origins. The most common are bacterial invasion of an auricular hematoma, thermal injury, postradiation effects, external otitis, dermatitis, and lacerations. Fever, pain, and a diffuse, red, doughy swelling that pits on digital pressure characterize this condition.

Treatment. This consists of keeping the involved areas disinfected, giving systemic antibiotics, and applying hot compresses. Pain medication may be indicated. The physician should be careful to rule out diabetes mellitus.

Complications. These are serious with this condition. Abscess formation requires incision and drainage. The pus should be cultured and the wound packed open. A light dressing is then applied. Loss of cartilage results in the collapse of the auricular framework and permanent disfigurement. Catheter insertion, with local antibiotic perfusion and débridement of necrotic debris, may be necessary. Septicemia is a possible complication.

External Ear Canal

FURUNCULOSIS

Furunculosis of the external auditory canal can be the result of an insect bite, trauma to the cartilaginous canal (improper ear cleaning or a foreign body), or chronic dermatitis with secondary bacterial invasion. The bacterial pathogen usually is gram-positive *Staph. aureus.* Furunculosis is marked by severe pain and trismus, swelling of cartilaginous hair-bearing portion of the external canal, and tenderness of the tragal cartilage to palpation. Cellulitis of the concha and pretragal regions may occur.

Treatment. This consists of penicillin or erythromycin, and pain medication, if necessary. Local heat (Hydroculator pack) is a good therapeutic measure. Insertion of an Ergophene ear wick in the canal aids in local treatment. If fluctuation of the ear is observed, incision and drainage is indicated.

EXTERNAL OTITIS

External otitis may be bacterial, fungal, noninfectious, or malignant. As a general rule, any refractory case of external otitis should be referred to an otolaryngologist. Patients must be impressed with the need to adhere to treatment programs accurately and to avoid water and contact allergens. Differential diagnoses of external otitis include otitis media, mastoiditis, temporomandibular joint arthritis, parotitis, lymph adenitis, furunculosis, psoriasis, tinea capitis, dermatitis, and neoplasia.

DIFFUSE EXTERNAL OTITIS

Diffuse external otitis, sometimes referred to as "swimmer's ear," is caused by gram-negative infection. Generally, the patient has a history of swimming, frequent showers, or other exposure to water. Manifestations include severe pain, pretragal and tragal tenderness, diffuse swelling of the external canal, and local adenopathy. The ear canal contains debris and white exudate. The tympanic membrane, if visible, is normal.

Treatment. This demands that all canal debris be evacuated and cultured. The ear canal is carefully cleaned and irrigated with a 2 per cent acetic acid or aluminum acetate solution. Ergophene is applied on a cotton wick and allowed to remain in situ for 12 hours. Antibiotic otic drops are then prescribed for use in the ear canal for ten days. Pain medication is usually indicated. Systemic antibiotics are prescribed for an infection that has spread beyond the confines of the ear canal.

FUNGAL EXTERNAL OTITIS

Fungal external otitis is usually caused by *Candida albicans* or *Aspergillus niger.* The ear canal is swollen and contains cheese-like debris; Candida will appear as gray debris, whereas black spots characterize Aspergillus. The patient experiences moderate pain with severe itching, and the history frequently indicates the chronicity of the disease.

Treatment. This again involves a culture and fungal stains. Frequent cleaning of the ear canal is imperative. The physician should irrigate the canal with Burrow's solution. A Mycolog ear wick should remain in situ for 48 hours, followed by frequent applications of merbromin solution to the canal wall skin, which should be dried with an air stream. Cresatin, gentian violet, and Tinactin are useful alternative medications.

NONINFECTIOUS OTITIS

Noninfectious otitis is difficult to diagnose and is dependent on a careful history and systematic elimination of other diseases. Contact dermatitis, neurodermatitis, psoriasis, or dermatitis medicamentosa characterize this category.

Treatment. This rests primarily with elimination of the underlying cause. Dermatitis medicamentosa is best treated by eliminating the offending medication. The use of topical steroids, accompanied by irrigation with Burrow's solution, is effective in all noninfectious types.

MALIGNANT EXTERNAL OTITIS

Malignant external otitis is caused by *Pseudomonas aeruginosa*, and is characterized by a progressive necrotizing granulomatous inflammation. The external ear canal is involved primarily. The patient complains of severe pain, is febrile, and generally has a positive history of diabetes mellitus.

Treatment. This is imperative, as malignant external otitis is a life-threatening disease. Progressive necrosis can lead to involvement of the entire temporal bone, temporomandibular joint, and parotid gland. Meningitis, brain abscess, sinus thrombosis, general toxemia, and even death eventually may result.

Middle Ear

ACUTE OTITIS MEDIA

Acute otitis media may present as one of three types: acute bacterial, acute viral, and acute serous. In acute bacterial otitis media, a frequent pathogen in patients below the age of 6 years is *Hemophilus influenzae*. Above the age of 6, the frequent pathogens are Pneumococcus and Streptococcus. Viral otitis media as a distinct entity is less common. Hemorrhagic blebs or bullae involving the tympanic membrane may occur secondary to viral infection.

Fever, otalgia (mild to severe), conductive hearing loss, and lethargy are all indicative of acute otitis media. In young children, symptoms include difficulty in nursing, agitation, ear pulling, and vomiting. The patient may have a history of a recent upper respiratory illness. Rare findings include tinnitus, vertigo, and facial nerve paralysis. Physical findings include a red, bulging tympanic membrane, loss of normal membrane landmarks, and, later, membrane perforation with mucopurulent exudate. Mastoid x-rays demonstrate a diffuse increased density of the mastoid air cell system and middle ear space without bony cellular destruction.

Serous otitis media may result as a residual disease after a viral or bacterial otitis media or as a sequela of an upper respiratory tract infection. Serous otitis media is characterized by a blue, relatively immobile tympanic membrane. Middle ear bubbles or air fluid levels and a conductive hearing loss without pain may be seen.

ACUTE NECROTIZING OTITIS MEDIA

Acute necrotizing otitis media is caused by beta-hemolytic streptococcus. This disease usually occurs during an exanthema in childhood. It is characterized by progressive, rapid destruction of the tympanic membrane and ossicles.

Type III pneumococcus causes a virulent, rapidly progressive middle ear infection that frequently results in mastoiditis, meningitis, labyrinthitis, and severe hearing loss.

A careful review of the history, with particular reference to previous upper respiratory and ear infections as well as to the exclusion of systemic disease, is mandatory before treatment.

Any unilateral or bilateral serous otitis in an adult suggests the possibility of a nasopharyngeal neoplasia.

Treatment. This should begin immediately with antibiotics. Below the age of 6 years, ampicillin is prescribed; above this age, penicillin is the favored therapy. A loading parenteral dose is recommended according to age and weight. This is followed by oral therapy for a minimum of ten days. Pain medication, antihistamine, and nasal decongestants may be indicated. If a perforation is present, antibiotic ear drops should be used for two weeks. Throat and ear cultures are recommended.

Pain, high fever (with or without convulsions), vertigo, and/or facial nerve paralysis can indicate the need for an immediate myringotomy. In children, general anesthesia usually is necessary when performing this operation, which should be undertaken only by physicians experienced and trained in the technique. Permanent and significant complications can occur. The patient should return for follow-up examination after treatment is complete.

Complications. These include bacterial otitis media, mastoiditis, labyrinthitis, meningitis, facial nerve paralysis, brain abscess, lateral sinus thrombosis, and generalized septicemia. Mastoiditis is the most common complication. It is characterized by progressive swelling and tenderness of the postauricular crease, forward projection of the pinna, spiking fever, progression of constitutional symptoms, and persistent ear pain, even if the tympanic membrane is perforated and draining. A conductive hearing loss may or may not be present. X-rays will show evidence of decalcification and destruction of the mastoid cell system.

CHRONIC OTITIS MEDIA

Chronic otitis media is subdivided into three types: chronic tuberculous, chronic osteitic, and chronic cholesteatomatous.

Chronic otitis media implies a continuous pathologic process of middle ear and mastoid infection. Its hallmark is a period of inactivity alternating with periods of active infection. The principal symptoms and signs are otorrhea, aural fetor, and hearing loss. Chronic perforation, middle ear epithelial debris, and granulation and perforation of the tympanic membrane are frequent findings in the osteitic and cholesteatomatous types.

Tuberculous otitis media is characterized by a painless, odorless otorrhea associated with granulation tissue and multiple perforations of the tympanic membrane. Pulmonary pathology may or may not be demonstrated. All cases of chronic otitis should be referred to an otolaryngologist.

BAROTRAUMA

Barotrauma is a nonbacterial inflammation of the middle ear space caused by a sudden change in middle ear pressure. It may occur while diving or during descent while flying. It is primarily due to improper eustachian tube function and subsequent failure of middle ear pressure equalization.

Recognition generally is not difficult. The patient will give a history of flying or diving, and will experience pain and a conductive deafness. Findings during examination include a retracted hemorrhagic tympanic membrane, air fluid levels in the middle ear space, and hemotympanum. Occasionally, the tympanic membrane may be ruptured.

Treatment. For severe cases, this should begin with a myringotomy and evacuation of all fluid. Nasal decongestants may be indicated. Adequate follow-up, including audiometry, is essential. Secondary infection is treated with antibiotics. Mild cases may be treated with decongestants without myringotomy, however.

PENETRATION INJURY

Penetration injury of the tympanic membrane can be caused by a foreign body such as a stick, welding spark, Q-tip, etc. The patient experiences sudden pain, vertigo (transient to permanent), and hearing loss. Blood will be present in the external canal, and the tympanic membrane will be perforated. Hemotympanum also is a symptom. Clinical findings include spontaneous nystagmus, positional nystagmus, and hearing loss.

Treatment. This is dependent on the patient's complaints. Because ossicular and inner ear injuries may be present, immediate otologic consultation is imperative. Antibiotics, antihistamines, and antinausea medication generally are in order as primary therapy.

Inner Ear

TINNITUS

Tinnitus is the sensation of spontaneous, internal sound without an external source. There are two types: subjective (heard only by the patient), and objective (heard by both the observer and the patient).

Differential diagnoses involving the external and middle ear are ceruminosis, patulous eustachian tube, eustachian tube dysfunction, acute and chronic inflammatory disease, hemorrhage, transudate or exudate into the middle ear space, otosclerosis, and neoplasia, especially glomus jugulare tumor. Inner ear or cochlear differential diagnoses for tinnitus are inflammatory conditions of any cause, Ménière's disease, degenerative cochlear disease of any cause, acoustic neuroma, and toxic cochlear degeneration, as with aspirin, neomycin, etc. Dysfunction of the central nervous system may be responsible for tinnitus, as in arteriosclerosis, degenerative demyelinating disease, aneurysm, and neoplastic lesions.

Treatment. This frequently is a multidisciplinary problem. Otologic, neurologic, audiologic, and radiologic investigations are minimal prerequisites. All treatable diseases must be ruled out.

It is an unfortunate fact that most forms of tinnitus cannot be treated. The best course of action is reassurance. Particular emphasis should be placed on the knowledge that tinnitus does not necessarily indicate impending stroke. Patients should be warned against false claims and treatments.

LABYRINTHITIS

Labyrinthitis is the result of bacterial or viral invasion of the inner ear space. It can be of a serous type or suppurative. It has many causes, among the most common being acute otitis media, chronic otitis media, syphilis, temporal bone fracture, mastoiditis, semicircular canal fistula communicating with inner ear space, meningitis, and septicemia of various causes.

Recognition of serous labyrinthitis involves detailed analysis of the patient's history and symptoms. Generally he has experienced vertigo with spontaneous nystagmus to the opposite ear, nausea and vomiting, and sensorineural hearing loss. Caloric function is present on testing, but may be abnormal. Suppurative labyrinthitis is characterized by most of the above-mentioned symptoms, but is progressive and of greater severity. In addition, it is characterized by fever, prostration, and confusion, total deafness of the sensorineural type, and no response to caloric testing.

Treatment. This should be preceded by a careful physical examination, audiogram, caloric testing, fistula testing, and mastoid x-rays.

Differential diagnoses are Ménière's disease, spontaneous otologic fistula, inner ear concussion, benign paroxysmal positional vertigo, temporal bone fracture, acoustic neurinoma, intracerebral vascular occlusion, CNS neoplasia, degenerative or demyelinating CNS disease, metabolic disease such as diabetes, anemia, drug toxicity, etc.

ACUTE SUDDEN HEARING LOSS

Acute sudden hearing loss may be of vascular, viral, or idiopathic origin, the latter being the most common. The patient may give a history of diabetes, hypertension, re-

cent upper respiratory infection, recent exertion, cerebrovascular disease, or hematologic disease. Vertigo sometimes is part of the symptom complex.

Treatment. This must be administered by an otologist. A complete audiometric and otologic evaluation, including caloric testing, is indicated.

SUDDEN FACIAL NERVE PARALYSIS

Sudden facial nerve paralysis is classified as either central or peripheral. Central paralysis occurs as the result of a cerebrovascular accident, neoplasia (especially of the cerebellopontine angle), poliomyelitis, meningitis, multiple sclerosis, or other demyelinating diseases. Peripheral facial paralysis is subdivided into intratemporal or extratemporal, depending on the location and type of pathologic process.

Intratemporal paralysis can be of infectious origin, as in otitis media, herpes zoster, varicella, rubella, mumps, and syphilis. Tumors also may be causative, as in facial nerve neuroma, acoustic neurinoma, metastatic tumor, leukemia, and glomus jugulare tumor. Other causes include Wegener's granuloma, sarcoidosis, tuberculosis, trauma (temporal bone fracture, surgical), autoimmune (Guillain-Barré syndrome), toxic (diabetes, uremia), and vasculitis (polyarteritis, Melkersson's syndrome). Extratemporal causes include trauma, parotid tumor, and sarcoidosis. Most frequently, no etiologic diagnosis is possible.

Radiographic evaluations include polytomography of the temporal bone, skull x-rays, posterior fossa myelography, carotid arteriography, and brain scan, as indicated clinically. The patient should undergo audiometric examination. Clinical tests will involve Schirmer's test for lacrimation, test for stapedial reflex, electrogustometry, submaxillary salivary gland testing, nerve excitability tests, and electromyography.

Treatment. This is so diversified that it is not within the scope of this discussion to examine all details of treatment for facial nerve paralysis. It is recommended that textbooks of otolaryngology and neurology be consulted. The Emergency Department physician should be aware of the implications of this finding, and should provide the patient with medical direction, urging immediate otolaryngologic and neurologic consultation.

NOSE AND PARANASAL SINUSES

ACUTE NASAL CONGESTION

Acute nasal congestion (acute rhinitis) may be of viral, bacterial (Pneumococcus, *Staphylococcus aureus*), allergic, chemical (caustic vapors, smoke, industrial pollutants), vasomotor, or medicamentosa types.

The etiologic diagnosis of acute nasal congestion requires studies of nasal secretion (microscopic examination for eosinophils, culture, sugar, and electrolyte determination), sinus transillumination, direct nasopharyngoscopy, and sinus x-rays. Findings will include diffuse edema and erythema of the nasal mucosa. Watery, clean secretions usually are associated with viral or chemical rhinitis, whereas bacterial rhinitis results in a mucopurulent exudate. Vasomotor rhinitis is characterized by engorged, pale turbinates productive of profuse nasal discharge. Nasal polyposis is found with either allergic or bacterial rhinitis. Findings in caustic rhinitis depend on the offending agent. Friable mucosa with submucosal hemorrhage is frequently seen.

Treatment. For viral rhinitis, this includes a short term nasal decongestant spray and an oral antihistamine. Bacterial rhinitis is treated with penicillin, steam inhalation, oral antihistamine and decongestant spray. In allergic rhinitis, the hypersensitive tissue is the nasal mucous membranes. Topical steroids in the form of a nasal spray, antihistamines, and a cool mist vaporizer are most effective. Severe cases require systemic steroids. Long term treatment of allergic rhinitis depends on an accurate determination of the offending inhalants. The patient should be urged to consult an allergist for subsequent evaluation. Treatment of chemical rhinitis, as of allergic rhinitis, depends in large part on avoidance of the irritant. A patient who presents with rhinitis medicamentosa should follow the same measures as one with allergic rhinitis. Also, all medication, especially nasal sprays, should be terminated.

The differential diagnoses of acute rhinitis include neoplasia, cerebrospinal fluid rhinorrhea, meningoencephalocele, associated sinusitis, and the presence of a foreign body.

NASAL CELLULITIS

Nasal cellulitis or abscess (vestibulitis) is the result of trauma, bacterial rhinitis (with or without sinusitis), neoplasia with infiltration and necrosis, dermatologic disease, or dental abscess with extension. The bacterial offenders are coagulase-positive *Staphylococcus aureus*, Pneumococcus, beta-hemolytic Streptococcus, and *Hemophilus influenzae*. The patient will present with diffuse erythema and edema of the nasal vestibule. Intense pain, malaise, and fever characterize nasal cellulitis.

Treatment. This is dependent on laboratory demonstration of the bacteria involved. A nasal culture and gram stain are essential. Other diagnostic studies should include a WBC (with differential), sinus x-rays, blood sugar, and a biopsy of neoplastic tissue, if present.

Laboratory results of the nasal culture and gram stain will indicate the appropriate antibiotic. Pain medication may be required. Local heat also is effective. Failure of adequate, early treatment can result in serious complications. Hospitalization is mandatory if cellulitis is extensive; if there is evidence of neoplasia; or if the patient complains of severe headache and has a high fever, with or without meningeal signs or visual symptoms. Careful and judicious handling of nasal cellulitis bears a direct relationship to the avoidance of severe complications, which can include meningitis, septal necrosis, osteomyelitis, and cavernous sinus thrombosis.

NASAL SEPTAL HEMATOMA

Nasal septal hematoma or abscess can result from trauma, the presence of a foreign body in the nasal cavity, or nasal infection. Facial and nasal x-rays will aid in establishing a correct diagnosis. A nasal culture is mandatory.

The clinical picture consists of pain, nasal obstruction, external evidence of trauma or infection, and widening of the nasal septum. Boggy mucosal edema may be visualized. Constitutional symptoms will be indicative of developing complications.

Treatment. This should include incision and drainage of the submucoperiosteal fluid collection. A small window of mucosa is removed and a Penrose drain sutured in place. Antibiotics should be prescribed in accordance with the culture results. Compressive nasal packing is of value, and the patient and physician should be impressed with the need for daily follow-up.

ACUTE SINUSITIS

Acute sinusitis sometimes is difficult to treat because of its various manifestations. It can be of allergic, viral, barotraumic, or bacterial (Pneumococcus or *Staphylococcus aureus*) origin. The most common locations are the ethmoid, frontal, and maxillary sinuses; on occasion, the sphenoid sinuses will be involved.

A careful history is important. The most common symptoms of sinus disease are nasal discharge and pain. It is important, however, to review carefully the history of discomfort or pain related to the various paranasal sinuses. Generalized headache usually is *not* a symptom of sinusitis. Pain from the frontal sinus can be present directly over the sinus or in the orbit. This pain appears each morning and progresses in severity until late afternoon, at which time is subsides spontaneously. Pain from the maxillary sinus can occur directly over the sinus, in the orbit, or at the roots of the upper teeth. Pain from the ethmoid sinus usually is in, or medial to, the orbit on the affected side. The pain resulting from sphenoid sinus disease is most difficult for the patient to describe. It usually is severe and persistent, and emanates from the "center of the head" or radiates to the ear. A change of head position may either worsen or relieve the pain.

There are numerous orbital manifestations of sinus disease. These include orbital pain, exophthalmos, enophthalmos, lid swelling, mass in the orbit, epiphora, orbital cellulitis, and abscess.

Examination of the sinuses should include palpation of the roof and floor of the orbits, of the ascending process of the maxillae, and of the canine fossae. Tenderness may be elicited in these areas, and masses or defects may be felt. Transillumination is of limited value, but should not be excluded: its use is limited to the diagnosis of frontal and maxillary sinus disease. For the frontal sinuses, the light is placed under the medial aspect of the supraorbital rim for observation

of the forehead; for the maxillary sinuses, it is placed above the infraorbital rim for observation of the hard palate. The test is of limited diagnostic value, for both the frontal and maxillary sinuses vary considerably in their degree of development. A sinus filled with clear liquid will transilluminate well. The presence of a mass, thickness, or reaction in the surrounding bone will interfere with transillumination. The procedure is most useful as a tool for following the patient's progress.

Diagnostic studies should begin with a culture of the nose and nasopharynx, and a gram stain of secretions. Dental examination may be indicated if the maxillary sinuses are the source of complaint. The patient should have a complete blood count and chest as well as sinus x-rays.

Treatment. This will be in accordance with the gram stain and culture results. Antibiotics should be used where indicated. Penicillin generally is the drug of choice, unless culture results show a resistant organism. A fundamental factor in healing is the drainage and ventilation of the infected mucosa; nasal decongestants (Neo-Synephrine, cocaine, etc.), antihistamines, and steam inhalation are therefore necessary. The patient should be cautioned that prolonged use of nasal decongestants (more than one week) is not advisable. Some relief may be gained by heat application to the painful areas.

Allergic rhinitis and sinusitis may be treated by the use of short term steroids systemically and locally. Careful diagnosis is mandatory before steroids are used.

Some cases of sinusitis may require surgical treatment, depending on the clinical severity or lack of response to treatment. The patient should be informed of possible complications such as osteomyelitis, orbital cellulitis, mucocele, or pyocele. Intracranial extension of infection can lead to meningitis, subdural abscess, brain abscess, and venous sinus thrombosis. Necrosis of the maxillary sinus wall with fistula formation (oral antral fistula) is a possible complication.

PHARYNX

ACUTE GLOSSITIS

Acute glossitis is characterized by progressive swelling of the tongue, progressive dysphagia, drooling, agitation, fever, pain, and trismus. Acute glossitis can be allergy-induced, or the causative agents can be bacterial, such as *Staphylococcus aureus*, Pneumococcus, Streptococcus, and *Hemophilus influenzae*.

Treatment. Treatment for allergic acute glossitis calls for immediate systemic epinephrine, intravenous fluids, and systemic steroids. Airway obstruction is not an uncommon complication with this entity.

Bacterial acute glossitis should be treated with intravenous antibiotics. Observation for airway obstruction again is indicated.

ACUTE PHARYNGITIS

Acute pharyngitis is a relatively common entity characterized by oral pain, fever and chills, otalgia, cervical adenitis, and oropharyngeal mucosal erythema and edema, with or without membrane involvement.

A number of infections are grouped together under the title "acute pharyngitis." This includes the nonmembranous types such as Streptococcus, Pneumococcus, influenzal, and viral, as well as the membranous types such as follicular tonsillitis, Vincent's angina, infectious mononucleosis, diphtheria, and fungal pharyngitis.

Diagnosis of acute pharyngitis generally is not difficult in the light of its obvious symptoms. Acute pharyngitis may be a symptom, rather than an isolated entity. For this reason, some further diagnostic tests may be indicated. These should include mononucleosis spot test, throat culture, gram and fungal stains, CBC, and possibly chest x-ray.

Treatment. This should be in accordance with the etiologic type of pharyngitis present. An antibiotic is prescribed if indicated by the culture results, or if the clinical condition is such that a delay while these results are awaited might be dangerous. Warm oral saline irrigation of the inflamed area aids significantly both in the comfort of the patient and in the cleansing of the infected area.

ACUTE TONSILLITIS

Acute tonsillitis is easily recognizable, as there is visible erythema and edema of the tonsillar tissue, with an accumulation of debris entrapped in the tonsillar crypts. The patient complains of dysphagia and may experience chills. Fever and cervical lymphadenitis are common.

The usual bacteria that cause tonsillitis are Streptococcus, *Staphylococcus aureus*, *Hemophilus influenzae*, and Pneumococcus. Tonsillitis also may be the result of a viral infection.

As with acute pharyngitis, diagnostic studies should include a throat culture, gram stain, CBC, mononucleosis spot test, and chest x-ray.

Treatment. This should be in accordance with the age of the patient and the results of the gram stain and culture findings. Antibiotic therapy initially should be parenteral, followed by a full oral course. Irrigation of the inflamed area with warm saline solution will add to the patient's comfort.

PERITONSILLAR ABSCESS

Peritonsillar abscess is a complication of untreated or inadequately treated tonsillitis. It generally is unilateral, with the tonsil medially displaced to the midline; however, 20 per cent of patients have bilateral involvement. There is marked edema and erythema of the tonsil, pillars, and ipsilateral soft palate. The patient experiences odynophagia, dysphagia, intense local pain, and referred otalgia. A high fever, chills, prostration, severe trismus, and painful cervical lymphadenitis also characterize this entity. Peritonsillar abscess is uncommon in children, and is rarely seen in patients under 10 years of age.

Necessary studies are a culture and gram stain of tonsillar exudate, a WBC with differential, and a chest x-ray.

When an abscess forms, it usually is necessary to drain it through an incision. This should be done by an otolaryngologist, in view of the serious potential complications, including aspiration and airway obstruction. Oral hot saline douches will aid in the comfort of the patient while parenteral antibiotics are taking effect. Since the swelling interferes with swallowing, intravenous feedings may be indicated.

LARYNX AND UPPER AIRWAY

ANGIONEUROTIC EDEMA

Angioneurotic edema is the manifestation of an allergy or of other hypersensitivity phenomena. It is characterized by a diffuse, rapidly progressive, pale mucosal edema of the laryngotrachea that also may involve the tongue. The patient will experience light-headedness and shortness of breath, wheezing, and inspiratory or expiratory stridor. The upright position will be the most comfortable.

If the clinical situation allows, chest and lateral neck x-rays, a complete blood count, eosinophil count, BUN, creatinine analysis, and a throat culture are indicated.

Upper airway obstruction may occur rapidly in these patients.

Treatment. Because of the danger of airway obstruction, this should commence with immediate hospitalization of the patient. Subcutaneous epinephrine, systemic steroids, and antibiotics (if bacterial etiology is suspected) should be prescribed. Intravenous fluid supplementation often is indicated. The use of a mist tent may be required. A tracheostomy set-up should be at the bedside in case of acute airway obstruction. The physician should rule out ingestion or inhalation of a foreign body, and the presence of laryngeal tumor, before making the diagnosis of angioneurotic edema.

EPIGLOTTITIS

Epiglottitis is viewed carefully through indirect mirror examination as a markedly swollen, erythematous epiglottis that sometimes is visible above the level of the base of the tongue. The most common bacterial organism cultured is *Hemophilus influenzae.* In adults, *Staphylococcus aureus* and Streptococcus also are frequently cultured. Occasionally, the bulbous epiglottis can be seen on direct examination.

The patient, often a child, will be very apprehensive, with a sense of fullness in the throat. History will reveal rapidly progressive dysphagia, progressive upper airway obstruction, and a very painful throat. The patient may insist on sitting up with the head extended and may experience fever, chills, and cervical adenopathy.

Since tracheotomy often is needed to relieve this serious airway obstruction, careful observation and rapid treatment are mandatory. Borderline airways are treated effectively by the temporary use of an endotracheal tube for 24 to 48 hours.

Treatment. As previously mentioned, this should be immediate. Intravenous antibiotics (ampicillin or tetracycline) and systemic steroids (Decadron) definitely are in order. Other supportive measures, such as oxygen, mist tent, and intravenous fluids, also are important. Since acute airway obstruction is a complication, a tracheostomy set-up should be at the patient's bedside. Sedation is not recommended until the patient's airway status is controlled.

LARYNGOTRACHEITIS

Laryngotracheitis, or "croup" as it is commonly called, is progressive subglottic edema with a viral or bacterial etiology. This entity is more frequent than epiglottitis. The patient presents with progressive dyspnea, hoarseness, difficulty in swallowing, and explosive bouts of sharp, barklike coughing. Inspiratory stridor, expiratory wheezing, supra- and substernal retractions, poor appetite, fever, chills, and a recent upper respiratory infection are additional symptoms and signs of laryngotracheitis. Severe cases are life-threatening.

Studies to confirm the diagnosis of croup should include a CBC, blood gases, chest x-ray, soft tissue x-rays of the upper airway, throat, and sputum, blood cultures, and gram stain.

Treatment. This necessitates constant and vigilant attendance by a physician. Careful monitoring of vital signs, blood gases, and difficulty with breathing is mandatory.

The patient should be placed in a steam room or mist tent with oxygen. He should be given fluids and Decadron and ampicillin intravenously. The Decadron is repeated every three hours for 12 hours if there is improvement. Possible airway obstruction requires that a tracheostomy kit be kept at the patient's bedside.

A gradual but progressive betterment in the patient's breathing and a decreasing pulse rate are the most important signs of improvement.

ACUTE LARYNGEAL STENOSIS

Acute laryngeal stenosis may occur following endoscopy, intubation, or any surgical procedure involved with the intrinsic larynx or its supporting cartilaginous structures.

Proper management is of utmost importance. The respiratory, phonatory, and deglutitory disabilities following laryngeal trauma frequently persist to the chronic stage.

Initial Treatment. This is dependent on the status of the airway. The necessity for an immediate tracheotomy should be obvious. A rapid evaluation of the patient will distinguish between obstruction at and above the larynx. With obstruction above the larynx, the stridor is of low pitch, and the patient's cheeks are retracted during attempted inspiration and blown out during expiration. The stridor at the laryngeal level is high-pitched (squeak). There may be suprasternal retraction during inspiration. The airway is re-established by inserting an endotracheal tube or performing a tracheotomy. Artificial respiration may be required.

Any one or all of the laryngeal functions can be disturbed. Usually, respiratory and phonatory functions are disturbed simultaneously. Deglutitory complications are manifested by aspiration, dysphagia, or odynophagia. Local pain may occur following laryngeal injury, especially during speaking or swallowing, and can be referred to the region of the ears (otalgia).

An accurate assessment of the phonatory and respiratory functions of the larynx can be accomplished readily by simply listening to the patient's speech and to quiet respiration with his mouth open. Laryngeal edema may cause the patient to swallow frequently. Observation will disclose disturbances of deglutition and the presence of aspiration.

If the patient is in no immediate respiratory distress, indirect laryngoscopy may be possible. During this examination, the following are assessed: the amount and location of laryngeal edema; the amount and degree of ecchymosis and/or hematoma; narrowing of the subglottic airway; decrease in or loss of laryngeal function; and asymmetry or a deviation of the vocal chink from its normal anteroposterior direction.

Radiographic evaluation of the larynx is essential prior to any definitive investigation or therapy. Routine anteroposterior and lateral neck x-rays often are of value, and may indicate an abnormality in the upper airway column. If, for some reason, indirect laryngoscopy cannot be undertaken, fluoroscopy will be helpful in evaluating the laryngeal function.

Direct laryngoscopy performed in the immediate period following the injury is hazardous, and usually adds little to the information obtained from indirect laryngoscopy and radiographic evaluation.

At times, it is difficult to decide whether to perform a tracheotomy, especially when subcutaneous emphysema is present and laryngeal functions appear to be normal. Careful observation certainly is not out of order, provided that emphysema is not increasing rapidly and the patient is not coughing frequently. A tracheotomy should be performed when subcutaneous emphysema and a large laceration within the larynx are present.

Treatment. The patient is put on complete bed rest and complete voice rest in a room with high humidity. Oxygen is administered as needed. Antibiotic therapy usually is indicated, except possibly when internal lacerations, subcutaneous emphysema, and hematomas are not present. Steroid therapy in maximum dosage should be instituted immediately. This has been shown to be of great value for rapid resolution of edema, which is at its maximum six hours following injury. The steroids slow formation of granulation tissue, reduce the degree of fibrosis, and are said to reverse the neuromuscular complications more rapidly than when they are not administered.

CAUSTIC INGESTION

Acid or alkali ingestion is common in children and in persons attempting suicide. Vesicles, degranulation and erythema of the lips, and oral, posterior pharyngeal and nasopharyngeal mucosa characterize this extremely painful entity. The patient coughs, drools, and has severe dysphagia and possible airway obstructive symptoms. There may be a fever and chills.

Careful history and examination will make this condition easily recognizable. Chest x-ray, CBC, and electrolyte determinations will aid in evaluating the extent of the damage.

TREATMENT

This should begin with immediate transfer of the patient to an intensive care unit. Antibiotics, and steroids (triamcinolone diacetate) should be administered intravenously immediately. Prompt attention should be paid to the airway. A nasogastric tube should be inserted carefully; stomach lavage may be indicated in accordance with the time of ingestion and the agent swallowed. Do *not* induce vomiting. The need for esophagoscopy at the proper time necessitates early otolaryngologic consultation.

SPACE INFECTIONS OF THE HEAD AND NECK

Space infections of the head and neck have markedly declined in frequency owing to the early and judicious use of antibiotics. The results of antibiotic therapy, however, can be misleading since a space infection may be suppressed but not eliminated. The facial space is subdivided into the canine, buccal, and mental spaces. Neck space infections are superficial or deep. Examples of deep space infections are retropharyngeal, prevertebral, pericarotid, pharyngomaxillary, submandibular, retromandibular, masticator, temporal, parotid, and peritonsillar spaces.

Dental disease is the cause of about 35 per cent of space infections in the head and neck; pharyngeal disease accounts for 40 per cent, and other sources, such as otologic disease and dermatologic disorders, for 25 per cent.

Space abscess formation requires drainage if the clinical response indicates continued sepsis after five days of antibiotic therapy. Indications of continued infection are low grade fever, fever spikes, sweats, persistent leukocytosis, trismus, torticollis, rigidity, persistent dysphagia, odynophagia, hoarseness, or CNS complications. Failure of adequate drainage can result in the erosion of the internal and external carotid vessels, jugular vein thrombosis, septicemia, and CNS complications.

Chapter 46

Chapter 46 # ENDOCRINOLOGIC EMERGENCIES

A. Diabetic Ketoacidosis and Hyperglycemic Hyperosmolar States
B. Hypoglycemia
C. Selected Emergency Endocrinologic Problems
D. Porphyrias
E. Pheochromocytoma

A. DIABETIC KETOACIDOSIS AND HYPERGLYCEMIC HYPEROSMOLAR STATES

John K. Davidson

INTRODUCTION

The death rate for uncomplicated severe diabetic ketoacidosis ($CO_2 < 10$ mEq./liter) is about 1 per cent, and for complicated severe diabetic ketoacidosis (i.e., that associated with overwhelming infection, renal failure, myocardial infarction, stroke, etc.) it is over 10 per cent. The death rate for the less common hyperglycemic hyperosmolar coma state is even higher. All of these conditions are bona fide medical emergencies that require immediate recognition and prompt, optimal therapy. An understanding of the pathogenesis in each case facilitates data collection (history, physical, laboratory) and planning for initial and follow-up therapy.

PATHOGENESIS

Table 1 outlines the pathogenesis of acutely decompensated diabetes mellitus as it may occur in a hypothetic 80 kg. adult. In the wake of an insulin deficit, substrate catabolism accelerates and substrate anabolism decelerates. Glucose production increases and the plasma glucose level rises; fatty acid release and ketone production increase, and the H^+ ion level rises accordingly.

The *rising plasma glucose level increases serum osmolality* (each 100 mg./dl. increase above normal in plasma glucose can increase serum osmolality by 5.5 mOsm./liter; see Table 3, *A*) and this in turn causes water to migrate from the intracellular to the extracellular compartment (the Donnan equilibrium requires that intracellular and extracellular osmolality be balanced, see Tables 2*A* and 2*B*). This initial migration of water from the intracellular to the extracellular compartment may account for dilutional hyponatremia (i.e., a plasma glucose

of 650 mg./dl. increases serum osmolality by 30 mOsm./liter and can account for a lowering of the serum Na^+ from 139.5 mEq./liter to 111.5 mEq./liter). The body tries to compensate for the hyperosmolar state by increased water intake (thirst) and by excretion of excess glucose by osmotic diuresis (kidney). Depending on the relative amount of water lost as compared to solute, the result could be isotonic, hypotonic, or hypertonic volume contraction. Because of the hypovolemia, renal plasma flow and glomerular filtration decrease, and BUN and uric acid typically rise out of proportion to creatinine; oliguria and acute renal failure may further complicate diabetic acidosis.

The body tries to compensate for the increasing H^+ ion level by hyperventilation to lower P_{CO_2} (lungs); by buffering the excess H^+ ions with bicarbonate and other buffering mechanisms (buffers, see Table 3, *B* and *C*); and by excreting more H^+ ions as free acid, titratable acidity, and NH_3 buffered ketone salts (kidney). Triglycerides and cholesterol may accumulate in the plasma compartment, and can displace plasma water and account for a spuriously low serum sodium (lipid content of plasma can rise as high as 5 per cent, and the measured serum sodium thus decreases spuriously). Electrolytes, especially Na^+ and K^+, are lost in large amounts with the osmotic diuresis. As the H^+ ion production increases, the buffer-kidney-lung compensatory mechanisms are progressively depleted, and the effects of the acidosis become more evident and ominous. The end-result of these events, if uninterrupted by appropriate therapy, is severe diabetic ketoacidosis and death.

Acutely decompensated diabetes mellitus varies from mild to moderate to severe. The pathogenic spectrum ranges from pure hyperglycemia without ketosis, to mixed hyperglycemia and ketoacidosis, to almost pure ketoacidosis with insignificant hyperglycemia. The latter occurs in association with protein and carbohydrate substrate deficits.

An audit at Grady Memorial Hospital from mid-1973 to mid-1975 of over 1000 cases of acutely decompensated diabetes mellitus revealed that about 67 per cent had mild (total CO_2 content > 20 mEq./liter) or moderate (total CO_2 content = 10 to 20 mEq./liter) ketoacidosis; about 25 per cent had severe ketoacidosis (CO_2 < 10 mEq./liter and serum osmolality < 350 mOsm./liter); about 2 per cent had a pure hyperglycemic hyperosmolar state (serum osmolality > 350 mOsm./liter without ketonemia or ketonuria); and about 1 per cent had almost pure severe diabetic ketoacidosis (CO_2 < 10 mEq./liter, glucose < 150 mg./dl.).

A thorough understanding of the pathogenesis of each case facilitates the planning of therapy so that metabolic homeostasis can be promptly re-established by replacing insulin, water, electrolyte, and substrate (i.e., glucose) deficits as needed.

DATA BASE AND ASSESSMENT

In the Emergency Department an *abbreviated data base* should be collected and a preliminary assessment made as quickly as possible (usually within ten minutes). The patient may or may not be comatose. Acutely decompensated diabetes mellitus usually can be recognized promptly, as outlined in Tables 4 and 5. Hypoglycemia, intoxications by beverages, drugs, or poisons, and other causes of coma and/or metabolic acidosis should be excluded.

TREATMENT PLAN

If the patient is comatose or has a plasma glucose > 500 mg./dl. and/or ketonemia or moderate to large ketonuria, he should be transferred to an Intensive Care Area with intravenous 0.9 per cent NaCl running in less than 30 minutes after arriving in the Emergency Department. The admitting treatment team should promptly collect a *defined data base*, such as that shown in Table 5, and should initiate insulin therapy either en route to or immediately upon arrival in the Intensive Care Area (Table 6).

A flow sheet (Table 7) should be maintained until the patient has completely recovered.

As early as possible in the course of therapy, the factor (or factors) that precipitated the acutely decompensated diabetes should be identified (Table 8). Complications (Table 9) should be noted and appropriately treated. Side-effects of therapy (Table 10) should be prevented if possible, or treated promptly.

Table 11 contains a list of the equipment and supplies needed to optimally diagnose and treat acutely decompensated diabetes mellitus. Equally important to optimal diagnosis and treatment is a well-trained team of professionals (M.D., R.N., R.D., and laboratory technician) who monitor the patient's progress continuously and who are capable of appropriately modifying standard therapy so as to avoid or minimize side-effects and/or complications.

EDUCATION AND POSTDISCHARGE FOLLOW-UP

Prior to the patient's discharge, he and his family should be educated in depth concerning the nature of diabetes and its acute and chronic complications. They should understand the manner of measuring and administering insulin, and should realize the importance of and be thoroughly knowledgeable concerning the manner of continuing optimal diet therapy. The patient should be followed at frequent intervals by persons conversant with diabetes. Education and appropriate behavior modification must be continued, and the diabetes must be regulated as carefully as possible.

THERAPY*

General

Optimally the patient should arrive in the Intensive Care Area within 30 minutes after arrival in the Emergency Department. Patients who are in coma or shock, who are hypotensive, or who have severe ketoacidosis or a hyperglycemic hyperosmolar state

Text continued on page 1073

---

*See outline, Table 6.

TABLE 1 Pathogenesis of Acutely Decompensated Diabetes Mellitus (Hypothetic 80 Kg. Adult)

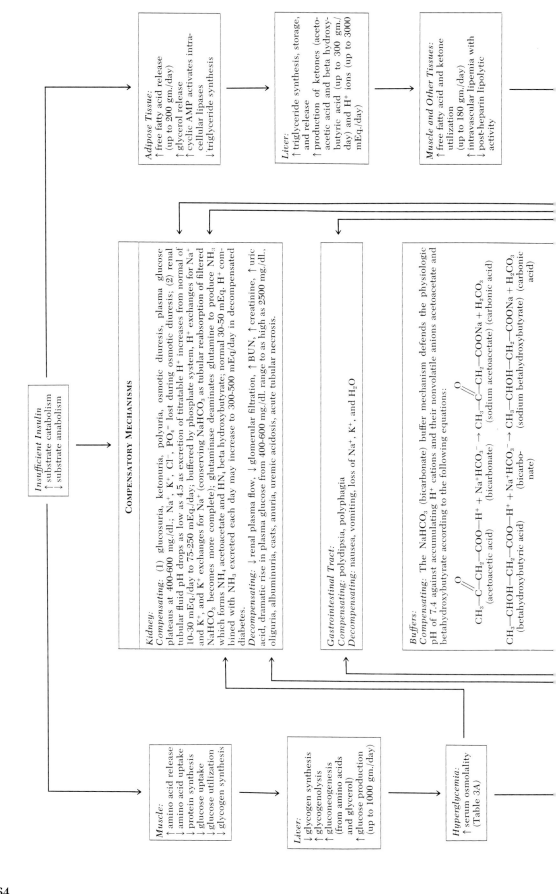

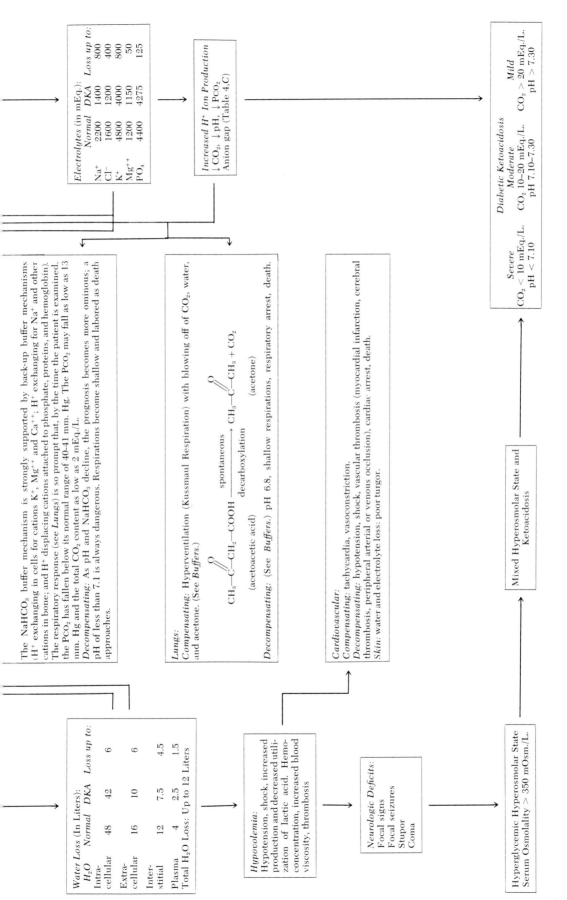

Electrolytes (in mEq.):

	Normal	DKA	Loss up to:
Na^+	2200	1400	800
Cl^-	1600	1200	400
K^+	4800	4000	800
Mg^{++}	1200	1150	50
PO_4	4400	4275	125

Increased H^+ Ion Production
$\downarrow CO_2$, $\downarrow pH$, $\downarrow Pco_2$
Anion gap (Table 4,C)

The $NaHCO_3$ buffer mechanism is strongly supported by back-up buffer mechanisms (H^+ exchanging in cells for cations K^+, Mg^{++} and Ca^{++}; H^+ exchanging for Na^+ and other cations in bone; and H^+ displacing cations attached to phosphate, proteins, and hemoglobin). The respiratory response (see *Lungs*) is so prompt that, by the time the patient is examined, the Pco_2 has fallen below its normal range of 40-41 mm. Hg. The Pco_2 may fall as low as 13 mm. Hg and the total CO_2 content as low as 2 mEq./L.
Decompensating: As pH and $NaHCO_3$ decline, the prognosis becomes more ominous; a pH of less than 7.1 is always dangerous. Respirations become shallow and labored as death approaches.

Lungs:
Compensating: Hyperventilation (Kussmaul Respiration) with blowing off of CO_2, water, and acetone. (See *Buffers.*)

$$CH_3-C(=O)-CH_2-COOH \xrightarrow[\text{decarboxylation}]{\text{spontaneous}} CH_3-C(=O)-CH_3 + CO_2$$

(acetoacetic acid) (acetone)

Decompensating: (See *Buffers.*) pH 6.8, shallow respirations, respiratory arrest, death.

Cardiovascular:
Compensating: tachycardia, vasoconstriction.
Decompensating: hypotension, shock, vascular thrombosis (myocardial infarction, cerebral thrombosis, peripheral arterial or venous occlusion), cardiac arrest, death.
Skin: water and electrolyte loss: poor turgor.

Mixed Hyperosmolar State and Ketoacidosis

Diabetic Ketoacidosis

Severe	*Moderate*	*Mild*
$CO_2 < 10$ mEq./L.	CO_2 10–20 mEq./L.	$CO_2 > 20$ mEq./L.
pH < 7.10	pH 7.10–7.30	pH > 7.30

Water Loss (In Liters):

H_2O	Normal	DKA	Loss up to:
Intracellular	48	42	6
Extracellular	16	10	6
Interstitial	12	7.5	4.5
Plasma	4	2.5	1.5

Total H_2O Loss: Up to 12 Liters

Hypovolemia:
Hypotension, shock, increased production and decreased utilization of lactic acid. Hemoconcentration, increased blood viscosity, thrombosis

Neurologic Deficits:
Focal signs
Focal seizures
Stupor
Coma

Hyperglycemic Hyperosmolar State
Serum Osmolality > 350 mOsm./L.

Cations	MEq.	MOsm.	Anions	MEq.	MOsm.
K^+	150°	150	Cl^-	15	15
Na^+	10	10	HCO_3^-	10	10
Mg^{++}	40	20	PO_4^-, $PO_4^=$, and $SO_4^=$	140	94.5
			Protein	35	5
Total	200	180		200	124.5

°Dependent on specific tissue analyzed.

TABLE 2B   Extracellular Electrolytes

In Serum (93% of Water Phase of Serum)						In Water Phase of Serum					
Cations	MEq.	MOsm.	Anions	MEq.	MOsm.	Cations	MEq.	MOsm.	Anions	MEq.	MOsm.
Na^+	139.5	139.5	Cl^-	102.3	102.3	Na^+	150	150	Cl^-	110	110
K^+	3.7	3.7	HCO_3^-	25.1	25.1	K^+	4	4	HCO_3^-	27	27
Ca^{++}	2.8	2.4	$PO_4^=$	1.9	1.0	Ca^{++}	5	2.5	$PO_4^=$	2	1
Mg^{++}	2.8	1.4	$SO_4^=$	1.0	0.5	Mg^{++}	3	1.5	$SO_4^=$	1	0.5
			Protein	14.9	2.0				Protein	16	2
			Organic acid	5.6	5.6				Organic acid	6	6
Total	148.8	147.0		150.8	136.5		162	158		162	146.5

Normal osmolality in intracellular water compartment: cations + anions = 180 + 124.5 = 304.5 mOsm.
Normal osmolality in the water phase of serum: cations + anions = 158 + 146.5 = 304.5 mOsm.
Intracellular water osmolality (304.5 mOsm.) = extracellular water osmolality (304.5 mOsm.).

TABLE 3   How to Calculate Serum Osmolality, pH, and Anion Gap

(A) To Calculate Serum Osmolality:
Normal: $2[Na^+ + K^+] + [glucose\ (mg./dl.)/18] + [BUN/2.8] = 285–305$ mOsm.
Example: $2[139.5 + 3.7] + [90/18] + [12/2.8] = 295.7$ mOsm.
Abnormal   (Hyperglycemic hyperosmolar state):
$2[Na^+ + K^+] + [glucose\ (mg./dl.)/18] + [BUN/2.8] > 350$ mOsm.
Example: $2[138 + 5.3] + [1080/18] + [60/2.8] = 368.0$ mOsm.

Measured serum osmolality (osmometer) may be 10-30 mOsm. higher than calculated serum osmolality, because some of the measured osmotically active particles are not calculated in the above formula.

(B) Henderson–Hasselbalch Equation:
$$pH = 6.10 + \log \frac{Na^+\ (HCO_3^-)}{dissolved\ CO_2 + H_2CO_3}$$

HCO_3^- is measured as CO_2 content. Dissolved $CO_2 + H_2CO_3$ may be calculated by measuring P_{CO_2} in mm. Hg and converting to mEq./L. of H_2CO_3 by multiplying P_{CO_2} (in mm. Hg) by 0.03.

Normal: $pH = 6.10 + \log \dfrac{CO_2\ content\ (mEq./L.)}{P_{CO_2}\ (mm.\ Hg) \times 0.03}$

$$= 6.10 + \log \frac{24\ mEq./L.}{40 \times .03}$$

$$= 6.10 + \log \frac{20}{1} = 6.10 + 1.30 = 7.40$$

Abnormal   (In severe diabetic ketoacidosis, the following may occur):

$$pH = 6.10 + \log \frac{2\ mEq./L.}{13 \times .03}$$

$$= 6.10 + \log \frac{5}{1} = 6.10 + 0.70 = 6.80$$

(C) To Calculate Anion Gap:
Normal: $[Na^+ + K^+] - [Cl^- + HCO_3^-] = 16 \pm 7$ (unmeasured anions)
Example: $[139.5 + 3.7] - [102.1 + 25.1] = 16$
Abnormal   (As may occur in diabetic ketoacidosis because of accumulation of acetoacetate and betahydroxybutyrate):
Example: $[139.5 + 3.7] - [100 + 5] = 38.2$ mEq. The *anion gap* is 38.2 mEq.

Collect *abbreviated data base* as quickly as possible (usually within ten minutes) consisting of immediately relevant subjective and objective data (see Table 5). In the *comatose* patient, maintain a *patent airway*; in the patient in *shock*, start intravenous infusion of *isotonic saline* immediately. Stat plasma glucose (preferably by the Beckman oxygen rate method) and serially diluted plasma ketones (preferably by the Denco "Acetone test") will confirm the diagnosis of decompensated diabetes mellitus (or hypoglycemia*) in a few minutes. If available *without catheterization*, quantitative urine glucose and ketones should be measured by the same methods.

If plasma glucose is <50 mg./dl. and patient is unable to swallow, give stat. 50 ml. 50 per cent glucose I.V. or 1 mg. glucagon I.M.

If plasma glucose is <50 mg./dl. and patient is able to swallow, give Coke, sweetened orange juice, or candy per os.

If plasma glucose is >50 mg./dl. and no ketonemia or ketonuria, or if plasma glucose >150 mg./dl. and moderate-to-large ketonuria and/or ketonemia, collect *venous* blood (red top tube) for SMA/6 (Na$^+$, K$^+$, CO$_2$, Cl$^-$, BUN, glucose), *venous* blood (in plastic syringe wet with heparin, rotate syringe, bend needle, place syringe on cracked ice) for pH† and *venous* blood (red top tube) for measurement of serum osmolality (osmometer).

Transfer all patients with acutely decompensated diabetes mellitus to an Intensive Care Area with intravenous isotonic saline running. This should be accomplished as soon as possible (usually within 30 minutes after arrival at the Emergency Department).

When laboratory data become available, *classify* acutely decompensated diabetes mellitus as *severe, moderate,* or *mild ketoacidosis* or *hyperglycemic hyperosmolar state* (see Table 5, Assessment).

In patients who are *comatose,* or who have *metabolic acidosis,* the following problems should be considered in the differential diagnosis:

(1) INTOXICATIONS
   A, *Beverages*
     1. Ethanol
       a, Hypoglycemia (with or without ketonuria).
       b, Alcoholic ketoacidosis (uncommon, history of protracted vomiting, prolonged abstention from food, chronic alcoholism, appreciable alcohol intake before admission, blood ethanol may be 50–500 mg./dl., ketonemia, frequent lactic acidemia, plasma glucose <150 mg./dl.).
       c, Without hypoglycemia or metabolic acidosis.
     2. Methanol (formaldehyde, formic acid, metabolic acidosis).
     3. Isopropyl alcohol (transient ketonuria, no acidosis).
     4. Smoke (hypoglycemia).
     5. Antifreeze (ethylene and diethylene glycol metabolized to oxalate, metabolic acidosis).
   B, *Drugs*
     1. Salicylates (plasma salicylate level >30 mg./dl., respiratory alkalosis with renal bicarbonate loss, hyponatremia, ketoacidosis, dehydration).
     2. Paraldehyde (characteristic odor, metabolic acidosis).
     3. Barbiturates.
     4. Opiates.
     5. Bromide.
     6. Chloral hydrate (metabolic acidosis, respiratory depression, acute hepatic necrosis).
     7. Other sedatives.
   C, *Poisons*
     1. Phenol and other cresols (white burns of mouth).
     2. Fluoride (tetany, hyperglycemia unresponsive to insulin).
     3. Milk sickness (from ingestion of milk or meat of animals poisoned by snakeroot, richweed, or rayless goldenrod; hypoglycemia, acidosis, ketonuria).

(2) OTHER CAUSES OF METABOLIC ACIDOSIS
   A, Lactic acidosis (anion gap otherwise unaccounted for, may be due to phenformin poisoning or shock; draw venous blood *without stasis*, allow it to clot, then separate and freeze serum until assayed for lactate and pyruvate; normal lactate 3.5–12.5 mg./dl. or 0.4–1.4 mEq./L.; normal pyruvate 0.6–1.2 mg./dl. or 0.07–0.14 mEq./L.; in lactic acidosis serum lactate is ≥63 mg./dl. or ≥7 mEq./L.
   B, Uremic acidosis (anion gap otherwise unaccounted for, elevated BUN, creatinine).

(3) OTHER CAUSES OF COMA
   A, Hypernatremia, hypercalcemia, hypoxia, hepatic coma, myxedema coma, adrenal cortical insufficiency.
   B, Severe systemic infection (pneumonia, gram-negative septicemia, typhoid, malaria, meningococcemia).
   C, Shock from any cause, cardiac failure (either may be associated with lactic acidosis).
   D, Hypertensive encephalopathy, eclampsia.
   E, Marked hyperthermia or hypothermia.
   F, Brain hemorrhage, thrombosis, embolism, or abscess.
   G, Epidural or subdural hemorrhage, brain contusion, subarachnoid hemorrhage.
   H, Brain tumor, acute bacterial meningitis, viral encephalitis, epileptic seizure.

(4) KETONURIA DUE TO STARVATION KETOSIS
This is common in individuals who are ingesting less than 100 gm. carbohydrate daily. It rarely, if ever, accounts for significant ketonemia or metabolic acidosis.

---

*See Hypoglycemia, page 1075.
†Venous pH closely approximates arterial pH in this setting.

TABLE 5   *Problem Statement: Acutely Decompensated Diabetes Mellitus (Subsets: Severe, Moderate, or Mild Diabetic Ketoacidosis; Hyperglycemic Hyperosmolar State)*

RECOGNITION (DEFINED DATA BASE):

SUBJECTIVE (HISTORY): *(a)*, known diabetes mellitus, previous episodes of acutely decompensated diabetes mellitus, insulin dose and type, missed insulin, diet prescription, gross dietary indiscretion, obesity, weight loss or gain, family history of diabetes mellitus; *(b)*, polyuria, glucosuria, ketonuria; *(c)*, thirst, polydipsia, polyphagia, vomiting, nausea, anorexia, abdominal pain; *(d)*, coma, stupor, drowsiness, listlessness, weakness; *(e)*, rapid breathing, shortness of breath, chest pain; *(f)*, shock, fever, infection, pregnancy, thyrotoxicosis, surgery, trauma, anesthesia; *(g)*, beverage (especially ethanol) or drug abuse, poisoning, medications (steroids, sulfonyluria, phenformin), emotional upset.

OBJECTIVE: (1) PHYSICAL EXAMINATION: coma, stupor, poor skin turgor, weak rapid pulse, hypothermia or hyperthermia, reclining and/or orthostatic hypotension, neck veins, dry dirty mouth and tongue, fruity odor of breath, rapid deep respirations (becoming shallow when death approaches), soft eyeballs, dilated pupils, lipemia retinalis, diabetic retinopathy, lung rales, pleural friction rub, abdominal tenderness, abdominal distention (dilated stomach), flaccid muscles, weak or absent tendon reflexes, skin or other infection, height, frame, body weight; (2) LABORATORY DATA: glucosuria, ketonuria (acetoacetic aciduria), possibly albuminuria and/or pyuria, hyperglycemia, ketonemia (acetoacetic acidemia: serially diluted plasma), decreased venous pH (avoid arterial puncture), decreased total CO_2 content, decreased P_{CO_2}, increased serum osmolality (measured, calculated), increased BUN and uric acid, elevated triglycerides, cholesterol, and fatty acids, abnormal (Fredrickson) lipoprotein typing (usually type V, IV, or III), leukocytosis, increased hematocrit, serum sodium, potassium, and chloride, plasma lactate and pyruvate, serum magnesium and calcium, amylase, bilirubin, EKG, chest x-ray.

ASSESSMENT: *(a)* severe diabetic ketoacidosis: $CO_2 < 10$ mEq./L. and/or venous plasma pH < 7.10; *(b)* moderate diabetic ketoacidosis: CO_2 10–20 mEq./L. and/or pH 7.10–7.30; *(c)* mild diabetic ketoacidosis: $CO_2 >$ mEq./L. and/or pH > 7.30; *(d)* hyperglycemic hyperosmolar state: osmolality > 350 mOsm./L. due primarily to hyperglycemia without ketonemia or ketonuria. Search for *concurrent problems:* infection, GI bleeding, acute myocardial infarction, congestive heart failure, arterial or venous thrombosis, uremic acidosis, lactic acidosis. Rule out other causes of *coma* and/or *metabolic acidosis* (see Table 4).

TABLE 6   Outline of Therapy of Acutely Decompensated Diabetes Mellitus*

A, FOR PATIENTS IN:

(a) Shock
(b) Coma
(c) Hypotension
(d) Severe ketoacidosis
(e) Hyperglycemic,
    Hyperosmolar state

BEGIN:

1. I.V. isotonic saline
2. Initiate insulin immediately
3. Maintain airway, give O$_2$
4. Urinary catheter if needed
5. NG tube if needed
6. Monitor continuously: cardiac monitor; hourly glucose; hourly potassium
7. CVP if needed

BEWARE OF: Congestive heart failure
Pulmonary edema
Cardiac or respiratory arrest
Hypokalemia, Hyperkalemia
Cerebral edema with deepening coma

B, USE OF INSULIN:

Unless insulin-resistant, use U-100 regular insulin. Dose must be individualized owing to possible wide range needed; however, average doses are:

Severe Ketoacidosis: 550 units in first 24 hr.
Moderate Ketoacidosis: 150 units in first 24 hr.

DETERMINE DOSE BY:
Rate of decline of blood glucose (hourly values of glucose). When value reaches 100–200 mg./dl., begin 5 per cent dextrose solution.
Clearing of ketonemia and ketonuria (hourly ketones).

METHODS OF ADMINISTRATION: (In severe cases, for adults, since children may need much less, dependent on body weight and response)
I.V. Infusion   3–12 units per hour
I.V. Bolus   100 units per hour [Method at Grady Memorial Hospital]
Intramuscular
Subcutaneous   (Avoid in dehydrated or hypotensive)

IN MILD OR MODERATE KETOACIDOSIS:
1. 25 to 50 units subcutaneously of U-100 regular insulin repeated every 1–3 hours until glucose falls to 100–200 mg./dl. and ketosis has cleared.
2. Oral liquids and food every 1–2 hours.
3. Use intermediate (NPH or lente) insulin when glucose falls to 100–200 mg./dl.

C, FLUIDS AND ELECTROLYTES

In severe ketoacidosis or hyperosmolar coma

FLUIDS

1. Initially start 0.9 per cent sodium chloride solution. If osmolality >350mOsm./L., next infusion should be with 0.45 NaCl.
2. If pH <7.10 use bicarbonate up to 166 mEq. (more needed if lactic acidosis).
   CAVEAT: Beware metabolic alkalosis with hypokalemia.
3. *Potassium:* Begin to replace with 2nd infusion— replace up to 20–40 mEq. per hour as long as urine flow is >40 ml./hour and there is no evidence of hyperkalemia.
   Replace half the potassium deficit (but no more than 400 mEq. potassium) in first 24 hours, then use oral route.
   CAVEAT: Watch for hypokalemia, renal failure, fluid overload.

Not usually necessary to replace magnesium and/or phosphate deficits.

In mild or moderate ketoacidosis

Give oral fluids with sodium chloride and potassium hourly, or more frequently if tolerated.

WHILE THERAPY IS PROCEEDING, TEST AND EXAMINE FOR:
(1) Infection—Check urine, sputum, blood, and skin (take suitable cultures). Sometimes dehydrated patients do not become febrile and pulmonary rales do not appear until rehydration has occurred.
(2) Take repeat chest x-ray even if initial x-ray is clear.
(3) Check for other causes of coma or acidosis, and evaluate for any other concurrent illness (Tables 4 and 5).

*See text for details.

TABLE 7, A   Diabetes Flow Sheet (Grady Memorial Hospital, Atlanta, Georgia)

Patient Identification:

DATE / /		PHYSICAL EXAM				URINE			PLASMA (1)			PLASMA (2)		SERUM							THERAPY H$_2$O (Liters) and SOLUTES (mEq.)					
HR	ECG	WT	T	P	R	BP	VOL	ACE	GLU	ACE	GLU	BUN	pH	pCO$_2$	Na	K	Cl	CO$_2$	MEAS mOsm	CALC mOsm	REG INS	H$_2$O	Na	K	Cl	HCO$_3$	GLU

TABLE 7, B   Diabetes Flow Sheet, Monitoring Schedule, and Therapeutic Indications*

EKG: Record every hour for first six hours from fixed monitoring V_2–V_3 electrode, then at indicated intervals thereafter.

Body Weight: Record initially, and at indicated intervals thereafter.

T. P. R. BP: Record every hour.

Urine Volume: Measure in polyethylene graduated cylinder, and record at hourly intervals.

Urine Acetone (Acetest or Ketostix) and *Urine Glucose* (Clinitest): Record at hourly intervals

Plasma Acetone, Glucose, and *Bun:* Determine initially, one hour later, then as indicated.
    Requires 5 ml. venous blood in gray top tube. At bedside, determine the highest serial dilution that is positive for acetone (undil., 1/2, 1/4, 1/8, 1/16).

Plasma pH, and *PCO_2:* Determine initially, one hour later, then as indicated. Collect 5 ml. venous blood in a plastic syringe that has been wet with heparin, rotate the syringe, bend the needle, place the syringe on cracked ice, and send immediately to the central laboratory.

Serum Na, K, Cl, CO_2, and *Measured Serum Osmolality;* Determine initially, one hour later, then as indicated. Requires 5 ml. venous blood in red top tube.

Calculate Serum Osmolality (in mOsm.) from the following formula:

$$2 \, (Na + K) + glucose/18 + BUN/2.8$$

Therapy: Record the number of units of *regular insulin* and the route of administration (I.V. or S.C.). Record administered *water* in liters (0.5 or 1) and *solutes* (Na, K, Cl, HCO_3, and glucose) in mEq. Therapeutic indications for frequently used solutions are as follows:

WATER	%	SOLUTE	MEQ./L.		MOSM./L.	THERAPEUTIC INDICATION
1 L.	1.4	NaHCO₃	Na HCO₃	166 166	332	pH below 7.1. *Use cautiously.* 0.5 to 1 L. of 1.4% solution usually sufficient.
1 L.	.45	NaCl	Na Cl	77 77	154	Osmolality above 350 mOsm. (Normal serum equals 280–290 mOsm.)
1 L.	.90	NaCl	Na	154	308	pH above 7.1, osmolality below 350 mOsm.
Ampoules (*Add to full liter of infusion fluid and mix thoroughly*)		KCl	K Cl K Cl	20 20 40 40	40 80	When urine flow reaches 40 ml./hr., or if EKG or clinical evidence of hypokalemia appear, infuse at rate of 20–40 mEq. K/hr.
1 L.	5.0	Glucose		278	278	Start glucose infusion when plasma glucose falls to 150 mg./dl. and continue infusion at rate sufficient to maintain glucose level at 100–200 mg./dl.
1 L.	10.0	Glucose		556	556	

  *This *diabetes flow sheet* was designed to *suggest* ways to collect data of diagnostic and therapeutic significance to the management of otherwise uncomplicated, acutely decompensated diabetes mellitus. The recorded *data base* should be modified to conform to the needs of each individual patient. When appropriate, additional physical examination data and laboratory data should be recorded. Additional laboratory data that are sometimes needed include hematocrit, white blood cell count and differential, complete urinalysis, plasma lactate and pyruvate, magnesium, calcium, amylase, cholesterol, triglycerides, lipoprotein typing (Fredrickson), and fatty acids. If lipid is present, measure the lipid layer in a hematocrit tube and correct electrolyte and glucose concentrations in plasma water accordingly.

Start oral fluid and food and NPH or lente insulin as soon as the patient can tolerate them. For the majority of patients, this should be within 12 to 24 hours after initiation of therapy.

TABLE 8   *Precipitating Causes of Severe Diabetic Ketoacidosis and Hyperglycemic Hyperosmolar State at Grady Memorial Hospital (1973–1975)*

VERY COMMON:

    Stopping insulin therapy (50%) – this occurred most commonly in emotionally immature juvenile diabetics, alcoholics, schizophrenics, or inadequately educated and/or supervised patients.

COMMON:

    Infection (30%) – urinary tract, pneumonia, other.
    Alcohol abuse (4%).

UNCOMMON:

    Excess caloric intake and obesity (2%).
    Immunologic insulin resistance (1%).
    Steroid medication (1%).
    Inadequate fluid intake with dehydration and inability to sustain osmotic diuresis (1%).
    Surgical and other types of stress (1%).
    Previously undiagnosed diabetes (10%).
    No apparent cause (10%).

TABLE 9   *Complications Encountered During the Treatment of Acutely Decompensated Diabetes Mellitus*

1. Malnutrition with substrate deficit (usually occurs in alcoholics and patients poorly nourished because of gastrointestinal surgery, etc.). Give insulin plus glucose to abort diabetic acidosis and to replace tissue glycogen; replace protein deficit later.
2. Acute tubular necrosis with renal shut-down.
3. Lactic acidosis.
4. Hypernatremia or hyponatremia.
5. Hypomagnesemia or hypophosphatemia.
6. Cardiac arrhythmias (due to K^+ deficit or excess).
7. Acute pancreatitis (due to prior alcohol intake or hypertriglyceridemia).
8. Immunologic insulin resistance.
9. Urinary tract infection (catheter).
10. Aspiration pneumonia due to vomiting and/or respiratory obstruction.
11. Vascular occlusions:
    a. Myocardial infarction
    b. Stroke
    c. Peripheral arterial thrombosis
    d. Mesenteric thrombosis
    e. Pulmonary embolus
    f. Peripheral thrombophlebitis or phlebothrombosis
12. Death:
    a. Cardiac
    b. Respiratory
    c. Metabolic (pH less than 6.8, fatal hypokalemia)

TABLE 10   *Side-Effects of Therapy for Acutely Decompensated Diabetes Mellitus*

COMMON:

    HYPOGLYCEMIA (PLASMA GLUCOSE <50 MG./DL.): Prevent by monitoring plasma glucose at bedside (Beckman glucose analyzer) at hourly intervals, and starting infusion of 5–10% dextrose in distilled water at appropriate rate when plasma glucose has fallen to 100–200 mg./dl. level. 25% of patients became hypoglycemic (most were asymptomatic) during the course of treatment of severe diabetic ketoacidosis or hyperglycemic hyperosmolar coma at Grady Memorial Hospital during the period 1973–1975.

    HYPOKALEMIA (SERUM K^+ ≤3 MEQ./L.): Due to giving too little K^+ or too much $NaHCO_3$ with resultant metabolic alkalosis with hypokalemia. The normal K^+ range is 4.0–5.4 mEq./L. Prevent hypokalemia by monitoring serum K^+ and EKG at hourly intervals; start K^+ replacement in second liter of fluids (unless contraindicated), or earlier if evidence of hypokalemia is available; and continue K^+ infusion to maintain serum K^+ between 3 and 6 mEq./L. 15% of patients became hypokalemic (most were asymptomatic) during the course of treatment of severe diabetic ketoacidosis or hyperglycemic hyperosmolar coma at Grady Memorial Hospital during the period 1973–1975.

UNCOMMON:

    METABOLIC ALKALOSIS: Due to giving too much $NaHCO_3$. Prevent by using $NaHCO_3$ sparingly, if at all, and by monitoring CO_2, pH, and Pco_2 at hourly intervals initially.

    FLUID OVERLOAD WITH CONGESTIVE HEART FAILURE: Due to giving too much fluid. Avoid by monitoring urine output, dyspnea, pulmonary rales, and if necessary, central venous pressure.

    RECURRENT KETOACIDOSIS: Due to failure to give adequate amounts of insulin at frequent enough intervals during the recovery phase. Avoid by giving appropriate amount of intermediate insulin (NPH or lente) when acidosis has cleared, and monitoring plasma glucose in post-recovery period so that small amounts of regular insulin can be given every 4 hours if hyperglycemia increases during that period.

RARE:

    CEREBRAL EDEMA: Occurs rarely in children, rarely if ever in adults. Prevent by starting 5–10% dextrose infusion when plasma glucose falls to 100–200 mg./dl., and keeping it at that level during the recovery period.

    CEREBRAL HYPOXIA: In addition to shock and inadequate ventilation, a hypothetic cause of cerebral hypoxia has received some attention of late. 2,3-diphosphoglycerate binds specifically to deoxyhemoglobin and lowers its affinity for oxygen; this in turn shifts the dissociation curve to the right and facilitates the delivery of oxygen to tissues. Acidosis lowers 2,3-DPG but shifts the dissociation curve to the right, so that the two opposing forces cancel each other. However, acidosis may be corrected in a few hours, but it may take up to 96 hours for 2,3-DPG to return to normal, especially if inorganic phosphate is in short supply. This sequence of events could cause hypoxia, and *may* justify more widespread use of phosphates and more restricted use of sodium bicarbonate in the treatment of ketoacidosis.

TABLE 11   *Equipment and Supplies Needed to Optimally Diagnose and Treat Decompensated Diabetes Mellitus*

IN EMERGENCY DEPARTMENT:
1. To measure plasma glucose stat
   a. Oxygen rate method glucose analyzer (Beckman) (1 minute)
   b. SMA/6 (Central Chemistry Laboratory)
   c. Dextrostix—less satisfactory than methods *a* and *b*. Deteriorates with aging and exposure to light and moisture. If used, check with 5% dextrose in D/W or with Coke for ability to react, and check plasma glucose (SMA/6) in Central Chemistry Laboratory.
2. To measure plasma ketones stat
   a. Acetone Test "Denco" (Denver Chemical Manufacturing Company, Stamford, Conn. 06904). Test plasma, serially diluted from undiluted to 1/16 dilution
   b. Acetest tablets, crushed (Ames Co., Elkhart, Indiana 46514). Less satisfactory than *a*. Test plasma serially diluted
   c. Ketostix (Ames Co.). Unsatisfactory for plasma
3. To measure urine glucose
   a. Oxygen rate method glucose analyzer (Beckman). Measures urine glucose accurately and quantitatively. Normal level 3–25 mg./dl., abnormal level >25 mg./dl.
   b. 2-drop and 5-drop Clinitest
   c. Testape and Clinistix
4. To measure urine ketones
   a. Acetone test "Denco"
   b. Acetest tablets
   c. Ketostix
5. Gray top tube (plasma for glucose and ketones), red top tube (serum for SMA/6 and serum osmolality), blood in plastic syringe with heparin on crushed ice (for pH)
6. Blood pressure cuff, stethoscope, and thermometer
7. 0.9% NaCl in 1000 ml. bottles for intravenous administration

IN INTENSIVE CARE AREA:
1. Disease Process Standard (Table 5)
2. Flow sheets (Table 7)
3. Gray top tube (plasma for glucose and ketones), red top tube (serum for SMA/6 and serum osmolality), plastic syringe, heparin, and crushed ice (for pH)
4. Oxygen rate method glucose analyzer (Beckman), acetone test "Denco," Clinitest tablets, possibly Acetest tablets, Ketostix, Testape, and Clinistix
5. Thermometer (rectal), blood pressure cuff, stethoscope, bedscales, tape-measure, EKG machine and monitor, polyethylene graduated cylinder (to measure urine volume), infusion pump (IVAC), sterile venous pressure tray with inside needle catheter (to measure central venous pressure)
6. U-100 regular insulin (rarely U-500 regular insulin and U-100 sulfated insulin are needed); U-100 NPH and U-100 lente insulin
7. 50 ml. vials of 7.5% $NaHCO_3$ (44.6 mEq.)
8. 1000 ml. bottles of 0.45% NaCl, 0.9% NaCl, 5% dextrose in distilled water, 10% dextrose in distilled water, and 50 ml. vials of 50% dextrose in distilled water
9. KCl vials containing 20 or 40 mEq. KCl
10. Cardiorespiratory arrest cart

IN CENTRAL CHEMISTRY LABORATORY:
1. Osmometer to measure serum osmolality
2. SMA/6 to measure Na^+, K^+, Cl^-, CO_2, BUN, and glucose
3. Equipment to measure pH
4. Equipment to measure other indicated chemicals (Tables 5 and 7), including enzymatic assay for lactate and pyruvate (on freshly drawn, heparinized arterial blood deproteinized promptly with cold perchloric acid and centifuged in the cold with assays being promptly performed, or on venous blood drawn without stasis clotted on ice with serum being separated and frozen until assayed), enzymatic assay for acetoacetate and betahydroxybutyrate, and suspected intoxicants, drugs, or poisons (collect serum and urine and store in freezer until analyzed by Central Chemistry Laboratory, or by The Poison Lab Inc., 1469 South Holly St., Denver, Colorado 80222)

should have intravenous isotonic saline running, and the admitting treatment team should initiate insulin therapy immediately either en route to or on arrival in the Intensive Care area. A clear airway should be established (using an endotracheal tube if necessary), secretions should be suctioned if necessary, and oxygen should be given if the patient is hypoxic or cyanotic. The patient should be checked for a distended bladder (catheterized if absolutely necessary) and a dilated stomach (rarely, a stomach tube must be inserted), and occasionally sideboards and restraints must be applied to prevent him from falling out of bed. The treatment team must be in *constant attendance* and must *continuously monitor* the patient (Table 7) until the diabetes has compensated and the patient is alert. Hypoglycemia (plasma glucose < 50 mg./dl.) should be prevented by hourly monitoring of the plasma glucose, and hypokalemia (serum K^+ < 3 mEq./liter) should be prevented by hourly monitoring of the serum potassium. Shock should be treated aggressively with prompt and adequate fluid replacement, but fluid overload with congestive heart failure should be avoided. Cardiac or respiratory arrest may occur either secondary to hyperkalemia or hypokalemia, and equipment should be maintained near the patient for either of these emergencies.

Insulin

U-100 *regular insulin* (rarely U-500 regular insulin or U-100 sulfated insulin in "insulin-resistant" patients) is used routinely; the dose must be individualized and should be sufficient to lower the plasma glucose at an optimal rate (monitor plasma glucose at hourly intervals using glucose analyzer—Beckman). The average dose required by over 300 cases of severe diabetic ketoacidosis and hyperosmolar coma at Grady Memorial Hospital over a two-year period was 550 units, but the dose range in individuals (without immunologic insulin resistance) was very large (from 10 units to 5000 units in 24 hours). The dose required by patients with moderate or mild ketoacidosis averaged 150 units, but the dose range again was large (from 10 units to 1000 units in 24 hours). It is impossible to predict in advance how much insulin will be "enough"; this must be determined by the rate of decline of the plasma glucose and the clearing of the ketonemia and ketonuria. In the early stages of treatment, there may be a paradoxical increase in ketonemia because of the conversion of large amounts of betahydroxybutyrate to acetoacetate, which in turn is responsible for a positive nitroprusside reaction as measured by the "acetone test."

At the present time there is controversy concerning the optimal manner of insulin administration, various authors preferring one of the following: (1) intravenous infusion using an IVAC or similar pump at a rate of 3 to 12 units per hour; (2) intravenous bolus administration at a rate of 100 units per hour (the dose being increased as treatment progresses in the unresponsive patient); (3) intramuscular administration; or (4) subcutaneous administration. The subcutaneous route should be avoided initially in the markedly dehydrated, hypotensive, or shocked patient because of poor absorption from that route; the intravenous route is preferable in these individuals. At Grady Memorial Hospital, the presently preferred methods of insulin administration are as follows.

(1) *In severe diabetic ketoacidosis and hyperosmolar coma:* 100 units insulin as a stat I.V. bolus, repeated at hourly intervals with the dose being adjusted to the rate of decline of the plasma glucose (the average adult is given 400 to 500 units in the first six hours, but some are given considerably more and some considerably less; depending on body weight, children are given one-twentieth to one-half as much); when the plasma glucose reaches a level of 100 to 200 mg./dl., an infusion of 5 per cent or 10 per cent dextrose in distilled water is started to maintain the plasma glucose at that level, and the patient is given an appropriate dose of intermediate insulin (NPH or lente) to prevent recurrence of significant hyperglycemia or ketoacidosis.

(2) *In mild or moderate ketoacidosis:* 25 to 50 units subcutaneously is given every one to three hours in adults (less in children) until the plasma glucose level falls to 100 to 200 mg./dl. and ketosis has cleared; oral fluids and food are given every one to two hours plus an appropriate amount of intermediate insulin (NPH or lente) to prevent recurrence of significant hyperglycemia or ketoacidosis.

Water and Electrolytes

(1) *In severe diabetic ketoacidosis and hyperosmolar coma.* The patient may have lost as much as 12 liters of water and as much as 800 mEq. Na^+ and as much as 800 mEq. K^+, somewhat less Cl^-, and smaller amounts of Mg^{++} and phosphate: the first clysis contains isotonic (0.90 per cent) NaCl; if the osmolality is > 350 mOsm./liter, 0.45 per cent NaCl should be given in subsequent clyses until the osmolality has fallen below that level; if the pH is < 7.10, up to 166 mEq. $NaHCO_3$ may be given to correct the acidosis (more may be needed if lactic acidosis is present, but carefully avoid inducing metabolic alkalosis with hypokalemia, which is very dangerous. Potassium replacement usually is started with the second clysis (with 20 to 40 mEq. routinely being mixed with *1 liter* of infusion fluid); usually 20 to 40 mEq. is replaced every hour (if urine flow is as much as 40 ml./hr. and there is no evidence of hyperkalemia); serum K^+ should be kept above 3 mEq./liter but below 6 mEq./liter; about half the K^+ deficit is replaced (up to 400 mEq. K^+) during the first 24 hours, the rest being replaced by the oral route during the next five to ten days. The patient should be carefully monitored for electrocardiographic or physical evidence of hypokalemia; the patient also should be carefully monitored for evidence of renal failure and/or fluid overload.

(2) *In mild or moderate ketoacidosis.* Oral fluids containing Na$^+$ and K$^+$ given at hourly or more frequent intervals usually are sufficient to replace the water and electrolyte deficit within 24 hours. It is rarely necessary to replace magnesium and/or phosphate deficits, since dietary replacement after recovery usually is sufficient.

Infection

Evidence of urinary tract, pulmonic, and other infection should be sought routinely, and if indicated blood, urine, sputum, or other cultures and bacterial sensitivity studies should be obtained. Sometimes dehydrated patients do not become febrile and pulmonic rales do not appear until rehydration has taken place.

Other Causes

Other causes of *coma* and/or metabolic acidosis and/or *concurrent illness* should be sought and appropriately treated if detected (see Tables 4 and 5, Assessment).

References

Arieff, A., and Carroll, H. J.: Nonketotic, hyperosmolar coma with hyperglycemia: clinical features, pathophysiology, renal function, acid-base balance, plasma-cerebrospinal fluid equilibria, and the effects of therapy in 37 cases. Medicine 51:73, 1972.

Beigelman, P., and Warner, N. E.: Thirty-two fatal cases of severe diabetic ketoacidosis, including a case of mucormycosis. Diabetes 22:844, 1973.

Cooperman, M. T., et al.: Clinical studies of alcoholic ketoacidosis. Diabetes 23:433, 1974.

Davidson, J. K.: Diabetes mellitus in adults. *In* Conn, H. F. (ed.): Current Therapy. Philadelphia, W. B. Saunders Co., 1974, p. 386.

Felts, P. W.: Current Concepts: Coma in the Diabetic. Upjohn Co., 1974.

Genuth, S. M.: Constant intravenous insulin infusion in diabetic ketoacidosis. J.A.M.A. 223:1358, 1973.

Posner, J. B., and Plum, F.: Spinal fluid pH and neurologic symptoms in systemic acidosis. N. Engl. J. Med., 277:605, 1967.

Young, E., and Bradley, R. F.: Cerebral edema with irreversible coma in severe diabetic ketoacidosis. N. Engl. J. Med. 276:12, 665, 1967.

B. HYPOGLYCEMIA

John K. Davidson

INTRODUCTION

The mean plasma glucose level in normal humans fasted overnight is 92 mg./dl. (range 78 to 115 mg./dl.). In such individuals, the glucose level fluctuates over a remarkably narrow range, rising modestly after feeding and falling modestly during fasting. When *glucose production* (primarily from glucose absorbed from the gastrointestinal tract after feeding and from liver gluconeogenesis during fasting) lags behind *glucose utilization* (primarily to provide substrate for energy production during exercise, or to be stored as glycogen when insulin levels are inappropriately elevated) for a significant period of time, hypoglycemia results.

The lowest level of plasma glucose that can be regarded as *normal* varies from person to person. Some patients are symptomatic when the plasma glucose falls as low as 50 mg./dl., whereas some are asymptomatic when the plasma glucose falls as low as 30 gm./dl. Thus, the level from three to five hours after a glucose load may fall as low as 35 mg./dl. in some asymptomatic individuals, and during fasting the level may fall as low as 30 mg./dl. in some asymptomatic females. Males are rarely asymptomatic if it falls during a fast below 50 mg./dl.

Since prolonged or repeated hypoglycemic episodes can result in permanent brain damage and death, it is prudent, as a general rule, to regard all patients with measured plasma glucose levels <50 mg./dl. as having hypoglycemia until proved otherwise. Individuals who have a plasma glucose level of 30 to 50 mg./dl. and who are asymptomatic when initially seen should be classified as *hypoglycemia suspects*, and they should be carefully studied to determine whether or not they develop symptomatic fasting hypoglycemia or symptomatic reactive hypoglycemia after a glucose load.

RECOGNITION

Symptoms and signs similar to those of hypoglycemia frequently occur in emotionally disturbed patients. Thus, a diagnosis of symptomatic hypoglycemia cannot be confirmed unless the timing of symptoms and signs coincides with the lowest plasma glucose levels. One should avoid an erroneous diagnosis of hypoglycemia because of improper blood specimen collection, preservation, or analysis ("desk-top hypoglycemia"). It is important not to confuse *asymptomatic* and *unrecognized* hypoglycemia. Many diabetics, especially those with neuropathy, have severe hypoglycemic episodes which neither they nor their peers recognize, and many patients with insulinomas have been confined to mental institutions because hypoglycemia was not suspected.

Over 95 per cent of hypoglycemic episodes seen in most Emergency Departments occur in patients known to have diabetes mellitus that is being treated with insulin or a sulfonylurea. About two-thirds of those affected have not eaten appropriately. Hypoglycemia of brief duration may cause cerebral malfunction, which can result in accidental injury or jail confinement, and more prolonged hypoglycemia (usually four or more hours) may result in irreversible brain damage (with paralysis and/or imbecility) or death. In a two-year audit (1973–1975) of 240 cases of hypoglycemia observed in the Grady Memorial Hospital Emergency Clinic, eight (3.3 per cent) terminated fatally. *Thus, all cases of hypoglycemia should be regarded as true medical emergencies that require prompt confirmation by a stat plasma glucose measurement and immediate treatment with oral or intravenous glucose.* A "Dextrostix" determination is useful only as a gross indicator and a control (using dextrose in water or a known normal) should be done, since deterioration of the testing sticks re-

---

TABLE 1   Pathogenesis of Symptomatic Hypoglycemia

(A) *Adrenal medulla overactivity with hyperepinephrinemia:*
  Subjective: Anxiety, palpitation, occasionally angina pectoris.
  Objective: Perspiration, pallor, hypothermia, tachycardia, hypertension, cardiac arrhythmias, dilated pupils.
(B) *Neurologic dysfunction:*
  Initially, the higher cortical centers malfunction because the glucose supply is insufficient to maintain normal metabolic activity; oxygen utilization decreases; later, centers in the midbrain and medulla are similarly affected. In fatal reactions there is cerebral edema, multiple petechial hemorrhages, and widespread necrosis of cortical ganglion cells. Prolongation of hypoglycemia (usually four or more hours), not depth to which the plasma glucose falls, is responsible for irreparable brain damage.
  Subjective: Headache, blurring of vision, transient diplopia, paresthesias, hunger, nausea, fatigue, drowsiness, irritability, vertigo.
  Objective: Mental confusion, bizarre behavior, speech difficulties, irrational agitation, combativeness, delirium, vomiting, lethargy, somnolence, aphasia, tremor, ataxia, nystagmus, paralysis, seizures, coma, Babinski reflexes, shallow respiration, bradycardia.

TABLE 2   Causes of Hypoglycemia in Patients Being Treated for Diabetes Mellitus

(A) Inadequate carbohydrate intake
(B) Vigorous exercise
(C) Insulin therapy
  1. Excess insulin dose:
    a. Erroneously prescribed
    b. Failure to match insulin potency with correct syringe (i.e., each should be U-100)
    c. Visual failure with inability to measure correct dose
    d. Attempted suicide or homicide
  2. Failure to reduce insulin dose when need for insulin decreases:
    a. During reduction of body weight
    b. Endocrine deficiency
      (1) Hypopituitarism
      (2) Adrenal cortical insufficiency
    c. Reduction in dose of corticosteroid
    d. Decreased rate of insulin degradation due to kidney failure or liver failure
    e. After recovery from stressful situations
      (1) Infection
      (2) Pancreatitis
      (3) Acutely decompensated diabetes
      (4) Surgery
    f. At termination of pregnancy
(D) Sulfonylurea therapy (tolbutamide, tolazamide, chlorpropamide, acetohexamide, glyburide, glipizide)
  1. Excess dose
  2. Diminished degradation or excretion, as in kidney failure
  3. Potentiation by other drugs (Table 3) that displace sulfonylureas from albumin combining sites
(E) Ethanol, drugs, and toxins that lower plasma glucose level

TABLE 3 Some Drugs that Lower the Plasma Glucose Level in Patients Being Treated for Diabetes Mellitus

(A) Potentiation of Sulfonylureas
  1. Barbiturates
  2. Bishydroxycoumarin
  3. Chloramphenicol
  4. Monamine oxidase inhibitors
  5. Phenylbutazone
  6. Salicylates
  7. Sulfonamides
  8. Thiazides
(B) Increased Insulin Production
  1. Alpha adrenergic blockers
  2. Beta adrenergic stimulators
  3. Monamine oxidase inhibitors
(C) Decreased Hepatic Glycogenolysis
  1. Propranolol
(D) Mechanism Unknown
  1. Antihistamines
    a. Antazoline phosphate
    b. Tripelennamine hydrochloride
  2. Morphine
  3. Probenecid
  4. Propylthiouracil
  5. Tuberculostatic drugs
    a. Isoniazid
    b. Aminosalicylic acid

TABLE 4 Disease Process Standard for Recognition and Assessment of Hypoglycemia Problem Statement: Hypoglycemia (Subsets: Reactive, Exogenous, Fasting)

RECOGNITION (DEFINED DATA BASE):

Subjective: (a) Neurologic dysfunction: headache, blurring of vision, transient diplopia, paresthesias, hunger, nausea, fatigue, drowsiness, irritability, vertigo. (b) Hyperepinephrinemia: anxiety, palpitation, occasionally angina pectoris. (c) Known diabetes mellitus. (d) Insulin therapy: type, dose, time. (e) Sulfonylurea therapy: type, dose. (f) Diet prescription: calories, grams of protein, carbohydrate, and fat, division. (g) Missed food: time. (h) Vigorous exercise: time. (i) Level of control of diabetes. (j) Previous hypoglycemia. (k) Weight loss. (l) Duration of symptoms (minutes). (m) Drugs: salicylates, steroids, other. (n) Ethanol. (o) Toxins. (p) Gastrectomy.

Objective: (a) Neurologic dysfunction: mental confusion, bizarre behavior, speech difficulties, irrational agitation, combativeness, delirium, vomiting, lethargy, somnolence, aphasia, tremor, ataxia, nystagmus, paralysis, seizures, coma, Babinski reflexes, shallow respiration, bradycardia. (b) Hyperepinephrinemia: perspiration, pallor, hypothermia, tachycardia, hypertension, cardiac arrhythmias, dilated pupils. (c) Venous plasma glucose <50 mg./dl. (absolute requirement).

ASSESSMENT:

Is hypoglycemia (a) Reactive?: early diabetes mellitus, dumping syndrome, leucine sensitivity, fructose intolerance. (b) Exogenous?: insulin, sulfonylurea, missed meal, excess exercise, ethanol, drug, toxin. (c) Fasting?: insulinoma, other neoplasm, malnutrition, hypopituitarism, adrenal cortical insufficiency, glycogen storage disease (I, III, VII), glycogen synthetase deficiency, galactosemia, congenital adrenal hyperplasia, cretinism, epinephrine deficiency, severe liver disease, transient neonatal hyperinsulinemia in infant of diabetic mother, ketotic, idiopathic (including familial), other.

sults in no or little color change which can be incorrectly interpreted.

PATHOGENESIS

An understanding of the pathogenesis of symptomatic hypoglycemia (Table 1) facilitates data base collection and therapy. Over 95 per cent of cases of hypoglycemia seen in a busy Emergency Department are exogenous in origin (Tables 2, 3, 4, and 5); reactive hypoglycemia of early diabetes (due to delayed hyperinsulinemia following a meal or glucose load) and hypoglycemia in infants of diabetic mothers (due to beta cell hyperplasia and transient hyperinsulinemia following birth) are seen occasionally; other causes of reactive and fasting hypoglycemia are rarely seen. Causes of exogenous hypoglycemia in patients being treated for diabetes mellitus are listed in Table 2, and some drugs that can lower the plasma glucose and precipitate hypoglycemia in patients being treated for diabetes mellitus are listed in Table 3. Alcohol-induced hypoglycemia can occur, which should be sus-

pected. Special thought should be given to the possibility of accidental ingestion of medications which are close in spelling. For example, "Ornade" and "Orinase."

TABLE 5 Audit of Causes of 240 Consecutive Cases of Hypoglycemia in Patients Known to Have Diabetes Mellitus (Grady Memorial Hospital Emergency Clinic, 1973–1975)

(1) Inadequate food (carbohydrate) intake	66%
(2) Excess insulin dose	12%
(3) Sulfonylurea therapy	12%
(4) Strenuous exercise	4%
(5) Ethanol intake	4%
(6) Other (kidney failure, liver failure, decrease in corticosteroid dose)	2%

TABLE 6   Treatment Plan

Initial (in Emergency Department): Initiate immediately after drawing stat venous plasma glucose. (a) If able to swallow: oral glucose, candy, Coke, orange juice, or food. (b) If unable to swallow: I.V. Glucose (25 gm.) or S.C. or I.M. glucagon (1 mg.). (c) Observe until complete recovery, repeat plasma glucose, and give additional food. (d) Additional diagnostic data: if delayed recovery, neurologic damage, or uncertain etiology of hypoglycemia, hospitalize. (e) Patient and family education: if prompt recovery, reinstruct on and/or revise as indicated: diet, insulin, and/or exercise. Omit ethanol, drugs, toxins. See (d) *Management After Hospital Discharge* below.

Follow-up (in Hospital and After Discharge): (a) *Abnormalities to be sought:* if *reactive* hypoglycemia: do oral 6-hour G.T.T. (after 300 gm. C/d for three days prior to test—abnormal in early diabetes and dumping syndrome), I.V. G.T.T. (normal in dumping syndrome); if indicated, leucine and/or fructose tolerance tests. If *fasting* hypoglycemia: up to 72-hour fast with plasma glucose every 6 hours; terminate test if hypoglycemia occurs. If indicated, collect data base to evaluate subsets under *Assessment* (c) in Table 4. Because of the rarity, complexity, and numerous causes of *fasting* hypoglycemia, their diagnosis and treatment will not be discussed here. Such information is available in References 1 and 4. (b) *Complications:* evaluate residual neurologic damage: motor, sensory, cerebellar, judgment, memory, I.Q.; cranial nerves: evaluate EKG and cardiac status. (c) *Predischarge Examination:* were precipitating factors identified and appropriately treated, and precautions taken to avoid recurrence? (d) *Management After Hospital Discharge:* if indicated, revise diet and/or insulin therapy and/or exercise pattern. Carry Lifesavers at all times; prescribe snack 60 minutes before hypoglycemia is prone to occur; prescription for and instruction of relatives on use of glucagon if recurrence of hypoglycemia and unable to swallow; give diabetes identification card, bracelet, and/or necklace; caution about driving motor vehicles and working around dangerous machinery and in unprotected high places; arrange continuing follow-up in ambulatory care facility such as Diabetes Clinic or physician's office.

DATA BASE AND ASSESSMENT

A data base should be collected as rapidly as possible (Table 4). A plasma glucose can be done in less than one minute using the Beckmann Glucose Analyzer, and in a few minutes using the SMA/6. Dextrostix are less accurate and frequently have given erroneous readings because of faulty methodology. Causes of hypoglycemia in the Emergency Department at Grady Memorial Hospital are shown in Table 5.

TREATMENT PLAN

Immediately after a stat plasma glucose is done (within one minute), treatment should be started (Table 6). If recovery is not prompt, the patient should be hospitalized for further evaluation and follow-up. In general, the more prolonged the period of hypoglycemia, the slower the response to glucose. Techniques of education and follow-up after hospital discharge are also outlined in Table 6.

References

Cornblath, M., and Schwartz, R.: Disorders of Carbohydrate Metabolism in Infancy. Philadelphia, W. B. Saunders Co., 1966.

Merimee, T. J., and Tyson, J. E.: Stabilization of plasma glucose during fasting. N. Engl. J. Med. *291:*1275, 1974.

Seltzer, H.: Drug-induced hypoglycemia. Diabetes *21:*955, 1972.

Steinke, J.: Hypoglycemia. *In* Joslin's Diabetes Mellitus. Philadelphia, Lea & Febiger, 1971, p. 797.

C. SELECTED EMERGENCY ENDOCRINOLOGIC PROBLEMS

Roberta Beckman Gonzalez

The growing body of students and practitioners who attend the patient at his earliest and often most chaotic entry into the medical delivery system has a pressing need to collect information rapidly and logically. The purpose of the problem-oriented medical record (Weed, 1969) was to categorize subjective and objective data, assess the accumulated facts and inferences, devise a plan, and initiate it with the least expenditure of time. The Weed method (modified by Bjorn and Cross, 1970) disciplines us to record our thinking in a format guided by the acronym S.O.A.P., which describes four steps in data collection and handling.

(1) *Subjective* information is that supplied by the patient or his close observers.

(2) *Objective* information is that which the examiner detects.

(3) *Assessment* is the step in which the

two first categories are used in concert with the experience and knowledge of the responsible practitioner, as he sifts through a differential diagnosis.

(4) The *plan* emanates reasonably from the assessment.

The endocrinologic emergencies to be discussed in this section—thyrotoxic storm, myxedema coma, thyroiditis, addisonian crisis, acute hypercalcemia, tetany, hypomagnesemia, and hypermagnesemia—are occurrences in which successful treatment demands brisk and logical thinking translated into effective action. They are presented in the problem-oriented format in order to recommend it and because the structure encourages just these goals. The findings in these endocrinologic problems frequently are so nonspecific or subtle as to muddy the proverbial waters. There is nothing quite so effective as "S.O.A.P." to clear them.

THYROTOXIC STORM (THYROID STORM)

SUBJECTIVE

The patient complains of weight loss, heat intolerance, nervousness, and agitation; perhaps a severe personality change with a lability of affect that makes him fear that he is "going crazy." There is muscle weakness, fatigue, inability to concentrate, almost constant motion, excessive perspiration, diarrhea, and palpitations of the heart.

There may be specific complaints of fever, abdominal pain, cough with sputum, dysuria, etc., which are important clues if an underlying infection precipitates hyperthyroidism into storm.

OBJECTIVE

Usually, one finds a thyrotoxic patient in severe distress. Dyspnea and hyperpyrexia almost always are prominent findings. Thin skin, a film of warm perspiration, warm moist palms, tachycardia, atrial fibrillation, wide pulse pressure with systolic hypertension, and hyperkinesis are frequent findings. Exophthalmos, when present, is evidenced by lid lag and/or infiltration around the orbit. With proptosis, incomplete closure of the eye decreases protection, and signs of conjunctivitis may be prominent. Extraocular muscle palsies often accompany these symptoms. The thyroid gland usually is diffusely enlarged, but may be nodular, and there often is an easily audible bruit. The hair is thin and there may be evidence of hair loss. Fine tremor and signs of muscle weakness, especially of the quadriceps, are seen, and true muscle atrophy occurs, notably in the temporal muscles. Abdominal pain and vomiting may be prominent, and a surgical abdomen may be suspected (Fig. 1).

Laboratory values in storm are not remarkably distinct from those of hyperthyroid-

Symptom	Per Cent	Symptom	Per Cent
Nervousness	99	Increased appetite	65
Increased sweating	91	Eye complaints	54
Hypersensitivity to heat	89	Swelling of legs	35
Palpitation	89	Hyperdefecation (without diarrhea)	33
Fatigue	88	Diarrhea	23
Weight loss	85	Anorexia	9
Tachycardia	82	Constipation	4
Dyspnea	75	Weight gain	2
Weakness	70		

Sign	Per Cent	Sign	Per Cent
Tachycardia*	100	Eye signs	71
Goiter†	100	Atrial fibrillation	10
Skin changes	97	Splenomegaly	10
Tremor	97	Gynecomastia	10
Bruit over thyroid	77	Liver palms	8

*In other studies thyrotoxic patients with normal pulse rate have been observed.

†The data shown in this table are taken from Williams, R. H.: *J. Clin. Endocr.* 6:1, 1946. In the experience of the present authors, enlargement of the thyroid is lacking in approximately 3 per cent of patients with thyrotoxicosis.

Figure 1 Incidence of symptoms and signs observed in 247 patients with thyrotoxicosis. (From Williams, R. H.: Textbook of Endocrinology, 5th ed. Philadelphia, W. B. Saunders Co., 1974.)

ism. A high serum T_4 (usually over 12 μg per cent), low serum cholesterol, high T_3 resin uptake or PBI, and low carotene are usual; these take some days to obtain, however, so the two-hour I-131 uptake can be most helpful (Menendez and Rivlin, 1963), and usually is over 19 per cent in severe hyperthyroidism. Occasionally a low T_4 and high I-131 uptake are a keynote for T_3 thyrotoxicosis, for which management is identical after the difficulties of recognition are overcome. (T_3 must be measured by radioimmunoassay.)

ASSESSMENT

Thyroid storm is hyperthyroidism that has been exacerbated by some factor—infection, thromboembolism, surgery, emotional trauma, drug reaction, or withdrawal of thyroid-blocking medication, into a life-threatening hypermetabolic state manifested by high fever, tachycardia, and circulatory, CNS, and hepatic dysfunction. Infection is the most common precipitating factor, but cardiovascular diseases, gastrointestinal disorders, vigorous palpation of an unblocked hyperfunctioning gland, toxemia of pregnancy, or parturition, radioiodine treatment for hyperthyroidism, and diabetic ketoacidosis all have been implicated etiologies for storm. There is an apparent relationship to the amount of circulating thyroid hormones, since ingestion of thyroxine or triiodothyronine has caused storm in untreated hyperthyroid patients. In some debilitated patients with untreated hyperthyroidism, the excessive tissue demands seem to culminate in a metabolic crisis without other predisposing factors.

The principles of successful therapy are as follows.

(1) Assisting the organism to defend itself against high levels of circulating thyroid hormone with fluids and electrolytes, cooling, treatment of infection, maximal caloric intake, vitamins, and digitalis if necessary (particularly in older age-groups).

(2) Inhibiting the release of thyroid hormone from thyroglobulin with iodide (Fig. 2).

(3) Inhibiting the biosynthesis of thyroid hormone with the thiourylenes methimazole (Tapazole) or propylthiouracil (Fig. 2).

(4) Blocking the adrenergic neurotrans-

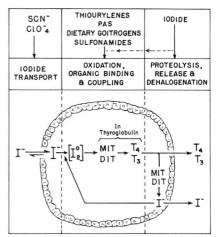

Figure 2 Diagram of the major steps in thyroid hormone biosynthesis. In this diagram, the follicular outline is intended merely to differentiate the intrathyroid from the interstitial compartment and should not be construed as indicating that the reactions shown necessarily occur in the follicular lumen. Note that the concentration of intrathyroid iodide maintained by the iodide transport mechanism is greater than that in the extracellular fluid. The processes of iodide oxidation, organic binding, and coupling of iodotyrosines are grouped together, since they appear to be closely related oxidative reactions. The precise proportions of the iodide liberated from iodotyrosines by dehalogenation that are reused or released into the extracellular fluid are unknown.

Shown above are the major inhibitors of the several steps in hormone biosynthesis. Large quantities of iodide inhibit organic binding and coupling (*dashed lines*), but this effect usually is transient. Although not shown, the lithium ion, like iodide, is an inhibitor of proteolysis and release. (From Williams, R. H.: Textbook of Endocrinology, 5th ed. Philadelphia, W. B. Saunders Co., 1974.)

mittor (Dratman, 1974) that mediates the effects of excessive thyroid hormones with propranol (Das and Krieger, 1969), guanethidine, or reserpine.

(5) Supplying glucocorticoid to cover the needs of a functional hypoadrenalism.

PLAN

(1) Draw blood for studies and start an I.V. using 5 per cent dextrose in normal saline solution, with 1 to 2 gm. of sodium iodide and 100 mg. of hydrocortisone.

(2) Administer propranalol, 1 to 5 mg. I.V. or 40 to 80 mg. orally, unless asthma or severe congestive failure not secondary to

thyrocardiac disease is present, in which case guanethidine 20 to 40 mg. every four to six hours is appropriate. Reserpine, 1 to 3 mg. I.M. every four hours may be given alternatively; in addition to depleting catecholamine stores, it has a sedative effect that can be helpful in the severely agitated patient. Both reserpine and guanethidine can cause significant postural hypotension, and doses smaller than the full recommended dose should be tested for a possible idiosyncratic response.

(3) Give Tapazole, 10 to 20 mg. every four to six hours orally or by gastric tube. Propylthouracil, 250 mg. every four to six hours, may be substituted if the patient has had no response or has a previous allergy to Tapazole. Blood counts must be watched with either antithyroid agent, because of bone marrow suppression that sometimes may be pronounced.

(4) If the patient remains in extremis and death seems imminent despite these measures, plasmapheresis or exchange blood transfusion to remove the high levels of circulating plasma and red cell thyroxine has been done effectively. Five hundred cc. of blood is removed at three-hour intervals, and the red blood cells are separated and returned to the patient, or whole blood is exchanged. Serum thyroxine values of 40 μg per cent have been successfully lowered to 13 μg per cent (Ashkar et al., 1970). Peritoneal dialysis also has been effective, but is slower.

(5) Steroid therapy is life-supporting in thyroid storm, with its 20 to 60 per cent mortality rate. Full doses commensurate with adrenal output in stress, i.e., 300 mg. of cortisol or its equivalent in analogues, are given to obviate functional hypoadrenalism caused by the shortened half-life of adrenal steroids secondary to hypermetabolism. It is well to remember that the use of steroids will mask the objective findings of underlying disease (pneumonia, appendicitis, empyema of the gall bladder, etc.). Specific treatment of any infection must be determined and initiated to *prevent* the progression of thyroid storm.

(6) Continue supportive measures, i.e., replenishment of fluids and electrolytes, antipyretics, cooling blankets, sponge baths, and sedatives. High caloric diet and vitamin B and C supplementation should be initiated.

MYXEDEMA COMA

SUBJECTIVE

The patient in myxedema coma frequently cannot give subjective impressions, but the family might attest to decreased energy, complaints of severe cold intolerance, apathetic muting of the patient's personality, with lassitude and little expression of enthusiasm or anger. True personality changes, reaching a point of psychosis accompany extreme hypothyroidism. Constipation is frequent, there is easy weight gain, the features and hair coarsen, and a noticeable yellow hue to the complexion may have developed. The physician's subjective note may be of an elderly female patient with these historical findings who, during her hospitalization, is either subjected to emergency surgery with anesthesia, or given narcotics, or exposed to cold, with subsequent consciousness changes leading to stupor and, finally, coma. Fifty per cent of myxedema coma patients develop this complication after admission to the hospital.

OBJECTIVE

The patient often is described as having a "leonine" facies, and has hoarseness of the voice, remarkably dry skin, and hyperkeratoses around the elbows and knees. Obesity is usual, as is a large tongue with dental impressions; alopecia; edema of the periorbital tissues; and often abdominal distention with hypoactivity of the bowel, fecal impaction, and sometimes ileus. Delayed tendon reflexes, bradycardia, and hypothermia, with extremes of body temperature as low as 75° F., may be found. The presence of a healed thyroidectomy scar is a good clue to diagnosis, especially when a history of thyroidectomy is not available. The EKG shows low voltage, with widespread depressed or inverted T waves and prolonged Q-T interval. Sinus bradycardia is the rule. Examination of the blood usually reveals an anemia that most often is normochromic and normocytic, but may be microcytic or macrocytic if iron or vitamin deficiency predominates. The serum may be lactescent, reflecting delayed clearing of chylomicrons, and hypercholesterolemia is present. There is elevation of the cerebrospinal fluid pressure and protein, and pleural, peritoneal, and

Symptom	Per Cent of Cases	Symptom	Per Cent of Cases
Weakness	99	Constipation	61
Dry skin	97	Gain in weight	59
Coarse skin	97	Loss of hair	57
Lethargy	91	Pallor of lips	57
Slow speech	91	Dyspnea	55
Edema of eyelids	90	Peripheral edema	55
Sensation of cold	89	Hoarseness or aphonia	52
Decreased sweating	89	Anorexia	45
Cold skin	83	Nervousness	35
Thick tongue	82	Menorrhagia	32
Edema of face	79	Palpitation	31
Coarseness of hair	76	Deafness	30
Pallor of skin	67	Precordial pain	25
Memory impairment	66		

Figure 3 Symptomatology of myxedema. (From Williams, R. H.: Textbook of Endocrinology, 5th ed. Philadelphia, W. B. Saunders Co., 1974.)

pericardial effusion fluid also is high in protein. The serum thyroxine level is low, as is the T_3 resin uptake. Low serum sodium with high urine osmolarity, compared to low serum osmolality, bespeak the syndrome of inappropriate antidiuretic hormone secretion, a frequent complication of myxedema coma (Fig. 3).

ASSESSMENT

Alveolar hypoventilation with hypercarbia and hypoxemia, hyponatremia, and hypothermia are key factors in the genesis of the coma in thyroxine deficiency. Retention of carbon dioxide occurs independent of the factors of obesity or underlying pulmonary disease, and is reversed after replacement of the hormone. There is a reduction in maximum voluntary ventilation reflecting diminished bellows action of the thorax, and impaired respiratory motion by pleural effusions and ascites. Decreased carbon dioxide diffusing capacity occurs secondary to lung parenchymal changes, and diminished ventilatory responses to breathing 7.5 per cent carbon dioxide demonstrate a defect in CNS regulation of respiration. When blood gas determinations indicate the need for respiratory assistance, tracheostomy, rather than simple intubation, is suggested, since the above expressions of thyroid hormone deficiency are not corrected for seven to ten days, and patients frequently relapse when extubated after three to four days (Senior et al., 1971).

Another factor in the genesis of coma is the hyponatremia resulting from inappropriate ADH secretion, which also is associated with seizures in about 25 per cent of these patients. Additionally, cerebral oxygen consumption is not diminished by thyroid hormone lack as in other tissues, and while cardiac output diminishes cerebral anoxia supervenes. Failure of adequate adrenal response to stress probably is a factor in the high mortality associated with myxedema coma. Although adrenal atrophy has not been demonstrated, diminished release of ACTH by the pituitary has (Menendez and Rivlin, 1963). High dose corticosteroids are given for a short period on this basis.

PLAN

(1) Thyroid replacement: intravenous levothyroxine, 0.4 to 0.5 mg., saturates the binding proteins, and significant signs of increased metabolism are evident by six hours, without the occurrence of cardiac arrhythmias that were frequent with the use of triiodothyronine.

(2) Steroid replacement: 100 to 200 mg. of cortisol or its equivalent are given I.V., to be repeated every eight hours and stopped abruptly the next day.

(3) Sodium replacement: hypertonic saline is given cautiously, for serum sodium values below 115 mg. per cent, and fluids are restricted for the hyponatremia of inappropriate ADH secretion. In adults, limitation to 1000 cc. of fluid daily might be necessary, or just the amount to replenish urine output plus insensible loss.

(4) EKG monitoring is done to signal the need to treat cardiac ischemia as tissue ox-

ygen requirements increase secondary to replacement of thyroxine.

(5) Respiratory assistance is given with oxygen administration, usually by way of tracheostomy, when symptoms and blood gases indicate respiratory failure. Ventilatory support may be needed.

(6) Treatment of any underlying infection is of extreme importance. Any patient with myxedema coma and a normal body temperature is probably toxic, and infections should be treated specifically and promptly to aid in reversing the comatose state.

(7) External warming for hypothermia is contraindicated, since already diminished cardiac output may be diverted from vital organs, and cardiovascular collapse can ensue.

THYROIDITIS

SUBJECTIVE

The patient has pain in the anterior neck that appears gradually or suddenly, usually following an upper respiratory infection. Pain is accentuated by turning the head or swallowing, and may radiate to the ear, the jaw, or the occiput. The patient may be hoarse of voice, and, when severely affected, is febrile. There may be nervousness and palpitations, but lassitude is the most frequent complaint.

OBJECTIVE

A rapid pulse, slight-to-moderate temperature elevation, and firm, tender, sometimes nodular thyroid gland are found. The overlying skin is occasionally rubrous and warm. The finding of a low I-131 uptake and normal or high T_4 is expected, as is a high sedimentation rate.

ASSESSMENT

Inflammation of the thyroid, or thyroiditis sufficient to bring the patient to the Emergency Department, would be acute and suppurative, or subacute (de Quervain's). Acute suppuration of the gland is rare; when present, it is caused by pyogenic bacteria with a septic focus elsewhere, and should be treated with specific antibiotics and with surgical drainage if fluctuation occurs. Subacute thyroiditis is more common; its causative agent is probably viral, with mumps, coxsackie, influenza, and ECHO viruses all implicated. Occasionally, the acute onset of autoimmune thyroiditis (Hashimoto's) may cause the same symptomatology, but circulating antibodies are very high in Hashimoto's and are present only occasionally with subacute thyroiditis, and in low titer.

PLAN

Aspirin and bed rest usually suffice. If severe discomfort continues, glucocorticoid therapy relieves symptoms, but does not alter the inflammatory process.

Propranolol will reduce the peripheral effects of elevated thyroid hormone in those few patients who present during this very transient phase. Subacute thyroiditis is self-limited and long term hypothyroidism is rarely encountered.

HYPERCALCEMIA

Any patient with a serum calcium level greater than 15 mg. per cent must be considered a medical emergency.

SUBJECTIVE

The patient complains of lethargy, anorexia, thirst, dryness of the nose, difficulty in swallowing, and personality changes ranging from apathy to depression or frank psychotic behavior. These signs usually have occurred for some weeks or months. In the acute condition, the patient has nausea and vomiting and depressed sensorium; he may be delirious, stuporous, or comatose. Abdominal pain of ulcer or pancreatitis is not an unusual finding.

OBJECTIVE

The general demeanor is that of a person disoriented and stuporous or comatose. A high BUN may be due to dehydration alone, or also may signify renal insufficiency, in which case the creatinine and potassium also will be elevated. Nephrocalcinosis or renal calculi may be apparent on abdominal flat plate. Calcium phosphate crystals may be visible in the conjunctivum of the palpebral fissures, and band keratitis occurs on the corneae. Depressed deep tendon reflexes are elicited, as is an unusual flexibility of the limbs secondary to hypotonicity of muscles. Decreased excitability of the neuromuscular apparatus can be demonstrated. Perivascular and periarticular calcifications and/or chondrocalcinosis may be seen on x-ray. Cardiac arrhythmias are frequent, and the EKG will show a shortened Q-T interval. Blood studies reveal a high serum calcium: levels above 15 mg. per cent represent a serious emergency. Alkaline phosphatase is high if there is associated or concomitant bone disease. The serum phosphorus may be normal, high, low normal, or low, depending on the cause of the hypercalcemia. High phosphorus usually distinguishes hypervitaminosis D; low levels suggest hyperparathyroidism or pseudohyperparathyroidism.

ASSESSMENT

The differential diagnosis is germane to the choice of therapies. Hyperparathyroidism or pseudohyperparathyroidism—the latter term being applied to that clinical state in which nonparathyroid tumor tissue ectopically produces a polypeptide with parathormone-like activity on bone and renal tubular function—generally are responsible for severe hypercalcemia. Vitamin D intoxication, acute adrenal insufficiency, sarcoidosis, hyperthyroidism, multiple myeloma, neoplasia with osseous metastases, or milk-alkali syndrome are other causes. Hypercalcemia occurs secondary to the immobilization of patients with fractures, poliomyelitis, Paget's disease, or acidosis. Measurement of the protein level and albumin/globulin ratio can be useful, since hyperglobulinemia occurs in multiple myeloma and sarcoid. A serum chloride level greater than 102 mEq./liter tends to distinguish the hypercalcemia of hyperparathyroidism, as does a low bicarbonate level, probably because of the citrate accumulation in hyperparathyroidism. The definitive measurement is the radioimmunoassay of parathormone.

PLAN

(1) Begin EKG monitoring. If the patient is taking digitalis, watch for toxicity. (Calcium has a synergistic action on the myocardium and conducting system with digitalis.) The T-wave flattening and QRS widening of an associated hypokalemia also must be noted. Draw blood for parathormone level, BUN, creatinine, electrolytes, calcium, phosphorus, and alkaline phosphatase.

(2) Rehydrate the patient with 1 liter of a normal saline solution infused every three to four hours. Potassium replacement and vasopressors should be used if indicated.

(3) Give furosemide at a dosage of 100 mg. per hour I.V. to effect renal tubular rejection of calcium with sodium, and to hasten calcium excretion.

(4) If the response to the above measures is inadequate in reversing the hypercalcemic symptoms and signs, give 1.5 gm. of phosphate I.V. every six to eight hours. This can be repeated daily, although more than two infusions are rarely needed.

Alternatively, calcitonin (if available) can be infused at a rate of 0.2 mg./hr., or mithramycin can be given acutely as a single dose of 25 μg./kg. I.V.; both of these effect a rapid and life-saving fall in excessive serum calcium levels.

A 50 mg./kg. EDTA infusion (sodium ethylene diamine tetra-acetate) can be very effective, but should not be continued longer than 24 hours, since renal tubular damage may ensue. In less dire situations in which the calcium level is less than 15 to 16 mg. per cent, a trial of corticosteroid suppression can be both therapeutic and diagnostically helpful. 150 mg. of hydrocortisone or 40 mg. of prednisone are given daily for five to seven days. Dramatic suppression of calcium indicates sarcoidosis or vitamin D intoxication, in which corticosteroids block an excessive gut absorption of calcium. Mild suppression has been seen with malignancies, myeloma, leukemia, and lymphomas. Occasionally, the hypercalcemia of increased parathormone is reported to be lowered by corticosteroids. Generally, the effect is too slow to be useful in a real hypercalcemic emergency, and the other measures are preferable. Emergency parathyroidectomy should be reserved until the patient is rehydrated and stable and the diagnosis has been confirmed.

ACUTE ADRENAL INSUFFICIENCY

SUBJECTIVE

The patient with Addison's disease that has been exacerbated to crisis gives a history of chronic fatigue, anorexia with nausea and vomiting, severe nonspecific abdominal pain, weight loss, weakness, and giddiness on standing. The presentation of the patient will depend on the relative deficiencies of glucocorticoid and mineralocorticoid (Figs. 4 and 5).

OBJECTIVE

The patient in crisis has fever, tachycardia, and a thready pulse. The initial presentation may be of a person in shock, and previous subjective history may not be available. When obvious causes of shock are not present, adrenal insufficiency must be considered. Orthostatic hypotension may be marked.

Mucocutaneous pigmentation, especially in areas of friction, are a good clue to excess MSH (melanin stimulating hormone) like activity in patients whose primary adrenal failure results in high ACTH levels. Hypoglycemia, hyponatremia, hyperkalemia, and hypercalcemia are frequent findings. Calcification of the adrenals on x-ray may suggest either tuberculosis or the sites of old calcified adrenal hemorrhage. A small cardiac silhouette also is suggestive.

A. Inability to conserve sodium
    Decreased extracellular fluid volume
    Weight loss
    Hypovolemia
    Hypotension
    Decreased cardiac size
    Decreased cardiac output
    Decreased renal blood flow
    Prerenal azotemia
    Increased renin production
    Decreased pressor response to catecholamines
    Weakness
    Postural syncope
    Shock
B. Impaired renal secretion of potassium and hydrogen ions
    Hyperkalemia
      Cardiac asystole
    Mild acidosis

Figure 4 Manifestations of aldosterone deficiency. (From Williams, R. H.: Textbook of Endocrinology, 5th ed. Philadelphia, W. B. Saunders Co., 1974.)

---

1. *Gastrointestinal:* anorexia, nausea, vomiting, hypochlorhydria, abdominal pain, weight loss
2. *Mental:* diminished vigor, lethargy, apathy, confusion, psychosis
3. *Energy metabolism:* impaired gluconeogenesis, impaired fat mobilization and utilization, liver glycogen depletion, fasting hypoglycemia
4. *Cardiovascular-renal:* impaired ability to excrete "free water," impaired pressor responses to catecholamines, hypotension
5. *Pituitary:* unrestrained secretion of ACTH and MSH, resulting in mucocutaneous hyperpigmentation
6. *Impaired tolerance to stress:* any of the above manifestations might become more pronounced during trauma, infection, or fasting

---

Figure 5 Manifestations of cortisol deficiency. (From Williams, R. H.: Textbook of Endocrinology, 5th ed. Philadelphia, W. B. Saunders Co., 1974.)

ASSESSMENT

In the past, tuberculosis, especially of the gastrointestinal and urogenital tract, was complicated by adrenal involvement. Addison's crisis was seen in newborns with bilateral adrenal hemorrhage and in patients with overwhelming sepsis—the Waterhouse-Friderichsen syndrome.

The widespread use of corticosteroids in recent times for the treatment of nonendocrinologic diseases has produced a sizeable number of patients with suppressed pituitary-adrenal reserve who are candidates for addisonian crisis if faced with the stress of trauma, surgery, or infection. Similarly, patients who have had hypophysectomy, adrenalectomy, or radiation to these structures in order to treat malignant disease or severe diabetic retinopathy also are at risk. During nephrectomy, the adrenal may be damaged inadvertently and may prove to be the sole adrenal in that patient, resulting in postoperative adrenal crisis. It is important to note that, as in thyrotoxic storm and myxedema coma, the patient with untreated Addison's disease may be catapulted into crisis while he is undergoing catharsis for GI studies or other stressful diagnostic procedures.

PLAN

The following protocol has been designed to be life-saving and at the same time to allow for firm diagnosis retrospectively. The use of 10 to 20 mg. of dexamethasone raises the serum cortisol level by only 2 to 3 μg. and the urinary measurement of corticosteroids by two to 4 mg., so these determinations will reflect deficiencies despite therapy.

(1) Draw blood for plasma cortisol assay, electrolytes, and blood count.

(2) Start a rapid intravenous infusion of physiologic saline; add 4 mg. dexamethasone phosphate (1 ml. of the pharmaceutic solution), and 25 I.U. corticotropin. This first liter of saline with dexamethasone and corticotropin should be infused within the first hour.

(3) At the end of the infusion, draw a second 10-ml. specimen of blood for plasma cortisol assay.

(4) Administer additional 5 per cent dextrose in saline as rapidly and as long as indicated for treatment of dehydration and shock.

(5) Start a 24-hour urine collection for 17-OHCS assay or urinary-free cortisol.

(6) Inject I.M. 80 I.U. of corticotropin or 0.5 mg. of synthetic ACTH (Cortrosyn, 0.25 mg., equal to 25 I.U. ACTH). As an alternative, one might add corticotropin to each liter of intravenous saline, so that at least 3 I.U. are infused every hour for at least eight hours.

(7) Obtain a third blood specimen for plasma cortisol assay between the sixth and eighth hours of treatment with corticotropin.

With Addison's disease, there should be rapid improvement with saline and dexamethasone treatment. All plasma cortisols should be less than 15 μg per cent, including those after administration of corticotropin. If adrenal stimulation occurs, the diagnosis was faulty, and steroids can be withdrawn rapidly.

In acute adrenal crisis, the dehydration usually is equivalent to 20 per cent of the patient's extracellular volume. The sodium deficit cannot be replenished by giving mineralocorticoid alone, so it is mandatory to replenish saline—up to 3 liters in a few hours. A CVP line or Swan-Ganz catheter should be used to avoid overhydration and precipitation of pulmonary edema.

Florinef acetate, 0.1 mg. three times a day, may be used in conjunction with the glucocorticoid if hypotension continues to be significant despite rehydration and dexamethasone administration.

TETANY

SUBJECTIVE

The patient who suffers an acute fall in his serum calcium—notably the ionized fraction—complains of a sensation of numbness and tingling of the extremities, with a "pins and needles" sensation around the mouth, cramping of the limb muscles, and carpopedal spasm. In the severest form, wheezing, true laryngeal stridor, and convulsions occur. There are psychiatric symptoms ranging from emotional lability and irritability to hallucinations, delusions, and other psychotic manifestations.

OBJECTIVE

The Chvostek sign—twitching of the upper lip in response to tapping the homolateral facial nerve anterior to the ear—is positive, as is the Trousseau sign. To elicit the latter, circulation in the arm is impeded by inflating a blood pressure cuff sufficiently to occlude pulsations for at least three minutes; the test is positive if carpal spasm occurs.

If the patient has had longstanding hypoparathyroidism, there will be thin and patchy hair on the head, axillae, pubis, eyelids, etc.; deformed and brittle nails are common, often with candidal infestation. Cataracts and dental deformities and cavities occur, and the bone density is increased on x-ray. The serum calcium is measurably low unless hyperventilation is the cause of the tetany, in which case the calcium is normal. The Q-T interval on the EKG is prolonged.

ASSESSMENT

The most frequent cause of tetany in patients presenting to the Emergency Department is hyperventilation, with its resulting respiratory alkalosis. The high pH affects membrane excitability, and tetany is seen in the face of a normal serum calcium and phosphorus; it is easily treated by having the patient rebreathe into a paper bag, thereby returning his expired carbon dioxide. Alkali ingestion similarly can cause tetany.

Tetany caused by a true decrease in the ionizable fraction of serum calcium occurs most frequently in a patient whose parathyroids have been damaged or removed in the course of thyroidectomy. Any patient with a past history of neck surgery who presents with vague symptoms of cramps, cataracts, lethargy, and emotional symptoms should be suspect. Pseudohypoparathyroidism, hypocalcemia associated with the hypokalemic alkalosis of aldosteronism, rickets, or osteomalacia are less common. Multiple blood transfusions can also result in a rapid decrease in ionized calcium.

PLAN

(1) Examine the patient carefully for cataracts, thyroidectomy scar, Chvostek's and Trousseau's signs, and past history of similar episodes with emotional upset.

(2) Have the patient rebreathe into a bag and draw blood for calcium, phosphorus, and serum protein determinantions, remembering that serum calcium is mostly bound to albumin and can be artifactually low in the face of hypoalbuminemia.

(3) Infuse 10 cc. of a 10 per cent gluconate, lactate, or chloride solution. A poor response to treatment of hypocalcemia may signify hypomagnesemia, in which case magnesium must be replenished. The infusion may be repeated later by slow intravenous drip, watching the Q-T interval for salutary effect. Oral calcium should be substituted as early as possible. Long term therapy necessitates administration of vitamin D and calcium, but this is not required during the time of acute emergency.

HYPOMAGNESEMIA AND HYPERMAGNESEMIA

SUBJECTIVE

The problem of deficiency or excess of magnesium ion usually occurs in the context of treatment for other conditions, and is rarely the cause of presentation of a patient for emergency care. In infants whose only dietary constituent is milk, and in patients on long term intravenous therapy without magnesium replacement, deficiency may result. It also may occur in malabsorption syndrome, alcoholism, cirrhosis of the liver, renal tubular necrosis in the diuretic phase, hypercalciuria, diabetic acidosis, chronic diuretic therapy, acute pancreatitis, and inappropriate secretion of ADH. Calcium and

potassium deficiencies frequently occur concomitantly, the renal conservation of these cations being impaired with magnesium deficiency.

OBJECTIVE

Objectively, these ion derangements cause tremor, tetany, convulsions, hallucinations, emotional lability, EEG changes, and cardiac arrhythmias.

ASSESSMENT

In assessing the necessary ions to replace, it is well to remember that magnesium must be replenished along with calcium or potassium in a mixed deficiency, since treatment with calcium or potassium alone may precipitate seizures and cardiac arrest secondary to the increased neuromuscular reactivity of magnesium deficiency.

PLAN

Treatment of acute hypomagnesemia is effected by replenishing 50 mEq of magnesium sulfate I.V. The intramuscular route also can be used, with 2.5 ml. of a 50 per cent $MgSO_4 \cdot 7H_2O$ supplying 5 mM. of magnesium. The dosages are empiric, since the appearance and regression of clinical signs do not follow serum levels in a direct relationship. Orally, magnesium can be given as chloride, citrate, acetate, or oxide salts, but diarrhea may be a complication.

Magnesium excess occurs with renal failure, when patients with diminished creatinine clearance are given large amounts of magnesium-containing antacids or cathartics. The objective findings, apart from high serum magnesium levels, are hypotension, nausea and vomiting, CNS depression with hyporeflexia, coma, respiratory depression, and cardiac arrest.

The treatment is to infuse calcium and to perform hemodialysis if necessary.

References

Ashkar, F. S., Katims, R. B., Smoak, W. M., III, and Gilson, A. J.: Thyroid storm treatment with blood exchange and plasmapheresis. J.A.M.A. *214*:1275, 1970.
Bjorn, J. C., and Cross, H. D.: The Problem-Oriented Private Practice of Medicine. Chicago, Modern Hospital Press, 1970.

Das, G., and Krieger, M.: Treatment of thyrotoxic storm with intravenous administration of propranolol. Ann. Intern. Med. 70:985, 1969.

Dratman, M. B.: On the mechanism of action of thyroxin, an amino-acid analog of tyrosine. J. Theor. Biol. 46:255, 1974.

Dumlao, J. S.: Thyroid storm. Postgrad. Med. 56:57, 1974.

Harrison, T. R.: Principles of Internal Medicine. 7th ed. New York, McGraw-Hill Co., 1974.

Holvey, D. N., et al.: Treatment of myxedema coma with intravenous thyroxin. Arch. Intern. Med. 113:39, 1964.

Menendez, C. E., and Rivlin, R.: Thyrotoxic crisis and myxedema coma. Med. Clin. North Am. 57:1463, 1963.

Senior, R. M., et al.: The recognition and management of myxedema coma. J.A.M.A. 217:6, 1971.

Weed, L. L.: Medical Records, Medical Education and Patient Care. Cleveland, Ohio, Western Reserve University Press, 1969.

Williams, R. H.: Textbook of Endocrinology. 5th ed. Philadelphia, W. B. Saunders Co., 1974.

D. PORPHYRIAS

Barbara H. Greene

Porphyrias are a group of rare disorders characterized by a primary abnormality in the metabolism of the porphyrins or their precursors. Some of these disorders are hereditary, but a few appear to be acquired. The porphyrias are classified as *erythropoietic, hepatic* or of *mixed types*, depending on the site of accumulation of the abnormal metabolites. Precise diagnosis of each of the porphyrias is based on identification of these metabolites in the tissues, or on a characteristic pattern of excretion in the urine or feces.

A detailed description of the signs and symptoms of each porphyria is not appropriate in this discussion: the reader is referred to several excellent reviews for this information. It is most important to recognize this diagnostic possibility in the Emergency Department so that diagnostic tests can be initiated.

Most porphyrias have skin manifestations, usually photosensitivity. These porphyrias include congenital erythropoietic porphyria, erythropoietic protoporphyria, erythropoietic coproporphyria, cutanea tarda and cutanea tarda variegata, and hereditary coproporphyria. More will be said about these latter two conditions under the heading of "acute intermittent porphyria." The skin's reaction to sunlight may vary from a mild burning or itching to urticaria and edema; from vesiculation or bullae to crusting, scarring, atrophy, and frank mutilation. The most disabling forms of photosensitivity are found in congenital erythropoietic porphyria. Systemic involvement includes erythrodontia (pink teeth), splenomegaly and hemolytic anemia in congenital erythropoietic porphyria, cholelithiasis associated with erythropoietic protoporphyria and erythropoietic coproporphyria, and hepatic enlargement with cutanea tarda. Treatment consists of shielding from the sunlight with clothing or creams, antihistamines for solar urticaria, and phlebotomy in the case of cutanea tarda.

Of much greater significance to the emergency physician is acute intermittent porphyria. Usually occurring in young adults but also seen in the middle-aged, the disease may present with abdominal pain, dark urine (especially on standing), severe constipation, peripheral or central nervous system neuropathy, or psychic disorders. The skin is not involved. The disorder is hereditary and probably transmitted as a mendelian dominant. Abdominal pain usually is colicky, moderate to severe in intensity, and associated with vomiting, constipation, or diarrhea. Fever, leukocytosis, and tachycardia may accompany the pain and lead to the mistaken diagnosis of an acute surgical abdomen. Labile hypertension, postural hypotension, sweating, and peripheral vascular spasm also may occur, and these, like the abdominal pain, have been attributed to instability of the autonomic nervous system.

Acute neuropathy may be sensory or motor, and may range from neuritic pain in an extremity to paraplegia or complete flaccid quadriplegia. It can be mistaken for poliomyelitis, encephalitis, or lead or arsenic poisoning. The disease may leave permanent nervous system damage.

Central nervous system involvement may produce bulbar paralysis, hypothalamic dysfunction, seizures, hallucinations, and coma. Inappropriate antidiuretic hormone secretion can occur, resulting in hyponatremia. Respiratory paralysis is the leading cause of death in acute intermittent porphyria. Psychiatric disorders range from vague neurotic complaints to organic brain syndrome, depression, and psychosis.

The diagnosis of acute intermittent porphyria is based on the demonstration of porphobilinogen in the urine. The qualitative technique of Watson-Schwartz should be supported by chromatography. Less frequently, porphyria cutanea tarda variegata and hereditary coproporphyrinuria present in a similar fashion. However, these latter two porphyrias may have a history of photosensitivity with skin involvement.

TREATMENT

Symptomatic treatment consists of opiates such as meperidine (Demerol) or the ganglioplegic drugs such as tetraethylammonium for the relief of pain. Chlorpromazine may be particularly helpful in relieving the abdominal pain. Chloral hydrate and paraldehyde may be used for sedation. Neostigmine is useful for the relief of constipation. Supportive therapy consists of correction of hyponatremia secondary to vomiting or inappropriate ADH secretion, respiratory support where necessary, and the early institution of physiotherapy. A diet high in glucose intravenously or orally is recommended to diminish the induction of delta-aminolevulinic acid synthetase. Prevention of further attacks is extremely important. A high carbohydrate diet is appropriate as mentioned above. Since menstrual periods and pregnancy may precipitate an acute attack, oral contraception also seems indicated in attacks temporally related to menses. The ingestion of various drugs also may precipitate an acute attack. Incriminated drugs are barbiturates, sulfonamides, griseofulvin, meprobamate, diphenylhydantoin, glutethimide, and chlordiazepoxide hydrochloride. The efficacy of these preventive measures and other therapeutic programs is very difficult to evaluate, as the disease may be latent for many years between attacks, and acute attacks may resolve spontaneously.

References

Goldberg, A.: Acute intermittent porphyria. Q. J. Med. New Series 28:110, 183, 1959.

Maruers, H. S.: The Porphyrias. In Stanbury, J. B., et al. (eds.): The Metabolic Basis of Inherited Disease. 3d ed. New York, Blakiston Division, McGraw Hill Book Co., 1972, p. 1087.

Tschudy, D. P.: Porphyrin Metabolism and the Porphyrias. In Bondy, P. K., et al. (eds.): Duncan's Diseases of Metabolism. 7th ed. Philadelphia, W. B. Saunders Co., 1974, p. 775.

Tschudy, D. P., et al.: Acute intermittent porphyria: Clinical and selected research aspects. Ann. Intern. Med. 83:851–864, 1975.

Waldenström, J.: The porphyrias as inborn errors of metabolism. Am. J. Med. 22:758, 1957.

E. PHEOCHROMOCYTOMA

Barbara H. Greene

Pheochromocytomas are rare catecholamine-producing tumors, arising most commonly from the chromaffin cells of the adrenal medulla, but also found in other sites of this neural crest-derived tissue. These tumors usually are detected around the fourth decade of life, but are seen also in children or in the elderly; they may be benign or malignant.

The tumors may be familial, in which case they have been associated with neurofibromatosis, hemangioblastomas of the central nervous system, medullary carcinoma of the thyroid gland, and other forms of neoplasia of the endocrine system. Elevated urinary levels of vanillylmandelic acid, metanephrine, and/or catecholamines establish the diagnosis.

CLINICAL PRESENTATIONS

The symptoms are a result of circulating catecholamines, and include palpitations, headache, flushing, diaphoresis, postural hypotension, and weight loss in association with paroxysmal or sustained hypertension.

THE ACUTE HYPERTENSIVE CRISIS

This may be precipitated by exercise, pressure on or palpation of the tumor, anesthesia, monamine oxidase-inhibiting drugs, surgery, ingestion of tyramine-containing compounds (notably cheddar cheese), and, rarely, by micturition when the tumor is located in the bladder wall.

COMPLICATIONS

Acute or sustained hypertension may lead to advanced retinopathy, renal disease, encephalopathy, cardiomyopathy with failure, pulmonary edema, cardiac arrhythmias, and death.

TREATMENT

Surgical removal of the tumor is the definitive therapy.

Medical management is aimed at the control of: (1) systemic arterial hypertension and its complications; (2) cardiac arrhythmias, prior to surgery or in patients with metastatic tumor; and (3) control or prevention of intraoperative hypotension following removal of the tumor, and control of intraoperative arrhythmias.

Treatment of Acute Hypertensive Emergencies.* An alpha-adrenergic blocking agent, such as phentolamine hydrochloride (Regitine), may be given intravenously, 2 to 5 mg. every five minutes, until blood pressure control is achieved. Thereafter, 2 to 5 mg. I.V. every two to four hours may be given to maintain control of blood pressure. Phenoxybenzamine hydrochloride (Dibenzyline), a long acting adrenergic blocking agent for oral use, may be used for long term control of hypertension, in preparation for

---

*See Chapter 42C.

surgery, or in the patient with metastatic tumor. An initial daily dose of 20 to 30 mg. (as a single or divided dose) may be increased by 10 to 20 mg. a day until blood pressure control is achieved and mild orthostatic hypotension is observed. A daily dose of 40 to 100 mg. usually is required. Drug therapy should be maintained until the day of surgery. Intraoperative hypertension should be controlled with phentolamine, as described above.

Treatment of Arrhythmias. Propranolol hydrochloride (Inderal), 1 to 2 mg. I.V., is given over a five- to ten-minute period for the control of severe sinus tachycardia, or atrial or ventricular arrhythmias. Constant monitoring of heart rate and rhythm is necessary. Oral propranolol, 20 to 40 mg. every six hours, usually will suffice in the long term control of these arrhythmias. Intraoperative arrhythmias also are managed with intravenous propranolol.

Intraoperative Hypotension. This condition, which is the result of chronically decreased intravascular volume, may be minimized by avoiding preoperative sodium restriction and by careful preoperative control of hypertension with Dibenzyline. The condition should be reversed by prompt intravenous administration of volume expanders in the form of saline, whole blood, plasma, or 5 per cent albumin and saline, with careful monitoring of central venous pressure and systemic arterial blood pressure.

References

Himathongkam, T., et al.: Pheochromocytoma. J.A.M.A. *230*:1692, 1974.
Levine, R. J., et al.: Catecholamines and the Adrenal Medulla. Pheochromocytoma. *In* Bondy, P. K., et al. (eds.): Duncan's Diseases of Metabolism. 7th ed. Philadelphia, W. B. Saunders Co., 1974, p. 1203.
Melmon, K. L.: Catecholamines and the Adrenal Medulla. *In* Williams, R. H.: Textbook of Endocrinology. 5th ed. Philadelphia, W. B. Saunders Co., 1974, p. 283.
Sjoerdsma, A. S., et al.: Pheochromocytoma: current concepts of diagnosis and treatment. Ann. Intern. Med. *65*:1302, 1966.

Chapter 47

NONTRAUMATIC GENITOURINARY EMERGENCIES

Lester Karafin
and A. Richard Kendall

URINARY RETENTION

ETIOLOGY

The physiologic act of micturition is taken for granted by all human beings until there is some disturbance in function. The actual inability to void is most often the final event, but is preceded by years of symptomatology such as hesitancy, dribbling, and a poor stream. However, men, women, and children can present in the Emergency Department with a complete inability to void, usually accompanied by abdominal discomfort—or the condition may be of the "silent" variety, so that the individual just gives a history of not voiding over the past 12 to 24 hours.

A detailed history will help delineate the actual cause. In the case of the adult male, a history of a previous urethral stricture with passage of sounds is a good clue that the retention may be due to a urethral stricture. The patient may state that he has had prostate gland trouble for some time with such signs and symptoms of obstruction as hesitancy and dribbling. He may state that he has had a growth in his prostate with hormone therapy and an operation on his scrotum (bilateral orchiectomy for carcinoma of the prostate). Clot retention may occur with hematuria secondary to a bladder tumor, prostatism, or upper tract disease. Neurogenic bladder disease usually is apparent and is associated with such other marked neurologic abnormalities as a cerebral vascular accident or chronic neurologic disease. However, we have seen acute urinary retention as the only presenting sign of multiple sclerosis. Medications (antihistamines) or parasympatholytic drugs (e.g., Banthine) may produce acute urinary retention. In children, such congenital anomalies as a urethral valve or a meatal stenosis can actually produce complete urinary retention. Finally in the differential diagnosis, hysterical retention may be seen in a young female. Foreign bodies (self-inserted) or bladder calculi that obstruct the vesical neck are much rarer causes of this problem.

DIAGNOSIS

Physical examination usually will reveal a large globular mass above the symphysis extending up to the umbilicus. It is amazing how many times an abdominal mass can disappear on simple insertion of a urethral catheter. Rectal examination may reveal a benign enlarged prostate or the typical stony-hard, irregular enlargement of carcinoma of the prostate. A normal-feeling prostate on rectal examination does not preclude prostatism as a cause of urinary retention. The absolute diagnosis as well as part of the initial management is made by passage of a small No. 16 or 18 urethral catheter. If the instrument passes easily through the urethra, stricture would be ruled out, and if a large amount of urine is obtained the diagnosis of urinary retention is made. Emptying the bladder via catheter and evacuating more than several hundred cc. of urine followed by disappearance of the abdominal mass makes an absolute diagnosis of urinary retention.

1091

MANAGEMENT

Nonoperative management is by the use of urethral catheters of one type or another. There are many factors to be considered in instrumentation. Initially we should use an aseptic technique, since the obstructed bladder provides a fertile field for bacterial growth. The genitalia should be washed thoroughly with soap and water or pHisoHex solution and an antiseptic sponge placed on the urethra, either on the glans or the vulva. Bacteria always are present in the urethra, and external cleansing will not preclude the possibility of introduction of bacteria.

Both the catheter and the urethra should be adequately lubricated. Ordinarily it is sufficient to lubricate the catheter with one of the tubes of water soluble jellies in use at the present time. Urethral catheterization should be done gently, without force. We are convinced that the discomfort experienced in a urethral catheterization is similar to that in a rectal examination when the examiner attempts to force his finger through the anal sphincter. Therefore, if the doctor forces a catheter through the urethral sphincter it will cause a great deal of discomfort. Instilling lubricant directly into the penis is helpful. Asking the patient to attempt to urinate on catheterization can be an aid, and in a patient with an enlarged prostate simply inserting your finger in the rectum and directing the tip over the median lobe while someone else inserts the catheter can be helpful. A soft rubber catheter should be used routinely. The calibration most often used is the French scale in which each number equals .33 mm. Thus a No. 30 French sound has a diameter of 10 mm. A No. 16 or 18 soft rubber catheter is the one used most often for diagnostic purposes, as this size should pass in the absence of a stricture. We believe that it is a mistake to attempt to pass anything smaller than a No. 16 French catheter in adult males as smaller sizes frequently lack the necessary stiffness and are apt to coil in the urethra. A No. 18 Foley is probably the best catheter to choose when you suspect urinary retention because it will not make it necessary to catheterize an individual twice.

If you are unable to pass the catheter and the area of hold-up is not in the urethra but back at the prostate, the next step is to use your finger in the rectum as described previously or to select a coudé catheter, which has a curved tip at the end that allows the catheter to slide over the median lobe of the prostate.

If this approach is unsuccessful, a lubricated catheter stylet placed within the lumen of the catheter before insertion can be used if it is a familiar instrument to the operator and he is careful in insertion. The technique is similar to that used in passing a sound, but we would caution again that it should be done only by those experienced in its use. A filiform and following sound will be described later in this chapter, and might be a safer instrument to use in this situation. The catheter is inserted like a sound, the stylet is removed, and the catheter remains in the bladder. The danger is perforation of the urethra or the bladder by the rigid instrument. If a Foley cannot be inserted, a straight rubber catheter can be placed and taped to the penis. It is important to allow for expansion of the penis and not to use tape around its entire circumference.

In the presence of a urethral stricture, filiforms and following sounds are indicated. The filiforms are made of woven silk-plastic material and come in sizes 3 to 6 French. There are various types of tips available, with a corkscrew or coudé being quite useful. The other end of the filiform is equipped with a female thread so that a following metal or woven catheter can be used from sizes 8 to 30. These catheters can be solid or hollow so that drainage can occur. Filiforms are inserted into the bladder, using two or three since some go into the false passages. It takes some experience to be certain that the filiform is completely within the bladder. Then the following sound is screwed on and dilatation of the urethral stricture is done in a progressive manner. Regular metal sounds without these filiforms are commonly used, chiefly in large caliber strictures. Sounds are curved at the end and come in sizes from 8 to 30 French. It is better to start with a sound about No. 22 so that the broad tip will not perforate the urethral wall. If it is necessary to use a size smaller than No. 20, it is better to use a filiform. Once the sound is introduced and reaches the external sphincter, the handle is brought down to a vertical position, which enables the sound to pass.

Occasionally the panendoscope is used

in order to find the way into a very tortuous urethra that resists all forms of catheterization.

Operative management is required when the urethra cannot be traversed and retention is not relieved. A suprapubic catheter can be inserted under local or field block anesthesia by direct visualization of the bladder and insertion of a large mushroom or Foley catheter from above. The Campbell punch cystotomy instrument can be used in the Emergency Department only if the bladder is definitely palpable. This allows the insertion of a No. 18 Foley through a trocar. The use of an Intracath inserted by suprapubic needle puncture is a temporary measure of suprapubic diversion that can be used for a period of up to 24 hours, but usually either pulls out or plugs in a relatively short time.

OLIGURIA AND ANURIA

ETIOLOGY

When the catheter is inserted as described in the previous section and either no urine or small quantities of urine are obtained, the possible diagnosis of supravesical blockage by ureteral obstruction or renal and prerenal disease must be considered. When the catheter is allowed to remain indwelling and the urinary output is so low that metabolites cannot be excreted, the patient must be said to be in a state of *oliguria*. The usual definition of the oliguric state is that a patient excretes less than 500 cc. of urine a day, but this is only applicable in one whose urine concentration approaches 1040 milliosmols. Another patient whose urine concentration is only 1006 milliosmols may be oliguric when he excretes more than 1000 cc. of urine.

The etiology of oliguria can be organic or can be due to renal lesions such as acute tubular necrosis, to severe fluid and electrolyte imbalance, or to a urinary tract obstruction such as bilateral ureteral calculi. The diagnosis of the first two problems usually is apparent in that the patient may have been through a period of shock or exposure to toxic chemicals or may be markedly dehydrated. The possibilities of bilateral obstructive disease from metastatic tumor, bilateral calculi, retroperitoneal fibrosis, or iatrogenic occlusion during gynecologic surgery must be considered. Cystoscopic examination and an attempt at bilateral ureteral catheterization should be done immediately to rule out the possibility of obstruction. Prior to instrumentation, a high-dose infusion pyelogram should be attempted. This may rule out obstruction, making instrumentation unnecessary. If obstruction is ruled out by the above procedures, the diagnosis is most likely a renal or a prerenal condition.

MANAGEMENT

Acute tubular necrosis most commonly occurs after shock, blood transfusions, or exposure to chemicals. Good management requires that fluid intake be limited, electrolytes corrected, and medical therapy instituted.

PHYSIOLOGIC IMBALANCES CAUSING OLIGURIA

Most commonly, poor renal output is caused by severe dehydration. Treatment is the administration of fluids, rather than restriction as in acute tubular necrosis. Oliguria also can be caused by diminished renal blood flow, as in cardiac failure and relative hypotension in normally hypertensive patients. Treatment is directed at the restoration of blood pressure. Uremia is a syndrome characterized by disturbances of electrolyte balance and retention of nitrogenous and other metabolic end-products. It is reversible when caused by decreased renal blood flow, dehydration, acute tubular necrosis, or urinary tract obstruction; but it is irreversible when due to destruction of the kidney itself. The serum creatinine rises with elevation of serum phosphate, sulfate, and other acid radicals, in turn producing a metabolic acidosis. The electrolyte abnormalities are hyperkalemia, hyponatremia, hypocalcemia, and hyperchloremia. Clinically the patient usually presents with markedly elevated creatinine and BUN and with electrolyte abnormalities. Weakness, drowsiness, and lethargy with generalized pruritus and uremic frosting may ensue. Coma can occur. Treatment is directed at the underlying cause, such as obstruction and dehydration.

INDICATIONS FOR DIALYSIS

Peritoneal dialysis can be used in all hospitals and in all patients except those with abdominal wounds or intestinal adhesions. Indications are:

(1) Uremic coma.
(2) Pericardial friction rub.
(3) Bleeding diathesis.
(4) Potassium intoxication.
(5) Blood urea nitrogen of 125 mg. per 100 ml. or over.
(6) Clinical deterioration.
(7) Severe infection.

ACIDOSIS

Metabolic acidosis is present in uremia. There is a decreased renal tubule excretion of ammonium and a retention of organic acids that may lead to a blood pH as low as 7.0. Thus, acidosis and Kussmaul breathing may present in the Emergency Department. The urine may have a pH of 5 to 5.5. Treatment is by sodium bicarbonate or one-sixth molar lactate I.V.

POTASSIUM INTOXICATION

Protein catabolism and metabolic acidosis increase extracellular potassium concentration. Elevated potassium is the leading cause of death in acute renal failure because of its cardiac toxicity. The diagnosis is made by EKG and must be treated promptly if there is an abnormality. Emergency Department treatment of potassium intoxication is by counterbalancing the effect of potassium ionically and effecting the removal of potassium. An intravenous infusion of 200 ml. of 3 per cent sodium chloride solution or 88 mEq. of sodium bicarbonate will reverse the potassium-induced conduction defects within 10 to 30 minutes. This only lasts several hours, and the use of cation exchange resins administered through retention enemas will help. The retention enemas at two-hour intervals, each containing 60 gm. of sodium polystyrene sulfonate (Kayexalate), will remove 10 to 50 mEq. of potassium per enema. Glucose and insulin infusions to bind potassium with glycogen in hepatic cells can be used, but carry greater hazards. If the potassium cannot be removed, dialysis should be resorted to.

CALCIUM INTOXICATION

Hypercalcemia is an infrequent complication of urologic problems. It may be seen in chronic renal failure with recurrent stone disease, and is a manifestation of renal cell carcinoma and other malignant tumors. It is also seen in hyperparathyroidism. The patients present with gastrointestinal symptoms with neurologic signs and symptoms and may become comatose. The treatment is by infusion of:

(1) Saline—adequate hydration is critical.

(2) Sodium sulfate continuously at the rate of 1 liter every three to six hours—no more effective than above.

(3) Corticosteroids in doses of 500 mg. every eight hours will lower serum calcium.

(4) Phosphate intravenously—500 cc of .1 molar solution of sodium phosphate and monopotassium phosphate over six to eight hours.

(5) EDTA is a powerful chelating agent, but there has been severe renal tubule damage noted with its use.

(6) Mithramycin is an actinomycin D-like antitumor agent that has a consistent hypocalcemic effect. It also causes a fall in urinary calcium. Apparently it blocks the peripheral action of the parathyroid on gut and bone, either by direct action or by making the patient vitamin D resistant.

(7) Calcitonin has been used with patients with hypercalcemia due to hyperparathyroidism and vitamin D intoxication.

(8) Cellulose phosphate may be given orally and can reduce serum calcium.

DYSURIA, PYURIA, AND SEPSIS

The urologic patient may present in the Emergency Department with severe burning and frequency of urination, with or without associated chills and fever. Urinalysis most often reveals pyuria and bacteriuria on staining or culture. This is a very common presenting symptom of many problems in the urinary tract.

The usual etiology is gram-negative rods (*E. coli, Proteus vulgaris*) and, occasionally, gram-positive cocci (Staphylococcus and Streptococcus). This is distinguished from such diseases as tuberculosis, gonorrhea, and actinomycosis. Occasionally Aerobacter, *Pseudomonas aeruginosa*, and *Streptococcus faecalis* are found.

ACUTE PYELONEPHRITIS

Clinically the patient will present with severe flank or back pain with associated chills and fever. At the same time such symptoms of lower urinary tract infection as frequency, nocturia, urgency, and dysuria occur. There may be associated gastrointestinal symptoms. The patient usually is quite ill with a great deal of tenderness over the affected kidney. Leukocytosis may occur with a shift to the left. The urine will show large numbers of pus cells and bacteria, but hematuria can also occur. A stained urinary sediment will reveal bacteria when the count is significant. The differential diagnosis includes any intraabdominal disease, such as pancreatitis, basal pneumonia, acute appendicitis, acute diverticulitis, and herpes zoster.

Management is supportive, with fluids, rest, and antibiotic therapy. The culture should be done, but the patient can be started immediately on one of the broad spectrum drugs such as ampicillin, 2 gm. per day in divided doses. The medication should be continued for at least seven to ten days, but can be cut down to 250 mg. four times a day once a clinical response occurs, usually by the second day. In 48 to 72 hours the patient is asymptomatic unless there is obstructive uropathy or stasis present.

A specific etiology, such as urinary retention or a calculus, must be ruled out by intravenous urogram within a reasonable period of time after the onset of the illness. These patients often may be managed on an ambulatory basis. The need for hospitalization depends on how ill they are clinically. Obviously the patients who are severely ill must be admitted to the hospital. This subject of gram-negative septicemia is treated elsewhere in this textbook. Obstructive uropathy must be ruled out in this clinical picture. Therefore, if the patient is in retention, he must have a catheter inserted, and if calculus disease is causing an obstruction, this must be determined and overcome. Obviously if there is a perinephric abscess, it must be drained.

Simple, uncomplicated acute pyelonephritis usually responds extremely well to therapy. Admission to the hospital is necessary only in the situation where you may be dealing with a perinephric abscess or gram-negative septicemia or in a patient who is not maintaining his vasomotor system and in those patients who cannot retain oral feedings. It is important to follow these patients to make sure that their urine clears and that they have no further bacteriuria. In all infections of the urinary tract cultures are necessary to detect resistant organisms.

Gram-negative septicemia with shock is an emergency. The shock usually is caused either by cardiac failure with an inadequate blood volume or by an enlargement of the vascular space. The patient is clouded mentally when the systolic blood pressure falls below 80 mm. Hg. Treatment should be aimed at combating the underlying cause, treating the infection, restoring the blood volume, and improving the cardiac output and perfusion. A urethral catheter is placed not only to monitor the flow but also to find out whether the patient is in retention. A central venous pressure catheter is inserted, and the patient should be treated vigorously with antibiotics (gentamicin and Keflin is one effective combination) in appropriate dosages by body weight. Cortisone in large doses of 1 to 2 gm. should be used and repeated periodically, I.V. fluids must be given in amounts determined by venous pressure readings, and the patient must be admitted to the hospital for other supportive measures. The mortality rate is still around 50 per cent, although this may be improving with increased supportive measures and earlier treatment.

RENAL CARBUNCLE

This is an abscess occurring in the periphery of the kidney, and usually is due to staphylococci. The findings are similar to those in acute pyelonephritis, but the urinalysis may be negative except for occasional showers of bacteria. Treatment is by antibiotics, and, if the presence of an abscess is established, drainage is necessary.

PERINEPHRIC ABSCESS

There may be a history of prolonged recurrent urinary tract infection or there may be a history of a skin infection a few weeks before the onset of symptoms. The febrile response can be either high or low grade, there is marked tenderness over the kidney, and a large mass may be felt or percussed. X-ray findings show the diaphragm on the involved side to be high, and the kidney does not move on respiration. There is obliteration of the psoas shadow. Because of spasm, scoliosis occurs in the spine, with concavity to the affected side. Treatment is by antibiotics and drainage.

ACUTE CYSTITIS AND PROSTATITIS

Cystitis is much more common in the female than in the male and usually occurs by ascent of bacteria from the urethra. Symptoms are burning on urination, with urgency often to the point of incontinence. Frequency, nocturia, and occasionally hematuria (usually terminal) are also present. Fever is not usually associated with cystitis. The symptoms may follow sexual activity in women. In men, the infection may be secondary to prostatism.

Examination does not reveal any specific findings, although the bladder may be tender suprapubically. The urinalysis does reveal pyuria and bacilluria. In the differential diagnosis of acute cystitis, the female urethral syndrome must be considered when the urinalysis is negative. Allergic responses, stones, and neoplasms of the bladder may produce cystitis-like symptoms.

Treatment is usually by drugs, such as nitrofurantoin or the sulfonamides. If these do not work within 48 hours, a culture should be used to ascertain the organism and sensitivities. A culture prior to institution of therapy should be obtained but it is not necessary to wait for results. Symptomatic measures, such as increased fluid intake, warm tub baths, and antispasmodics, can be used. In women, the first episode does not require a complete urologic work-up.

Acute prostatitis in the male does occur and usually is associated with an acute cystitis. The diagnosis is made when rectal examination reveals a very tender prostatic bed. Moderate to high fever is usual, and WBCs are in the prostatic fluid. The patient may go into urinary retention. The treatment is by antibiotics. Initial therapy can be with a sulfa combination such as Septra or with a tetracycline antibiotic. Instrumentation is contraindicated. If there is a frank abscess, drainage is necessary. General measures such as bed rest and plenty of fluids are indicated. Chronic prostatitis is mentioned only to condemn this "wastebasket" diagnosis for several psychosomatic ills that too many physicians place in the realm of chronic prostatitis.

ACUTE URETHRITIS (NONGONOCOCCAL)

The patient may present himself in the Emergency Department with a urethral discharge associated with burning and frequency of urination. The leading symptom is a urethral discharge. There may be itching or a burning sensation in the urethra. The discharge should be examined, stained, and cultured. Many times the condition is a nonspecific urethritis and prostatitis. Once again, treatment is by antimicrobial therapy. The new Trimethoprim-sulfonamide combination seems to be the drug of choice. Tetracyclines and erythromycin also are effective.

ACUTE EPIDIDYMITIS

In acute epididymitis the patient presents with a very swollen, tender enlargement of the scrotum, frequently following a severe physical strain, urethral instrumentation, or prostatectomy. The pain develops suddenly in the scrotum, radiating along the spermatic cord. It is severe and is accompanied by a high temperature. The swelling may be rapid, causing the organ to become two to three times its normal size. On examination there is tenderness along the spermatic cord and the scrotum is enlarged. The overlying skin may be reddened and, if seen quite early, the enlarged epididymis may be palpable. The differential diagnosis will be discussed later under masses of the scrotum. Treatment is antibiotic therapy, bed rest, and support to the scrotum. The acute epididymitis resolves within one to two weeks, but the epididymis may take four to six weeks to return to normal size.

ACUTE ORCHITIS

The testicle may become inflamed from a hematogenous source, such as a virus. Mumps orchitis can occur associated with mumps parotitis. The clinical findings are approximately the same as for epididymitis. The treatment once again is antibiotics, bed rest, and support.

General Remarks Concerning Treatment of Urinary Tract Infections

The goals of treatment in urinary tract infection are symptomatic relief, clearing of the bacteriuria, return of normal function to avoid sequelae, and, finally, prevention of recurrences. Ancillary methods of treatment of urinary tract infection are to increase oral fluids; adjust the urinary pH to a more acid state; restrict activity; and treat the associated fever, pain, dysuria, and bladder spasm. The ideal antibiotic is one that is effective across a wide antibacterial spectrum, rarely leads to development of resistance, and is effective for either short or long term use and for acute or chronic infection. It should be safe, with no toxicity, no side-effects, and no allergic reactions. It has to be accepted by patients, and it should be oral (a small tablet or capsule) and have no objectionable odor or taste. Few doses per day should be required, and the drug should be inexpensive and readily available. Appropriate antibiotics during pregnancy would be nitrofurantoin, ampicillin, penicillin, or sulfonamides in the first two trimesters. The antibiotics not to use during pregnancy would be streptomycin, chloramphenicol, sulfonamides in the third trimester, and tetracycline—particularly after the fourth month of the pregnancy. The appropriate antibiotic in renal failure would be ampicillin, cephalosporin, penicillin, nalidixic acid, sulfonamides (if urinary output is over 1000 cc. per day), and reduced dosages of gentamicin and kanamycin. Remember that there is a normal defense mechanism consisting of the bladder wash-out immunoglobulins, urea, acid urine, and intrinsic antibacterial substances.

ANTIMICROBIAL DRUGS

SULFONAMIDES

The soluble sulfonamides are bacteriostatic, have a wide spectrum, are inexpensive, and cause very few side-effects. They are an excellent first line of drugs where the patient is not excessively toxic. The newer combination with Trimethoprim allows for better tissue penetration, particularly in urethritis and prostatitis.

PENICILLIN

The penicillins are bactericidal. Ampicillin is a broad spectrum drug which has excellent activity against E. coli and Proteus and is the choice for infections caused by Streptococcus faecalis. It can be used in doses of 250 to 500 mg. every six hours.

CEPHALOSPORINS

These are semisynthetic drugs that are bactericidal against E. coli and Proteus.

They are ineffective against Pseudomonas and Proteus vulgaris. These drugs can be used intravenously, and cephalexin is an effective oral cephalosporin. The dosage is 250 to 500 mg. every six hours. Those patients allergic to penicillin may also be allergic to the cephalosporins (with approximately 10% cross-reactivity).

TETRACYCLINES AND CHLORAMPHENICOL

Tetracyclines are bacteriostatic agents. They may be used for gram-negative and coccal infections in dosages of 250 to 500 mg. every six hours.

Chloramphenicol is an excellent bacteriostatic antibacterial drug, but should be reserved for patients with serious infections unresponsive to other agents. Aplastic anemia is a side-effect of chloramphenicol and a potentially dangerous one.

STREPTOMYCIN

Streptomycin is a bactericidal drug that can sterilize the urine rapidly, but because of its toxicity it is rarely used.

COLYMYCIN AND KANAMYCIN

Colymycin and kanamycin are bactericidal drugs particularly useful against Pseudomonas aeruginosa, but both agents are nephrotoxic and cause deafness and skin rash. They should be used only to combat the most serious infections.

GENTAMICIN

Gentamicin is a drug similar to kanamycin and is particularly useful in severe infections caused by E. coli, Proteus, and Klebsiella.

NITROFURANTOINS (MACRODANTIN)

In the area of urinary antiseptics, nitrofurantoin is an excellent drug to be used in nonserious infections. Dosage is 50 to 100 mg. four times a day. It is not effective against Pseudomonas. Instances of allergic pneumonitis have been reported.

METHENAMINE (MANDELAMINE)

Methenamine with organic acid (Mandelamine) is an old drug that is useful in the treatment of some cases of urinary tract infection. The urine must be acid. The dosage is 1 gm. four times a day, and the agent is used in nonserious disease. It may be useful in long term prolonged suppressive therapy.

NALIDIXIC ACID (NEGRAM)

Nalidixic acid is effective against gram-negative rods, except Pseudomonas. It is an excellent drug, but does have some toxic side-effects, such as skin rash, nausea, drowsiness, photophobia, and, rarely, convulsions.

HEMATURIA

A patient presenting in the Emergency Department with the complaint of bloody urine is both quite common and important to evaluate. The initial problem is to determine whether the condition is truly blood in the urine. In the female, it may be a bloody vaginal discharge; in the male, bleeding can be from varices on the scrotum or a bloody urethral discharge.

A history in the female usually will reveal that the bleeding occurred spontaneously and was not associated with urination if it is vaginal bleeding. However, women are not used to looking at their urinary stream while they are voiding, and may find it difficult to tell from where the blood is coming. In the male, spontaneous bleeding from varices on the scrotum can occur, and the patient awakes with blood on his pajamas. Hematospermia will be discussed in a different section. The history is important to determine whether the patient has had a prostatectomy within the last several weeks, whether urination is painful, and if blood was seen throughout the entire urinary stream.

Of course, if the patient has renal colic, this would certainly suggest bleeding from the upper tracts secondary to a calculus. However, a clot from a renal tumor can cause the same type of pain. It is always important to consider that hematuria may be due to a tumor of the bladder or the kidney, particularly when it is unassociated with other complaints. The fact that bleeding may stop and not return cannot be used as an excuse to forget about it. Initial hematuria suggests an anterior urethral lesion. Terminal hematuria usually arises from the posterior urethra, bladder neck, or trigone. Total hematuria is usually from the upper tracts or bladder.

Remember that all red urine is not necessarily hematuria. Certain individuals will pass red urine after eating beets or taking laxatives like phenolphthalein, and there are coloring agents in foods that can cause red urine. Hemoglobinuria can occur in hemolytic syndromes.

MANAGEMENT

Post-Prostatectomy or Urethral Manipulation Bleeding. It is common to see hematuria approximately ten days to two weeks after a prostatectomy. This may be minimal, and usually subsides spontaneously. However, the patient's bleeding may be severe enough to cause clot retention, and he will become uncomfortable and present himself at the Emergency Department. Management is by insertion of an adequate sized Foley catheter (No. 24 to 26 and either a 5-cc. or 30-cc. bag). The bladder is emptied and irrigated copiously with a large amount of fluid, using a Toomy irrigating syringe, until all clots are removed from the bladder. If the irrigations then become crystal clear, the patient may be sent home with or without his catheter. However, if the irrigations continue to be bloody, the patient should be kept in the hospital for continued observation. Bleeding usually persists only a day or two and clears spontaneously. Rarely will a patient have to be taken back to the operating room for hemostasis in delayed postoperative bleeding. Bleeding can also occur after instrumentation, as in a cystoscopy, where dilated veins over an enlarged prostate can rupture and bleed. This is easily handled by insertion of a Foley catheter. A hemoglobin test should be made to establish that the patient has not lost a lot more blood than you think and may need replacement. If there is any question of shock, the patient should not be sent home.

Bleeding Associated With Renal Colic

The diagnosis is most likely a ureteral calculus but could be a piece of tumor, and the patient should be evaluated for any anatomic problems. If the gross hematuria is not severe, the patient does not have to be hospitalized, and studies can be carried out on an outpatient basis. If renal colic is found, its management is discussed under stone disease.

Bleeding Associated with Cystitis

Bleeding will frequently occur associated with burning and signs and symptoms of cystitis. This infection can be bacterial or viral. The bleeding can be profuse, but is easily diagnosed by the associated signs and symptoms of bladder infection. As long as the patient is emptying his bladder adequately, there is no need for catheterization. The treatment is that as for cystitis. Complete urologic evaluation is indicated, including intravenous pyelogram and cystoscopy, but after control of symptoms.

Sickle Cell Disease

Sickle cell trait can be associated with hematuria and usually is of the total, painless variety. Depending on the degree and severity of bleeding, the patient may or may not have to be hospitalized. Remember that this type of bleeding is intermittent and can originate from either side. On some reported occasions bleeding has been so severe that the patient required hospitalization and transfusion, and in life-threatening situations even nephrectomy has been considered. However, the warning that bleeding in sickle cell disease may originate from either side must be considered if surgery is ever considered.

Drug-Induced Hematuria

Some of the drugs used in the treatment of blood dyscrasias (e.g., Cytoxan) cause a chemical cystitis that may produce a great deal of bleeding. This may be prevented by increased fluids and alkalinization of urine. Catheterization may be needed if the patient is unable to urinate, but otherwise use supportive management only. Heparin and Dicumarol frequently cause microscopic hematuria. When there is gross hematuria, urologic evaluation must be performed. The yield of urologic pathologic studies has been significant, making them well worth doing.

Bleeding Secondary to Radiation Cystitis

Patients with carcinoma of the cervix or carcinoma of the bladder or prostate who have received irradiation may develop radiation cystitis with severe bleeding. The situation is most distressful, the patient requiring hospitalization with bladder irrigations via catheter until the bleeding subsides. It has at times been necessary to go as far as cystectomy to control this bleeding. Formaldehyde and fulguration have been suggested.

Carcinoma of the Prostate

Carcinoma of the prostate may present with gross hematuria. This finding is not uncommon in association with neoplasms of the prostate, and once again must be treated as previously described, depending on the severity of the presenting symptom.

Neoplasms of the Urinary Tract

Neoplasia in the urinary tract will present with gross hematuria, and these patients should be evaluated with complete urologic studies.

In any case of gross hematuria, if the etiology is not specifically determined a complete urologic evaluation is indicated. We would repeat for emphasis that intermittent hematuria does *not* preclude the possibility of serious urologic disease. In general, patients with gross hematuria think that they are losing a lot more blood than they are, since a small amount in a large amount of urine will give the appearance of passing a tremendous amount of blood. A significant amount *is* lost when patients pass blood clots or go into clot retention. These provide more important diagnostic criteria, as do hemoglobin and hematocrit studies.

RENAL COLIC

The patient may present in the Emergency Department with a typical severe colicky pain originating in the costovertebral angle in the flank and radiating down to the right or left lower quadrant into the testicle or vulva. It is not unusual for the pain actually to radiate into the leg. The pain frequently is not typical and can simulate biliary colic, ovarian disease, appendicitis, or ruptured ulcer. The pain is due to distention of the ureter and renal pelvis above the point of obstruction and is not caused by spasm.

DIFFERENTIAL DIAGNOSIS AND MANAGEMENT

Any intra-abdominal pathology may produce pain that simulates renal colic. The drug addict will describe a typical story for stone disease that will perhaps get him the sedation he wants. The diagnosis is suggested by history of passing stones before, by the association of gross or microscopic hematuria, and by an intravenous urogram, which may show the calculus or the secondary obstruction. There have been many cases of "acute appendicitis" that were found at operation to be a ureteral calculus. Gastrointestinal complaints frequently are associated with renal colic.

Management is primarily to make the diagnosis in the Emergency Department and then to give the patient pain relief with either morphine, 15 mg. subcutaneously, or intravenous morphine, Demerol, or Dilaudid. There is no real place in the management of renal colic for atropine or any of the antispasmodics. If the patient is having continued colic, admission to the hospital is indicated. However, patients frequently will be relieved by sedation and be perfectly comfortable. They may have passed their calculus by the time they have reached the Emergency Department, even though the pain continues. The patient can be managed on an ambulatory basis as long as he is not septic nor in severe discomfort.

Colic can be due to the passage of blood clots or any type of acute obstruction, such as passage of renal papillae. A stone can be as small as a piece of gravel or very large. Calculus size is unrelated to the severity of the pain. The position of the stone, however, has some relationship to where the pain is felt. If it is near the bladder, patients can have frequency, urgency, and dysuria. Their pain usually is abrupt in onset. These patients are usually restless, move around in the Emergency Department, and have associated gastrointestinal symptoms. A stone at the ureteropelvic junction gives flank pain; a stone in the mid-ureter above the iliac vessels produces right lower or left lower quadrant pain; finally, a stone at the ureterovesical junction may radiate to the vulva or scrotum.

The cessation of pain does not necessarily mean that the stone has passed, and urologic evaluation and management must still be carried out.

MASSES OF THE SCROTUM AND PENIS

The patient may present in the Emergency Department with a swelling on either or both sides of the scrotum. This is a common phenomenon, and its exact etiology must be differentiated.

Torsion of the Spermatic Cord (Torsion of Testicle)

Most commonly this occurs in a child or young man who presents with a sudden onset of severe pain and swelling on one side of his scrotum. It may well occur during physical activity, but does not have to be associated with this. There will be some nausea and frequently vomiting. There has been no preceding urethral discharge or fever. The diagnosis is made by examination of a tense swollen mass in the scrotum in which the epididymis cannot be outlined. The testicle usually is riding high in the upper part of the scrotum. The cord, if palpable, is edematous; the overlying skin can be edematous and reddened. There may be a history of previous temporary occurrences of this problem with complete cessation of symptoms after a short period.

The condition almost always occurs in prepubertal boys, and we have seen at least one case in the newborn. There usually is an underlying congenital abnormality of the tunica vaginalis with a "bell-clapper" type of deformity. This allows the testicle to rotate within the tunica. The pain may be increased by lifting the testicle, as does not occur in the case of epididymitis. If the child is seen early, it is easier to make the diagnosis because the epididymis may be palpable anteriorly, whereas later on there is swelling of the entire area and nothing distinct can be palpated.

Torsion of the testicle must be differentiated from epididymitis, orchitis, tumors, and trauma. The use of a Doppler stethoscope to determine blood supply has been found useful in management. Recently a testicular scan study has proved helpful in determining viability of the organ.

In treatment, if the child is seen early we have tried manual detorsion, and this has worked in a number of cases. It usually is best to twist gently in either direction. If this does not work, immediate operation should be done. Reported time limits of four to six hours are not necessarily true. We have seen individuals who have had signs and symptoms of torsion for several days but whose testicles have remained viable. This probably occurs because the testicle detorts intermittently and some blood gets through. It is always important to pex the other gonad. Operation is indicated in all torsions, whether intermittent or manually detorted, in order to pex both testicles.

Torsion of the Appendices of the Testis and Epididymis

Instead of torsion of the entire spermatic cord, the appendices can twist. Once again this usually occurs in children and is noted by the sudden onset of severe testicular pain. On examination, a small, tender lump may be felt in the upper anterior pole of the testicle or epididymis. However, later in the disease, the entire testicle is swollen and tender. Surgical exploration is usually done in order to make the diagnosis and relieve the torsion. The use of the Doppler stethoscope may make operations unnecessary in certain cases.

Hydrocele

A hydrocele is a collection of fluid within the tunica vaginalis. Approximately 15 per cent of testicular neoplasms present as hydroceles, but most often no etiology is found or the hydrocele is found secondary to inflammatory disease or trauma. Many infants are born with hydroceles, and these disappear during the first or second years of life. Most hydroceles occur in men past 40. If a hydrocele changes in size, as it frequently does in children, there may well be a patent processus vaginalis and an associated hernia.

There is no pain involved and the patient will present with a mass, occasionally quite large. Examination reveals a round intrascrotal mass that is not tender and in which the testicle usually is not palpable. Transillumination is easily performed, but may not be practicable in patients with pigmented skin. Occasionally, if the testicle is not palpable, it is important to aspirate the fluid and make sure that the testicle itself is normal.

Management usually is nonoperative unless the patient believes that a very large hydrocele is causing him a great deal of difficulty because of its size. We do not believe in aspirating a hydrocele routinely, as complications can outweigh the beneficial effects. Hydrocele fluid is clear.

Spermatocele

This is a painless cystic mass containing sperm. It lies above and posterior to the testis but is separated from it. The testicle is easily palpable, as is the epididymis. On examination these are small and nontender, and no correction is necessary unless the patient insists.

Varicocele

This condition is quite common in young, sexually active men and is actually a dilatation of the pampiniform plexus of the spermatic cord. It usually is seen on the left side, but can occur on the right. The left drains into the internal spermatic vein and then directly into the renal vein. On the right it empties into the vena cava. Because of incompetent valves in the internal spermatic vein, leading to poor drainage, the veins gradually dilate and elongate. A symptomatic varicocele is one that develops secondary to a renal tumor invading the renal vein and does not disappear on recumbence. Diagnosis is made by examination of the scrotum, where a mass of veins is felt above the testicle. On recumbency the mass disappears. The only indication for surgical correction would be as a factor in an infertility problem. Treatment is by ligation of the internal spermatic vein at the internal inguinal ring or above.

Tumor of the Testicle

This disease usually occurs in men in their second or third decades and will present as a painless mass in the scrotum. However, there may be hemorrhage into the tumor, and the patient may present with typical painful sudden swelling that mimics an inflammatory testicle. Examination will reveal a very hard mass involving the testicle and a normal epididymis. The association of trauma is incidental and probably is the event that draws the patient's attention to a mass already present. This should be treated as an emergency, with admission to the hospital, followed by surgical exploration of the mass as soon as possible.

Epididymitis

An epididymitis usually presents as a very painful mass on one side of the scrotum. If examined early, the enlarged tender epididymis can be palpated, but later on there is a very tender scrotal mass. It usually lies in the bottom half of the scrotum and the patient is made more comfortable by scrotal elevation. A history of previous urethral dilatation, catheterization, operation, or urethral discharge is often present. The inflammation may be associated with a high fever and generalized sepsis. The differential diagnosis between torsion and tumor can be difficult. The overlying skin is red and edematous and it may be bilateral at times.

Management is by supportive therapy, with bed rest and antibiotics, depending on the presence of urinary tract infection. A scrotal suspensory or elevation of the scrotum while the patient is in bed relieves pain. Some have advocated infiltration of the spermatic cord with an anesthetic to alleviate the severe distress. The only indication for operation is if the diagnosis cannot be determined or if an abscess develops.

Cryptorchidism

An undescended testis sometimes presents as a mass in the inguinal region with an absence of a testicle in the scrotum. Diagnosis is made by history and by the palpation of the inguinal testicle. Management should be by a course of gonadotropins to see whether the testis will descend; if unsuccessful, surgery is required. If an undescended testis is found in an adult, we believe that exploration and removal are indicated.

Scrotal and Penile Edema

In congestive heart failure, massive swelling of the entire scrotum and penis can occur. This is easily differentiated, as the swelling is in the scrotal skin and there is pitting edema. Sometimes the penis disappears within the mass, and it may be difficult to catheterize the patient.

Hernia

A scrotal mass may be a hernia. This is important to determine prior to needling any scrotal mass. Peristalsis can be heard on auscultation, and the mass does not transilluminate. The mass frequently is reducible and a normal testicle can be felt below. In children, herniograms may be useful in the differential diagnosis.

Paraphimosis

In the uncircumcised male, the prepuce may be caught behind the glans, leading to the development of a great deal of swelling with a collar ring deformity. Diagnosis is made by a history of no circumcision and the typical picture of massive swelling behind the glans. Management is by reduction of the paraphimosis manually by pulling the foreskin beyond the glans. This may be helped by squeezing the edema fluid out, or it may require anesthesia with a dorsal slit and eventual circumcision.

Tumor of the Penis

This occurs only in uncircumcised males and will present as a mass usually palpable underneath the foreskin. If the prepuce cannot be pulled back and a mass is felt, biopsy is indicated. Occasionally a patient will wait too long, and a completely eroding ulcerative lesion of the penis can be seen. This must be considered as carcinoma until proved otherwise by biopsy. Any lesion of the penis not of a specific etiology should be biopsied. A number of precancerous skin lesions, such as erythroplasia of Queyrat, Bowen's disease, and leukoplakia may occur and must be treated.

VENEREAL DISEASE AND SKIN DISEASES OF THE GENITALIA

Gonorrhea

This is primarily a urethritis and is usually self-limiting. A creamy white discharge occurs approximately three days to a week after sexual exposure. There is associated burning on urination. Staining the sediment will reveal gram-negative intracellular diplococci, and a culture will be positive for gonococcus. The differential diagnosis is between nonspecific urethritis and Trichomonas urethritis. Treatment is easily done by antibiotics. Penicillin, 4.8 million units I.M. plus 1 gm. of probenecid will cure 90 per cent of cases. Tetracyclines (1.5 gm. STAT 0.5 gm. QID for four days) are a good alternative. It is important to reassure the patients and to follow them to make sure that there are no longer any gonococci present. A VDRL report is necessary.

Syphilis

This will present with a painless sore on the penis or vulva several weeks after sexual contact. The ulceration has indurated edges and is not painful on pressure. The diagnosis is made by dark field examination and a positive syphilis blood test. Treatment is by penicillin given over a two-week period intramuscularly.

Chancroid (Soft Chancre)

This is a common venereal disease usually accompanied by inguinal adenopathy. It is caused by the *Hemophilus ducreyi* and usually occurs a few days after sexual exposure. The inguinal nodes may suppurate and drain spontaneously. The diagnosis is established by examination of the discharge and a positive skin test. Biopsy may be required. Management is by tetracycline.

Lymphogranuloma Venereum (Lymphopathia Venereum)

This venereal infection is caused by a virus. There is a transient genital lesion followed by lymphadenopathy and, in the female, a rectal stricture. In the male the inguinal and subinguinal nodes become matted, suppurate, and form sinuses. The lesion usually occurs one to three weeks after sexual exposure and may be papular or vesicular. Later, painful nodes develop. The Frei test is positive in about 66 per cent of patients, and the complement fixation test also can be positive. Treatment is by the tetracyclines.

Granuloma Inguinale

This is a chronic venereal infection of the skin and subcutaneous tissue of the genitalia, perineum, or inguinal region. It is caused by the *Donovania granulomatis* organism. The first sign of the disease is swelling of the skin of the genitalia, which ulcerates and is moderately painful. Identification of the Donovan body in large monocytes on a stained smear confirms the diagnosis. Complement fixation and skin tests are not reliable. Treatment is by the tetracyclines.

Erosive and Gangrenous Balanitis

This is caused by a Vibrio and spirochete. There are small single or multiple ulcerations that become deep and painful. Small nodes may occur. Diagnosis is by dark field examination.

Herpes

Herpes progenitalis is caused by a virus. Multiple or superficial vesicles are seen on the foreskin or the glans. Slight local burning or itching may occur. Treatment is difficult and the disease prolonged.

SEXUAL EMERGENCIES IN THE MALE

Priapism

Priapism, by definition, is a sustained erection of the penis not relieved by ejaculation. It is usually associated with discomfort. The etiology of priapism can be specific or idiopathic. The patient will present in the

Emergency Department with an erection of long term duration that has now become painful and that may or may not have started with sexual arousal. The association of sickle cell disease as the etiologic agent is moderately frequent. Tumor infiltration, leukemia, and hematologic or neurologic disorders may be associated. However, a large number of cases are idiopathic. We have seen several instances of priapism in children, one a diabetic.

Management initially in the Emergency Department is sedation for pain. If the erection persists, the patient is scheduled for the operating room, at which time spinal or caudal anesthesia is used. Under anesthesia the erection may disappear. If not, we then recommend the use of a 15-gauge needle, introduced into each corpora cavernosa. The dark, viscid blood is removed by massage and aspiration. A heparin solution is irrigated through the needles, and the penis will become completely flaccid. On irrigation it will become tumescent once again.

The deflated phallus is compressed against the perineum with a catheter in place and held there with adequate dressings. This is probably one of the most important aspects of nonsurgical management—making sure that the compression dressing is secure and adequate. This has been highly effective treatment in our experience and has succeeded 90 per cent of the time.

If the erection recurs, an operative procedure such as the corpora-saphenous shunt or the corpora-spongiosum shunt should be used. The operation is done by either anastomosing the saphenous vein through a window in the tunica albuginea, or a cavernosum-spongiosum shunt is done between the two corpora. It has been our experience that if the patient is managed with any of the above types of therapy, impotence may not result. However, if priapism is allowed to continue for a sufficient time, many patients complain of an inability to achieve erections.

Hematospermia

Many middle-aged men will present with blood in their semen. Many times the wife will complain that she has bleeding, but then the couple realize that it is the man. It must be ascertained whether the semen was bloody or whether this was blood coming from scrotal varices. Management in the Emergency Department is strictly reassurance. If the condition recurs, urologic investigation is indicated. Almost always the etiology is non-neoplastic and probably arises from varicosities near the verumontanum.

Peyronie's Disease

This is a fibrous plaque of the corpora cavernosa that produces chordee and pain on erection, the so-called "bent spike" syndrome. The patient may present in the Emergency Department because of difficulty in intercourse because of the bent erection. The important thing to remember is that there is considerable psychologic overlay with this problem. Such patients require a great deal of reassurance and support and avoidance of operative intervention. There is no medication that is effective. Through examination and discussion of the mechanism of the curvature, the problem is usually managed satisfactorily.

Chapter 48

MUSCLE AND JOINT EMERGENCIES

A.   Neuromuscular Diseases
B.   Acute Arthritis

A. NEUROMUSCULAR DISEASES

Linton C. Hopkins

INTRODUCTION

Neuromuscular diseases do not constitute a large percentage of cases seen in most Emergency Departments today. Since these diseases frequently are severe, however, their importance far exceeds their numbers. The symptom that all have in common is muscular weakness, which may be generalized and can involve extremity muscles and extraocular and bulbar muscles. Occasionally, one of those muscle groups is involved alone. When a patient is severely or acutely weak, rapid assessment and appropriate management are essential, and this chapter will provide a brief review of neuromuscular diseases likely to be seen in Emergency medicine practice.

MYASTHENIA GRAVIS AND OTHER CAUSES OF ACUTE WEAKNESS

Since the time of Sir Thomas Willis (Willis, 1672) in the 17th century, myasthenia has been known as a disease likely to confuse even the most knowledgeable physician.

RECOGNITION

Historical features that strongly suggest myasthenia gravis are: (1) weakness that varies from hour to hour and day to day, frequently more severe late in the day; (2) a strong history of muscle fatigue with a need for frequent periods of rest; (3) a history suggestive of difficulty with extraocular muscles, diplopia, or difficulty with bulbar muscles, dysphagia, or dysarthria. In the mildest form of the disease, the history may reflect only nonspecific muscle fatigue. The physical examination is likely to vary tremendously from one patient to another, as some will have weakness only of extraocular muscles, or of extraocular muscles and bulbar muscles, whereas others will have a severe generalized muscle weakness syndrome. However, there are some features of the examination that might be called typical. It is unusual for a patient with generalized myasthenia gravis to have a totally normal ocular examination with normal extraocular movements, strength of eye closure, and absence of ptosis. The weakness of extraocular movement is likely to be disconjugate. Weakness in the extremities is more proximal than distal, and power frequently is normal in the hands and feet. Although an asthenic appearance is common, there usually is no great loss of muscle bulk or wasting. Muscle tone is diminished in a weak extremity, and a remarkable finding is that, despite the presence of severe generalized myasthenia with flaccid quadriplegia, deep tendon reflexes usually are normal to slightly brisk. Some other neuromuscular diseases that will be discussed may have preserved reflexes in the face of profound weakness, but myasthenia is by far the most common.

The response to anticholinesterase medication is so typical of myasthenia gravis that it has become a major diagnostic tool. Before proceeding with edrophonium injection (Tensilon), the physician should examine the muscular system and make an objective measurement of respiratory function. Since Tensilon may provoke a different response in different muscle groups in patients with myasthenia, it is most important to follow those muscles that are most important to the patient's survival, namely respiratory muscles and those used in swallowing. After the initial evaluation, 0.2 cc. (2 mg.) of a 10 per cent solution of edrophonium is injected rapidly I.V. The physician then immediately measures all modalities of strength that he has tested prior to the injection, with particular emphasis on the important muscles mentioned above. Most patients with myasthenia gravis will show a response to this 2-mg. dose. If the patient is quite elderly, or has heart disease, or is quite young and has a very low body weight, the 2-mg. dose might be sufficient. On the other hand, if no response is obtained and there has been no change in pulse or blood pressure from the 2-mg. injection, an additional 8 mg. is given over a period of about 30 seconds, and the response to that is monitored as above. Only an unequivocal change in muscle power is diagnostic of myasthenia gravis. Many neuromuscular diseases causing vast weakness will have a transient mild increase in strength following injection of edrophonium; only an unequivocal dramatic response is diagnostic.

TREATMENT

Currently, oral anticholinesterase medication is the treatment of choice in myasthenia gravis. The usual medication is pyridostigmine (Mestinon), 60-mg. tablets, one or two every four hours. Treatment with parenteral medication is rarely required unless the patient is in crisis (see below), but if parenteral medication is to be substituted for Mestinon, neostigmine (Prostigmin), 1.5 mg. I.M., is roughly equivalent to one 60-mg. tablet of pyridostigmine orally and to 15 mg. of neostigmine orally. An important principle of treatment is to start the patient on a low dose, 60 mg. of Mestinon q4h, and adjust the dose to the patient's requirements thereafter. Chronic treatment of myasthenia gravis with oral administration of corticosteroid hormones has been widely discussed recently (Warmolts and Engel, 1972; Seybold and Drachman, 1974). Most patients with generalized myasthenia improve remarkably when given corticosteroids, but if a patient is already taking oral anticholinesterase medication and doing poorly, introduction of corticosteroids at full dosage can be expected to *increase* his weakness before there is any improvement; for that reason, hospital admission is required for any myasthenic in whom major medication changes are anticipated. Thymectomy is indicated as the treatment of choice in all myasthenics regardless of sex or duration of symptoms, with the exception of those who are poor anesthetic risks for medical reasons. Since patients over 70 frequently have an involuted thymus, the surgery may not be indicated in that age group. Whereas other forms of therapy cause suppression or control of the disease, thymectomy may cause cure in as many as 40 per cent of patients after five years (Papatestas, et al., 1971).

MYASTHENIC CRISIS

When a patient with myasthenia has severe oropharyngeal and/or respiratory weakness, he is in "crisis." A vital capacity below 15 ml./kg. or 1 liter indicates the need for respiratory assistance; intubation and artificial ventilation should be carried out promptly. The most common cause of mortality in an acutely ill and weak patient with myasthenia is delay in recognition of the need for artificial ventilation. Any myasthenic who becomes acutely weak should not be managed with drugs, but should be intubated and assisted. Although classic papers sharply differentiate between "myasthenic" and "cholinergic" crisis, the difference is of little practical importance except that the latter seems to be rather uncommon. In both types of crisis, all drugs should be discontinued after respiratory assistance is attained; the patient should be allowed to rest on artificial ventilation for a few days; and therapy should then be resumed in small doses. If a patient has difficulty in swallowing, it is preferable to maintain him on intravenous fluid or gastric intubation than to attempt to feed him normally.

A large majority of myasthenics who become acutely ill and are therefore in "crisis" have neither clear-cut myasthenic crisis with an exacerbation of the disease nor "cholinergic" crisis as a result of too much medication; the greatest number have a "crisis" of resistance. In other words, no matter what medication the patient takes, it does not have the expected effect and the patient deteriorates. The most common cause of this state is an upper respiratory infection that usually is viral, but may be bacterial. Vigorous efforts should be instituted to diagnose and effectively treat any such infection. No attempt should be made to determine if the patient needs more or less drugs, e.g., by giving Tensilon, when the patient is in a crisis situation. Some muscles might get better, others might get worse, and the situation becomes far too confusing; all that is needed initially is respiratory assistance, time, and treatment of infection.

COMPLICATIONS

The complications of the disease are obvious and reflect the effect on the patient of severe bulbar muscle weakness and respiratory muscle weakness. Aspiration pneumonia and the resulting hypoxia is the most common cause of death in myasthenia gravis. Patients who take anticholinesterase drugs commonly have muscarinic side-effects of excessive lacrimation, salivation, and abdominal cramping, and these should be treated by carefully reducing the dose or by adding atropine. Recently, evidence has been introduced that long term anticholinesterase therapy might be toxic to neuromuscular junctions (Engel et al., 1973). This is still being defined and should not concern the clinician at present. Complications of long term, high dose corticosteroids, either in daily dosage or in alternate-day dosage, are well known and need not be reiterated here. One that particularly affects myasthenics is the potassium-depleting effect of corticosteroids, and this can accentuate myasthenic weakness markedly. All myasthenics on prednisone therefore, should receive adequate potassium supplementation.

OTHER FORMS OF ACUTE WEAKNESS

In addition to myasthenia gravis, there are other important causes of flaccid weakness that will be encountered in an Emergency Department setting. *Botulism* (Tyler, 1963), which usually causes extraocular, bulbar, and upper extremity proximal muscle weakness, may appear very much like acute onset myasthenia, but the reflexes are commonly depressed in botulism. Characteristically, patients have facilitation of muscle power with exercise. In this disease, as in any disease causing flaccid paralysis, maintenance of the airway is a primary concern, and specific treatment comes later. Once the presumptive diagnosis of botulism has been made by obtaining a history of ingestion of contaminated food, followed within hours by weakness (especially, if present in more than one member of the family), treatment should be undertaken with antitoxin obtained from the Center for Disease Control, U.S. Public Health Service, Atlanta, Georgia.

Patients with *idiopathic polyneuropathy*, or the *Guillain-Barré syndrome*, commonly present at an Emergency Department. Early recognition is important, not to initiate any specific therapy but to support the patient during a potentially dangerous illness. These patients normally present with one or two days of tingling paresthesias at the tips of the toes and fingers, gradually ascending to involve a stocking-glove distribution. An ascending paralysis develops that is areflexic, and usually associated with some peripheral sensory findings. Spinal fluid protein is elevated out of proportion to any

cellular reaction. Supportive treatment is all that usually is required.

Tick paralysis (Schmitt et al., 1969) is an odd syndrome associated with tick bite and the presence of the tick on the body. It is a flaccid ascending paralysis usually starting in the legs; it may be limited to the legs, and improves when the tick is removed from the body. The tick commonly is embedded in scalp hair; the only treatment is removal.

ACUTE MYOSITIS AND MYOPATHY (POLYMYOSITIS, ALCOHOLIC POLYMYOPATHY, AND MYOGLOBINURIA)

The inflammatory myopathies, polymyositis, dermatomyositis, and childhood dermatomyositis, usually do not present a major problem in diagnosis when modern EMG and muscle histology and histochemistry are available. In the Emergency Department, however, these patients may present as profoundly weak, very toxic, and obviously acutely ill, and some characteristics need to be emphasized.

RECOGNITION

Polymyositis usually presents as a subacute painless illness over a period of a month or more, but exceptionally can present over a week with severe muscle pain, swelling of the muscles, and marked weakness. Usually, neck flexion is involved particularly, but facial muscles and extraocular movement muscles generally are spared. Sensory examination, of course, is normal. Deep tendon reflexes usually parallel the degree of weakness, and may well be absent in a patient who is totally flaccid and paralyzed. The usual chronic type of polymyositis does not have muscle pain, tenderness, and swelling, but simply presents with a syndrome of proximal muscle weakness.

Rhabdomyolysis or *acute muscle destruction* usually associated with *myoglobinuria*, is a syndrome that has many causes (Rowland and Penn, 1972). Alcoholic rhabdomyolysis, the type most commonly seen in Emergency Departments, is a disease that occurs in the setting of chronic alcoholism, usually with an acute increase in alcohol intake. Onset is with muscle pain (usually more severe in the legs), rapidly progressive weakness, and dark urine. If the patient has tender, swollen muscles (which depends on the severity of the muscle destruction), he may be quite toxic. Rhabdomyolysis also can arise from rarer diseases such as muscle phosphorylase deficiency or McArdle's disease, or an even rarer disease, phosphofructokinase deficiency. Rhabdomyolysis, of course, can occur from an unknown cause, so-called "idiopathic recurrent rhabdomyolysis," and has been reported to be associated with influenza and other viral illnesses. Barbiturate poisoning and carbon monoxide poisoning are other causes.

TREATMENT

Corticosteroids are the treatment of choice in inflammatory myopathy. The dose selected depends on the severity of disease. A typical starting dose is prednisone, 50 or 60 mg. daily, or 100 mg. every other day.

Emergency Department management of rhabdomyolysis involves immediate assessment and protection of urine output. The patient with severe destruction of muscle will have myoglobinuria and can be expected to develop hyperkalemia and hypocalcemia, because of the release into the circulation of potassium and phosphorus when muscle is destroyed. Urine output is the major concern, and the urine should be alkalinized to increase the solubility of the myoglobulin and thereby aid in its excretion.

CHRONIC DISORDERS OF MUSCLE

These diseases cause patients to come to the Emergency Department only at the later stages of the disease. However, if a patient with one of these diseases presents for other causes, the disease should be recognized.

By far the most common and most severe of the muscular dystrophies is *Duchenne's muscular dystrophy*, which is an X-linked recessive disease that affects boys before the age of 5 and usually causes death by the age of 20. Classicially, it presents with proximal muscle weakness in the lower extremities, with hypertrophy of the calf muscles. Later on, proximal arm weakness develops. The disease is symmetric and is associated with a definite and marked rise in serum muscle enzymes, particularly CPK, which is frequently greater than 5000 and usually greater than 1000. *Facioscapulohumeral muscular dystrophy* is a disease that usually is asymmetric, starting with face and shoulder weakness and usually presenting with asymmetric facial weakness and upper extremity proximal muscle weakness. Later in the course, distal leg weakness with foot drop may develop, but it can be recognized most easily by an abnormal smile, weak eye closure, and usually scapular winging. *Limb-girdle dystrophy* is a chronic proximal myopathy, usually inherited as an autosomal recessive, rarely dominant, and occasionally sporadic. It normally is a symmetric proximal muscle weakness disorder, and can be differentiated from inflammatory myopathy mainly by its very chronic course. *Myotonic dystrophy* is unique among the dystrophies: patients present with distal muscle weakness, particularly in the hands, and have a peculiar response to percussion or forced contraction of the muscle, in that there is delayed relaxation that electromyographically consists of repetitive firing of crescendo-descrescendo volleys of biphasic waves. There is a very characteristic facial appearance, sleepy-appearing facies with ptosis and bifacial weakness. Patients have distal muscle weakness as well as proximal muscle weakness. *Congenital muscular dystrophy,* a much rarer condition, is a progressive myopathy beginning at or before birth, associated with progressive proximal muscle weakness in infancy. Patients present with hypotonia and have a variable course: some slowly progressive and associated with several decades of life, others more rapidly progressive and ending in death by the age of 5 to 10.

Progressive degenerative disease of anterior horn cells may occur at any age. In infancy it is called *infantile spinal muscular atrophy*, or *Werdnig-Hoffmann disease*, and is characterized by hypotonia and symmetric generalized areflexic weakness, clinically distinguished also by the presence of fasciculations in the tongue. It usually is fatal before the age of 2. In adults, the most common anterior horn cell disease is *amyotrophic lateral sclerosis*, which characteristically presents as an asymmetric distal wasting disease associated with fasciculations and bulbar muscle weakness. All anterior horn cell diseases, no matter what the age of presentation, are characterized by the total absence of sensory findings and by the sparing of extraocular muscles. *Poliomyelitis* is another example of anterior horn cell disease that is no longer common, of course; however, in view of the very poor immunization status of many children reported recently, it needs to be thought of occasionally. It is a febrile illness presenting with asymmetric, usually distal muscle weakness progressing to generalized muscle weakness, respiratory muscle weakness, and bulbar paralysis. There is a cellular reaction in the spinal fluid that is predominantly lymphocytic; deep tendon reflexes usually are lost asymmetrically, and the patient frequently has signs of meningitis with nuchal rigidity, and of a viral illness with fever and myalgias.

In summary, patients with any neuromuscular disease, whether acute, subacute, or chronic, may present at any Emergency Department at any time. Emergency treatment is life-saving only in those diseases associated with acute deterioration, but it is important to be aware of the more chronic causes of generalized muscle weakness so that accurate diagnosis, treatment, or genetic counseling can be instituted.

References

Engel, A. G., Lambert, E. H., and Santa, T.: Study of long-term anticholinesterase therapy. Neurology 23:1273, 1973.

Papatestas, A. E., et al.: Studies in myasthenia gravis: effects of thymectomy. Am. J. Med. 50:465, 1971.
Rowland, L. P., and Penn, A. S.: Myoglobinuria. Med. Clin. North Am. 56:1233, 1972.
Schmitt, N., Bowmer, E. J., and Gregson, J. D.: Tick paralysis in British Columbia, Can. Med. Assoc. J. 100:417, 1969.
Seybold, M. E., and Drachman, D. B.: Gradually increasing doses of prednisone in myasthenia gravis. N. Engl. J. Med. 290:81, 1974.
Tyler, H. R.: Botulism. Arch. Neurol. 9:652, 1963.
Warmolts. J. R., and Engel, W. K.: Benefit from alternate-day prednisone in myasthenia gravis. N. Engl. J. Med. 286:17, 1972.
Willis, T.: De Anima Bruturum. London, 1672, pp. 286–288.

Suggestions for Further Reading

GENERAL

Walton, J. N.: Diseases of Voluntary Muscles, 3d ed. London, Churchill-Livingstone, 1974.

MYASTHENIA GRAVIS

Osserman, K. E.: Myasthenia Gravis. New York, Grune & Stratton, 1958.
Osserman, K. E.: Myasthenia gravis. Proc. 3rd Int. Symp. Ann. N.Y. Acad. Sci., vol. 135, 1966.

B. ACUTE ARTHRITIS

C. H. Wilson, Jr.

The following discussion is intended to emphasize some considerations that the emergency physician should keep in mind early in the presentation of a patient with acute arthritis. If he proceeds properly, he will quickly highlight problems that might require emergency or immediate action and will begin structuring a data base which can be added to in orderly fashion to properly diagnose and manage the problem.

The most important immediate consideration is the exclusion of an acute presentation of *septic arthritis* because of the need to diagnose this early and begin treatment in order to prevent the destruction of cartilage and the invasion of bone. Following this are the considerations as to whether one is dealing with a *traumatic injury to the joint*, *acute gout*, or *acute pseudogout*, since these conditions can be diagnosed quickly and

appropriate therapy can be instituted immediately. Finally, it is important to consider the possibility of an *acute presentation of a systemic problem* that might pose a more serious threat to the patient by involvement elsewhere in the body; such problems include acute rheumatic fever or an acute presentation of rheumatoid arthritis, systemic lupus erythematosus, or one of the other collagen vascular diseases.

In collecting data, one should keep several diagnostic questions in mind:

1. Is the problem monarticular or polyarticular? (See Table 1.)

2. Is this an inflammatory or noninflammatory problem? (See Table 2.)

3. What is the relative importance of the problem of arthritis with respect to the other problems with which the patient might present?

TABLE 1 Significant Signs in Arthritis*

1. Number of joints involved
   a. Monarticular—suggests septic arthritis, acute gout, osteoarthritis, traumatic arthritis
   b. Polyarticular
      Few joints—gonococcal arthritis, juvenile RA
      Many joints—RA and variants
2. Distribution of involved joints
   a. Small peripheral joints (metacarpophalangeal, proximal interphalangeal, metatarsophalangeal)—RA
   b. First metatarsophalangeal joint—gout
   c. Symmetric involvement—RA
3. Onset
   a. Rapid (30 minutes to two hours)—acute gout, septic arthritis, ARF
   b. Insidious—chronic nonspecific inflammatory arthritis (e.g., RA and variants)
   c. Migratory—ARF
      Early phase of gonococcal arthritis
   d. Recruitment—as in (b) above
4. Pain
   a. Severe throbbing pain—gout, septic arthritis
   b. Pain (aching) at rest—any of the inflammatory arthritides
   c. Pain on motion, relieved by short periods of rest—noninflammatory arthritides
5. Fever
   a. Fever associated with chills—highly suggestive of septic arthritis
   b. Low-grade fever—suggestive of any of the inflammatory arthritides

*The above data are nondiagnostic alone but are highly suggestive and, when used in conjunction with other data, will lead to the proper problem formulation and diagnosis. Key: RA = rheumatoid arthritis; ARF = acute rheumatic fever; SLE = systemic lupus erythematosus.

SUBJECTIVE DATA (See also Table 1)

With these considerations in mind, one should quickly collect historical data. In questioning the patient, the physician should note (1) which joint(s) are involved, (2) the distribution of involvement, and (3) whether this involvement is symmetric, as in rheumatoid arthritis. The rapidity of the onset of the arthritis, as well as the description of the pain, is important. If more than one joint is involved or has been involved, it is important to know whether this is a migratory arthritis or whether it has been characterized by persistence in the original joint with recruitment of other joints. Finally, in describing the specific, involved joints it is important to know whether there was associated trauma with the precipitation of the acute joint problem.

The patient should be asked about problems that might be associated with the acute arthritis. Is there a history of fever or skin rash? Has there been a recent infection in a contiguous or remote area, such as an infected puncture wound in the vicinity or a history of pneumonia, urinary tract infection, or pharyngitis? Are there associated symptoms of a more widespread systemic illness, such as weight loss or anorexia? Is there an associated urethral discharge or evidence of a pelvic inflammatory problem? Is there evidence of a recent or more remote inflammatory eye problem, and is there a history of recent sexual exposure? Has the patient been on medication that might be implicated in a hypersensitivity reaction?

A quick review of past problems should be made. Have there been similar episodes in the past, as one might expect in gout or acute rheumatic fever? Is there a history of skin rash that is no longer present, as sometimes occurs in acute systemic lupus erythematosus? Is there a history of serositis in the past or is there previous history of a hypersensitivity problem? The patient should be asked whether there is a family history of similar problems (e.g., gout, ankylosing spondylitis, Reiter's disease).

OBJECTIVE DATA (See Tables 2 and 3)

During the physical examination one should note specifically those signs that would differentiate between acute inflammatory arthritis and a noninflammatory joint problem. Is there redness on observation? If there is swelling, is it limited to the joint, or does it involve the surrounding structures, such as the tendon sheaths? By palpation can one differentiate swelling due to synovial thickening, bony enlargement, or effusion within a joint capsule? Is there increased warmth, tenderness to pressure, pain on motion? When the joint is moved, is there palpable crepitus? Is there an attitude of deformity? Is there limitation of motion? If so, is the limitation due to pain or to structural damage?

After one has adequately evaluated the specific findings in the joint, it is important to look at the remainder of the physical examination for associated data. Is the patient febrile? Is there evidence of current or past inflammatory disease of the eye? Is there an associated skin rash? Is there a pharyngitis?

TABLE 2   Differential Diagnosis of
Inflammatory and Noninflammatory Arthritis

NONINFLAMMATORY ARTHRITIS

SUBJECTIVE
  Pain on motion relieved by short period of rest
OBJECTIVE
  Physical Examination
  1. Palpable bony enlargement about margin of joint
  2. Soft-tissue swelling about joint does not have the "doughy" consistency of inflamed synovium
  Laboratory Findings
  1. Usually normal sedimentation rate (unless elevated as a result of some other problem)
  2. Noninflammatory findings on synovial analysis (see Table 3)
  X-ray Examination
  1. Loss of articular cartilage, which appears as narrowing of the joint space
  2. Reactive changes in subchondral bone, with
    a. Eburnation (increased density of subchondral bone)
    b. "Spurring" – exostosis at margin of joint, appearing as a spur on x-ray, but actually due to a reactive bony ridge at margin of cartilage.

INFLAMMATORY ARTHRITIS

SUBJECTIVE
  Pain at rest
OBJECTIVE
  Physical Examination
  1. Redness
  2. Soft-tissue swelling (palpable, "doughy" inflamed synovium suggestive of chronic inflammatory arthritis, e.g., RA or rheumatoid variant)
  3. Increased warmth to palpation
  4. Tenderness to pressure and pain on motion
  Laboratory Findings
  1. Elevated sedimentation rate
  2. Anemia suggests a more chronic inflammatory arthritic disease
  3. Inflammatory findings on synovial analysis (see Table 3)
  X-ray Examination
  1. Soft-tissue swelling may be the only early sign
  2. Juxta-articular osteoporosis
  3. Erosion into juxta-articular bone may suggest RA, gouty tophi, or septic invasion of bone

Is there evidence of pneumonia or pleural problems or a cardiac problem with a valvular lesion or a conduction defect? Is urethritis present with urethral discharge or is there evidence of inflammation in the pelvis on abdominal and pelvic examination?

Joint Fluid Examination. Examination of the *joint fluid* can furnish the most quickly definitive diagnostic information (Table 3). During arthrocentesis it is important that one observe absolute sterile technique in order to avoid introducing organisms with the needle. Once the fluid is withdrawn, one should immediately obtain as much data as possible from its examination. It is important to note the color and the clarity. Some indication of the quality of the mucin within the fluid can be obtained by doing a string test and by an acetic acid clot test, which will help differentiate between an inflammatory and noninflammatory fluid. A fresh specimen of the fluid should be examined on a slide in order to determine an approximate white blood cell count, whether "ragocytes" are present, and whether there is cartilage debris. The presence of fat would indicate a fracture adjacent to the joint with some extrusion of marrow contents. This fresh joint fluid sample can be examined in polarized light, using a first-order red compensator for identification of urate or calcium pyrophosphate crystals.

The next most important test on the joint fluid is the total white blood cell count. In doing the WBC count, it is important to remember that normal saline should be used as the counting fluid, since acetic acid in the usual white blood counting fluid will cause the mucin to precipitate and will give an erroneous count. The smear should be Wright-stained for a differential WBC count. On the Wright-stained slide one can also look for LE cells and for Pekin-Zvaifler cells.

In the chemistry laboratory the most important early test result is the joint fluid sugar. Other tests that are important later in the differential diagnosis include the joint fluid protein and complement level. A culture should always be made on joint fluid when it is obtained and a Gram stain should be done immediately to look for bacteria.

Joint fluid examination done by the physician in the acute situation may allow early diagnosis and institution of treatment, which not only saves time, and reduces a patient's pain, but may prevent long-term disability.

In the *clinical laboratory* the blood study that is most helpful immediately is a complete blood count to indicate whether there is a leukocytosis with a shift to the left, as one would see in an infection. An anemia may indicate that one is dealing with a more chronic illness. The sedimentation rate can be done within an hour and is helpful in differentiating between an inflammatory problem and a noninflammatory problem.

TABLE 3 *Differential Diagnostic Data—Joint Fluid*

I. COLOR
  Technique: direct observation
  Data obtained
    a. Straw-colored—noninflammatory
    b. Yellow → green—Inflammatory of varying degrees
    c. "Milky"—gout or pseudogout
II. CLARITY
  Technique: hold tube in front of newsprint
  Data obtained
    a. Clear (can read newsprint easily)—noninflammatory
    b. Slightly cloudy → cloudy—inflammatory of varying degrees
    c. Purulent—septic arthritis
    d. Bloody—trauma
III. VISCOSITY
  Technique: "string test"
    a. Allow fluid to drip from end of needle and observe the string formed before drop separates. The longer the string, the higher the viscosity.
  or
    b. Place a drop of fluid on the thumb. Touch index finger to fluid and slowly spread thumb and index finger, observing the length of the string formed before it breaks, as above.
  Data obtained
    a. High viscosity—noninflammatory
    b. Decreased viscosity—inflammatory with the viscosity varying inversely with the degree of inflammation
IV. MUCIN CLOT
  Technique
    a. "Ropes test"—add a small amount of synovial fluid to 5 per cent acetic acid in a test tube or beaker
    b. Add a few drops of glacial acetic acid to a test tube containing the synovial fluid
  Data obtained
    a. Tight clot—noninflammatory
    b. Flocculant dispersion on mild agitation—inflammatory
V. WHITE BLOOD CELL COUNT
  Technique
    Cells of joint fluid counted by same technique as circulating peripheral WBCs (saline should be used for diluent to prevent precipitation of mucin by acetic acid)

Data obtained
    a. < 2000—noninflammatory
    b. >5000—inflammatory varying directly with severity of inflammation (≥100,000/cu. mm. pathognomonic of infection)
VI. WET PREPARATION FOR MICROSCOPIC EXAMINATION
  Technique
    A drop of fresh fluid or fluid collected in a heparinized tube is placed on a slide and covered with a coverslip. It is then examined microscopically in plain transmitted light and then in polarized light with a first-order red compensator in the system for crystal identification.
  Data obtained
  Plain transmitted light
    a. Cartilage debris—degenerative
    b. Fat globules—fracture into joint with marrow elements in fluid
    c. "Ragocytes" (WBCs with cytoplasmic inclusions)—suggestive of, but not pathognomonic of, RA
  Polarized light with first-order red compensator in optic system
    a. Strongly negatively birefringent, needle-like crystals = monosodium urate crystals—pathognomonic of gouty arthritis.
    b. Weakly positively birefringent needle-like or rhomboid crystals = calcium pyrophosphate crystals—diagnostic of pseudogout ("chondrocalcinosis")
VII. DIFFERENTIAL WBC
  Technique
    Direct smear of joint fluid on slide is allowed to dry and then stained with Wright's stain. If cell count is low, fluid may be spun down before making smear.
  Data obtained
    a. ≤25 per cent polymorphonuclear leukocytes—noninflammatory
    b. ≥50 per cent polymorphonuclear leukocytes—inflammatory
    c. LE cells are pathognomonic of systemic lupus erythematosus
    d. Pekin-Zvaifler cells (macrophage with ingested poly)—suggestive of (but not diagnostic of) Reiter's disease

Other laboratory tests that should be made immediately and may be of help later are tests for rheumatoid factor, LE cell preparations, antinuclear antibodies, liver and muscle enzymes, and serum uric acid.

On *x-ray examination* one should look for evidence of fracture adjacent to or into the joint and erosions adjacent to the joint (which might be produced by invasion of the bone with synovium or urate tophi or invasion of the bone by a septic process producing an osteomyelitis). One may also obtain helpful

points in the differential diagnosis by noting reactive changes such as thinning of the cartilage (loss of joint space) and reactive bone changes (such as eburnation beneath the cartilage surface and spurring at the margin of the joint). Calcification is sometimes seen in the cartilage, indicating chondrocalcinosis with pseudogout.

Certain other studies are of prime importance: (1) An *EKG* may indicate some conduction or pericardial problems in such disorders as acute rheumatic fever or systemic lupus erythematosus with pericarditis. (2) A *chest x-ray* should be obtained to look for infiltrates (possibly associated with a septic arthritis) or pleural reaction (as in SLE). (3) A *Gram stain and culture* should be made of the urethral discharge, if present, and cultures should be taken from the pharynx, cervix (in a female), and the rectum.

Having obtained the initial data, it is important to realize that observation over a period of time is as important as any other diagnostic procedure once an emergency or threatening situation has been ruled out. The patient should be made as comfortable as possible, using codeine or other narcotics for short-term control of pain. One should keep in mind that immobilizing a joint by splinting is very effective in controlling joint pain, as is the application of heat or, at times, ice. Aspirin or other antipyretic drugs that might alter the temperature curve should be withheld until the temperature pattern has been observed over a period of 24 to 48 hours for the presence of fever and the pattern of the fever if the diagnosis is in doubt. No antibiotics should be administered until the diagnosis is clear. As soon as enough data are available to substantiate the diagnosis, one should begin appropriate therapy at that time.

CHARACTERISTIC FEATURES OF COMMON INFLAMMATORY ARTHRITIDES

Several common inflammatory arthritic problems are listed below, and the characteristic subjective and objective data supporting the diagnoses are outlined.

Septic Arthritis
Subjective
1. Usually monarticular
2. Rapid onset
3. Frequently associated with fever and chills
4. History of recent infection highly suggestive
5. Pain at rest frequently described as throbbing
Objective
1. Physical signs of inflammatory arthritis (see Table 2)
2. Joint fluid analysis consistent with inflammatory arthritis (see Table 3); may be purulent

3. Gram stain of joint fluid may or may not reveal organisms
4. Joint fluid culture positive
5. X-ray not helpful early, usually showing only soft-tissue swelling and effusion

Gonococcal Arthritis
Subjective data are the same as for other septic arthritides, plus the following:
1. Usually monarticular, but may have two or even three joints involved
2. Often a history of migratory arthritis for several days at outset
3. May obtain history of
   a. Sexual exposure
   b. Urethral discharge
   c. Pelvic inflammatory disease
4. In female, frequently occurs at end of menstrual period
Objective:
1. At times discrete, red maculopapular lesions progressing to vesicles, pustules and central necrosis seen on skin, usually in small numbers
2. Often one sees tenosynovitis adjacent to involved joint, particularly on dorsum of wrist and ankle
Note: If one has reason to suspect this problem, blood cultures should be drawn and cultures should be obtained from pharynx, urethra, cervix, and rectum as well as joint fluid. These should be planted as quickly as possible (preferably in examining room) on Thayer-Martin medium.

Gout
Subjective
1. 90 per cent of patients are male
2. Monarticular (although may be polyarticular later in disease)
3. Severe throbbing pain
4. Early episodes affect first metatarsophalangeal joint in approximately 70 per cent of cases
5. May be history of renal stones
6. Family history often reveals relatives with gout
Objective
1. Signs of inflammatory arthritis (see Table 2)
2. Frequently there is significant periarticular swelling
3. Redness overlying joint may be so deep as to appear violaceous
4. Tophi may be seen or palpated over elbows or tendon sheaths or in ear

5. Inflammatory joint fluid (see Table 3) may appear "milky" if many crystals are present
6. Strongly negatively birefringent crystals on polarized light examination of joint fluid with first-order red compensator in optic system
7. X-ray may show punched-out juxta-articular lesions with overhanging edge

Pseudogout
  Subjective
    1. Sex distribution approximately equal (male/female ratio of 1:1)
    2. Most often seen beyond age of 50 (but may occur in young)
    3. Knee more frequently involved, but may involve any joint
  Objective
    1. Physical signs of inflammatory arthritis (see Table 2)
    2. Synovial analysis consistent with inflammatory arthritis (see Table 3)
    3. Weakly positive birefringent crystals on microscopic examination in polarized light with first-order red compensator in optic system
    4. X-ray often shows characteristic calcification in cartilage

Acute Rheumatic Fever
  Subjective
    1. Most frequently seen in children
    2. May be a history of preceding sore throat
    3. Past history of acute rheumatic fever helpful
    4. Symptoms of systemic disease (fever and malaise)
    5. Acute onset
    6. Often symptoms of cardiac disease
  Objective
    1. Fever
    2. Signs of inflammatory arthritis (see Table 2)
    3. Synovial analysis consistent with (usually) mild inflammatory arthritis (see Table 3)
    4. Rash of erythema marginatum may be present
    5. Possible cardiac murmurs, rubs
    6. Choreoathetoid movements may be present
    7. EKG may show conduction disturbance or evidence of myopericarditis
    8. X-ray of joints reveals only soft tissue swelling with or without effusion
    9. X-ray of chest for possible enlargement of cardiac shadow

Rheumatoid Arthritis
  Subjective
    1. Polyarticular
    2. Symmetric
    3. Small peripheral joints (proximal interphalangeal, metacarpophalangeal, metatarsophalangeal)
    4. Insidious onset
    5. Recruitment to involve other joints
    6. May have symptoms of systemic illness
       a. Fever (usually low grade)
       b. Weight loss
       c. Anorexia
  Objective
    1. Signs of inflammatory arthritis (see Table 2)
    2. May have subcutaneous nodules over olecranon
    3. Laboratory evidence of inflammatory arthritis (e.g., elevated sedimentation rate and anemia) (see Table 2)
    4. Inflammatory joint fluid on analysis—"ragocytes" may be present in large numbers (see Table 3)
    5. Rheumatoid factor present in serum in approximately 85 per cent of cases (drawn in emergency room, but reported later)

Systemic Lupus Erythematosus
  Subjective
    1. Frequently a history of rash, or sun sensitivity
    2. Serositis in the past or with present episode
  Objective
    1. May have typical discoid LE skin rash
    2. Signs of inflammatory arthritis, usually subacute (see Table 2)
    3. Synovial analysis reveals a (usually) mild inflammatory arthritis (see Table 3)
    4. Wright stain smear of synovial fluid may reveal LE cells
    5. May have microscopic hematuria and proteinuria on urinalysis
    6. X-ray of joints shows only soft-tissue swelling and possible effusion
    7. Chest x-ray may demonstrate serositis of pleura or pericardium
    8. EKG may reveal evidence of myopericarditis

Suggestions For Further Reading

Cohen, A. S., and Kim, I. C.: Acute suppurative arthritis. In Hill, A. G. S. (Ed.): Modern Trends in Rheumatology. Vol. 1. New York, Appleton-Century-Crofts, 1966.

Erlich, G. E.: Total Management of the Arthritic Patient. Philadelphia, J. B. Lippincott, 1973.

Hollander, J. L., and McCarty, D. J., Jr. (Eds.): Arthritis and Allied Conditions, 8th ed. Philadelphia, Lea & Febiger, 1972.

Kelly, P. J., Martin, W. J., and Coventry, M. B.: Bacterial (suppurative) arthritis in the adult. J. Bone Joint Surg. (Am) 52A:1595, 1970.

Klinenberg, J. R. (Ed.): Gout and purine metabolism. Arthritis Rheum. (Suppl.)18(6):659, Nov.–Dec. 1975.

McCarty, D. J., Jr. (Ed.): Pseudogout and pyrophosphate metabolism. Arthritis Rheum. (Suppl.)19(3):275, May–June 1976.

Moskowitz, R. W.: Clinical Rheumatology. Philadelphia, Lea & Febiger, 1975.

Rodnan, G. P. (Ed.): Primer on the Rheumatic Diseases, 7th ed. Reprinted from J.A.M.A. 224, No. 5 (Suppl), distributed by The Arthritis Foundation, New York, 1973.

Chapter 49

HEMATOPOIETIC EMERGENCIES

A. Bleeding Disorders
B. Disorders of Leukocytes
C. Disorders of the Red Blood Cells
D. Splenomegaly

A. BLEEDING DISORDERS

Milton Corn

Because current concepts of hemostasis are complicated, "bleeders" can be clinically confusing and often are mismanaged. The complexities of the system should not, however, be overemphasized.

PHYSIOLOGY OF HEMOSTASIS

Analysis and emergency treatment can be simplified by considering hemostasis to be composed of four component systems: blood vessels; clotting; platelets; and fibrinolysis (Goulian, 1966).

BLOOD VESSELS

Abnormalities of the vessel itself (as in allergic vasculitis or hereditary telangiectasia) or of the supporting tissue (as in scurvy) can lead to leakage of blood. Hemorrhage tends to be from small vessels and commonly manifests itself as purpura (petechiae and ecchymoses).

PLATELETS

Platelets form plugs at vessel rents and make available a phospholipid, platelet factor 3, which accelerates clotting. When the endothelial surface is disrupted, platelets adhere to the exposed collagen and release adenosine diphosphate, a platelet-clumping agent, which rapidly induces the formation of an aggregated platelet mass at the site of the leak. Abnormalities of platelet number (thrombocytopenia or significant thrombocytosis) or of platelet function (failure of adsorption, release, or aggregation) can, like vessel disease, cause purpuric bleeding.

CLOTTING

Blood clots through the sequential interaction of a number of substrates and enzymes, with the eventual production of thrombin, an enzyme capable of converting fibrinogen into insoluble fibrin. The clot consists of a tangled web of fibrin enmeshing variable quantities of serum, red cells and platelets. Detailed knowledge of the clotting sequence is not essential for most clinical applications, but it is useful to note that two major pathways are available for the production of thrombin: an intrinsic pathway activated by the contact of blood with foreign surfaces (measurable by the partial thromboplastin time) and a more rapid extrinsic pathway, activated by the admixture of blood with certain tissue juices (measurable by the prothrombin time). The prothrombin time is not affected by alterations of factors VIII, IX, XI or XII, while the partial thromboplastin time does not detect changes in factor VII. Since both sequences have a final common pathway, abnormalities of the later stages of clotting can affect both tests.

Defects at any point in the clotting sequence can cause a hemorrhagic diathesis, which tends to involve larger vessels than the purpuric disorders and is often manifest as joint and deep intramuscular hemorrhages or as delayed bleeding after trauma or surgery.

FIBRINOLYSIS

Perhaps because persistent thrombi are undesirable, most clots dissolve hours or days after formation. Plasminogen, a normal component of plasma, can be converted to plasmin by the clotting process itself and by other agents. Plasmin is a proteolytic enzyme that lyses fibrin into a number of split products. Excessive fibrinolytic activity can attack several clotting factors other than fibrinogen-fibrin and lead to a hemorrhagic tendency resembling the clotting abnormalities.

SOME REPRESENTATIVE HEMOSTATIC DISEASES

Purpuric Disorders

ALLERGIC PURPURA

The term allergic purpura is applied to a non-thrombocytopenic purpura for which no other cause can be found (Cream, et al., 1970). The condition often is accompanied by skin rash and edema. An inciting "allergen" such as a drug, insect bite, infectious organism or certain foods can be incriminated only in a minority of patients. When the purpura coexists with arthralgias and gastrointestinal symptoms the syndrome is referred to as Henoch-Schönlein purpura. Hemostatic function tests usually are normal.

IDIOPATHIC THROMBOCYTOPENIC PURPURA (ITP)

An unexplained decrease in platelet count, sometimes to extremely low levels, is a common acquired disorder. Although usually self-limited in children, the disease may persist for years in some adults (chronic ITP). The onset of purpura may be gradual or explosive. The illness is believed to have an immunologic basis, but no reliable confirmatory test is available. The physician investigating thrombocytopenia must rule out the presence of a host of platelet-depressing disorders, with particular attention to such entities as infection, drug or alcohol toxicity, deficiency of vitamin B-12 or folic acid, bone marrow diseases, collagen-vascular syndromes, thrombotic thrombocytopenic purpura, and hypersplenism (Baldini, 1966).

QUALITATIVE PLATELET DISORDERS

Drugs (particularly aspirin) and uremia are common causes of acquired functional platelet defects. Subdividing terms such as "thrombasthenia" and "thrombocytopathy" are not needed for most clinical purposes. A qualitative platelet disorder should be suspected when increased bleeding time is found in the presence of normal platelet number and normal clotting tests. Specific tests of platelet function are not usually available in hospital laboratories (Weiss, 1972).

DYSPROTEINEMIC BLEEDING

Cryoglobulin, monoclonal gammopathy (as in myeloma or macroglobulinemia), or occasionally polyclonal gammopathy may cause bleeding by unknown mechanisms perhaps involving interference with platelet function, vessel integrity or clotting factors. The hemorrhagic tendency may be puzzling because hemostatic function tests are often normal (Gottlieb, 1972).

Clotting Disorders

HEMOPHILIA

A sex-linked defect of the intrinsic clotting pathway, hemophilia is caused by deficiency of factor VIII (classic hemophilia) or, less commonly, factor IX (Christmas disease). Found almost exclusively in males, the illness usually is manifest by age five, although an occasional mildly deficient patient may remain asymptomatic until stressed by trauma or surgery in adult life. The diagnosis can be suspected when an isolated prolongation of the partial thromboplastin time is found, since the hemophilias constitute 90 per cent of the congenital disturbances of the intrinsic pathway. Specific factor assays are necessary to distinguish between the two hemophilias and to rule out such other causes of isolated prolongation of the partial thromboplastin time as deficiencies of factor XI or factor XII (Goulian, 1966).

FIBRINOLYSIS

Plasmin can cause a severe coagulation disorder by destruction of various clotting factors as well as fibrinogen and fibrin (Pechet, 1965). Primary fibrinolysis is rare, however, and excessive fibrinolytic activity usually should be assumed to indicate an underlying inciting coagulation process. Fibrinolysis is accompanied by hypofibrinogenemia, abnormally prolonged clotting tests, and the presence of split products. Fibrinolysis itself usually does not affect the platelet count significantly.

COUMARIN TOXICITY AND HEPARIN TOXICITY

An overdose of coumarin drugs can cause severe depletion of factors II, VII, IX, and X, with prolongation of both prothrombin time and partial thromboplastin time. Heparin prolongs the partial thromboplastin time and, in large doses, may also prolong the prothrombin time. Hemorrhage with both types of anticoagulants may present with bleeding at single or multiple sites.

CIRCULATING ANTICOAGULANTS

If an apparent clotting defect fails to respond to appropriate therapy the physician may suspect the presence of inhibitors to some stage of clotting (Bidwell, 1969). Special tests are necessary for confirmation.

Hybrid Disorders

VON WILLEBRAND'S DISEASE (VASCULAR HEMOPHILIA)

A congenital disorder found in both sexes, von Willebrand's disease affects both platelet function (poor adsorption) and clotting (deficient factor VIII production). Clinical severity is variable, and some patients may not be detected until late in life. Diagnosis is based on the laboratory triad of prolonged bleeding time, poor adsorption of platelets to glass beads, and a prolonged partial thromboplastin time (or preferably, the more sensitive specific assay of factor VIII). Repeated testing may be necessary, since the abnormalities fluctuate. In some patients transfusion temporarily stimulates the patient's own production of factor VIII.

DISSEMINATED INTRAVASCULAR COAGULATION (DIC)

An acquired disorder in which coagulation proceeds abnormally within the vascular tree, DIC can cause a severe hemorrhagic tendency by depleting essential hemostatic elements. Platelets and such clotting factors as V, VIII, and fibrinogen are consumed so rapidly that replacement processes are unable to maintain normal levels. The bleeding tendency is enhanced by the anticoagulant properties of split products of fibrinolysis, a process that usually accompanies DIC and may be responsible for the relatively low incidence of thrombotic complications. DIC is a reaction, not a primary disease, and may be initiated by a variety of events among which infection, shock, severe tissue damage, and obstetric complications

are common. The diagnosis should be suspected in any patient who simultaneously develops thrombocytopenia, clotting disorders, and fibrinolysis. Microangiopathic hemolytic anemia, sometimes associated with DIC, is probably due to the mechanical trauma imposed on red cells forced through the intravascular fibrin mesh (Colman, 1972).

WHEN TO SUSPECT A HEMOSTATIC DEFECT

In most bleeding patients hemorrhage can be attributed to local injury, which should be diligently sought. However, the possibility of an underlying hemostatic disorder should be kept in mind and will usually be suggested by certain clinical findings. Evaluation of hemostasis should be considered when the physician encounters:
1. Bleeding at multiple sites or in several body systems concurrently.
2. "Spontaneous" deep hematomas or hemarthrosis.
3. Unusually prolonged bleeding after local injury.
4. Disproportionately large hemorrhage after a minor insult.
5. Late bleeding which follows a period of apparently normal hemostasis after surgery or trauma.
6. Inability to find an organic cause for hemorrhage in a specific area or organ system.

EVALUATION OF A SUSPECTED BLEEDER

Since hemorrhagic tendencies, particularly in adults, may be associated with a variety of diseases, clinical judgment must determine the extent of the general evaluation. Furthermore, bleeding tendencies often express themselves through an organic lesion for which a thorough search is indicated. Certain types of information, however, are particularly helpful in establishing the presence and character of a bleeding tendency per se.

HISTORY

A bleeding disorder that appears early in life is likely to be congenital and an intrinsic clotting abnormality. (Thrombocytopenia is probably the most common acquired disorder). In obtaining the history, specific attention should be given to the patient's response to such hemostatic stresses as healing of the umbilical stump, circumcision, eruption of teeth, minor trauma, surgery, and dental extraction. A history of uneventful dental extraction rules out all but the mildest congenital coagulation defects.

A family history of bleeding disorders may be helpful, but the label of "bleeder" is often bestowed casually, and detailed questioning may be necessary to identify clinically plausible cases. Exposure to radiation, drugs, and toxins must be determined. The patient may be taking anticoagulants, drugs that affect platelet count or function, or agents capable of inducing allergic vasculitis.

The site of present or past bleeding may indicate the type of disorder. Petechiae, epistaxis, gum bleeding, and menorrhagia suggest vascular disease or platelet abnormalities, including von Willebrand's disease. Large hematomas and joint bleeding suggest disorders of clotting. Skin ecchymoses and bleeding into the head, gastrointestinal tract, or urinary system may occur with either the purpuric or the clotting disorders.

PHYSICAL EXAMINATION

Skin and mucous membranes are particularly likely to exhibit hemorrhage, but fundi, joints, and, large muscle groups also should be examined. The lesions of hereditary hemorrhagic telangiectasia may be found on the lips, mucous membranes, fingers, or under the nails. Hemorrhages around hair follicles, gums and at pressure areas are seen in scurvy. Bleeding into the lids and pinch bleeding suggest amyloid infiltration. Petechiae in the palms or soles imply allergic vasculitis. Hemarthrosis is seen almost exclusively in clotting disorders.

LABORATORY EVALUATION

History and physical examination can suggest the presence of a bleeding tendency and often will permit a guess as to the type of defect (Leslie and Ingram, 1971). Definitive evaluation, however, usually requires laboratory confirmation. Of the dozens of tests applicable to this area, five widely available procedures (Table 1) provide a rapid, efficient screening set that can help elucidate the great majority of bleeding problems: bleeding time (BT), platelet count (Plat.), partial thromboplastin time (PTT), prothrombin time (PT), and fibrinogen concentration (Fib.). This simple battery usually will detect a defect if present, and in most instances will permit tentative identification.

Bleeding time, tested on the forearm by the Ivy method or with a template, will be prolonged in the presence of significant thrombocytopenia or functional platelet disorders, including von Willebrand's disease. A platelet count can establish the presence of thrombocytopenia or thrombocytosis (both conditions can cause bleeding), but electronic counting methods do not eliminate the value of examining the stained periph-

TABLE 1   Interpretation of Five-Test Screening Battery

ABNORMAL TEST PATTERN°	ABNORMAL COMPONENT	SOME POSSIBLE CAUSES
↓ Plat. or ↓ Plat., ↑ BT	Thrombocytopenia	ITP, others
↑ Plat.	Thrombocytosis	Myeloproliferative disorders, others
↑ BT	Platelet dysfunction	Aspirin, uremia, von Willebrand's †
↑ PTT	Intrinsic clotting pathway	Hemophilia (rarely ↓ XI or ↓ XII), heparin
↑ PT	Extrinsic clotting pathway	↓ Factor VII (rare)
↑ PT, ↑ PTT	Extrinsic clotting pathway	Vitamin K deficiency, coumarin drugs, liver disease, heparin
↓ Fib.	Hypofibrinogenemia	↓ Fibrinogen (rare)
↓ Fib., ↑ PT (± ↑ PTT)	Fibrinolysis	Underlying DIC, primary fibrinolysis
↑ BT, ↑ PTT	Hybrid disorder	von Willebrand's
↓ Plat., ↑ PT, ↓ Fib. (± ↑ PTT)	Hybrid disorder	DIC, liver disease
All tests normal	?	Normal hemostasis, allergic vasculitis, scurvy, dysproteinemia, others

° ↓ Signifies decrease, ↑ signifies increase or prolongation
†Mild cases of von Willebrand's disease may not affect the PTT

eral blood smear as a rapid and useful estimate of platelet number.

Intrinsic and extrinsic clotting pathways are measured by the partial thromboplastin time and prothrombin time, respectively. Fibrinolysis is not evaluated specifically, but if suggested by severe hypofibrinogenemia and abnormal clotting tests in the presence of relatively normal platelet count, may be tested for by procedures such as the plasma thrombin time or other methods of detecting split products. For detecting marked fibrinolysis, the simple technique of observing a whole blood clot for dissolution within a four-hour period is relatively insensitive, but occasionally helpful. The whole blood clotting time, as an over-all test of coagulation, is grossly insensitive and has no value as a function test.

No reliable method of testing vessel function is available. The well-known tourniquet test, although occasionally positive in vascular disorders as well as platelet disorders, is imprecise and affected by so many variables that useful information is rarely obtained.

EVALUATION OF LABORATORY DATA

INTERPRETING THE DEGREE OF ABNORMALITY

Data obtained from the screening battery can be analyzed as in Table 1, but the physician must take into account the extent of the abnormality. Minor deviations from the normal range should not be assigned unwarranted significance. "Spontaneous" bleeding usually is not encountered unless the platelet count is less than 50,000/cu. mm. or greater than 1,000,000/cu. mm., or the timed clotting tests are more than twice normal, or fibrinogen is less than 100 mg. per cent. In the presence of multiple defects or stress, however, even modest abnormalities may become clinically significant. Purpuric lesions, for example, are more likely to develop in the presence of fever. A prothrombin time greater than four times the normal value suggests coumarin toxicity. DIC should be considered when the triad of platelet count less than 150,000/cu. mm., prothrombin time greater than 15 seconds and fibrinogen less than 160 mg. per cent is

found. If only two of the three abnormalities are present, a thrombin time or other test for lysis or split products can be used for confirmation.

INTERACTION OF THE TESTS

Proper interpretation of the screening battery also requires recognition of some unavoidable redundancy in the tests. In the presence of platelet counts less than 100,000/cu. mm., a prolonged bleeding time merely reflects thrombocytopenia and adds no additional information. Similarly, because all factors (except VII) that influence the prothrombin time also affect the partial thromboplastin time, a prolonged partial thromboplastin time is difficult to interpret when the prothrombin time is known to be prolonged. PT and PTT may have imprecise end points and become uninterpretable when fibrinogen is less than 50 mg. per cent.

DIC AND LIVER DISEASE

Recognizing DIC in the presence of severe liver disease is difficult because both conditions may cause similar abnormalities of hemostatic function tests, including evidence of fibrinolysis. A superimposed DIC may be suspected if a patient with liver disease shows rapid progression of the thrombocytopenia and clotting abnormalities and a depression of factor VIII (which is not made in the liver), but no consistently reliable differentiating test is available.

SIGNIFICANCE OF NORMAL SCREENING BATTERY

A normal screening battery effectively rules out any significant hemostatic abnormality if history and physical examination are essentially benign. However, if clinical data strongly suggest a hemorrhagic tendency, a number of conditions not detectable by the screening battery must be considered. Purpura in the presence of normal tests suggests a vascular disorder such as allergic vasculitis, scurvy, dysproteinemia, or amyloidosis. Self-induced (factitial) purpura may be recognized by restriction of lesions to accessible areas on the limbs or breasts. Small ecchymoses limited to the superficial layers of the skin may be found in skin which has lost elasticity through age or the effects of corticosteroid therapy. Simple purpura remains a catch-all term for unexplained benign easy bruisability.

A clotting disorder, often manifested by delayed hemorrhage and poor wound healing, may be due to deficiency of factor XIII, a fibrin-stabilizing factor that must be tested for specifically if suspected. Occasionally, hemostatic lesions too mild to affect the screening tests must be sought later by special tests not usually available in emergency situations.

EMERGENCY MANAGEMENT

Most forms of hemostatic therapy carry some risk and should not be initiated precipitously merely to correct abnormal test data (Greenwalt, et al., 1970). The decision to treat should be based on the clinical judgment that present or imminent bleeding threatens death or serious injury. When corrective therapy seems necessary, informed interpretation of the screening battery will usually permit selection of an appropriate blood component or drug. Fresh whole blood, despite its widespread use, is not a universal remedy for bleeding problems because significant correction of platelet or clotting defects usually cannot be achieved without intolerable volume overload.

GENERAL MEASURES

The application of pressure to accessible bleeding points and meticulous attention to volume replacement are as important in "bleeders" as in patients with hemorrhage from organic lesions. However, cautery, sutures, and other trauma-inducing procedures should be delayed if possible until the hemostatic defect has been ameliorated. Intramuscular and subcutaneous injections should be avoided when possible and prolonged pressure should be applied to injection and venipuncture sites.

THROMBOCYTOPENIA

Bleeding attributed to thrombocytopenia is best controlled with platelet concentrates. Each 25-ml. unit of concentrate contains approximately 70 per cent of the platelets found in a unit of fresh whole blood. Although formulas for calculating correct dosage are available, it usually is suf-

ficient to assume that a single platelet unit can raise the platelet count by 5000/cu. mm. in an adult of average size. In smaller patients a unit will, of course, be more effective. A total dosage calculated to produce a final platelet count of 40,000 to 60,000/cu. mm. should be infused. The dose may be doubled if surgery is imminent. Although the expected platelet rise is usually obtained in patients with thrombocytopenia caused by poor platelet production, platelet transfusions may fail to increase the count significantly in patients suffering from increased platelet destruction as in ITP. On the presumption that at least some of the transfused platelets may escape destruction, most clinicians believe a trial of transfusion therapy is worthwhile, even when platelet counts are unlikely to improve.

If platelet transfusions fail to improve the count or are unavailable, prednisone (or equivalent) in dosage of 1 mg./kg./day in divided doses may be instituted on the basis of a widely-held belief that corticosteroids in some manner partially protect the blood vessels from the effects of thrombocytopenia.

Platelet transfusions should not be given casually, since platelets carry HLA antigens and repeated transfusions may eventually result in destructive antibody formation, even if the infused units are ABO and Rh compatible. In asymptomatic patients, prophylactic transfusions usually are not justified unless the platelet count is less than 10,000/cu. mm. and the depletion is expected to be temporary.

QUALITATIVE PLATELET DEFECTS

If clinical bleeding is severe, functional defects due to aspirin can be treated with platelet concentrates (6 to 8 units for an adult). In uremia the defect is secondary to an abnormal plasma environment and can be relieved temporarily by dialysis.

INTRINSIC CLOTTING DISORDER

The patient known to have factor VIII deficiency is most conveniently treated with cryoprecipitate. An initial priming dose of two bags per 12 kg. of body weight should be followed by a maintenance regimen of half the primary dose every 12 hours.

A commercial concentrate containing

factors II, VII, IX, and X may be used for treatment of factor IX deficiency, but carries a high risk of conveying hepatitis. Dosage should be guided by the manufacturer's recommendations, with a goal of raising the depressed component to about 40 per cent of the normal average value.

If the nature of the intrinsic clotting defect is unknown, treatment requires the infusion of fresh or fresh-frozen plasma in an initial volume approximately equal to 20 per cent of the predicted total blood volume. The patient must be observed for evidence of fluid overload.

The risk of permanent knee damage from hemarthrosis may be reduced if the joint is aspirated aseptically *after* corrective therapy has been given.

HEPARIN OVERDOSE

Since the heparin blood levels are rarely calculable, a bleeding patient may be treated with a single course of 50 mg. protamine sulfate injected over a ten-minute period. Residual heparin, if any, will be eliminated over the next few hours by normal excretory routes.

EXTRINSIC CLOTTING DISORDERS

"Prothrombin problems" are almost always caused by coumarin drugs, vitamin K deficiency, or liver disease. If the patient with coumarin overdosage is not bleeding and coumarin therapy is to be resumed, simply stopping the drug for several days is the preferred treatment, since vitamin K administration will cause temporary resistance to coumarin drugs. Under all other circumstances, and particularly if the patient is bleeding, vitamin K-1, 10 to 25 mg. given orally or intramuscularly is indicated and will provide correction in 12 to 24 hours. If the bleeding problem is serious, vitamin K-1 given intravenously will provide correction more quickly, but with a slight risk of adverse reaction. Only in acute emergencies does the patient need immediate replacement therapy with infusion of either fresh frozen plasma, as in intrinsic clotting disorders, or commercial concentrates of factors II, VII, IX, and X. The concentrates are more effective, but carry a much higher risk of hepatitis.

Even in patients known to have liver disease, a prolonged prothrombin time should not be attributed to liver injury until a trial of vitamin K-1 has proved to be ineffective. The hemostatic abnormalities of liver disease, when not correctable by vitamin K, are not usually treatable. Replacement therapy gives transient improvement at best and may precipitate an acute episode of DIC or fibrinolysis.

DISSEMINATED INTRAVASCULAR COAGULATION

DIC is best managed by intensive therapy of the underlying disease, whether shock, infection, obstetric catastrophe, or some other. Heparin, by inhibiting the coagulation process, can lead to replenishment of the depressed hemostatic elements, but is rarely necessary and may be dangerous in a vigorously bleeding patient. If the underlying process is unknown or requires extended therapy for control, intravenous heparin by drip or by intermittent dose every four hours to provide 400 to 600 I.U./kg./day may be tried. If successful, a significant rise in fibrinogen should be noted within 24 to 36 hours.

When hemorrhage in DIC is life-threatening, replacement therapy to correct severe thrombocytopenia and/or severe hypofibrinogenemia frequently is effective, but must be given concurrently with heparin to avoid accelerated clotting and thrombosis. Significant correction of hypofibrinogenemia requires the infusion of 3 to 6 gm. of concentrated fibrinogen (plasma alone is ineffective) and carries an extremely high risk of transmitting hepatitis. Cryoprecipitate and fresh plasma can be added to the replacement regimen, but are probably of less value.

In patients with hemorrhagic DIC superimposed on liver disease, heparin may cause catastrophic bleeding and is almost never helpful.

FIBRINOLYSIS

Fibrinolysis can be inhibited by epsilon-aminocaproic acid (EACA) in dose of 18 to 24 gm./day, but drug therapy is rarely necessary since most cases of fibrinolysis are secondary to DIC and will subside if the DIC is treated. If EACA seems indicated to control fulminating fibrinolysis, it is wise to assume underlying DIC and administer heparin simultaneously to minimize the risk of thrombosis. In addition, replacement therapy, if indicated, may be given as for DIC.

VON WILLEBRAND'S DISEASE

This disorder may be treated with cryoprecipitate as in the therapy of factor VIII deficiency.

HEMORRHAGE WHEN SCREENING BATTERY NORMAL

Scurvy responds quickly to vitamin C. Allergic vasculitis occasionally responds to prednisone 1 to 2 mg./kg./day in divided doses. Dysproteinemic bleeding has no remedy available under emergency conditions and must usually be managed with replacement of lost blood. Treatment for other conditions in this category depends on specific identification.

References

Baldini, M.: Idiopathic thrombocytopenic purpura. N. Engl. J. Med., 274:1245, 1966.

Bidwell, E.: Acquired inhibitors of coagulants. Ann. Rev. Med., 20:63, 1969.
Colman, R. W., et al.: Disseminated intravascular coagulation: An Approach. Am. J. Med., 52:679, 1972.
Cream, J. J., et al.: Schönlein-Henoch purpura in the adult. J. Med., 39:461, 1970.
Gottlieb, A. J.: Nonallergic Purpura. In Williams, W. J., et al. (eds.): Hematology. New York, McGraw-Hill, 1972, pp. 1176–1179.
Goulian, M.: A guide to disorders of hemostasis. Ann. Intern. Med., 65:782, 1966.
Greenwalt, T. J., et al. (eds.): Management of Hemorrhagic Diseases, Chapter X (pp. 59–66), In General Principles of Blood Transfusion. Chicago, American Medical Association, 1970.
Holmberg, L., and Nilsson, I. M.: Two genetic variants of von Willebrand's disease. N. Engl. J. Med., 288:595, 1973.
Leslie, J., and Ingram, G. I. C.: The diagnosis of long-standing bleeding disorders. Seminars Hematol., 8:140, 1971.
Pechet, L.: Fibrinolysis. N. Engl. J. Med., 273:966, 1965.
Weiss, H. J.: Acquired Qualitative Platelet Disorders. In Williams, W. J., et al. (eds.): Hematology. New York, McGraw-Hill, 1972, pp. 1171–1175.

General References

Biggs, R.: Human Blood Coagulation, Haemostasis and Thrombosis. Oxford, Blackwell, 1972.
Williams, W. J., et al. (eds.): Hematology. Part IV, Hemostasis. New York, McGraw-Hill, 1972.

B. DISORDERS OF THE LEUKOCYTES

James W. Keller

Leukocyte or white blood cell disorders encompass a variety of diseases with many presentations. For the purposes of this chapter, these disorders will be approached in two ways: (1) common modes of presentation; and (2) a short treatise on some of the common diseases with emphasis on rapid diagnosis and immediate treatment, and the complications of chemotherapy.

PRESENTATIONS

(1) Fever with stomatitis/pharyngitis.
(2) Bleeding.
(3) Lymphadenopathy.
(4) Bone pain and abnormal skeletal x-rays.

(5) Chest x-ray abnormalities.
(6) Abnormalities of white blood cell count and differential.
(7) Hyperviscosity syndrome.

Fever with Stomatitis/Pharyngitis

Fever obviously may be associated with a variety of diseases, but, when it is accompanied by stomatitis and/or pharyngitis, profound granulocytopenia should be strongly suspected. An absolute granulocyte count (WBC times percentage of segmented neutrophils and bands) of 1000 or less signifies an increased susceptibility to infections, especially bacterial ones. The presence of fever in association with significant granulocytopenia is tantamount to a life-threatening infection, and is a true medical emergency. The patient should be promptly and thoroughly cultured, and then immediately placed on broad spectrum antibiotics, and later the etiology of the granulocytopenia can be evaluated. Delay in starting antibiotics is a serious omission, since death may occur within 24 hours.

Bleeding

The subject of bleeding was covered in Chapter 49A. However, bleeding secondary to thrombocytopenia may be a presentation of certain leukocyte disorders, especially diseases that infiltrate the marrow or processes that produce marrow hypoplasia. Platelet transfusions are helpful in the treatment of this type of bleeding.

Lymphadenopathy

Lymph node enlargement can be found in many disorders. The ones of most interest here include Hodgkin's disease, non-Hodgkin's lymphomas, chronic lymphocytic leukemia, acute leukemias, and infectious mononucleosis.

Normal nodes should not be palpable, but palpable lymphadenopathy does not necessarily imply a neoplastic or life-threatening disease. It is not unusual for youngsters to have mild adenopathy (shotty, shot-like, 0.5 to 1.0 cm. in diameter). Frequently, adenopathy in certain anatomic sites may be secondary to chronic skin or nail infections, e.g., inguinal and axillary nodes. Enlargement of the deep cervical nodes located below the jaw angles almost invariably accompanies pharyngitis, tonsillitis, and other infections of the throat and face. Lower cervical, supraclavicular, and femoral nodes are more likely to be pathologic, as are large, matted nodes, which may be fixed to adjacent structures. Node tenderness frequently is a sign of inflammation, whereas painless adenopathy is more suggestive of neoplasia, but one must not be too rigid in interpretation of this rule. Hodgkin's disease commonly presents with superficial adenopathy, especially in the cervical-supraclavicular areas. Non-Hodgkin's lymphomas, chronic lymphocytic leukemia, and acute lymphocytic leukemia frequently are associated with generalized adenopathy. Infectious mononucleosis often is accompanied by diffuse adenopathy, but posterior cervical adenopathy is nearly always present in this disease. Node biopsies are needed to diagnose Hodgkin's disease and non-Hodgkin's lymphoma, but studies of blood and marrow aspirates can establish the diagnosis of infectious mononucleosis, acute lymphocytic leukemia, and chronic lymphocytic leukemia without resorting to excisional biopsy.

Bone Pain and Abnormal Skeletal X-rays

Bone pain, especially without antecedent trauma, may present in a variety of disorders. Skeletal x-rays taken for other reasons may demonstrate abnormalities that are clues to other diseases. Plasma cell myeloma frequently presents with bone pain and accompanying lytic lesions on x-rays, with or without compression fractures. Obviously, lytic lesions and compression fractures may be related to metastatic solid tumors and lymphomas as well. Osteoblastic bone lesions not uncommonly can be found in Hodgkin's disease, as well as metastatic solid tumors, such as cancers of the breast or prostate. A patient with myelofibrosis may demonstrate bony sclerosis.

Spinal cord compression is an uncommon initial presentation for patients with lymphomas, but it can occur. More frequently, lymphoma of the spinal epidural space may be a complication during the course of the disease. Complaints of back or radicular pain, with or without motor dysfunction and superficial sensory loss, in a patient with lymphoma should make one suspect cord compression. Prompt evaluation is mandatory, usually with myelography. If the condition goes unattended, it may progress to full paraplegia and loss of sphincter control, which is a true emergency that usually requires immediate myelography and decompression laminectomy.

Chest X-ray Abnormalities

This test is performed commonly in Emergency Departments. In most cases, specific symptoms prompt the physician to order a chest x-ray, but occasionally it is done blindly for evaluation of a difficult diagnostic problem. The important findings in disorders of white blood cells include mediastinal and hilar adenopathy secondary to lymphoreticular neoplasms. Sometimes a patient will present with the superior vena cava syndrome (SVCS), which is caused by blockage of venous drainage from the upper part of the thorax, which secondarily increases venous pressure. The syndrome usually is manifested by engorgement of collateral veins of the upper thorax and neck, with swelling of the face and upper torso, edema of the conjunctiva, and central nervous system symptoms, such as headache, distorted vision, and altered mental states. Occasionally, SVCS may be accompanied by airway or esophageal obstruction. Although this syndrome most commonly is related to bronchogenic carcinoma (75 per cent of patients), lymphomas are the next largest category (15 per cent). Chest x-ray usually reveals a mediastinal mass.

SVCS sometimes presents as an emergency. Immediate therapy may be required to alleviate the symptoms and prevent further complications. Potent diuretics may offer dramatic help in emergency situations prior to initiation of radiation therapy, which is the treatment of choice.

Other clues to mediastinal disease might be a brassy-sounding cough or hoarseness secondary to recurrent laryngeal nerve palsy. Disorders of leukocytes also may be associated with opportunistic lung infections with parenchymal infiltrates.

Abnormalities of White Blood Cell Count and Differential

Although patients do not "present" with an abnormal WBC, certain symptoms and signs, such as adenopathy, bone pain, unexplained bleeding, stomatitis/pharyngitis, gum hyperplasia, splenomegaly, and pallor, indicate the need for a complete blood count (CBC). Currently, a CBC is ordered as part of the initial evaluation of the ill patient. Abnormalities, if found, should be pursued with further tests; they may consist of leukocytosis, granulocytopenia, immature white blood cells, atypical lymphocytes, eosinophilia, or basophilia. Concomitant anemia and/or thrombocytopenia provide helpful clues to differential diagnosis and usually indicate more serious disorders.

Hyperviscosity Syndrome

This is a complex of symptoms that is quite rare and frequently goes undiagnosed for a long time. The signs and symptoms usually are centered around ocular, hematologic, and neurologic manifestations. Eye changes range from minor disturbance in vision to almost complete blindness, which may be acute at onset. Features diagnosed ophthalmoscopically include distention and tortuosity of the retinal veins, with beading and dilatation creating a "string of sausage" appearance and flame-shaped hemorrhages. Hematologic changes normally are related to bleeding, especially from mucous membranes of the mouth and gums and from epistaxis, as well as from other sites, such as the gastrointestinal and genitourinary tracts. Neurologic changes include headache, dizziness, vertigo, and somnolence progressing through stupor to coma, with an occasional patient manifesting a convulsive disorder. Rarely, there may be cardiovascular manifestations related to expanded plasma volume and increased viscosity, producing congestive heart failure.

SPECIFIC DISEASES

Granulocytopenias

As mentioned above, granulocytes are extremely important in combating bacterial infections. An absolute granulocyte count of 500 to 1000 signifies an increased risk of infection, and depression to less than 500 increases the risk factor even further.

Reduction in peripheral granulocytes may be associated with thrombocytopenia and anemia (pancytopenia), or may present as a single abnormality (agranulocytosis). Granulocytopenia can be secondary to increased peripheral destruction or utilization, such as may occur with (a) hypersplenism; (b) sepsis; (c) antibodies in association with certain diseases; or (d) antibodies related to drugs. Similarly, reduction of granulocytes may be secondary to decreased production, such as (a) maturation defects (vitamin B_{12} and folic acid deficiency); (b) infiltrative processes in the marrow, e.g., metastatic carcinoma, leukemia, myeloma, and myelofibrosis; and (c) hypoplasia related to radiation, drugs, or as yet undetermined causes.

Drugs currently are an extremely important cause of agranulocytosis or aplastic anemia, i.e., pancytopenia. The common drugs producing agranulocytosis include phenothiazines, antithyroid drugs (thiouracils and methimazole), sulfonamides and derivatives, pyrazolones (phenylbutazone and dipyrone [Pyralgin]), and antibiotics (e.g., methicillin). These reactions are of the idiosyncratic type that occur only in susceptible individuals.

Aplastic anemia is a predictable event with anticancer drugs, and usually is related to drug dosage; however, the damage is transient and recovery ensues. Other drug-induced aplastic anemias normally are not transient, and may indeed progress long after the drug has been discontinued. Recovery, if it does happen, may take years. In general, the mechanism of drug-induced aplastic anemia is unknown. The most common offenders include chloramphenicol, sulfonamides, pyrazolones (e.g., phenylbutazone), hydantoins (e.g., diphenylhydantoin), sulfonylureas (e.g., oral hypoglycemic agents), and gold compounds.

Many cases of aplastic anemia are idiopathic, and it appears that more are being reported in association with hepatitis. From an emergency point of view, the patient with granulocytopenia should be promptly hospitalized and evaluated. Fever in this setting is a medical emergency.

Lymphomas

HODGKIN'S DISEASE

This disease presents in most cases with superficial lymphadenopathy, the supraclavicular area being the most common site. In addition to adenopathy, a percentage of patients will present with systemic symptoms, such as weight loss (greater than 10 per cent of body weight in the preceding six months), night sweats, fever, pruritus, and alcohol-induced pain. Biopsy of a node is essential for diagnosis. Once the latter is established, the patient must be staged carefully (often with laparotomy) to determine the exact extent of the disease. Proper staging is extremely important in planning therapy with curative intent. Treatment usually includes radiation or chemotherapy, or both.

NON-HODGKIN'S LYMPHOMA

Included in this category are all other lymphomas. The old classification consisted of such entities as reticulum cell sarcoma, lymphosarcoma, and giant follicular lymphoma. These have now been divided into nine different categories, with the general division between nodular and diffuse types. Unlike Hodgkin's disease, this group frequently presents with more generalized adenopathy and visceral disease. Again, biopsy is essential for diagnosis. Staging laparotomies in these types of lymphomas usually are not performed, in view of the multifocal nature of the disease. Bone marrow and liver biopsies are undertaken commonly, since these organs frequently are involved and establish unequivocal dissemination of the lymphoma. Treatment usually consists of chemotherapy. Localized disease, when found, is treated with radiation. Total body irradiation is employed with some success currently in certain non-Hodgkin's lymphomas, even when the process is generalized.

Infectious Mononucleosis

Infectious mononucleosis (IM) is an extremely common disease in young adults, usually manifesting in one of three symptom complexes, although it may present with atypical symptoms, including those of a predominantly neurologic nature. The most common (80 per cent) consists of pharyngitis, fever, diffuse adenopathy with special involvement of posterior cervical and postauricular nodes, and a soft, but enlarged, spleen. Less common signs might include also eyelid edema, as well as a palatal enanthema. The second type is the so-called typhoidal form (occurring in about 12 per cent of patients), with high fever the important manifestation; adenopathy is present, but not pharyngitis. A third type of presentation is jaundice (8 per cent). The striking abnormality in the peripheral blood is seen in increased lymphocytes (higher than 50 per cent, more than 20 per cent of these being atypical lymphocytes). The total WBC often is normal. The diagnosis is confirmed by a positive monospot test followed by a positive heterophil antibody test. The heterophil antibody titer should be ≥ 1:56 without absorption, with a titer of at least 1:28 after absorption with guinea pig kidney, and no agglutination after the beef cell antigen absorption. It must be appreciated that the monospot and heterophil antibody tests may not be positive during the early course of the disease. Atypical lymphocytes are not absolutely specific for this disease, and may be found in a variety of other conditions, including infectious hepatitis, drug hypersensitivity, and a host of viral diseases. Occasionally, a patient may present with all the signs and symptoms of IM without a positive heterophil antibody test. In some cases, there may be a true heterophil-negative case of IM, as determined by a rise in the Epstein-Barr (E-B) virus titer. Cytomegalic virus disease and acquired toxoplasmosis may behave clinically like IM. The treatment is symptomatic. It must be stressed that ampicillin should not be given in cases of suspected IM, because of the high incidence of skin reactions.

Plasma Cell Dyscrasias

PLASMA CELL MYELOMA

In the past it quite often was not uncommon for a patient with plasma cell myeloma to present with back pain and skeletal x-rays revealing lytic areas or diffuse osteolytic lesions. Currently, routine testing might reveal such clues as rouleau formation on a blood film, anemia or pancytopenia, extreme elevation of the sedimentation rate, or significant elevation of the total serum protein on a chemical profile. The presence of proteinuria might lead to a work-up culminating in the diagnosis of myeloma, because of the presence of Bence-Jones proteinuria. Other diagnostic tests are important in establishing the diagnosis. Besides the presence of lytic bone lesions, there should be bone marrow plasmacytosis, and the presence of an "M"-protein in the blood serum, and/or Bence-Jones proteinuria. The presence of "M"-protein is not diagnostic of myeloma, since it may occur in lymphoma, and, indeed, there is a condition of benign monoclonal gammopathy. Bone marrow plasmacytosis is seen in many disorders, but, in general, a bone marrow containing more than 20 per cent plasma cells is strongly suggestive of myeloma. Once the diagnosis is established, the patient customarily is treated with chemotherapy. Occasionally, radiation therapy is used for localized, extremely painful bony lesions or localized plasmacytoma. Complications of this disease include a susceptibility to infection (especially pneumococcal), bone fractures, cord compression, and bleeding.

WALDENSTRÖM'S MACROGLOBULINEMIA

Macroglobulinemia is a rare disease found mainly in patients over the age of 50. Nonspecific symptoms of fatigue and weight loss are present at onset, and generalized lymphadenopathy and hepatosplenomegaly are noted on examination. The disease is quite similar to myeloma in its hematologic and protein abnormalities, except that the "M"-protein is invariably IgM, and the bone marrow usually demonstrates increased numbers of small atypical "plasmacytoid lymphocytes." Osteolytic bone lesions are rare. Symptoms of hyperviscosity usually occur at some time in the course of the disease (see above). In 85 to 90 per cent of cases of hyperviscosity syndrome, the cause is related to Waldenström's macroglobulinemia; the remaining cases involve plasma cell myeloma. The diagnosis of this hyperviscosity syndrome rests on determination of the serum viscosity, using either an Ostwald viscosimeter or, more simply, a red blood cell hemacytometer pipette. A measure is taken of the time required for a constant volume of serum and water at a given temperature to flow through a capillary tube. The relative viscosity of the serum is obtained by dividing the flow time of serum by the flow time of water. Nearly all individuals with a relative viscosity greater than 8 are symptomatic, as are many with a viscosity between 5 and 8. Initial treatment is accomplished by plasmapheresis, if the full syndrome is present, and in some situations this can be life-saving. Chemotherapy usually is administered, in an attempt to decrease the production of the protein.

Leukemias

ACUTE LEUKEMIA

Lymphoblastic leukemia is more common in the younger age-groups, whereas myeloblastic and monoblastic leukemias are found more classically in older patients. As the name implies, the acute leukemias usually are of short duration and are heralded by prominent symptoms. Onset is accompanied normally by bleeding, symptoms secondary to anemia, or high fever usually associated with some type of bacterial infection. Physical examination generally shows pallor, adenopathy and/or splenomegaly (especially in the lymphoblastic type), and evidence of a bleeding tendency. The WBC may be strikingly elevated, normal, or depressed; but the hallmark is the presence of immature white blood cells (lymphoblasts, myeloblasts, or monoblasts) in the peripheral blood. A concomitant anemia or thrombocytopenia frequently is present, and may be a helpful clue to the diagnosis. Occasionally, a patient may have only pancytopenia without immature cells in the peripheral blood, but the leukemic cells can be detected in the bone marrow (so-called aleukemic leukemia).

Acute leukemia should be considered a medical quasi-emergency, especially in the presence of fever or bleeding. A bone marrow usually is essential to establish the diagnosis in most cases. Fever generally is tantamount to an infection (almost always bacterial initially), and it is most appropriate to obtain cultures of blood, urine, and sputum, and to start on broad spectrum antibiotics while awaiting the results of these cultures. Bleeding almost invariably is related to thrombocytopenia (especially with platelet counts of less than 20,000/cu. mm.), and this can be managed effectively with platelet transfusions, usually given as eight platelet concentrates at one time. One unit of platelet concentrate/m.^{2} should raise the peripheral platelet count of an adult 12,000/cu.mm. when the platelet count is measured one hour after infusion. Factors that may decrease the yield include infections, splenomegaly, bleeding, fever, and platelet antibodies. Bleeding also may be a manifestation of disseminated intravascular coagulation, such as is present commonly with promyelocytic leukemia. Treatment with chemotherapeutic agents is usually initiated promptly after the diagnosis is established. The prognosis in these groups of diseases has improved significantly, to the point where childhood acute leukemia has a cure rate approaching 50 per cent. Unfortunately, adult types of acute leukemia do not have so good a prognosis, but great strides are being made in treatment.

CHRONIC LEUKEMIA

These types of leukemias often are insidious in onset, and their course covers a period of years, not months. There are two varieties: chronic lymphocytic leukemia and chronic granulocytic leukemia. The former is not difficult to diagnose. Frequently, the diagnosis is made incidentally on demonstration of an elevated WBC with an absolute lymphocytosis (WBC times percentage of lymphocytes) usually greater than 15,000/cu.mm. Generalized adenopathy and splenomegaly frequently are found on physical examination. A bone marrow examination confirms the presence of increased numbers of well-differentiated lymphocytes. Chronic granulocytic leukemia (CGL) also may be detected on a routine WBC, which shows an extreme elevation (frequently greater than 100,000/cu.mm.) with a significant number of mature and immature granulocytes. Fatigue and malaise, as well as low grade fever, are not unusual presenting symptoms, and the spleen generally is enlarged, frequently extending below the umbilicus. The bone marrow in CGL demonstrates myeloid hyperplasia. A portion of the marrow aspirate should be reserved for chromosome analysis, to ascertain the almost invariable presence of the Philadelphia chromosome. In general, these diseases do not present as emergency disorders unless there is a secondary complication of infection or bleeding. Chemotherapy is the current treatment of choice.

Myeloproliferative Disorders

Classically, six disorders are included under this heading: idiopathic myelofibrosis with myeloid metaplasia; acute and chronic granulocytic leukemia; polycythemia rubra vera; erythemic myelosis (Di Guglielmo's syndrome); and idiopathic thrombocytosis. Erythemic myelosis frequently behaves like acute leukemia. Idiopathic thrombocytosis will be discussed with problems of bleeding and platelets. Idiopathic myelofibrosis with myeloid metaplasia may present in a very similar fashion to chronic granulocytic leukemia. An enlarged spleen almost invariably is present, and frequently is the massive type extending below the umbilicus. The WBC usually is elevated (but generally less than 100,000/cu.mm.), and again the left shift in the white blood cell maturation will be noted. Myelofibrosis usually does not present as an emergency, except for an occasional patient with an infection or symptoms referable to a ruptured spleen. The differentiation of this disease from chronic granulocytic leukemia is made on the basis of bone marrow aspirate and biopsy, as well as culture of the bone marrow for the presence of abnormal chromosomes. Treatment is not specific and may include chemotherapy, androgens, corticosteroids, and splenectomy, depending on the major hematologic problem.

Leukemoid Reactions

Leukemoid reactions are peripheral blood counts resembling leukemia, and generally are quite rare. The term implies an elevation of the WBC to a degree not seen with the usual diseases (perhaps over 30,000/cu.mm.), with or without immature granulocytes or abnormal numbers of other white blood cells. It may occur with a variety of diseases, such as disseminated tuberculosis, overwhelming sepsis, chronic liver disease with acute exacerbations, tissue necrosis, carcinoma, subacute bacterial endocarditis, burns, trauma, Hodgkin's disease, or severe hemorrhage or hemolysis. In general, the WBC is less than 100,000/cu.mm., and myeloblasts or monoblasts are absent or infrequent in the peripheral blood. Concomitant anemia and thrombocytopenia are not present in leukemoid reactions, unless produced by the underlying disease. The leukocyte alkaline phosphatase almost always is elevated. Generally, the spleen is not enlarged except as related to the basic disease, and a bone marrow test may be helpful in differentiating leukemoid reactions from leukemia. Leukemoid reactions may be of the granulocytic type, which are the most common, but monocytic and lymphocytic types sometimes occur.

Eosinophilia and Basophilia

Mild degrees of eosinophilia may be seen in a variety of conditions, and extensive evaluation frequently does not reveal a cause. Common conditions to be considered include allergic states, such as hay fever, asthma, and drug reactions; parasitic diseases, especially tissue invaders; skin disorders, such as pemphigus or dermatitis herpetiformis; myeloproliferative disorders; occasionally, Hodgkin's disease; and a variety of other conditions, such as periarteritis nodosa, eosinophilic granuloma, eosinophilia collagen vascular disease, and eosinophilic leukemia.

Basophilia of any significant degree is extremely rare. It usually is associated with one of the myeloproliferative syndromes.

Complications of Chemotherapy

It is obvious from the above information that many disorders of white blood cells are treated with chemotherapeutic agents, and it is not uncommon at present to see patients in Emergency Departments with a known disease undergoing treatment. Most chemotherapeutic agents have significant hematologic toxicity, which can result in bleeding related to thrombocytopenia and increased susceptibility to infections related to granulocytopenia. Since chemotherapeutic agents affect normally dividing cells as well as tumor cells, it is not unusual to find accompanying alopecia, mucositis (involving the mouth, vagina, and rectum), nausea, vomiting, and diarrhea. Infertility, either transient or permanent, also may be found. Certain drugs have certain unique toxicities, and a few are listed below:

(a) cyclophosphamide – hemorrhagic cystitis;

(b) vincristine – peripheral neuropathy and constipation;

(c) bleomycin and busulfan – pulmonary fibrosis;

(d) adriamycin and daunomycin – cardiac toxicity resulting in congestive heart failure and arrhythmias;

(e) methotrexate, nitrosoureas, mithramycin, and mercaptopurine – liver toxicity;

(f) mithramycin – bleeding abnormalities not necessarily mediated by platelets.

References

Becker, G. A., and Aster, R. H.: Platelet transfusion therapy. Med. Clin. North Am. 56:81, 1972.

Bloch, K. J., and Maki, D. G.: Hyperviscosity syndromes associated with immunoglobulin abnormalities. Semin. Hematol. 10:113, 1973.

Bodey, G. P., et al.: Quantitative relationship between circulating leukocytes and infection in patients with acute leukemia. Ann. Intern. Med. *64*:328, 1966.

Hoagland, R. J.: The clinical manifestations of infectious mononucleosis. Am. J. Med. Sci. *240*:21, 1960.

Huguley, C. M., Lea, J. W., and Butts, J. A.: Adverse hematologic reactions to certain drugs. Progr. Hematol. 5:105, 1966.

Jones, S. E., et al.: Non-Hodgkin's lymphomas. IV.

Clinicopathologic correlation in 405 cases. Cancer *31*:806, 1973.

Kaplan, H. S.: Hodgkin's Disease. 1st ed. Cambridge, Mass., Harvard University Press, 1972.

Lokich, J. J., and Goodman, R.: Superior vena cava syndrome. J.A.M.A. *231*:58, 1975.

Mullins, G. M., et al.: Malignant lymphomas of the spinal epidural space. Ann. Intern. Med. *74*:416, 1971.

Williams, W. J., et al.: Hematology. 1st ed. New York, McGraw-Hill Co., 1972.

C. DISORDERS OF THE RED BLOOD CELLS

Alan O. Feingold

ANEMIA

Anemia may be caused by many disease processes, and a patient with anemia may present with one or many of a myriad of signs or symptoms. Furthermore, there is no clinical means of diagnosing or excluding anemia other than the hemoglobin and hematocrit. Thus, the hemoglobin and hematocrit are among the most frequently used laboratory tests. In this discussion of anemia from the standpoint of the emergency physician, the broad outlines of the diagnostic approach to assessing anemia and discovering its etiology will be followed by a brief discussion of the emergency treatment of anemia.

DEFINITION

Anemia is usually defined as a lower than normal hematocrit or hemoglobin level. The *hematocrit* measures the volume of red blood cells as a fraction (percentage) of the total blood volume. The *hemoglobin* is expressed as a concentration in grams per 100 ml. of whole blood. These tests do not measure the volume of blood in the body, the total amount of hemoglobin in the body, or the total body mass of red blood cells. A change in blood volume due to acute bleeding does not change hemoglobin and hematocrit values until compensatory mechanisms come into play. Changes of blood volume due to fluid shifts can cause great increases or decreases in hemoglobin and hematocrit values without any change in total body hemoglobin or red blood cell mass. Thus dehydration may cause an anemic person to have a normal hematocrit. Overhydration can produce a low value for hemoglobin or hematocrit that otherwise would be normal. To avoid serious clinical errors, the physician must use the hemoglobin and hematocrit as information about the clinical situation and must not define the clinical situation in terms of the hemoglobin and hematocrit.

BLEEDING AND ANEMIA

Bleeding is an important cause of anemia but should never be confused with anemia. A patient with substantial bleeding can still have a normal hemoglobin. Acutely, bleeding causes loss of blood volume, but hemoglobin values are lowered only as hemodilution occurs as a compensatory mechanism to restore blood volume. While changes are often marked in the first four hours, hemodilution and equilibration take 24 to 48 hours to be completed, although they will occur faster with I.V. fluid administration. Therefore, a single hemoglobin determination is never a good way to determine *blood loss* in the acute situation. Furthermore, if a man with a hemoglobin level of 17.6 gm. per 100 ml. should lose a liter of blood, his hemoglobin level after hemodilution occurred would be about 14.4 gm. per 100 ml. (still normal!), but a man with a usual hemoglobin of 14.1 gm. per 100 ml. needs to lose only a small quantity of blood to cause his hemoglobin value to drop below normal limits.

In the *acute situation*, decreases in blood volume caused by bleeding (or other fluid loss) must be detected by *orthostatic changes in pulse and blood pressure*. Ordinarily there is a small increase in blood pressure in the standing position, 2 to 5 mm. Hg more than in the supine position. In situations of loss of blood volume, blood pressure will drop and pulse rate will increase on assumption of the standing position. A drop of more than 5 mm. Hg in the diastolic pressure and 10 mm. Hg in the systolic pressure, or a rise in pulse rate of 10 beats per minute or more indicates significant loss of blood volume (unless peripheral vasodilatation is occurring or there is a neurologic abnormality). Whenever bleeding is suspected, orthostatic changes in blood pressure and pulse should be looked for, and the patient should be questioned about symptoms of orthostatic hypotension: dizziness, fainting, visual disturbances, rapid heart beat.

DIAGNOSIS

It is best to base the diagnosis of anemia on the *hemoglobin level* because microcytic anemias may have a *normal red blood cell count*, and some anemias with abnormal red blood cell shape may have a normal *packed cell volume* due to false elevation of the value by plasma trapping. As a practical matter, however, the microhematocrit method is fast, accurate, and inexpensive and is only rarely falsely negative. The fingerstick method should be used with caution in an edematous or vasoconstricted patient, as lymph dilution may cause false lowering of the hematocrit.) The normal values of hemoglobin are lower for women and children and tend to decrease slightly with advanced age. It is important to remember that normal values are statistical 95 per cent limits and that 2.5 per cent of normal people will have an "anemia" if defined on such a basis. To complicate matters, normal values depend on the methods used. The microhematocrit method yields a value 1 to 2 percentage points higher than the Coulter counter method because of plasma trapping. Different chemical methods of hemoglobin determination will yield different values. Finally, venous blood hemoglobin concentrations are higher than those of arterial blood because of loss of plasma to the lymph. The most common normal hemoglobin values usually cited are 12 to 16 gm. per 100 ml. for women and 14 to 18 gm. per 100 ml. for men, but values as low as 11 gm. per 100 ml. in women and 13 gm. per 100 ml. in men may occur in healthy people. When a hemoglobin value occurs in the range of 11 to 12 gm. in women and 13 to 14 gm. in men, it must be interpreted carefully because it is in this range that normal and abnormal overlap.

CLINICAL PRESENTATION

Patients with anemia usually present with the symptoms of the disease causing the anemia. Often anemia is discovered fortuitously when a complete blood count (CBC) is ordered as a routine procedure. Anemia rarely causes symptoms until the hematocrit drops below 30 per cent, unless the drop is acute. The explanation for this is that oxygen delivery is not substantially decreased until the hematocrit is less than 30 per cent. Several compensatory mechanisms may act to increase O_2 delivery: (1) viscosity decreases as hematocrit decreases, and tissue blood flow increases proportionally; (2) 2,3-diphosphoglycerate increases, causing increased O_2 dissociation at any given Po_2. Patients who engage in strenuous activity will probably report decreased exercise tolerance with small decreases in hematocrit. At hematocrits below 30 per cent, patients begin to report exertional dyspnea and tachycardia with normal activities. Weakness, tiredness, and dizziness may be reported. On the other hand, the patient may often have no symptoms referable to anemia even with a hematocrit as low as 18 to 20 per cent, particularly if the anemia is slowly progressive and of long duration. Below 18 per cent, patients may have resting dyspnea and tachycardia. Paleness may be present at any degree of anemia, but most patients with mild anemia and many patients with severe anemia will have pink nailbeds and conjunctivae. Absence of paleness should never be a reason to omit hemoglobin and hematocrit tests.

Anemia may provoke symptoms of other disease or may serve as a precipitating factor. Congestive heart failure, angina pectoris, myocardial infarction, stroke, and transient cerebral ischemic attacks all may be precipitated by anemia if there is underlying vascular disease. Also, discovery of an anemia may be the clue that serious disease is present in a patient who has what appear to be minor complaints. For example, anemia in a patient with gastrointestinal symptoms may mean possible ulcer or cancer.

DETERMINING THE ETIOLOGY

Anemia is caused by either a decrease in production of hemoglobin by the bone marrow or an increase in blood loss. The usual classification of anemias is outlined as follows:

Decreased Production (reticulocyte count normal or low)
  Microcytic hypochromic—iron deficiency, thalassemia
  Macrocytic hypochromic—vitamin B_{12} and folate deficiencies
  Normochromic normocytic systemic disease, bone marrow suppression due to toxins and specific diseases
Increased Loss (reticulocyte count high, usually normochromic normocytic)
  Blood loss due to bleeding
  Hemolytic
    Intravascular
      1. Immune mechanisms
      2. Red blood cell defects
      3. Red blood cell enzyme deficiencies
      4. Hemoglobinopathies
      5. Toxic agents
      6. Mechanical destruction
    Extravascular
      1. Hypersplenism
      2. Red blood cell abnormalities

Any anemia may be quickly characterized by the hemoglobin, hematocrit, and red blood cell count, red blood cell indices, and a reticulocyte count. Adding to this information the white blood cell count and differential, looking at a peripheral smear for red blood cell morphology, and correlating with the patient's clinical situation will almost always sufficiently resolve the approximate etiology on which to base initial therapy. The definitive diagnosis will then be based on findings of specific tests.

The first step is to classify the anemia as *microcytic, normocytic,* or *macrocytic. Microcytic hypochromic anemias* are almost always caused by iron deficiency but are occasionally caused by thalassemia, lead poisoning, or other less common entities. The reticulocyte count should be low if this anemia is caused by decreased red blood cell production due to lack of iron. A history of bleeding or occult blood in the feces is circumstantial confirmation of the cause. Starch or clay eating can also cause iron deficiency by binding iron and making it unavailable for absorption. In any patient presenting with microcytic hypochromic anemia without an obvious source of blood loss such as heavy menstrual bleeding or

epistaxis, a careful search for a GI source of bleeding must be done. Thalassemia minor can be recognized by a mildly increased reticulocyte count and target cells on the blood smear. This diagnosis should be suspected in blacks and ethnic groups of Mediterranean origin.

Normochromic normocytic anemias are most commonly due to chronic disease, particularly chronic renal failure, rheumatoid arthritis, diabetes, and infections. Leukopenia and thrombocytopenia in a patient with a normochromic normocytic anemia or the presence of abnormal white blood cells or platelets indicates a possible toxic etiology or a primary bone marrow dysplasia.

Macrocytic anemias are usually due to folate or vitamin B_{12} deficiencies, although mild macrocytic indices are often seen in liver disease. Vitamin B_{12} deficiency should be suspected in older patients and patients with gastric or small bowel surgery, malabsorption, or neurologic symptoms (particularly numbness or burning paresthesia in the legs). Folate deficiency is common in alcoholics, pregnant women, and those with poor nutritional status and may be caused by drugs. Definitive diagnosis is based on serum levels of folate and vitamin B_{12} and on the Schilling test for vitamin B_{12} absorption. Bone marrow aspiration may be useful in proving that the anemia is megaloblastic.

In all anemias, a bone marrow aspiration may help provide a definitive diagnosis. Bone marrow study may prove very useful in a complicated acute situation, although it is usually reserved for cases in which simpler noninvasive techniques fail to provide a definitive etiology.

Every anemia must be considered to be caused by bleeding until conclusively proved otherwise. *Bleeding can mimic many types of anemia:*

1. *Hypochromic microcytic anemia* is usually caused by blood loss. Deficient dietary iron may be a problem in a milk-fed infant, but in an adult only 1 mg. of iron a day is needed to replace non-blood losses, and bleeding must be considered to be the cause. Menstrual blood loss is the most common etiology (sometimes complicated by decreased iron absorption because of starch or clay eating). Occult GI blood loss is next in frequency. This may be due to cancer, polyp,

gastritis, peptic ulcer, parasites, or other causes. In the over-40 age group, the discovery of an iron deficiency necessitates a search for a gastrointestinal malignancy, even if another possible cause is present.

2. *Normochromic normocytic anemia* can result from acute blood loss. A reticulocyte response may not appear for 3 to 10 days, particularly if a concomitant illness is present.

3. Blood loss is the most common cause of a misdiagnosed *"hemolytic anemia"* that is actually a normochromic normocytic anemia with an increased reticulocyte count due to the blood loss.

4. Bleeding may mimic a macrocytic anemia because a high percentage of reticulocytes, which are larger than mature red blood cells, will falsely elevate the mean cell volume.

THERAPY FOR CHRONIC ANEMIAS

Emergency treatment of a chronic anemia is rarely necessary. Emergency blood transfusion is indicated only for serious symptoms attributable to the low hemoglobin level *per se.* Possible indications for transfusion are acute myocardial infarction, severe angina, severe congestive heart failure, acute cerebrovascular insufficiency, and severe dyspnea. Transfusion, if necessary, should be accomplished with packed red blood cells, since blood volume is usually normal in chronic anemias. To avoid volume overload, each unit should be transfused over two hours or longer unless the severity of the problem necessitates a faster rate. Ordinarily a hematocrit of 28 to 30 per cent is sufficient and any transfusion to levels above that not only is wasteful but increases the likelihood of an adverse transfusion reaction without corresponding benefit.

Each unit of packed cells (about 250 cc.) will increase the hematocrit in an average person by approximately 3 per cent. The number of units of blood needed can be calculated easily, but a hematocrit should be determined after every 2 units to monitor the transfusion. If the etiology of the anemia is not known, then before any transfusion is given, sufficient blood should be drawn for future testing and possibly a bone marrow aspiration done so that the etiology may be determined. Tests done after transfusion may be inaccurate because of the transfused blood.

In most cases, chronic anemia should be treated specifically as determined by the underlying etiology. Response to specific therapy then confirms the diagnosis. Chronic anemia secondary to chronic renal disease usually stabilizes at a hematocrit of 19 to 24 per cent, which is well tolerated, so transfusion is almost never justified in such patients. Anemia of chronic systemic disease is usually stable at a hematocrit level to 25 to 30 per cent; again, transfusions are almost never justified, and therapy should be directed to the associated disease.

HEMOLYTIC ANEMIA

The hallmark of a hemolytic anemia is a significantly increased reticulocyte count. However, a patient may present with severe hemolysis but a normal or low reticulocyte count. Furthermore, an occasional patient may have severe hemolysis with a reticulocytosis but a normal hematocrit. On the other hand, there are several situations in which a reticulocytosis does not indicate hemolysis.

Reticulocytosis is a response to hemolysis. At least a 48-hour time lag occurs between the bone marrow stimulus of falling hematocrit and a noticeable rise in newly formed red blood cells in the circulation, so that with an acute hemolytic event the reticulocyte count will be normal for at least 48 hours. If bone marrow suppression is produced at the same time, reticulocytosis will not occur until the marrow recovers. When hemolysis is an ongoing process, a steady state will occur in which red blood cell loss due to hemolysis is balanced by newly formed red blood cells. In this situation, the hematocrit will usually be stable and the rate of hemolysis can be gauged by the degree of reticulocytosis. Rarely, the bone marrow response may be great enough to maintain the hematocrit at normal levels.

The diagnosis of hemolysis cannot be based solely on the presence of reticulocytes. As already discussed, bleeding will produce a brisk reticulocytosis, and chronic blood loss will produce continuing reticulocytosis. Other situations that produce a reticulocytosis not associated with hemolysis are cases of recovery from anemia in which red blood cell production has been suppressed. Treatment with iron, folate or vitamin B_{12} in the respective deficiency anemias produces marked reticulocytosis as the hemoglobin level rises to normal.

CLINICAL PRESENTATION

Patients with hemolytic anemia may present with the symptoms of their underlying disease, or with symptoms caused or provoked by the low hemoglobin level itself. The only common sign or symptom caused by the hemolytic process itself is jaundice (with increased indirect bilirubinemia) produced by increased bilirubin formation from increased hemoglobin turnover. Rarely with acute intravascular hemolysis, acute renal failure can occur from free hemoglobin in large amounts affecting the renal tubules. Also in chronic hemolytic anemias, bilirubin gallstones may be formed and the patient may present with acute cholelithiasis.

DIAGNOSIS

Reticulocytosis and jaundice occurring in an anemic patient are clues that hemolysis is producing the anemia. Other associated changes that may be produced as part of the hemolytic process, but which are not in themselves diagnostic of hemolysis, are increased serum LDH (from red blood cell lysis), and increased urinary urobilinogen (from increased bilirubin metabolism). Leukocytosis, thrombocytosis, and nucleated red blood cells can occur from increased bone marrow turnover produced by the stimulus of anemia. In acute hemolysis, brown urine may be due to the products of hemoglobin metabolism. All these findings are helpful indications of hemolysis, but the diagnosis of hemolysis must be based on direct evidence of red blood cell destruction. Changes in the plasma indicating red blood cell hemolysis are increased free hemoglobin, decreased haptoglobin, decreased hemopexin, and increased methemoglobin. The urine may contain hemoglobin, methemoglobin, or hemosiderin. If bleeding has been rigorously excluded, decreased survival of labeled red blood cells is the definitive test to demonstrate continuing hemolysis. However, these tests are not usually available on an emer-

gency basis. A quick, although not very accurate or sensitive method of testing for free plasma hemoglobin is to inspect the plasma of freshly centrifuged blood such as that in a microhematocrit tube. Pink plasma indicates free hemoglobin. Free hemoglobin may be demonstrated in the urine with benzidine. It is also easy to use the test for occult blood on a urine dipstick. If the microscopic examination of the urine reveals no blood cells, a positive test for occult blood is strong indication of free hemoglobin in the urine, particularly if the patient has recently noticed pink or brown urine. Fresh urine must be examined because red blood cells may lyse in hypotonic urine. (Myoglobinuria must also be considered and excluded in patients with dark urine.)

Careful distinction must be made between evidence for the occurrence of hemolysis and evidence of an etiology of the hemolysis. Many patients may have abnormal red blood cells, red blood cell enzymes, hemoglobins, and Coombs' tests. Such abnormalities do not represent the cause of an anemia, and it must be stressed that they do not even indicate that hemolysis is occurring. For example, about 10 per cent of all black men have glucose-6-phosphate dehydrogenase (G-6-PD) deficiency. The presence of G-6-PD in a patient with anemia in no way indicates that hemolysis is occurring or that the anemia is caused by G-6-PD deficiency. First, the existence of hemolysis must be proved, and then other possible causes must be excluded.

Discovering the etiology of a hemolytic anemia may involve complicated laboratory testing. The rest of this section will consider

***TABLE 1 Some Causes of Acute
Hemolytic Anemia***

---

1. Paroxysmal nocturnal hemoglobinuria
2. Red blood cell enzyme deficiencies: e.g., glucose-6-phosphate dehydrogenase (G-6-PD) deficiency
3. Hemoglobin abnormality: e.g., sickle cell anemia
4. Transfusion reaction
5. Infections
6. Drugs
    a. Direct toxic hemolysis
    b. Enzyme deficiency
    c. Allergic immune hemolysis
7. Chemicals and venoms
8. Heat
9. Microangiopathic causes
    a. Thrombotic thrombocytopenic purpura
    b. Disseminated intravascular coagulation

TABLE 2 *Some Causes of Chronic Hemolytic Anemia*

1. Red blood cell membrane abnormalities
   a. Spherocytosis
   b. Elliptocytosis
   c. Lipid abnormalities
2. Hemoglobin abnormalities
   a. Sickle cell disease
   b. Unstable hemoglobins
   c. Thalassemia
   d. Hemoglobin C–C, D–D, E–E diseases
3. Autoimmune anemia
   a. Idiopathic
   b. Infections
   c. Lymphoma and other malignancies
   d. Collagen vascular diseases
   e. Drugs (Aldomet, etc.)
   f. Cold hemagglutinins
4. Microangiopathic: e.g., prosthetic heart valves
5. Hypersplenism

only the more common causes and the diagnostic steps that a physician should take on an emergency basis once he has established the likelihood of a hemolytic anemia (see Tables 1 and 2).

One of the most important steps in evaluating the etiology of a hemolytic anemia is the history. Careful questions should be asked about any drug ingestion (both prescription and over-the-counter drugs), exposure to any toxic agent or chemical at home or at work, and any history of travel to endemic malaria areas. Past episodes of similar conditions and a family history of similar problems indicate the possibility of a hereditary red blood cell defect. Any existing or past medical problems could be linked to the present problem. Physical examination may provide general clues to the etiology. Fever should stimulate a search for an infectious etiology. Splenomegaly may implicate a hemoglobinopathy, spherocytosis, or lymphoma but also raises the possibility that the anemia is *due* to the enlarged spleen (hypersplenism). One would then investigate the causes of splenomegaly (see p. 1144). Joints, particularly those of the hands, should be inspected for signs of synovitis and inflammation of systemic lupus erythematosus and for Raynaud's phenomenon. Subungual hemorrhages may be a sign of subacute bacterial endocarditis, disseminated intravascular coagulation or thrombotic thrombocytopenic purpura and can also occur with sickling.

Finally, a stained peripheral blood smear must be inspected. Target cells indicate a hemoglobinopathy. Heinz bodies and other red blood cell inclusions are signs of an unstable hemoglobin. The finding of sickle cells, spherocytes, or elliptocytes would be diagnostic. Schistocytes, red blood cell fragments, and bizarre red blood cell shapes all may be found in a microangiopathic anemia. Malaria parasites should be looked for in the febrile patient who has traveled in endemic malaria areas, and leukemia may be diagnosed on the basis of abnormal leukocytes. Much time may be saved and the diagnosis simplified by knowing what to look for and having a good microscope readily available in the emergency facility.

THERAPY

Treatment of a hemolytic anemia is aimed at correcting the underlying disease or causative factor. Usually no treatment is needed for the anemia itself, particularly if it is chronic or compensated and stable. For acute hemolysis, particularly if the hemoglobin drops below 6 gm. per 100 ml., severe symptoms may occur. Oxygen delivered by mask will increase the amount of oxygen carried in solution in the blood, even though it will not increase the O_2 carried by the available hemoglobin. At low hemoglobin levels, this additional O_2 is helpful. Transfusions must be considered very cautiously, since transfused blood may be hemolyzed and may increase the problem. If the hemolysis was acute from exposure to a toxic agent, then transfusion, if needed, would be safe once the agent had been eliminated. Immune-mediated hemolysis would probably be a contraindication for transfusion. In long-term treatment, measures such as splenectomy or steroid therapy are indicated for hemolysis of certain etiologies, but this discussion is beyond the scope of a text on emergency management.

POLYCYTHEMIA AND ERYTHROCYTOSIS

Erythrocytosis is an increase in total body red blood cell mass. Definitive diagnosis must be made by a tracer dilution method. An increase in hemoglobin or hematocrit or red blood cells may be caused by an increase of total body red blood cell mass (true erythrocytosis) or a decrease in plasma volume (dehydration); the latter should be easily recognizable by the patient's clinical state. Polycythemia is either a *primary disorder* of the bone marrow, polycythemia rubra vera (PCRV), or a *secondary response* of the erythrogenic bone marrow to physiologic stimulation. PCRV is characterized by an increase of all marrow elements—platelets and neutrophils as well as red blood cells—although all three need not be elevated at the same time during the course of the disease. An erythrocytosis secondary to other factors is characterized by elevation of red blood cell mass alone, with normal numbers of white blood cells and platelets.

The patient with PCRV may present with a hyperviscosity syndrome—transient ischemic attacks, cerebrovascular accident, visual problems—with facial plethora, or paradoxically, with bleeding. The patient with secondary erythrocytosis usually presents with symptoms of his underlying disease, and the erythrocytosis is an incidental finding.

Causes of secondary erythrocytosis include (1) chronic hypoxia from any source—right-to-left shunts, lung disease, high altitudes—as well as from abnormal hemoglobin with decreased oxygen dissociation; (2) neoplastic production of an erythropoietic factor; (3) increased hormonal stimulation, as in Cushing's syndrome or virilizing syndromes in women; or (4) occasionally

TABLE 3 *Causes of Erythrocytosis*

1. Hypoxia
   a. Cardiac right-to-left shunts
      (1) Cyanotic congenital heart disease (e.g., tetralogy of Fallot)
      (2) Congenital heart disease with pulmonary hypertension (Eisenmenger physiology)
      (3) Pulmonary arteriovenous fistula
   b. Pulmonary
      (1) Chronic obstructive pulmonary disease/emphysema
      (2) Pneumoconiosis
      (3) Fibrotic lung syndromes
      (4) Cancer
   c. High altitude
   d. Mechanical interference with breathing (e.g., massive obesity)
   e. Hemoglobin abnormality
2. Tumors
   a. Renal tumors
   b. Cerebellar hemangioblastoma
   c. Neoplasms of different types (rarely)
3. Renal disease
   a. Polycystic kidney
   b. Renal cyst
   c. Hydronephrosis

increased erythropoietin production in otherwise benign renal disease (see Table 3).

DIAGNOSTIC EVALUATION

If a hemoglobin over 18 gm. per 100 ml. or hematocrit over 54 per cent in a man or over 16 gm. per 100 ml. and over 48 per cent in a woman is discovered, further evaluation can usually be completed on an outpatient basis. Examination for presence of an enlarged liver or spleen and a white blood cell and platelet count will uncover evidence in favor of PCRV. Evidence for a secondary cause will be gathered by auscultation of heart and lungs, a chest x-ray, arterial blood gases for diagnosis of hypoxia, and urinalysis. If these simple procedures do not establish a diagnosis, total red blood cell mass should be studied to confirm actual polycythemia, since a few people will have normal values above the conventionally defined limits. If red blood cell mass is elevated and a cause is not apparent from the initial tests, intravenous pyelogram, bone marrow aspiration, and hemoglobin oxygen dissociation curves may be necessary to complete the diagnostic evaluation.

THERAPY

Often no specific therapy is needed for secondary erythrocytosis. Indeed, the increased hemoglobin level is often physiologically helpful in increasing oxygen-carrying capacity in hypoxic situations. Treatment should be directed at the underlying disease. However, if symptoms occur due to the increased viscosity associated with a very high hematocrit, then cautious phlebotomy may be indicated.

In a patient with PCRV, phlebotomy may be required as emergency treatment, but long-term treatment is usually accomplished with ^{32}P (radiophosphorus) or alkylating agents.

SICKLE CELL ANEMIA

Sickle cell anemia is a chronic hemolytic anemia caused by the inheritance of hemoglobin S (Hb S). Persons who are homozygous for hemoglobin S develop sickle cell *anemia*. Heterozygosity for Hb S results in sickle *trait*, in which the patient's blood contains both Hb S and Hb A. The red blood cells of persons with sickle trait can be shown to sickle under low oxygen pressure. However, sickle trait does not usually produce any clinical disease unless another abnormal hemoglobin (e.g., Hb S–C disease) or thalassemia (sickle cell disease–thalassemia) is simultaneously inherited. Definitive diagnosis is made by the finding of 90 to 100 per cent Hb S by Hb electrophoresis. Quick screening tests are available for demonstrating the presence of Hb S, but these tests do not distinguish between sickle trait and homozygous Hb S–S. The presence of sickled red blood cells on a peripheral smear is an excellent means of quick, although not definitive, diagnosis.

CLINICAL PICTURE

Sickle cell anemia produces both chronic and acute problems. Chronically the patient may suffer the debility of a chronic anemia, cardiomegaly, chronic heart failure, pulmonary disease, hepatomegaly, leg ulcers, joint degeneration, and retinal disease. Characteristically the patient has many acute problems. The most common is the *sickle cell crisis,* which causes the sudden onset of pain in muscles, bones, chest, and abdomen. Some patients have typical crises in which their pain is located in the same places each time, but the pains can be located in any combination of areas. Many crises will be mild and require only aspirin for analgesia. At other times the pain may be excruciating and will require narcotics for relief. Crises are caused by occlusion of small blood vessels by sickled red blood cells. Severe crises can be precipitated by hypoxia such as during anesthesia or unpressurized airplane ascents. Crises may also be precipitated by fever, infection, dehydration, or acidosis. For most crises, no specific cause can be identified; however, every patient presenting with sickle cell crisis must be thoroughly evaluated for a precipitating cause. A search for infections is mandatory because these patients are prone to a variety of infections, particularly in the lungs, urinary tract, and bones.

Before diagnosing a sickle cell crisis in a patient with sickle cell anemia, the physician must exclude all other acute complications of sickle cell anemia that may mimic a sickle crisis. Bone infarctions are common and may also produce aseptic necrosis of the femoral head. Osteomyelitis is not uncommon. Cholelithiasis and infarctions of the liver and spleen may produce acute abdominal symptoms. Acute pulmonary disease may occur from pulmonary infarctions or bacterial infection. Other serious complications include convulsions, cerebral infarction, priapism, hematuria, and vascular complications in the eye.

TREATMENT

Treatment of sickle cell crises is mainly symptomatic in addition to correction of any precipitating causes. At our institution, a combination of *meperidine* (Demerol) and *promethazine hydrochloride* (Phenergan) is commonly used for relief of severe pain. Hypoxia should be corrected with appropriate levels of *oxygen;* dehydration is corrected by administration of intravenous *fluids.* The role of bicarbonate is controversial – some clinicians recommend administration of $NaHCO_3$ even if no acidosis exists. Others find it of no value. We do not routinely administer bicarbonate unless the patient is acidotic. Recent hopes for urea or sodium cyanate as antisickling therapy have not been translated into clinical utility. Their use at this time is still limited to the experimental situation.

TRANSFUSION REACTIONS

Blood transfusion can cause a wide variety of adverse effects, ranging from immediate life-threatening hemolytic crises to a long-delayed infection of serum hepatitis. Although excellent blood banking procedures and standard precautions keep these problems to a minimum, the physician must always bear in mind these potential complications when he is weighing the relative merits of giving a blood transfusion. Table 4 outlines the basic reactions that may occur, either acutely or delayed.

Acute Hemolytic Crises

The inadvertent transfusion of mismatched blood can be catastrophic. Symptoms may begin after only a few milliliters of blood or may not appear until a substantial amount has been transfused. The patient may

TABLE 4   Acute and Delayed Transfusion Reactions

Acute Reactions
  Hemolytic
    ABO incompatibility
    Other blood group incompatibilities
    Overheating of transfused blood
    Inadvertent freezing of transfused blood
    Transfusion under pressure through a small bore
      needle
    Patient with paroxysmal nocturnal hemoglobinuria
  Febrile
    Acquired antibodies to histocompatibility loci
      Leukocytes
      Platelets
    Bacterial contamination
    Pyrogens
  Urticaria and anti-IgA antibodies
    Passive transfer of allergy
    Platelet and leukocyte antibodies
  Asthma
  Pulmonary edema
  Air embolism
  Hyperkalemia
  Hemorrhagic tendency
  Hypocalcemia
  Acidosis
  Hypothermia

Delayed Reactions
  Hemolytic
    Rh incompatibility
    Minor blood group incompatibility
    Old blood
  Infection
    Hepatitis
    Cytomegalovirus
    Malaria and other parasites
    Syphilis
  Allergic: urticaria and asthma
    Passive transfer of antibodies in serum
  Thrombophlebitis
  Hemosiderosis

---

become anxious and restless and may feel a sense of oppression in the chest. Pain in the chest, back, and muscles occurs and may be accompanied by flushing, headache, vomiting, or diarrhea. Sometimes pulmonary symptoms are more prominent, with cough, dyspnea or wheezing. Fever to 105°F. may be accompanied by violent chills and shaking. Soon afterward, red urine may appear. If the reaction is not identified and corrected early enough, it may progress to shock and cyanosis. A hemorrhagic diathesis may develop, and occasionally the syndrome of disseminated intravascular coagulation may be precipitated.

Acute renal failure can develop. Although the specific cause has not been identified, hemoglobin precipitating in the renal tubules is thought to be an important part of the pathogenesis of the renal failure. In any given hemolytic reaction, not all of these problems may develop and the reaction may be of only mild degree.

Blood group incompatibility is not the only cause of acute hemolysis. Thermal damage to the blood before transfusion can result in hemolysis. Occasionally, freezing may have occurred by malfunctioning refrigeration or because of contact with dry ice in shipment. Overheating can occur if the blood has been placed inadvertently near a lighting fixture or radiator or has been purposely heated. The common practice of using pressure to speed transfusion can cause hemolysis, especially if a needle bore less than size 18 is used.

DIAGNOSIS OF ACUTE HEMOLYTIC REACTIONS

The diagnosis of an acute hemolytic reaction must be made as soon as any of the symptoms occur, and *the transfusion should be stopped immediately* before laboratory confirmation. Blood should immediately be drawn for repeat cross-matching, free hemoglobin, bilirubin, haptoglobin, and methemalbumin. Any remaining blood from the transfusion should be returned immediately to the blood bank for investigation. The next voided urine should be tested for free hemobglobin and hemosiderin. Without waiting for these laboratory tests, a hematocrit should be done immediately. Pink plasma and a drop in the hematocrit from the pretransfusion level confirms significant hemolysis. However, clear plasma and no drop in the hematocrit do not constitute evidence against a hemolytic reaction.

THERAPY

To treat a transfusion reaction, *immediately stop the transfusion.* For minor symptoms, no other treatment is needed except perhaps an analgesic. Fever may be treated with acetaminophen. Pulmonary symptoms, if severe, may be treated with oxygen and, if there is wheezing, epinephrine. If the problems progress to shock, administration of fluids and drug support of blood pressure will be necessary, and further careful assessment must be done. Transfusion may be necessary if much hemolysis has occurred, and blood must be cross-matched with a freshly obtained specimen of the patient's blood. Some clinicians have advocated use of corticosteroids in such cases, but benefits have not been proved.

Acute renal failure is always a danger when hemolysis occurs, and a large fluid intake to maintain adequate urinary output is indicated whenever a hemolytic reaction occurs. If oliguria occurs, mannitol in a dose of 20 gm. (100 ml. of 20 per cent mannitol solution) may produce an osmotic diuresis. If no diuresis occurs within one hour, the dose should be repeated or a dose of furosemide, 40 to 80 mg., given intravenously. Also, sodium bicarbonate should be given for 24 hours by mouth or intravenously in a dose sufficient to keep the urine alkaline for the theoretical benefit of aiding the solubility of hemoglobin in the renal tubules. If oliguria continues, treatment for acute renal failure should be started.

Other Acute Transfusion Reactions

Febrile reactions to leukocytes and platelets in the transfusion may occur but are common only in patients who have received many previous transfusions and have developed antibodies to leukocyte or platelet antigens. *Urticaria* may also occur. These reactions are easily treated with antihistamines and antipyretics. If *bronchospasm* is part of the reaction, then epinephrine may also be needed. In a patient who is known to be sensitized, the reaction may be prevented by using buffy-coat-poor packed red blood cells and using an antihistamine prophylactically. Febrile reactions due to pyrogens or bacterial contamination of the transfused blood have become very rare.

Pulmonary edema can be precipitated by volume overload of the circulatory system. In chronic anemia, packed red blood cells should always be used in order to keep volume expansion to a minimum. Whole blood should only be used for acute blood loss when volume expansion is needed. Treatment for pulmonary edema precipitated by transfusion essentially consists of removal of excess fluid with diuretics and perhaps phlebotomy, along with standard measures, including morphine and, if needed, aminophylline.

Air embolism is a danger when using pressure to speed transfusion. Because pressure can also cause hemolysis, every effort should be made to use a large bore needle and not to use pressure. If pressure must be used, it should only be applied outside a closed transfusion system that has no air within the system.

Stored red blood cells slowly lose potassium, so the plasma of stored blood may contain relatively large amounts of potassium. If whole blood is transfused quickly, temporary *hyperkalemia* may result and may cause cardiac arrhythmias. In patients with renal failure, hyperkalemia is a danger, even with slow transfusion. The use of fresh whole blood or packed red blood cells will lessen the danger of producing hyperkalemia in patients with compromised renal function.

Hypocalcemia and *acidosis* can be caused by acid citrate anticoagulant when large amounts of whole blood are transfused quickly. Calcium gluconate and sodium bicarbonate may be used to correct these imbalances. The amounts used should be determined by titrating the results with frequent pH and serum calcium determinations.

Hypothermia can result when multiple units of cold blood are transfused quickly. Hypothermia may complicate the clinical situation and cause cardiac arrhythmias. The blood should not be warmed except by careful methods especially designed for warming blood (if available) because of the danger of thermal degradation of the blood and subsequent hemolysis when transfused.

DELAYED TRANSFUSION REACTIONS

Jaundice can develop several days following blood transfusion as a result of a gradual hemolysis from a minor blood group incompatibility or because old blood was transfused. Serum hepatitis (hepatitis associated antigen–positive) is a well-known delayed complication that is seen much less frequently with the identification and elemination of HAA-positive donor blood.

Infectious (short incubation) hepatitis A may also be transmitted. Cytomegalovirus has been identified as a cause of some of the delayed febrile illness following multiple blood transfusions. Transfusion-induced malaria is quite rare in this country but occasionally occurs and should be considered in a patient who develops fever a few days following a transfusion. Syphilis is now almost never transmitted by blood transfusion because of reagin testing and the spirocheticidal effect of cold storage of blood.

A patient may temporarily acquire an allergic tendency of the blood donor. Urticaria, rash, or asthma may then be provoked by food, contact allergens, or animal dander that the patient has never reacted to before. These allergic phenomena are temporary and may be treated with the usual regimen of an antihistamine and epinephrine. Phlebitis not uncommonly occurs in the vein used for transfusion. Conservative treatment is usually all that is required. Long-term multiple transfusions for chronic anemia may eventually cause hemosiderosis. Keeping transfusions to a minimum can help delay this problem.

METHEMOGLOBINEMIA

Methemoglobin is hemoglobin with an iron atom in the ferric state rather than the usual ferrous state. Methemoglobin results from oxidation of the hemoglobin iron and is normally present at levels less than 1 per cent of circulating hemoglobin. Methemoglobin is not capable of carrying oxygen reversibly as is hemoglobin. Cyanosis occurs when concentrations of methemoglobin are greater than 2 gm. per 100 ml.

CAUSES

Methemoglobinemia can be inherited or may be acquired from toxic exposure. The hereditary form can be due to the inheritance

of an abnormal hemoglobin, which allows easier oxidation of the iron in hemoglobin, or to a decreased activity of the NADH-methemoglobin reductase system, which is not able to reduce the small, naturally occurring amounts of methemoglobin. Acquired methemoglobinemia may result from exposure to a variety of agents (see Table 5). Nitrites and nitrates (which are converted to nitrites in the GI tract) are perhaps the most common causes of acquired methemoglobinemia. Infants and children are especially vulnerable to nitrates in the water supply, and cases may occur where the local water supply has naturally high concentrations of nitrate or when contamination occurs from water runoff containing fertilizers used in agriculture. Sodium nitrite, which is used as a preservative, has also caused many cases of methemoglobinemia through accidental poisoning—either through excess use or inadvertent substitution for ordinary table salt.

Drugs, particularly antimalarials, are another frequent cause of acquired methemoglobinemia. Most of these drugs produce methemoglobinemia only rarely. When they do, it may be because of individual sensitivity, unusually large doses, or in the case of topical drugs, an unusual increase in absorption. Finally, aniline dyes may be the cause. Infants have developed methemoglobinemia from skin absorption of the dye from laundry marks on diapers or from ingesting crayons.

CLINICAL PRESENTATION

Patients with methemoglobinemia present with *cyanosis*. In the congenital varieties cyanosis is usually present from early infancy. The acquired forms are usually acute and follow toxic exposure. With low levels of methemoglobin, there may be no symptoms

TABLE 5   *Acquired Causes of Methemoglobinemia*

INORGANIC AGENTS	DRUGS		MISCELLANEOUS
Bivalent copper	Acetanilid	Primaquine	Alloxons
Chlorates	Phenacetin	Chloroquine	Aniline
Chromate	Para-aminosalicylic	Dapsone	Naphthalene
Nitrates	acid (PAS)	Nitroglycerin	Nitrosobenzene
Nitrites	Phenazopyridine	Amyl nitrite	Quinones
	Sulfonamides	Silver nitrate	
	Prilocaine	Resorcinol	
	Lidocaine	Menthol	
	Benzocaine	Guaiacol	

other than cyanosis. With increasing amounts, dyspnea, tachycardia, and nonspecific symptoms may appear, and finally stupor and coma may occur. Toxic symptoms of the offending agent may also be present.

DIAGNOSIS

Methemoglobinemia should be suspected whenever cyanosis occurs in a patient with normal arterial oxygen saturation. A quick and easy test is to draw a few milliliters of blood and shake it with air. If the blood does not become red, the cyanosis is not due to hypoxia. Definitive diagnosis must be done by the clinical laboratory. Recent ingestion of a drug or toxin known to produce methemoglobinemia is highly suggestive of the diagnosis in a cyanotic patient with normal arterial oxygen saturation.

TREATMENT

No treatment is needed unless the patient is symptomatic. Lower levels of methemoglobin will revert to normal without treatment in one to three days. Oxygen administration may be helpful, as will efforts to aid elimination of the toxic agent (gastric lavage, catharsis). Methylene blue will reverse the methemoglobin to hemoglobin. The dosage of methylene blue is 1 to 2 mg./kg. I.V., given slowly; repeated doses may be needed. Extravasation of the drug should be avoided, since skin slough has occurred. It may also be given orally in a dose of 3 to 5 mg./kg.

D. SPLENOMEGALY
Alan O. Feingold

The detection of an enlarged spleen is an important clinical finding in many disease states. The most frequent causes of splenomegaly will differ greatly according to the geographic area and the age and ethnic composition of the population. A useful way to categorize the etiologies is to group them under infectious agents, portal hypertension, hemolytic anemias, infiltrative processes, and lymphoproliferative diseases (see Table 1).

CLINICAL PRESENTATION

Splenomegaly usually produces no symptoms per se, although rarely, an infarction may occur in any enlarged spleen and cause left upper quadrant abdominal pain. Thus, splenomegaly is usually discovered in the clinical setting of the underlying disease producing the enlargement. It is important for the emergency physician to automatically examine for an enlarged spleen in certain situations (see Table 2). For example, a patient with mild lymphadenopathy and symptoms of a viral syndrome will have a simple viral syndrome 99 times out of 100. The presence of splenic enlargement, however, will alert the physician to the possibil-

ity of infectious mononucleosis, toxoplasmosis, cytomegalovirus, or a more serious infectious process. Patients who present with viral symptoms and fever may often have heart murmurs because of the fever and accompanying hyperdynamic state. However, the additional finding of an enlarged spleen may suggest the possibility of subacute bacterial endocarditis. An enlarged spleen in a patient presenting with GI bleeding will suggest the presence of portal hypertension and a possible diagnosis of bleeding esophageal varices.

In addition, careful palpation for an enlarged spleen should be made whenever an anemia or a low white blood cell or platelet count is discovered. Splenomegaly from any cause may by itself (through splenic trapping and sequestration) lead to lowered values of one, two, or all three blood cellular components (see Table 3).

APPROACH TO DIAGNOSTIC EVALUATION

Often the etiology of the splenomegaly will be obvious from the associated clinical findings. In the young patient with a viral syndrome, pharyngitis, and minimal spleno-

TABLE 1 Causes of Splenomegaly

I. Infectious agents
  A. Viruses and virus-like agents
    1. Infectious mononucleosis
    2. Cytomegalovirus
    3. Viral hepatitis
    4. Psittacosis
    5. Rocky Mountain spotted fever
  B. Bacterial
    1. Tuberculosis
    2. Subacute bacterial endocarditis
    3. Typhoid
    4. Brucellosis
    5. Syphilis
    6. Meningococcemia
    7. Abscess
  C. Parasitic
    1. Toxoplasmosis
    2. Malaria
    3. Kala-azar
    4. Trypanosomiasis
    5. Echinococcosis
  D. Fungal
    1. Histoplasmosis

II. Infiltrative processes
  A. Sarcoidosis
  B. Gaucher's disease
  C. Niemann-Pick disease
  D. Hunter and Hurler syndromes
  E. Amyloidosis

III. Increased portal pressure
  A. Cirrhosis of the liver
  B. Splenic vein thrombosis, stenosis, or aneurysm
  C. Portal vein obstructions or thrombosis
  D. Schistosomiasis
  E. Congestive heart failure

IV. Hemolytic anemias
  A. Thalassemia
  B. Hemoglobin C disease
  C. Hemoglobin S–C disease
  D. Autoimmune hemolytic anemias
  E. Other hemolytic anemias

V. Lymphoproliferative disease
  A. Lymphoma
  B. Leukemia
  C. Reticulum cell sarcoma
  D. Histiocytosis X
  E. Myeloma
  F. Polycythemia rubra vera
  G. Myelofibrosis with myeloid metaplasia

VI. Neoplastic disease
  A. Benign tumors
  B. Cysts
  C. Metastatic cancer

VII. Miscellaneous causes
  A. Systemic lupus erythematosus
  B. Felty's syndrome
  C. Idiopathic thrombocytopenic purpura

TABLE 2 Conditions Suggested by an Enlarged Spleen

SYMPTOM OR SIGN	CONDITION
Sore throat	Infectious mononucleosis
Lymphadenopathy	Infection
	Cytomegalovirus
	Toxoplasmosis
	Lymphoma
Heart murmur	Subacute bacterial endocarditis
Jaundice	Portal hypertension
	Hemolytic anemia
GI bleeding	Portal hypertension
Fever	Bacterial or parasitic disease

megaly only a WBC and differential blood count plus a mono-spot test or heterophil titer are needed to diagnose infectious mononucleosis. The person with acute onset of jaundice and mild hepatosplenomegaly requires only bilirubin, SGOT and alkaline phosphatase for confirmation of viral hepatitis. When the etiology is not obvious from the clinical setting, the basic evaluation of a patient with splenomegaly should include questions about alcohol intake, travels, and medical history. Examination should include temperature, cardiac auscultation, and careful palpation of lymph nodes and liver as well as inspection for subungual splinter hemorrhages, jaundice, and arthritic changes. Laboratory tests should include chest x-ray, complete blood count with WBC differential, platelet count, and reticulocyte count. If this basic evaluation does not yield a diagnosis, further testing should be based on the clinical situation. Presence of fever indicates a probable infection and the need for testing for a presumed infectious agent. A child with splenomegaly may require investigation for a lipid storage disease. An afebrile adult would need a hemoglobin electrophoresis, biochemical profile including bilirubin, SGOT, alkaline phosphatase, and serum proteins, possibly followed by liver scan and bone marrow aspiration and biopsy.

TABLE 3 Conditions Caused by an Enlarged Spleen

Thrombocytopenia
Leukopenia
Abdominal (left upper quadrant) pain
Hemolytic anemia

THERAPY

Treatment is directed at the underlying disease. Only rarely would the splenomegaly itself be treated. Splenomegaly is curative for some cases of idiopathic thrombocytopenic purpura. In early stages of Hodgkin's disease, the presence or absence of splenomegaly is an adjunct to diagnosis and treatment, serving to "stage" the disease process. Occasionally in advanced lymphoproliferative disease, splenic irradiation will be palliative for massive splenomegaly. Splenic rupture is a danger with any greatly enlarged spleen and, of course, necessitates surgical repair.

SPLENIC INFARCTION

Splenic infarction may occur in any greatly enlarged spleen. Usually this event is silent and is discovered only at autopsy. However, in sickle cell disease it is common ("autosplenectomy"). In children with homozygous S hemoglobin it occurs almost universally. In patients with hemoglobin S–C disease or sickle cell disease–thalassemia, the sickle cell disease is usually much milder, and these patients may have few or no problems until adulthood. Splenic infarction in hemoglobin S–C disease is often precipitated by hypoxia, such as occurs in an unpressurized aircraft or during surgery, but will often be spontaneous. The patient presents with acute left upper quadrant pain which may have a pleuritic component and may radiate to the left shoulder. The spleen will usually be enlarged and tender but may not be palpable if previous infarctions have reduced its size. A rub may be heard. A spleen scan may provide definitive evidence of an infarction. A positive sickle cell test and target cells on the blood smear provide a presumptive diagnosis, but hemoglobin electrophoresis is needed for definitive evaluation of the hemoglobinopathy. Therapy is conservative with analgesics and bed rest. Oxygen is needed only if there is hypoxia.

Suggestions for Further Reading

Arena, J. M.: Poisoning. Springfield, Ill., Charles C Thomas, Publisher, 1974.

Conn, H. F. (Ed.): Current Therapy 1977. Philadelphia, W. B. Saunders Co., 1977.

Costea, N.: The differential diagnosis of hemolytic anemias. Med. Clin. North Am. 57(2):289, March 1973.

Harris, J. W., and Kellermeyer, R. W.: The Red Cell (Production, Metabolism, Destruction: Normal and Abnormal). Rev. Ed. Cambridge, Mass., Commonwealth Fund, Harvard University Press, 1970.

Wintrobe, M. W., et al.: Clinical Hematology. Philadelphia, Lea & Febiger, 1974.

Chapter 50

NEUROLOGIC EMERGENCIES

Thomas D. Sabin

INTRODUCTION

Many neurologic problems have been covered in other chapters of this text, but a number of disorders of compelling relevance for the Emergency Department physician have been left for discussion here. Rather than selecting a list of diseases, an attempt has been made to retain an orientation to problems that cause patients to come to the Emergency Department. For this reason, the common chief complaint of "acute weakness" has been arbitrarily selected for diagnostic analysis.

Most patients complaining of "weakness" are describing the lassitude that accompanies systemic disease or emotional disorders. Patients with actual paralysis more often describe their impaired functions and will state: "My leg is dragging;" "I am short of breath;" "Liquids run from the corner of my mouth;" or "I can't write." All such patients, however, require meticulous and systematic examination of muscle strength, tone, coordination, and gait. The term, "diffuse weakness" so often found in medical records is nearly always incorrect and reflects a failure to exploit the distinctive patterns of weakness associated with dysfunction at the various anatomic levels of the motor system.

In every patient with weakness the physician should determine whether the process involves the pyramidal system, anterior horn cells, nerve roots, peripheral nerves, neuromuscular junction, or muscles. The following is a brief account of some of the acute paralytic or paretic disorders encountered in the Emergency Department.

1146

MUSCLE DISEASE

The common pattern of weakness seen in the primary muscle diseases is a symmetrical paresis of the proximal limb girdles and axial musculature. The patient will complain of difficulty in arising from a chair or bathtub, climbing stairs, rolling over in bed or in activities requiring elevation of the arms such as shaving or grooming the hair. The most common varieties of muscle disease (dystrophies and polymyositis) allow time for thorough investigation and do not constitute true emergencies. Occasionally, however, chronic muscular weakness can result in respiratory failure if there is sudden strain on the muscles of respiration due to infection, asthma, or pulmonary diseases with increased airway resistance.

PERIODIC PARALYSIS

Acute widespread myopathic paralysis is seen in the rare hereditary conditions known as *periodic paralysis*. Hypokalemic periodic paralysis is characterized by acute attacks of flaccid quadriplegia that begin in the second decade of life. The individual attacks tend to occur after heavy meals or after a rest which followed vigorous physical activity. The paralysis lasts six to 48 hours and is associated with hypokalemia. A history of prior attacks and similarly affected relatives is most helpful in establishing the diagnosis. The cranial nerve and the respiratory musculature usually are spared. Oral potassium preparations may be used to abort or avert attacks.

The hyperkalemic form of periodic paralysis also follows an autosomal dominant pattern of inheritance. Attacks are milder than in the hypokalemic type, and exposure to cold is the most effective precipitant of the paralysis. Myotonia, especially of the eyelids, is a characteristic finding. Thiazide diuretics are used to lower serum potassium levels. Varieties of periodic paralysis without abnormal serum potassium also have been described.

A loss of direct muscle excitability can be demonstrated in paralyzed muscles in all three forms of periodic paralysis. A brisk tap of the reflex hammer on a normal muscle belly mechanically initiates depolarization of the muscle membrane, and contraction occurs. When paralysis is due to primary muscle disease no contraction occurs. If the muscle is paralyzed because of denervation, direct muscle excitability will be normal or enhanced, even though the tendon reflexes are absent.

A myopathic pattern of paralysis may be a prominent feature of hyperthyroid storm (see Chapter 46).

Myoglobinuria results from disruption of muscle membranes with release of myoglobin into the circulation. The myoglobin is rapidly cleared into the urine, which then develops a pink-red hue and becomes guaiac or benzidene positive. While the test for blood is strongly positive in the urine, few or no red blood cells are seen. The serum should be examined to distinguish this event from hemoglobinuria. Since hemoglobin is bound to proteins, the serum remains pink, but myoglobin is unbound and so rapidly excreted that the serum remains clear.

The most common cause of myoglobinuria seen at the Boston City Hospital is pressure necrosis of muscles due to the prolonged immobility of drug overdose. Intense repetitive exercise by formerly sedentary individuals is an occasional cause of myoglobinuria usually reported at military training centers. The same factor is present in myoglobinuria seen after a bout of status epilepticus. Crushing or thermal ("trench foot") injuries may be sufficient to cause disruption of muscle membranes. Alcohol, the glycyrrhizic acid in licorice, carbon monoxide poisoning, and sea snake venom have all been cited as toxic causes of myoglobinuria. In hereditary muscle phosphorylase deficiency (McArdle's disease) exertion causes painful, electrically silent cramps which have been occasionally associated with myoglobinuria.

Once myoglobinuria is recognized, the most urgent problem is to avert renal failure due to accumulation of myoglobin in the renal tubules (see Chapter 7).

DEFECTS IN NEUROMUSCULAR TRANSMISSION

Motor nerve impulses result in a release of acetylcholine from the nerve terminals. The acetylcholine diffuses across the synaptic cleft and initiates depolarization of the muscle membrane. Interference with this chemical mediation between nerve and muscle results in paralysis even though the nerve and muscle are normal. Paralysis of the extraocular and bulbar musculature is a prominent feature in most of the diseases of the neuromuscular junction.

Myasthenia Gravis*

The cause and exact nature of the neuromuscular transmission defect in myasthenia is unknown, but increasing the available acetylcholine at the neuromuscular junction by the use of anticholinesterase agents usually improves the excessive fatigability and delayed recovery of muscle strength that characterize the disease. The disorder is rare (1:20,000) but may occur at any age, although onset in the second and third decades is usual and females are more commonly affected than males. The initial symptoms characteristically relate to fluctuating weakness in the extraocular, facial, masticatory, or pharyngeal muscles.

The patient notes intermittent diplopia, nasal voice, dysphagia, weakness in chewing, nasal regurgitation, or change in appearance due to ptosis and flattening of facial features. The symptoms are clearly increased because of the affected muscles. Normal functions may be present after sleep, but progressive weakness often develops during the day's activities. Weakness often affects limb and respiratory muscles, but paralysis "below the neck" without obvious weakness in the cranial musculature is extremely rare.

The examination of strength before and after muscular activity will reveal the characteristic abnormal fatigability and delay in

---

*See also p. 1106.

recovery of strength. For example, the patient may be asked to sustain upward gaze, and progressive ptosis or failure in maintaining the position of the eyes will become apparent. When the limb muscles are affected, repetitive tapping of a tendon may show a fatigue of the reflex as neuromuscular transmission fails. Repetitive squeezing of an ergometer or a partially inflated blood pressure cuff may also be used at the bedside, but the electromyographer can eliminate subjective factors by directly stimulating the nerve at a rapid rate and displaying the declining muscle potentials on the cathode ray tube.

TENSILON TEST

A transient improvement in strength with I.V. administration of a short-acting anticholinesterase agent such as edrophonium chloride (Tensilon) is diagnostic. A total of 10 mg. (1 cc.) is drawn up into the syringe, but only 2 mg. is administered initially and the patient is observed for changes in strength. If no clear change occurs after one minute, the remaining 8 mg. is given. The dosage is staged in this manner to avoid cholinergic weakness in patients extremely sensitive to anticholinesterase agents. Increased weakness with Tensilon is characteristic in a "cholinergic" crisis.

MYASTHENIC CRISES

Patients with myasthenia are subject to sudden bouts of profound weakness which are life-threatening because of respiratory paralysis. Such "crises" are not a usual presenting feature of the disease, so that most patients in crisis will be known to have myasthenia and will have been taking oral anticholinesterase medications. The patient may have tried to combat his progressive weakness by increasing his medications. When this has occurred the physician must be aware that *the crisis may be due either to worsening of the myasthenia or to the neuromuscular blockade caused by excess anticholinesterase agents (known as cholinergic crisis).* Overdose of anticholinesterase drugs increases available acetylcholine to levels capable of causing continued depolarization of the muscle membrane and blocking neuromuscular transmission (depolarization blockade). *The distinction between myasthenic crisis and cholinergic crisis is of critical importance in the early management of these patients.* A Tensilon test will worsen the weakness in cholinergic crisis and is apt to be accompanied by crampy abdominal pain and showers of fasciculations, especially around the eyelids. Patients with myasthenic crisis may show improved strength or no change with Tensilon. When no change occurs with Tensilon, the patient is in an anticholinesterase-resistant phase of the disease.

Too often the emergency physician ponders too long over vaguely recalled neuromuscular pharmacology and fails to take the prompt measures to secure an airway and adequate ventilation that he would for a patient with a similar degree of respiratory distress due to other diseases. The myasthenic is in jeopardy, not only from decreased tidal volume, but also because the faulty swallowing mechanism allows aspiration of secretions. Tracheal intubation and frequent suctioning may be necessary. Some cause for the occurrence of the crisis, such as an infection (especially aspiration pneumonia), another systemic disease, or a harmful drug should be serached for.

Treatment of Cholinergic Crisis. When cholinergic crisis is present most clinicians simply support the patient until the anticholinesterase effects abate. This time will vary according to the amount and type of medication the patient has taken. Many patients are now taking long-acting preparations of pyridostigmine bromide (Mestinon Timespaans) which have a half-life of six hours. Atropine (1 mg. I.V.) is useful in reducing the parasympathetic overactivity (abdominal cramps, excessive secretions, nausea, and lacrimation), but has no effect on the weakness in striated muscle.

Treatment of Myasthenic Crisis. When cholinergic crisis has been ruled out, the patient may be given neostigine (Prostigmin), 1 mg. I.V., which may be repeated, but not to exceed a dose of 2 mg. per hour (1 mg. I.V. is equivalent to 15 mg. S.C. or 30 mg. P.O.).

If weakness is unresponsive to increasing amounts of neostigmine, the patient is classified as anticholinesterase-resistant. Resistance may abate when an underlying infection, hypoxia, or endocrine or metabolic disturbance is treated. Otherwise such patients may have anticholinesterase medication withdrawn and be treated supportively for several days until the weakness again becomes responsive to these agents. Frequent Tensilon testing is invaluable in determining the presence of anticholinesterase resistance and in adjusting neostigmine dosage.

MEDICATIONS THAT MAY WORSEN MYASTHENIA

Medications that are potentially harmful to the myasthenic include: opiates, barbiturates, muscle relaxants, quinine and quinidine, and some antibiotics (most of the aminoglycosides). ACTH and steroids in large doses may precipitate or worsen myasthenic crises. Although these agents are sometimes tried despite this problem because a remission may follow the steroid-induced exacerbation, steroids and ACTH should not be used for the patient who presents with crisis.

Neurologic opinion should be sought to plan long term management. This may involve thymectomy, a change in drug regimen or steroid therapy.

Botulism

This rare disorder is discussed fully in Chapter 53, but is mentioned here because each of the immunologically distinct toxins produced by the six types of *Clostridium botulinum* blocks transmission in cholinergic nerve terminals. These heat-labile toxins usually are ingested with improperly canned foods and produce symptoms within a few hours in severe cases. Dysfunction of the cholinergic autonomic terminals causes fixed, dilated pupils, dry mucous membranes, urinary retention, abdominal distention, and postural hypotension. The striated muscles supplied by the cranial nerves usually develop weakness first, and the patient notes diplopia, nasal voice, and difficulty with chewing and swallowing. Weakness often becomes widespread and paralysis of respiration may ensue, leading to rapid death. Gastric gavage may be used to remove unabsorbed toxin. Antitoxin is administered, and every effort is made to sustain life during the period of respiratory paralysis because full neurologic recovery can be anticipated in survivors. An important diagnostic point in botulism is the maintenance of a clear sensorium.

PERIPHERAL NEUROPATHY

The differential diagnosis of the neuropathies is a formidable problem, but in fact there are only a few acute life-threatening neuropathies relevant to the emergency physician.

LANDRY-GUILLAIN-BARRE SYNDROME (LGBS)

Since poliomyelitis has become rare in the U.S. the most common acute paralytic disease of young adults is now LGBS. This disorder has been associated with infectious mononucleosis, the collagen-vascular diseases, porphyria, and diabetes; but in 95 per cent of cases no specific associated illness is present. In most cases there is a history of a nonspecific viral illness or surgical procedure 10 to 14 days prior to onset of the polyradiculoneuropathy. The pathology of the neuropathy consists of widespread loss of myelin in the nerve roots and peripheral nerves, with a relative preservation of axons. A similar disorder can be produced in animals by creating an immunity to peripheral nerve myelin (acute experimental allergic neuritis), but the role of autoimmunity to myelin in man is less clear.

A prodrome of tingling in the extremities is followed by the appearance of a symmetrical paralysis and loss of deep tendon reflexes. The pattern of evolution of the paralysis is variable, but usually the weakness appears in the distal lower extremities, then in the thighs, forearms, proximal limb girdles, and finally in respiratory and bulbar musculature (so-called "ascending paralysis"). Other patients may develop bilateral facial paralysis at the outset and have a descending spread of paralysis. The usual onset is acute or subacute, with maximal paralysis developing within a few hours to six weeks. Progression may cease at any stage, but about one-half of the cases will develop severe weakness of the respiratory muscles. Sphincter function is spared in 90 per cent of patients. Although rare, chronic and relapsing forms of this syndrome have been delineated.

Examination reveals symmetric weakness, loss of deep tendon reflexes, and preserved direct muscle excitability in paralyzed muscles. Fasciculations are absent, and wasting occurs only in proportion to disuse, because the demyelinated but otherwise preserved axon maintains its trophic influence on muscle, although the conduction of impulses is blocked. Although early sensory symptoms are common, the sensory examination is normal or reveals only a moderate loss of vibration and position sense.

The spinal fluid is clear, colorless and acellular. A significant elevation of CSF protein (80 to 250 mg. per cent) occurs within 21 days, but even when the CSF protein is quite elevated xanthochromia is absent.

The major error in the Emergency Department is to misdiagnose the healthy appearing patient with "floppy legs" or bizarre gait as hysterical. Although specific therapy is not available, the cornerstone of management is meticulous general medical support during a period of days or weeks of respiratory paralysis. This is especially crucial, because the outlook for eventual full neurologic recovery is excellent.

Steroids have been useful in some of the chronic and relapsing forms of LGBS, but their effectiveness in the acute or subacute forms is equivocal.

DIPHTHERITIC NEUROPATHY

Diphtheria toxin may cause paralysis of individual or multiple specific peripheral nerves or nerve roots, but infrequently causes an acute or subacute polyradiculoneuropathy with widespread proximal and distal weakness. There is more intense sensory loss to all modalities than is usually seen in the Guillain-Barre syndrome. Early paralysis of the palate and ocular accommodation are highly characteristic of diphtheria. If the patient survives the bout of diphtheria, the prognosis for nerve recovery within several months is excellent. (See Chapter 53.)

TICK PARALYSIS

A toxin released from the gravid tick, *Dermocenter andersoni*, is capable of causing a rapidly developing ascending flaccid quadriplegia that resembles the Guillain-Barre syndrome. Tick paralysis is seen most often in children, and a search for a tick, particularly at the hairline of the nape of the neck, should be made in cases suspected of having acute motor polyneuropathy. Removal of the tick is rewarded by prompt recovery.*

PARALYTIC SHELLFISH POISONING (RED TIDE)

Marine protozoans of the genus Gonyaulax proliferate massively when certain temperature, salinity, and nutrient conditions occur in the sea and cause a reddish luminescent discoloration on the surface of the water. These organisms produce a poison known as saxitoxin, which is ingested by clams, oysters, snails, cockles, and starfish. Lobsters and finned fish do not retain the poison. The shellfish are not themselves harmed, but birds and mammals feeding upon the contaminated shellfish suffer an acute and potentially fatal illness. The lethal dose of saxitoxin in man has been estimated at 1000 to 2000 μg. The toxin prevents propagation of nerve impulses by interfering with neuronal membrane permeability to sodium ions. Within 30 minutes to four hours after ingestion of saxitoxin, the patient experiences a prodrome of intense paresthesias in the distal extremities that rapidly spread proximally. There is vertigo and numbness of the scalp and mouth. Examination at this stage shows severe sensory loss especially to position and vibration sense, dysarthria, dysphagia, and intention tremor. In severe cases the sensory symptoms are soon followed by flaccid quadriplegia and respiratory paralysis. The spinal fluid is normal. Treatment is supportive; most patients surviving the first 24 hours of the illness will start to improve.*

NERVE ROOTS

The motor nerve roots emerge from the ventrolateral sulcus of the spinal cord and extend through the subarachnoid space into the root sleeves of the meninges. The most common problem affecting nerve roots is impingement on individual nerve roots by ruptured intervertebral lumbar or cervical disks. These syndromes are not usually true emergencies if the spinal cord is not affected. An important exception is the occasional midline protrusion of a lumbar disk that impinges upon the cauda equina. The patient experiences low back pain and radicular radiation of pain into the perineal region. There is acute paralysis of bladder and rectal sphincters. Examination reveals a patulous anal sphincter, loss of the anal

*See p. 810.

*See p. 813.

scratch and bulbocavernosus reflexes, and a sensory loss in the "saddle" region. The prognosis for recovery from this syndrome is very dependent on how rapidly surgical decompression of the roots can be accomplished.

The so-called "acute disk syndrome" involves a herniation of a disk, usually lumbar, with generally unilateral weakness, sensory changes, and reflex decrease. Neurologic consultation is vital in such cases.

PYRAMIDAL SYSTEM DYSFUNCTION

The major central pathway for voluntary movement is known as the corticospinal or pyramidal pathway and arises from cells in the motor cortex of the frontal lobe. The axons of these cells course into the capsule, cerebral peduncle, base of the pons, and medulla. At the junction of the medulla and spinal cord, 90 per cent of these fibers cross to the opposite side into the lateral columns of the spinal cord, where they descend to influence the anterior horn cells.

Damage to this system results in the characteristic weakness, spasticity, hyperreflexia, and Babinski response of the upper motor neuron lesion. When pyramidal tract damage is partial, only certain movements may become weak; others may remain normal. This predilection pattern produces most marked weakness in the extensors and abductors of the upper extremity and the flexors (including dorsiflexion of the foot) and abductors of the lower extremity. For this reason the common practice of screening for weakness by testing the hand grips should be abandoned. The emergency physician must also recall that acute extensive damage to the pyramidal system presents with a flaccid, areflexic paralysis. This resemblance to a lower motor neuron type of weakness is not confusing when the patient is hemiplegic, but when weakness develops bilaterally with acute spinal cord damage, an incorrect diagnosis such as an acute polyneuropathy is often suspected.

PARAPARESIS AND QUADRIPARESIS

Bilateral limb weakness due to pyramidal system damage may result from bilateral lesions in the cerebral hemispheres or brainstem, but when neurologic function rostral to the medulla is normal, spinal cord disease is most likely. Because bilateral paralysis is the most common feature of spinal cord disease, the problem will be discussed at this point. However, spinal cord disease may present without weakness; weakness may be unilateral (as in the Brown-Sequard syndrome) or predominantly of the lower motor neuron type, as in poliomyelitis or some types of motor neuron disease. When strength is normal, sensory, pain, or autonomic dysfunction alone may direct attention to spinal cord disease.

SPINAL CORD COMPRESSION

Spinal cord compression is a true emergency, and every physician should be capable of assessing this problem. The duration of the patient's history will depend on the underlying disease process. If an inflammatory or neoplastic lesion involves the vertebrae, local pain at the level of the lesion may be prominent. This pain may worsen at night and changes with posture. When nerve roots are also compressed, radicular pain may occur. This pain may be an important clue to the level of a compressive lesion. Radicular pain radiates out into the region of sensory distribution ordinarily supplied by that root and is often exacerbated by coughing, sneezing, or the Valsalva maneuver. Compression of the cord itself causes difficulty in urination and defecation and sensory-motor signs that begin in the distal lower extremities and progress up to the level of the lesion as the spinal cord is further compromised. For obscure reasons, some patients with rapidly evolving quadriparesis show a relative indifference to this calamity, and the misdiagnosis of hysteria is not uncommon!

The neurologic examination seeks to determine the longitudinal and transverse extent of cord dysfunction. Signs related to the dorsal columns (ipsilateral position and vibratory loss), lateral spinothalamic tracts (contralateral pin and temperature loss), and corticospinal (ipsilateral weakness) tend to begin in the distal lower extremities and ascend toward the level of the lesion. The upper level of these tract signs may therefore be significantly below the actual level of a compressive lesion. However, segmental signs, such as an absent deep tendon reflex, focal atrophy, and fasciculations or radicular sensory loss will accurately determine the true level of a compressive lesion. General medical examination may uncover signs of lung, breast, prostatic, or other neoplastic disease that may have metastasized to the epidural space. A healing furuncle may be a clue to the presence of an epidural abscess.

In any case with progressing spinal cord signs consistent with cord compression, emergency spine x-ray films and myelography must be performed. The diagnostic examination of the *spinal fluid* should be done *at the time* of myelography. If a lumbar puncture is performed below a complete spinal block, it is often impossible to do a second puncture for the myelogram owing to the collapse of the dural sac. The myelogram will demonstrate whether the mass is extradural (disk, spondylosis, abscess, metastasis, lymphoma), extramedullary, intradural (meningioma neurofibroma), or intramedullary (glioma, ependymoma, syrinx).

Decompression of the cord is nearly always accomplished by immediate neurosurgical intervention. In certain cancers, however, where the longitudinal extent of disease and associated destruction of vertebrae make surgery technically inadvisable, emergency radiation or chemotherapy may be tried. Steroids are used to reduce edema of the cord and tumor during initial radiotherapy.

NONCOMPRESSIVE ACUTE SPINAL CORD SYNDROMES

Compressive myelopathy does not encompass all the urgent or all the treatable disorders of the spinal cord. The subacute combined systems disease of *vitamin B-12 deficiency* should be regarded as an emergency. These patients complain of intense tingling paresthesias in the hands and show loss of position and vibration sense with pyramidal weakness in the lower extremities. The knee and ankle jerks are lost but the Babinski response is present. A serum B-12 level should be drawn, and the patient given B-12 immediately. A Schilling test also serves both to treat and diagnose the disorder. *Acute postinfectious or postimmunization transverse myelitis should be treated with steroids.* Schistosoma hematobium and mansoni may embolize via Batson's venous plexus to the cauda equina or thoracolumbar cord and produce a painful acute paraplegia, sensory loss in the lower limbs, and sphincter disturbance. Specific anti-schistosomal and steroid treatment should be instituted for this syndrome in a patient who has lived in endemic regions and who has eosinophilia and characteristic lesions on cystoscopy or sigmoidoscopy. Biopsy of the rectal mucosa or complement fixation tests support the diagnosis. *Meningovascular syphilis* may produce a rapid, extensive cord syndrome that is halted by penicillin therapy.

Hemiplegia

Acute paralysis of the face, arm, and leg on one side of the body is most commonly caused by cerebrovascular disease. If we accept the limitations that the full differential diagnosis of acute hemiplegia cannot be discussed here and that many strokes are not accompanied by hemiplegia, it would nevertheless be useful to discuss the principles of early evaluation and management of cerebrovascular disease utilizing the paradigm of acute hemiplegia.

FOCUS OF HISTORY IN ACUTE HEMIPLEGIA

The patient's history is directed toward discovering: (1) preexisting disorders which predispose to stroke; (2) symptoms that localize the affected brain areas; (3) the mode of onset and evolution of the neurologic symptoms. Thrombotic stroke often is associated with hypertension, hyperlipidemias, diabetes mellites, cigarette smoking, and the occurrence of the atherosclerotic process in other organ systems, as indicated by a history of angina pectoris, myocardial infarction, or intermittent claudication. Patients with thrombotic strokes may also have a history of prior transient ischemic attacks often affecting the same brain regions that ultimately become infarcted. In order to be labeled as a transient ischemic attack, a bout of neurologic deficits must fully resolve within 12 hours, but the most common types last only a few minutes. A *thrombotic stroke* frequently occurs in the early morning and takes several minutes or hours for the full neurologic syndrome to appear. *Cerebral embolus is usually more sudden,* and the maximal neurologic deficit is present at the onset. The dramatic reversal of deficits sometimes observed with cerebral embolism has been attributed to the fragmentation of the embolus. The history usually will provide evidence for the most common sources of emboli. Over 80 per cent of cerebral emboli occur in patients with mitral valvular disease, atrial fibrillation, or recent myocardial infarction. Emboli also arise from subacute bacterial endocarditis, marantic endocarditis, prosthetic heart valves, and atheromatous material and thrombus on the walls of the aorta and carotid arteries. Prior headache and visual symptoms in patients over 50 years old suggest the possibility of giant cell arteritis. Stroke in young adults direct the history toward the pesence of migraine, symptoms of one of the collagen-vascular diseases, or recent trauma to the carotid artery in the neck.

Most patients with primary nontraumatic intracerebral hemorrhage have a history of established significant hypertension. The remainder are found to have deficits in the clotting mechanism (anticoagulant therapy, blood dyscrasias, hepatic disease, etc.). Characteristically, with intracerebral hemorrhage there is a severe headache at the onset followed by focal neurologic defects and progressive deterioration in the level of consciousness (see Chapter 23).

LOCALIZATION OF INFARCTION

Complete neurologic examination usually will define the region of infarction, and the constellation of deficits often will point to the territory supplied by a specific artery. In some instances the clinical examination will define pathogenesis and prognosis quite accurately. For example, the small 2 to 10-mm. infarctions that occur at the termination of small penetrating arteries in hypertensive patients have been associated with several characteristic acute clinical syndromes including: (1) pure motor hemiplegia; (2) pure hemisensory loss; (3) dysarthria and unilateral clumsiness of the hand; (4) weakness of the leg and ipsilateral cerebellar ataxia. There is good recovery, and recurrence of stroke can be prevented by control of hypertension. Nuchal rigidity will develop within one to two hours of a massive intracerebral bleed or subarachnoid hemorrhage. Acute hemiplegia with nuchal rigidity may also point to a meningitis with an inflammatory vasculitis as the cause of a stroke.

VASCULAR CAUSES

Blood pressure should be measured in both arms. A marked decrease in the left is seen with occlusion of the subclavan artery. If the occlusion is proximal to the mouth of the left vertebral, signs of vascular insufficiency may be caused by reversal of flow in the vertebral, which now provides collateral circulation for the arm (the so-called subclavian steal syndrome). Examination of the heart may reveal a potential source of emboli such as arrhythmia, valvular disease, or left atrial myxoma. Bruits over the neck vessels and palpation of the volume of the carotid preauricalar and facial pulses may assist in localizing the vascular disease.

LABORATORY TESTS AND SPECIAL DIAGNOSTIC PROCEDURES

Blood Tests. The initial laboratory investigation is aimed at uncovering remediable conditions and confirming the diagnosis. The CBC may reveal an anemia sufficient to precipitate cerebral ischemia. Conversely, the hematocrit may be elevated enough to result in a critical hyperviscosity in states of severe dehydration of polycycthemia. The white count may point to systemic or intracranial infection. Hypoglycemia may produce focal signs that arise from the territory of supply of a stenosed vessel. Derangements in electrolytes, acid-base equilibrium, and arterial blood gases may also cause focal signs which disappear when the metabolic disorder is remedied. An erythrocyte sedimentation rate should be done immediately when temporal arteritis is suspected.

Frequently hospital laboratories will not do an ESR on off-hours, so the emergency physician should know how to perform this simple test. *Lumbar puncture* is always necessary to ascertain the presence of increased pressure, blood, white cells, protein, and Wasserman reaction. Bland cerebral infarctions do not usually cause a protein elevation above 100 mg. per cent.

An *electrocardiogram* may reveal an otherwise silent myocardial infarction that produced a stroke by causing a fall in cardiac output or was the source of an embolus. A *chest x-ray* should be examined for alterations in the size and shape of the heart; widening of the mediastinum is seen when a dissection of the aorta has produced signs by occluding the origins of the carotid arteries. *Angiography* is not necessary in most acute thrombotic strokes, but is useful in finding the source of bleeding in subarachnoid hemorrhages or in searching for a surgically accessible clot in cases of intracerebral hemorrhage. *Brain scans* are of limited use as cerebral infarctions often do not become positive on isotope brain scans until four to five days after the episode. *Computerized axial tomography* of the brain shows an area of decreased density within 24 hours.

TREATMENT OF CEREBRAL INFARCTION

The early treatment of cerebral infarction is aimed at minimizing the amount of brain tissue that will be permanently destroyed. In many cases postmortem study will show partial narrowing of a cerebral vessel without actual occlusion. This implies that dynamic circulatory events act to precipitate cerebral infarctions. Hypotension, congestive heart failure, and cardiac arrhythmias should be promptly corrected. Adequate ventilation should be insured. Severe hypertension should be cautiously normalized as too rapid lowering can increase ischemia. Anemia, dehydration, and metabolic derangements must be corrected. Significant temperature elevations should be lowered to decrease the metabolic demands of the brain. Cerebral hypothermia has been suggested, but is still experimental.

Use of Anticoagulants. Anticoagulation is not useful in completed strokes, but should be started in patients with strong clinical evidence for cerebral emoblus who do not have bloody spinal fluid, subacute bacterial endocarditis, or other contraindications to anticoagulant therapy. The high risk of a second embolus in such clinical settings as mitral stenosis with atrial fibrillation probably outweighs the risk of causing a bland infarction to become hemorrhagic by starting anticoagulation therapy immediately. For this reason a coumarin derivative and heparin may be started at the time of diagnosis, and the heparin tapered once the prothrombin time reaches therapeutic range.

Anticoagulants also reduce the number of transient ischemic attacks (TIA's) in some patients; the prognosis for ultimate stroke is not so clearly affected.

The enthusiasm evoked by the occasional dramatic improvement of acute stroke with carotid endarterectomy has been dampened by several controlled series demonstrating a consistently poorer prognosis in the surgically treated groups. Surgery for the acute stroke has been abandoned at most centers. In a patient with TIA's and a significant unilateral carotid stenosis, endarterectomy reduces the frequency of TIA's.

The use of inhaled CO_2 and other cerebrovasodilators is also becoming less common. Brain ischemia is the most potent stimulus for local vasodilatation, and the production of generalized cerebral vasodilatation may actually shunt blood from the ischemic region.

Aspirin has become widely used in prevention of TIA's, based on its effect of reducing platelet adhesiveness, but the merit of this practice is unproved.

Steroids are useful in treating patients with giant cell arteritis and some of the collagen-vascular diseases that affect the brain.

Brain swelling with progressive obtundation and signs of herniation, which may occur two to five days after cerebral infarction, can be controlled with osmotic agents such as mannitol, urea, or glycerol. Parenteral steroids in high dosages also control brain edema effectively without the problem of rebound edema seen when urea and mannitol are used. Dexamethasone may be started with an initial I.V. dose of 10 mg., followed by 4 mg. q 6 hours for 48 hours and then tapered according to the patient's response. The vigorous treatment of cerebral edema has not been proved to alter the survival or ultimate disability of the stroke patient.

References

Browne, J. R., and Poskanzer, D. C.: Treatment of Strokes. N. Engl. J. Med., 282:594, 1969.

Dyck, P. J.: Peripheral neuropathy. Postgrad. Med., 41:279, 1967.

Glaser, G. H.: Crisis, precrisis and drug resistance in myasthenia gravis. Ann. N.Y. Acad. of Sci., 135:335, 1966.

Haymaker, Webb: Bing's Local Diagnosis in Neurological Diseases, 15th ed. St. Louis, C. V. Mosby Co., 1969.

New, P. F. J., et al.: Computerized axial tomography with the EMI scanner. Radiology, 110:109, 1974.

Osserman, K. E.: Myasthenia Gravis. New York, Grune and Stratton, 1959.

Seybold, M. E., and Drachman, D. B.: Gradually increasing doses of prednisone in myasthenia gravis. N. Engl. J. Med., 290:81, 1974.

Walton, J. N. (ed.): Disorders of Voluntary Muscle. Boston, Little, Brown & Co., 1969.

Chapter 51

NONTRAUMATIC OPHTHALMIC EMERGENCIES

George L. Spaeth, and John Purcell

SPECIAL CONSIDERATIONS REGARDING THE MANAGEMENT OF OCULAR DISORDERS

The dictum of all physicians is "primum non nocere." Specialized technique is required in the evaluation and treatment of disorders of the eye, and help should be sought if there is any doubt concerning the diagnosis. The urgency of treatment of the most common serious problems is shown in Table 1 of Chapter 15 (p. 399). The majority of cases coming to the Emergency Department with an ocular complaint can, however, be perfectly well managed by the trained and thoughtful emergency physician.

The use of topical medications in treating the eye requires stressing. Topical anesthetics are dangerous when used chronically, and should not be given to patients for their personal use to relieve pain at home; severe corneal damage including perforation has been caused by such a practice. Topical corticosteroids or steroid-antibiotic combinations also are potentially dangerous. Steroids can cause the intraocular pressure to rise (painlessly) in susceptible individuals, and blindness may result. Steroids also facilitate the growth and ocular penetration of herpes simplex, leading to corneal perforation and blindness. Wound healing may be retarded, saprophytic or fungal elements may overgrow and cause severe ocular damage, and serious eye inflammation may be masked by steroids. Dilating drops should be used with caution. Long-acting dilating drops should be avoided (atropine, scopolamine) as they cause prolonged blurring of near vision (up to 14 days with atropine 1 per cent); their use also increases the difficulty of reversing an angle closure attack. Short-acting agents such as tropicamide 0.5 per cent or homatropine 2 per cent are preferred.

All patients with significant eye disorders should be followed by an ophthalmologist. Corneal abrasions may heal poorly and break down continuously, leading to troublesome corneal erosions; glaucoma can ensue after blunt trauma; retinal detachment may be a late sequela of trauma; and severe superinfections or chronic conditions may develop from the use of topical drugs.

SUDDEN LOSS OF VISION

CENTRAL RETINAL ARTERY OCCLUSION

Complete occlusion of the central retinal artery causes sudden, painless loss of vision in one eye. Visual acuity is typically limited to light perception and the pupil is sluggish or even nonreactive to the stimulation of a direct light. The posterior pole of the ocular fundus is edematous and white, except for the macula, which has a "cherry red" appearance due to the edema surrounding the fovea. The retinal arteries are narrowed (Fig. 1). When occlusion affects a branch rather than the main vessel, loss of vision occurs in the field corresponding to the vessel occluded, and ophthalmoscopic findings will be limited to the area served by that vessel. Causes of occlusion include arteriolarsclerosis, embolus (platelet, arteriosclerotic, septic, etc.), giant cell arteritis, trauma, sickle cell disease, and disease of the carotid arteries.

In the Emergency Department the patient should immediately be given carbon dioxide 5 per cent and oxygen 95 per cent by inhalation therapy. If the patient has called in or such inhalation therapy is not available, he should be instructed to breathe into a paper bag. The carbon dioxide dilates the retinal arterioles. Some recommend administration of low molecular weight dextran 10 per cent (Rheomacrodex, Gentran 40) intravenously. This is thought to reduce whole blood viscosity, have a disaggregating effect on erythrocytes, and interfere with thrombus formation. It has not been proved beneficial. Aspirin may offer some benefit, but this too is unproved. The eye should be vigorously compressed digitally for five seconds and then suddenly released in an effort to move any embolus further out in the arteriolar tree and to reduce the intraocular pressure. This should be repeated three to five times, firmly. The intraocular pressure should always be measured digitally, as promptly as possible, to be certain that an acute glaucoma is not present. In addition, some recommend lowering of intraocular pressure in all cases by prompt administration of glycerol, 1 cc./kg. body weight. This usually should be done.

Others recommend lowering of intraocular pressure by performing anterior chamber paracentesis. Probably this is best performed only by an ophthalmologist. Retrobulbar injection of tolazoline causes vasodilatation and has also been advised, though is not routinely carried out in all ophthalmic Emergency Departments. An ophthalmologist should be consulted for further treatment and hospitalization to determine the etiology of the occlusion if indicated. A sedimentation rate should be obtained in the Emergency Department on all branch or central arteriole occlusions. If this is elevated, a strong suspicion of giant cell arteritis should be entertained; hospitalization is probably indicated. Disease of the carotids can be recognized by decreased pulsation, the presence of a bruit, or other symptoms of cerebrovascular insufficiency. Whatever treatment is given, however, the prognosis for recovery of useful vision following central retinal artery occlusion is extremely poor.

CENTRAL RETINAL VEIN OCCLUSION

Complete occlusion of the central retinal vein of the eye causes a sudden, severe, painless loss of vision. The acuteness and the density of visual loss usually are less than with central retinal artery occlusion. The fundus is filled with hemorrhages; dilatation and tortuosity of the retinal veins add to the dramatic picture (Fig. 2A). The optic disk often appears swollen, and exudates are present about the posterior pole. The process is usually unilateral. The most common cause is hypertensive-arteriosclerotic disease, although various conditions such as polycythemia or cryoglobulinemia causing blood hyperviscosity, or leukemia, multiple myeloma, diabetes mellitus, and carotid disease must be considered. In most patients with severe visual loss an element of arteriolar occlusion is also present, and thus treatment must be vigorous. If acute, these patients may be hospitalized under the care of an ophthalmologist during which time an evaluation of the etiology of their vein occlusion is carried out. Around half these patients have underlying glaucoma. Aspirin may be useful treatment in some cases. Anticoagulation was widely employed in the past, but its value is not established. When the occlusion has occurred at high altitudes there has been a suggestion that return to sea level should be considered.

Branches of the retinal vein may also occlude (Fig. 3). Symptoms are less prominent and are related to edema of the posterior pole of the fundus. Treatment of such cases is not urgent. However, all should be referred for ophthalmic diagnosis and management as the likelihood for future visual loss is significant.

OPTIC NEURITIS OR RETROBULAR NEURITIS

Inflammation of the optic nerve causes variably rapid diminution of central visual acuity. Visual acuity may be only very slightly reduced, perhaps only to 20/25, or may even be normal. Comparison of the visual acuity of the two eyes gives a clue that the vision has indeed been affected. Recognition of color is especially helpful in this regard. In some cases a different response of the two eyes to a red object may be the only observable finding. In other cases the visual acuity may be only light perception or even less.

Pain is frequent. This is described as an ache behind the involved eye made worse by moving the eyes. Such pain almost always accompanies optic neuritis in patients less than 20 years old, but is uncommon in the elderly. Photophobia may be noted by some patients. A central scotoma is almost always present.

When inflammation affects the most anterior portion of the optic nerve, the examining physician may observe papillitis with edema and hemorrhages of the optic disk. Visual field changes occur; the blind spot is enlarged. Arcuate scotomas are not rare, and other field loss also may be present (Figs. 4 and 5). In retrobulbar neuritis it is said that "the patient sees nothing (central scotoma) and the doctor sees nothing" (no evidence of inflammation within the eye). However, the presence of an afferent pupillary response (Marcus Gunn) (see p. 402) is *objective* evidence of optic nerve damage. There is a variable relationship to multiple sclerosis, and controversy as to the treatment. Ischemic optic neuropathy is a frequent cause of "acute optic neuritis" in the elderly, and may occur in younger patients as well. The role of oral contraceptives is uncertain but they appear to be a predisposing factor. Generally, these patients should be hospitalized under the care of the ophthalmologist or neurologist; some favor treatment with steroids or ACTH.

RETINAL DETACHMENT

Visual symptoms vary from vague blurriness to vision limited to perception of light. The loss of vision that may be complete or sectoral is usually in the lower field. Frequently, there are previous brilliant flashes of light (photopsias) due to traction on the retina. The patient will often describe a "cloud" coming over the vision. If the retina is detached only in the periphery, the central vision (visual acuity) may be normal. Detachment may be caused by trauma, a hole in the retina (rhegmatogenous), traction (proliferative vasculopathy), tumors, or exudate from inflammation. When examined through a dilated pupil, the retina will be elevated, billowing, and frequently floating (Fig. 6). However, if the detachment is in its early stages the retinal elevation will be slight and is not easily observed. These patients need admission to the hospital for complete evaluation. The great majority will require surgical intervention. If visual loss has been present for longer than one week there is usually no urgency regarding treatment. However, if the macula is threatened or if the macula has just become detached, then referral to an ophthalmologist should be as prompt as possible. Preferably such patients should be hospitalized immediately and placed on bed rest on the back with the head flat.

VITREOUS HEMORRHAGE

Bleeding into the vitreous is associated with sudden loss of vision described as a "cloud." Underlying causes may be trauma, diabetes, hypertension, tumor, inflammatory process, vitreous retinal traction, hematopoietic disorders, or retinal detachment. If marked bleeding has occurred, the fundus will not be visible; the vitreous will be but a red-black haze. Such patients may develop an acute glaucoma with severe pain. When bleeding is slight the site of origin may be seen. These patients need evaluation by an ophthalmologist. No treatment need be given in the Emergency Department unless glaucoma is present.

ACUTE GLAUCOMA

A sudden rise of the pressure inside the eye produces painful "smoky" loss of vision with an associated hazy cornea, congested eye, and dilated pupil. Acute glaucoma may be extremely painful, mimicking systemic disease (rigid abdomen, chest pain, headache, etc.). Surprisingly, many cases, especially in the elderly in whom pain may be poorly localized, are misdiagnosed as acute cholecystitis. *Pain, however, need not be present.* The degree of pain correlates well with the degree of inflammation in the eye but poorly with the actual level of intraocular pressure (Figs. 7, *A* and *B*). For example, patients with acute glaucoma due to a disintegrating melanoma of the choroid may have severe pain and inflammation with intraocular pressures of 30 to 40 mm. Hg, whereas cases in whom there have been recurrent episodes of incomplete angle closure will often have intraocular pressure above 50 mm. Hg but white, quiet eyes. The presenting symptom of these latter cases is slightly

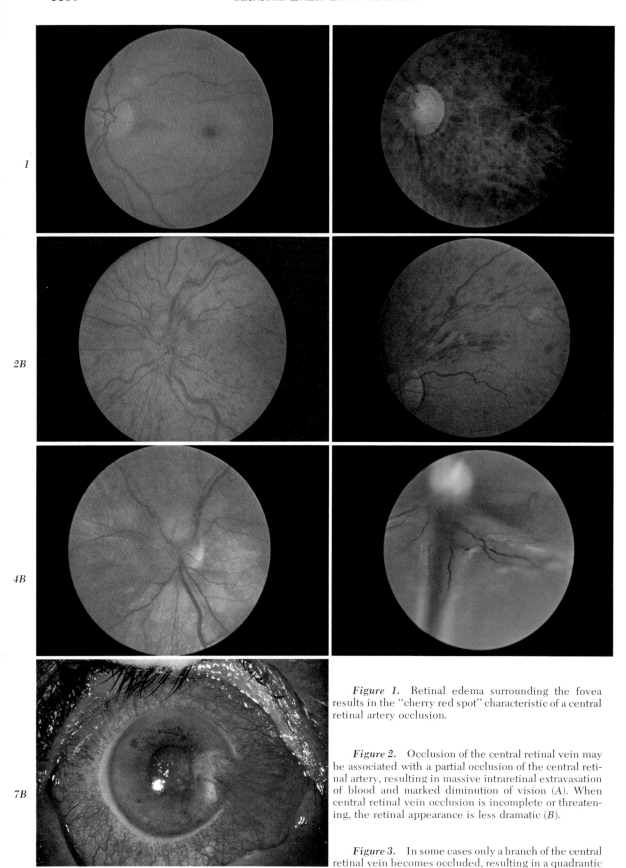

Figure 1. Retinal edema surrounding the fovea results in the "cherry red spot" characteristic of a central retinal artery occlusion.

Figure 2. Occlusion of the central retinal vein may be associated with a partial occlusion of the central retinal artery, resulting in massive intraretinal extravasation of blood and marked diminution of vision (A). When central retinal vein occlusion is incomplete or threatening, the retinal appearance is less dramatic (B).

Figure 3. In some cases only a branch of the central retinal vein becomes occluded, resulting in a quadrantic retinal abnormality (Fig. 2B).

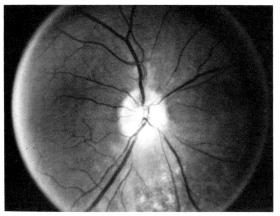

Fig. 4A

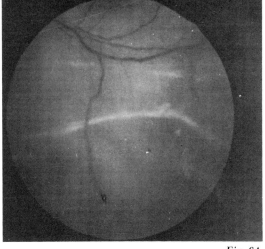

Fig. 6A

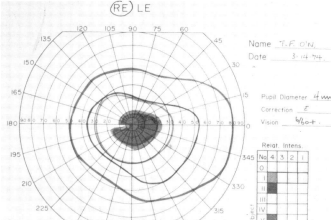

Fig. 5

Figure 4. Edema of the optic nerve head due to inflammation is characteristic of papillitis. Hemorrhages and vascular congestion may be present (A). Optic neuritis may involve only a sector of the disc (B).

Figure 5. Optic neuritis is associated with reduction of visual acuity; a central scotoma is most characteristic, as shown here.

Figure 6. Retinal detachment usually starts in the far peripheral portion of the retina. It may be easily overlooked unless the pupil is widely dilated and indirect ophthalmoscopy utilized. As the detached retina is often translucent, its elevation from the underlying retinal pigment epithelium may be difficult to detect. Anterior deviation of retinal blood vessels is a helpful sign, as is a white demarcation line (A). When total, as in B, the detachment is easily recognized by the wavy grayish surface of the retina protruding into the vitreous cavity.

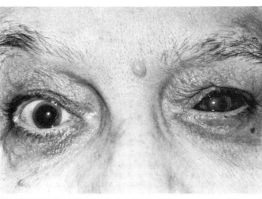

Fig. 7A

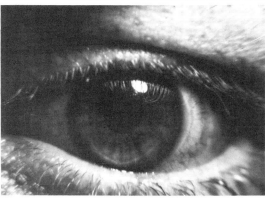

Fig. 7C

Figure 7. Acute primary angle closure is most typical when associated with sudden onset of severe pain, redness of the eye, dilation of the pupil, and blurring of the vision (A). The cornea will be hazy, the iris may be partially atrophic, and early cataractous changes take place in the lens (B). On the other hand, angle-closure glaucoma can be chronic, in which case intraocular pressure may be greatly elevated (50 to 60 mm. Hg) and yet the eye may appear grossly normal.

1159

blurred vision or colored halos. It is to be emphasized that pain and inflammation need *not* be present in patients with serious, even potentially blinding glaucoma.

The classic signs of acute glaucoma are a dilated fixed pupil in a severely inflamed eye with a hazy cornea (Fig. 7, *A*). Sector iris atrophy, fine pigment deposits on the corneal endothelium and milky opacities of the anterior capsule of the lens are even more specific indications of a rapid rise in intraocular pressure. Severe glaucoma may, however, be present in an eye that appears grossly normal (Fig. 7, *B*).

Once the diagnosis is suspected, consultation should be sought to determine the etiology and treat the process. If the intraocular pressure is nearing the usual mean pressure of the retinal vessels, that is, above 50 mm. Hg, then treatment must be promptly started, for permanent blindness caused by ischemia may be caused by delay. If arterial pulsations are present the treatment is urgent, and if retinal arteries are filling poorly the treatment is emergent. Patients not allergic to sulfonamides should be given intravenous acetazolamide, 500 mg.; glycerol, 1 cc./kg. body weight should also usually be administered. Referral to the ophthalmologist should take place as rapidly as possible. There are different modes of therapy and surgery that may be indicated. Where pain is severe, analgesia should be afforded the patient.

Miotics should not be given unless the emergency physicians are certain of the diagnosis *and* have examined the fundus completely. It may be very difficult to visualize the fundus once miotics have been administered. The hazy cornea may be cleared for gonioscopy and fundoscopy by topical administration of anhydrous glycerol. This is painful unless the eye has been well anesthetized previously. Several drops of glycerol may need to be used. As the dehydrating effect is transient the fundus should be examined as thoroughly as possible, specifically looking for tumor, retinal detachment, and central retinal vein occlusion. The presence of glaucomatous cupping or atrophy of the optic nerve head is a strong suggestion that the patient has had prior glaucoma.

A good general rule for the treatment of glaucoma is, "the redder the eye and the whiter the disk, the more urgent the treatment."

VISUAL LOSS DUE TO INTRACRANIAL DISEASE

Central nervous system visual loss usually is sudden, painless, and may be associated with other neurologic deficits. The usual etiology is vascular and may involve either the anterior middle, or posterior cerebral arteries as well as the vertebral system. Characteristic field defects outline the area involved. Anterior to the chiasm the loss is usually uniocular. Posterior to the chiasm the typical homonymous hemianopia is observed, becoming more congruous the more posterior the lesion is located. This is a "stroke" in the traditional sense, although it may only involve those cortical areas associated with vision and the field loss may be surprisingly small in area. Patients with hemianopic types of visual loss should be referred to a neurologist or neurosurgeon. No emergency treatment is indicated.

Papilledema may cause a mild reduction of visual acuity. This may be transient and intermittent. There is an enlargement of the blind spot. Certainly the optic disk should be carefully examined for signs of papilledema where headache is present, especially when associated with visual symptoms (Fig. 8).

MIGRAINE

Migraine can be limited to the visual system. The symptoms are highly characteristic. The patient complains of scintillating lines, usually in a zigzag, "Maginot Line" formation, off to one side. This may be accompanied by severe reduction of acuity, although this is unusual. Headaches and other symptoms of migraine are often absent. The attack passes spontaneously after a few minutes, but leaves the patient anxious. In most instances no treatment other than reassurance is needed. The differential diagnosis includes conditions such as retinal detachment that cause unilateral "flashing lights."

MALINGERING OR HYSTERIA

Nonorganic causes of a sudden loss are common. The visual field examination is usually the best way to discriminate between the causes of such nonorganic causes of visual loss. It is important to distinguish between the malingerer trying to give the impression of visual loss and the hysterical patient in whom visual loss is "real," although emotionally caused.

In the normal individual a test object can be seen at a measurable distance from the point of fixation of gaze; when tested at twice the distance (say 2 meters instead of 1 meter) the same test object will be able to be seen almost twice as far away from the point of fixation. That is, the normal field is cone-shaped, and enlarges as the distance between the subject and the testing screen is increased. The patient attempting to "fake" a field loss usually (though not always) is unaware of this physiologic fact and reports seeing the object the same distance from fixation no matter how great the distance between him and the test screen. Thus the field is "tubular," rather than conical.

Hysterical patients are not, in contrast, consciously trying to "fake" field loss, but will still often give the tubular type of field just described. Many times the field will be "spiral" in nature, or even unobtainable because of inconsistency of response.

A highly valuable clue is given by the functional visual field as opposed to the tested field. The patient's actual visual field is tested by asking him to follow the examiner into a room for a special test. It usually becomes readily apparent whether the patient's alleged field loss is "real" or feigned, for in the former case the patient will stumble over chairs, miss corners, etc., whereas the patient trying to mislead the examiner will perform satisfactorily.

Examination of cases who are malingering or have hysterical visual loss will disclose no findings to accompany the apparent insult to vision. Many of these patients have deep-seated emotional problems. They should be evaluated by a neurologist. *Placebo medications in the Emergency Department should not be given as they may actually reinforce the symptoms.* The emergency physician should be extraordinarily cautious in what he says and records regarding the patient in whom there appears to be discrepancy between symptoms and objective findings. The Emergency Department records may well later prove to be important issues in litigation. Malingering is in many ways an accusation. The diagnosis is difficult to prove. The physician should suspect malingering, but should not be satisfied with that diagnosis unless the evidence is overwhelmingly clear.

EVALUATION OF THE RED EYE

One of the commonest presenting symptoms of an ocular disorder is an inflamed eye. Conjunctivitis, uveitis, corneal ulcer, glaucoma, and orbital cellulitis may all cause red inflamed eyes. The differentiation of these difficult conditions is crucial for the proper management of the patient (Table 1).

CONJUNCTIVITIS

Conjunctivitis may be bacterial, viral, fungal, parasitic, allergic, or chemical. Generally, conjunctivitis is not painful, although when acute it may be mildly so; the eye is red; tearing, discharge, and itching may occur. The lids are stuck together when the patient awakens. Vision is blurred when copious amounts of discharge are present. The disease may be bilateral, but generally begins with one eye.

Table 2 enumerates the important factors present with the most common types of conjunctivitis.

With allergic conjunctivitis, chemosis (swelling of the conjunctiva) and papillae often are present (Fig. 9). The major symptom is usually itching. There may be a history of contact with an allergen. Mild allergic conjunctivitis is treated best by no therapy other than removal of the offending agent. If more severe, a decongestant or vasoconstrictor topically every four to six hours and cold compresses may be added. If severe, antihistamines systemically or steroids topically may be needed. However, steroids have serious complications, including activation of herpes simplex and induction of glaucoma.

Bacterial conjunctivitis is usually of acute onset; a mucopurulent or purulent discharge is present. There is intense congestion of the conjunctival vessels, and papillae are present on the tarsal conjunctiva of the lids (Fig. 10). In mild cases it usually is not necessary to culture the organism. Use of antibiotic combinations such as neomycin, polymyxin and bacitracin is adequate in most cases. This constitutes one of the few places in medical practice where such a "shot-gun" approach may be warranted. If the therapeutic response is not very prompt, however, the case should be referred to an ophthalmologist, who may have a difficult time defining the responsible organism. In severe cases a gram stain, culture, and sensitivity should be done and the patient placed on

TABLE 1   Differential Diagnosis of the "Red Eye"

	PAIN	PHOTOPHOBIA	VISION	OCULAR INJECTION	OCULAR DISCHARGE	LID SWELLING	PUPIL
1. Conjunctivitis (See Table 2)	minimal	none to mild	slightly blurred by discharge	lid and eye	marked (except allergic type)	varies	normal
2. Episcleritis	moderate	none	normal	deep vessels of sclera often focal	minimal	none	normal
3. Corneal ulcer	none to severe	varies	decreased markedly	diffuse	present	none to mild	normal
4. Uveitis	mild to severe	mild to severe	normal or moderately reduced	next to limbus	none	none	small
5. Glaucoma acute	severe or mild	moderate	decreased by corneal edema	diffuse	none	none	dilated
chronic	none	none	normal	none	none	none	normal
6. Orbital cellulitis	none to severe	none	normal or reduced	diffuse with chemosis	none	diffuse (confined to orbit)	normal

TABLE 2 *Various Features of Commonly Occurring Conjunctivitis*

	DISCHARGE	TEARING	ITCHING	INJECTION	PAPILLAE	FOLLICLES
Allergic	+	+++	+++	+	++	0
Bacterial	+++	+	+	++	+	+−
Viral	+ (watery)	+	+	++	0	++

appropriate antibiotic drops at least every four hours and given warm compresses. Appropriate systemic antibiotics also may be needed. The infection should resolve in three to five days; if marked clinical improvement is not seen the patient should be referred to an ophthalmologist. If the cornea is involved the situation is extremely serious and immediate referral should be made; a smear and culture should be taken and treatment started if examination by the opthalmologist will be delayed.

Viral conjunctivitis is frequently acute in onset, has a watery discharge, mild infection, and follicles on the tarsal conjunctiva (Fig. 11). A preauricular enlarged lymph node may be present. Treatment is symptomatic with warm compresses. A topical sulfa or antibiotic solution has been recommended by some, allegedly to prevent a superinfection with bacteria. Others believe that no medication should be used.

Both bacterial and viral conjunctivitis share a most characteristic symptom, specifically, sticking together of the eyelids on awakening.

Other types of conjunctivitis than these three just discussed are less often seen and should usually be referred.

Topical corticosteroids or combination corticosteroid-antibiotic drops or ointments are fraught with hazard and should be used sparingly, if at all, by the emergency physician. Steroids may cause the intraocular pressure to rise and provoke rampant spread of herpes simplex infection of the cornea; they prevent corneal healing in injuries, allow overgrowth of bacteria and fungal elements, and may mask underlying inflammatory conditions.

UVEITIS

Uveitis is an inflammation of the uveal tract. The iris (iritis), iris and ciliary body (iridocyclitis), the choroid (choroiditis), or the entire uveal tract (panuveitis) may be affected. One or all of these areas of the uvea may be involved at the same time. Traumatic iritis is discussed in Chapter 38. Patients who present with photophobia, miosis, injection over the ciliary body, flare and inflammatory cells in the anterior chamber have iridocyclitis and deserve further evaluation by an ophthalmologist. The potential etiologies are manifold and may be systemic or local in origin. The precise cause is rarely found. Immediate treatment may be given if the diagnosis is sure and includes analgesics, sunglasses to reduce photophobia, and cycloplegia (scopolamine 0.25 per cent or homatropine 5 per cent three or four times daily). Care should be taken not to dilate patients with shallow anterior chambers.

CORNEAL ULCER

Ulcerative lesions of the cornea are an emergency. Prompt identification of the bacterial or fungal agent and rapid institution of correct therapy are necessary. The cause may be chronic or acute; pain may be absent or severe. An opaque, gray-white area on the cornea is noted. The conjunctiva and episcleral vessels are injected, and purulent discharge is present. The anterior chamber often contains a hypopyon (Fig. 13). An ophthalmologist should be consulted and the patient hospitalized after specialized scraping, staining, and culture techniques have been employed.

ACUTE GLAUCOMA

The signs and symptoms of acute glaucoma are discussed in detail on page 1157. Briefly, the patient may give a history of episodes of hazy vision associated with "colored rings around street lights" (due to edema of the cornea caused by the transient elevation of the intraocular pressure). The first attack often causes pain, injection of the conjunctiva and ciliary vessels, a cloudy cornea, a dilated pupil, and an elevated intraocular pressure (Figure 7, A). The disease

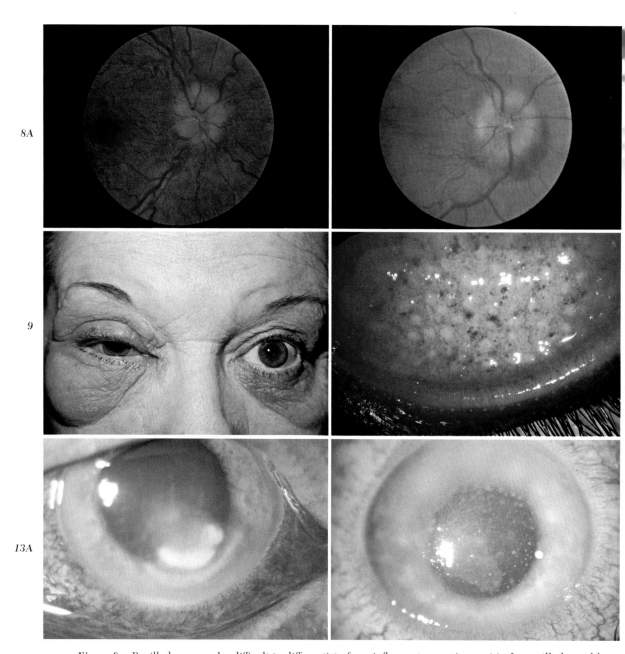

Figure 8. Papilledema may be difficult to differentiate from inflammatory optic neuritis. In papilledema dilatation of the veins may be marked as seen in the papilledema associated with a posterior fossa tumor illustrated in A. Retinal folds are noted in *B* as well as a fresh hemorrhage along the disc margin. Haziness of the disc margins is usual (*C*). The field defect usually consists of enlargement of the blind spot rather than the central scotoma typical of optic neuritis.

Figure 9. Allergic conjunctivitis and blepharitis may follow a variety of contacts, including ocular medication such as epinephrine (shown here) and neomycin.

Figure 10. Bacterial conjunctivitis induces a purulent discharge as well as the four classic signs of inflammation. Severe conjunctivitis may lead to corneal abscess and perforation, especially when caused by gonococcus.

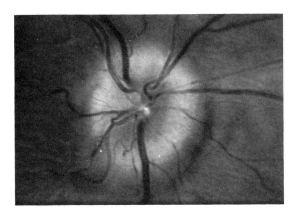

Fig. 8C

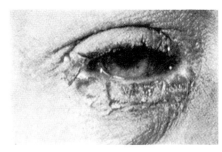

Fig. 10

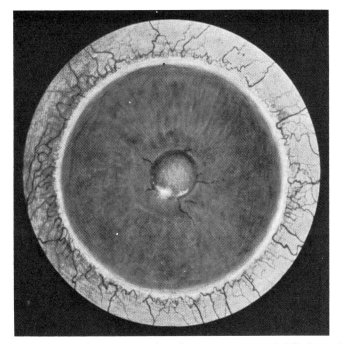

Fig. 12

Figure 11. Follicular changes are characteristic of viral conjunctivitis. Both follicles and papillae are seen in this case of epidemic keratoconjunctivitis due to an adenovirus.

Figure 12. The hallmarks of uveitis are photophobia, limbal flush, and a small pupil. Slit lamp examination shows an anterior chamber reaction. When uveitis is secondary to glaucoma or itself causes a glaucoma, the pupil may be large.

Figure 13. Bacterial corneal ulcers may penetrate rapidly. The frequently noted hypopyon usually is sterile. However, treatment must be prompt, vigorous, and appropriate for the organism, most often a pneumococcus (*A*). Pseudomonas is a less frequent but even more virulent cause. Fluorescein can be used to demonstrate loss of epithelium as in this case with herpes simplex uveitis and a corneal erosion (*B*). Corneal erosions, even when apparently trivial, predispose to bacterial ulcers. When initially seen, the pupil is small because of anterior uveitis. In eyes with wide anterior chamber angles dilatation is an important aspect of therapy.

may mimic systemic disease. No drops should be instilled in the eye; an ophthalmologist should be consulted promptly regarding hospitalization and therapy of the patient. Intraocular pressure may need immediate lowering (p. 1156), especially if arterial pulsations are noted or the pressure is above 50 mm. Hg.

ORBITAL CELLULITIS

Infection within the orbit is a life-threatening process. If extension into the cavernous sinus or the epidural space occurs severe neurologic deficits, seizures, and death may result. Concurrent ethmoid or pansinusitis is the most common etiology. The patient presents with an erythematous, edematous area outlined by the orbital septum. The conjunctiva is chemotic; ocular motion is limited due to edema. The affected area is warm and focally tender. The patient may appear toxic and is febrile. The pupil is spared unless swelling is so severe as to involve the third nerve, producing the "orbital apex syndrome," or there is an extension into the cavernous sinus. Patients with orbital cellulitis usually should have x-ray examinations of the sinuses and orbits, cultures of the nasopharynx and blood, and should be hospitalized for intensive antibiotic therapy and observation.*

*Thanks are given to Doctor W. Annesley of the Retina Service, Doctor G. Shannon of the Oculoplastic Service, and Doctor P. Laibson of the Cornea Service of Wills Eye Hospital, who supplied many of the photographs illustrating Chapters 38 and 51.

Chapter 52

PSYCHIATRIC EMERGENCIES

A. The Psychiatric Emergency
B. The Depressed Patient
C. The Assaultive Patient
D. The Floridly Psychotic Patient
E. The Organically Confused Patient
F. Psychiatric Emergencies in Childhood and Adolescence
G. Overdosage with Psychotropic Drugs
H. Emergencies in Medical, Surgical, or Obstetric Patients Who Are Severely Ill
I. The Physically Abused Patient

A. THE PSYCHIATRIC EMERGENCY

Jean-Pierre Lindenmayer and Nathan S. Kline

DEFINITION AND CONCEPT

Often a psychiatric emergency is seen simply as a situation in which a patient is regarded as suicidal or homicidal and for which immediate psychiatric attention is required. For our purposes, however, such an emergency could be defined more broadly as the sudden occurrence of a behavioral or emotional response which, if unresponded to, will result in life-threatening or psychological harmful consequences. This usually occurs in situations in which the patient has undergone overwhelming emotional stress and his usual coping mechanisms have broken down. The patient's resulting behavior is different from his usual pattern, and generally not in proportion to the event that presumably has set off the reaction. He may appear acutely fearful and panicky, enraged and destructive, or confused and disoriented. Again, he may be withdrawn or depressed and may talk about suicide. A major hallmark of a psychiatric emergency is emotional distress.

Such emergencies also usually affect quite severely those people close to the patient. In our experience, it is often the family or friends who define what constitutes the psychiatric emergency for the given patient. This is mainly when their own abilities to accept the patient's disordered or unusual behavior are overtaxed after a particular socially unacceptable or frightening event has taken place. For example, a euphoric manic patient who had been hyperactive and expansive for several weeks was brought to the Psychiatric Emergency Department after he was found directing the traffic at a busy intersection. Up to that point the family had been able to accept his eccentricities. Frequently, then, the request for treatment is made by someone acting on the patient's behalf (Detre and Jarecki, 1971). Clearly, psychiatric emergencies have to be considered not only from the individual patient's point of view, but also in the context of his immediate family, his community, and other social factors.

GENERAL PRINCIPLES OF ASSESSMENT AND MANAGEMENT

INITIAL ASSESSMENT

The first task is the assessment of the nature of the problem and its severity. The immediately preceding facts that led up to the crisis, and the possible precipitating events, will have to be gathered from the patient. Often he will not be able to communicate well enough, making it mandatory that family and friends be interviewed to add further information. The gathering of these facts from the patient and others constitutes an important management step, and actually is already a part of the treatment. The way the physician conducts his interview will help to decrease the patient's emotional distress; on the other hand, if this is not well done, the interaction between the patient and the interviewer can augment the difficulty.

Except for a few special situations, it is important to let the patient tell his story and intervene only when he is blocking or when important details have to be learned. The physician should appear calm and unhurried and provide a flexible structure in the interview, but not without setting clear limits. In other words, a patient should not be allowed to ramble on, but should be redirected to the question asked. For patients who are confused or very withdrawn, more active and goal-directed questioning will be necessary.

The setting for the examination should be as quiet as possible, and disturbing friends, relatives, or others should be removed. Nevertheless, help should be nearby, particularly with an aggressive or agitated patient in case he should lose control. It is advisable to talk to the relatives or friends in the presence of the patient in order to reduce his suspiciousness. However, if the patient does not wish to be present, this request too should be respected.

In learning the history of the crisis, the physician will have to look particularly at three questions that will help him to arrive at an appropriate disposition: (1) why has the crisis occurred now? (2) who labeled the situation as a crisis? (3) what are the expectations of the patient?

(1) *Why now?* The interviewer will have to explore what event precipitated the present crisis for the patient or the patient's surroundings. Often a pathologically stressful situation has existed for a long time, but a new element suddenly disrupts a labile equilibrium. Management measures, therefore, will have to be directed at the crisis and toward returning the patient to his precrisis condition or reaching a resolution.

(2) *Who labeled the situation as a crisis?* As pointed out above, the crisis sometimes is not experienced by the patient himself, but possibly by his family, associates, or the referring agency. In that case, the crisis might be more a sign of distress evoked by that particular surrounding, and interventions will have to be geared toward relieving the anxieties inherent in that particular surrounding of the patient.

(3) *What are the expectations of the patient?* Every patient seen by a physician has a certain set of expectations about the kind of help he will receive. It is important to clarify some of these expectations and to attempt to modify them if they are unrealistic. One of the more common ones is that many patients expect to be hospitalized as a result of their crisis presentation, when other treatment modalities possibly might be more helpful. Plans for disposition, therefore, should take this into account.

In addition to ascertaining the history of the crisis, the physician will have to examine carefully the patient's mental state. The degree of anxiety, the contact with reality, the degree of orientation, the impulse control, and the suicidal potential will have to be evaluated. It also will be important to assess the degree of cooperation and insight the patient shows, since this in part will influence the type of management chosen. In particular, the degree of seriousness of the problem will have to be evaluated in order to help the physician select the proper treatment modality.

Most of the time, the physician will find it difficult to establish an exact diagnosis in an emergency situation, since there will not be enough time for a full diagnostic evaluation. It will be easier, therefore, to describe the patients according to their perceived abnormal behavior. In addition to determing which behavior pattern is most prevalent, the physician must decide whether he is dealing with a functional problem or an underlying organic disorder that presents with behavioral symptoms. For example, a patient was brought to the general Emergency Department and admitted to Psychiatry with a diagnosis of catatonic stupor. It turned out, after careful neurologic examination, that the patient almost had been electrocuted and had extensive brain damage. Clues to the presence of an underlying organic illness are clouding of the sensorium, disorientation, confusion, recent memory losses, and sometimes visual hallucinations. If an organic diagnosis is established, the patient should be referred for the appropriate neurologic or metabolic work-up.

MANAGEMENT OF THE ACUTE SYMPTOMS

In managing functional disorders, some general guidelines can be established.

(1) The first step consists of helping to reduce the anxiety of the patient by providing a few empathic statements, by helping him relax, by providing a flexible interview structure, and by removing him temporarily from the crisis situation. In acutely psychotic patients, it will be important to indicate where the patient is and what is the purpose of the examination.

(2) It always will be helpful to appeal to the remaining healthy aspects of the patient's thinking, feeling, and behaving.

(3) It is wise to insist on firm limit-setting, if the patient is about to lose control.

(4) It is unwise to agree or disagree with a patient's particular delusions, but important to accept them as a fact *for the patient.* If a disagreement arises, the physician should not let himself be seduced into an argument, but simply should point out the difference of views.

(5) Throughout the interview, the physician may have to explain what is being done for the patient. Particularly at the end, whenever possible he should give clear and

straightforward explanations of the patient's condition and the proposed treatment, which will help the patient to trust the physician and also to receive from him a sense of firmness, purposefulness, and decision. In an acutely psychotic patient, however, such discussion might be deferred until some of the agitation has been controlled by tranquilizers. This is especially necessary if the patient is aggressive and requires physical restraints.

DISPOSITION

Specific decisions will have to be made soon after the evaluation of the patient, and sometimes even before a clear diagnosis has been made. In the emergency setting, the crisis generally assumes primary importance. One of the first decisions will be whether to hospitalize the patient or to treat him outside. The physician evaluating such a patient on an emergency basis must assess whether the patient is likely to hurt himself or others — often an extremely difficult decision since, if the patient is considered a threat, he may require hospitalization in a locked facility against his will. When there is a clear-cut suicidal or homicidal threat, the decision for hospitalization is not difficult. In many cases, however, the situation is more complex and requires a careful balancing of the patient's impulsivity, the psychologic effects of psychiatric hospitalization on the patient, and the family's ability and willingness to supervise the patient effectively if he remains on the outside. Another important step will be the decision for psychiatric referral. Once this decision is made, it should be explored briefly with the patient in terms of his expectations and possible fear at being seen by a psychiatrist. He should be clearly told why he is referred and to whom. Whatever the disposition, it should be presented to the patient, as far as possible, in a way that he can accept. It also is important to involve the family or friends in the treatment plans and to secure their cooperation, if they have brought the patient to see the physician in the first place. At the end of the interview, the patient should know the treatment proposed and have a specific plan for the follow-up after the crisis. If possible, the physician should remain available for consultation or phone calls from the patient and the family until the former has made contact with the recommended follow-up.

INVOLUNTARY HOSPITALIZATION

As mentioned previously, psychiatric hospitalization at times may be necessary in order to protect both the patient from himself, and the people around him. Most of the time, the decision for hospitalization will be made by the psychiatric consultant. There will be situations in which the patient is unwilling to see the consultant to be evaluated for hospitalization, despite a clear need. To enable the physician to send the patient against his will to the hospital, the former has to be familiar with the criteria for involuntary hospitalization and with the commitment procedures applicable in the state in which he is practicing.

The critiera for commitment vary from state to state, but a few basic ones usually are included in the laws of each state.

(1) Persons dangerous to self or others. Suicidal or homicidal behavior usually is the major reason for commitment.

(2) Persons "in need of treatment and care." This category can be quite extensive, and therefore also rather vague.

(3) Cases of drug and alcohol addiction. Although states differ on the definition of addiction, treatment for drug addicts or alcohol addicts can be obtained in many states through civil involuntary commitment.

In most states, involuntary patients can be hospitalized by the physician on an emergency basis or a temporary/observational basis with a formal application. These commitments usually are only for a limited period; those for a prolonged period are achieved by two processes.

(1) Judicial commitment, involving an application to the court, a hearing, and a judge making the decision as to the presence of mental illness and the need for hospitalization.

(2) Medical certification. In this situation, an application for involuntary hospitalization usually is made by a family member of the patient, and one or two physicians establish that the patient is mentally ill. The examining physician(s) have to be licensed in the state in which the hospital is located, and often need not include a psychiatrist. The patient usually has the right to have this

certification reviewed by a court hearing or, in other states, has to be released after submitting a request to that effect, following a brief hospitalization for observation. For all these procedures, it is important that the physician be familiar with the local laws when managing an involuntary patient. These regulations can usually be obtained from a local police station or mental hospital or by writing to the state department of mental health or hygiene.

References

Anderson, W. H., and Kuehnle, J. C.: Strategies for the treatment of acute psychosis. J.A.M.A. 229:1884, 1974.

Bellak, L., and Small, L.: Emergency Psychotherapy and Brief Psychotherapy. New York, Grune & Stratton, 1965.

Detre, T. P., and Jarecki, H. G.: Modern Psychiatric Treatment. Philadelphia, J. P. Lippincott Co., 1971.

Gwartney, R. H., et al.: Panel discussion on psychiatric emergencies in general practice. J.A.M.A. 170:1022, 1959.

Hankoff, L. D.: Emergency Psychiatric Treatment. Springfield, Ill., Charles C Thomas, 1969.

Klein, D. F., and Davis, J.: Diagnosis and Drug Treatment of Psychiatric Disorders. Baltimore, Williams & Wilkins Co., 1969.

Kline, N. S., and Lehman, H. E.: Psychopharmacology. Boston, Little, Brown & Co., 1965.

Lindenmayer, J. P., and Grad, G.: The psychiatric emergency room: a study of patient treatment requests. Int. J. Soc. Psychiatry. (In press.)

Linn, L.: Other Psychiatric Emergencies. In Freedman, A. M., and Kaplan, H. I., and Sadock, B. J. (eds.): Comprehensive Textbook of Psychiatry. II. Baltimore, Williams & Wilkins Co., 1975, p. 1785.

MacKinnon, R. A., and Michels, R.: The Psychiatric Interview in Clinical Practice. Philadelphia, W. B. Saunders Co., 1971.

Resnik, H. L. P., and Ruben, H. L.: Emergency Psychiatric Care: The Management of Mental Health Crises. Bowie, Md., Charles Press, 1975.

Slaby, A. E., Lieb, J., and Tancredi, L. R.: Handbook of Psychiatric Emergencies. New York, Medical Examination Publishing Company, Inc., 1975.

Ungerleider, T.: The psychiatric emergency. Arch. Gen. Psychiatry 3:593, 1960.

B. THE DEPRESSED PATIENT

Jean-Pierre Lindenmayer
and Nathan S. Kline

RECOGNITION

Depressed patients seen by the physician on an emergency basis usually suffer from rather severe states of depression that are not difficult to recognize. Their sad, melancholic expression, combined with either retardation or agitation, are practically pathognomonic of depression (Beck, 1967). They complain of feelings of sadness and hopelessness, of a reduced or absent capacity for enjoyment; they show a gloomy outlook on life and they suffer from slowed-down thinking and indecisiveness. Their depressive ruminations often show ideas of self-accusation that sometimes can assume psychotic proportions, with delusions of worthlessness. The patient may think that he has committed a terrible crime for which he deserves punishment. Rarely, he also may report hallucinations, particularly of an auditory nature, such as voices accusing him of his various sins. In elderly patients, delusions of poverty or the belief that they have some fatal somatic disorders are observed frequently. In milder states, hypochondriacal preoccupations are quite common. Suicidal ideation almost always is present in more severe depressions, and must be evaluated carefully.* Suicide threats, gestures, or attempts probably are the most frequent emergencies encountered in association with depression. Vegetative signs also are present in almost every depression. Easy fatigability, loss of appetite, and insomnia, particularly early awakening, frequently are reported. Loss of libido and constipation also are common complaints. At times the physical symptoms are so predominant that the depression is overlooked. Such "masked depressions" were first described about 30 years ago (Schick, 1947).

The agitated depressive patient may be more difficult to recognize. Motor restlessness, pacing up and down, wringing of

---

*See Chapter 34.

hands, and severe anxiety will be prominent. The patient tends to be both demanding and clinging. The agitation can be so severe as to lead to physical exhaustion, which itself represents an emergency. The patient, when first seen, may have been anorexic for several weeks and may have lost a great deal of weight, leading to malnutrition. Occasionally, he may hide his feelings behind a cheerful facade that will require careful interviewing to reach the underlying depression (Beck, 1967).

EVALUATION OF THE SUICIDAL PATIENT*

All states of depression may be accompanied by various degrees of suicidal preoccupation and action. The patient may express these in active or passive terms. A lesser suicide risk may be indicated by wishes expressed in a passive way, such as the wish "not to wake up in the morning," to be killed by an accident, or ambivalence about the wish to die. A severe risk is represented by the patient who has thought out suicide plans, has the instruments of destruction (pills, gun, etc.), or who reports impulsive suicidal wishes. The physician also should be alert to pick up indirect suicidal communications: the patient who reports with little affect that he has been driving his car recklessly, or that he has begun to put his financial affairs in order, communicates serious suicidal intentions. In very retarded depressions suicidal preoccupation may be constant, but patients are too inhibited by their retardation to carry out the suicide attempt. The physician should ask every depressed patient directly about his suicidal thoughts and intentions during the initial assessment; more often than not, he will give quite accurate answers. All too frequently, physicians are uneasy or hesitant to ask questions like these because of their erroneous belief that this may "give the patient wrong ideas." Actually, quite the opposite is true; most patients are relieved to discuss their thoughts. Although there is no exact way to predict a patient's suicidal intentions, a number of factors can be isolated during an

interview that contribute to the suicide potential of a patient.

(1) *Age and sex.* At high risk in terms of age are older men and young female adults. Men commit suicide more often, but women more often make the unsuccessful attempt.

(2) Previous suicide attempts and completed suicides in the family.

(3) Recent suicide of a famous person given newspaper and T.V. publicity.

(4) A detailed suicide plan that the patient describes.

(5) Stressful precipitating events that have not been resolved. Most of these will involve losses of persons close to the patient or of important material goods. Since these losses may be irreversible, the patient may feel there is no way to adapt to the new situation other than through suicide. There are feelings of hopelessness, and the feeling of being "at a dead end." There may be reactions occurring on the anniversary of the loss of a loved person.

(6) Provocative statements about how much he will be missed—how others will be sorry or angry or glad.

(7) Abrupt lessening of the depth of the depression, with a sudden feeling of relief when the decision has been made to go through with the suicide.

(8) Auditory hallucinations giving the patient self-destructive orders.

(9) Concomitant severe or chronic medical illness which the patient feels has totally exhausted his physical and psychologic resources or a condition which the patient judges to be fatal, whether it is or not, regardless of reassurances from the patient's physician.

MANAGEMENT
Initial Steps

Contact with the patient often may be difficult because of his withdrawal and state of inhibition. The physician will first have to attempt to create an empathic rapport between himself and the patient in order to be able to assess the nature, conditions, and severity of the depression. He will have to be tolerant, and be willing to wait for the patient and must avoid any critical statements. Possible precipitating events should be explored, such as the recent or threatened loss of a beloved one. One of the most important

*See also p. 34.

aspects of the initial assessment will be the evaluation of the suicide risk, as outlined previously. If a patient has attempted suicide, the question must be asked whether he still has suicidal wishes. If this is denied, one will have to examine carefully whether the suicide attempt has produced any change in the patient's environment. If the situation that precipitated the attempt is unchanged the suicide risk is still high.

The patient's relationship to the people with whom he is in closest contact should be examined to determine how much support the patient will be able to get from them. They also may provide helpful information about the patient's clinical state and suicide potential.

Psychologic Management

The physician should offer his help in a noncritical and empathic fashion, since the patient perceives his need for help as a blow to his self-esteem (Bellak and Small, 1965). It therefore is important to convince the patient that coming to see a physician is *not* a sign of weakness, but rather a sign of strength. Statements exhorting him "to straighten out," "to pull himself together," should be avoided, since they are liable to increase the patient's guilt or hostility (Kline, 1974).

During his interview the physician should help the patient to express and ventilate some of the pent-up feelings, and possibly to identify the loss which precipitated the depression—if it is of psychologic origin. In many depressions the origin appears to be biochemical and there is no specific environmental or psychologic "cause."

A brief explanation of the illness and its basically favorable prognosis will contribute to relieve some of the patient's anxieties and to build up his trust in the physician. If the basis of the depression is an acute grief reaction to the loss of a loved one, it is important to point out that this is normal (MacKinnon and Michels, 1971). The patient should be given support and helped to ventilate some of his feelings of sadness over his loss. The physician should explore with the patient other possible sources of emotional support, and help him to accept them. Bland reassurance often has a negative effect, since the patient may perceive it as indifference.

Disposition

If the suicide risk has been evaluated as high, someone should be with the patient constantly, preferably a nurse. The decision will have to be made whether psychiatric consultation and hospitalization are necessary. As a rule, every patient admitted to an Emergency Department after an attempted suicide should be seen by the psychiatric consultant as soon as the patient is medically cleared. If the suicide risk is only minor, the patient can be discharged home with psychiatric follow-up; however, the family should be made aware of the risk, and somebody should monitor the patient at home constantly. They also should be asked to remove from ready access all available medication and dangerous objects in the house. Prescribed medication may have to be given in a quantity that cannot be used for suicidal purposes. The patient also should be told that he can call the physician day or night, if he should feel that his suicidal urges are not under control. If the suicide risk is considerable, immediate hospitalization is indicated, directly or through psychiatric referral. This decision is best explained to the patient and the family as a protective measure against the patient's suicidal urges. If no real suicide risk appears to be present, psychiatric referral is also indicated in order to have treatment instituted and possible future suicide risks monitored.

In addition, in depressions with vegetative and/or psychotic symptoms, patients should be placed on antidepressant medication. The physician should explain the rationale of the treatment and the kind of medication to be used in pharmacotherapy. In particular, it will be important to stress the fact that the effect of antidepressant medication will not appear before two to three weeks. The most frequent side-effects to be anticipated also should be explained briefly.

For retarded depressive syndromes, the patient should be treated with tricyclic antidepressants at sufficiently high dosages (150 mg. or more, or 20 to 30 mg. of protriptyline) on an increasing dosage schedule. In order to minimize sedative side-effects during the day, the major part of the daily dosage can be given before the patient retires. This also will help to treat any sleep disturbance present. Patients who have not responded to tricyclics in the past can be treated by MAOIs in similarly adequate amounts (30 to 60 mg. per day).

For agitated depressive syndromes, when adequate sedation is needed, we recommend an effective minor tranquilizer such as diazepam in combination with a sedative tricyclic antidepressant (doxepin or amitriptyline). In some cases, levomepromazine can be used. High dosages of tricyclic antidepressants, if necessary in combination with a nonsedative antipsychotic drug in lower dosages, should be used for depressed patients with delusions and hallucinations.

The kind of treatment and disposition on which the physician has decided should be briefly discussed with the patient as well as with his family. There should be an opportunity for them to ask any questions about the further course of action. Their response to the treatment plan and referral can be checked, and possible complications can be prevented in this fashion.

COMPLICATIONS

Suicide

As pointed out above, suicidal preoccupation is to a greater or lesser degree a constant feature of depressive states. The careful appraisal of suicide risks therefore is particularly important.* This is necessary not only at the initial evaluation of the patient, but also later on, when the psychomotor retardation starts to lift. This is a particularly dangerous phase, since the patient begins to become more active and is able now to put suicidal thoughts into action. When hospitalization and drug therapy are insufficient to remove the imminent and severe danger of suicide, electroconvulsive therapy may be indicated. A short series of shocks may be sufficient (up to eight) to lift the worst part of the depression to eliminate the constant danger of suicide.

Refusal of Hospitalization

Occasional depressed patients may refuse hospitalization once this course has been chosen by the physician. It is impor-

tant not to try to convince the patient immediately, but rather to try to explore his fears of hospitalization. Most often, it will be regarded as another blow to self-esteem, generating guilt, particularly about failure to fulfill the usual role in the family. The fact of having to become temporarily dependent is seen as a weakness by the patient, and therefore something he wishes to avoid. Psychiatric hospitalization also may be feared because of the real and imagined stigmas attached to it by the patient's family and social environment. It also may mean to the patient that he "must be crazy," and that he will never be able to leave the hospital if the doctor recommends his going there. The physician should explore these various fears and remain firm in his decision, and usually will be successful in his approach. There may be situations, however, where involuntary commitment is necessary. At any event, it will be important for the physician to explain his rationale for hospitalization and possible commitment openly, rather than be vague or secretive about it. In our experience, it is most helpful to have the cooperation of the family in this matter and to gain their support. If the family also is undecided as to the value and need for hospitalization, it will be almost impossible to convince the patient. If, in spite of all the discussion, hospitalization is still refused, the physician should insist on discharging the patient if he fails to comply. Usually, this threat is sufficient to persuade the patient and the family to follow the recommendations.

Failure of the patient to follow recommendations as to hospitalization are not essentially different from the situation in which a patient has a myocardial infarction. If the physician continues to care for the patient outside the hospital, he is assuming a medico-legal responsibility of which he should be aware. At the very least, an immediate psychiatric consultation should be insisted upon.

Pharmacologic Complications

Patients with glaucoma and prostatic hypertrophy present a partial contraindication to the use of tricyclics because of the anticholinergic properties of these agents. If the decision is made to use a tricyclic, the patient should be checked regularly. Also, patients with serious cardiac disease should

---

*See also Evaluation of Suicide Potential, Chap. 34.

be followed carefully because of possible arrhythmias and EKG changes.

Patients may report excessive initial sedation, dryness of mouth, sweating, and constipation. Postural hypotension also is not uncommon. More detailed discussion of side-effects and contraindications for each of the compounds can be found elsewhere.

ACUTE GRIEF REACTIONS

Recognition

Acute grief reaction is the normal, though painful, process through which individuals must go after having lost a close relative, and to a lesser degree after divorce, separation, or break-up with a lover. The bereavement process has been characterized by Lindemann (1944) as having five distinct features.

(1) Sensations of somatic distress with lack of strength, feelings of exhaustion, anorexia, and insomnia.

(2) Intense preoccupation with the image of the deceased.

(3) Feelings of guilt, with the individual accusing himself of negligence, and exaggerating minor omissions.

(4) Feelings of hostility, often displaced onto the physician.

(5) A change in conduct pattern, such as restlessness, moving about in an aimless fashion, or the feeling that all customary activity has now lost its significance.

The acute grief reaction usually lasts four to six weeks, but its duration will depend on the success with which an individual resolves this ultimate separation from the lost person and readjusts to the environment and the changes brought on by the loss. The individual will first attempt to deny the reality of the loss, but ultimately will have to accept the disappearance of the deceased. This separation process is a very painful one, and strains the individual's usual coping mechanisms considerably. If this process is avoided, or if the coping mechanisms of the individual fail, pathologic grief reactions are encountered.

It is important that the physician be able to recognize pathologic grief reactions, since if these are treated adequately he can help prevent prolonged and serious social and psychologic maladjustments. Examples of pathologic grief reactions are set out below.

(1) Bland acceptance of the loss, with delayed grief reaction, the delay ranging from weeks to months, or sometimes occurring at an anniversary of the death.

(2) Overactivity without a sense of loss, sometimes resembling those activities formerly carried out by the deceased.

(3) Taking on the symptoms belonging to the last illness of the deceased.

(4) Progressive social isolation, with lack of initiative and inactivity.

(5) Strong hostility against persons in the patient's environment, such as the physician, who is accused of having neglected the deceased.

(6) Self-punitive behavior, e.g., becoming involved in poor business transactions and other actions detrimental to the patient's economic existence.

(7) Agitated depression (Lindemann, 1944).

A number of factors will determine in part the kind of grief reaction any given individual will show. Certainly, the quality of the relationship with the deceased is very important. The sex and age of the bereaved, the age of any surviving children, the timeliness of the loss, other crises occurring at the same time, and the presence of supportive relatives are other factors affecting the grief reaction (Parkes, 1972).

Management

(1) The patient should first be allowed to ventilate his or her feelings about the suffered loss. Through emphatic listening, the physician will be able to evaluate the quality of the grief reaction. Over-reaction or the lack of an appropriate emotional response to the loss should warn the physician of possible difficulties later on. The nature of the loss and its meaning to the patient should be explored, as well as it circumstances. Patients with pathologic grief reactions should be referred for psychiatric consultation.

(2) The suicide risk of the bereaved person should be evaluated. If the lost relative has provided the patient's only rewarding and important relationship or if the latter feels responsible for the death of the relative, suicidal risk can be particularly high. Under these circumstances, psychiatric con-

sultation is mandatory, and hospitalization may be indicated.

(3) The bereaved should be encouraged to seek support from relatives insofar as they are available. If the patient is alone, relatives or friends should be encouraged to stay with him during the first few days after the loss of the deceased.

(4) If the death of the relative occurred in an accident, the bereaved and the family should be given the opportunity to view the body. This also is important for mothers who lose a child pre- or postnatally. Preventing the bereaved from viewing the body fosters a state of partial denial (Kubler-Ross, 1975).

(5) A hypnotic medication may be given for the first few nights to combat insomnia (e.g., Dalmane, 15 to 30 mg., by mouth when retiring). Antidepressant medication should be given only for pathologic grief reaction, such as states of agitated depression.

(6) Follow-up appointments should be made in order to continue to give support to the patient and to help him accept the pain of the bereavement and ultimately to resolve it. If pathologic grief reactions appear subsequently, psychiatric referral should be instituted. In addition, the physical health of the bereaved should be monitored carefully during the year following the bereavement, since there often is a tendency for marked deterioration of health following the loss of a close relative.

References

Beck, A. T.: The Diagnosis and Management of Depression. Philadelphia, University of Pennsylvania Press, 1967.
Bellak, L., and Small, L.: Emergency Psychotherapy and Brief Psychotherapy. New York, Grune Stratton, 1965.
Farberow, N. L.: Suicide. Morristown, N.J., General Learning Corporation, 1974.
Kline, N. S.: Depression: Its Diagnosis and Treatment. New York, Brunner/Mazel, 1969.
Kline, N. S.: From Sad to Glad. New York, G. P. Putnam, 1974.
Kübler-Ross, E.: Crisis management of dying persons and their families. In Resnik, H. L. P., and Ruben, H. L. (eds.): Emergency Psychiatric Care. Bowie, Md., Charles Press, 1975.
Lindemann, E.: Symptomatology and management of acute grief. Am. J. Psychiatry 101:141, 1944.
MacKinnon, R. A., and Michels, R.: The Psychiatric Interview in Clinical Practice. Philadelphia, W. B. Saunders Co., 1971.
Parkes, C. M.: Bereavement: Studies of Grief in Adult Life. New York, International University Press, 1972.
Schick, A.: On a physical form of periodic depression. Psychoanalytic Rev. Vol. 34, No. 4, Oct. 1947.
Shneidman, E. S., Farberow, N. L., and Litman, R. E.: Psychology of Suicide. New York, Science House Inc., 1970.

C. THE ASSAULTIVE PATIENT

Jean-Pierre Lindenmayer and Nathan S. Kline

RECOGNITION

Acutely assaultive patients usually present emergencies that are difficult and challenging in their management. Often the violence already has been acted out or is in the process of being discharged when the physician arrives at the scene, so that recognition is not very difficult. The patient already may be restrained by family or attendants, or may be handcuffed and sitting in a wheelchair. However, there usually is little time to establish the underlying cause or diagnosis of the violent behavior: the physician will have to intervene immediately. This also illustrates how recognition and management of this kind of emergency are very closely interrelated. The recognition can be more difficult with a patient who has not yet actually assaulted anyone but who is on the verge of losing control. The patient appears tense and agitated, pacing up and down, and unable to sit for any length of time. He may be uttering or shouting threatening remarks toward people around him, and may become even more agitated if he feels that he is being trapped by a closed door or by the physician who positions himself between the patient and the door.

These states of assaultiveness can be due to a number of underlying conditions. The most frequent cause is an acute paranoid schizophrenic state in which the patient appears guarded and suspicious. He will interpret ordinary facts, such as the presence of the physician, and ordinary reactions of other people in a delusional way, thinking them directed intentionally against him in a persecutory fashion. He may feel that the physician is out to kill him, or is part of an elaborate organization of persons who are persecuting him. Sometimes, he also may experience hallucinations, mainly auditory ones of a threatening or accusatory nature. He may feel that he has to defend himself from these multiple imaginary threats, and therefore will become violent and assaultive. Close family members and other people who try to intervene are seen as potential persecutors who must be attacked. Delusions of grandeur also may be present.

Other syndromes to be considered in the differential diagnosis are acute organic brain syndromes caused by CNS disease or acute intoxications. Included in these may be alcoholic hallucinosis, with predominantly auditory hallucinations, amphetamine psychosis, with delusions of persecution, and reactions to LSD.

Convulsive disorders, such as temporal lobe epilepsy, also should be considered. Rarely, acute manic states can present as an emergency with violent behavior. Hyperactivity, logorrhea, and ideas of grandeur will help to establish the diagnosis.

MANAGEMENT

Initial Steps

The most important first step in managing the assaultive patient is to help him to bring his violence under control, and thus to protect both him and the people around him. It is essential to understand that, although those around the patient are frightened about his violence, the patient who perceives himself out of control is even more so. Any delay or half-hearted attempts to control his violence, therefore, result in even more violence, since the patient realizes that the physician is unable to control him. It may be necessary to use attendants in sufficient numbers to overpower the patient — efficiently and without hurting him. This demonstration of force usually suffices to help the patient regain control over his aggressive impulses (MacKinnon and Michels, 1971). If the patient already is restrained and sitting in a wheelchair, the physician should con-

duct his initial assessment under these conditions until he is completely sure that the patient is in control of his impulses. The patient should be consulted directly by the physician about this, and in particular should be told to indicate if he feels that he is about to lose control again.

Patients who have not yet lost control but seem to be on the verge of doing so should be approached in a calm but firm manner. Here again, the physician should keep in mind the need to protect both himself and the patient. The door of the room should be kept open to reduce the patient's possible feeling of being trapped, which would provoke more fear and therefore increase the possibility of violence; there should be help nearby to cover this contingency. The manner of the physician should be firm and decided; if the patient believes the physician to be afraid or indecisive, he may react with aggressive behavior.

Psychologic Management

Communication with the patient should be made in a clear and firm fashion from the start, and should be directed at two main points. First, it should aim at exploring the cause of the patient's loss of control and of his ensuing rage, and it should point out that anger to the patient. Second, if the patient is confused about his present environment, this should be pointed out to him by indicating repeatedly his surroundings, the purpose of the examination, and the identity of the people attending to him at the moment. Throughout the interview, care should be taken to explain every procedure or action of the physician in order to minimize any possible misinterpretation by the patient. At times, communication cannot be established without administering tranquilizers, which should enable the physician to conduct the interview in a calmer fashion.

Communication with a paranoid patient presents special problems, since usually he has been brought for treatment against his will, and does not consider himself to be sick. The patient's position is characterized by suspiciousness, mistrust, anger, denial of feelings, and projection of these onto others. Most of the time this results in a state of negativistic and angry withdrawal, with silence. In order to establish rapport with the patient, this anger should be recognized and pointed out to him; for example, the physician can acknowledge that the patient was brought to him against his will. The patient then may go into a long tirade about the harmful things his family is doing to him. The physician should permit the patient to give his account. Particularly, he should abstain from challenging the delusional state, since it would be fruitless. It is more important to ask the patient the reasons for his being the focus of his perceived persecutions. If the patient directly asks the interviewer to agree with his delusions, the latter should respond that he can understand the interpretation of the facts by the patient, but that his own interpretation might be different.

Once communication with the patient is established and some of the factors that brought on the loss of control are discussed, a more detailed history usually can be gathered. This should be compared with the history given by the family, which often may differ significantly. In particular, the patient may want to minimize past violent behavior and psychopathology, since it is difficult for him to see himself as sick.

During the interview a careful mental status examination should be performed. If the patient is calm enough to tolerate a physical examination, this should also be done. In the case of a paranoid patient, consideration also should be given to possible drug-induced states, such as amphetamine psychosis; during the physical examination, attention should be directed toward possible self-injection sites. These procedures together with the history, should help the physician to arrive at an appropriate disposition.

Disposition

In most cases, psychiatric consultation will be necessary. One of the exceptions may be when there is a clear-cut underlying somatic cause that can be treated specifically. Again, the patient should be told clearly and briefly about the disposition and the treatment plan, and the physician's reasons for them. This is particularly important with the assaultive patient, who may deny any need for treatment or psychiatric consultation. It then may be necessary to help the patient to get treatment against his will through psychiatric hospitalization, in order to protect him and the people around him. Again, the physician's rationale should be explained in the hope of securing voluntary cooperation by the patient. As mentioned in a previous chapter, if hospitalization is refused, there should be first an attempt to explore the patient's reasons, which usually are based on his fears that he will be trapped and never able to leave the hospital. It is particularly helpful if the patient's family or friends support the physician's recommendation; sometimes a person more familiar to the patient is better able to help him accept the recommendation.

In terms of pharmacotherapy, major tranquilizers are very helpful. If rapid sedation is indicated, intramuscular chlorpromazine is most effective. For a physically healthy individual, the dosage should range between 50 to 100 mg., according to approximate body weight. This dose can be repeated every four hours. The most untoward side-effect is an occasional severe hypotensive response, which requires immediate treatment (see below). This should be particularly kept in mind with elderly patients, and with hypertensive and arteriosclerotic patients, for whom the dose should be reduced to 25 mg. If chlorpromazine is contraindicated for some reason, 8 to 10 cc. of paraldehyde, I.M., or amobarbital, 65 to 500 mg., I.V., can be administered slowly. Once the acute agitation has subsided, the underlying cause should be treated. If the patient has been diagnosed as schizophrenic, major tranquilizers of the sedative type should be used: e.g., chlorpromazine, haloperidol, or chlorprothixene. Other causes should be treated specifically also. If the patient's state of agitation is due to withdrawal or ingestion of an unknown drug, it is wise not use any other drug, since there is always a possibility of unpredictable and dangerous interaction from a combination of drugs.

If psychiatric consultation is not immediately available and the patient can be discharged home in the meanwhile, the family members and/or friends should be alerted as to the risk for further possible violent behavior.

COMPLICATIONS

The Barricaded Patient

The most important step here is to establish rapport with the patient in any possible way, and to keep negotiating with him. This obviously includes listening to his demands and conditions for release. It should be pointed out to him that the physician is offering help, and therefore is not one of his persecutors. Rather than engage in a gunbattle, police should surround and isolate the person, and then allow him time to think and become hungry and thirsty (Zusman, 1975).

Pharmacologic Complications

As mentioned above, one of the more severe side-effects of tranquilizers, particularly phenothiazines, is hypotension, especially after parenteral use. For acute hypotension the patient should be put in Trendelenburg position, and I.V. sympathicomimetic medication should be administered. Orthostatic hypotension is not an infrequent complaint. Patients should be instructed to get up slowly from a seated or recumbent position.

Other impressive side-effects are the extrapyramidal symptoms manifested by: (a) pseudoparkinsonism; (b) akathisia; and (c) dystonias or dyskinesias. Of these, the most rapid to occur is dystonia (oculogyric crisis, torticollis, opisthotonos). These symptoms respond effectively to I. M. injections of benztropine, 1 to 2 mg., or 50 mg. of diphenhydramine. In severe reactions Benadryl can be given I.V. Antiparkinsonian agents should then be continued by mouth. Autonomic nervous system effects usually are easily manageable: among these are drowsiness, dry mouth, blurred near vision, and constipation. Patients with prostatic hypertrophy can present difficulties because of possible urethral spasm. Possible atonic intestinal reactions require that bowel movements be charted.

Unrecognized Somatic Causes For Violent Behavior

Certain acute organic brain syndromes can present with violent behavior as the most visible symptom, which actually is a manifestation of an underlying physical disorder. If the underlying condition is recognized, specific treatment can be instituted.

Transient ischemic episodes with confusion, disorientation, and transient neurologic symptoms may lead the patient to react with perplexity, depression, hostility, and assaultiveness.

Cerebral vascular accidents may cause confusion and, occasionally, aggressive behavior. The presence of permanent neurologic deficits assists in making the diagnosis.

Seizure disorders, particularly temporal lobe epilepsies, also may be mistaken for purely psychologic disorders. A history of identical episodes and of an aura preceding the fit will contribute to the correct diagnosis.

Infections of the CNS may be the correct diagnosis when the rest of the clinical picture and a lumbar puncture confirm their presence.

Metabolic disorders, such as hypoglycemic episodes or severe azotemia in elderly patients, also can produce aggressive and assaultive behavior.

The presence of intracerebral pathology such as a subdural hematoma, tumors, or infections can alter behavior substantially. Upon suspicion of organicity, a careful neurologic examination should reveal evidence of some focal signs.

Careful attention to the language used can assist differentiation between confused states, in which thought is difficult, and schizophrenic states characterized by bizarre speech patterns.

References

Bullard, D. M.: Psychotherapy of paranoid patients. Arch. Gen. Psychiatry 2:137, 1960.

Cameron, N.: Paranoid Conditions and Paranoia. In Arieti, S. (ed.): American Handbook of Psychiatry. New York, Basic Books, 1959.

Connell, P. H.: Amphetamine Psychosis. London, Chapman & Hall, 1958.

Lion, J., Bach-y-Rita, G., and Ervin, F.: Violent patients in the emergency room. Am. J. Psychiatry 125:1706, 1969.

MacKinnon, R. A., and Michels, R.: The Psychiatric Interview in Clinical Practice. Philadelphia, W. B. Saunders Co., 1971.

Shader, R. I., and DiMascio, A.: Psychotropic Drug Side-effects. Baltimore, Williams & Wilkins Co., 1970.

Zusman, J.: Recognition and Management of Psychiatric Emergencies. In Resnick, H. L. P., and Ruben, H. L. (eds.): Emergency Psychiatric Care. Bowie, Md., Charles Press, 1975.

D. THE FLORIDLY PSYCHOTIC PATIENT

Jean-Pierre Lindenmayer and Nathan S. Kline

RECOGNITION

The central feature of this syndrome is the patient's loss of contact with reality. The normal boundaries between him and his surrounding world have broken down. As a result, he may feel that other people know all about him and even his thoughts. His thinking appears confused and illogical. He may show looseness of associations, tangentiality, and at worst incoherence. He may feel that things are put into his mind, and at other times that his thoughts are "snatched" away so that his mind suddenly goes blank. At times, the feeling exists that someone or something apart from himself is controlling his actions. Alternatively, he may believe that he is able to influence the thoughts and actions of people around him, and therefore is the center of the universe. The patient also may experience delusions (fixed false beliefs), often of persecutory or grandiose content. Hallucinations may be reported— usually auditory, less frequently visual. The voices he hears may repeat aloud his thoughts or comment on them. They are frequently of an accusatory nature, or can give frightening orders to the patient, e.g., to kill himself. Such "command" hallucinations can be very dangerous if the patient feels he must obey.

As a consequence of these false perceptions and his misinterpretations of reality, the patient is agitated and anxious. He may be pacing the floor with a bewildered facial expression, or may sit expressionless in his chair and stare into empty space, possibly listening to his inner voices.

The patient or his family may report that he has been unable to sleep for several nights and that he has not been eating for days. The syndrome may represent the beginning of a schizophrenic illness or may be a one-time psychotic reaction to an emotionally stressful event. In younger patients, one also has to consider the ingestion of hallucinatory substances, such as mescaline, hashish, cocaine, peyote, and LSD, as causative agents. The hallucinations in these patients usually are visual, not auditory, and often the patient knows the effect is from drugs, but mind-altering drugs may precipitate an incipient psychosis. Finally, hallucinations also may be seen in women as a feature of postpartum psychosis.

Sometimes it may be difficult to differentiate this syndrome from an acute organic brain syndrome. This is discussed in more detail later in this chapter.

MANAGEMENT

Initial Steps

Communication with the acutely psychotic patient usually is very difficult because of his illogical thinking and disorganized ways of expressing himself, which make sense only to him. His state of panic and lack of trust present added difficulties in establishing rapport. In attempting to establish this rapport, the physician should be very active, explicit, and firm during the whole interview. Repeatedly, he may have to point out to the patient where he is and what the purpose of the interview is. He should actively help structure the patient's productions and gently keep him on the track of the current focus of his questions. Again, after exploring what brought the patient to see the physician, the question *"Why now?"* will have to be asked. A history of possible precipitating events should be elicited, with specific questions about recent changes in the patient's life, since the patient often will not volunteer such information spontaneously. If drugs are etiologic factors, a careful history should be taken of the the types and quantity of drugs used. This may help to prevent unexpected withdrawal reactions or incompatibilities between the ingested drug and medications prescribed for the present emergency.

The initial assessment also should include a brief evaluation of the patient's resources for support, such as his family or available friends.

Psychologic Management

Since disorganization is one of the hallmarks of an acute psychotic episode, the physician's interventions should aim at attempting to reorganize and structure as much as possible the patient's communications and perceptions. The interviewer must reveal his difficulty in understanding the patient, rather than responding, as in most social situations, with feigned understanding (MacKinnon and Michels, 1971). He must assist the patient continuously in following a more or less logical course of thought.

A second major set of interventions should be directed toward the patient's acute feelings of anxiety and emotional turmoil. The physician can pick up on the affect displayed by the patient and verbalize in an empathic fashion the feelings he thinks the patient is experiencing. In so doing, he can explore the patient's frightening hallucinatory perceptions and establish rapport. It also reassures the patient to realize that the physician is familiar with the kind of "crazy" experiences he has. In exploring briefly these delusional and hallucinatory perceptions, attention also should be given to their suicide potential, such as "command" hallucinations with the order to commit suicide. The risk of danger to others also should be evaluated along these lines.

In handling the patient's delusions and hallucinations, the same guidelines should be followed as for the paranoid patient. If asked to agree, the physician should remark that he can understand the patient's perceptions but that he does not necessarily share them.

If restraints are necessary to control assaultive behavior, they should be used decisively and with sufficient staff to overpower the patient effectively.

Although the patient may not seem able to understand, his condition should be briefly explained to him, as well as the further course of action, which should be outlined clearly in order to minimize paranoid interpretation and to further communication.

Disposition

Psychiatric consultation usually will be indicated, and should be presented openly to the patient and his family or companions. The consultation in most cases probably will lead to psychiatric hospitalization in order to provide safeguards against the patient's suicidal or homicidal tendencies. If the patient has to wait for this consultation, he should be put in as quiet and safe an area as possible in order to minimize environmental stimulation. Also, unobtrusive measures should be taken to prevent his possible escape. Often this can be achieved by having a trustworthy family member or companion sit with him. If the patient attempts to leave, the physician or an attendant should try to persuade him to stay. If the patient continues on his way and if the physician lacks the necessary help to detain him effectively, there should be no attempt at forceful restraint. Instead, the family and, if necessary, the police should be notified to return the patient to the hospital.

Pharmacologic management includes the use of sedative major tranquilizers, such as chlorpromazine or chlorprothixene, for patients who show marked agitation. Those with less or no agitation may be given less sedative phenothiazines, such as perphenazine or fluphenazine. If rapid action is required, phenothiazines can be given in liquid form or parenterally. At first, the phenothiazine may have to be given at frequent intervals and in increasing amounts, such as 50 to 75 mg. of chlorpromazine every hour, until the patient is sleepy, yet arousable. Daily maintenance dosage schedules should amount to chlorpromazine, 100 to 200 mg., four times daily; perphenazine, 4 to 6 mg., four times daily; or fluphenazine, 2 to 8 mg., four times daily.

Most drug-induced psychoses also respond well to the administration of phenothiazines, such as chlorpromazine. A word of caution is in order if there is suspicion that an anticholinergic agent has been mixed with the ingested drug. In such instances, phenothiazines can potentiate the anticholinergic effect and lead to a dangerous cholinergic crisis. In such situations, or when in doubt, minor tranquilizers used parenterally are the drugs of choice. Similarly, if the psychoses might be drug-precipitated, caution should be exercised in the use of phenothiazines. Although an LSD reaction is effectively treated thereby, untoward effects have been reported with the amphetamine derivative hallucinogens, particularly the one street-named "STP."

COMPLICATIONS

Suicide Attempts

Patients with floridly psychotic states not uncommonly show suicidal ideation as a result of bizarre delusional ideas or as a response to hallucinated commands. They are particularly prone to act on these suicidal impulses, since their hold on reality is minimal. They therefore present at times a rather severe suicide risk, and should be evaluated carefully for such a possibility, as mentioned above. If such suicidal ideation is present, psychiatric hospitalization is always mandatory.

Unrecognized Acute Organic Brain Syndrome

At times, acute psychotic states due to underlying organic factors may be overlooked and mistaken for a functional psychosis. In these cases, the disorientation, confusion, and perplexity of the patient, his visual hallucinations, and possibly his difficulties in recent memory will help in establishing the correct diagnosis. The cirrhotic with hepatic pre-coma, the uremic in renal failure, and the diabetic in hypoglycemic pre-coma are typical examples. Other states of toxic delirium due to iatrogenic interventions also have to be recognized: corticosteroid-psychosis; postoperative delirium; psychotic reactions after heart surgery and transplant surgery; and isolation reactions in intensive care units. Whenever possible, specific treatment should be directed at the underlying cause.

Pharmacologic Complications

As mentioned earlier, major tranquilizers can show a number of side-effects, of which the two major ones are: (1) severe hypotensive reactions; and (2) extrapyramidal symptoms. Further details are given in an earlier chapter in this section.

Postpartum Syndromes

Since childbirth is a major physical and emotional stress for the mother, it is not surprising that the period following can present the physician with various types of emergencies.

(1) Acute organic brain syndromes. These usually develop a few days after delivery, and are due to toxic or infectious causes. The patient's state of consciousness is impaired, and there can be visual hallucinations and delusions with disorientation. This state usually lasts for several days only, and should be treated along the lines described in the chapter for the organically confused patient.*

(2) Postpartum psychosis. This syndrome usually develops some time after the delivery, with symptoms of depression and anxiety. The woman feels overwhelmed by her new tasks of having to take care of the newborn child; she feels inadequate and is continously afraid of making a mistake. She ruminates obsessively over her helplessness, may have crying spells, and experiences profound sadness. In addition, she may have episodes of severe panic, with breaks with reality, paranoid ideation, and mostly auditory hallucinations. These experiences often focus on persecutory themes, and even can "command" the mother to kill her baby. This, together with the patient's impulsiveness, always constitutes a serious emergency, particularly if she is left alone with her baby. Bizarre attempts at hurting the infant may be tried, and the consequences can be severe both for the mother, who upon recovery may not be able to live with her guilt, and for the child, who may be maimed.

Psychiatric referral is always indicated, and psychiatric hospitalization will be required in most cases in order to arrest further disorganization of the patient and to restrain her possible destructive urges.

*See page 1183.

References

Bellak, L., and Small, L.: Emergency Psychotherapy and Brief Psychotherapy. New York, Grune & Stratton, 1965.
Hamilton, J. A.: Postpartum Psychiatric Problems. St. Louis, C. V. Mosby, Co., 1962.
Jacobsen, E.: Clinical pharmacology of the hallucinogens. Clin. Pharmacol. Ther. 4:480, 1963.
Klein, D. F., and Davis, J.: Diagnosis and Drug Treat-

ment of Psychiatric Disorders. Baltimore, Williams & Wilkins Co., 1969.

MacKinnon, R. A., and Michels, R.: The Psychiatric Interview in Clinical Practice. Philadelphia, W. B. Saunders Co., 1971.

Waskow, I. E., et al.: Psychological effects of tetrahydrocannabinol. Arch. Gen. Psychiatry 22:97, 1970.

Wolbach, A. B., Jr., Miner, E. J., and Isbell, H.: Comparison of psilocin and psilocybin, mescaline and LSD-25. Psychopharmacologia 3:219, 1962.

E. THE ORGANICALLY CONFUSED PATIENT

Jean-Pierre Lindenmayer and Nathan S. Kline

RECOGNITION

This syndrome at times may be difficult to recognize, because of the great phenomenologic variation found in the organically confused patient. In its *acute and reversible form*, this disorder can take different forms, depending on the severity of the confusion. Sometimes there is only minor confusion, with a mild degree of distractability, reduced attention span, and some difficulty in recognizing familiar faces and environments. There may be difficulties in orientation, particularly with respect to time. In more advanced forms, the disorientation is classically more severe and also extends to place and person. Along with this, the patient shows fluctuating disturbances of consciousness. He may not be able to grasp what is going on or may not remember where he is and who the people are around him. He may misidentify people who are strangers to him, such as the physician, believing them to be persons he knows. But above all, and as a result of the sudden loss of cognitive capacities, the patient will exhibit either an expression of perplexity and of fear or, on the contrary, an absent-minded withdrawal. States of panicky agitation can alternate with stuporous mutism. The patient's affect is markedly labile and often disinhibited. Trivial events easily provoke him to tears or anger. Since the sensory and perceptual systems are impaired, these patients usually are even worse at night when appropriate sensory input is normally reduced, and this often is the time when they are found to wander about aimlessly and to present emergencies.

In its most severe form, there may be hallucinations and delusions of simple but frequently changing content. The hallucinations are typically visual and are based on some misidentification of objects or sensory perceptions in the patient's view. Shadows on the wall are seen as threatening people, objects on the floor as crawling animals or insects. The patient, as a result, may be extremely agitated and fearful, or may even become assaultive. At other times, he may be depressed or oblivious to the events around him. Almost as a constant feature, however, his clinical state is a fluctuating one, changing states of confusion alternating with more lucid intervals. In any event, the clinical state represents a medical emergency, since the underlying causes can lead to permanent brain damage if not treated. Recognition and diagnosis of the underlying medical illness, therefore are very important. Possible neurologic findings may help in this diagnosis, such as aphasia, bilateral asterixis, and the presence of slowing of the EEG. History and additional information from the family will help establish the diagnosis. The more frequent underlying causes can be summarized as follows.

(1) *Toxic—metabolic causes.* Liver failure; renal failure; cardiac failure; endocrine disturbances; hypoxia; atropine intoxication; withdrawal from alcohol, barbiturates; isoniazide intoxication; carbon monoxide intoxication.

(2) *Infectious causes.* Toxic states during periods of high fever in acute infectious diseases.

(3) *CNS-related causes.* Increased intracranial pressure; brain tumor; hematomas; cerebral infarct; CNS infections.

Acute brain syndromes occasionally may be confused with acute forms of schizophrenia, particularly with catatonic stupor. The history of a severe medical illness or of trauma, plus the disorientation and fluctuating level of awareness, usually distinguish this organic syndrome from a functional one. Psychotic reactions to certain drugs, such as mescaline, hashish, cocaine, peyote, or LSD, may appear, resembling those seen in an organic brain syndrome; but the level of disorientation and awareness is not reduced to the same degree. On the contrary, the reaction to such drugs may produce heightened levels of awareness, often accompanied by vivid and rich visual hallucinations.

Some forms of dissociative hysterical reactions also may simulate symptoms of an acute brain syndrome. Usually, disorientation, decrease in the level of awareness, and memory disturbances are either too complete or too erratic and will help in ruling out an organic brain syndrome. Amnesia for one's own identity almost always is an hysterical phenomenon (Engel and Romano, 1959).

The *chronic irreversible form* of the organic brain syndrome appears less often as a psychiatric emergency than does the acute form. Often, the patient's symptoms have developed slowly over several months. Less frequently, they may have emerged after a sudden trauma to the CNS, such as a stroke. Impaired memory and affective changes are the main features of this syndrome. The patient shows difficulties in retaining and recalling information. Events from the recent past cannot be remembered, and there are various degrees of disorientation; but these are less obvious than with the acute syndrome. Such patients become easily confused in new and unfamiliar situations. Their capacity for abstract and more complex thinking is greatly reduced. There will be irritability and affective lability, but again it is less conspicuous than in the acute syndrome. Angry outbursts or states of depression may occur in response to partial awareness of deterioration. Since these patients have suffered for some time from these defects, they often have been able to develop some ways to mask their deficiency, such as negativism, vagueness, denial, and confabulation. Another result of such deficiency may be lethargy and apathy which, together with social isolation, lead to neglect of physical appearance and hygiene.

The most frequent examples of this syndrome are senile dementia and arteriosclerotic dementia, both occurring in the elderly

patient. The emergency usually is caused by some new change in the environment of the patient which suddenly has become too demanding, stimulating, or unfamiliar, and which compounds the patient's already limited coping mechanisms. The resultant feeling of helplessness and alienation can lead to depression. This, together with forgetfulness, may represent at times a serious suicide risk that manifests itself by a patient's leaving the gas jets open or starving himself. Sometimes patients who already have a pre-existing, slowly extending dementia develop an acute medical illness, which in turn produces an acute brain syndrome.

These dementias also have to be differentiated from states of retarded depression, particularly in the elderly. A history of prior depressions, hypochondriacal complaints, relatively intact memory, and orientation can help establish the correct diagnosis.

Here, as well as in the acute brain syndromes, a finding of focal neurologic symptoms and aphasias, agnosias, or apraxias will point to the underlying etiologic factors of the syndrome.

MANAGEMENT

Initial Steps

Since the patient has suffered a significant loss in his intellectual capacities, it is important from the first contact onward to limit cognitive stimulation and to simplify the demands made by his environment. The initial evaluation, therefore, should be relatively brief, but not rushed, in order not to overtax the patient's limited coping abilities. Support and structure may have to be given to the patient because of his difficulties in communicating intelligibly. This initial evaluation may be best conducted in the presence of the relative or companion who usually accompanies the patient. Seeing a familiar face will help diminish the patient's perplexity and anxiety. After the chief complaint and present illness have been explored, particular attention should be focused on possible precipitating events, such as recent changes in the patient's current life situation, recent change of residence, or loss of people close to him. A careful mental status examination often can be integrated smoothly into these lines of inquiry. Here, particularly, the degree of orientation, retention, and recall of recent events is important. Specific tasks, such as the calculating and repeating of digits, may have to be given to the patient. The physician should always ask these questions in a noncritical and reassuring fashion, since the patient almost always has some awareness of his deficits. Often, those dealing with the patient underestimate the degree of his awareness of these deficits and of what is going on around him.

The relatives, too, should be asked for their observations and about possible recent changes in the family's situation. Particularly with elderly patients, it is important to get a good picture of the over-all family situation and to understand the family's motivation in bringing the patient to a physician at this particular time. It then may be apparent that the patient's condition has not really changed, but that the family's coping abilities have been exhausted.

Psychologic Mangement

Organically confused patients have very short attention spans and rapid fatigability. As mentioned above, it is important to keep the interview short and also to allow time for the patient to find his answers. Impatience on the physician's part increases the patient's disorganization. If the patient becomes too disorganized despite the physician's care, the latter must provide structure by asking clearly focused questions. It also is helpful to indicate to the disoriented patient where he is, what the purpose is of the examination, and who the interviewer is, in order to reduce his perplexity. Allowing the patient as much as possible to be with people with whom he is familiar and keeping his environment constant also contribute to his ability to compensate for his cognitive deficiencies.

Often patients are very much ashamed of their deficits and try desperately to hide them. As far as possible, the physician should respect this and try to stress intact areas of functioning in which the patient is able to perform independently. A brief explanation of the underlying organic factors that produced the deficits can be reassuring to the patient.

These patients can present particularly serious suicide risks, which have to be evaluated carefully. The distortions of reality in the acute brain syndrome can be so frightening that the patient would rather be dead than continue to experience them. The chronic organically confused patient may be very aware of the loss of his intellectual and mental abilities, and will respond with depression. Living alone and in isolation from his family may add to his hopelessness and suicide potential. Inquiries about suicide plans and general plans for the future may help clarify this point.

Disposition

Treatment plans depend not only on the patient's clinical status, but also on the family's cooperation and coping capacities. Hospitalization, for example, must be weighed carefully in terms of its advantages and disadvantages for both the patient and the family.

ACUTE ORGANIC BRAIN SYNDROME

Hospitalization is necessary for most of these patients. If the patient's level of agitation or suicidal risk permits, he should be admitted to a medical ward where further diagnostic tests can be done, such as skull x-rays, EEG, brain scan, lumbar puncture, and metabolic tests. Until treatment of the underlying medical illness has been initiated, supportive measures should be provided, such as maintenance of adequate hydration and of the patient's electrolyte balance. Psychologic support should include frequent reassurance, and the creation of an atmosphere that contains minimal stimulation but avoids monotony. A night light should be provided. If the patient's agitation and fearfulness are overwhelming and particularly if they prevent him from cooperating in medical treatment, psychopharmacologic agents should be used. Particular care must be exercised in using these agents, since they all can hide organic signs.

The patient's vital signs and neurologic status therefore should be stable when such treatment is instituted. Low doses of a phenothiazine of sedative type, such as chlorpromazine, should be given parenterally. A dosage schedule beginning with 25 mg. I.M., every four hours should be established, increasing the dose by 25-mg. steps every four hours until the patient is sufficiently sedated, yet fully arousable. In view of the hypotensive effect of chlorpromazine, bed rest should be ordered and the blood pressure should be taken before and after each dose, and the next dose withheld if there is a significant drop in blood pressure. Once the dose is reached that gives the required effect, the physician should give that dose orally on a six-hour basis. If there are reasons to anticipate seizures, paraldehyde can be used I.M. instead of a phenothiazine. With elderly patients and patients with cerebrovascular problems for which hypotensive effects are particularly undesirable, a butyrophenone like haloperidol can be given, starting with 0.5 to 1.0 mg. four times daily.

If the patient is depressed, possibly having even expressed self-destructive preoccupations, psychiatric consultation is in order, together with the institution of suicide prevention precautions such as: (1) having a person stay with the patient 24 hours a day; (2) removing all sharp objects; (3) locking all reachable windows; and (4) possibly transferring the patient to a psychiatric ward.

CHRONIC ORGANIC BRAIN SYNDROME

The treatment plan will depend to a large extent on the degree to which the underlying factors are correctible, as well as the rehabilitative capacity of the patient. The plan has to be placed in the context of the patient's over-all life patterns, and particularly of his family situation. In order to achieve this, psychiatric consultation will be necessary. A social worker may be needed to assess the family's strengths and their wishes for the disposition of the patient. The family should be helped to accept the irreversible character of the patient's illness, and the patient in turn should be supported to maximize his coping mechanisms in dealing with his impairments. Careful attention must be paid to the question whether the patient should be maintained at home or in an institution, such as a nursing home. As a rule, hospitalization is not indicated.

In more specific terms, the patient should be encouraged to do as many things as possible for himself, to maintain social stimulation, and to remain in his familiar environment as long as possible. Psychotropic drugs, when indicated, should be used in moderate amounts, because these patients have increased sensitivity to such drugs. States of anxiety can be treated with minor tranquilizers or with nonsedating phenothiazines, e.g., 4 mg. of perphenazine or 2 mg. of trifluoperazine, three to four times daily. Depressive states with marked psychomotor retardation can be treated with low doses of imipramine, 10 to 25 mg. three times daily. Because of these drugs' anticholinergic properties, side-effects such as prostatic obstruction, increased intraocular pressure, and constipation can occur. These medications, therefore, should be handled with particular care in the elderly.

COMPLICATIONS

The Elderly Patient

The physical, physiologic, psychologic, and environmental changes that are a consequence of old age can create specific emergencies that require a good understanding of the specific problems of the elderly. Physical factors, such as diminished visual acuity and hearing, mild-to-severe organic brain syndromes, and other somatic problems reduce the elderly patient's coping abilities and resistance to stress. Changes in his occupational status — mainly retirement with its ensuing role changes — can bring significant loss of self esteem if there are no other resources to fill the gap. The over-all negative view of society about aging also can contribute to undermining the patient's self esteem and also can reinforce his already prevalent fears of death and dying. Isolation from family through loss of loved ones or because of rejecting attitudes of family members may compound all these difficulties for the elderly. However, the single most important factor determining the way the elderly patient will cope with these various changes is the individual's pre-existing character style and personality structure. Difficulties in coping with particular problems arise when there have been premorbid personality disturbances and maladaptive coping mechanisms in the individual. Old age brings an intensification of such maladaptive traits and even a caricaturization of these patterns. Those who are isolated become withdrawn and depressed; suspicious individuals become paranoid; those with somatic concerns may become hypochondriacal.

These reactions can be precipitated by changes in the environment, together with impaired intellectual capacities. The patient may misinterpret and not fully understand what is happening around him and to him. He may react with intense anxiety and present various emergency situations, particularly: (1) acute depression, agitation, or withdrawal; (2) paranoid reactions, with possible assaultiveness; (3) hypochondriacal reactions, with obsessive concern about various body functions or malfunctions; (4) exacerbation of a chronic brain syndrome into an acute one.

As far as treatment goes, the approach should be along the same lines as described for the acute and chronic organic brain syndromes. The first concern again should be about a possible underlying correctible medical condition. It often is surprising to observe a significant improvement after the patient's cardiac decompensation has been stabilized by appropriate medical management. Once the patient is medically cleared, the final disposition depends not only on the patient's psychiatric status, but also on the over-all family situation. Usually, the adult children or other family members will be quite involved with the patient, and any successful treatment plan must include them. Often it will be apparent to the physician that the family is holding on to the care of the elderly at home for far too long, and in situations that they are not equipped to handle. In those circumstances, the family must be helped to arrive at an appropriate placement of the patient.

If psychopharmacologic agents are necessary, special caution must be used, since any sedative or tranquilizing agent may lower the cerebral blood supply, and patients with organic brain syndromes generally have a lower tolerance to drugs. One should start with low doses and increase them slowly. Barbiturates should be avoided because of their depressant effect on the cardiovascular system, their prolonged action, and their cumulative effect.

Postconvulsive Confusion (Postictal Twilight State)

These states usually occur after one or several grand mal seizures or a temporal lobe seizure and can last from several hours to several days. The patient shows perplex-ity and confusion and replies to questions in a distant and absent-minded fashion; at other times there may be agitation and hallucinations. A history of seizure disorder, complete amnesia for the episode, and a positive EEG with diffuse slow activity will guide the physician to the correct diagnosis. These states usually clear spontaneously, but they can result in psychiatric emergencies if prolonged or accompanied by agitation.

After the physician has established the diagnosis and made sure that the patient is on an anticonvulsant regimen, phenothiazines in moderate dosages can be used. Higher doses should be avoided, since phenothiazines can lower the seizure threshold. Fluphenazine or (if severe agitation is present) chlorpromazine can be used.

Psychomotor Seizures

The correct underlying cause of these emergencies often is difficult to diagnose correctly. These seizures either are preceded by grand mal seizures or replace them entirely, and occur without loss of consciousness. Vegetative, olfactory, or psychic auras are reported by the patient. The seizure itself can lead to hallucinatory experiences, most often in the auditory sphere, and to feelings of depersonalization, with "déjà vu" impressions and simple or complex stereotyped automatisms. If these automatisms are more complex, they are experienced as alien to the patient and have an impulsive character that the patient reports he cannot control. Such automatisms may range from simple movements to exhibitionistic, kleptomaniac, suicidal, homicidal, or fuguelike actions. Typically, they are inappropriate to the situation and are stereotyped. A careful history from the patient and his family, a complete physical examination, and positive EEG findings will help establish the diagnosis.

If raising the dose of anticonvulsant agents does not bring the seizures under control, phenothiazine given in slowly increasing dosages may be useful.

References

Ayd, F. J., Jr.: Tranqulizers and the ambulatory geriatric patient. J. Am. Geriatr. Soc. 8:909, 1960.
Brain, W. R., and Walton, J. N.: Brain's Diseases of the

Nervous System. London, Oxford University Press, 1969.

Busse, E. W.: Geriatrics today—an overview. Am. J. Psychiatry 123:1226, 1967.

Detre, T. P., and Jarecki, H. G.: Modern Psychiatric Treatment. Philadelphia, J. B. Lippincott Co., 1971.

Engel, G. L., and Romano, J.: Delirium, a syndrome of cerebral insufficiency. J. Chron. Dis. 9:260, 1959.

Glaser, G. H.: The problem of psychosis in psychomotor temporal lobe epileptics, Epilepsia 5:271, 1964.

Goldfarb, A. I., and Sheps, J.: Psychotherapy of the aged: brief therapy of interrelated psychological and somatic disorders. Psychosom. Med. 16:209, 1954.

Goldstein, K.: Functional Disturbances in Brain Damage. In Arieti, S. (ed.): American Handbook of Psychiatry. Vol. 1. New York, Basic Books, 1959.

Plum, F., and Posner, J. L.: Diagnosis of Stupor and Coma. Contemporary Neurology Series. Philadelphia, F. A. Davis Co., 1966.

Slater, E., Beard, A. W., and Glithero, E.: The schizophrenia-like psychoses of epilepsy. Br. J. Psychiatry 109:95, 1963.

F. PSYCHIATRIC EMERGENCIES IN CHILDHOOD AND ADOLESCENCE

Gary J. Grad, Jean-Pierre Lindenmayer, and Nathan S. Kline

DEFINITION AND CONCEPTS

As with adult patients, emergencies in children or adolescents can be seen as sudden behavioral or emotional responses to overwhelming anxiety. The child's or adolescent's usual coping mechanisms have broken down or are inadequate to deal appropriately with his anxiety. However, much more so than with adult patients, the parents define what constitutes a "psychiatric emergency" for their child, as children and adolescents seldom seek out physicians when acutely anxious or upset. The parents are the ones who are presented with the child's distress, and they request treatment when their own anxiety over their child's unusual behavior has become so overwhelming that they feel helpless. Also again much more than with the adult patient, the parents' presentation of the child as an "emergency" actually may be an expression of internal family distress, not of the child's pathology. It therefore will be particularly important in these situations to explore carefully how the "emergency" came to be labeled as such and by whom.

Psychiatric emergencies in children and adolescents differ in another major way from those in the adult. The child or adolescent patient is limited in his ability to register complaints about upset feelings and situations in affects or words, unlike the adult. Distress most often is manifested by action and changes in behavior that are either developmentally deviant or disordered for the given child. The younger patient, for example, may begin to play with much younger children than himself, or an adolescent may react by running away from home rather than expressing his depression. As children become older they differentiate along developmental lines, and the ways in which they express their reactions to stress become more like those of the adult. Therefore, specific syndromes differ more among adolescents than among younger children, whose abnormal behavior is more difficult to recognize and diagnose correctly.

Another aspect, differing from emergencies with adult patients, is represented by acute difficulties related to the lack of mastery of a developmental step. The normal psychologic development of children can be seen in the context of the mastery of new and more complex situations. If difficulties in handling these situations arise, they should be resolved as quickly as possible, since they otherwise may lead to further developmental problems. One example of such a situation is that of the school-phobic child (often afraid of separation from his mother), who warrants emergency care.

Another differentiating aspect from adult patients who show acute behavior difficulties is reflected in the frequent overlapping of organic and functional difficulties. It may be difficult to differentiate the effects of underlying "soft" neurologic signs, or of a seizure disorder, from the effects of psychologic problems related, for example, to a disturbed family situation. Generally, these aspects will have to be explored through specialized consultations once the immediate emergency situation has been handled.

GENERAL PRINCIPLES OF ASSESSMENT AND MANAGEMENT

Evaluation of the Problem

It is important to realize that the establishment of contact with the patient and the parents and the gathering of facts about the problem constitute a therapeutic step. The firm, knowledgeable, and open way with which the physician conducts himself will help to decrease the patient's emotional distress and will aid the parents through providing support and direction.

In taking the history of the younger child, the physician usually talks with the parents first, but may decide to interview the adolescent before seeing his parents, especially when the issue is an anxiety- or guilt-provoking one. In either case, both parents and child should be interviewed, and their feelings about the problem should be noted. If the physician can assure the child of some confidentiality, his history-taking probably will be more fruitful. It is important to realize that the child who is brought to a physician on an emergency basis is likely to be confused as to why he is being seen, and fearful about the outcome of the visit. This is especially true when the symptoms are behavioral in nature; his own complaints may be far different from those for which he is being presented by the adults concerned. Seeing the doctor may be viewed as only another step in a continuum of punitive actions by his parents. Depending on his sophistication and on what he has been told about the visit, he may even fear that he is "crazy" and will be removed from his home and placed in an institution. Adolescents may view being taken to the doctor even more as a punitive act. The physician therefore, must be aware of the reasons why the child is being brought and the child's own view of the problem and his feelings about both of these.

Physicians often find it difficult to establish rapid contact with the child patient. Even the younger child should be spoken with privately in an open, respectful, and nondemeaning way—and at a level that he can understand. It may be necessary to allow the child to familiarize himself with his surroundings, and even to permit him to touch objects in the office (without risk of danger, of course). He may not respond to direct questioning, or may do so only after some period of time. The older child and adolescent may be angry about his presentation to the physician. If the latter indicates awareness of this, is respectful of the patient's view of the situation, and allows for ventilation of some anger, the patient may be more approachable.

In interviewing both the parents and the child, three important questions should be answered.

(1) *Why did the crisis occur now?* Recent changes in the child's environment should be noted (including recent moves, changes in the composition of the household, death or illness of close relatives and friends, changes in school), because the child may be sensitive to these, and the problem may be directly related to such occurrences.

(2) *Who labeled the situation as a crisis?* The physician should explore here whose anxiety tolerance has been over-taxed—the child's or the parents'—or was the situation identified by community agencies? Once this has been clarified, the physician must address himself specifically to the main participant in the emergency situation.

(3) *What are the expectations of the patient and the parents?* This is particularly important with children and families, as pointed out above. These expectations should be taken into account when formulating the management plan.

(4) Finally, careful attention should be paid to the *psychologic and physical developmental history*, as this will give the physician an idea of the acuteness and extent of the problem, as well as of the possibility of an underlying organic basis. Comparison by the physician with childhood norms will aid this process.

If a physical examination is indicated, it must be geared to the presenting complaints. Physical findings, developmental anomalies, and hard and "soft" neurologic signs (Chamberlain, 1975), as well as a mental status indicating cognitive deficits, help point to organic factors in the etiology of the physical or behavioral complaint. After the presenting situation has been fully evaluated, constellations of symptoms and signs may point to specific diagnoses and/or lead to further evaluations through specialized consultations.

Handling the Parents

The parents of the child with an organic deficit, especially if it is severe and irreversible, may feel that some deficit in themselves caused the disorder. In most instances this is not true, and the doctor should indicate this to the parents through a complete and thoughtful presentation. Where organic deficits exist, the parents may withdraw from the child and/or deny the existence of the organicity. These reactions tend to perpetuate the difficulties of the child, who already has been compromised in his adaptive ability. Parents can be counseled that organic deficits do not place an absolute limit on a child's development and that there are many agencies that can help them and their child. Finally, the parents may not want to believe the physician and may seek further consultation with other experts. This may be necessary and cannot be denied to the family, but the sooner accurate and adequate treatment for the child begins, the greater is the possibility that he will be helped. Continuous consultations may maintain unreasonable hopes and stave off feelings of guilt, fear, and depression—but not really help the family or the child.

If the difficulty is seen as being primarily psychologic, the parents again may be prone to react with withdrawal and denial. The physician may reassure them that not all psychologic problems indicate insanity in the child or themselves and that they are not necessarily to blame. They may want to find some organic disease to reassure them, and may attempt to do so through additional consultations rather than through appropriate psychiatric help. Again, this may delay help for the child and lead to a worsening of the situation.

We have focused on the reactions of the parents, but the physician also should explain his findings to the child in an age-appropriate, nonpatronizing way that should help enlist the child's cooperation in the management of his problem.

Psychopharmacologic Management

There are many times when the physician will use a psychotropic medication to help alter the situation. Medication use should be target-symptom-directed, and the physician should be familiar with the medication used. Patients placed on medication for behavioral problems should be referred for follow-up evaluation at frequent intervals. Initial emergency management may require medication, but since the child's problem may be situational or due to some resolving developmental issue, it is useful to reduce medication, discontinue it after three to six months, and re-evaluate the problem (except in a very few syndromes). If the problem still exists, psychiatric consultation should be sought. A basic notion about medication use is that, whereas it may be the treatment of choice for specific syndromes and indispensible for certain emergency situations, "psychiatric complaints in children require psychological methods of management to a greater or lesser degree and drugs do not cure, educate, or unlearn the basic causes of the disorder but only alleviate the most prominent symptoms" (Conners, 1975). However, this often may be sufficient to induce a significant improvement.

SYNDROMES AND THEIR MANAGEMENT

Suicide Threats and Attempts

Depression is difficult to identify in children but may be manifested by sadness, feelings of inadequacy, loneliness, eating and sleeping disturbances, chronic whining and crying, fatigue, and concentration difficulties. These symptoms are somewhat similar to those of the adult, but antisocial behavior (destruction of property and animals or stealing), running away from home, and accident proneness also may signify depression. Therefore, when a child makes a serious suicide attempt, it often may come as a surprise. Another factor contributing to the difficulty in predicting suicide potential in children is that when they are angry and wish either to punish their parents or themselves, they may verbalize a wish to be dead (Prugh and Kisley, 1972). Younger children do not perceive the finality of death cognitively, and the threat may be idle, although it indicates unhappiness. When a child of this age is seen after such a threat, its seriousness may be evaluated by assessing the child's general level of functioning and symptomatology.

If the child with suicidal threats shows either symptoms of depression and/or difficulties in various areas of functioning, he and his parents should be referred for psychiatric consultation.

If the presenting complaint is that of a serious suicide attempt, immediate psychiatric consultation should be sought, after the safety of the child is assured. If the child must be hospitalized owing to the medical complications of the attempt, the pediatric ward should be alerted so as to preclude another attempt and avoid placing additional stress on the child. For example, if an argument with a parent was a precipitating factor, visiting may have to be limited.

Suicide threats and attempts are more common in adolescence. The adolescent who attempts suicide should be evaluated and medically treated as the adult, but psychiatric consultation has to be sought even more rapidly, as those in this age-group are less likely than the adult to seek such help on their own. The depressed adolescent may present symptoms similar to the depressed adult, but complaints and behaviors such as boredom, restlessness, bodily preoccupation, antisocial behavior, flight to or from others, excessive self-criticism, drug use and abuse, pregnancy, and somatic complaints also may signify depression. If a teenager comes to the attention of the physician with one or more of these complaints, especially repeatedly, depressed feelings and suicidal notions usually may be elicited.

In evaluating these patients, particular attention should be paid to precipitating events, such as recent losses among the patient's family or loss of friends, and possible difficulties in the relationship of the patient's parents. Adolescents are at particular risk for suicide attempts, and this risk therefore, must be evaluated carefully.

Since the family often will be seen as being a factor in the production of the depression, the patient may be reluctant to inform them of what is going on. However, in the context of a good patient–doctor relationship, the physician may be able to work with the adolescent toward notifying the parents and enlisting their cooperation. If a suicide attempt has been made, the parents should be informed directly by the physician. At any event, psychiatric consultation will be needed and both patients and parents should be adequately prepared for this by the physician.

Destructive and Bizarre Behavior

The child who is brought on an emergency basis because he has manifested bizarre and/or destructive behavior deserves a most careful evaluation. Causes of such behavior are many and varied, ranging from the organic to the psychologic. The behaviors differ also from the younger child to the adolescent.

THE PRESCHOOL CHILD

The preschool child may show self-preoccupation, lack of communicative skills, lack of relatedness to others, stereotyped affect and activities, mutilation of self and others, and sleep disturbances. He often has a history of developmental lag, and, if without mental retardation and physical abnormalities, may be suffering from one of the variants of childhood psychosis.

THE SCHOOL AGE CHILD

The school age to pre-teenage child may present destructive behavior together with periods of lack of awareness of his surroundings, destruction of property, continuous fighting, homicidal threats and attempts, learning problems, clumsiness, accident proneness, and destruction of pets. The most frequent cause here may be an underlying hyperactive syndrome, which will be discussed in detail below.

THE ADOLESCENT

The adolescent may manifest eating disturbances, severe weight fluctuations, panic states, and somatic symptoms, as well as symptoms similar to those of the depressed or psychotic adult. Most frequently, the underlying cause is an incipient schizophrenic process.

Other causes for destructive behavior less related to the patient's age can be central nervous system disorders, such as a seizure. This should be investigated particularly if the bizarre or destructive behavior includes alterations of consciousness or involuntary motor movements not preceded by emotional upsets. Also, a child with acute lead poisoning may present with symptoms of irritability and agitation; lead poisoning also has been associated with the hyperkinetic syndrome (David, 1973).

MANAGEMENT

If firm limit-setting by the physician and the parents has not brought the acute destructive and agitated behavior under control, medication will be needed to remedy, at least temporarily, the loss of control. Effective medications include diphenhydramine, 5mg./kg./24 hours in three or four doses, but not to exceed 300 mg. each day; chlorpromazine, 50 to 100 mg. and 200 mg. daily in divided doses in younger and older children, respectively; and thioridazine in similar doses as chlorpromazine (but not in children under 2). The piperazine group of phenothiazines and butyrophenones are not indicated for general use, as the incidence of dyskinesias is high in children. Minor tranquilizers, specifically chlordiazepoxide and diazepam, may lead to "paradoxical" reactions including rage and temper tantrums, especially in those under 6 and in children with "soft" signs of neurologic damage (Conners, 1970; Conners, 1975). Generally, medications should be begun at low doses and maintained at the lowest doses necessary to alleviate symptoms. The major side-effect of note with diphenhydramine is tiredness. Parkinsonian syndromes as a consequence of phenothiazines may be corrected with antiparkinsonian drugs, as in adult patients. Tardive dyskinesia is manifested in children more often in the trunk, arms, and legs than periorally, as in the adult. It should be remembered that other commonly used medications also may lead occasionally to psychiatric emergencies in children, e.g., the aggressive behavior in children placed on barbiturates, cold or allergy medications, or methylphenidate and amphetamine.

Depending on the severity and degree of the destructive and agitated behavior, and on how much it inhibits the child in school, leads to familial unhappiness, and stops him from having normal peer relationships, child psychiatric consultation will have to be sought. Supportive counseling for the parents, with emotional support for the child (as provided through the family, school counselor, or religious affiliate) may be adequate in the instance of a family crisis, as long as serious injury to the child or others is not threatened. The child also will require increased supervision. This not only helps control the situation, but also increases the attention the child receives from his parents, which probably was decreased as a result of the crisis. If the situation is dangerous and under insufficient control, or if the child is homicidal, psychiatric hospitalization will be necessary.

INCIPIENT SCHIZOPHRENIA IN ADOLESCENCE

A psychotic process that begins in adolescence is a difficult syndrome for the physician to distinguish, owing to the fact that many adolescents experience considerable distress and may manifest psychiatric symptoms. The notion of incipient schizophrenia has been briefly mentioned previously. This syndrome may be seen in the young adolescent, but is more common after the age of 15. More specifically, the young adolescent who is beginning to become schizophrenic may present to the physician with the already-mentioned eating disturbances, panic states, and somatic symptoms; but more important for the recognition of this syndrome are: (1) the slow but continuous withdrawal from contact with family and friends (this lack of contact, not anger or belligerence, may be noted by the physician while interviewing the patient); (2) onset of failure in, or refusal to attend, school; (3) failure to master developmental tasks (dating, work, and recreational activities, inability to progress to college, and others); and (4) the fading of the sense of self. These adolescents also may present with suicide attempts or unusual patterns of antisocial behavior, engaged in alone or as a peripheral group member. Caution should be maintained in diagnosing an adolescent as psychotic or schizophrenic without the presence of a thought process disorder, hallucinations, delusions, or inappropriate affect. Of course, the adolescent patient who presents as more grossly psychotic should be examined for the presence of an organic brain disorder—especially one secondary to infection, trauma, metabolic disorder, seizure disorder, and drug and alcohol abuse.

Several other psychogenic states may present with psychosis in adolescence and mimic schizophrenia. These include confusional and homosexual panic states. They usually develop rapidly and may be related to specific stressful situations. The first of these is marked by anxiety, confusion, and depersonalization; the second may be manifested by guilt-laden homosexual hallucinations, delusions, and verbal preoccupation. If the development of schizophrenia is suspected, psychiatric consultation should be sought, since psychotherapy, family intervention, medication, special education, and possibly residential treatment may be necessary to alter the course of the disease. If an adolescent presents as psychotic, and medical illness can be ruled out, psychiatric consultation should be sought. The physician, of course, must manage the acute situation as discussed previously.

THE HYPERACTIVE SYNDROME

School-age children who present with variations of the dangerous behaviors described above, in addition to learning difficulties, may be suffering from the hyperactive syndrome. A history of birth difficulties, injury to the central nervous system, and/or lead intoxication, as well as parental and school reports of excessive activity, distractability, restlessness, and short attention span, strengthen this diagnosis. These children can be medicated with either amphetamine sulphate (Benzedrine), dextroamphetamine sulphate (Dexedrine), or methylphenidate hydrochloride (Ritalin), 2.5 mg. b.i.d. in those under 5, or 5 mg. b.i.d. in older children. This medication can be doubled weekly until 60 mg. daily is reached for Ritalin and 40 mg. daily for the amphetamines. Behavioral alterations should occur rapidly if the medication is effective. Side-effects other than the toxic ones, but not dose-related, include anorexia and insomnia, which can be reduced by giving the medication before school and at lunch time on school days only, and only during the school year. Phenothiazines and imipramine also have been used for this syndrome. Often, parents are not willing to have their children placed on medications for long periods; the physician should elicit the parents' feelings about medication use so that their negative reactions do not lead to the child's symptoms persisting through parental noncompliance. The physician may decide to seek child psychiatric or neurologic consultation if the amphetamines and methylphenidate do not control the symptoms.

Fire-setting and Running Away From Home

Fire-setting by a young child, especially if it does not endanger property or the child, may be seen as natural curiosity about exciting natural phenomena. Education by the parent may be adequate to handle the situation. A nonpunitive approach may be suggested. Fire-setting by the school-age child may be part of a syndrome including enuresis and hyperkinesis (Linn, 1975). The medications indicated for hyperkinesis may be used, but child psychiatric consultation is more appropriate. In the adolescent, it may be part of vengeful, group antisocial, or homosexual activity, which again requires psychiatric consultation.

Often, running away from home is not serious, in that usually the child is easily found and not absent long. This may not even come to the attention of the physician unless he specifically asks, although the child's feelings of rejection by the parent may be involved. When the child endangers himself or does not seem to intend to be found, severe family conflict or rejection should be suspected, and child psychiatric consultation is recommended.

School Phobia

School phobia is most common in kindergarten and in the first grade, in the third to fourth grades, and in junior and senior high school (Berlin, 1975). In the first few years of school, it usually is related to the child's concerns about leaving home and also to the mother's anxiety about separation from her child. Later on, it can be related to greater learning demands made on the child.

The child may present to the physician at the point of entering school with multiple, minor physical complaints that lead to his inability to attend school. When the physician notices this, he should reassure the mother that the child is not ill (usually the case), limit his examinations unless illness is quite probable, and help set a date with the school for the child's return. The father may be brought in more actively to provide support, especially for his wife. If school attendance still does not proceed, more severe pathology may be suspected and psychiatric consultation should be sought. The third- to fourth-grade child who will not go to school should have adequate psychologic tests to rule out retardation or other causes of school failure. A hyperactive syndrome may be discovered, for which the medication previously indicated is necessary. The child who will not attend high school after successful previous attendance should receive psychiatric consultation, especially since more severe psychopathology can be suspected.

Anorexia

The anorexic child may present at times as a true medical emergency requiring immediate hospitalization. However, more frequently, the patient will come to the attention of the physician because of severe weight loss, requests for special diets to lose weight, amenorrhea, or concerns by the parents for their child's dieting or food fads. The patient usually is a girl and may be a young teenager, although the syndrome is most common in young women in their late teens and early 20s.

The syndrome is best treated, if noticed very early, before the point of medical emergency or before a severe, overt family conflict over eating develops. Psychiatric consultation is necessary. The treatment approach may include the physician, psychiatrist, and other professionals who attempt to intervene through the family's patterns as well as the individual's problems. Antidepressants, and especially the monoamine oxidase inhibitors, have been claimed to be useful, although prolonged administration for several months usually is needed.

Sexual Promiscuity and Pregnancy

Promiscuous behavior is difficult to define. The physician's role may be to intervene only when the adolescent is being self-destructive. Parental reactions may be extremely punitive and nonproductive. The physician may be of help in modulating parental responses, noting the adolescent's behavior, and developing a working relationship with the parents and teenager that will allow them to seek psychiatric help. The physician should be aware of punitive attitudes on his part also, which could drive his patient away from professional help.

The adolescent who becomes pregnant does so for a variety of reasons, ranging from being in love to wanting to be loved by a baby. She may consult the physician and show tremendous ignorance about her body and about pregnancy. A variety of issues may arise, including adequate care of the pregnant woman, decisions about termination of the pregnancy, the desire for and possibility of marriage, keeping or giving up the child, and parental responses of anger and withdrawal from the adolescent. The physician can be most helpful in preliminary counseling of the parents and their daughter, and helping find adequate gynecologic, pediatric, and (if necessary) psychiatric facilities.

Rape and Incest

The raped child or adolescent presents the physician with multiple problems and issues. He must first determine whether rape has occurred and, if so, determine the extent of any bodily damage, and the possibility of pregnancy or infection. Rapport should be established with the victim and her parents. If penetration has occurred, examination should proceed only after parental consent has been obtained. Vaginal aspirate can be examined for sperm and can be used for bacterial culture. Treatment for gonorrhea may be necessary, and an anti-implantation pill may be used. A VDRL is necessary several weeks after the rape. Adequate records for police use are appropriate, if they are to be informed. In some areas this is not an automatic procedure, but depends on the parents' decision.

The parents may be as upset and angry as the victim, and she may feel angry, violated, and guilty. The physician should help the patient in a supportive way to ventilate her upset feelings about this extremely frightening experience. Immediate psychiatric help may be indicated by the degree of upset experienced by the victim and/or parents. In some instances, more severe psychologic reactions may occur some time after the rape. Contact should be maintained for up to three months, and psychiatric help should be made available, if and when necessary (Lewis and Lewis, 1973; Burgess and Holstrom, 1974). Hospitalization may be needed for very young victims. Often the rapist is known to the family, and they must be counseled against any attempt at retribution other than through legal channels.

Incest probably is more common than suspected. It may come to the attention of the physician on routine examination of a child patient with frequent vaginal infections or as part of a pattern of parental abuse or neglect. In some areas it must be reported, and legally constitutes abuse. The most common pattern is father-daughter incest. Surprisingly often, the mother knows of the incestuous relationship. Its existence is greatest in disturbed families where the daughter has, in a sense, taken the mother's place or where there is severe psychopathology in family members. Psychiatric consultation is imperative if the physician has proof of the existence of incest.

Abuse and Neglect

The abused or neglected child comes to the attention of the physician when presented for medical care following the abuse. The infant may not be developing at a normal rate, and may show failure to thrive without any renal, cardiac, or CNS defects. The child may have injuries that cannot be explained adequately by the parents, such as multiple skin lesions, old and new fractures, and retinal hemorrhages. There also may be delay in seeking medical attention. The abused child is often that one in the family who is seen as "different": the youngest; the oldest; the only one of a particular sex; one having physical deformities; and/or one who creates a nuisance. The parents often are immature, have problems controlling their anger, are not gratified in their own lives (unemployed or drug or alcohol users), and cannot satisfy a wide variety of their partner's needs in the marital relationship. Patterns of abuse may have been present in their own parents' homes.

The physician's role in situations of child abuse and neglect is well defined. He documents the possibility of abuse, and begins the attempts necessary to guarantee the child's future safety. If the physician suspects abuse, and if the child is under 5 and in possible danger if allowed to go home, the child should be hospitalized (Helfer, 1975). Necessary laboratory tests and specialty consultations should be obtained, both to treat the child and to document the abuse as accurately as possible. This should be done in either the inpatient or outpatient situation. The home circumstances and the parents should be evaluated as soon as possible. This usually is accomplished through the child welfare agency that is designated to do so in each area. It is advisable to obtain psychiatric consultation for the parents. In situations of possible abuse, it often is difficult to maintain a neutral, helpful attitude toward the parents. They must be advised of the physician's suspicions and that welfare agencies will be involved. The physician may have to wait before discharging the hospitalized child until he is notified by these agencies whether the child will be placed or allowed to be sent home. Most of the responsibility falls on social agencies and psychiatric facilities after the diagnosis is made, but physical care of the child may continue to be the responsibility of the physician.

Situational Reactions

Throughout the discussion of emergency situations in childhood and adolescence, we have mentioned the possibility of symptoms demanding emergency treatment stemming from the child's reaction to stressful situations. In this section, several situations will be briefly mentioned that are particularly stressful to the child and that may warrant special attention. In all these situations, the child may regress in his behavior. Additional support and appropriate concern for the child can be helpful in mastering these periods of stress.

The first of these is the death of a close relative, parent, or sibling. The child should be gently informed of the death and allowed to ask questions. These are determined by the attachment of the child to the dead person, the child's level of cognitive development, and his ongoing personality patterns. It should be made clear to the child that he is not responsible for the death. Severe behavioral symptoms should lead to psychiatric consultation.

Children, especially those in the age-group 5 to 6, are particularly sensitive to the separation necessitated by hospitalization. Parents should be allowed as much contact as possible with the child through visiting. The child should be stimulated by ward staff through play, books, etc. The older child may react to hospitalization or chronic illness with antitherapeutic behavior. In all instances, the child should be told as much as possible in advance about the hospitalization, when this can be anticipated, and the treatment of the illness should be explained in terms the child can understand.

Adolescent Drug Use

Adolescent drug use is very common today. Patterns include occasional experimentation, addiction, attempts at self-medication, psychologic distress, and suicide attempts. It is most important for the physician to attempt to discover why drug use is occurring. If the adolescent patient presents himself, he may do so because of acute intoxication or overdose, for which emergency measures will be indicated. The adolescent also may consult a physician in an attempt to find out what effect a medication will have, with physical symptoms due to chronic drug use, or as a method of informing his parents and/or physician of his drug use in order to get help or to create a difficult situation. The physician should attempt to determine the patterns or use, as well as the reasons why the patient is presenting at that time. The patient with an addiction problem who seeks help voluntarily should be directed to appropriate, nonpunitive agencies. A psychologically distressed youth may require psychiatric consultation. The informed physician can educate the adolescent about drugs, their effects, and their use.

A most important aspect of adolescent drug use is the handling of the patient's parents. The latter may present as if an emergency exists, and if so may be reassured that the adolescent (if he is willing, and the physician feels competent) will be seen by the physician and his situation evaluated. The occasional use of nonaddicting drugs should not be viewed as an emergency, but still should be evaluated. Such occasional use, if nonprogressive and occurring without antisocial behavior or psychiatric disturbance, may best be handled nonpunitively. The most important aspects of the consultation are the maintenance of trust with the adolescent and his parents, and the avoidance of involvement in a family argument. If there is severe mistrust between parents and child or severe family discord (especially with the occurrence of violence), psychiatric — most probably child psychiatric — consultation should be recommended.

In the emergency setting, it is particularly important to evaluate the young person in the context of his environment. Frequently, if the adolescent is brought in by the police, the officers apply pressure on the physician not only to take blood and urine tests, but also to provide details regarding former usage. Naturally, this sort of action destroys all confidence. Furthermore, bearing in mind the highly variable child detention facilities and the possibilities of extreme psychic trauma for an adolescent placed in such a holding facility, it may be best to defer discussion or to seek psychiatric opinion without actually referring the patient. It is difficult to counsel in a crisis environment.

It is essential that the emergency physician should have a broad perspective of drug use in our society, in order to evaluate the individual patient, and to differentiate between the adolescent who is simply experimenting with drugs and those who already are addicted or who are becoming addicted.

References

Berlin, I. N.: Psychiatry and the School. *In* Freedman, A. M., Kaplan, H. T., and Sadock, B. J. (eds.): Comprehensive Textbook of Psychiatry. II. Baltimore, Williams & Wilkins Co., 1975, pp. 2251–62.

Burgess, A. W., and Holstrom, L. L.: Rape trauma syndrome. Am. J. Psychiatry *131*:981, 1974.

Chamberlain, H. R.: Mental Retardation. *In* Farmer, T. W. (ed.): Pediatric Neurology. Hagerstown, Md., Harper & Row, 1975, pp. 90–117.

Conners, C. K.: Organic Therapies. *In* Freedman, A., Kaplan, H. T., and Sadock, B. J. (eds.): Comprehensive Textbook of Psychiatry. II. Baltimore, Williams & Wilkins Co., 1975, pp. 2240–46.

Conners, C. K.: Psychopharmacological Treatment of Children. *In* DiMascio, A., and Shader, R. I. (eds.): Clinical Handbook of Psychopharmacology. New York, Science House, 1970, pp. 281–87.

David, O.: Personal communication, 1973.

Helfer, R. E.: Child Abuse and Neglect: The Diagnostic Process and Treatment Programs. Department of Health, Education and Welfare Publication No. (OND) 75–69, U.S. Government Printing Office, 1975.

Lewis, M., and Lewis, D. O.: Pediatric management of psychologic crises. Curr. Probl. Pediatr. 3:12, 1973.

Linn, L.: Other Psychiatric Emergencies. *In* Freedman, A. M., Kaplan, H. T., and Sadock, B. J. (eds.): Comprehensive Textbook of Psychiatry. II. Baltimore, Williams & Wilkins Co., 1975, pp. 1785–98.

Morrison, G. C., and Smith, W. R.: Emergencies in Child Psychiatry: A Definition. *In* Morrison, G. C. (ed.): Emergencies in Child Psychiatry. Springfield, Ill., Charles C Thomas, 1975, pp. 13–20.

Prugh, D. G., and Kisley, A. J.: Psychosocial Aspects of Pediatrics and Psychiatric Disorder. *In* Farmer, T. W. (ed.): Pediatric Neurology. Hagerstown, Md., Harper & Row, 1975, pp. 564–96.

G. OVERDOSAGE WITH PSYCHOTROPIC DRUGS

Jean-Pierre Lindenmayer and Nathan S. Kline

INTRODUCTION

Physicians in Emergency Departments often are presented with patients who have taken an acute overdose of a psychotropic drug. Most of these patients have suicidal intentions, although there may be an occasional accidental overdose. Immediate treatment often is required in order to eliminate the drug and to stabilize basic vital functions. Most of these treatment measures will depend on the type and amount of drug ingested. It is therefore important to have some information about the kind of drug and to be able to recognize the clinical picture of the particular drug intoxication. This is quite difficult at times, because several drugs may have been taken simultaneously, but whatever drug has been taken by the patient, certain priorties must be observed in emergency management of any such patient (Kline, et al., 1974):

(1) adequate pulmonary ventilation should be assured;

(2) adequate blood pressure must be maintained;

(3) convulsions and abnormally high or low temperature must be treated immediately.

The specific supportive treatment designed to achieve these points can be found in detail elsewhere in this book.

A fourth priority is to ensure that, after vital functions are stabilized, measures to increase the excretion, elimination, or breakdown of the ingested drug are taken.*

Once all these measures have been taken and the patient has become responsive, proper psychiatric management is the next step. Patients who have taken drug overdosages have an unusually high incidence of recidivism. It therefore is important to evaluate the exact circumstances of the overdose and the patient's mental state. In all such situations, psychiatric consultation is indicated.

*See also Management of Poisonings, Chap. 58A.

MAJOR TRANQUILIZERS (PHENOTHIAZINE VARIETIES)

Recognition

There will be somnolence, confusion, restlessness, dryness of mucosa, blurred vision, diaphoresis, hyperactive tendon reflexes, tachycardia, and at times an extrapyramidal syndrome such as the following:

(1) Pseudoparkinsonism: tremors, various degrees of rigidity, excessive salivation.

(2) Dystonia and dyskinesia: perioral spasms, oculogyric crisis, tonic and myoclonic muscular twitches.

(3) Akathisia: motor restlessness, inability to keep still.

Postural hypotension may be present, and may be complicated by cardiovascular insufficiency, cardiac arrhythmias, EKG changes, and shock.

Convulsions usually appear late. Bladder and bowel paralysis also may occur. Temperature regulation disturbances can include hyperthermia or hypothermia. Finally, respiratory depression and coma follow.

Management

(1) Maintain adequate pulmonary ventilation.

(2) Maintain adequate blood pressure:

(*a*) elevate feet;

(*b*) administer vasopressors: Levophed 0.2 per cent solution, 4 ml./1000 ml. of 5 per cent dextrose; or Neo-Synephrine, 10 mg./500 ml. 5 per cent dextrose in water or saline;

(*c*) *do not use epinephrine or related compounds because of possible paradoxical reaction.*

(3) Control convulsions with short-acting barbiturates. Remember that their sedative effect is potentiated by phenothiazines.

(4) Promote elimination of drug:

(*a*) induce vomiting if patient is conscious and has adequate gag reflexes;

(b) use gastric aspiration and lavage, even hours after ingestion (if semicomatose or comatose, endotracheal intubation is necessary to avoid aspiration);

(c) leave solution of sodium sulfate in stomach as cathartic (30 gm./250 ml. water);

(d) induce diuresis by slowly giving 100 to 250 ml. 25 per cent mannitol intravenously.

(5) Treatment of extrapyramidal syndrome:

(a) Use antiparkinsonian agents, such as Cogentin, 1 to 2 mg. I. M.; Akineton, 2 to 4 mg. I.M.; Kemadrin, 5 to 10 mg. I.M.; or diphenhydramine (Benadryl), 50 to 100 mg. I.V.

(6) Control patient's temperature.

Peritoneal dialysis and hemodialysis have not been found to be very effective.

TRICYCLIC ANTIDEPRESSANTS

Recognition

(1) *Atropine-like signs (anticholinergic syndrome):* dry mouth, mydriasis with blurred vision, and bowel and bladder paralysis may be observed. Sinus tachycardia also may be present.

(2) *Cardiovascular signs:* these appear 30 minutes to 24 hours after drug ingestion. Cyanosis and a rapid, weak pulse may be noted. Hypertension or hypotension leading to shock may be present. Cardiac conduction and rhythm disturbances are typical characteristics of tricyclic overdosage (atrial fibrillation, atrioventricular block, intraventricular block, ventricular flutter). These are related to the tricyclic's anticholinergic properties, as well as to a direct myocardial depression.

(3) *CNS signs:* ataxia, agitation, dysarthria, hyperreflexia, and extrapyramidal rigidity are observed, and later may culminate in delirium and, finally, coma. This is a light, arousable coma that may be interrupted by typical myoclonic convulsions and epileptic states. If it does not recede within 12 hours, combinations of drugs should be suspected.

Respiratory depression with irregular, weak, and rapid respirations may be present.

(4) *Disturbance of temperature regulation:* severe sweating or hyperpyrexia can be present, and may be one of the few causes of death.

Management

(1) Maintain adequate pulmonary ventilation. Intubate the unconscious patient with cuffed endotracheal tube.

(2) Maintain adequate blood pressure, and correct arrhythmias and conduction disorders immediately.

Avoid quinidine. Do not use vasopressors.

(3) Promote elimination of drug:

(a) induce vomiting, if patient is conscious;

(b) use gastric aspiration and lavage;

(c) leave solution of sodium sulfate in stomach as cathartic (30 gm./250 ml. water); save aspirate and washings for laboratory study.

(d) continue stomach lavage because of low plasma levels; high rate of drug secretion into stomach, and the atropinic effect of the drug, which inhibits peristalsis; this may be effectively done with a double lumen tube.

(e) prolonged diuresis to wash out metabolites may be useful, since tricyclics are essentially eliminated by the kidneys;

(f) catheterize periodically; there may be bladder paralysis.

(4) Convulsions should be controlled by diazepam, 5 to 10 mg. I.M., or short-acting barbiturates. *No barbiturates should be used if the patient has also been on monoamine oxidase inhibitors.*

(5) Use physostigmine, 1 to 4 mg. I.M. or I.V., in order to reverse the tricyclic-induced central anticholinergic syndrome. If symptoms persist, doses should be repeated at 30-minute intervals.

Peritoneal dialysis and hemodialysis have not been found particularly useful.

MONOAMINE OXIDASE INHIBITORS (e.g., PARNATE, MARPLAN, etc.)

Recognition

Clinical signs of overdosage may not appear for up to 12 hours after drug ingestion.

On the other hand, overdosage signs may continue for eight to ten days after ingestion.

(1) *Atropine-like signs:* dry mouth, mydriasis, photophobia, and bowel and bladder paralysis are present.

(2) *CNS-signs:* excitability, hypertonia, and spasticity (neck, face, and jaw) are observed, finally resulting in convulsions. Agitation can progress from confusion and incoherence to stupor and, finally, to coma.

(3) *Cardiovascular signs:* postural hypotension and tachycardia leading to shock can be noted.

Hypertensive crisis is manifested by flushed face, occipital headache radiating frontally, neck stiffness, nausea, vomiting, and photophobia. Hypertensive crisis occasionally may occur concurrently with postural hypotension.

(4) *Hyperpyrexia and increase in respiratory rate.*

Dangerous combinations:

(a) Monoamine oxidase inhibitors with large doses of drugs that may precipitate a hypertensive crisis: amphetamine; epinephrine; norepinephrine; methyldopa or dopamine; large/parenteral doses of dibenzepine derivatives, such as desipramine (Norpramin), amitriptyline (Elavil); large doses of drug combinations containing a sympathomimetic agent (cold, hay fever, and diet pills); food high in tyramine, such as beer, wines, certain fermented cheeses, pickled herring, chicken livers, yeast extract; and food high in tryptophan, such as broad beans;

(b) with drugs possibly causing serious hypotension, if used in high doses: barbiturates; narcotics; analgesics; alcohol; thiazide diuretics; phenothiazine compounds.

Management

(1) Maintain adequate pulmonary ventilation.

(2) Maintain adequate blood pressure. Give vasopressors very cautiously, and only when all other measures have been used and found inadequate. Remember that tissues already are saturated with epinephrine.

Hypertension: use phentolamine (Regitine), 5 mg. I.V., or pentolinium (Ansolysen), 3 mg. s.c. *Do not give parenteral reserpine.*

(3) Promote elimination of drug:

(a) induce vomiting if patient is conscious;

(b) use gastric aspiration and lavage;

(c) force diuresis.

(4) Control convulsions by correcting shock or hypotension if present. Cautiously administered short-acting barbiturates help relieve myoclonic reactions. Phenothiazines (I.V.) are helpful for sedation. Succinylcholine, 10 to 15 mg. I.V., should be administered very slowly under strictly controlled ventilation in order to control convulsions, if other measures have failed.

(5) Follow patient for at least ten days; toxic effects may be prolonged. Liver function tests should be performed and repeated in four to six weeks.

Use cautiously and only if necessary:

(a) CNS depressants such as narcotics, Demerol, ethanol, anesthetics, atropine, papaverine, scopolamine;

(b) cocaine or local anesthetics containing sympathomimetic vasoconstrictors.

MINOR TRANQUILIZERS (e.g., DIAZEPAM, CHLORDIAZEPOXIDE, MEPROBAMATE, etc.)

Recognition

Initially there will be drowsiness and lethargy, accompanied possibly by lassitude and muscle relaxation. Vision may be blurred, and pupils are pinpoint. Nystagmus or diplopia and tinnitus may be present. Reflexes will be diminished, and mental confusion and hallucinations are noted. Finally, hypotension/shock and respiratory depression lead to coma with cyanosis.

In some cases, hyperactivity and convulsions or paradoxic excitation can be observed.

These drugs are potentiated by narcotics, monoamine oxidase inhibitors, tricyclics, barbiturates, and phenothiazines.

Management

(1) Maintain adequate pulmonary ventilation.

(2) Maintain adequate blood pressure by maintaining fluid balance with intravenous fluids. It should be kept in mind,

however, that these patients are susceptible to congestive heart failure and pulmonary edema. *Do not give epinephrine.* Its action may be paradoxic.

(3) Promote elimination of drug:

(*a*) retard drug absorption by giving tap water or milk, 100 to 500 ml. (usually two or three times), or use activated charcoal (50 gm. in 500 ml. water);

(*b*) induce vomiting in conscious patients;

(*c*) use gastric lavage; leave solution of sodium sulfate (30 gm./250 ml.) in stomach as cathartic; meprobamate and diazepam (Valium) are not water-soluble, so that best results are obtained if gastric elimination attempts are started soon after drug ingestion;

(*d*) if coma does not respond to routine measures, osmotic diuresis, mannitol diuresis, peritoneal dialysis, or hemodialysis may be tried;

(*e*) with meprobamate overdose, the drug may not be absorbed entirely from the intestinal tract during coma and hypotensive state; the residual drug therefore is absorbed with return of normal circulatory function, thus causing a reappearance of the overdose syndrome, and the patient should be observed and carefully monitored for at least 72 hours after drug ingestion.

Do not administer barbiturates to patients who show signs of overstimulation.

LITHIUM

Lithium carbonate has become the treatment of choice for the patient with manic depressive illness, manic phase. Overdosage usually is due to accidental ingestion of inappropriate amounts of lithium, rather than to suicidal intentions. Since lithium is almost exclusively excreted in the urine, overdosage also can be a result of reduced excretory capacity of the kidneys or, less frequently, of abnormal lithium retention in certain tissues (Agulnik, et al., 1972). The degree of toxicity usually correlates with the serum lithium level, although this may not always be the case. Particularly during illnesses that cause a loss of fluid or in some other way affect the kidney's excretory capacity, serum lithium levels are less reliable. It also should be explored if the patient has been taking diuretics or has been placed on a low salt diet, since these measures may significantly alter his salt balance, with a resulting abnormality in lithium clearance.

Recognition

(1) Mild overdose: signs usually occur with serum lithium levels above 1.6 mEq./liter and 48 hours after the ingestion of the overdose. Patients experience thirst, nausea, and vomiting. Abdominal pain and diarrhea are reported. Polyuria also is noted.

(2) Moderate overdose: in addition to the previous symptoms, confusion, dysarthria, coarse tremors, and muscle fasciculations are observed. Later on, muscle twitching, ataxia, nystagmus, and hyperreflexia are present.

(3) Severe overdose: a stuporous state appears, with epileptic seizures and transitory neurologic asymmetric symptoms simulating cerebral hemorrhage. Finally, there is coma with complete unresponsiveness.

Management

(1) Maintain adequate pulmonary ventilation.

(2) Maintain adequate blood pressure.

(3) Promote elimination of drug:

(*a*) induce vomiting if patient is conscious;

(*b*) perform gastric lavage with physiologic saline or tap water;

(*c*) force diuresis with fluids; mannitol or urea may be used if necessary;

(*d*) alkalinize urine;

(*e*) administration of aminophylline will also increase elimination;

(*f*) administer isotonic sodium chloride solution to facilitate elimination.

(4) Regulate kidney function, since lithium is excreted by the kidneys. Correct fluid and electrolyte balance. Obtain frequent serum electrolyte and lithium levels.

With normal kidney function, serum lithium concentration decreases by one-half every 24 to 36 hours.

(5) Treatment of coma: be alert to pulmonary complications (e.g., atelectasis, pneumonia) while patient is in this state.

In severe overdoses hemodialysis is indicated.

References

Agulnik, P. L., DiMascio, A., and Moore, P.: Acute brain syndrome associated with lithium therapy. Am. J. Psychiatry 129:621, 1972.

Detre, T. P., and Jarecki, H. G.: Modern Psychiatric Treatment. Philadelphia, J. P. Lippincott Co., 1971.

Heiser, J. F.., and Wilbert, D. E.: Reversal of delirium induced by tricyclic antidepressant drugs with physostigmine. Am. J. Psychiatry 131:1275, 1974.

Kline, N. S., Alexander, J. F., and Chamberlain, A.: Psychotropic Drugs. A Manual for Emergency Management of Overdosage. Oradell, N.J., Medical Economics Co., 1974.

Shader, R. I., and DiMascio, A.: Psychotropic Drug Side-effects. Baltimore, Williams & Wilkins Co., 1970.

H. EMERGENCIES IN MEDICAL, SURGICAL, OR OBSTETRIC PATIENTS WHO ARE SEVERELY ILL

Jean-Pierre Lindenmayer and Nathan S. Kline

INTRODUCTION

Severe medical, surgical, or obstetric illness presents a major psychologic and physical stress for the patient, and requires the mobilization of a maximum of coping abilities. The patient must adapt to the loss of function that results from his illness, to the demands of confinement in a hospital, and to the demands of multiple diagnostic or surgical procedures. Cooperation with the treatment recommended by the physician is not always easy, but is essential. If these coping strategies are called on too abruptly, or if the patient fails to respond to these many demands, an emergency situation can result wherein the patient's psychologic or physical health is acutely endangered.

In addition, other factors associated with the patient's lack of coping abilities may lead to emergency situations. The attitudes and reactions of the physician, and also those of the family, may contribute to creating an emergency, and therefore also will have to be considered.

PSYCHOLOGIC RESPONSES TO PHYSICAL ILLNESS

Reactions to the Illness

Disruption of somatic well-being causes anxiety in every normal human being and brings about various degrees of feelings of helplessness; in particular when the condition occurs suddenly, reactions tend to be more severe. In order to cope with this anxiety, less mature forms of behavior may appear that can be more or less adaptive. The main reaction is in the area of dependency, with some patients reacting in an overly dependent fashion. Others, fearful of dependency, feel they may be made helpless by their illness, and therefore will try to minimize its reality and the need for treatment. Other reactions may be depression, denial, lack of cooperation, agitated anxiety, exaggerated pain reactions, prolonged convalescence, and drug dependence. The degree with which these forms of behavior appear depends on the severity and nature of the illness, the patient's pre-existing level of psychologic functioning, and the psychosocial environment (including the medical staff and the patient's family). All these reactions are used by the patient to reduce anxiety about his physical illness and what it represents. At times, illness can pose a major threat to the patient's self-image as an independent, self-sufficient individual, or it may revive strong underlying wishes to be taken care of. The physician then is seen as a protective, omnipotent authority who will take care of the patient.

The anxieties related to illness obviously are the greatest when the patient is threatened by, for example, terminal cancer. Such patients are brought to Emergency Departments as the progression of the disease results in severe pain or a medical crisis. The prospect of death, a universal fear, can be overwhelming to the patient, producing a helpless and lonely feeling, particularly if his family and physician shy away from him through their own fear of death. Patients cope with this fear in various ways, depending on previous experience, and particularly often in a manner similar to the way they have handled previous separation experiences. Doctor–patient relationships in these circumstances are particularly important.

The difficulties related to illness also are significant when they force the patient to change his life-style radically. A patient with myocardial infarction compelled to reduce activities may develop a depression. A patient in chronic renal failure who has to reorganize life around frequent dialysis may respond by becoming negligent of his diet.

Other factors influencing the patient's reaction to illness are his expectations and anticipations about treatment. These attitudes may include both negative and positive aspects. This applies particularly to surgical procedures for which the patient may have unrealistic expectations that can lead to disappointment and more severe reactions.

Reactions to the Hospital

Anxieties also in part determine reactions to the hospital environment and to the medical procedures related to the illness. The two extreme reactions are: (1) the patient who wants to sign out against medical advice; and (2) the patient who tries to postpone discharge in direct or indirect ways. Both reactions are extreme positions on the spectrum of dependence: the former patient cannot tolerate dependence and is afraid of losing his personal freedom; the latter's dependency needs are satisfied by the hospital, and he doesn't want to give up this gratification. All other reactions can be placed between these two extremes. Some patients make continuous special demands, and are easily annoyed and critical of the staff, picking fights with them in every available situation. Other patients may be overly clinging and dependent, exaggerating their physical complaints without clear organic causes, and may turn the staff against them through their excessive demands and over-utilization of available services. Other factors that contribute to anxieties over hospitalization can be the temporary separation from family and the newness and strangeness of the environ-

ment of the hospital, with its particular and peculiar pattern combining sensory deprivation and overstimulation.

Reactions to Surgery

Anxieties related to the surgical experience are certainly common and appropriate, but if they provoke an exaggerated emotional response or are handled by the patient inappropriately, they can lead at times to emergency situations necessitating intervention by the physician. These anxieties usually are related to the real or symbolic meaning of the particular organ involved in surgery, to the loss of control resulting from anesthesia, or to other underlying fantasies and expectations. The reactions can be classified conveniently into (1) preoperative and (2) postoperative syndromes.

PREOPERATIVE SYNDROMES

These can range from utter and supreme calmness to panic and overt psychosis (Abram, 1975). Such reactions are related to the anticipation the patient feels about the surgery, usually a mixture of hope and despair (Hackett and Weisman, 1960).

POSTOPERATIVE SYNDROMES

These consist of a heterogeneous group of reactions, such as depressions, anxiety states, paranoid states, and various forms of psychosis. These latter reactions are, in large part, acute or chronic organic brain syndromes (including postoperative delirium). Accurate prognosticators for postoperative psychiatric complications are the patient's unrealistic expectations of surgery, the major use of denial, and excessive preoperative anxiety (Abram and Gill, 1961). Other factors involved are age (those over 65 being more susceptible), the duration and depth of anesthesia, the type of surgical intervention, and the degree of organic impairment caused by the surgery.

Family's Reaction to Patient's Illness

The patient's illness also represents an additional stress for the family, for whom this new situation can create a variety of problems. If the family's coping abilities fail in dealing with these, the result certainly can provoke an emergency situation for the patient. These problems depend on the nature of the relationship the patient has with his family, the nature and duration of the illness, and the family's cohesiveness. Frequent reactions of family members are feelings of guilt for not having sent the patient earlier for medical attention or feelings of resentment for being deprived of the patient's support and help. Even the inconvenience of hospital visits at times can produce considerable irritation, leading the family to minimize the patient's complaints, possibly leading to premature discharge from the hospital. The withdrawal of family support can contribute to exacerbations of the illness or can create emergency situations. In one case, a young woman with lupus erythematosus had been stabilized successfully with appropriate medical treatment. When her discharge was planned, it became clear that her mother did not want to take her back into her family because of various negative feelings she had about her daughter and the illness. The daughter subsequently developed an acute psychotic reaction that required psychiatric intervention.

Physician's Reaction to Patient's Illness

An emergency situation may be a result not only of the nature of the patient's condition and the ways he deals with it, but also of some sudden reaction or change in the physician's attitude toward the patient or his illness. A particularly dependent and demanding patient, turned away by an impatient physician, may resort to bizarre behavior in order to gain the physician's attention. Another chronically ill patient may react with intense depression and withdrawal after his house staff physician has been rotated to another floor or has taken an unannounced vacation. At times, it is actually the physician who determines whether an emergency situation will or will not result. For example, a 23-year-old woman with chronic renal failure had been treated on a medical floor for several weeks. Her hospital course was punctuated by several minor psychotic episodes during which she would wander off the floor, show severe paranoid ideation, and cause considerable disruption in ward routine. Unwisely, psychiatric consultation was delayed and finally requested on an emergency basis only when she attempted suicide.

GENERAL PRINCIPLES OF MANAGEMENT

Psychologic Management

The most important factor is the quality of the doctor–patient relationship. The physician should be compassionate and understanding toward the patient, showing that he is an ally, not an antagonist. Communications should be in terms the patient can understand. It may be necessary to repeat to the patient several times *who* the physician is, *where* the patient is, and *what* the purpose of the examination is. This is particularly important if the patient is paranoid or delirious.

Once initial contact has been established, the physician should discuss some of the facts relevant to the present illness and gradually inquire about the patient's feelings toward the illness and how it has affected or will affect his present and future life. Realistic and unrealistic expectations about the illness and its treatment should be discussed. This is especially important for patients involved in surgical procedures. If the patient shows excessive denial of underlying feelings of anxiety, *this should be left untouched.* In other words, the patient should *not* be forced to "face" his illness if he chooses to deal with the problem by denial.

In contrast, other patients may wish to know all the details. In any case, questions the patient may ask about the diagnostic and therapeutic procedures he is undergoing should be answered, whenever possible and appropriate, in a straightforward and open fashion: this often helps to reduce his anxiety considerably. Throughout the interview, the physician will be able to gather data in this more or less "unstructured" fashion to judge the patient's mental status. Questioning also should include inquiries into the possibility of suicidal ideation, and in all cases should be directed toward an assessment of the patient's state of orientation. This last point, together with the evaluation of the patient's memory function may help establish the presence of an organic brain syndrome.

In addition to gathering information

from the patient, it is important to ask the nursing staff for their observations of his behavior. Since they are in constant contact with the patient, they usually have valuable information to contribute. It may be important to interview the family if the emergency has been precipitated by some change in the domestic situation.

Disposition

Evaluation of the patient's medical and mental status leads to a decision about disposition. The physician may decide that additional support and clarification, together with sedative medication, is sufficient to bring the situation under control. On the other hand, psychiatric consultation may be required.

If suicide risks are prominent, precautions must be taken, such as 24-hour nursing, removal of sharp objects, and locking of windows. A patient who is violent or who wanders off the ward may have to be restrained. It should be kept in mind, however, that restraints sometimes increase, rather than decrease, the agitation. Often, when restraints are required, they can be discontinued after a relatively brief period in certain patients. The patient should be evaluated after a half hour or so to determine whether restraints need to be continued. A patient with acute brain syndrome should have his environment simplified as much as possible. It is helpful to have one nurse, familiar to the patient, take care of him, rather than rotate nurses automatically according to hospital routine.

Considerations in Psychiatric Consultation

When requesting a psychiatric consultation, it is imperative for the physician to be clear about two points so that both the physician and the patient may receive maximal benefit. (1) What are the reasons for psychiatric consultation, and are they spelled out clearly for the psychiatrist? (2) Has he adequately prepared the patient to be seen by a psychiatrist?

INDICATIONS FOR PSYCHIATRIC CONSULTATION

It is important that the physician decide what the objectives of such a consultation should be and what kind of problems he wants solved by the psychiatrist, who otherwise might focus on aspects with which the physician is less concerned. Here are the major indications for such a request, limited to the context of emergency care.

(a) If the patient has a mental condition that substantially interferes with necessary medical treatment.

(b) If the patient has an acute pre- or postoperative syndrome that interferes with proper surgical treatment, e.g., pulling out transfusion needles.

(c) If the patient is suicidal or homicidal.

(d) If the patient is acutely psychotic, and presents major management problems on the ward, such as wandering off the floor, going into other patients' rooms, and picking fights with the staff.

PREPARATION OF PATIENT FOR CONSULTATION

Adequate preparation is important for several reasons. Usually, the consultation is requested by the physician and, therefore, is an involuntary procedure for the patient. The latter may have various ambivalent feelings about seeing a psychiatrist, ranging from indifference to anxiety to total refusal to speak to the consultant. These feelings should be clarified as much as possible by discussing them with the patient and by informing him of the purpose of the consultation.

Psychopharmacologic Management

If severe panic and agitation are present, sedation with a psychotropic agent may be necessary. Acute psychotic productions, such as delusions and hallucinations, should be controlled by medication. In the use of these drugs, the patient's medical condition and possible side-effects must be taken into careful account. In addition, the patient's vital signs and neurologic status should be as stable as possible when such treatment is instituted.

Low doses of phenothiazines of the sedative type, such as chlorpromazine, should be given parenterally. If the medical status permits it, a dosage schedule beginning with 25 mg. I.M. every four hours should be established, increasing the dose, if necessary, by 25 mg. steps every four hours until the patient is sufficiently sedated, yet fully arousable. Because of the hypotensive effect of chlorpromazine, the blood pressure should be taken before and between each dose, and the next dose withheld if there is a significant drop in blood pressure. Once the dose is reached that gives the required effect, the physician should give that dose orally on a six-hour basis. If there are reasons to anticipate seizures, paraldehyde I.M. can be used instead of a phenothiazine. With elderly patients and those with cerebrovascular problems for whom hypotensive effects are particularly undesirable, a butyrophenone like haloperidol can be given, starting with 0.5 to 1.0 mg. four times daily. Benzodiazepines such as chlordiazepoxide are suitable for short term use: 10 mg. I.M. every two to four hours usually is sufficient in the acute stage, with transfer to oral dose as soon as the patient is stabilized.

The more frequent side-effects of the phenothiazines are extrapyramidal symptoms, such as dyskinesia, pseudoparkinsonism, and akathisia. An antiparkinsonian agent (benztropine, procyclidine, or biperiden) effectively helps control these effects. Postural hypotension is another not infrequent side-effect, although this usually does not consitute a problem, since these patients are kept at bed rest. Occasionally, more severe hypotension can develop, particularly with high doses of intramuscular medication. For a patient with cardiovascular disease, the doses should be increased more slowly and the blood pressure monitored more frequently. If a hypotensive episode develops, vasopressor medication such as norepinephrine may be indicated. *Epinephrine, however, is contraindicated* since it may accentuate the hypotension.

No specific teratogenic effects arising from the use of phenothiazines during pregnancy have been reported. These medications, therefore, can be used during pregnancy when essential. However, both an extrapyramidal and a postnatal depression syndrome, followed by agitation in the newborn, have been noted (Appleton and Davis, 1973).

SYNDROMES AND THEIR MANAGEMENT

Acute Reactions in Intensive Care Units

Medical and surgical intensive care units present for most patients a rather new and frightening environment: isolation from familiar persons, and sensory monotony with transient overstimulation and sleep deprivation due to the constant activity of staff and the various monitoring devices. Stabilizing natural day and night patterns are smiliarly altered, particularly when there are no windows in the I.C.U. Patients usually react to these new demands with anxiety and, to a greater or lesser degree, with denial (Hackett, et al., 1968). The effect of the confinement in such units, together with the physiologic defects arising from the underlying illness, can lead to acute psychiatric emergencies. In addition, staff in I.C.U.s themselves may contribute to patient problems through overconcern with technical aspects and avoidance of interpersonal contact with the patient.*

The most severe reactions are acute organic brain syndromes characterized by disorientation as to time, place, and person; fluctuating states of consciousness; and disturbed mood, ranging from severe agitation to depression. These syndromes occur particularly after cardiac surgery and in the elderly patient.

Other acute reactions include paranoid reactions in which the patient may feel that the staff and the physician are against him, or that the treatment he is receiving is actually detrimental to him—e.g., medication is poisoned, food is contaminated, and he is "being experimented with." At times this may lead the patient to refuse necessary procedures or treatment. Acute states of depression and anxiety states also are encountered occasionally. If the patient is not in contact with reality, the physician must help him to appraise the situation more correctly by reducing overstimulation, explaining carefully and simply whatever is being done, and providing appropriate information and reassurance. When agitation and high levels of anxiety are present, tranquilizing medication and night-time sedation should be used carefully. Sudden decreases in such

---

*See Chapter 76.

agitation may result in excess physiologic depression because formerly adequate doses of medication now become excessive. If the patient's mental state interferes in a major way with his medical or surgical treatment, psychiatric consultation should be requested.

Acute Reactions to Renal Dialysis and Transplantation

RENAL DIALYSIS

For patients with progressive end-stage kidney disease, maintenance hemodialysis usually is the major treatment modality that will prolong life. Adaptation both to the disease itself and to the treatment can be very demanding and difficult for the patient, as well as for the family. The treatment usually requires that the patient spend six to eight hours, two or three times a week, attached to the dialysis machine. This invariably leads to feelings of intense dependence toward the machine, which the patient perceives on the one hand as life-saving and sustaining, yet on the other hand as severely limiting his freedom and constantly reminding him of his extreme fragility. The illness and treatment also require from both patient and family drastic changes in their usual life pattern in order to adjust to the new situation. In addition, there is the constant hope for an eventual kidney transplant or, if this has already been done, the continuous fear of possible rejection. If adaptation to these multiple demands and stresses fails, various acute psychiatric problems can develop that may aggravate the already difficult situation significantly, such as: (1) acute organic brain syndromes; (2) depressive states; and (3) anxiety states (Levy, 1976).

Acute Organic Brain Syndrome. The patient will present states of confusion in various degrees that alternate with more lucid intervals, and that usually are accompanied by cognitive impairments, such as problems in orientation, reduced attention span, and difficulties in recognizing familiar faces and environments. In more severe forms there will be hallucinations, mainly of the visual type, and delusions, often of the persecutory type. There always is some lability of affect, ranging from agitated perplexity to absent-minded withdrawal.

Renal and extrarenal factors, such as infections or cardiac and pulmonary decompensations, can lead to this syndrome. It is important to recognize the underlying organic cause and to correct it, since usually this syndrome is reversible. In his approach to these patients, the physician should help them to appraise reality correctly, e.g., by repeating *where* the patient is, *who* the physician is, and *what* his function is. Reassurance, structure, and support should be provided for the patient. If agitation is severe and prevents proper medical treatment, a phenothiazine or benzodiazepine may be indicated, and should be used as described in the previous section.

Acute Depressive States. These states are seen most commonly in association with acute medical and social problems (Levy, 1976). Patients express feelings of hopelessness and helplessness, and sometimes anger at the physician or at the staff, because of the need to endure chronic dialysis and to accept overdependence. Suicidal preoccupation, with actual direct or indirect suicide attempts, is particularly frequent among patients on maintenance dialysis (Abram, et al., 1971).

The physician should attempt to clarify in a supportive fashion some of the underlying reasons for the patient's depression, since often there are real family, social, and financial difficulties. The physician also should carefully explore suicidal preoccupations that may be quite indirect, such as the deliberate neglect of dietary restrictions. For continuous supportive treatment, psychiatric consultation usually is required. Antidepressant medication can be used to alleviate some of the symptoms of the depression.

Anxiety States. Acute anxiety reactions or panic states often are related to the sense of danger produced by the dialysis procedure, in which the patient sees his blood continually flowing out and back again through a complex system of machinery (Levy, 1976). The physician can be of great help to the patient by identifying such fears in a supportive fashion and correcting them through appropriate information if they are a result of distortions of reality. Also, speaking to other patients who have adapted to the procedure successfully can help reduce the anxieties of the patient. Minor tranquilizers also can contribute to overcoming a transiently difficult situation. If the fears and anxieties continue to be manifested, psychiatric consultation is indicated.

RENAL TRANSPLANTATION

Acute reactions after the transplantation procedure are rather infrequent, particularly compared to reactions after cardiac transplantation. Acute organic brain syndromes are rare. Occasionally, depressive states can be observed related to a constant concern over possible rejection, or ambivalence over accepting the donor's kidney (living or cadaver transplant). These depressive states can be particularly severe and accompanied by suicidal ideation in patients who have rejected their transplant and are awaiting new ones, and thus forced to resume chronic dialysis (Abram, 1972). Another factor that can affect the patient's adaptation to the transplant is steroid medication used for immunosuppression, which may produce a steroid psychosis or the typical Cushing "moon face."

If such difficulties arise, psychiatric consultation usually is indicated to help the patient achieve better psychologic acceptance of his transplant. This is especially important if the patient has to go back on chronic dialysis.

Acute Reactions to Heart Surgery

PREOPERATIVE REACTIONS

Cardiac surgery, with its threat to life and its symbolic implications, represents a major challenge to the patient's coping abilities. The heart certainly occupies a central position in the patient's conception of his body, and is directly related to his very existence. Particular coping mechanisms are mobilized by the patient in order to deal with the stress related to cardiac surgery. Immobilization, hysterical amnesia or depersonalization, belligerence, excitement, and denial are used (Fox, et al., 1954). Other reactions, such as preoperative depression and anxiety states, have been correlated with the postoperative course. The highest mortality has been found in preoperatively depressed patients, and the greatest morbidity in preoperatively anxious patients (Kimball, 1969).

Adequate preoperative preparation of the patient is very important in order to reduce the intensity and frequency of these reactions. A good patient–doctor relationship is vital. The physician should help to clarify some of the patient's preoperative expectations. Psychiatric intervention may be needed if the reaction is severe and endangers the postoperative course.

POSTOPERATIVE REACTIONS

The most common psychiatric complication after cardiac surgery is a postoperative psychosis, usually an acute organic brain syndrome. It is characterized by impairment of orientation, memory, intellectual function, and judgment, and by lability of affect (Blachly and Star, 1964). Sometimes, a schizophrenia-like psychosis can be observed; these states are related etiologically to a number of factors, ranging from organic factors causing CNS dysfunction to the particular I.C.U. environment, to factors related to the intensive anxiety of having an operation on the heart, and to the fear of death. Most of these states are transient and usually clear up after a few days.

Another postoperative reaction is a "catastrophic"-type response, the patient lying immobile with an affectless mask, cooperating passively with the staff, and responding monosyllabically to questions (Kimball, 1969). These reactions clear after four to five days, with amnesia for the episode.

The physician must provide reassurance and support during this difficult period. If the patient is disoriented, it is helpful to indicate where he is, what the purpose of the medical procedures are, and who the physician is. It also is important to keep the environment as simple and constant as possible, since the patient's cognitive capacities are greatly impaired. If suicidal ideation is present, precautions should be taken to protect the patient, and psychiatric consultation should be requested. Psychotropic medication should be used very cautiously and sparingly, in view of the delicate cardiovascular and pulmonary situation.

Reactions to Plastic Surgery

Acute psychologic reactions after plastic surgery are not infrequent, particularly after interventions that involve the face. Acute psychotic states of a schizophrenic type and depressions with feelings of hopelessness may be encountered. These reactions can be understood as resulting from abrupt changes in the body image that the patient cannot tolerate. On the other hand, the patient may have had unrealistic expectations about the results of the surgery, hoping that it would solve all his interpersonal problems. As a rule, the less prominent the preoperative disfigurement and the more it is used to cover severe personality difficulties, the greater is the likelihood of adverse psychologic reactions (Taylor, et al., 1966).

In most cases, psychiatric consultation is necessary. This is especially important if further plastic surgical interventions are contemplated.

Reactions to Amputation

The loss of a body part through amputation occasionally can result in psychologic reactions similar to those seen with other significant losses. These patients can present the physician with postoperative depressions characterized by feelings of hopelessness and helplessness, preoccupation with death, and not infrequently with suicide (Caplan and Hackett, 1963). This syndrome is seen particularly in elderly patients for whom amputation "seems to symbolize the encroachment of death" (Caplan and Hackett, 1963). Other reactions to amputation include defiance, regression, and fears resulting from nonacceptance (Kelham, 1958). Later, patients commonly report phantom sensations or the perception of a phantom limb. These phenomena are related to the persistence, after the amputation, of the mental representation of the intact model of the body. Such patients are rarely seen on an emergency basis unless pain is a component of their sensation.

The depressive reactions are in part due to unrealistic preoperative expectations; patients have either tended to minimize the effect of the amputation or to hope that the amputation would be a total cure for their illness. It therefore is important, if possible, to clarify the expectations of the patient preoperatively and to rectify them in a nontraumatic way. In handling postoperative reactions, the physician should support and repeatedly point out that the reality of the situation does not correspond with the gloomy picture the patient may paint. Antidepressant medication, such as doxepin, amitryptyline, or imipramine, also may be indicated. If the depression interferes with

the proper postoperative progress, or if suicidal ideation is present, psychiatric consultation should be requested.

Acute Reactions to Colostomy

A patient after colostomy undergoes serious changes in body form and function that cause new, often stressful, challenges to his coping abilities. He must adapt to the loss of a psychologically valued organ; to the loss of a basic body control function; to a radically changed body image; and to the colostomy training, with its possible restrictive family and social implications. These stresses can threaten or disrupt the patient's usual coping abilities and lead to acute psychiatric difficulties.

The most frequent acute reaction is a postoperative depression, characterized by feelings of personal inadequacy and helplessness and by disturbances of eating and sleeping patterns and of sexual function. It often is precipitated by the initial sight of the colostomy, which is perceived as a mutilation and disfigurement (Sutherland, et al., 1952). The patient becomes concerned and fearful about possible spillage and other problems related to the colostomy, and how the environment will react to it; he also may show suicidal ideation. Later on, a marked sense of weakness out of proportion to the patient's physical state can be found and may lead to severe restrictions of activities and social withdrawal (Sutherland, et al., 1952).

If possible, time should be spent by the surgeon in the preoperative phase—establishing a supportive and trusting patient–doctor relationship. The patient should be helped to verbalize preoperative expectations and fears about the surgery, and accurate information should be given, when appropriate. Fears and distorted preoccupations expressed in a postoperative depression should be corrected in a supportive fashion by the physician. The effect of the colostomy on the patient's family, work situation, and other social involvements also must be explored. Other staff members can help the patient to regain some degree of self-esteem through bowel control by colostomy training. If the depression continues in spite of these supportive approaches, psychiatric intervention will be necessary. After the initial crisis has been resolved, the patient also may benefit from participation in colostomy clubs, which provide continuous support on a long term basis.

Acute Reactions to Eye Surgery

A patient whose eyes have been bilaterally bandaged after some form of eye surgery not infrequently presents a postoperative psychosis ("black patch delirium"). He appears restless, anxious, and suspicious. He is disoriented as to time and place and may misidentify people around him and replace them with familiar figures from his home or work environment. Sometimes there may be delusions with persecutory content, auditory and visual hallucinations, and (rarely) suicidal ideation. This syndrome usually begins early in the postoperative period, and often is worse at night, when auditory cues that helped the patient to orient himself are less available. Elderly patients are particularly susceptible.

In the management of such a syndrome, the quality of the doctor-patient relationship is of central importance (Weisman and Hackett, 1958). The physician should offer some of the correct appraisal of the visual reality that the patient is unable to provide for himself any longer owing to his temporary blindness. He can begin by explaining preoperatively to the apprehensive patient both the operative procedures and what is to be expected once the bilateral masking has been applied. Postoperatively, the physician must help the patient in a very literal sense to reorient, since reality orientation is temporarily severely limited. This can be done by using other perceptual channels that are not impaired and by providing the patient with auditory, gustatory, tactile, and olfactory perceptual cues (Weisman and Hackett, 1958). It should be pointed out repeatedly to the patient where he is and who the people are around him, and his room and surroundings should be described. Other steps in the management will include the following.

(1) Psychiatric consultation. The psychiatrist will be able to support the patient more extensively with respect to deficient reality evaluation.

(2) If possible, arrangements should be made to have a family member stay at the bedside. It also is helpful to have the same nurse take care of the patient, as far as possible.

(3) If severe agitation, active delusions, and hallucinations are present, phenothiazines may be helpful and should be used as indicated under "General Principles of Management."

Reactions to Death and Dying

ATTITUDES TOWARD DEATH AND DYING

Facing and, to the extent possible, accepting death is a difficult and frightening task for the terminally ill patient and all those involved in his care. How it is accomplished is determined largely by the attitude toward death of the patient, the family, and the physician as well as the surrounding staff. These attitudes, to a large extent, are related to the underlying fear of death present in every human being and to the meaning a given individual attaches to death. For some patients it may mean isolation and loneliness, for some it may represent a punishment, and for others it may awaken repressed childhood fears of abandonment. The intensity of the fear of death, together with pre-existing personality traits, determines the way each individual deals with death and dying. One of the chief coping mechanisms is denial. By stating "this doesn't happen to me, only to my neighbor," by becoming feverishly busy with medical machinery around dying patients, by avoiding talk with terminally ill patients, some physicians and nurses attempt to deny their own fear of death and the finality of the end of life.

Other attitudes toward death and dying may include the view that death represents a reunion with beloved ones in a world after death, and that it represents a relief, a reward, or an act of cosmic retribution (Weisman, 1975). It is very important that the physician first examine his own attitudes toward death when dealing with terminally ill patients. This, in turn, will help him better to understand his patients' attitudes and fears and to assist them through their terminal illness and to death with dignity. Avoiding these issues and avoiding the patient only increase the latter's despair and sense of isolation, sometimes to the point of precipitating a crisis situation.

REACTIONS TOWARD DEATH AND DYING

Kübler-Ross (1969) has described a sequence of five stages of dying that can be seen as typical coping mechanisms of patients dealing with death. They can occur in sequence, or may be present to various degrees at the same time. After an initial temporary state of shock, the patient attempts to deny his fatal illness, and then may postpone seeking help. This denial is replaced by feelings of anger, rage, envy, and resentment over the fatal, uncontrollable course that life is taking. This anger often is projected on the outside, on family and staff, which may increase the patient's isolation. This is followed by the "bargaining" stage in which patients try to have some special favor fulfilled by God, usually some extension of life, in return for good behavior. Depression is the next stage, with feelings of sadness over the impending loss of loved ones and everything achieved in life. During this phase of genuine mourning, the patient should be allowed to express his sorrow, and should be given support rather than encouraged superficially to "cheer up." Finally, if the patient has been able with some help from the outside to work through the previous stages, he reaches the stage of acceptance. This should not be confused with a hopeless "giving up;" it is rather a stage characterized by acceptance of fate without anger or depression.

DEALING WITH THE DYING PATIENT

How to Tell the Patient? In an extreme emergency situation, patients often ask whether they are going to die. Usually they should be reassured that this will not happen, even when the situation, in fact, is grave. However, the family should be informed of the critical nature of the illness. In contrast, it is important to realize that most patients with terminal illness actually know the truth without being told. A relative or someone else in the patient's environment will give the nonverbal message that there is something seriously wrong by the way he deals with the patient. Therefore, the question "whether or not to tell" is less of an issue. The question, "How do I share this knowledge with my patient?" is really the crucial one (Kubler-Ross, 1969). The physician must devote some time to deciding how ready and willing his patient is to hear the truth. If the patient indicates verbally or nonverbally that he is ready, the physician should present the facts in a simple, but emphatic, way, pointing out any hopeful aspects of the treatment, and particularly stressing that everything possible will be done in order to provide the best and most appropriate treatment. It is important to let the patient know that he will not be "dropped." The physician should take enough time to stay with the patient for awhile after he has been told the facts about his illness in order to give him support and evaluate his reactions. Preferably, he should communicate all this to the patient in a place where some degree of privacy is assured, rather than in the hallway with a group of medical students around him.

Helping the Patient to Cope with Terminal Illness. Weisman (1975) has listed a few guidelines to help the physician in dealing with the terminally ill. Patients of this sort frequently are seen on an emergency basis when home care becomes difficult or sudden deterioration occurs.

(1) *Adequate relief of pain.* The patient should be given sufficient and appropriate pain-relieving medication and sedation if he desires it, but not to the point that he is dehumanized. Customary concern about addiction dangers are no longer relevant.

(2) *Open and Candid Communication with Patient and Family.* Diagnosis and treatment should be dealt with as described above. The patient should be involved as much as possible in important decisions about his treatment. The physician also should be available to the family and open to their needs for information, advice, and support.

(3) *Preservation of Self-Esteem and Autonomy.* The physician can support and stress those aspects of the patient's functioning that are still intact or still rewarding to the patient. He also can try to give the patient control over his daily functions and routines, so far as this is medically and practically feasible.

(4) *Genuine Courage to Accept What Cannot Be Changed.* The patient does not expect superficial reassurance, but rather wants to know that the physician is willing and ready to share his concern about the inevitable and to provide help in accepting it.

Psychiatric consultation may be required if some of the reactions described above become excessive and destructive. This may be the case if the patient's depression becomes severe or even of psychotic proportions, or if his anger over his terminal illness alienates all those around him, staff and family included.

Helping the Dying Patient in the Emergency Department. Critically ill or injured patients seen in the Emergency Department present a particular problem, since typically there is little time or leisure available to give attention to their emotional needs. The various members of the medical team have to concentrate first on attempting to stabilize the vital functions and to save the patient's life. However, if the patient is conscious, he usually is quite anxious, possibly in a state of emotional shock, or at times even quite aware of the seriousness of the situation. Once the patient's vital functions are stabilized, it is important for the physician or a member of the treatment team to communicate with the patient in order to allay his anxieties. A few guidelines should be followed.

(1) The patient should be told where he is, who the physician and the people around him are, and what is being done to him.

(2) If the patient was brought alone, assurance should be given that all efforts will be made to notify his family and that they will be asked to come immediately.

(3) The patient should be informed about his state in a simple and honest way, but only if he appears to be ready for this. Hope should always be included in any such statement. If a patient asks if he is dying, he should *not* be told so. Instead, he can be told that the physician does not know, but that everything possible will be done to save his life and that he should not give up (Kubler-Ross, 1975).

(4) If the patient is conscious, he should be involved in important decisions related to his treatment. This is particularly true for necessary major surgical interventions. If he is not conscious, his family will have to be involved.

(5) If other family members or companions of the patient have been killed in the same accident, this should not be communicated to the patient until his vital functions are well stabilized or his critical condition is under control. The moment to communicate further bad news should be chosen with great care since the patient is already in emotional shock over his own injuries.

(6) Once inititial care has been given to the patient and his medical needs have been temporarily met, family members or friends should be allowed to see him for a short time and in a restricted number. This is particularly important if the patient is dying. The family or the patient, if conscious, may want to exchange last concerns, give some last reassurance, or ask for forgiveness (Kübler-Ross, 1975).

Helping the Family of the Patient. The family, in anticipating loss, also goes through phases similar to those of the patient. Their initial reactions are of denial and disbelief regarding the fatal outcome. Later on, they may show anger at the doctor for not having diagnosed the illness earlier, and may have a guilty feeling that in some ways it is their fault that the patient is going to die. The family also will have to cope with practical problems such as changed and possible increased financial demands, or the care and raising of children in the case of a dying parent. Loneliness will have to be faced. In order to be able to deal with these many demands, it is important that the family maintain a balance between serving the patient and respecting their own needs. Once death has occurred, the family become involved in the mourning process itself and have to work through their feelings of loss, anger, and guilt to an acceptance of the loss. During the anticipatory grief phase and during the mourning phase, the physician can be helpful in providing support and understanding. He also can spot and identify particular difficulties the family may have in dealing with the terminal illness, and he can initiate appropriate professional contacts, such as psychiatric consultation, referrals to the social worker, and contacts with the chaplain.

Some special problems arise for families who have a member admitted to an Emergency Department in critical condition. They may themselves be in a state of emotional shock, and may need support from the staff and the chance to ventilate their feelings. Since they want to remain close to a critically ill or dying patient, family members should be able to wait in a place not too far from the patient where some privacy is assured. The hospital chaplain or another person trained in dealing with grief-stricken relatives can be very helpful in staying with the family. If the patient is dead on arrival or dies during emergency procedures, the family should have the opportunity to see the body if they request it (Kübler-Ross, 1975). This can help them to face, and ultimately accept, the reality of the death of their relative.

Acute Reactions to Mastectomy

RECOGNITION

Women who undergo mastectomy for carcinoma of the breast have to adjust to the loss of an important organ that has various meanings to them; to a significant change of their body image; and to the frightening possibility of having a deadly disease. These adjustments are difficult, and can lead at times to acute psychiatric problems. A frequent reaction is a post mastectomy depression, characterized by anxiety, insomnia, feelings of shame and worthlessness, and occasional ideas of suicide, or actual attempts (Renneker and Cutler, 1952). Underlying themes to this depression are mainly twofold: (1) the mourning over the loss of the breast, which is the most visual and most valued evidence of the woman's sexuality; (2) the fear of having lost major attributes of the mothering role, since the breast represents the nurturing function. The younger woman still in her childbearing years is more prone to this syndrome than is the older, postclimacteric woman. For the latter, the difficulties lie more in adjusting to the possible malignant disease and the threat of death. The depression is most extreme in women who have invested irrational, disproportionate pride or shame in their breasts (Renneker and Cutler, 1952).

MANAGEMENT

The proper management of the surgeon–patient relationship is of great importance. The surgeon must take time to discuss with the patient some of her anxieties and fears in regard to her perceived loss of femininity and to the presence of a possible malignant tumor. He should approach the patient with support and understanding, pointing out the reality when the patient appears to distrust it. If he does not feel comfortable in doing this, a psychiatric consultation may be more appropriate. In addition, antidepressant medication can be helpful at times.

The patient's husband also should be involved, if he is available. He should be told about the pre- and postoperative feelings his wife will have to deal with: particularly that she may be afraid that he may reject her because of her mastectomy. He should be encouraged to focus, in his interactions with his wife, on her past and still-present feminine achievements. He also should be instructed and prepared for the sight of the operative scar, and should learn to treat it in a casual way.

The other major issue for the mastectomy patient is coping with the prognosis of her illness, which in turn depends on how far it has progressed when treatment is begun. If the prognosis is compromised, the question of how to deal with terminal illness will involve both patient and physician. This is discussed in the preceding section of this chapter.

Patients Who Refuse Treatment

Severely ill patients who refuse lifesaving treatment or necessary diagnostic procedures present a major challenge and frequently create feelings of frustration and helplessness in the physician and staff. Because of these feelings, both the physician and patient often become entrenched in their mutually opposed opinions, and communication breaks down completely, preventing further discussion that might have helped change the patient's mind. There are ways of handling such situations of refusal that can help the patient to change his position and accept treatment.

Fear is one of the most important factors in contributing to the patient's refusal of procedures or to his wish to leave the hospital. Lack of communication between patient and doctor or disorganized thinking due to some organic process may be other factors. In handling these patients, it is helpful to distinguish two types of situations (Himmelhoch, et al., 1970).

REFUSAL WITH COEXISTING PSYCHOPATHOLOGY

Patients may refuse treatment because of irrational fears related to an underlying psychosis with an active delusional system. Other patients may be in a state of panic and may refuse treatment because their cognitive capacities are severely impaired by an acute organic brain syndrome.

REFUSAL WITHOUT COEXISTING PSYCHOPATHOLOGY

In this situation, a patient may refuse treatment because he has not been adequately involved by the staff in important decisions concerning his treatment, or because his family has been avoided by the physician and has not been informed appropriately about the procedures. Divergent opinions among the staff as to the advisability of a particular procedure can also contribute to the patient's refusal. Religious or philosophic beliefs can be the reason for refusing certain types of treatment. In the emergency setting the patient has not had time to prepare and often is fearful of unfamiliar physicians. Also, he may deny the seriousness of the problem. Bringing in familiar physicians or staff members when possible is of utmost help.

MANAGEMENT

It is important to realize that the patient's refusal is not necessarily final. It therefore is helpful to take time to listen to the patient's reasons for his refusal. The physician should inquire into possible underlying fears of real or imaginary dangers about the procedures, and particularly should ensure that the patient understands the purpose and nature of the treatment or procedure. One of the crucial questions to be answered through this investigation is whether there is significant psychopathology, and if so, how it interferes with the patient's adjustment. For example, if the patient has an acute organic brain syndrome, attention and treatment must be focused on its cause, which in turn will ameliorate the patient's mental status. Psychiatric consultation is indicated in most cases in which psychopathology is present.

Other steps to be taken involve family and staff. If possible, the family should be informed about what is at stake and about the nature of the procedure. This is obligatory in the case of children or adolescents, for whom the parents' attitudes may have a

significant influence on the patient's acceptance or refusal of procedures. The position of the staff also should be examined briefly in terms of the agreement of different staff members on the course of treatment. Especially with a large staff, with various hierarchical, levels, any disagreement about the treatment or procedures planned is communicated to the patient and increases his ambivalence.

Finally, the physician must be able to review his treatment plan (Himmelhoch, et al., 1970) and determine whether an alternative, more acceptable approach is available, or if a postponement of the procedure to a more appropriate time might be feasible.

If, despite all efforts, the patient continues to refuse the procedure and wants to leave the hospital, the physician should carefully record on the chart: (1) the treatment or procedure indicated; (2) the fact that the patient has refused all advice; and (3) the action taken to help him to accept the physician's recommendation. If the patient is intoxicated, or otherwise mentally incapacitated, attempts should be made to keep him in the hospital until the altered state of consciousness clears. Actual physical restraint, however, is dangerous and has legal implications that must be considered.* Police may have to be involved if the patient presents indications that he might hurt himself or others.

---

*See page 1499.

References

Abram, H. S.: The psychiatrist, the treatment of chronic renal failure, and the prolongation of life. III. Am. J. Psychiatry 128:1534, 1972.

Abram, H. S.: Psychiatry and Surgery. In Freedman, A. M., Kaplan, H. T., and Sadock, B. J. (eds.): Comprehensive Textbook of Psychiatry. II. Baltimore, Williams & Wilkins Co., 1975.

Abram, H. S., and Gill, B. F.: Predictions of postoperative psychiatric complications. N. Engl. J. Med. 265:1123, 1961.

Abram, H. S., Moore, G. L., and Westervelt, F. B.: Suicidal behavior in chronic dialysis patients. Am. J. Psychiatry 127:1199, 1971.

Appleton, W. S., and Davis, J. M.: Practical Clinical Psychopharmacology. New York, Medcom, Inc., 1973.

Blachly, P. H., and Star, A.: Post-cardiotomy delirium. Am. J. Psychiatry 121:371, 1964.

Caplan, L. M., and Hackett, T. P.: Emotional effects of lower-limb amputation in the aged. N. Engl. J. Med. 269:1166, 1963.

Castelnuovo-Tedesco P.: Psychiatric Aspects of Organ Transplantation. New York, Grune & Stratton, 1971.

Fox, H. M., Rizzo, N. D., and Gifford, S.: Psychological observations of patients undergoing mitral surgery. Psychosom. Med. 16:186, 1954.

Hackett, T. P., Cassem, N. H., and Wishnie, H. A.: CCU: appraisal of its psychologic hazards. N. Engl. J. Med. 279:1365, 1968.

Hackett, T. P., and Weisman, A. D.: Psychiatric management of operative syndromes. The therapeutic consultation and effect of non-interpretive intervention. Psychosom. Med. 22:267, 1960.

Himmelhoch, J. M., et al.: Butting heads: patients who refuse necessary procedures. Psychiatr. Med. 1:241, 1970.

Kelham, R. L.: Some thoughts on mental effects of amputation. Br. Med. J. 1:334, 1958.

Kemph, J. P.: Renal failure, artificial kidney and kidney transplant. Am. J. Psychiatry 122:1270, 1966.

Kimball, C. P.: Psychological responses to the experience of open heart surgery. I. Am. J. Psychiatry 126:348, 1969.

Kübler-Ross, E.: On Death and Dying. London, Macmillan, 1969.

Kübler-Ross, E.: Crisis Management of Dying Persons and their Families. In Resnik, H. L. P., and Ruben, H. L. (eds.): Emergency Psychiatric Care. Bowie, Md., Charles Press, 1975.

Levy, N. B.: Coping with maintenance hemodialysis — psychological considerations in the care of patients. In Massry, S. G., and Sellers, A. L. (eds.): Aspects of Uremia and Dialysis. Springfield, Ill., Charles C Thomas, Publisher, 1976.

Pasternak, S. A.: When a patient wants to sign himself out. Hosp. Physician 5:120, 1969.

Renneker, R., and Cutler, M.: Psychological problems of adjustment to cancer of the breast. J. Am. Med. Assoc. 148:833, 1952.

Sutherland, A. M., et al.: The psychological impact of cancer and cancer surgery. Cancer 5:857, 1952.

Taylor, B. W., Litin, E. M., and Litzow, T. J.: Psychiatric considerations in cosmetic surgery. Mayo Clin. Proc. 41:608, 1966.

Titchener, J., et al.: Psychological reactions of the aged in surgery. Arch. Neurol. Psychiatry 79:63, 1958.

Weisman, A. D.: Thanatology. In Freedman, M., Kaplan, H. T., and Sadock, B. J. (eds.): Comprehensive Textbook of Psychiatry. II. Baltimore, Williams & Wilkins Co., 1975.

Weisman, A. D., and Hackett, T. P.: Psychosis after eye surgery. N. Engl. J. Med. 258:1284, 1958.

I. THE PHYSICALLY ABUSED PATIENT

Jean-Pierre Lindenmayer and Nathan S. Kline

THE VICTIM OF RAPE

Victims of forcible rape, who have been reported in increasing numbers over the past several years, present the physician with several issues when they arrive at the Emergency Department or his office. Usually, the victims are female and vaginal intercourse has been completed or (less frequently) attempted by the rapist. Occasionally, anal intercourse or oral sex also is reported. The victim has been both physically and emotionally traumatized, and often appears in a state of shock or disbelief, with feelings of humiliation, anxiety, anger, and self-accusation. She may express these feelings by crying or agitation, or may hide them under a withdrawn affect. A prominent fear mentioned is that of physical violence and death. The victim's body may show bruises and lacerations on arms, neck, throat, legs, and around the genitals. This acute phase of disorganization is observed during the hours immediately following the rape.

A second phase of reorganization begins about two to three weeks after the attack. This two-phase reaction has been identified and described as the "rape trauma syndrome," and is seen as an acute stress reaction to a life-threatening situation (Burgess and Holmstrom, 1974). It is important to understand that rape is primarily an aggressive, rather than sexual, act and the victim reacts to it with anger but is helpless to do anything about it. During the first phase, the victim tends to blame herself for having contributed in some way to the attack, by not having been careful enough; during the second phase, however, she often suffers anxiety attacks, phobias, hypochondriasis, or depression.

Only rarely does the rape occur in response to a provocative woman, yet this explanation continues to dominate, and often prevents professionals involved in rape cases from giving nonjudgmental and appropriate treatment. As far as possible, the physician should be objective and compassionate in his approach. In particular, careful physical and psychologic data should be gathered and documented for possible subsequent presentation in court if legal proceedings are initiated by the victim. In any event, the physician should be aware of the local laws pertaining to the reporting of rape cases to the authorities.

Management

(1) *Establish rapport with the victim.* The physician should first attempt to create an atmosphere of calm and privacy in which the patient feels safe and can ventilate her feelings. A room should be found where doctor and patient can be undisturbed, and overzealous policemen who may be involved in the case should be kept away. Interrogations by the police should be delayed until the patient has calmed down sufficiently to tolerate them.

(2) *Establish the circumstances of what happened.* The physician should ask for the details of the rape in a noncritical and empathic fashion. The patient should be encouraged to express her feelings about what has happened. An important area to clarify is what the victim means by "rape" and if it really has occurred. Other areas of the patient's life also should be explored briefly, such as her sexual and social functioning and her relationship with her family. The patient's fears and apprehensions about how the rape will affect her life also should be inquired into. Finally, the patient should be prepared for the physical examination. She should be told what kind of examination she will be given and what its purpose is. Written permission usually is required. If photographs are required as evidence, the victim should be so informed and should be told why they are needed (Polak, et al., 1975).

(3) *The physical examination.* A careful and tactful physical examination should be carried out, and all findings fully recorded. Bruises and lacerations in the genital area should be noted carefully, as well as the findings of the vaginal examination. Smears should be made to test for the presence of sperm and gonorrhea.

(4) *Medical treatment.* Preventive treatment against venereal disease and pregnancy should be discussed with the patient. If such measures are indicated, they should not be instituted until written consent has been obtained from the patient, and should in-include:

(*a*) appropriate antibiotic therapy to prevent venereal disease;

(*b*) diethylstilbestrol, 50 mg. daily for five days, to abort the possible pregnancy;

(*c*) a pregnancy test.

If the anxiety of the patient has not been sufficiently relieved by the interview with the physician, a minor tranquilizer may bring relief (e.g., benzodiazepam, 10 mg. p.o., chlordiazepoxide, 25 mg. p.o., or meprobamate, 800 mg. p.o.).

(5) *Legal implications.* It is understandable that victims often are reluctant to report the offense to the authorities, but the physician should encourage them whenever possible to do so. He also should be aware of the additional burden these contacts with the law create for the patients. Furthermore, since the physician may be called to testify in court, he should obtain consent for all his measures, and carefully record the history and all findings. It also is important to document in writing all transfers of specimens. All slides should be marked with an etching pencil; a fresh slide should be examined for the presence of spermatoza, and a note made of their mobility.

(6) *Disposition.* The patient should be informed of the results of the examination in a tactful fashion. In particular, she should be reassured that she is physically intact and that she will be able to enjoy normal intercourse at some future date (Halleck, 1962). She also should be advised of the need for medical follow-up, if indicated. On the emotional side, the patient should be referred for crisis counseling, if this is available. If there is evidence of serious psychopathology, either as a reaction to, or present before the rape, psychiatric consultation definitely is indicated.

Throughout the physician's contacts with the patient, her family or companions should be involved and kept informed, subject to her agreement. In particular, the follow-up plans should be discussed with them, and it should be emphasized that the patient will need support in the weeks to come. If the rapist is known to them, they may have to be counseled against any retribution other than through legal channels.

THE VICTIM OF VIOLENCE

There often is little time in busy Emergency Departments to care for the emotional needs of victims of violence. It is obvious that surgical and medical interventions have priority in order first to stabilize vital functions. However, once this is accomplished, it is important that the physician's attention should focus also on how the patient is coping with the impact of the crisis. Often, the patient who has been exposed to violence may be in a state of shock or emotional numbness, showing apathy and withdrawal. There can be a feeling of helplessness, a sense of utter fragility, and the dread that one will remain in fear continuously. The patient also may manifest self-accusation or express rage and the wish to take revenge. In the older age-groups, patients may be puzzled and frightened by what has happened to them. Except for this latter group, most of these reactions are usually self-limited and require only some immediate crisis intervention.

Management

The patient should have an opportunity to ventilate his feelings about the attack and its circumstances. Through appropriate interventions by the physician, there should be clarification of the *real* and *imagined* impact on the patient's life by the attack and the injuries from it. The physician also should make certain that the police have been appropriately notified. The family or friends should be informed when appropriate in order to arrange for them to come to the Emergency Department to assist the patient. If the patient lives alone, other arrangements should be made so that he can spend the first few days and nights after the assault with relatives or friends. If the patient has not been able to regain emotional control, immediate psychiatric consultation should be considered. This is particularly indicated for the elderly patient, who may remain confused and perplexed and develop a depression. Follow-up of these patients is important, either through the psychiatric consultant or through social service.

References

Burgess, A. W., and Holmstrom, L. L.: Rape trauma syndrome. Am. J. Psychiatry *131*:9, 981, 1974.

Halleck, S.: The physician's role in management of victims of sex offenders: J.A.M.A. *180*:273, 1962.

Polak, P. R., Reres, M., and Fish, L.: The Management of Family Crises. *In* Resnik, H. L. P., and Ruben, H. L. (eds.): Emergency Psychiatric Care. Bowie, Md., Charles Press, 1975.

Chapter 53

EMERGENCY DIAGNOSIS AND MANAGEMENT OF INFECTIOUS DISEASE

Frank Calia and Theodore Woodward

GENERAL CONSIDERATIONS

Patients with symptoms and signs of infection present frequently at Emergency Departments. Proper diagnosis and management of such patients are among the most formidable challenges faced by the Emergency Physician. While most infectious conditions are minor and many are self-limited, clinical judgment must be developed to detect the patients whose conditions may be life-threatening.

Also, assessment of the dynamics of an infectious condition is essential to identify those patients whose condition will worsen without more extensive treatment, or hospitalization in some instances. For example, of the many children presenting with a "croup" condition (larnygo-tracheo-bronchitis), a decision must be made as to which case might increase in severity to the point of severe respiratory embarrassment, requiring hospitalization or even tracheostomy. Similarly, of the many adults presenting with a complaint of "sore throat," it is essential to detect the more serious peritonsillar abscess, life-threatening Ludwig's angina, or epiglottitis. To illustrate further, while identification and initiation of treatment for an underlying source of infection (e.g., kidney, lung) may be all that are necessary, it can be life-saving to identify those patients—albeit rare—with gram-negative bacteremia or sepsis.

Such clinical decisions must be made after necessarily limited patient contact and a relatively limited data base. Results of cultures are rarely available for the Emergency Physician, although it is his responsibility to initiate suitable testing and cultures. Because initiation of treatment, based on limited data, might be necessary, reasoning as to the likely organism involved and its antibiotic sensitivity is often required.

Throughout this chapter the "problem-oriented" approach is used. This involves a sequence of initial description followed by a sequence of subjective symptoms, objective signs, assessment, and treatment plan. This format is particularly applicable in this section, since such patients present at emergency units with nondifferentiated symptoms and signs.

Some specific organ system infections are covered elsewhere in the book. Such discussions include cardiovascular infections (p. 952), central nervous system infections (pp. 506, 518, and 1362), and gastrointestinal infections (p. 988). Of course, infectious disease is so ubiquitous that it overlaps most other areas.

UPPER AIRWAY INFECTIONS

Infections of the upper airway can cause great discomfort and morbidity. Wherever these infections produce obstruction of the respiratory tract, they may also threaten life.

Laryngo-tracheo-bronchitis

Laryngo-tracheo-bronchitis, commonly occurring in childhood, is caused by a variety of viruses, including the parainfluenza and respiratory syncytial (RS) viruses. Infection with RS virus is especially common in children under 1 year of age. On occasion, influenza virus, adenovirus, and the enterovirus have been implicated. This syndrome is especially dangerous in young children because their upper airway is narrow and may become obstructed suddenly.

SUBJECTIVE FEATURES

Fever and breathlessness are typical. Parents note that the child has noisy respiration, cough, and wheezing. Coryza and hoarseness occur frequently.

OBJECTIVE FEATURES

Temperature elevation, tachypnea, respiratory stridor, cyanosis, and intercostal, supersternal, and supraclavicular retractions may be prominent. Pharyngeal inflammation and a boggy, swollen nasal mucosa with copious discharge are also common. Wheezing, rhonchi, and rales may be heard on auscultation of the chest. Chest roentgenograms may reveal atelectasis and/or pulmonary infiltrates.

ASSESSMENT AND PLAN

The diagnosis is based on the clinical findings. This syndrome must be distinguished from other conditions that present with breathlessness including epiglottitis, diphtheritic laryngitis, and peritonsillar abscess. The causative organism may be isolated from respiratory tract secretions or pharyngeal washings, and specific viral antibody titers are elevated in convalescent serum. These laboratory tests are usually unnecessary and are rarely useful to the clinician.

Therapeutic efforts are aimed at maintenance of an adequate airway and hydration. Humidification of the inspired air is helpful in preventing inspissation of tracheobronchial secretions. A portable humidifier that produces an aerosol spray may be used in the home. Children who appear cyanotic, physically exhausted, or moribund should be hospitalized. Such patients should be placed in a croup tent, which provides oxygen and humidification. If adequate oxygenation is not achieved, the use of an intermittent positive pressure respirator may be necessary. Rarely, nasotracheal intubation or tracheostomy must be performed. If dehydration is prominent, intravenous administration of fluids is indicated. Antibiotics are ineffec-

tive. Glucocorticoids and epinephrine have been used to relieve airway obstruction, but their value has not yet been proved. Racemic epinephrine given by nebulizer offers some symptomatic relief.

Peritonsillar Abscess

Peritonsillar abscess is an infrequent complication of streptococcal pharyngitis and tonsillitis. The infection extends from the palatine fossa through the tonsillar capsule into the surrounding connective tissue of the neck. Once this loose connective tissue is infected, suppuration and abscess formation follow. Although the initial infection is caused by group A streptococcus, the abscess results from secondary invasion with anaerobic organisms, including *Bacteroides*, *Fusobacterium*, and *Peptostreptococcus*.

SUBJECTIVE FEATURES

The patient has symptoms compatible with pharyngitis, i.e., sore throat, pain on swallowing, fever, and large tender anterior cervical lymph nodes. With the development of a peritonsillar abscess, pain and fever increase abruptly and swelling of the neck on the affected side appears. Patients have difficulty opening their mouths because of pain. Dizziness and syncope are occasionally seen.

OBJECTIVE FEATURES

The patient's breath has an offensive, putrid odor. The involved tonsil and anterior pharyngeal pillar are markedly swollen and extend toward the midline. An area of fluctuance may be palpated within this swollen mass. The anterior cervical nodes are markedly enlarged and tender.

ASSESSMENT AND PLAN

Group A streptococcus may be isolated by throat culture. Attempts to isolate anaerobic bacteria by culture are of little value. These organisms constitute the normal pharyngeal flora, and their recovery from purulent material does not distinguish colonization from actual invasion. Treatment should be directed to the group A streptococcus and the anaerobes that are sensitive to penicillin. Procaine penicillin G, 1.2 million units given

I.M. twice daily for a minimum of 10 days, is the treatment of choice. Benzathine penicillin is effective therapy for streptococcal pharyngitis but inadequate treatment for peritonsillar abscess.

Fortunately, most abscesses drain spontaneously. On occasion, incision and drainage are required. Surgical and spontaneous decompression prevent the development of a serious complication–septic thrombophlebitis of the deep cervical veins.

Ludwig's Angina

Ludwig's angina, a gangrenous cellulitis of the floor of the mouth, may be initiated by a number of conditions. The most common are dental infection, mandibular fractures and other maxillofacial injuries, and lacerations of the floor of the mouth. The infection originates in the area around the submaxillary gland and extends into the sublingual or submaxillary spaces without salivary gland or lymph node involvement. Because the cellulitis spreads along the fascial planes of the head and neck, there is the potential for acute upper respiratory tract obstruction. For this reason, Ludwig's angina has been known historically as *morbus strangulatorius*.

SUBJECTIVE FEATURES

A recent history of a facial injury or of a dental procedure, usually involving the molars, is typical. The patient complains of fever and the rapid onset of swelling of the neck and face, which may cause difficulty in breathing.

OBJECTIVE FEATURES

There is massive cervical-facial swelling, especially anteriorly. The swelling tends to be brawny; fluctuance is uncommon. The tongue enlarges and protrudes, and the floor of the mouth is elevated. Evidence of a recent dental extraction or an injury may be present. Visualization of the posterior pharynx is usually impossible. Cyanosis, dyspnea, and stridor may be prominent.

ASSESSMENT AND PLAN

This is a life-threatening situation necessitating the immediate establishment of an airway. Distortion of the upper respiratory tract is usually so severe that direct laryngoscopy and intubation may produce severe laryngeal spasm and sudden death. Immediate tracheostomy should be performed under local anesthesia. In the event that purulent material is available at the focus of infection, a specimen should be obtained for aerobic and anaerobic cultures. Needle aspiration of a tooth socket or the subperiosteum may yield an appropriate specimen. Contamination of this specimen with oral secretions invalidates the culture results. Bacteria recovered from purulent material from patients with Ludwig's angina include *Staphylococcus aureus*, group A streptococcus, oropharyngeal anaerobic organisms, and aerobic gram-negative bacilli.

Once the airway is established, antimicrobial therapy should be instituted. A combination of clindamycin, 600 mg. 3 times daily, and gentamicin, 5 mg./kg. B.W./day administered I.M., provides adequate coverage. If aerobic gram-negative bacilli are not isolated, gentamicin may be discontinued. The early institution of antibiotic therapy may obviate the need for incision and drainage. *It should be emphasized that the critical part of early management is the establishment of an adequate airway.* A delay in the performance of a tracheostomy in order to administer antibiotics or obtain culture material may result in death.

EPIGLOTTITIS

Epiglottitis, an acute bacterial infection of the epiglottis, typically is a disease of childhood, with a peak incidence in children between 2 and 7 years of age. On occasion, the infection is encountered in adults and as such is a life-threatening infection. The enlarged edematous epiglottis acutely obstructs the upper airway. A delay in diagnosis and treatment results in death from anoxia. *Hemophilus influenzae* type B is the most common etiologic organism; occasionally, *Staphylococcus aureus* and *Streptococcus pneumoniae* have been incriminated.

SUBJECTIVE FEATURES

Sore throat, dysphagia, and low-grade fever develop acutely. At this point, the disease is indistinguishable from many other types of upper respiratory tract illness. These symptoms may persist for 3 to 4 days.

Dysphagia grows worse, saliva leaks from the side of the mouth, and the child's voice becomes muffled. The parents note the rapid development of respiratory stridor.

OBJECTIVE FEATURES

The child is agitated and has a muffled cry. Respirations are labored, and stridor is audible without a stethoscope. Cyanosis and drooling may be prominent. A "bull neck," the result of soft tissue swelling, may be evident, as may erythema and edema of the oropharynx and the base of the tongue. Indirect laryngoscopy reveals an enlarged, boggy, reddened epiglottis with diminution of the glottic aperture. On occasion, the swollen epiglottis is visualized without a laryngoscope.

ASSESSMENT AND PLAN

If the mortality rate of epiglottitis is to be lowered, it is critical that the clinician entertain the diagnosis, perform the necessary laryngoscopy, and rapidly implement medical and surgical therapy. Lateral roentgenograms of the neck may substantiate the presence of edema; however, attempts to obtain roentgenograms needlessly delay treatment. Once this diagnosis is ascertained by physical examination and laryngoscopy, tracheostomy should be performed immediately. Blood cultures usually are positive, and the causative organisms may also be isolated on culture of the larynx. These cultures should be obtained but only after tracheostomy. Intravenous ampicillin, 200 mg./kg. B. W./day, is the treatment of choice. Chloramphenicol, 50 mg./kg. B. W./day, given intravenously may be substituted for ampicillin in patients allergic to penicillin or in communities where ampicillin-resistant *Hemophilus* strains are encountered. Methicillin or other penicillinase-resistant penicillins should be used if *Staphylococcus aureus* is recovered from blood cultures. Any of the manifestations of bacteremia may be encountered, including hypotension. Therapy for this is outlined in the section on gram-negative bacteremia.

DIPHTHERIA

Most of the clinical manifestations of diphtheria are due to a potent exotoxin, which is elaborated by the causative organism, *Corynebacterium diphtheriae*. This toxin is lethal to mammalian cells following absorption and penetration into the cell. Antitoxin blocks absorption but is ineffective once penetration has occurred. Toxin production occurs at the site of bacterial multiplication and disseminates by way of the blood stream. Initially, a patchy exudate develops at the site of infection, most commonly in the oropharynx. Infection also may arise in the nasopharynx and skin wounds. The exudate is transformed rapidly into a membrane composed of necrotic tissue, inflammatory cells, blood, and fibrin. Membrane formation may extend to involve the tonsils, the nasopharynx, the larynx, and the trachea. The membrane is associated with considerable local edema and hemorrhage. If the edema and the membrane encroaches on the respiratory passages, lethal anoxia is a potential danger. Following dissemination, the toxin also affects the neurologic and cardiovascular systems, but this occurs relatively late.

SUBJECTIVE FEATURES

Previously immunized patients may have few symptoms such as low-grade fever and mild throat pain. The unimmunized patient has a moderate fever, moderately severe to severe pharyngeal pain, swelling of the neck with cervical adenopathy, and a nonproductive cough. If the primary site of infection is the nasopharynx, the patient may complain of a serosanguineous nasal discharge. In the infant and child, stridor is a clue to impending obstruction of the upper respiratory tract.

OBJECTIVE FEATURES

The oropharynx is edematous and mildly erythematous. Severe pharyngeal erythema suggests a concomitant group A streptococcal infection. The extreme cervical lymphadenopathy may produce a "bull neck" appearance. The classical lesion is the diphtheritic membrane, which is gray to black. Removal of a portion of this membrane results in considerable bleeding from the bed of the ulceration. The membrane may be restricted to the nasopharynx in the nasopharyngeal form of the disease or may spread there from the oropharynx. When the membrane extends into the larynx, there is severe hoarseness. If the trachea is involved, respiratory embarrassment becomes evident with tachypnea, sternal retractions, respiratory stridor, and cyanosis.

ASSESSMENT AND PLAN

Microscopic examination of the exudate obtained with a throat swab or of a piece of membrane may reveal the etiologic organism; a methylene blue or toluidine blue stain can be used. Pleomorphic, deep blue bacilli containing metachromatic granules are characteristic. Because this is an uncommon disease in the United States, few clinicians are sufficiently experienced in identifying *C. diphtheriae*. Consequently, culture of the exudate utilizing an appropriate medium, i.e., Loeffler's tellurite agar, should be performed.

Maintenance of an airway and institution of antitoxin and antimicrobial therapy are basic to treatment. Any compromise of the airway necessitates the performance of an emergency tracheostomy. Antitoxin therapy serves to neutralize unfixed toxin and prevents additional local tissue necrosis. Since antitoxin is derived from horse serum, allergic reactions develop in at least 10 per cent of patients. Fortunately, serum sickness and delayed hypersensitivity reactions are more common than is anaphylaxis. Prior to antitoxin administration, a conjunctival or skin test for hypersensitivity to horse serum should be performed. An immediate wheal-and-flare reaction should identify those patients likely to develop anaphylaxis. Epinephrine should always be on hand at the bedside whenever antitoxin is administered. In the event that the conjunctival or skin test is positive, desensitization must be performed. Patients with mild to moderate disease should receive 30,000 to 40,000 units of antitoxin injected intramuscularly. In severe disease, twice this dose is required, half of which should be given in a slow I.V. infusion. Procaine penicillin G, 600,000 units, should be given intramuscularly daily for 2 weeks. Erythromycin, 2 gm./day orally for a period of 2 weeks, is also effective.

LUNG INFECTIONS

Bacterial Pneumonia

Bacterial pneumonia is an infection of the lung caused by bacterial invasion. Evidence suggests that the infection develops following aspiration of infected secretions from the upper respiratory tract. Normally, the lung is protected from aspiration and infection by the epiglottal reflex, cilia, respiratory tract mucus, the cough reflex, and phagocytic cells (fixed and mobile). Conditions that alter or overwhelm these defenses and predispose to pneumonia include cerebrovascular disease, neuromuscular disease involving the chest, general anesthesia, alcoholism, soporific drugs, viral respiratory infections, cystic fibrosis, pulmonary edema, prolonged bed rest, cigarette smoking, inhalation of noxious gases, uremia, and immunodeficiency disease.

The clinical manifestations of bacterial pneumonia are determined by the nature of the invading organism, the condition of the host, and the host-parasite relationship. The classical expression of pneumonia is that kindled by *Streptococcus pneumoniae*. Improved techniques for identifying the etiologic organism have shown that many other species of bacteria, including several once considered nonpathogenic, are capable of causing pneumonia.

SUBJECTIVE FEATURES

One or more of the many predisposing conditions may be present. The symptoms associated with these conditions, e.g., coryza, sore throat, and malaise, precede those of pneumonia; however, an abrupt alarming change occurs with the development of pneumonia. The patient is aware of the sudden onset of a striking, shaking chill and sustained fever. Rigor may be recurrent. A productive cough develops shortly after the chill. The sputum may be frankly purulent, rust-colored, or bloody. If the inflammatory process extends to the pleural surface, pleuritic chest pain is prominent. As the infection evolves, shortness of breath may progress to air hunger.

OBJECTIVE FEATURES

An elevated temperature is most often present, although fever may be absent in the chronic alcoholic or the patient receiving corticosteroids. Splinting of the chest accompanies pleuritic pain. Flaring of ala nasi during inspiration indicates respiratory distress. With lobar involvement inspiratory rales and signs of consolidation (i.e., bronchial breathing, increased tactile fremitus, and dullness to percussion) are present. Findings of consolidation are absent in bronchopneumonia, but inspiratory rales are prominent. Evidence of pleural fluid, dullness to percussion, decreased tactile fremitus, and absent breath sounds may be noted when empyema or a sterile effusion complicates the pneumonia. A pleural friction rub is heard when the inflammatory process extends to the pleural surface, and when the sign is accompanied by an effusion, empyema can be suspected. Cyanosis becomes prominent as more of the lung becomes involved. A putrid odor of the patient's breath and sputum suggests a necrotizing pneumonia and/or lung abscess.

Posteroanterior and lateral chest roentgenograms reveal opacification of the lung in a lobar, segmental, or patchy distribution. Whereas the chest film is seldom diagnostic of a specific organism, it may be suggestive. In infants under 1 year of age, the presence of single or multiple pneumatocoeles suggests *Staphylococcus aureus* pneumonia. In the adult, lung abscess and empyema are common in staphylococcal pneumonia. Beta-hemolytic streptococcal pneumonia commonly is associated with the rapid development of a pleural effusion. *Klebsiella* pneumonia typically involves the upper lobes, and because of the gelatinous nature of the exudate, there is a gain in volume of those segments. On the lateral chest roentgenogram, a characteristic convex bulging of the major fissure may be seen. Single or multiple abscesses are characteristic of necrotizing pneumonia, which may be caused by aspiration of oral aerobic and anaerobic organisms and aerobic gram-negative bacilli (e.g., *Pseudomonas aeruginosa*, *Serratia marcescens*).

Leukocytosis is common but not invariable. With extensive lung involvement, respiratory acidosis and hypoxia may be present.

ASSESSMENT AND PLAN

Identification and isolation of the etiologic organism are mandatory if the physician is to select an antibiotic rationally. Microscopic examination of a Gram stain of an adequate sputum specimen allows the rapid, tentative identification of the organism. A preponderance of buccal squamous cells in the specimen suggests that saliva has been stained. Such specimens contribute nothing of interpretable value. The presence of polymorphonuclear and broncial epithelial cells in the specimen assures the clinician that the material is from the lower respiratory tract.

Gram-positive, lancet-shaped diplococci are suggestive of *Streptococcus pneumoniae*; clusters of large gram-positive cocci suggest *Staphylococcus aureus*; small pleomorphic gram-negative coccobacilli, indicate *Hemophilus influenzae*; large encapsulated gram-negative bacilli indicate *Klebsiella pneumoniae*; and a mixture of gram-positive cocci and gram-negative bacilli, with or without tapered ends, suggests upper respiratory tract aerobic and anaerobic organisms which are believed to cause aspiration-induced pneumonia. A specimen of sputum should be forwarded to the diagnostic microbiology laboratory to corroborate the impression gained on viewing the Gram stain. Unfortunately, many of the organisms that are capable of causing pneumonia may be part of the normal oropharyngeal flora. Therefore, isolation of the organism from sputum does not confirm its pathogenic role. Not infrequently, patients are severely dehydrated and adequate sputum may be difficult to obtain. Rapid rehydration may be of considerable help; however, valuable time may be lost when the patient is moribund. Percutaneous transtracheal aspiration may provide an adequate sputum specimen from such patients. There are dangers associated with the use of this procedure, and it is contraindicated in the patient with a bleeding tendency, marked hypoxia, or an uncontrollable cough. This procedure also may be helpful with patients with suspected superinfection pneumonia or those who fail to respond to antibiotics. Transtracheal aspiration allows specimens to be obtained from the lower respiratory tract uncontaminated by secretions and flora of the upper respiratory tract. Although this procedure has been recommended for patients with aspiration pneumonia and/or lung abscess, it is not mandatory, since the causative organisms are usually penicillin-sensitive.

A minimum of two blood cultures should be obtained from all patients with suspected bacterial pneumonia. Because pleural fluid may reveal the organism on Gram stain and may yield it on culture, thoracentesis should be performed on all patients with pneumonia and pleural effusion. This has therapeutic value as well. Recovery of an organism from blood or pleural fluid establishes its etiologic role.

Posteroanterior and lateral chest roentgenograms should be performed routinely. In this way, the diagnosis of pneumonia can be substantitated, important clues as to the etiologic agent identified, and the presence of pleural effusion ascertained. Pneumonic tularemia should be suspected in hunters, trappers, and laboratory workers, especially when bronchopneumonia is accompanied by severe headache and a normal white blood cell count. Sputum examination is not helpful, but *Francisella tularensis* may be recovered from cultures of sputum, blood, and gastric washings. Special media are required; routine media will not support the growth of this organism. The diagnosis of this disease is usually based on the development of agglutination titers.

TREATMENT

Pneumococcal pneumonia in young adults without significant underlying disease may not require hospitalization. The majority of patients, however, are at the extremes of age and have underlying complicating diseases; these patients should be hospitalized. Proper hydration and aeration are important aspects of therapy which frequently are overlooked. Intravenous fluid replacement and oxygen supplementation may be necessary. Significant empyema should be drained by a chest tube. The development of antimicrobials had a major impact on the morbidity and mortaility rates associated with pneumonia. The selection of an antibiotic is determined by the species of bacteria causing the infection. Pneumococcal pneumonia may be treated with aqueous procaine penicillin G, 600,000 units intramuscularly every 12 hours for 7 to 10 days. This is adequate therapy as well for meningococcal, beta-hemolytic streptococcal, and aspiration pneumonia. The presence of empyema calls for higher doses of aqueous penicillin. Cephalosporins or erythromycin may be used in patients allergic to penicillin. *Staphylococcus aureus* pneumonia should be treated with a penicillinase-resistant penicillin; methicillin, 12 gm./day, or nafcillin, 8 gm./day, intravenously. A cephalosporin antibiotic may be substituted in patients allergic to penicillin. *Hemophilus influenzae* pneumonia is treated with ampicillin, 4 to 6 gm./day intravenously. With usual precautions, chloramphenicol, 3 gm./day orally or intravenously, may be used for penicillin-allergic patients or when ampicillin-resistant strains are encountered. *Klebsiella* pneumonia is treated with gentamicin, 5 mg./kg. B.W./day in 3 divided doses given intramuscularly. Another antimicrobial may be given in addition to gentamicin. Chloramphenicol, 3 gm./day, or cephalothin, 6 to 8 gm./day in combination with gentamicin, may have synergistic activity against this organism. This presupposes that the organism is sensitive to the cephalosporin or chloramphenicol. *Pseudomonas* pneumonia is treated with a combination of gentamicin, 5 mg./kg. B.W./day intramuscularly in 3 divided doses, and carbenicillin, 30 to 40 gm./day intravenously.

Nonbacterial Pneumonia

Pneumonia may be caused by a variety of nonbacterial microorganisms including viruses, mycoplasmas, rickettsiae, fungi, and chlamydiae. The manifestations of infection with any of these organisms are so similar as to be indistinguishable on clinical grounds alone. The symptom complex is sufficiently different from that encountered in bacterial pneumonia, however, as to be recognizable as a distinct clinical entity. For this reason, the syndrome is referred to as primary atypical pneumonia to distinguish it from bacterial pneumonia. The most common etiologic organisms are *Mycoplasma pneumoniae*, adenovirus, parainfluenza virus, influenza virus, respiratory syncytial virus, *Coxiella burnetii*, and *Chlamydia*. Primary atypical pneumonia is acquired by the respiratory route.

SUBJECTIVE FEATURES

The illness occurs most frequently in young adults, especially under conditions of crowding as encountered in boarding schools and military installations for training recruits. There is an insidious onset of malaise, sore throat, nasal congestion with rhinorrhea, and low-grade fever. A chilling sensation may be prominent, but a frank rigor is unusual. A nagging nonproductive cough develops early. As the infection evolves, scanty quantities of sputum are produced. The sputum tends to be mucoid but may be purulent. Blood streaking of sputum may be noted, but true hemoptysis is uncommon. Pleuritic chest pain is unusual, although substernal burning is a frequent complaint. Certain clues may point to the etiologic agent. Q fever occurs in those who have contact with domestic animals or following laboratory exposure. Ornithosis follows exposure to a wide variety of birds, including psittacine birds (parrots, parakeets) as well as ducks, pigeons, turkeys, and chickens. Adenovirus and mycoplasmal infections are common in military recruits. Pneumonia due to *Histoplasma capsulatum* may develop following exposure to bird droppings, and *Coccidioides immitis* occurs in individuals exposed in the proper geographic setting (California, Utah, New Mexico, Arizona, Texas, and areas in Central and South America). Erythema nodosum may accompany pulmonary infection with these fungi.

OBJECTIVE FEATURES

In contrast to patients with bacterial pneumonia, the patient does not appear to be acutely ill, and the temperature is elevated only modestly. The nasal mucosa and pharynx may be edematous and erythematous. Examination of the lungs may be unremarkable, although scattered, moist, inspiratory rales are common. Evidence of consolidation is found rarely. The chest roentgenogram is usually more impressive than the physical examination. Extensive infiltration may be present on the x-ray despite normal physical findings. Patches of bronchopneumonia radiating from the hilus and involving one or more lobes are typical. The lower lung fields tend to be more involved than the upper. Minimal pleural effusions are present in a small percentage of patients. The white blood cell count may be elevated, normal, or depressed.

ASSESSMENT AND PLAN

The identification of the specific cause of the primary atypical pneumonia syndrome is based on the serologic response to infection. Approximately 50 per cent of patients with *Mycoplasma* pneumonia develop significant cold agglutination titers and may develop also a false positive biologic test for syphilis. The more specific tests are based on the development of positive indirect immunofluorescent and complement fixation antibody titers. The organism may be isolated from nasopharyngeal cultures, but it is fastidious and grows slowly. For this reason, the diagnosis is based on specific serologic tests.

Patients with ornithosis develop a significant rise in the specific complement-fixing antibody titer. Although the organism, a chlamydia, may be recovered on culture, few clinical laboratories are capable of isolating it. Q fever produces a rise in the complement-fixing and agglutinating antibody titers. Although the rickettsia, *Coxiella burnetii*, may be recovered on culture, it is extremely contagious and presents a hazard in the clinical laboratory. The fungal diseases caused by *Histoplasma capsulatum* and *Coccidioides immitis* are confirmed by identifying a rise in complement-fixing antibody titers. The viral pneumonias may be detected by isolation of the virus or the serologic response to infection. Because chemotherapy of viral pneumonias is ineffective, neither procedure is helpful to the clinician in treatment.

TREATMENT

The majority of patients are young adults without underlying disease and not severely ill. Most may be treated without hospitalization and many without chemotherapy. An attempt should be made to distinguish *Mycoplasma* pneumonia, Q fever, and ornithosis from other causes of primary atypical pneumonia syndrome. These organisms are sensitve to the broad-spectrum antibiotics tetracycline and chloramphenicol. In addition, *Mycoplasma pneumoniae* is sensitive to erythromycin. These drugs shorten the period of convalescence. Response to chemotherapy is frequently dramatic in patients with early ornithosis but not in patients with *Mycoplasma* pneumonia or Q fever. Antibiotics are ineffective in the treatment of primary atypical pneumonia caused by viruses or fungi. The syndrome produced by *Histoplasma* and *Coccidioides* is usually an acute self-limited disease and does not require therapy with antifungal agents. The overall prognosis for patients with primary atypical pneumonia is excellent.

INTRA-ABDOMINAL INFECTIONS

Peritonitis

Inflammation of the peritoneum may be induced by chemical irritation or bacterial invasion. Chemical peritonitis may follow the introduction of bile, gastrointestinal fluid, pancreatic secretions, or blood into the peritoneal cavity. Primary bacterial peritonitis is a consequence of hematogenous seeding of the peritoneum with organisms from an inapparent source. Predisposed are patients with ascites due to cirrhosis or nephrotic syndrome. Primary peritonitis usually is caused by a single species of bacteria, most commonly *Streptococcus pneumoniae*, members of the Enterobacteriaceae, *Pseudomonas*, or alpha- and beta-hemolytic streptococci. Secondary bacterial peritonitis, which is the more common, is due to entry into the peritoneal cavity of organisms from within the gastrointestinal tract or from the external environment. Any process that interrupts the integrity of the gastrointestinal tract or the abdominal wall may give rise to secondary bacterial peritonitis. Therefore, trauma, intra-abdominal infection, mesenteric vascular insufficiency, gastrointestinal neoplasms, and the postoperative state are common predisposing factors. The most common entities are perforated peptic ulcer, appendicitis, cholecystitis, intestinal obstruction, diverticulitis, colonic carcinoma, salpingitis, and abdominal trauma. A mixed chemical and bacterial peritonitis may occur when both irritants are introduced into the peritoneal cavity, e.g., perforated peptic ulcer. Secondary bacterial peritonitis invariably is caused by multiple species of organisms that usually are derived from the gastrointestinal tract. These include the anaerobes *Bacteroides*, *Fusobacterium*, peptostreptococcus, peptococcus, and *Clostridium* and the aerobes *Escherichia coli*, *Proteus*, *Klebsiella*, *Enterobacter*, *Pseudomonas*, and group D streptococcus. Peritonitis arising from the female genital tract may be due to any of the above-mentioned organisms in addition to *Neisseria gonorrhoeae* and various strains of aerobic streptococci.

SUBJECTIVE FEATURES

Patients note the acute onset of abdominal pain, fever, and chills. Symptoms associated with the underlying cause of the peritonitis are also typical, e.g., nausea, vomiting, and jaundice with acute cholecystitis; chronic constipation and weight loss with carcinoma of the colon. The location of the pain may suggest the underlying cause, e.g., right lower quadrant pain in acute appendicitis.

OBJECTIVE FEATURES

Findings include elevated temperature, abdominal distention, diffuse and/or localized tenderness, rebound tenderness, rigidity of the abdominal wall, and decreased or absent bowel sounds. Such findings tend to be less prominent in infants, the elderly, alcoholics, and patients who are receiving steroids or who have ascites. Localized tenderness may be elicited on vaginal or rectal examination as well as abdominal examination and suggests involvement of an underlying viscus. Leukocytosis is typical but may be absent.

ASSESSMENT

Results of simple laboratory procedures may help determine the underlying cause. Examination of the stool for gross or occult blood, studies of liver function, determination of serum amylase concentration, and a supine and an upright flat plate roentgenogram of the abdomen are helpful. The roentgenograms may reveal free air in the peritoneal cavity, gas in an abdominal abscess, evidence of ileus, obliteration of the psoas shadows, calcification within the gallbladder, or evidence of peritoneal fluid. Paracentesis should be performed when physical findings are consistent with the diagnosis of peritonitis in a patient with ascites. Ascites tends to dilute the inflammatory nature of the response to infection. The protein concentration and cell count in ascitic fluid may be lower than expected with peritonitis. Nevertheless, the fluid usually contains a white blood cell count in excess of 300/cu. mm., a predominance of polymorphonuclear cells, and an elevated protein concentration. The amylase concentration in ascitic fluid is elevated in patients with pancreatitis. Microscopic examination of a Gram stain of fluid sediment may reveal the causative organism. The fluid should be cultured in aerobic and anaerobic media. Blood cultures also may yield the organism.

PLAN

Primary peritonitis is best treated with antibiotics alone. This is a diagnosis by exclusion; evidence of inflammation and/or infection of an intra-abdominal structure other than the peritoneum must be absent.

Since the organisms most commonly incriminated are the pneumococcus and aerobic gram-negative bacilli, the treatment of choice is a combination of penicillin G, 4 million units in divided doses every 6 hours given intravenously, and gentamicin, 5 mg./kg. B.W./day in 3 divided doses given intramuscularly. Once the specific etiologic organism is identified, the unnecessary drug may be discontinued.

Secondary peritonitis requires surgical intervention, rehydration, and chemotherapy. Because enteric anaerobes and aerobes usually are involved in the inflammatory process, a combination of clindamycin or chloramphenicol and gentamicin is the treatment of choice. The dosage of gentamicin is the same as that for primary peritonitis; for chloramphenicol the dosage is 3 gm./day given intravenously every 6 hours, and for clindamycin it is 1.8 gm./day given intramuscularly every 8 hours. Surgery should be performed as soon as fluid replacement and antimicrobial therapy have been initiated and the patient is stabilized. The objective of surgery is to excise, drain, or isolate the source of the infection.

Subdiaphragmatic Abscess

Subdiaphragmatic abscesses are closed space, suppurative processes that usually follow spread of infection from within the peritoneal cavity. The right subdiaphragmatic space is involved more frequently than the left. An abscess may be a complication of abdominal surgery, intra-abdominal infection, or intestinal perforation. Common underlying diseases are perforated peptic ulcer, appendiceal abscess, biliary tract infection, and pelvic inflammatory disease. Rarely, an abscess is secondary to hematogenous spread of organisms from an extra-abdominal focus.

SUBJECTIVE FEATURES

The onset is insidious. Complaints may be minimal and include low-grade fever, anorexia, weight loss, pain in the upper abdomen or lower chest and singultus. With diaphragmatic irritation shortness of breath, cough, and shoulder pain are prominent. Recent surgery or symptoms consistent with peptic ulcer or gallbladder or pelvic inflammatory disease should alert the clinician.

OBJECTIVE FEATURES

Findings are usually unimpressive. Fever is low-grade to moderate, sustained or intermittent. Examination of the lungs on the involved side may reveal rales or findings consistent with a pleural effusion or an elevated diaphragm. Upper quadrant abdominal tenderness may be noted. Leukocytosis is common.

ASSESSMENT

A subdiaphragmatic abscess always must be suspected in a patient with unexplained fever and recent intra-abdominal surgery or infection. Chest and abdominal flat plate roentgenograms frequently are helpful. An elevated diaphragm on the involved side, pleural effusion, or gas-fluid level may be seen. When the abscess is on the left side, an upper gastrointestinal series may demonstrate displacement of the stomach. Fluoroscopic examination of the chest may reveal immobility of the diaphragm. A simultaneous liver-lung scan can identify the location of the abscess by defining a significant space between the liver and lung.

PLAN

A subdiaphragmatic abscess may be life-threatening when there is a delay in diagnosis and treatment. Transperitoneal or transthoracic drainage of the pus must be accomplished. Chloramphenicol or clindamycin and gentamicin should be administered. The dosages and schedules are identical to those recommended for secondary peritonitis. Aerobic and anaerobic cultures of exudate obtained at surgery may yield the causative organisms. Determination of the antibiotic sensitivity of these bacteria may dictate a modification of chemotherapy.

Cholangitis

Inflammation of the bile ducts is the result of bacterial invasion following ductal obstruction. Choledocholithiasis, strictures of the bile duct, or carcinoma of the ampulla or head of the pancreas may be the cause of this obstruction. The etiologic organisms are usually those that reside in the gastrointestinal tract.

SUBJECTIVE FEATURES

The symptoms are those of biliary obstruction and infection. Patients complain of acute severe right upper quadrant colicky pain, jaundice, frank rigors, and fever. Dark urine and acholic stools also may be noted.

OBJECTIVE FEATURES

Fever is marked and paroxysmal. Jaundice is usually prominent. Hepatomegaly is accompanied by extreme right upper quadrant tenderness and guarding. The presence of a palpable gallbladder suggests carcinoma of the ampulla or head of the pancreas (Courvoisier's sign). Shock and other signs consistent with vasomotor collapse indicate bacteremia. Laboratory abnormalities include leukocytosis and elevated serum concentrations of transaminase, bilirubin, and alkaline phosphatase.

ASSESSMENT

The high mortality rate of acute cholangitis underscores the need for immediate therapy. Diagnostic procedures should be completed rapidly, since surgery cannot be delayed. Liver function studies and blood cultures should be obtained on admission. Roentgenographic studies are seldom of value. A flat plate roentgenogram of the abdomen may reveal calcification within the gallbladder or gas bubbles in the biliary tree. Contrast studies usually fail to visualize the biliary tract, and their performance needlessly delays surgery. As soon as the diagnosis is established clinically, surgical drainage must be performed after stabilization of the patient with antibiotics and fluids. The extent of the surgery should be kept to a minimum, the objective is to establish drainage of the biliary tract. Definitive surgery can be performed at a later date. Fluid and electrolyte replacement is critical, especially in the hypotensive patient. Antibiotic therapy should be instituted prior to surgery. Chloramphenicol or clindamycin plus gentamicin is the treatment of choice. If organisms are isolated from blood cultures or from purulent biliary drainage, unnecessary antimicrobials may be discontinued. It must be re-emphasized that treatment is surgical; medical therapy alone should not be attempted.

Hepatic Abscess

Liver abscesses may be caused by enteric bacteria or amoebae, although the latter have become less common in the United States in recent years. Pyogenic liver abscesses may complicate biliary tract infections, penetrating or nonpenetrating abdominal trauma, systemic bacteremia, and pylephlebitis in the appendiceal area or arise by direct extension from contiguous areas of infection. Amoebic liver abscesses are a complication of intestinal amoebiasis.

SUBJECTIVE FEATURES

The history and symptoms may reflect the underlying cause, e.g., recent abdominal trauma or surgery, biliary colic, or right lower quadrant pain. Presenting complaints are shaking chills, right upper quadrant pain of an aching quality, and fever. Nausea, vomiting, weakness, malaise, dyspnea, cough, night sweats, and pleurisy may be present. In addition, patients with amoebic liver abscess may complain of chronic diarrhea which may be bloody.

OBJECTIVE FEATURES

A sustained or intermittent fever is associated with an enlarged, tender liver. Icterus may accompany an amoebic or pyogenic liver abscess. Signs of pleural effusion, rales, abdominal distention, and ascites are found on occasion. A hepatic friction rub is characteristic but noted in only a small percentage of cases.

ASSESSMENT AND PLAN

As the mortality rate of liver abscess is considerable, prompt diagnosis and therapy are mandatory. A series of diagnostic tests is necessary to confirm the diagnosis. The chest roentgenogram, particularly a lateral view, may reveal an elevated and immobile diaphragm. Liver function abnormalities are common and include elevated serum concentrations of hepatic enzymes and bilirubin. Radioisotope liver scans utilizing gallium or technetium and abdominal angiography are most helpful. Liver abscesses may be multiple and small, however, and difficult to visualize even with these techniques. When an abscess is identified by scanning and/or angiography, a needle aspiration may be attempted. Liquid material, if obtained, should be subjected to careful analysis and cultured in aerobic and anaerobic media. A foul smell suggests the presence of anaerobes. Examination of a Gram stain of the aspirate may reveal polymorphonuclear cells and bacteria. If bacteria are identified, the diagnosis of pyogenic liver abscess is established. Although the aspirate of an amoebic liver abscess classically resembles anchovy paste, it at times may be serosanguineous or purulent. Amoebae should be sought in an unstained specimen, but unfortunately, they are demonstrated in fewer than 50 per cent of cases of amoebic liver abscess. The presence of trophozoites of *Entamoeba histolytica* in the stool is suggestive but does not establish the diagnosis of amoebic liver abscess. Elevated antibody titers for *E. histolytica* are always present in patients with invasive amebiasis including liver abscess. The diagnosis is based on a positive liver scan and elevated specific antibody titers. On occasion, amoebae and bacteria may be recovered from the same abscess.

Pyogenic liver abscesses should be treated surgically. Abdominal exploration and transperitoneal drainage of the abscess as well as surgical treatment of the underlying condition (e.g., gallbladder disease, appendicitis with pylephlebitis) are required. The organisms usually incriminated in pyogenic liver abscesses are aerobic and anaerobic enteric organisms including *Clostridium* species, *Bacteroides*, microaerophilic streptococci, and Enterobacteriaceae. Liver abscesses arising hematogenously may yield *Staphylococcus aureus* or group A streptococci. A combination of clindamycin or chloramphenicol and gentamicin begun at the time of surgery is appropriate therapy. Cultures of abscess fluid aspirated prior to surgery may yield the causative organisms and allow the clinician to select specific antimicrobials. Similarly, postoperative culture results may dictate changes in chemotherapy. Multiple small pyogenic abscesses do not lend themselves to aspiration, surgical drainage is impossible, and empiric antibiotic therapy may suffice. Definitive surgery of the underlying cause, however, may be required.

Small amoebic abscesses do not require aspiration and respond well to chemotherapy. Large amoebic abscesses may require

needle aspiration as well as antiamoebic drugs. The drug of choice is metronidazole, 750 mg. given 3 times a day for 10 days. For children, the dosage is 35 to 50 mg./kg. B.W./24 hours in 3 divided doses for 10 days. Emetine hydrochloride is also effective and gives reliable results. Surgery is seldom indicated and may be dangerous in the event the abscess fluid spills into the peritoneal cavity.

Pancreatic Abscess

Pancreatic abscesses are severe, life-threatening infections which may follow a number of intra-abdominal events. An abscess may be a complication of pancreatitis due to alcoholism or gallbladder disease, may be a sequela of perforated duodenal ulcer, may follow abdominal trauma including pancreatic and peptic ulcer surgery, or may arise from secondary infection of an existing pseudocyst. Organisms reach the pancreas by contiguity or hematogenously. The bacteria in a pancreatic abscess are predominantly enteric organisms.

SUBJECTIVE FEATURES

A history consistent with pancreatitis or abdominal trauma is common. In addition, patients note the acute onset of high fever, severe abdominal pain, nausea, and vomiting. These symptoms may represent an exacerbation of pancreatitis or a pancreatic abscess.

OBJECTIVE FEATURES

Temperature elevation usually is marked. Signs of ileus and abdominal tenderness over the abscess are typical. The serum amylase, alkaline phosphatase, and bilirubin concentrations may or may not be elevated.

ASSESSMENT AND PLAN

An elevated diaphragm, atelectasis, and/or pulmonary effusion may be noted radiologically. When gas-forming organisms are present in the abscess fluid, abdominal roentgenograms may reveal a "soap bubble" suggestive of retroperitoneal abscess. Radiologic contrast studies may be helpful. An upper gastrointestinal series may demonstrate displacement of the stomach anteriorly, widening of the duodenal loop, or duodenal obstruction. A barium enema may silhouette displacement of the transverse colon or splenic flexure. Depression of the left kidney may be evident on intravenous pyelography. Ultrasonography may identify a collection of fluid within the pancreas. None of these findings distinguish a pancreatic abscess from a pseudocyst. High fever, leukocytosis, and positive blood cultures are highly suggestive of pancreatic abscess. Since bacteremia may accompany pancreatic abscess, blood cultures should be obtained routinely. Occasionally, abscesses rupture into the peritoneal cavity causing generalized peritonitis. Perforation into a hollow viscus including the colon, duodenum, stomach, biliary tree, or bronchus also occurs. This complication is attended by considerable hemorrhage. Erosion into a major vessel in the abdomen also may produce intra-abdominal hemmorrhage. Death commonly follows all these complications. Rupture of an abscess into the pleural space may produce empyema.

Early surgical intervention is critical. Drainage through a transperitoneal approach may prevent the development of potentially lethal complications. The recovery of enteric organisms in over 90 per cent of cases suggests that the combination of clindamycin or chloramphenicol and gentamicin is the treatment of choice. In the event that *Staphylococcus aureus* is involved, an antistaphylococcal penicillin is recommended as well. Pancreatic abscesses cannot be treated with antibiotics alone. Surgical decompression is necessary to prevent rupture.

INFECTIONS OF THE KIDNEY

Acute Pyelonephritis

Acute pyelonephritis is an inflammatory reaction involving the renal parenchyma and pelvis and is initiated by bacterial invasion. The kidney becomes infected by one of several mechanisms. Most frequently, pyelonephritis is the result of an ascending infection arising in the lower urinary tract. Normally, bacteria colonize only about the urethra and its distal third. Under certain circumstances, these organisms may migrate into the bladder. Evidence suggests that these bacteria usually are opposed by local defenses and are voided. Occasionally, however, these resistance mechanisms are ineffective and lower tract infection is established. Women are especially prone to infection because the urethra is short and subjected to repeated trauma during intercourse. Hematogenous spread of bacteria to the kidney is also an established mechanism of infection, although it is less common than the ascending route. Occasionally, pyelonephritis results from extension of infection from the contiguous area Finally, lymphatic spread of bacteria to the kidney has been postulated but not documented.

Numerous factors promote urinary tract infection. Obstruction to urinary flow, be it anatomic or physiologic, is an extremely important predisposing factor. In infancy, pyelonephritis is more common in males, reflecting the greater incidence of congenital abnormalities with resultant obstruction of the urinary tract in neonatal males. Benign prostatic hypertrophy, bladder neck obstruction, neurogenic bladder, congenital ureteral and urethral valves, stones, cystoceles, urethral strictures, and neoplasms are common predisposing conditions for the same reason. The presence of a foreign body within the urinary tract is another common predisposing factor. Catheterization and instrumentation of the urinary tract frequently introduce infection. Finally, diabetes mellitus, multiple pregnancies, and hypertension have been associated with an increased incidence of pyelonephritis.

The common causative organisms are those that normally reside in the gastrointestinal tract and colonize the perineum. *Escherichia coli* is recovered from the urine of 85 to 90 per cent of patients with urinary tract infection. This is followed in frequency by *Klebsiella, Proteus, Enterobacter, Pseudomonas*, group D streptococcus, *Staphylococcus aureus*, and *S. epidermidis*. Despite the fact that anaerobic organisms compose the major flora of the gastrointestinal tract, they are uncommon causes of urinary tract infections and pyelonephritis.

A positive correlation has been found between clinical manifestations and pathologic findings when the concentration of enteric organisms in urine is in excess of 100,000 organisms per milliliter, and therefore, this level is considered indicative of significant bacteriuria. The concentration that constitutes significant "bacteriuria" in staphylococcal and candidal infections has not yet been established. Significant bacteriuria is not synonymous with pyelonephritis. Bacteriuria establishes the presence of a bacterial infection of the urinary tract; it does not reflect the site of infection (upper or lower tract).

SUBJECTIVE FEATURES

Patients may be asymptomatic or gravely ill. Typically, fever, shaking chills, and pain in the involved costovertebral angle are present. Nonspecific symptoms such as nausea, vomiting, and headache may be prominent. Complaints referable to lower tract involvement—i.e., urgency, frequency, dysuria, pyuria, hematuria, and nocturia—may also occur. Indeed, patients may present exclusively with lower urinary tract symptoms despite involvement of the kidney. Colicky costovertebral pain and high fever in patients with diabetes suggest acute papillary necrosis associated with pyelonephritis.

OBJECTIVE FEATURES

Temperature elevation and tenderness to percussion over the costovertebral angle or angles may be noted. Bacteria may gain entry into the circulation and produce the clinical manifestations of gram-negative bacteremia including hypotension; cold, clammy skin; and oliguria. Patients with papillary necrosis especially are prone to this complication.

ASSESSMENT AND PLAN

Examination of the urine must be performed. Mild proteinuria is typical. Microscopic examination of the urinary sediment reveals an increased number of white blood cells, often occurring in clumps. Microscopic hematuria may also be noted and is customary with diffuse involvement of the bladder. White blood cell casts in the sediment suggest pyelonephritis. Pieces of renal medullary tissue may be seen in the urinary sediment of patients with papillary necrosis.

The diagnosis of urinary tract infection is based on the presence of significant bacteriuria. A clean midstream urine specimen should be obtained for culture. Quantification of organisms in this specimen is easily performed by the clinical laboratory. However, speciation and quantification may require a minimum of 48 hours. The clinician himself should perform a simple laboratory procedure that may identify significant bacteriuria prior to the culture report. A Gram stain of fresh, clean, unspun urine should be examined microscopically. A good positive correlation has been found between the presence of organisms in a Gram stain of an unspun urine specimen with a colony count of greater than 10^5 bacteria per milliliter of urine.

Intravenous pyelography should be performed on males of any age and on females with recurrent infection in order to identify predisposing factors such as obstruction. Pyelography usually is not required during the first few days of therapy unless an acute obstruction is suspected. Roentgenologic findings vary considerably; excretory urography may be unremarkable, or one of the many causes of urinary tract obstruction may be apparent. A history of recurrent infections usually is associated with dilatation and blunting of the calyceal system and perhaps with repeated attacks a reduction in the size of the renal cortex and kidney itself. The excretory urogram in acute papillary necrosis reveals reduced kidney size as well as cavities and sinuses in the areas of the renal papillae.

TREATMENT

The goal of therapy is to eliminate the causative organism and to relieve obstruction and other predisposing factors. Antimicrobial therapy is aimed at the former. Patients whose urinary tract infections arise in a nonhospital setting are assumed to be infected with E. coli or other antibiotic-sensitive organisms. A variety of antimicrobials administered orally can be recommended. These agents include ampicillin, 2 to 4 gm./day, tetracycline, 2 gm./day, or chloramphenicol, 2 to 3 gm./day, in 4 divided doses given every 6 hours. If the organism may have been acquired in the hospital or the patient has a history of multiple urinary tract infections, then drugs with a wider spectrum of antibacterial activity should be used. It is likely that the infecting organisms in such circumstances will be resistant to the more commonly used antibiotics. Gentamicin, 3 to 5 mg./kg. B. W./day in 3 equal divided doses given every 8 hours intramuscularly, is recommended. Once the organism has been identified and its sensitivity pattern has been determined, modification of therapy may be required. This may involve changing to a drug to which the organism is sensitive or changing to a less toxic drug.

Elimination of obstruction is of considerable importance. Insertion of a catheter or performance of a nephrostomy or other surgical procedures may be required. The ultimate objective is to relieve obstruction permanently.

Renal Carbuncle

A renal carbuncle is an abscess occuring within the kidney. Most commonly, it arises following hematogenous spread of *Staphylococcus aureus* from a distant focus. Infections of the skin, endocardium, or lungs are the most common foci. On occasion, infections may be due to enteric aerobic bacilli or rarely to anaerobes.

SUBJECTIVE FEATURES

Patients usually complain of fever, chills, and pain in the lumbar or flank areas. Typically lower urinary tract symptoms are absent. Symptoms referable to the underlying focus, e.g., painful furuncle, may be present.

OBJECTIVE FEATURES

A temperature elevation with tachycardia and localized pain over the costovertebral angle are usually the only findings.

ASSESSMENT AND PLAN

Clinically, renal carbuncle mimics acute pyelonephritis. In contrast to acute pyelonephritis, however, the urinary sediment is unremarkable. Unless the carbuncle ruptures into the renal pelvis, urine cultures are sterile. The absence of pyuria and bacteriuria in this symptom complex should alert the physician. Blood cultures may yield the etiologic agent and should be obtained in all suspected cases. Radiologic studies are required to establish the diagnosis. A flat plate roentgenogram of the abdomen may be unremarkable and may reveal intact psoas shadows and normal appearing diaphragms. The kidney border may be obscured, however; and on occasion, a gas-fluid level is seen within the renal parenchyma when the carbuncle is caused by gas-forming, gram-negative aerobic or anaerobic bacilli. Intravenous pyelography may demonstrate an intrarenal mass resembling a tumor or cyst with blunting, dilatation, and stretching of the pelvocalyceal system. Renal angiography will distinguish a carbuncle from other renal masses.

TREATMENT

Early incision and drainage of the carbuncle are mandatory. Administration of antimicrobials is important adjunctive therapy. If the distant focus of infection is consistent with a staphylococcal infection, e.g., furuncle, then a penicillinase-resistant penicillin, e.g., methicillin, 12 gm./day or a cephalosporin or cephalothin, 8 gm./day, given intravenously, is recommended. A gas-fluid level in the carbuncle suggests gas-forming organisms. Such patients should receive a combination of clindamycin or chloramphenicol and gentamicin. In the absence of an obvious focus or a gas-fluid level, clindamycin and gentamicin provide adequate coverage for the potential pathogens. Once the etiologic organisms are identified from cultures obtained at surgery, the unnecessary drug may be discontinued, or therapy altered accordingly.

Perinephric Abscess

A perinephric abscess is a suppurative infection within the perirenal fascia external to the renal capsule. Infections usually arise hematogenously, and a primary focus of infection is usually obvious. Carbuncles and infections of the tonsils and prostate are typical primary foci. *Staphylococcus aureus* and group A streptococcus are the more common etiologic organisms. Recently, gram-negative bacilli and anaerobes including *Escherichia coli*, *Proteus*, *Klebsiella*, *Enterobacter*, *Bacteroides*, peptostreptococcus, and *Clostridium* species have been incriminated in increasing frequency. Perinephric abscesses may also arise following rupture of a renal carbuncle into the perinephric space. Direct extension of infection from a nearby source, such as an appendiceal abscess or infected gallbladder, may also produce a perinephric abscess. Predisposing factors include obstructive renal disease, diabetes mellitus, and glucocorticoid therapy.

SUBJECTIVE FEATURES

The onset is usually insidious. Patients complain of low-grade fever occurring over several weeks accompanied by pain and a bulging mass in the flank. The pain may radiate anteriorly into the right upper and lower abdominal quadrants or may be referred to the hip or thigh. Characteristically, it is aggravated during extension of the thigh while walking and is relieved by flexion of the hip. Nausea, vomiting, and weight loss are common, whereas lower urinary tract symptoms such as dysuria, frequency, and urgency are uncommon.

OBJECTIVE FEATURES

There is evidence of fever and localized flank tenderness. A bulging mass may be palpated on the involved side. If the abscess drains spontaneously, a cutaneous sinus tract may be evident. Spasm of the paravertebral muscles may result in scoliosis.

ASSESSMENT AND PLAN

Microscopic examination of the urinary sediment usually reveals pyuria but is unremarkable in up to one-third of the cases. Fifty per cent of patients will have significant bacteriuria, i.e., 10^5 or more organisms per milliliter of urine. As a consequence, urine cultures should be obtained.

Radiologic studies help to establish the diagnosis. A flat plate roentgenogram of the abdomen may reveal absence of the psoas shadow and blurring of the renal outline. Gas-forming organisms will produce air bubbles within the abscess. Intravenous pyelography demonstrates immobility of the kidney, incomplete filling of the calyces, pelvocaliectasis, poor renal function, or displacement of the kidney and ureter. Leakage of contrast material into the perinephric space during intravenous or retrograde pyelography is virtually diagnostic. Occasionally, a fistula between the perirenal space and the related infected focus, e.g., appendiceal abscess, is visualized. Chest roentgenograms may reveal an elevated diaphragm on the involved side with or without associated pleural effusion and pulmonary atelectasis.

TREATMENT

Despite its insidious onset, perinephric abscess is life-threatening. Often the abscess ruptures into the peritoneal space of the pleural cavity and produces diffuse peritonitis or empyema. Early incision and drainage prevent such catastrophic complications. Surgical therapy of the source of infection or of urinary tract obstruction may also be required. Occasionally nephrectomy must be performed. As *Staphylococcus aureus*, streptococcus, Enterobacteriaceae, and anaerobes are the most common organisms recovered from perinephric abscesses, clindamycin and gentamicin in combination provide effective therapeutic coverage. The results of Gram stain and culture of purulent material obtained at surgery may dictate a modification of the antimicrobial regimen.

PELVIC INFECTIONS IN THE FEMALE

Salpingitis and Oophoritis

Salpingitis and oophoritis, bacterial infections of the fallopian tubes and ovaries respectively, are commonly associated with infections of the endometrium and pelvic peritoneum. Multiple recurrences and relapses are common. Eventually pathologic alterations of the tubes, ovaries, and uterus develop, consisting of edema, anatomic distortions, and loss of peristalsis of the fallopian tubes, which become filled with purulent material and obliterated with adhesions, resulting in eventual scarification and loss of function. These changes may extend to the ovaries. Abscess formation within the tubes and ovaries is common. The adnexa become large, swollen, and amorphous, occasionally rupturing and causing peritonitis. As a result, the entire pelvic region may become matted with adhesions.

Several species of bacteria may cause salpingo-oophoritis, and infection may arise by one of several mechanisms. *Neisseria gonorrhoeae* are involved in approximately 40 per cent of these infections. The remainder are caused by *Bacteroides* species, peptococci, peptostreptococci, aerobic streptococci, and *Staphylococcus aureus*. Mixed infections are common. Nongonococcal infections may be acquired venereally. *Neisseria gonorrhoeae* may have initiated the inflammatory reaction and pathologic-anatomic changes. Subsequent to the elimination of this organism by normal body defense mechanisms, there is a secondary infection with organisms that are part of the vaginal flora. Infections may also develop postpartum or after abortion. Also, they may arise by hematogenous spread from a distant focus or contiguous spread from a nongenital infection, e.g., ruptured appendix, diverticulitis, perforated peptic ulcer, or infected Meckel's diverticulum.

SUBJECTIVE FEATURES

The usual complaints are fever, generalized malaise, severe bilateral lower quadrant abdominal pain, and dyspareunia.

OBJECTIVE FEATURES

Fever, tachycardia, and bilateral lower quadrant tenderness are present. Pelvic examination reveals marked tenderness, and indistinct masses may be palpated in the adnexal regions. Movement of the cervix and uterus produces exquisite pain. If endometritis accompanies salpingo-oophoritis, considerable purulent material may be seen in the cul-de-sac.

ASSESSMENT AND PLAN

The diagnosis is a clinical one. The endocervix and rectum should be cultured for *Neisseria gonorrhoeae* on selective media. Blood cultures should also be obtained. Cultures of vaginal secretions for anaerobes are valueless, since these organisms are part of the normal flora. If surgery is required, purulent material aspirated from the abscess should be cultured for aerobic and anaerobic organisms.

Prompt antimicrobial therapy minimizes the destructive effect of infection on the tubes and ovaries. Infertility and ectopic pregnancies may be prevented. A delay in treatment may result in the development of hydro- and pyosalpinx, tubo-ovarian abscess, pelvic thrombophlebitis, peritonitis, infertility, or multiple relapses. Hospitalization usually is warranted for all patients except those with mild disease. This latter group may be treated effectively with oral tetracycline, 2 gm./day, or ampicillin, 2 to 4 gm./day, for 7 to 10 days. Usual initial treatment for gonorrhea is 4.8 million units of procaine penicillin, I.M., and probenecid (Benemid), 1 gm. orally. Patients with moderate to severe infections require more intensive therapy. Penicillin G, 8 to 12 million units/day given intravenously, plus clindamycin, 1.8 gm./day, or chloramphenicol, 3 gm./day, provide adequate coverage. Large

pelvic abscesses require surgical incision and drainage. Surgery should be accompanied by antimicrobial therapy.

Acute Endometritis

Acute endometritis, an infection of the uterine lining, varies considerably in its clinical course. At one end of the spectrum, it is a life-threatening infection; at the other end, it progresses to chronicity leading to intrauterine adhesions, infertility, and menstrual irregularities. The fallopian tubes and ovaries may be infected secondarily. Infection may spread from the endometrium to the uterine lymphatics and ultimately to the blood stream. In severe infections, the myometrium becomes involved and pelvic thrombophlebitis is common.

The infection may be acquired venereally (e.g., *Neisseria gonorrhoeae* endometritis) or may complicate a number of gynecologic procedures including dilatation and curettage, endometrial biopsy, insertion of intrauterine contraceptive devices, hysterosalpingography, and uterine sounding. Infection also may follow induced abortions or parturition. Clostridial species are important pathogens in those infections that complicate criminal abortions.

SUBJECTIVE FEATURES

A careful gynecologic history should be taken. Patients complain of fever, chills, and a purulent and/or bloody vaginal discharge. Occasionally irregular uterine bleeding, severe pelvic pain, and dyspareunia are prominent.

OBJECTIVE FEATURES

There is high fever, tachycardia, and marked uterine and cervical tenderness. Purulent or bloody material may fill the cul-de-sac. With florid bacteremia, there may be hypotension and other evidence of hypoperfusion. Pelvic thrombophlebitis may result in septic pulmonary emboli. Tachypnea, wheezing, hemoptysis, a pleural friction rub, and signs of pulmonary consolidation may develop in such patients.

ASSESSMENT AND PLAN

The history and physical findings establish the diagnosis. The endocervix and rectum should be cultured for *Neisseria gonorrhoeae*. Because, in the majority of cases, the causative organisms are those found in the normal vaginal flora, identification of bacteria in vaginal secretions is of no value. Blood cultures should be obtained.

Mild cases of endometritis may subside spontaneously. However, those cases that present to the clinician may be moderately severe or life-threatening. Such patients should be hospitalized. The treatment of choice consists of large doses of intravenous penicillin G plus oral chloramphenicol or clindamycin. Several investigators suggest that gentamicin be administered as well. Gentamicin always is indicated in the presence of shock. Treatment of pelvic thrombophlebitis and pulmonary emboli are discussed in the following section. Occasionally, curettage of the uterine cavity is necessary. Hysterectomy rarely is required.

Septic Pelvic Thrombophlebitis

Septic pelvic thrombophlebitis is a severe life-threatening complication of endometritis. Myometritis and salpingo-oophoritis are common in this group of patients. In addition to vaginal floral organisms, groups A and B streptococci have been implicated. Bacteremia is the rule, and septic pulmonary emboli are common.

SUBJECTIVE FEATURES

Patients present with symptoms consistent with endometritis, i.e., fever, vaginal discharge, menstrual irregularities, pelvic pain, and dyspareunia. Complaints secondary to bacteremia and pulmonary embolism are prominent, including rigor, shortness of breath, wheezing, cough with or without hemoptysis, and pleuritic chest pain.

OBJECTIVE FEATURES

Examination reveals high fever, tachycardia, and tachypnea. With frank pulmonary infarction, ascultatory findings consistent with consolidation and/or pleural effusion are present. Pelvic examination elicits severe pain on motion of the uterus and cervix. Bacteremia may be associated with hypotension and cold, clammy skin. Shock may be due to sepsis or pulmonary emboli.

ASSESSMENT AND PLAN

Blood cultures are usually positive and may reveal multiple organisms. Cultures of the vaginal discharge are of no value. Chest roentgenograms may demonstrate a wedge-shaped area of infiltration and/or pleural effusion. A lung scan showing an area of hypoperfusion in the absence of an infiltrate is diagnostic of pulmonary infarction. When the area of hypoperfusion is superimposed on an infiltrate, angiography is required to distinguish a pulmonary infarct from pneumonia.

Therapy as recommended for endometritis should be instituted, i.e., large doses of intravenous penicillin G plus chloramphenicol or clindamycin. In severely ill or hypotensive patients, gentamicin should also be administered. Treatment of shock is reviewed in the section on gram-negative bacteremia at the end of this chapter. If the diagnosis of septic pulmonary emboli is established, anticoagulation with heparin should be instituted.

Septic Abortion

The syndrome of septic abortion is not limited to criminal abortions but may follow those done under hospital precautions as well. Following removal of the intrauterine contents, endometritis and eventually parametritis may develop. The resident vaginal flora, including *Clostridium perfringens*, aerobic and anaerobic streptococci, and aerobic and anaerobic gram-negative bacilli, is commonly involved. Septic shock and renal failure are frequent complications. Sudden, massive hemolysis of red blood cells, associated with *Clostridium perfringens* and due to a potent exotoxin produced by this organism, contributes to the acute renal failure. Attempts at criminal abortion utilizing the injection of chemical substances including soaps, detergents, and lye into the cervical canal can contribute to the pathologic process.

SUBJECTIVE FEATURES

The abortion precedes the first symptoms by at least 48 hours. The incubation period may be shortened considerably when chemical substances have been used to induce abortion. Patients complain of the acute onset of fever, shaking chills, lightheadedness or syncope, vaginal bleeding, dark urine, and lower abdominal pain.

OBJECTIVE FEATURES

The manifestations of septic shock, including cold, clammy skin, hypotension, fever, tachycardia, and oliguria, are common. Pelvic examination may reveal evidence of attempted instrumentation. Chemical substances may be found in the vagina. A serosanguineous discharge may be present in the cul-de-sac. The uterus is enlarged and extremely tender. Palpable masses in either lower quadrant may represent a tube-ovarian abscess. Peritonitis, a common sequela to uterine puncture during instrumentation, may be evidenced by ileus, guarding, and rebound tenderness.

ASSESSMENT AND PLAN

Air under the diaphragm noted on an upright roentgenogram of the abdomen indicates uterine puncture. Paralytic ileus also may be identified radiologically. Blood cultures should be obtained. A Gram stain of the vaginal discharge revealing organisms consistent with *Clostridium* does not establish the diagnosis because these organisms may be part of the normal flora. Serum electrolytes must be monitored closely, since hypo- or hyperkalemia may develop. Rises in BUN and creatinine concentrations accompany renal failure. The potential for sudden hemolysis requires that hemoglobin concentrations be followed closely. Studies for coagulation defects, including platelet count, prothrombin and thrombin time, fibrin split products and fibrinogen concentrations, are also important. Blood gas determinations are helpful in quantifying metabolic acidosis and anoxia.

Therapy should include fluid replacement for hypovolemia and hypoperfusion, the use of antibiotics, and the removal of retained products of conception from the uterine cavity. Rapid fluid replacement should be monitored with a central venous catheter. A rapidly decreasing hematocrit due to hemolysis signals the need for whole blood replacement. Intravenous penicillin G, 20 to 40 million units/day, intravenous chloramphenicol, 3 to 4 gm./day, and intramuscular gentamicin, 5 mg./kg. B.W./day in 3 divided doses, should be instituted.

Acute renal failure may respond to intravenous mannitol, furosemide, or ethacrynic acid. Once the patient is stabilized, usually within 6 to 12 hours, a careful curettage of the uterus should be performed. This must be done even when most of the retained products have been expelled spontaneously. Septic pulmonary emboli dictate treatment with heparin. Disseminated intravascular coagulation also may be treated with heparin, although the efficacy of anticoagulants in treatment of this entity has not been established. Large intravenous doses of hydrocortisone, 1 to 2 gm., may be given if hypotension does not respond to fluid replacement. This dose may be repeated in 2 to 3 hours. Vasoconstrictors are not recommended, although in the face of persistent hypotension despite adequate fluid replacement and steroid treatment, dopamine may be tried. Oxygen therapy is indicated when hypoxia is prominent. Hyperbaric oxygen therapy has been used in clostridial pelvic infections, but its efficacy has not been established. Care must be taken to maintain renal output. Occasionally, dialysis must be performed. Correction of metabolic abnormalities including hypokalemia may be necessary.

INFECTIONS OF THE SKELETAL SYSTEM

Osteomyelitis

Acute bacterial sepsis of bone may arise by (1) hematogenous spread of infection from a distant focus such as soft tissue or the gastrointestinal, urinary, or respiratory tract, (2) contiguous spread occurring after trauma or surgery, or (3) infection of devitalized tissue produced by vascular insufficiency. The blood-borne route is the most common. Hematogenous osteomyelitis usually develops in rapidly growing bones; consequently, 85 per cent of cases occur in persons under 16 years of age. Infection starts in the metaphysis of long bones as a consequence of the anatomy of the blood supply. Bacteria enter the bone through metaphyseal capillaries and are contained by the epiphyseal growth plate. An acute pyogenic inflammatory response results. A combination of local pH changes, leukocyte migration, microvascular obstruction, and bacterial growth causes necrosis of bone, and secondary infection follows. Organisms also spread through haversian and Volkmann canals. The infection extends laterally and, as pressure builds, perforates the bony cortex, lifts the periosteum, and then spreads subperiosteally. Resulting ischemic necrosis of underlying bone is followed by secondary infection of the damaged bone. The periosteum itself responds by laying down new bone, the involucrum. In the hip and shoulder the synovial capsule reaches beyond the epiphyseal plate. Infection no longer limited by the growth plate may spread into the joint. In infants under 1 year of age, metaphyseal capillaries perforate the epiphyseal growth plate, and infection may spread to the epiphysis. Consequently, septic arthritis and destruction of epiphyseal growth are common in this age group. Coliform organisms commonly cause hematogenous osteomyelitis during the neonatal period; Hemophilus influenzae is responsible in children from about 6 months to 6 years of age; beyond these ages Staphylococcus aureus accounts for greater than 50 per cent of cases; Streptococcus pneumoniae and group A streptococci are incriminated throughout childhood. Patients with sickle cell disease are predisposed to salmonella osteomyelitis.

Osteomyelitis arising from contiguous spread of infection is commonly caused by Staphylococcus aureus. However, mixed infections are common. Enterobacteriaceae, Pseudomonas, group A streptococci, or Staphylococcus epidermidis are recovered from the site of infection with some frequency.

Osteomyelitis complicating peripheral vascular disease typically yields coagulase-negative and -positive staphylococci, many species of streptococci, or members of the Enterobacteriaceae.

SUBJECTIVE FEATURES

The symptoms of acute hematogenous osteomyelitis are attributed to the associated bacteremia and include chills, fever, irritability, and delirium in the young. A history of trauma to the long bones is common. Pain may be well localized and may lead to loss of function of the involved extremity. Patients with osteomyelitis due to trauma or contiguous infection give relevant histories. Erythema, pain, and occasionally purulent exudate are noted at the injury site. A history of claudication, diabetes mellitus, and/or hyper-

tension is typical in patients with osteomyelitis due to peripheral vascular disease. Patients with a history of hypertension usually present with low-grade fever and weight loss.

OBJECTIVE FEATURES

Fever and tachycardia may be the only abnormal physical findings. Localized swelling, tenderness, erythema and/or heat may occur over the area of involvement. Tenderness may be considerably localized and a careful search for it must be conducted. When septic arthritis complicates osteomyelitis, there may be erythema, swelling, and joint effusion. Occasionally, in the absence of septic arthritis, a sympathetic effusion in a nearby joint may be provoked. Local soft tissue infection may be evident when osteomyelitis arises by direct extension. When bone sepsis complicates peripheral vascular disease, a decreased blood supply may be detected by diminished peripheral pulses, rubor, thinning of hair, or superficial ulceration of the extremity.

ASSESSMENT

Bacteremia is present in over 50 per cent of cases of acute hematogenous osteomyelitis. Roentgenograms of bone show few abnormalities early in infection, but within 10 days to 2 weeks changes become manifest. Periosteal elevation and new bone formation occur early; lysis of bone occurs later.

PLAN

Early treatment with antibiotics is mandatory. As S. aureus accounts for the majority of cases of hematogenous osteomyelitis, a penicillinase-resistant penicillin is the drug of choice. Methicillin given intravenously, 200 mg./kg. B.W./day (child) or 12 gm./day (adult), in six divided doses, is appropriate. Other semisynthetic penicillins, such as oxacillin and nafcillin, may be used. For penicillin-allergic patients, cephalothin, 50 mg./kg. B.W./day intravenously, may be substituted. Clindamycin and lincomycin are effective alternative drugs. If the causative organism is penicillin sensitive, Staphylococcus aureus, Streptococcus pneumoniae, or group A streptococcus, then penicillin G, 100,000 units/kg. B.W./day given intravenously, is the treatment of choice. Because *Hemophilus influenzae* is a common pathogen in very young children, ampicillin, 100 to 200 mg./kg. B.W./day given intravenously, should be administered with methicillin until the etiologic organism is identified. For penicillin-allergic children, chloramphenicol, 50 mg./kg. B.W./day given intravenously, may be substituted for ampicillin. When osteomyelitis occurs in the neonatal period, Enterobacteriaceae organisms are suspected and coverage for these groups is required. Gentamicin, 1.5 mg./kg. B.W. given intramuscularly, followed by a maintenance dose of 3 to 5 mg./kg. B.W./day, is appropriate. Chloramphenicol or ampicillin in the above-mentioned dosages is effective treatment for *Salmonella* osteomyelitis. When osteomyelitis arises from a contiguous focus, cultures from local exudate should be obtained. A Gram stain may be helpful in selection of antibiotics. As *Staphylococcus aureus* and gram-negative bacilli are commonly recovered, methicillin and gentamicin provide appropriate coverage pending culture results. A similar selection may be made for patients whose infection complicates underlying vascular disease.

Additional therapy may include needle aspiration of the subperiosteum to remove subperiosteal accumulation of pus. This procedure should be performed under aseptic conditions. Occasionally, when large accumulations of pus are present, incision and drainage of the periosteum may be helpful. Immobilization of the involved extremity relieves pain. In treating patients with contiguous infections, debridement of decubitus ulcers and necrotic tissue or incision and drainage of a soft tissue infection may be helpful. Patients with osteomyelitis caused by vascular disorders frequently must undergo amputation of the affected extremity.

Septic Arthritis

Infections of the joint represent invasion of the synovial membrane and space by bacteria or viruses. Joints are usually infected by hematogenous spread. Occasionally, septic arthritis may complicate contiguous infections, including osteomyelitis. The most common cause of septic arthritis is *Neisseria gonorrhoeae*; the genital tract, rectum, or pharynx serves as the portal of entry. *Staphylococcus aureus* is another common cause of septic arthritis resulting from hemato-genous spread from the endocardium or infected tissue or from contiguous spread from osteomyelitis or soft tissue infections. Meningococcal arthritis may complicate meningococcemia with or without meningitis. *Streptococcus pneumoniae*, *Hemophilus influenzae*, and group A streptococci occasionally cause septic arthritis, and in neonates, gram-negative enteric organisms are causative. Septic arthritis may follow trauma or instillation of contaminated material into the joint space. Patients receiving intra-articular injections of steroids for treatment of rheumatoid arthritis are especially at risk. Salmonella may be recovered from septic arthritis in patients with sickle cell disease. Septic arthritis may complicate acute bacterial endocarditis.

SUBJECTIVE FEATURES

The classical manifestations of inflammation are pain, heat, swelling, loss of function of the joint, fever, and chills. Gonococcal arthritis occurs most often among male homosexuals and women; initiating events may be pregnancy or menstruation. A painful exanthema on the extremities is common. Patients with nongonococcal septic arthritis often manifest an infective site such as pneumonia, endocarditis, or meningitis.

OBJECTIVE FEATURES

Swelling, heat, tenderness, and loss of joint function are present. Two clinical varieties of gonococcal arthritis consist of a septic form and a nonseptic form. The septic form is a migrating polyarthralgia without significant objective articular findings, associated with fever and characteristic skin lesions. Lesions are small, erythematous, tender maculopapules, usually less than 10 in number, occurring on the extremities characteristically in the periarticular regions. These lesions may eventually become vesicular or pustular and ultimately develop into small necrotic ulcers. Hemorrhagic bullae may accompany gonococcal arthritis. The nonseptic form is characterized by a true arthritis, usually attacking one or two joints. Systemic manifestations of infection may be absent, and skin lesions are uncommon. Tenosynovitis occurs with either type of gonococcal arthritis. Large joints that are involved include the wrists, ankles, and elbows.

Patients with nongonococcal septic arthritis have similar joint findings and fever with tachycardia, indicating sepsis. Occasionally the presence of serious underlying causes of infection may be suggested by disseminated petechial rash in meningococcemia, peripheral signs of bacterial endocarditis, or clinical findings consistent with meningitis or pneumonia.

ASSESSMENT

Blood cultures, which may yield the etiologic agent, are positive in about 50 per cent of cases of septic forms of gonococcal arthritis. After scraping the surface, skin lesions occasionally yield organisms by smear or culture. Gram stains of exudate may reveal intracellular gram-negative diplococci. Whenever gonococcal arthritis is suspected, cultures of the cervix, rectum, and pharynx should be taken on Thayer-Martin or other selective media.

Arthrocentesis is a most important diagnostic step. Gram staining of synovial fluid often gives preliminary identification of the causative organism, although culture is required for definitive identification. A leukocyte count should be performed by diluting synovial fluid in normal saline; acetic acid should not be used because a mucin clot will be produced and the results will be uninterpretable. In septic arthritis, the synovial fluid count usually exceeds 10,000 cells per cu. mm., with a preponderance of polymorphonuclear leukocytes. A decrease in the glucose concentration is characteristic. Addition of synovial fluid to 2 per cent acetic acid usually produces a small and friable clot (mucin clot test). Microscopic examination of the fluid by polarizing light differentiates crystalline joint disease, i.e., gout or pseudogout, which may mimic septic arthritis. Crystalline joint disease and septic arthritis may coexist in the same joint. A distant focus of infection may yield the etiologic organism in nongonococcal septic arthritis, e.g., meningococci in spinal fluid, staphylococci in soft tissue infection.

PLAN

Early antimicrobial therapy slows, limits, and often arrests the destructive process. The low pH of metabolic end products and proteolytic enzymes of bacteria and leuko-cytes cause lysis of cartilage and ultimate destruction of the joint. Thus, multiple arthrocenteses can be helpful in removing leukocytes and enzymes and will allow the physician to monitor the response to antimicrobial therapy.

Antibiotics are not administered intra-articularly but should be given parenterally. Penicillin is the drug of choice for gonococcal arthritis. Aqueous penicillin G, 10 million units given intravenously for 3 days, followed by ampicillin, 500 mg. 4 times a day orally for a total of 7 additional days, has been used with considerable success. Ampicillin, 3.5 gm. given orally, plus 1 gm. probenecid followed by oral ampicillin, 500 mg. 4 times a day for an additional 7 days, may also be used. For patients allergic to penicillin, tetracycline, 1.5 gm. given orally, followed by 500 mg. 4 times a day for at least 7 days, or erythromycin, 0.5 gm. given intravenously every 6 hours for 3 days, is effective. In treating nongonococcal septic arthritis, the nature and sensitivity of the organism determine which antimicrobial agent should be selected. Meningococcal arthritis should be treated with high doses of penicillin. *Staphylococcus aureus* infections require methicillin or other penicillinase-resistant penicillins. Cephalothin is an effective alternative drug in the face of penicillin allergy. Penicillin is the drug of choice for pneumococcal and group A streptococcal arthritis; ampicillin is preferred for *Hemophilus influenzae* arthritis. For arthritis caused by gram-negative rods, sensitivity testing is especially critical. Gentamicin or tobramycin probably should be started early and continued until sensitivity testing of the organism has been completed. Chloramphenicol is the drug of choice for *Salmonella* arthritis; ampicillin is a reasonable alternative. Surgical incision and drainage of the joint are required only when medical therapy is ineffective or in patients encountered late in the course of the illness with purulent synovial fluid too thick for adequate needle aspiration. An unexplored form of therapy is the use of short-term corticosteroids to cause the inflammatory reaction and the consequent damage to abate. Steroid use requires absolute antibacterial control of the specific microorganism.

Splinting of the joint may ease pain, provided that the cast does not foster neglect by the physician and that there be constant assessment of the therapeutic response.

SOFT TISSUE INFECTIONS IN WHICH ANAEROBIC ORGANISMS HAVE A ROLE

Certain soft tissue infections with specific clinical manifestations on culture yield anaerobic organisms, although aerobic bacteria often are recovered as well. Since bacteremia infrequently accompanies these infections, there is difficulty in ascertaining the causative organisms. Conceivably, aerobic and anaerobic organisms act in concert in generating the soft tissue infections which display a considerable overlap in clinical manifestations. Thus, the majority of these syndromes are probably arbitrary steps in a pathogenetic continuum. The most distinct clinical entity is clostridial myonecrosis, which is usually referred to as gas gangrene.

Gas Gangrene

This syndrome may be caused by several species of *Clostridium; Cl. perfringens* is the most common. These saprophytes are large, gram-positive, anaerobic bacilli, which may contain spores when grown in synthetic media, and are found in soil, dust, the excreta of animals, and the gastrointestinal tract of man. They are usually noninvasive, but given the proper circumstances, these opportunists can initiate infection. The typical setting is tissue necrosis due to trauma, ischemia, or infection with other organisms, especially extensive trauma with soft tissue contamination by soil or excreta (e.g., automobile accidents, war injuries, septic abortions, ischemic vascular disease of the lower extremities or bowel, and surgery of the gastrointestinal tract). Lowering of the oxidation-reduction potential in tissues to a level that supports growth of these bacilli is a major requirement.

Cl. perfringens often is recovered from tissues and may be mixed with other organisms, including anaerobic and aerobic streptococci, staphylococci, Enterobacteriaceae, and *Bacteroides* species. Clostridia produce exotoxins, which facilitate the spread of infection through tissue. They may lyse erythrocytes. Some gram-negative anaerobic and aerobic bacteria produce gas in tissues. Consequently, the presence of gas in soft tissue is not pathognomonic of clostridial infection. Clostridia may colonize wounds without inducing sepsis, indicating that the mere recovery of these organisms does not establish the presence of wound sepsis. The combination of a characteristic clinical syndrome and identification of the organism in exudate does establish the diagnosis. The most life-threatening clostridial infection is myonecrosis (gas gangrene).

SUBJECTIVE FEATURES

Symptoms may develop within several hours, days, or weeks following injury, septic abortion, or surgery of the gastrointestinal tract. The patient notes increased swelling and pain at the site of injury or surgical wound. Serous or serosanguineous material may ooze from the wound.

OBJECTIVE FEATURES

Extremity wounds are the most common site, although incisional wounds following abdominal surgery may be the initial infective site. The gravely ill patient appears diaphoretic and pale. Delirium is common. Fever, if present, is usually low grade. Hypotension and jaundice may occur any time during the clinical course. The wound is very tender on palpation and is edematous; crepitation indicative of gas may or may not be detected, and the quantity of gas is rarely impressive. Bright red or dark brown serosanguineous exudate, occasionally having a sweet odor, may ooze from the wound. Eventually the exudate becomes green or black and the wound may become covered with blebs or bullae. Muscle tissue under the wound is pale and edematous and does not contract normally. When the muscle surface is cut, it has the appearance of fish-flesh and bleeds very little. When there is significant hemolysis, hemoglobinuria occurs.

ASSESSMENT

Gram stain of serosanguineous exudate from the wound usually reveals typical, large, gram-positive rods. Polymorphonuclear cells are absent unless there is superinfection with other organisms. Aerobic and anaerobic cultures of exudate and blood cultures should be obtained. Bacteremia resulting from clostridial soft tissue infections is usual. The hematocrit should be determined both early and frequently, since a precipitous drop may occur at any time. BUN, creatinine, and electrolyte concentration must be evaluated closely. Acute renal failure may result from hypotension or rapid hemolysis.

PLAN

Immediate surgical and medical intervention is necessary. Antibiotics are efficacious. Penicillin G, 10 to 20 million units a day given intravenously, is the drug of choice. Cephalothin, 8 to 12 gm./day, or erythromycin, 4 gm./day, given intravenously may be used in penicillin-allergic individuals. When other potential pathogens are present in the wound, e.g., gram-negative bacilli and gram-positive cocci, clindamycin and gentamicin or chloramphenicol and gentamicin are useful to supplement penicillin.

Surgical treatment is essential and consists of rapid removal of all necrotic and infected tissue. This may require amputation of an extremity or extensive debridement of the anterior abdominal wall. Hysterectomy may be required in septic abortion. The use of hyperbaric oxygen in the treatment of gas gangrene remains controversial. Many surgeons use hyperbaric oxygen prior to surgery in order to decrease the amount of devitalized tissue to be removed. In no circumstances should difficulty in initiating hyperbaric oxygen treatment delay surgical removal of dead tissue. Edema of muscle tissue tightly contained within fascia may further compromise blood supply. Fasciotomy in such situations may protect viable tissue and decrease the extent of debridement or amputation. It is important to distinguish *clostridial myonecrosis* from anaerobic cellulitis, which requires less drastic surgical intervention. Polyvalent antitoxin has been used in the treatment of gangrene, but its efficacy has not been established. Because antitoxin is prepared in horses, serum sickness is a common complication; thus, use of antitoxin is not recommended.

Anaerobic Cellulitis

Anaerobic cellulitis is a superficial infection of connective tissue, characterized by excessive gas formation but associated with very little systemic toxicity. The infection may arise subsequent to a soft tissue injury, such as a human bite, when multiple organisms including anaerobes are inoculated into the trauma site. Mixtures of numerous species of organisms, clostridia, and other anaerobes including peptostreptococci, *Bacteroides* species, and Enterobacteriaceae have been recovered from infected tissues.

SUBJECTIVE FEATURES

The incubation period is longer than in myonecrosis, usually 3 to 4 days. The patient has few constitutional complaints except for edema and local pain.

OBJECTIVE FEATURES

The wound appears dirty and erythematous and exudes a profuse seropurulent exudate with a foul, unpleasant odor. Gas in the soft tissues is evident by crepitation; it diffuses into the subcutaneous tissues and separates muscle groups, although muscle itself is not involved. There is very little pain or wound tenderness. Temperatures may be normal or slightly elevated, but unlike clostridial myonecrosis, there is no delirium and the patient appears generally well.

ASSESSMENT

Gram stain and cultures of the exudate and blood cultures should be obtained. The Gram stain usually reveals a mixture of organisms including gram-negative bacilli, gram-positive cocci, and gram-positive bacilli if clostridia are involved.

PLAN

This infection must be distinguished from myonecrosis in order to avoid unwarranted debridement or amputation. Muscle tissue remains viable in anaerobic cellulitis. The wound should be opened and drained. Occasionally, a fasciotomy is necessary to decompress swollen tissue. Antibiotic therapy is efficacious. Aqueous penicillin G, 10 to 20 million units daily given intravenously, in combination with chloramphenicol or clindamycin should provide appropriate coverage. If gram-negative bacilli are prominent in the Gram stain of exudate, gentamicin or tobramycin should be administered. Fluid and electrolyte abnormalities are less obvious but may merit attention.

Necrotizing Fasciitis

Necrotizing fasciitis is a severe, life-threatening infection of subcutaneous tissues and fascia and may follow surgical procedures or minor perforation of the skin or may arise spontaneously in patients with vascular disease or diabetes mellitus. Although the infection may develop at any site, involvement of the anterior abdominal wall and perineum is common. Aerobic and anaerobic streptococci and *Staphylococcus aureus* are commonly recovered.

SUBJECTIVE FEATURES

Usually there is a rapid onset of fever following trauma or surgery, the incubation period being less than 72 hours. Numbness and hyperesthesia of the skin over the involved fascia are common.

OBJECTIVE FEATURES

The temperature is usually elevated. With the shift of fluid and electrolytes into affected tissues, hypotension and edema of the involved area may be prominent. Delirium is uncommon. Occasionally there is wound crepitation. The overlying skin is necrotic, often with blebs, and may slough off or be lifted away from necrotic fascia, resulting in denudation of skin and subcutaneous tissue.

ASSESSMENT

Basically, the diagnosis is based on the clinical findings. Blood cultures and Gram stain and cultures of the necrotic tissue should be obtained in order to identify the etiologic agents.

PLAN

Early wide excision of all necrotic fascia, skin, and subcutaneous tissue must include the total extent of infection to the point where skin is not undermined. Antibiotic therapy should include large doses of penicillin and/or a penicillinase-resistant penicillin, e.g., 12 to 16 gm. of methicillin and/or 20 million units of penicillin daily. Cephalothin, 8 to 12 gm., may be used in penicillin-allergic individuals. Fluid and electrolyte balance must be maintained.

Synergistic Gangrene

Synergistic gangrene, a slowly progressive indolent infection of skin and subcutaneous tissue, usually follows abdominal surgery. Consequently, the anterior abdominal wall is most commonly involved, although infection may arise in other areas following trauma. Combinations of anaerobic or microaerophilic streptococci, *Staphylococcus aureus*, and gram-negative aerobic bacilli have been incriminated. Indeed, the synergistic contribution of several species of organisms characterizes this type of infection.

SUBJECTIVE FEATURES

A history of recent abdominal surgery or trauma with an extremely painful wound and few systemic complaints typifies this infection.

OBJECTIVE FEATURES

There is a central ulceration of the wound, with gangrenous margins surrounded by a violaceous induration ringed by erythema. The ulceration progresses centrifugally and is exquisitely tender to palpation. Fever, if present, is low grade, and systemic manifestations are uncommon.

ASSESSMENT

Gram stain and culture of the wound should be performed, and blood cultures should be obtained. Large and small gram-positive cocci and gram-negative rods may be noted in stained exudate.

PLAN

Necrotic tissue must be excised. Antibiotic therapy is helpful; a penicillinase-resistant penicillin or cephalosporin may be used. If gram-negative bacilli dominate the Gram stain, gentamicin or tobramycin should be added.

Tetanus

Tetanus is caused by a potent exotoxin elaborated in soft tissue infections by *Clostridium tetani*, an anaerobic spore-forming bacillus. This ubiquitous organism is found in soil, excreta from man and animals, household dusts, and narcotics distributed illicitly. Spores of this organism are capable of resisting some antiseptics and extremes of temperature. Given a favorable environment (i.e., a proper oxidation-reduction potential), spores introduced into injured soft tissue germinate to their vegetative form, which elaborates the exotoxin. Hence, soft tissue trauma, vascular ischemia, and foreign bodies in tissue are predisposing factors. Once elaborated into the circulation the exo- or neurotoxin rapidly binds to gangliosides in the central nervous system and acts much like strychnine. Inhibitory pathways of the motor neurons and interneurons are suppressed, allowing uninhibited excitatory responses of the central nervous system particularly in the brain, spinal cord, and sympathetic nervous system. Any external and certain internal stimuli produce marked neurologic activity affecting muscles and the sympathetic nervous system. Clinical manifestations of tetanus may be generalized or local or may involve only the head.

SUBJECTIVE FEATURES

The incubation period varies from 3 days to 3 weeks (commonly 7 to 10 days after injury) but may be briefer or much longer (several months). A history of penetrating injury is often difficult to elicit with an uncommonly long incubation period. The patient may complain of irritability, headache, and low-grade fever. Local spasm of muscles at the wound site may be unaccompanied by systemic complaints. There may be marked rigidity of the muscle groups involved. Cephalic tetanus usually follows injuries to the head or chronic otitis media. The cranial nerves most often involved are III, IV, VII, IX, X, and XII. Patients may complain of trismus, with an inability to open the mouth or swallow (the so-called "hydrophobia"). Cephalic and local types may progress to generalized tetanus characterized by widespread muscle spasms following any kind of external stimulus.

OBJECTIVE FEATURES

Patients with local tetanus demonstrate obvious spasm of muscle groups about the wound. Similarly, in the cephalic forms, spasm of the facial muscles is obvious. In generalized tetanus, there is trismus charac-

terized by a grotesque distortion of the facial muscles and inability to relax the masseters. A peculiar grin, *risus sardonicus*, often ensues. All muscle groups may be involved, including the abdominal and back muscles. Severe contraction of paravertebral muscles may produce opisthotonos. Painful, exhausting contractions, separated by periods of relaxation, occur in waves lasting from seconds to minutes. These paroxysms are produced by many kinds of external stimuli such as noise, lights, touch, or changes in temperature or internal stimuli produced by a full bladder or distended bowel. Patients may become cyanotic when the thoracic musculature is involved during paroxysms. Involvement of the larynx and glottis may produce severe cyanosis and asphyxia. Characteristically, the patient remains conscious during paroxysms and experiences intense pain accompanied by diaphoresis, fever, and tachycardia. There may be massive sympathetic discharge with severe tachycardia, a labile blood pressure, and arrhythmias.

ASSESSMENT

The diagnosis is based on clinical findings and not on isolation of the etiologic agent. Paroxysms of muscular contractions, trismus, muscle hypertonicity, hyperactive deep tendon reflexes, normal sensory examination, and low-grade fever are characteristic. Isolation of the organism from a wound does not establish the diagnosis, since *Clostridium tetani* may be only a contaminant. Wound cultures may yield *C. tetani* when grown under strictly anaerobic conditions. However, the organism is very fastidious and not commonly isolated. Blood cultures should be obtained, but recovery of the organism is uncommon. There are no significant spinal fluid changes; indeed, lumbar puncture should not be performed on patients with tetanus, since major paroxysms may be stimulated by the procedure. A careful history of previous toxoid immunization should be obtained, since tetanus is uncommon in persons who have been adequately immunized previously.

PLAN

Major treatment objectives are to maintain vital functions, remove the source of neurotoxin by surgical excision of the wound site, and when possible, neutralize circulating, unbound neurotoxin. Patients require constant monitoring and should be placed in a quiet, darkened room. Maintenance of an airway is critical. When generalized tetanus is present, early tracheostomy is warranted. Adequate sedation with diazepam, chlorpromazine, barbiturates, or meprobamate is essential to reduce the response to external stimuli. All drugs should be given parenterally. Chlorpromazine may cause hypotension and requires constant monitoring. Neuromuscular blocking agents, such as curare, may be helpful in selected cases; constant observation is required.

Diligent nursing care is extremely important to prevent decubiti, aspiration, atelectasis, and hypostatic pneumonia. Fluid and electrolyte balance and caloric intake must be maintained. Nasogastric tubes for maintenance of nutrition may be necessary, but aspiration penumonia may complicate their use. Intravenous hyperalimentation may be required. If tetanus persists for longer than 2 to 3 weeks, a gastrostomy may be required for feeding. The colon should be evacuated daily; tap water enemas may be indicated. Urinary retention requires insertion of an indwelling catheter.

Mild or local cases of tetanus may be treated with sedation and supportive care alone, reserving extensive surgery for more severe cases. The use of antimicrobial agents is recommended, but their relationship to the outcome has not been formally assessed. Because *C. tetani* is sensitive to penicillin G, 16 million units of penicillin given intravenously for 10 days has been recommended. Tetracycline, 2 gm./day orally or 1 gm. intravenously, can be used in patients sensitive to penicillin.

An early attempt to neutralize unbound toxin is indicated. Human tetanus immune globulin given intramuscularly in a single dose of 3000 to 6000 units is recommended. Some have suggested that a portion of the dose be injected into the wound site. When human immune globulin is unavailable, horse serum antitoxin may be given. A total dose of 100,000 units is recommended. Skin and conjunctival tests to rule out sensitivity to horse serum should be performed prior to administration. One-half of the total dose is given intramuscularly, and if tolerated, the remainder is given in a slow intravenous drip. Since the disease does not confer immunity, unimmunized patients should be immunized with tetanus toxoid administered

at a site distant from that used for administration of the antitoxin.

Treatment of patients with excessive sympathetic discharge must be individualized. Severe hypertension may require intravenous nitroprusside therapy, whereas hypotension may require exogenous catecholamines and/or fluid replacement. Tachycardia and arrhythmias are best treated with parenteral propranolol.

DISSEMINATED GRANULOMATOUS INFECTIONS

Miliary Tuberculosis

Miliary tuberculosis results from the unchecked dissemination of *Mycobacterium tuberculosis* throughout the body and, untreated, can be rapidly fatal. On very rare occasions, two other species of tubercle bacilli, *Mycobacterium bovis* and *Mycobacterium avium*, may cause a similar entity. In patients who are severely immunosuppressed, atypical mycobacteria may cause a similar syndrome.

M. tuberculosis infections are acquired by inhalation of infected droplets into the alveoli. Transmission by fomites, if it occurs at all, is unusual. Rarely are these organisms acquired by ingestion. In the lung, *M. tuberculosis* organisms are phagocytized by macrophages and multiply intracellularly. The inflammatory reaction that ensues is characterized by infiltration of small numbers of neutrophils mixed with fibrin and desquamated macrophages. Occasionally a lobular pneumonia with an outpouring of polymorphonuclear cells and a heavy concentration of organisms may be produced which histologically resembles any bacterial pneumonia. However, in most instances, the inflammatory response is modest. Early in the course, the organisms drain through the lymphatics and produce an inflammatory response of the hilar lymph nodes. From the hilar nodes, the organisms enter the thoracic duct and the blood stream for systemic dissemination. This pathogenic sequence probably most commonly occurs in those who acquire the tubercle bacillus, but most of the organisms die or become metabolically quiescent. Cellular immunity develops, resulting in phagocytosis of bacteria by macrophages, although some may continue to multiply within macrophages. Typical tubercle formation with epithelioid cells develops in response to induction. Some inflammatory cells in the central portion of the lesion die and produce caseous necrosis, which consists of a mixture of disintegrated cells and bacteria in a homogeneous coagulum. Calcium salts may be deposited in these granulomatous lesions. Such calcifications are common in the primary lesion and the associated lymph nodes and are referred to as the Ghon complex. Common areas for dissemination of the organism include the apices of the lung, bone, kidney, spleen, meninges, and liver. Following dissemination of the organism, few patients become symptomatic. The classical manifestations of miliary tuberculosis may become manifest in a very small percentage of persons following hematogenous dissemination after primary infection. In other infrequent instances lesions may remain quiescent after infection and reactivate later with bacteremia, dissemination, and metastatic focal infections. Thus, miliary tuberculosis may immediately follow the initial infection; within a few months or later endogenous reinfection may develop after a prolonged quiescent period. Delayed hematogenous dissemination occurs in the elderly, the malnourished, or persons with malignant disorders or defects of cellular immunity.

SUBJECTIVE FEATURES

The patient may be asymptomatic or may manifest acute toxic or chronic signs. Fever may be low or moderately elevated for days, weeks, or even months. There may be pleuritic chest pain, delirium, stiff neck, or abdominal pain. There may be only low-grade fever, headache, and malaise without pulmonary symptoms. Signs referable to serosal involvement of the peritoneum, pericardium, pleura, and meninges may be present. Rarely, tuberculosis may present as tuberculous meningitis without pulmonary symptoms. These patients present a difficult and puzzling clinical problem that can cause rapid death unless treatment is rapidly instituted.

OBJECTIVE FEATURES

There may be fever, weight loss, and tachypnea. Children or adults may appear acutely ill with meningeal signs. Other findings may be absent. However, if serosal surfaces are involved, specific clinical manifestations are evident. These include pericardial and pleural friction rubs, tenderness and spasm of the anterior abdominal wall, and stiff neck with positive Kernig's and Brudzinski's signs. Tubercles in the choroid occur as small, gray-white, oblong patches with indistinct margins. Lung findings are usually unremarkable. Splenomegaly is noted in half the cases.

ASSESSMENT

The important clinical sign is a positive chest roentgenogram. In children hilar adenopathy is common, and typical millet seed lesions are disseminated throughout the lung fields. These lesions may be as large as a centimeter but are typically 5 to 6 mm. in diameter. Other disorders such as disseminated fungal infection and lymphangitic spread of carcinoma mimic this pattern. In adults, hilar adenopathy is not ordinarily present. Occasionally, the chest roentgenogram is normal initially but manifests miliary patterns several days later.

If sputum is produced, the organisms may be identified by acid-fast stain (about one-third of cases) or recovered by culture (about two-thirds of cases). Gastric washings may yield the organism on culture. Their presence in an acid-fast stain is confusing because commensal acid-fast bacteria may be recovered from gastric washings. Whenever clinical evidence suggests meningitis, a lumbar puncture is essential. Characteristically, spinal fluid contains an elevated protein, a low to normal glucose, and a pleocytosis of approximately 100 to 200 cells. Most cells are lymphocytes, although neutrophils may predominate initially. Acid-fast stains may show organisms in centrifuged sediment; or in the pellicle (the membranous-like layering) that forms in cerebrospinal fluid after standing for several hours.

Tissue diagnosis is most helpful. Hepatic biopsy specimens reveal noncaseating and caseating granuloma, and occasionally, the organism may be identified. Unless the organism is identified, liver specimens are not diagnostic, since granulomatous hepatitis occurs in sarcoidosis, histoplasmosis, berylliosis, ornithosis, Q fever, and Hodgkin's disease, with caseous changes in some. Similarly, bone marrow biopsy may reveal granuloma with stainable organisms. Culture of liver and bone marrow tissue should be performed. Bone marrow aspiration is not as helpful. Although the organism may be isolated by culture, granulomas are not specifically identified histologically. Biopsy of serosal surfaces such as the pleura, in the presence of effusion, may aid in diagnosis. The diagnosis may be confirmed by brush biopsy or by percutaneous needle biopsy of the lung.

A tuberculin skin test should be performed, utilizing 5 tuberculin units (intermediate strength PPD) injected intradermally. The results are interpreted in 48 hours. Induration of 8 mm. or greater is considered a positive test, although approximately 10 per cent of patients with miliary tuberculosis are anergic. The elderly, the malnourished, and patients with concomitant viral diseases often accompanied by anergy, such as lymphoma or sarcoid, may not react to tuberculin. The diagnosis should always be suspected when prolonged fever of undetermined cause is associated with a positive tuberculin test.

In severely ill patients, a major arterial alveolar oxygen gradient or alveolar capillary block may be noted.

Hematologic abnormalities such as pancytopenia and rare leukemoid reactions have been reported; miliary tuberculosis may present as aplastic anemia or a leukemia-like illness.

PLAN

Early treatment with antituberculous drugs has reduced the mortality rate significantly. Isoniazid is the drug of choice. Since this drug readily crosses the blood-brain barrier, it is effective for treatment of miliary tuberculosis associated with meningitis. Isoniazid, 5 to 10 mg./kg. B.W., is given in a single daily oral dose, or intramuscularly in comatose patients. A second drug such as rifampin, a new, potent antituberculous drug, is recommended. This medication also crosses the blood-brain barrier. A single daily 600 mg. dose is recommended. Because rifampin is available only for oral administration its use in extremely ill or comatose patients is limited. Other useful drugs are ethambutol, 25 mg./kg. B.W. in a single oral daily dose, or streptomycin, 15 mg./kg. B.W. intramuscularly.

Supportive care is essential. Oxygen therapy is required in patients with significant alveolar capillary block. Occasionally, in very toxic patients, glucocorticoids are help-ful. Certain patients have adrenocortical insufficiency and replacement with mineralocorticoids and glucocorticoids is necessary. Dexamethasone may be helpful in patients with tuberculous meningitis who have evidence of increased intracranial pressure from cerebral edema. These patients often require dietary supplementation.

DISSEMINATED FUNGAL DISEASES

Deep fungal infections caused by the dimorphic fungi, *Histoplasma capsulatum*, *Coccidioides immitis*, and *Blastomyces dermatitidis* may on occasion be clinically indistinguishable from miliary tuberculosis.

Coccidioides immitis

This organism has a specific distribution to semiarid, low altitude regions of the Western Hemisphere and is typically found in southern California, particularly the San Joaquin Valley; New Mexico; southern Arizona; Utah; southwestern Texas; Mexico; and some areas in central and western South America. Fungi propagate in the soil, and their highly infectious mature arthrospores are disseminated during the hot, dusty dry spells in these regions. Spores blown about in airborne dust are inhaled. Organisms deposit in alveoli or bronchioles and initiate an inflammatory response, producing an acute pulmonary syndrome. The arthrospores enlarge and evolve into spherules with internal spores (endospores). These endospores are dispersed during rupture of the mature spherule, which may be phagocytized. Once inside viable phagocytes, the organisms may spread to local lymph nodes or to the blood vessels. The latter is less common. Dissemination from the primary pulmonary focus usually occurs within weeks to months after infection; the resultant clinical syndrome resembles primary disseminated tuberculosis. Dissemination many years after the initial infection, such as in endogenous reinfection tuberculosis, has been described but is rare. Fungi may spread to any tissue in the body including bone, kidney, spleen, and meninges. The typical host response is a granulomatous reaction with central microabscess formation. Caseous necrosis of the granuloma followed by calcification may also develop.

SUBJECTIVE FEATURES

In 1 to 3 weeks, after aerosolization of infected dusts, a typical flu-like syndrome develops, including fever, malaise, chest pain, headache, night sweats, anorexia, and a nonproductive cough. Chest pain may be pleuritic.

OBJECTIVE FEATURES

Within the first 2 days of illness, an erythematous exanthema, which can be macular and can resemble the rash of scarlet fever, may develop. Erythema nodosum or erythema multiforme may develop 3 days to 3 weeks after the first symptoms. With dissemination, there is persistence of fever. The patient may appear toxic and may show meningeal signs. Pulmonary abnormalities, including rales and friction rubs, may be evident. In summary, the findings may be indistinguishable from miliary tuberculosis.

ASSESSMENT

Suspicion is aroused whenever a patient from an endemic area manifests a recent episode of fever, chest pain, erythema nodosum, arthralgia, and/or pneumonitis. The organism may be identified in a wet mount of sputum digested with potassium hydroxide. Isolation of the organisms from sputum or demonstrating them in tissue also establishes the diagnosis. Extreme care must be taken in culture procedures. Culture bottles must remain stoppered, and laboratory personnel must not be exposed to the highly contagious spores.

Occasionally, the organism may be identified in spinal fluid. Serologic tests are helpful in establishing the diagnosis; precipitin antibodies usually appear within several weeks of illness. Complement-fixing antibodies appear later in the illness. Serologic cross reactions may occur with *Histoplasma* and *Blastomyces* antigens, although the specific titer is higher. Skin tests cross-react with those for other fungal infections. Although they become positive early in illness, they are not helpful in establishing the diagnosis.

PLAN

Patients with acute, self-limiting types of the illness should not be treated with an-

tifungal agents. However, disseminated form of the disease is usually fatal if not treated. Even with specific chemotherapy, it is attended by a high mortality rate. Amphotericin B is the drug of choice and is first given in a 1 mg. intravenous test dose. If the patient tolerates this dose, 5 mg. may be given intravenously over 4 to 6 hours. The dose is doubled each day until the patient is receiving approximately 35 mg./day. Amphotericin B must be dissolved in 1 liter of 5 per cent glucose in water for administration and will cause tissue necrosis if allowed to infiltrate. The incidence of phlebitis may be reduced by adding 25 mg. of hydrocortisone to each liter of fluid. Heparin in low doses also may be added. Glucocorticoids, aspirin, chlorpromazine, and antihistamines may be very helpful in patients who experience systemic drug reactions such as fever, chills, and headache. Therapy should be continued for at least 10 weeks. Other reactions that are noted as the drug is continued include anemia, hypokalemia, peripheral neuropathy, albuminuria, and azotemia. Patients with meningitis should receive amphotericin B intrathecally; this may require regimens of weeks to months. The initial dose is usually 0.025 mg., which is dissolved in 5 per cent glucose to which dexamethasone has been added. The dose is doubled every 2 days until an 0.5 mg. dose is achieved. This maximum intrathecal dose is administered twice weekly and may require the insertion of a subcutaneous Ommaya reservoir attached to an intraventricular catheter.

Histoplasmosis

Histoplasma capsulatum is a dimorphic fungus that is universally distributed but heavily seeded in states bordering the Mississippi and Ohio Rivers. The organism is found in soil, especially that which has been fortified by bird droppings and bat guano. Unlike *Coccidioides immitis* infection, the progressive, disseminated illness only occasionally follows the acute, primary disease. Pathogenically, histoplasmosis closely resembles endogenous, reinfection miliary tuberculosis. The early clinical signs of anorexia, weight loss, fever, night sweats, adenopathy and hepatosplenomegaly simulate other disseminated granulomatous diseases. In histoplasmosis, ulcerated lesions of mucosal surfaces, especially of the gastrointestinal and respiratory tracts, are more common.

ASSESSMENT

The organism with a characteristic morphology may be identified histologically in macrophages, bone marrow aspirates, sections of lymph nodes, liver biopsy specimens, oral or mucosal ulcerations, and occasionally spinal fluid. Gomori's methenamine silver stain and periodic acid–Schiff stain are most useful. Cultures of infected tissues on Sabouraud's medium should be performed. A positive skin test indicates prior infection and is of little diagnostic use. Serologic tests including complement fixation tests are available and may be helpful when a rising titer is obtained in the serum of a patient with a compatible syndrome.

PLAN

Therapy for disseminated histoplasmosis is very similar to that for *coccidioidomycosis* and includes *amphotericin B* in the same dosage. The intravenous dose of amphotericin B should not exceed 50 mg./day. Meningitis occurs less often, but when present amphotericin B given intrathecally and the insertion of an Ommaya reservoir should be considered. Some investigators have recommended that the minimal inhibitory concentration of the infecting strain of *Histoplasma capsulatum* and serum levels of amphotericin be determined. If such assays are available, it is recommended that the patient receive a dose of amphotericin B sufficient to achieve a serum concentration twice that of the minimum inhibitory concentration. Once this dose is achieved, it is recommended that the treatment continue for 10 weeks. These regimens are less toxic.

Blastomyces dermatitidis

Blastomyces is another dimorphic fungus capable of producing a deep-seated infection, which on occasion disseminates hematogenously. Such cases have been found throughout North America but are more prevalent in the southeastern United States and in the Mississippi River Valley. The source of the organism is unknown; although assumed to be derived from the soil, the organism has never been isolated from this source. Evidence suggests that the organism enters the respiratory tract and produces a primary subclinical pulmonary infection from which the fungus is probably carried by the circulation to other organs. The common sites of dissemination are the skin, bone, and genitalia, although any organ may be involved. The histologic lesion of mixed granuloma and suppuration is similar to that of coccidioidomycosis and histoplasmosis.

SUBJECTIVE AND OBJECTIVE FEATURES

The cutaneous disease is characterized by lesions on exposed parts of the body, especially the hands and face. Lesions begin as small, erythematous macules or papules, which become raised or verrucous. They may ulcerate and weep serous material. Typically, lesions are nonpruritic and painless. The borders of the lesions may become scalloped and may expand progressively over several months. Draining fistulae and ulcerations are common. Genital lesions may involve the prostate, epididymis, and testes, producing painful swelling of the testes or epididymis and vague, deep perineal pain. Occasionally, there may be spontaneous drainage from the scrotum. Bone involvement presents as a lytic lesion typically in the sacrum, vertebrae, long bones, pelvis, ribs, or skull. Bone lesions are painful and are associated with swelling of the overlying soft tissue, which may break down and form draining fistulae. Rarely, the disseminated form of the disease resembles miliary tuberculosis and may include meningitis and cerebral abscess.

ASSESSMENT

The diagnosis is established by cultivation of the organism from the material obtained from such areas as skin, mucosal lesions, sputum, and draining sinuses. The fungus may be identified microscopically in potassium hydroxide–treated pus, sputum, or skin scrapings. Histologic sections of biopsy material stained with Gomori's methenamine silver or Schiff's periodic acid stain may reveal the organism. Skin tests are frequently negative, and serologic tests cross-react; therefore, neither are of diagnostic help.

PLAN

Amphotericin B is the drug of choice and is given in dosages recommended for histoplasmosis. A 10-week course of therapy is usually sufficient. Hydroxystilbamidine is effective in treating nonprogressive, dermatologic blastomycosis. It is given in a dose of 5 to 8 mg./kg. B.W./day for a total of 8 gm. It should not be given to patients with evidence of multiple organ involvement.

GRAM-NEGATIVE BACTEREMIA

Gram-negative bacteria may produce a variety of well-defined clinicopathologic changes by invading the blood stream. Common complications of gram-negative bacteremia include hypotension or shock, acute renal failure, tissue anoxia due to hypoperfusion and vasoconstriction, disseminated intravascular coagulation, and metabolic changes such as lactic acidosis. Species of Enterobacteriaceae, *Pseudomonas*, *Neisseria*, *Hemophilus*, and other gram-negative aerobes as well as gram-negative anaerobes including *Bacteroides* have the ability to produce these complications.

All these organisms contain endotoxin, a lipopolysaccharide material, which is part of the bacterial cell wall. When administered to animals parenterally, this substance effects major hemodynamic, hematologic, and metabolic changes. Evidence suggests that endotoxin is responsible for many of the manifestations of gram-negative bacteremia. Experimentally, endotoxin has been found to initiate a chain of interrelated events. Following parenteral administration, it stimulates the release of a number of physiologically active substances including catecholamines, histamine, steroids, endogenous pyrogen, and vasoactive peptides (kinins). By activating Hageman factor and stimulating the release of platelet factor 3, endotoxin may also initiate blood clotting. Hageman factor, in turn, activates the plasminogen-plasmin system, which leads to fibrinolysis. Additional hematologic effects of this lipopolysaccharide include alterations in leukocyte migration, induction of leukocytic endothelial sticking, and reticuloendothelial cell blockade. Finally, the classical complement pathway, as well as the alternative (properdin) pathway, is activated. These multiple events, acting in concert, produce the varied clinicopathologic syndromes.

By inducing vasoconstriction of arterioles and venules, endotoxin, directly and in conjunction with catecholamines and kinins, shunts blood away from capillary beds supplying parenchymal cells of major organs. The lungs, kidney, skin, and liver are severely affected. Although the heart, brain, and muscles are spared initially, eventually they are also subjected to hypoperfusion. The intense vasoconstriction increases peripheral resistance and decreases cardiac return and output. Vasoconstriction also induces stasis of blood in the capillaries, resulting in anoxia of the vascular endothelium. Ultimately, the integrity of the endothelium is lost, and plasma and red blood cells leak into tissues, intensifying the local anoxia. The decrease in intravascular volume that ensues causes an additional decrease in cardiac output and blood flow to major organs. Because Hageman factor is activated by endotoxin, the clotting cascade may be initiated and disseminated intravascular coagulation produced. The development of multiple microthrombi within capillaries results in further tissue anoxia. This lack of oxygen augments the production of lactic acid, which in sufficient quantity causes metabolic acidosis. As the pH drops, there is dilatation of arteriolar but not venous sphincters. Capillary beds become engorged, resulting in further loss of plasma and red blood cells into tissue. This intensifies the anoxia and further decreases the cardiac return and output. Vicious hemodynamic and metabolic circles ensue. Finally, anoxia results in cellular autolysis with the release of lysozymes, which potentiates more cellular destruction.

Shock is one of the most dramatic complications of gram-negative bacteremia. Clinically, the systolic blood pressure falls below 80 mm. Hg and the urine flow decreases to less than 20 ml./hour. Tissues and organs are inadequately perfused with oxygenated blood because of hypovolemia. There are two components to this hypovolemia: (1) constriction of visceral arterioles and venules and (2) a decrease in circulating blood volume. Consequent to the decrease in intravascular volume, renal blood flow and glomerular filtration decrease. If severe enough, acute renal failure develops. Passage of fluid and erythrocytes into the lungs gives rise to pulmonary edema and the "stiff lung syndrome." Consumption of clotting factors during disseminated intravascular coagulation may lead to the development of a significant bleeding tendency. Renal failure, hemorrhage, lactic acidosis, and anoxia contribute to the high mortality rate in this syndrome. The ultimate prognosis, however,

TABLE 1   Factors Predisposing to Gram-Negative Bacteremia

A. Urinary tract
   1. Infection
   2. Instrumentation
B. Gastrointestinal tract
   1. Surgery
   2. Infection
C. Gynecologic tract
   1. Abortions
   2. Dilatation and curettage
   3. Pelvic sepsis
D. Neoplastic diseases
   1. Solid tumors
   2. Leukemia
   3. Lymphoproliferative disease
E. Respiratory tract
   1. Infection
   2. Respirators
F. Burns
G. Intravascular catheters
H. Wounds
I. "Compromised host"
   1. Broad-spectrum antibotics
   2. Immunosuppression
   3. Congenital or acquired immune defects
   4. Granulocytopenia
   5. Extensive trauma

is very often determined by the underlying state of the host. Over 80 per cent of patients without major underlying illnesses survive, whereas a similar proportion of individuals with severe underlying disease die. The most frequent predisposing conditions and sources from which gram-negative bacteria gain entry into the circulation are listed in Table 1.

The most common organisms include *Escherichia coli, Neisseria meningitidis, Klebsiella, Enterobacter, Proteus, Pseudomonas,* and *Bacteroides* species. It is important to note that certain gram-positive bacteria, *Staphylococcus aureus,* group A streptococci, and *Streptococcus pneumoniae* may cause a clinical syndrome indistinguishable from gram-negative bacteremia. Certain underlying conditions predispose to infection with specific organisms. Patients with burns, leukemia, or granulocytopenia are prone to become infected with *Pseudomonas.* *Bacteroides* bacteremia is more common among obstetric and gynecologic patients or following colonic perforations or gastrointestinal surgery.

SUBJECTIVE FEATURES

Symptoms referable to the predisposing condition or underlying source are usually present. The syndrome is ushered in by a shaking chill followed by fever. Shortness of breath, weakness, and a feeling of lightheadedness may occur.

OBJECTIVE FEATURES

The source of infection may be clinically apparent. Hyperpyrexia is typical, although occasionally a normal temperature or hypopyrexia is noted. Rigors and tachypnea may be obvious. The blood pressure may be stable or may fall to hypotensive levels. The skin is cold, clammy, and pale and may be cyanotic and/or icteric. Petechiae and purpura may cover the skin. Occasionally, in *Pseudomanas* bacteremia, characteristic skin lesions appear (ecthyma gangrenosum), characterized by a black macule approximately 1 cm. in diameter with a necrotic or ulcerated center surrounded by erythema. These lesions occur in the anogenital area, axillary folds, and extremities.

Initial laboratory data may reveal an elevated, normal, or low white blood cell count, anemia, and thrombocytopenia. The BUN and serum creatinine may be elevated.

ASSESSMENT AND PLAN

Care in the handling of burns, frequent changing of intravenous catheters, incision and drainage of collections of purulent material, the use of clean respirators, and discretion in the use of urinary catheters are important measures that may prevent the development of gram-negative bacteremia. Once it occurs, however, the truly emergent situation demands prompt attention to a number of objectives. There should be rapid recognition of the syndrome, immediate institution of effective antimicrobials, control of the hemodynamic alterations and the underlying anoxia, proper management of the source of infection, and finally, optimal management of underlying diseases.

Treatment must be aimed at the bacteremia and the underlying focus. Consequently, the source of the bacteremia must be established. Blood cultures should be obtained in order to identify the organism and determine its antibiotic sensitivity pattern. Other appropriate cultures (e.g., urine, sputum, pus) should also be obtained, depending upon the suspected focus.

ANTIBIOTICS IN BACTEREMIA

The aminoglycoside gentamicin has a wide spectrum against gram-negative aerobic organisms and is considered the keystone to antibiotic therapy. Five mg./kg. B.W./day in 3 divided doses given intramuscularly should be instituted. In the presence of shock the drug should be administered intravenously with caution over one-half hour. If there is evidence of renal failure, reduction in total daily dosage is appropriate; however, the initial dose should be at least 1.5 to 2 mg./kg. B.W. Because some gram-positive organisms may cause a similar syndrome, antibiotic coverage for these organisms is recommended. A penicillinase-resistant penicillin or cephalosporin such as methicillin, 12 gm./day, or cephalothin, 6 to 12 gm./day, given intravenously meets this recommendation. If *Bacteroides* bacteremia is suspected because of infection arising in the female genital tract or the gastrointestinal tract, treatment against this organism should also be instituted. Chloramphenicol, 3 to 4 gm./day given intravenously, or clindamycin, 600 mg. 3 times a day given either intravenously or intramuscularly, is effective. Once the etiologic agent is identified and the sensitivity ascertained, the unnecessary antimicrobials should be discontinued.

TREATMENT

Management of hemodynamic changes is of paramount importance. There must be restoration of the intravascular volume and an attempt made to overcome vasoconstriction. Fluid replacement may be in the form of normal saline, dextran, or plasma or whole blood if there is significant blood loss. Administration of fluid in and of itself helps to overcome intense vasoconstriction. In order to monitor the quantity of fluid required to restore the circulating blood volume and cardiac output, the central venous pressure (CVP) should be monitored with a CVP catheter. Fluids should be administered rapidly until the intense vasoconstriction is overcome as evidenced by a return of renal output, warm skin, and normal mentation and the blood pressure is restored to normal levels or until the CVP exceeds 12 cm. of saline. If venous pressure exceeds this level, congestive heart failure is imminent. Rapid intravenous digitalization may be necessary. Once the CVP drops below this level, fluid administration may be continued until normal hemodynamics are restored.

Several investigators have recommended the use of pharmacologic doses of glucocorticoids. In large doses steroids induce vasodilation and are ionotropic. In addition, they block the release of catecholamines and kinins and stabilize lysozymal membranes. One to 2 gm. of hydrocortisone may be administered in an intravenous bolus. This dose may be repeated in 1 to 2 hours if necessary.

The use of beta-receptor stimulators such as isoproterenol have been recommended but are controversial. Although isoproterenol induces peripheral vasodilatation, it may produce severe tachycardia and ectopic contractions. The use of vasoconstrictors such as norepinephrine should be avoided. Endogenous vasoconstriction plays a major role in the development of the syndrome, and administered vasoconstrictors serve only to accelerate the chain of events. Dopamine recently has been released for use in the treatment of shock. Unlike other pressor agents, dopamine does not reduce renal blood flow. The place of this drug in the management of gram-negative bacteremia with shock, however, has not been established. When there is no response to fluid replacement, steroids, and antibiotics, then dopamine may be used.

Intravascular coagulation may occur at any time. The diagnosis of disseminated intravascular coagulation is established in the presence of multiple bleeding sites; thrombocytopenia; fibrin split products in serum; a reduction in serum prothrombin, Factor V, and Factor VIII; and a prolongation of the thromboplastin and thrombin time. In the face of disseminated intravascular coagulation, heparin or dextran can be used, although their efficacy has not been established.

Incision and drainage of collections of purulent material to remove the source of the bacteremia are of the utmost importance.

Because anoxia is a very important component of the syndrome, adequate oxygenation must be assured. Considerable interstitial pulmonary edema may exist in the absence of rales. Oxygen therapy via a nasal catheter or a Venturi mask may suffice. To combat the "stiff lung syndrome," end expiratory positive pressure has been recommended. However, this decreases the cardiac return and, consequently, is a two-edged sword.

The effectiveness of leukocyte transfusions in patients who are granulocytopenic has not been firmly established and is currently being investigated.

Chapter 54

EMERGENCIES ASSOCIATED WITH ATMOSPHERIC POLLUTION

C. Stuart-Harris

Acute respiratory tract illnesses due to exposure to harmful substances inhaled from the air have long been recognized. Such are the acute conditions resembling pulmonary edema or acute bronchial infections that followed the exposure of servicemen to chlorine or phosgene gas during the first World War. Occasionally also an industrial accident resulting in the release of an irritant gas such as nitrogen dioxide has led to acute chest illnesses in those unfortunate enough to have inhaled the polluted air. These events led long ago to legislation stating the maximum permissible atmospheric concentrations in industrial undertakings of substances such as sulfur dioxide (SO_2). Yet the ambient atmosphere, though blamed for centuries as a source of unpleasant effects when polluted, was not generally regarded as hazardous to health until 1930. In December of that year an episode occurred in the Meuse valley in Belgium during fog in which a large number of persons developed respiratory symptoms such as coughing, dyspnea and retrosternal pain. Asthmatic symptoms, signs of pulmonary edema and cardiac insufficiency also were noted. More than 60 persons died on the fourth and fifth days of the fog, the death rate rose to 10 times the average and during the fog many cattle died and others were driven up hillsides to safety (Firket, 1931). Investigations suggested that SO_2 and sulfuric acid caused the disaster.

A similar episode occurred in 1948 in a steep-sided valley in Donora, Pennsylvania. As many as one-third of those exposed complained of cough. Sputum and dyspnea occurred in the most severely affected persons, and 18 deaths were attributed to the fog. Again, SO_2 or its oxidation products and particulate matter were blamed (Schrenk, et al., 1949). It was, however, the four-day London fog of December 1952 that dwarfed all previous episodes and led to more than 4000 deaths (Report of the Ministry of Health, 1954). A large number of persons became ill with minor symptoms, others developed acute illnesses requiring hospital admission. During the fog, the leaves of plants at Kew Gardens in southwestern London were blackened, cattle confined in central London during a livestock exhibition died, and women's nylon stockings were damaged. The fog was caused by anticyclonic conditions leading to an inversion of warm upper air holding down cold air in the Thames valley. It was accompanied by an increase in concentrations of smoke particles and SO_2 in the air to ten times average winter levels. The peak concentrations in a 48-hour period were 4460 μgm./cu. m. of smoke and 3830 μgm/cu. m. of SO_2 (Holland, 1972). These pollutants, as in the case of the earlier episodes, were attributed to coal-burning domestic and industrial appliances. The disaster led to an intensive study of the harmful effects of SO_2 on healthy persons, to extensive monitoring of air pollution in London and other British cities, and to legislation directed toward a limitation of the emission of smoke into the atmosphere. This has resulted in a virtual elimination of smog conditions from British cities, the last episode in London being in 1962, when a four-day fog resulted in high concentrations of SO_2 accompanied by much lower concentrations of smoke than in 1952. An excess mortality of 700 deaths was attributed to this episode.

THE MORTALITY DURING SMOG EPISODES

The autopsies carried out in Belgium in 1930, in Donora in 1948, and in London in 1952 all emphasize two important findings. Acute effects were largely confined to the mucosa and submucosa of the trachea and larger bronchi, with congestion, cellular infiltration, desquamation, and excessive mucus production. These changes, though slight, were consistent. Alveolar edema or hemorrhage sometimes were present. Chronic lesions of the lungs and heart were almost invariable in the London autopsies, as also in Donora (Report of the Ministry of Health, 1954). The certificates of deaths in London in relation to the 1952 episode stated that the commonest chronic pulmonary conditions were chronic bronchitis, emphysema, and bronchiectasis. Cardiovascular conditions including hypertension and coronary artery disease also were present in excess, although not to the same degree, and a few reports were made of combined chest and cardiac disease. The autopsy findings, although based largely on coroner's cases of unexpected deaths, thus indicated that the persons chiefly at risk during smogs were those suffering from previous chronic disease. Only a few previously healthy persons and young babies died, although the contributory effect of infections in the latter cannot be denied. Many of the unexpected deaths, even in those with chronic disease, occurred at home during sleep. The deaths from respiratory causes continued to be excessive for some days after the fog. It was surprising that cases of fatal pneumonia, although more numerous during the fog, did not increase proportionately with the total mortality. This finding contrasts strikingly with that of mortality during an epidemic of infection, such as influenza.

THE CLINICAL PICTURE OF ACUTE CHEST ILLNESSES DURING SMOGS

It is remarkable that relatively few good clinical records have been published based upon an analysis of patients observed during a pollution episode. This can be attributed, at least in part, to the relatively undistinctive character of these illnesses, for the patients resemble those admitted in any ordinary winter season except in number. The picture is one of acute exacerbation of illness familiar to those dealing with patients with chronic bronchitis accompanied by generalized airway obstruction (chronic obstructive bronchitis). Admission to the hospital is prompted chiefly by the development of increased dyspnea, which may be experienced at rest by those who were previously dyspneic only on exertion. At the same time increased cough of a particularly irritating character and increased volume of sputum indicate the mucosal action of the smoggy air. In some patients there may be complaint of watering of the eyes, sore throat, or substernal chest pain. The sputum, which was previously white, may become yellow or green and contains increased numbers of polymorphonuclear leukocytes and black particles.

On examination, patients with acute exacerbations of illness belong to one of two principal clinical types, the first of which consists of those who exhibit obvious respiratory distress with increased respiratory effort and rate. There may be wheezing on expiration, suggesting bronchial obstruction. In spite of the increased respiratory effort there is cyanosis, central in type and exhibited by the tongue as well as the lips. The chest has the character of the person with chronic airway obstruction, being distended even on expiration to a position of full inspiration, and the accessory muscles of respiration contract vigorously with each breath. There may be abundant rales and rhonchi in all zones. Such patients are unlikely to exhibit bronchial breathing or radiologic evidence of consolidation. Nor will there usually be evidence of congestive heart failure. Yet evidence of respiratory insufficiency exists in that the arterial oxygen tension (Pa_{O_2}) is reduced below normal and the arterial carbon dioxide tension (Pa_{CO_2}) is increased, although not usually in excess of 50 torr.

The second chief clinical variety is that of a deeply cyanosed, somnolent, or semiconscious patient who appears to be making little extra respiratory effort. Yet the deep cyanosis of tongue and lips indicates a serious degree of hypoxemia and the Pa_{O_2} may be 50 torr or less. The arterial blood shows hypercapnia with $PaCO_2$ of from 50 to 100 torr. Thus there is a more severe degree of respiratory failure than in the patients belonging to the group described above. The chest signs may be less prominent than in the grossly dyspneic patient, but feeble breath sounds and many rales are likely. The patient may exhibit distended jugular veins, hepatomegaly, and edema of the legs and back—the full picture of right-sided congestive heart failure. This is secondary to chronic pulmonary disease, and thus there will be other features of anoxic cor pulmonale. A right ventricular cardiac impulse, gallop rhythm of the heart sounds, and electrocardiographic changes such as "P" pulmonale in standard leads II and III and a right ventricular strain pattern in right-sided chest leads may be present. The latter changes indicate long-standing cardiac involvement and acute alterations may not, therefore, be easily recognized unless the patient has been under observation before admission to the hospital.

If the patient has been suffering from previous systemic hypertension or ischemic heart disease, then findings concordant with these may be present. But such cardiac patients do not resemble those described above as chronic cor pulmonale. In particular central cyanosis may not be so prominent, nor may there be drowsiness or alteration in consciousness. Chest signs are indicative of pulmonary edema due to left ventricular failure, but diffuse rhonchi or rales other than at the lung bases will indicate bronchial involvement precipitated by the environmental exposure.

Yet a further clinical variety revolves around a picture resembling asthma. Accounts of smog episodes clearly suggest that in some patients the picture may resemble an attack of spasmodic asthma including a clinical response to bronchodilator inhalants. The name "Yokohama asthma" given to the nocturnal syndrome occurring in Japan in the Yokohama area reinforces this concept. It appears that this syndrome is provoked by atmospheric pollution which, because of meterologic factors, builds up during the night. Experience of the syndrome in U.S. servicemen (Phelps and Koike, 1962) suggests that persons who develop the syndrome have either had chronic chest disease or have been heavy cigarette smokers. There is certainly no clear evidence that persons who have previously suffered from ordinary bronchial asthma are predisposed to the attacks by exposure to chemical pollutants. The account of the health of Japanese residents in the Tokyo–Yokohama area by Oshima and others (1965 a and b) suggests that chronic bronchitis is prevalent in the area and that ordinary asthma patients do not suffer from the pollution syndrome. The fact that U.S. servicemen who have suffered from the syndrome continue to experience symptoms and exhibit evidence of pulmonary dysfunction even after return to the U.S. suggests that there is no justification for regarding Yokohama "asthma" as being other than chronic obstructive bronchitis exacerbated by environmental exposure.

POSSIBLE MECHANISMS OF THE ADVERSE EFFECTS OF ATMOSPHERIC POLLUTION

Many minor symptoms, which are exhibited after exposure to smog conditions, occur in those with previous chronic chest disease. They were documented over several winter periods in London by Lawther, Waller, and Henderson (1970), who persuaded patients attending a clinic to keep diaries in which they recorded their health as the same, better, or worse than on the previous day. Summation of the replies enabled an index of health to be prepared, and graphic comparison of the findings with measured daily average concentrations of smoke and SO_2 revealed a remarkable degree of correlation. A "critical level" of SO_2 of 500 μgm./cu. m. accompanied by smoke of 250 μgm./cu. m. was found, above which exposure was accompanied by a sharp deterioration of health of the patients with chronic bronchitis during 1957 to 1965. Such concentrations of pollutants are substantially exceeded by those encountered during smog episodes and are unlikely to lead to emergency situations unless other exacerbating circumstances are also present. For instance, there is sometimes an epidemic of respiratory infection such as influenza during the winter season when pollution may rise above the so-called critical levels. Influenza is particularly likely to cause chest complications including pneumonia, in those with previous chronic lung disease. It is possible, therefore, that even a minor pollution episode during the period of an epidemic of influenza will at times create a dangerous situation.

The precise mechanism whereby pollution by smoke and SO_2 creates a deterioration in those with chronic obstructive bronchitis is not known. The airways of normal persons are sensitive to the inhalation of SO_2 gas alone, but only in concentrations such as 5 parts per million or more (15,000 μgm./cu. m.). Although some normal persons react to lesser concentrations, such as 1 to 2 parts per million, bronchitic subjects are not necessarily more sensitive. Nevertheless a degree of bronchoconstriction which is inappreciable in normal persons may worsen the disordered alveolar ventilation of such patients. Combined with excessive production of mucus, such airway narrowing enhances the existing imbalance of the ventilation and perfusion of the alveoli, particularly when it affects the peripheral bronchioles. Increased hypoxia results, and the secondary consequence of this is an increase in the pulmonary blood pressure. A critical effect is thus readily created between the airways supplying oxygen and the arterioles supplying blood. This results in respiratory failure, with or without right ventricular involvement, and ultimate heart failure. This appears to be the underlying reason for sudden exacerbations of illness in patients with chronic obstructive bronchitis or emphysema, however these are precipitated.

The mechanism for the occasional instance of acute pulmonary edema following the exposure of normal persons to very high concentrations of industrial gases such as nitrogen dioxide is probably different. An asphyxiating condition gradually leading to death has been traced to an organizing alveolar exudate which follows on the heels of the oedema (Darke and Warrack, 1958).

PRINCIPLES OF TREATMENT OF EMERGENCIES

The treatment required by patients following exposure to adverse environmental conditions depends to some extent on the clinical presentation. It is therefore only possible in this section to describe the principles which ought to be followed and which will now be listed.

RESTORATION OF AN ADEQUATE AIRWAY

This may require merely the use of bronchodilator drugs in those with mild bronchospasm. But patients with pre-existing chronic airway obstruction may already have been taking nebulized bronchodilator drugs such as isoproterenol, and more vigorous attempts to relieve obstruction will then be required. Aminophylline should be given by slow intravenous injection (250 mg.) and continued as a slow intravenous drip (500 mg. in 1 liter of normal saline). Patients whose airways are choked by quantities of sputum which cannot be expectorated, whether by reason of its extreme viscidity or because coughing has become feeble, will require mechanical assistance. Intubation permits the aspiration of secretion, and it may then prove possible for the patient to maintain adequate ventilation with humidified oxygen controlled at a rate determined by the arterial blood gases. Positive pressure ventilation may be required but, in general, tracheostomy is better avoided. The full description of the treatment of ventilatory failure is beyond the scope of this section.* In all patients other than those receiving assisted ventilation, sedatives of any sort should be forbidden.

MONITORING THE ARTERIAL BLOOD GASES

Relief of hypoxia is an essential ingredient in therapy, but although this is readily accomplished by giving oxygen, the patient likely to succumb to exposure to pollution is in risk of developing increased hypercapnia as a consequence of the reduced ventilation that follows too much oxygen. This sequela can be extremely hazardous because the patient may develop stupor or actual coma when the Pa_{CO_2} exceeds a certain level. The latter differs from patient to patient, and though a level in excess of 100 torr is usually critical, some patients may become unconscious at even lower levels. It is probable

_____

*See Chapter 10.

that the speed of rise is more important than the absolute level.

Controlled oxygen therapy at a rate of 2 liters per minute is safe in most patients, but if given by intranasal catheter may not suffice to raise the oxygen tension adequately. If the $PaCO_2$ is in the range of 45 to 55 torr on admission, it is probably safe to give oxygen at 3 to 4 liters per minute, but the CO_2 must be monitored after half-an-hour's treatment. A PaO_2 in excess of 55 torr is the minimum level at which to aim.

TREATMENT OF ACCOMPANYING BACTERIAL INFECTION

Antibiotic treatment is used on the assumption that secondary bacterial infection of the airway will almost certainly be present. This, however, must be verified by culture of the sputum, and until the result is available broad spectrum antibiotics such as tetracycline or ampicillin are preferred. Oral treatment at a rate of 500 mg four times daily is adequate unless the patient is unable to swallow capsules. The intramuscular route should then be used. There is still much to be said for initial therapy with penicillin combined with streptomycin intramuscularly. Therapy appropriate to the flora found in the sputum will later be substituted.

TREATMENT OF CARDIOVASCULAR COMPLICATIONS

Right-heart failure requires use of diuretics with or without the addition of digitalis. Even when peripheral edema is absent, a raised jugular venous pressure or findings in the electrocardiogram of "P" pulmonale or right ventricular strain pattern indicate a need for diuretic therapy. Furosemide (Lasix) is the drug of choice, combined with

an oral potassium supplement. If there are chest signs suggesting widespread pulmonary edema, furosemide should be given intravenously. Care must be taken to monitor the electrolytes.

References

Darke, C. S., and Warrack, A. J. N.: Bronchiolitis from nitrous fumes. Thorax, 13:327, 1958.
Firket, J.: Fog along the Meuse Valley. Trans. Faraday Soc., 32:1192, 1936.
Holland, W. W.: Episodes of High Pollution in Great Britain. In Air Pollution and Respiratory Disease. Westport, Conn., Technomic Publishing Co. Inc., 1972, p. 27.
Lawther, P. J., Waller, R. E., and Henderson, M.: Air pollution and exacerbations of bronchitis. Thorax, 25:525, 1970.
Oshima, Y., et al.: Air pollution and respiratory diseases in the Tokyo–Yokohama asthma. Am. Rev. Resp. Dis., 90:572, 1964a.
Oshima, Y., et al.: A study of Tokyo–Yokohama asthma among Japanese. Am. Rev. Resp. Dis., 90:632, 1964b.
Phelps, H. W., and Koike, S.: Tokyo–Yokohama respiratory disease. Arch. Environ. Health., 10:143, 1962.
Report of the Ministry of Health: Mortality and Morbidity During the London Fog of December 1952. Reports on Public Health and Medical Subjects, No. 95, H.M. Stationery Office, 1954.
Schrenk, H. H., et al.: Air pollution in Donora, Pa. U.S. Publ. Health. Bull, 306, 1949.

General References

Beaver Committee Report on Air Pollution, Cmnd. 9322. H.M. Stationery Office, London, 1954.
Holland, W. W.: Air Pollution and Respiratory Disease. Westport, Conn., Technomic Publishing Co., Inc., 1972.
Lee, D. H.: Environmental Factors in Respiratory Disease. New York, Academic Press, Inc., 1972.
Respiratory failure. Ann. N.Y. Acad. Sci., 121:651, 1965.
Royal College of Phsyicians: Air Pollution and Health. First Report. London, Pitman Medical, 1970.
U.S. Dept. H.E.W.: Air Quality Criteria for Sulfur Oxides. Washington, D.C., U.S. Government Printing Office, 1969.
U.S. Dept. H.E.W.: Air Quality Criteria for Particulate Matter. Washington, D.C., U.S. Government Printing Office, 1969.

Chapter 55

ALCOHOL AND DRUG ABUSE

David G. Levine

Alcohol and drug abuse are responsible for precipitating a variety of acute reactions requiring prompt medical intervention. *Drug abuse refers to the use, generally by self-administration, of psychoactive substances in a manner which adversely affects medical, psychosocial, or economic well-being.* So defined, the term encompasses alcohol abuse, which affects more people than all other forms of drug abuse combined. The need for emergency services for alcohol-related medical and behavioral problems has long been recognized. The expanding use of other mind-affecting substances has created additional demands for skilled treatment of drug-induced crises.

The term "addict" is derived from the Latin *addictus,* literally "given over," describing an individual who is awarded to another as a slave. In common parlance, addiction denotes an established pattern of compulsive drug abuse occurring at the expense of all nondrug-related activities. It is the extreme form of drug dependence. *Psychologic dependence* is characterized by variable degrees of obsessive preoccupation with drugs, preference for the intoxicated state, and chronic or recurrent abuse. *Physical dependence* is an altered physiologic state produced by repeated drug use and requiring continued drug use to prevent the emergence of withdrawal symptoms. This vulnerability to abstinence phenomena is often included in the concept of addiction. *Tolerance* is manifested by a diminished response to a constant dose of a drug, reflecting changes in pharmacodynamic and cellular mechanisms. Cross-tolerance is observed between different drugs of the same class.

Drugs of abuse are commonly categorized as follows: narcotics; sedatives; stimulants; psychedelics; inhalants; and alcohol. Clinically significant physical dependence occurs only with narcotics (morphine-type drug dependence) and with sedatives and alcohol (CNS depressant drug dependence). Psychologic dependence is seen in connection with all of these agents.

WHO ARE THE ABUSERS?

Alcohol and drug abusers are a heterogeneous group who represent a spectrum of subcultures ranging from extreme deviance to unalloyed conventionality. Skid-row derelicts and inner-city junkies compose only a small fraction of the affected population, which extends deeply into the working and affluent classes. These individuals are subject to an increased risk of both acute and chronic medical problems. Chronic ill health results as much from poor nutrition and hygiene as from direct drug toxicity. Frequent and recurrent use of the intravenous route also contributes significantly to addicts' morbidity. Diseases of long standing may retard recovery from alcohol- and drug-related emergencies.

Crises occur during intoxication and withdrawal. Intoxication may lead to adverse physiologic or psychologic reactions and, in cases of severe overdose, to coma and death. Withdrawal phenomena also require timely assessment, and may in certain circumstances progress to a fatal outcome. "Polydrug abuse," which refers to the habitual abuse of a variety of drugs, depending primarily on availability, has become increasingly prevalent and seriously complicates both the clinical presentation and proper management of drug abuse emergencies. It is conservatively estimated that 2 million

Americans are chronic polydrug users. Non-users, including children, are also subject to accidental intoxication.

Conducting an orderly and systematic history, physical, and laboratory examination is frequently impractical in patients with acute alcohol and drug reactions. More often, diagnosis and treatment must proceed concurrently. Coma, delirium, convulsions and psychoses are common presenting symptoms. Differential diagnostic possibilities must include exogenous poisons of all varieties; metabolic disorders; infections, injuries, and other diseases of the CNS; and psychiatric disorders. Historical data should be obtained from the patient whenever possible, as well as from family, friends and others, concerning the drugs involved, dose, route of administration, and time of last use. Particularly in the case of illicit drug abuse, reliable histories may be unobtainable. Occasionally, alcohol, drugs, prescriptions, or paraphernalia may be found among the patient's possessions, providing clues to the agents involved. Physical examination should be directed toward evaluating (a) the patient's status and requirements for support of vital functions, (b) diagnostic signs suggesting specific intoxication or withdrawal syndromes, (c) sequelae of chronic alcoholism or drug abuse, and (d) evidence of concurrent illness or injury.

The constellation of historical and physical findings determines which laboratory and x-ray examinations are appropriate. Gross metabolic, hepatic, and renal diseases may be revealed by routine screening tests. Serum electrolytes should be monitored in patients requiring intravenous hydration. Serial measurement of arterial blood gases is necessary for precise evaluation and control of respiratory status. Toxicologic analysis may finally confirm the diagnosis, although the results generally are unavailable during the initial management of the patient. Samples of blood, urine, vomitus, and other specimens should be saved for future toxicologic study.

DRUG ABUSE

NARCOTIC ANALGESICS

The narcotic analgesics comprise naturally occurring, semisynthetic and synthetic substances with pharmacologic properties similar to those of morphine, the principal alkaloid of opium. All drugs in this group have CNS effects, including analgesia, sedation, mental clouding, and changes in mood. Other effects are suppression of the cough reflex and suppression of gastrointestinal motility. In addition, narcotics regularly produce a dose-related centrally mediated respiratory depression.

ABUSE PATTERNS

An estimated 500,000 Americans are addicted to heroin, the preferred drug for most narcotics users. Heroin addiction is most prevalent among the urban poor, and a significant heroin-related subculture exists in the ghettos. The illicit status of this drug subjects the addict to adverse social and toxicologic consequences. Heroin is commonly adulterated with quinine, lactose, and mannitol, and occasionally with barbiturates.

Habitual users typically experience a profound euphoria after a "fix." The acute state is characterized by satiation of motivating drives. Repeated use leads to tolerance, requiring higher doses to achieve the desired effects—doses in the lethal range for nontolerant individuals. An invariable concomitant is the development of a morphine-type physical dependence. Psychologic dependence is manifested by compulsive drug-seeking behavior which often remains undiminished even after prolonged abstinence.

Depending on the particular preparation, narcotics may be used in many ways. Smoking, sniffing ("snorting"), ingesting, and injecting subcutaneously ("skin popping"), intramuscularly or intravenously ("shooting up") are all common practices. Intravenous injection is the preferred method in most parts of the world because the high cost of narcotics dictates an efficient method of administration. Furthermore, the intravenous technique produces a sudden "rush" of intensely pleasant sensations in addition to the drowsy euphoria which follows.

Physicians, nurses, and other health professionals engage in illicit narcotics use with a higher frequency than occurs among the

TABLE 1 Commonly Abused Narcotics

Opium	
Morphine	
Codeine	
Heroin	
Hydromorphone	(Dilaudid)
Oxymorphone	(Numorphan)
Levorphanol	(Levo-Dromoran)
Oxycodone	(Percodan)
Meperidine	(Demerol)
Methadone	(Dolophine)
Pentazocine	(Talwin)

general population. In such cases meperidine (Demerol), pentazocine (Talwin), and other legitimate pharmaceutical products are diverted for self-administration. Pentazocine is a synthetic analgesic with properties of both narcotics agonists and antagonists. When administered to an opiate-dependent individual, pentazocine evokes withdrawal symptoms. Psychotomimetic effects, such as visual hallucinations, depersonalization, and dysphoria occur at high doses.

Methadone is an orally-effective long acting synthetic narcotic used as a maintenance narcotic in rehabilitation programs for heroin addicts. Inevitably, some methadone is diverted into illicit channels. Methadone's longer duration of action, 24 to 48 hours, is an important consideration during both intoxication and withdrawal. An even longer acting congener, acetylmethadol, has a duration of 72 to 96 hours.

COMMON MEDICAL PROBLEMS

Except for their addictive properties, narcotic analgesics are relatively innocuous when administered in nontoxic doses. The physiologic and psychologic hazards of chronic narcotics use are not well understood. Nevertheless, addicts are subject to an increased prevalence of a variety of maladies. Much of the morbidity is a result of hypodermic needle use, particularly needle sharing, unsterile technique, and injection of particulate matter. Hepatitis is endemic among addicts. Pulmonary hypertension may result from emboli representing accumulations of cotton fibers and undissolved debris. Bacterial endocarditis may occur in both left and right heart valves. Tetanus appears with increased frequency where heroin is "cut" with quinine (eastern U.S.), and malaria is transmitted by needle where

quinine is not used (western U.S.). Cellulitis and skin abscess are very common, especially among "skin poppers." Some unusual cases of Guillain-Barré syndrome (acute polyneuritis) have also been observed that were believed to be related to intravenous opiate abuse. Other factors contributing to the ill health of narcotics addicts are the substandard nutrition, hygiene, and medical care prevalent among the lower socioeconomic strata.

Intoxication

The syndrome of narcotic overdose, particularly following intravenous injection of heroin, is a puzzling phenomenon which cannot be explained solely in terms of an excessive intake of the drug. Analyses of body fluids and residual drug samples usually do not point to an actual pharmacologic overdose. One addict may "OD" while another sharing the same syringe is unaffected. Death may occur suddenly—sometimes immediately after injection. Fulminant pulmonary edema often is evident. Such observations have led to considerable speculation concerning the mechanisms underlying the overdose syndrome. Acute hypersensitivity reactions, effects of quinine and other adulterants, and synergism with alcohol and barbiturates may contribute significantly to its genesis. At present, the evidence for any of these hypotheses is inconclusive.

The typical presentation of heroin overdose is (a) depressed level of consciousness, (b) depressed respiration, and (c) constricted pupils. In severe cases the patient is comatose and apneic. Frothy pulmonary edema is present on initial examination in more than half the cases. Temperature may be normal, elevated, or subnormal. Vomiting often occurs. The clinical picture is variable, depending in large measure on the degree and duration of hypoxia. With severe hypoxia, the skin changes from pale to cyanotic, the pulse becomes weak and slow, hypotension advances to shock, and grave neurologic signs appear: depression of deep tendon reflexes; emergence of pathologic reflexes; and paralytic dilatation of the pupils.

The first consideration in the treatment of narcotic overdose is the maintenance of adequate respiration. An obtunded or comatose patient must be evaluated to determine the frequency and depth of spontaneous res-

pirations, the degree of pulmonary congestion, and the presence of cyanosis. When
there is evidence of respiratory failure, a patent airway must be established, preferably
by endotracheal intubation with a cuffed
tube, and positive-pressure ventilation with
an oxygen-rich mixture instituted. Patients
with pulmonary edema are at high risk and
require careful management. Diuretics, digitalis preparations, corticosteroids, and antihistamines are of dubious efficacy in combating this complication. Assisted ventilation
with oxygen administration is crucial, and in
advanced cases when secretions cannot be
cleared sufficiently, tracheostomy is indicated.

Along with the institution of respiratory
support, cardiovascular status should be assessed. Hypotension and cardiac arrhythmias frequently improve when hypoxia and
acidosis are corrected. Severe hypotension
may require volume expansion, administration of vasopressors, and measures employed in treating shock from other causes.

Samples of blood, urine, and other
fluids should be obtained for toxicologic
analysis. A diagnosis of heroin intoxication is
confirmed by detection of morphine, its
major metabolite. Tests for other narcotics
are available in most laboratories and should
be requested in appropriate cases. Analysis
for CNS depressants and alcohol are indicated when clinical findings suggest multiple drug abuse. Gastric lavage should be
performed after intubation, and stomach
contents should be saved for subsequent
analysis. Routine laboratory data should be
supplemented by liver function tests. After
blood is drawn, 50 cc. of 50 per cent glucose
solution should be given I.V., since hypoglycemia may be present. Analysis of arterial
blood gases in stuporous or comatose patients assists in evaluation of respiratory depression and monitoring of treatment effectiveness. Chest x-rays provide a gauge of the
extent of pulmonary congestion. Skull films
should be obtained in comatose patients and
when trauma is suspected.

NARCOTIC ANTAGONISTS

Narcotic antagonists provide specific
treatment for narcotics poisoning. The antagonist of choice is naloxone (Narcan). In the
recommended dosage range, naloxone has
no morphine-like activity and cannot further
depress respiration. Other antagonists, such
as nalorphine (Nalline) and levallorphan
(Lorfan), have agonistic properties as well
and are for that reason less desirable for
treating respiratory depression when the
cause is uncertain. Naloxone has the additional advantage of effectively counteracting
the depressant activity of other narcotic antagonists, including pentazocine.

The usual initial dose of naloxone is 0.4
mg. I.V. If the diagnosis of narcotic intoxication is correct, an improvement in respiratory rate and depth should be observed after
one-half to two minutes. Recovery is often
dramatic, but care is required at this point.
Patients may emerge from a narcotic-in-
duced coma into an agitated state characterized by delirium and combativeness.
Hypoxia, pulmonary edema, polydrug
intoxication, and the precipitation of an
opiate withdrawal syndrome may all contribute to the problem. Attendants must be prepared to control a confused and struggling
patient. It is important to bear in mind that
the *target symptom is respiratory depression.* Treatment with antagonists should be
restricted to the lowest dose which effectively corrects respiratory inadequacy. They
should not be used to facilitate the return to
consciousness of a patient who is breathing
adequately without assistance. An an-
tagonist-induced withdrawal syndrome cannot be treated with narcotics until the antagonist has been eliminated from the body.

If the patient fails to respond to the administration of an antagonist, one or two additional doses should be given at five-
minute intervals. Unresponsiveness to repeated doses casts doubt on the diagnosis
and requires further evaluation for other
causes of coma and respiratory depression
(see *Coma,* Chapter 23). Patients who demonstrate a satisfactory response should remain under close observation, ideally on an
in-patient basis for 24 hours. Severe respiratory depression may recur within several
hours, necessitating further treatment with
antagonists, since they are eliminated more
rapidly than most opiates. In cases of poisoning with methadone and other long-acting
narcotics, antagonist administration every
two to three hours must continue until
recovery is complete.

Patients who have been resuscitated
from a narcotic overdose should be hospitalized for further observation and general
medical assessment—particularly when pulmonary edema, fever, or convulsions compli-

cate the acute episode. Pulmonary edema may be a late development, especially in cases of intoxication with long-acting opiates. Pneumonia, often secondary to aspiration, is another frequent pulmonary complication. Many other causes of fever must be considered, and body fluids should be cultivated to identify the pathogen. Staphylococcal infections are common. Seizures may result from codeine, pentazocine, and meperidine toxicity. Meperidine poisoning is characterized by respiratory depression, pupillary dilatation, tremor, hyperactive reflexes, and convulsions. Concurrent intoxication with stimulants or withdrawal from depressants may account for seizures in this setting. In cases of severe poisoning, catheterization of the bladder may be indicated to relieve urine retention. Rarely, myoglobinuria, acute renal failure, and transverse myelitis occur.

Prior to discharge, recovered patients should be encouraged to enroll in a rehabilitation program. Some addicts will be more receptive to referral after an overdose experience, and the opportunity should not be lost.

Withdrawal

An interruption of regular narcotic administration in an individual who has a morphine-type physical dependence leads to the development of an abstinence syndrome. The rapidity of onset of symptoms depends primarily on the particular narcotic and the usual daily dose. Drugs with short durations of action, like heroin or meperidine, are associated with brief and intense withdrawal syndromes. Withdrawal from methadone and other long-acting preparations is milder but more prolonged.

The narcotics abstinence syndrome is a stereotyped physiologic reaction characterized by autonomic disturbances, CNS hyperexcitability, and emotional liability, generally accompanied by persistent drug-seeking behavior. In the case of heroin withdrawal, the first symptoms appear about eight hours after the last dose and include lacrimation, rhinorrhea, diaphoresis, yawning, and sneezing. As the syndrome unfolds the addict experiences malaise, restlessness, irritability, depression, insomnia, and anorexia. Gastrointestinal symptoms may include nausea, vomiting, abdominal cramps,

and diarrhea. Myalgias, arthralgias, tremors, and twitches are often prominent. Pupils are moderately dilated. Episodes of pilomotor erection are seen: the term "cold turkey" denoting the untreated syndrome derives from this sign. Mild "rebound phenomena" such as hyperpnea, hyperpyrexia, and hypertension regularly occur. All but the most inexperienced addicts are aware that the administration of a narcotic will promptly and completely suppress the symptoms of withdrawal. If they remain abstinent, their symptoms peak in two or three days and then gradually subside in a week or so. Subtle physiologic abnormalities can be detected for many months after withdrawal, but the significance of these protracted abstinence phenomena is unclear.

In general, emergency services should not assume responsibility for detoxification of narcotic addicts but should refer them to specialized facilities. Medically supervised detoxification is directed toward reversing physical dependence while minimizing the discomfort and drug-craving experienced during withdrawal. The common methods of detoxification involve a stepwise reduction in daily opiate intake until abstinence is achieved. Because of cross tolerance, any narcotic other than one with antagonist properties may be used for this purpose. Substitution of methadone is recommended because of its longer duration of action and its reliable gastrointestinal absorption. Withdrawal may be carried out slowly over many months, or rapidly in several days. Acceptance of the regimen is increased when the addict has some control over the pace of detoxification. Unpleasant symptoms, primarily the flu-like illness of early withdrawal, are less prominent when the dosage reduction is gradual. Symptomatic treatment of the abstinence syndrome is an alternative to gradual detoxification. Sedatives may be prescribed to reduce irritability and insomnia. Mild analgesics provide some relief from muscle and joint pains. Gastrointestinal symptoms may respond to non-narcotic remedies. *Detoxification by whatever method is followed in most cases by a return to regular narcotics use.*

SEDATIVE–HYPNOTICS

The sedative–hypnotics include the barbiturates and a variety of other sub-

TABLE 2   Commonly Abused CNS Depressants

Barbiturates
  Pentobarbital (Nembutal)
  Amobarbital (Amytal)
  Secobarbital (Seconal)
  Secobarbital & Amobarbital (Tuinal)
Nonbarbiturate sedatives
  Chloral hydrate (Noctec)
  Paraldehyde
  Ethchlorvynol (Placidyl)
  Glutethimide (Doriden)
  Methyprylon (Noludar)
  Methaqualone (Quaalude)
Antianxiety agents
  Meprobamate (Miltown)
  Chlordiazepoxide (Librium)
  Diazepam (Valium)
  Oxazepam (Serax)

stances with general CNS depressant activity. Antianxiety agents (minor tranquilizers) are considered under this heading because of numerous similarities in pharmacologic properties and patterns of abuse. Cross-tolerance occurs among most of the sedatives. By these criteria, ethyl alcohol is also a member of this class, but because of its unique significance as a drug of abuse, it will be considered separately. Barbiturates and other depressants can produce relaxation, somnolence, stupor, and coma. In sufficient doses all cause respiratory depression. Sedatives are used in the treatment of a variety of psychiatric disturbances and convulsive disorders and as adjuncts to anesthesia.

ABUSE PATTERNS

While the true extent of abuse of barbiturates, tranquilizers, and other sedatives is unknown, there is no doubt that these substances constitute a public health problem of the highest magnitude. Abuse patterns vary from occasional episodes of self-medication to entirely drug-oriented life styles. Habitual use of sedatives frequently begins iatrogenically, especially among individuals who have no identification with drug-using subcultures. Prescribed for their tension-reducing or sleep-inducing properties, these drugs are often ingested in increasing doses, until physical dependence develops. Recreational use of sedative drugs by adolescents and young adults resembles in many respects periodic binges of alcohol intoxication. The desired effect is a "disinhibition euphoria." Some users indulge in the hazardous prac-

tice of intravenous injection of barbiturates. With this technique the addict experiences a "rush" of sensations not obtained when the drugs are taken by mouth.

Barbiturate abusers characteristically prefer the short acting compounds, such as amobarbital, pentobarbital, and secobarbital. These drugs may be taken orally or parenterally, either alone or in combination with other drugs and alcohol. Intermediate and long acting barbiturates such as butabarbital and phenobarbital do not produce a comparable degree of euphoria and consequently are rarely sought for this purpose. As with the barbiturates, certain non-barbiturate sedatives are favored above others by virtue of their effects, reputation, and availability. Chloral hydrate, glutethimide, methyprylon, and methaqualone are among the more commonly abused drugs in this group. Meprobamate and the benzodiazepines, particularly chlordiazepoxide and diazepam, also have abuse potential. Diazepam is a favored drug of some youthful abusers as well as many of their more conventional elders. The tranquilizers by themselves rarely cause fatal reactions, but may contribute to acute poly-drug toxicity.

COMMON MEDICAL PROBLEMS

Chronic intoxication with sedative–hypnotics appears to be considerably more deleterious than addiction to opiates when measured in terms of impairment of mental and physical function. The habitual user often neglects his personal hygiene and nutrition with adverse consequences to health maintenance. The risk of automotive and industrial accidents is increased as well. Barbiturate addicts who use hypodermic needles are subject to the same serious health hazards as are heroin "mainliners." In addition, because of their alkalinity, barbiturate solutions are extremely irritating if inadvertently injected intra-arterially. In such instances, a prolonged intensely painful vasoconstriction is precipitated which can result in severe ischemic damage to the affected extremity. Immediate hospitalization for anticoagulant treatment is necessary.

Intoxication

Acute barbiturate or other sedative poisoning is most often a consequence of deliberate ingestion of an overdose, although accidental poisoning clearly occurs as well. Tolerance to the euphoric effects of barbiturates is not accompanied by a proportionate elevation in the lethal dose. This reduction in the margin of safety, along with the common practice of ingesting multiple CNS depressants including alcohol, probably accounts for most cases of accidental overdose. "Drug automatism," in which intoxication leads to confusion and repeated ingestion, does not appear to be a significant cause of barbiturate poisoning.

Intoxication with sedative–hypnotics resembles alcoholic inebriation and may include dysarthria, ataxia, emotional lability, and a clouded sensorium. Sustained horizontal and vertical nystagmus usually are demonstrable. Severe intoxication is characterized by a progressive depression of consciousness along with respiratory and cardiovascular failure. Respirations may be slow or may be rapid and shallow. Ventilation is often further compromised by pulmonary edema, atelectasis, or pneumonitis. Blood pressure drops as a result of a centrally mediated vasomotor depression and direct cardiac and peripheral vascular effects, and secondarily as a result of hypoxia. Renal failure may develop if adequate perfusion is not maintained. Pupils may be constricted or dilated with advanced hypoxia. Deep tendon reflexes are often depressed, and pathologic reflexes may appear. Glutethimide has also been reported to cause sudden apnea and acute laryngeal spasm, effects not associated with other sedatives.

Treatment is primarily supportive. Good nursing care is essential and may be all that is required if cardiopulmonary functioning remains relatively normal. When spontaneous respirations are inadequate and gag and cough reflexes are suppressed, an airway should be established with an endotracheal tube. Insufficient respiratory exchange is treated with mechanical ventilation and oxygen administration and monitored by arterial blood gas analysis. Tracheostomy may be necessary when coma is profound and prolonged. Severe hypotension and shock generally respond to volume expansion with intravenous fluids. Prompt correction is required to avoid renal failure and other sequelae. Vasopressors and fluids may be administered to support blood pressure at about 90/60 mm. Hg, and central venous pressure should be monitored. Induction of vomiting should not be considered except for fully conscious patients. Because of the dangers of aspiration in obtunded patients, gastric lavage should be undertaken only after endotracheal intubation. The value of lavage depends on how soon it is performed after drug ingestion. Gastric half-life (when half of an ingested substance passes through the pylorus) is approximately 30 to 45 minutes, although the presence of food in the stomach can change this considerably.

Body fluids should be analyzed for barbiturates and other CNS depressants as indicated. Lethal blood levels of the commonly abused CNS depressants are generally in the range of 1 to 3 mg. per 100 ml., although tolerance and other factors account for considerable variability from case to case. Baseline values for serum electrolytes should be obtained along with other routine laboratory determinations. Measurements of body weight and fluid balance are important in comatose patients.

Forced diuresis accelerates the elimination of longer acting barbiturates. Excretion of short acting barbiturates and of most nonbarbiturate sedatives is only slightly enhanced. If renal function is adequate, mannitol infusion at a rate of 1 liter per hour, with sodium bicarbonate and potassium chloride added to the solution, should produce optimal output of urine. Alkalinization minimizes the tubular reabsorption of weak acids, particularly phenobarbital. Close monitoring of fluid and electrolyte balance, including potassium and magnesium levels, is required for periodic adjustment of the composition of the infusate. Hemodialysis is rarely indicated, but in extreme cases or when renal failure supervenes it may be lifesaving. Virtually all sedative–hypnotics are dialyzable, although short acting barbiturates, benzodiazepines, and glutethimide are less efficiently removed. Consultation with a dialysis team should be sought when clinical deterioration continues in the face of sound medical management.

Analeptics are generally not helpful in the treatment of sedative poisoning and may have adverse effects. Only clinicians experienced with their use should consider administering stimulants in this setting.

Whenever possible, recovered patients should be evaluated to assess the extent of their drug abuse, suicidal intent, and psychologic instability. Appropriate referral for follow-up care can then be made.

Withdrawal

Drug dependence of the barbiturate type is associated with a characteristic abstinence syndrome which in its severest form can be fatal. Following an initial period of apparent improvement, which may last for eight to 16 hours as the intoxication clears, symptoms of withdrawal emerge. Anxiety, tremulousness, insomnia, and weakness intensify as the syndrome progresses. These symptoms are often accompanied by nausea, vomiting, abdominal cramping, and anorexia. Postural hypotension is typically present. Coarse tremors, muscular twitches, excessive blinking, exaggerated startle responses and hyperactive deep tendon reflexes indicate a heightened degree of neurologic irritability which generally reaches a peak in two to three days. Convulsions of the grand mal type are most likely to occur at this time, although they may appear as much as a week after withdrawal, particularly in the case of long acting substances.

Improvement may begin as the seizures subside, or a slowly progressive delirium may develop. This organic brain syndrome is characterized by disorientation, vivid visual and auditory hallucinations, paranoid delusions, and overwhelming anxiety. In the course of the delirium, which may continue for several days, most patients display hyperventilation, tachycardia, hypertension, and fever. Marked hyperthermia can lead to cardiovascular failure and death. Usually, however, even the untreated syndrome clears in about a week.

Recognition of the sedative–hypnotic withdrawal syndrome is important. It must be remembered that withdrawal can begin shortly after recovery from an overdose. Because of the potential severity of the syndrome and the large doses of barbiturates which must be administered to treat it, detoxification should be performed on an inpatient basis.

Addicts may be stabilized on an adequate dose of a barbiturate and then receive decreasing daily doses until a drug-free state is achieved. Stabilization doses are estimated from the history and from the clinical response to trial intoxicating doses. Pentobarbital may be substituted for any barbiturate and for most other CNS depressants (including alcohol). Phenobarbital substitution is based on the same principles, but the longer duration of action allows for a smoother decline in blood levels. Withdrawal from lesser known sedatives should be done without substitution. Generally the dose cannot be reduced by more than 10 per cent daily without the emergence of symptoms. Close observation for signs of excessive or inadequate dosing is necessary throughout the course of detoxification, which may require several weeks to complete.

Seizures should be treated with a short acting barbiturate. Diphenylhydantoin and other nonbarbiturate anticonvulsants are ineffective in this instance. Delirium, once developed, is generally refractory to further barbiturate administration, although aggressive treatment with parenteral sedatives may shorten the duration and decrease the intensity of the reaction.

CNS STIMULANTS

The central nervous system stimulants are sympathomimetic substances which elicit states of heightened alertness, elevated mood, and enhanced psychomotor activity. The principal drugs of abuse in this group are the amphetamines and cocaine. Amphetamines have powerful stimulant effects which last for several hours. Appetite suppression and respiratory stimulation are centrally mediated. Peripheral effects include blood pressure elevation and bronchial dilatation. Cocaine is a local anesthetic obtained from the leaves of the South American plant, *Erythroxylon coca*. Cocaine has systemic and central nervous system effects similar to those of the amphetamines.

ABUSE PATTERNS

Amphetamines are taken by mouth, absorbed through the nasal mucosa, and injected intravenously. Habituation may occur following the prescription of amphetamines for obesity or mild depressions. In other cases, the drug is self-administered to allay fatigue and to improve performance of arduous tasks. Recreational use of amphetamines specifically for their energizing effects occurs primarily among polydrug abusers.

TABLE 3 Commonly Abused CNS Stimulants

Amphetamines
  Amphetamine (Benzedrine)
  Dextroamphetamine (Dexedrine)
  Dextroamphetamine + Amobarbital (Dexamyl)
  Methamphetamine (Desoxyn, Methadrine)
  Methamphetamine + Pentobarbital (Desbutal)
Phenmetrazine (Preludin)
Methylphenidate (Ritalin)
Cocaine

The transition from intermittent to sustained use marks the emergence of psychologic dependence. Tolerance develops with repeated use, necessitating substantial increases in dosage. Intravenous injection of methamphetamine is a particularly destructive practice in which the primary goal is to experience the intense "rush" following injection. "Speed freaks" typically repeat these injections every few hours for several days until supplies run out or exhaustion and paranoia supervene. Such "runs" are followed by a prolonged sleep. Subsequently, symptoms of lethargy and depression may persist until another "run" begins.

Cocaine is highly prized by drug abusers for its ability to induce a state of mental clarity and physical vitality. It is rapidly absorbed through the nasal mucosa, producing a euphoric state of brief duration. Sniffing is repeated periodically to maintain the intoxication. Oral ingestion is relatively ineffective. Intravenous injection of cocaine is most prevalent among those who also use other drugs by this route.

Phenmetrazine, methylphenidate, and other stimulants have similar effects and are subject to similar patterns of abuse. Users of CNS stimulants often seek relief from the agitation they produce by using opiates, barbiturates, and alcohol. These drugs may be taken alternately or simultaneously, evoking complicated psychophysiologic responses.

COMMON MEDICAL PROBLEMS

Chronic stimulant abuse is associated with nervousness, tremulousness, sleeping difficulties, anorexia, and weight loss. Common cardiovascular side-effects are arrhythmias and impaired blood pressure regulation. A variety of gastrointestinal, respiratory, and dermatologic symptoms are seen in connection with abuse of these drugs. Signs of mental deterioration, such as memory impairment, shortened attention span, and emotional instability have been observed among long term high-dose users.

Intravenous use of stimulants carries with it the morbidity resulting from injection of allergens, particles, and pathogens. An additional hazard of intravenous methamphetamine use is a generalized necrotizing angiitis resembling polyarteritis nodosa that produces hypertension, pulmonary edema, pancreatitis, and renal failure. Bacterial endocarditis and septic emboli occur with higher frequency in these groups, particularly when tablets are ground and mixed with water before injection. Subacute bacterial endocarditis occurs more commonly with methylphenidate injection, owing to insoluble components in the tablets. "Speed freaks" characteristically neglect their personal hygiene and nutrition to an alarming degree, even in comparison with other drug abusers.

Overdose

Acute overdose reactions reflect an accentuation of the usual pharmacologic effects of stimulants: anxiety, irritability, tachycardia, other arrhythmias, hypertension, headache, chest pain, and abdominal cramps. The skin is often moist and flushed. Bruxism and gnawing at the lips also are commonly seen. Pupils are dilated. Confusion and panic frequently lead to assaultive or self-destructive behavior. A toxic psychosis may develop, manifested by delirium, auditory and visual hallucinations, and paranoia. Life-threatening doses produce hyperthermia, convulsions, and cardiovascular collapse. Sudden deaths presumably are the result of acute cardiac arrhythmias. Toxicologic studies can detect amphetamines or other stimulants in the body, but the findings will not be available until after the acute reaction has passed.

In less severe intoxications, calm surroundings and mild sedation with a short acting barbiturate or a benzodiazepine may be sufficient treatment. With more extreme reactions, chlorpromazine or thioridazine may be useful for their antipsychotic and sedative effects. In addition, phenothiazines counteract the peripheral adrenergic effects of amphetamines, tending to reduce temperature, pulse, and blood pressure, although an occasional paradoxic hyperthermia has been reported. Anticholinergic reactions requiring physostigmine treatment occasionally result from synergistic reactions between common adulterants and the phenothiazines. Haloperidol also is useful for controlling acute psychotic symptoms and recently has been advocated as the pharmacologic agent of choice in amphetamine poisoning, owing to its dopaminergic activity. If the drugs have been taken by mouth, induced vomiting or gastric lavage may be of value, since stimulants tend to delay gastric emptying. Acidification of the urine by oral administration of ammonium chloride will significantly hasten renal clearance of amphetamines.

Severe hypertension occasionally develops and can cause intracranial bleeding. Sustained systolic pressures above 200 mm. Hg should be brought under control with an alpha-adrenergic blocking agent such as phenoxybenzamine or phentolamine. Hyperthermia should be controlled when temperatures rise above 102°F. A hypothermic blanket may be effective. Phenothiazines can be employed to suppress shivering and reduce fever. Convulsions tend to occur in connection with a rapid rise in body temperature. Seizures may reflect stimulant toxicity, sedative withdrawal, or both conditions simultaneously. Intravenous barbiturate administration is indicated and should be continued as needed to suppress seizure activity. In extreme cases, status epilepticus develops and vigorous treatment is required.

Acute cocaine poisoning differs from amphetamine toxicity primarily in that it runs a more rapid course. Parenteral barbiturate administration is required to control the accelerated progression of symptoms. Otherwise, the same general supportive measures are appropriate. Severe tachycardias or other arrhythmias can be controlled with propranolol.

STIMULANT PSYCHOSIS

Amphetamine psychosis is a distinctive paranoid psychosis which develops in a setting of chronic amphetamine abuse. Similar psychophysiologic reactions are associated with abuse of cocaine, methylphenidate, phenmetrazine, and other CNS stimulants. The syndrome may include paranoid thinking, often with persecutory delusions; auditory, visual, or haptic hallucinations, the latter sometimes leading to excoriation of the skin from attempts to remove imagined parasites; hyperactivity, especially stereotyped compulsive behavior; and a labile affective state in which anxiety and hostility generally predominate. In the typical presentation there is no confusion, disorientation, or memory impairment, distinguishing this syndrome from most toxic psychoses. Amphetamine psychosis should be considered in the differential diagnosis of acute paranoid schizophrenia, for which it is frequently mistaken on initial evaluation. A history of stimulant abuse, physical sequelae such as emaciation, or signs of acute intoxication strongly suggest the diagnosis. Toxicologic analysis of body fluids provides confirmation.

A tranquil and reassuring environment is vital in the management of amphetamine psychosis and may be all that is required in some cases. An accompanying acute intoxication should be treated as described above. Benzodiazepines or other sedatives may be administered for agitation; phenothiazines or haloperidol should be used for more extreme paranoid behavior. Hospitalization is advisable if the psychosis persists or progresses. The symptoms will abate as the drug is excreted. Hallucinations rarely continue for more than one or two days after cessation of amphetamine use. Patients usually sleep excessively for several days and manifest a confused dreamlike state while awake. With no further use of stimulants, the psychosis generally clears within a week.

Chronic "speed" users commonly undergo a progressive psychosocial disintegration. Referral for supportive services is often necessary.

Withdrawal

Although CNS stimulants do not induce physical dependence of a degree comparable to that seen with narcotics and sedatives, withdrawal is not symptom-free. Hypersomnia occurs for the first few days. Depression, fatigue, and apathy are typical and may persist for weeks or months, depending in part on the extent of drug abuse preceding withdrawal. These symptoms may reflect the unmasking of an underlying exhaustion resulting from chronic overstimulation. Relief is often sought through renewed use of stimulants. Emergency treatment is not required. Referral for psychiatric evaluation and counseling is appropriate. In addition, some clinicians recommend prescription of a brief course of tricyclic antidepressants.

HALLUCINOGENS AND CANNABIS

The hallucinogens are a heterogeneous group of substances which produce characteristic "psychedelic" alterations in perception, thought, and affect. Although there are differences in potency, route of administration, somatic side-effects, and duration of action, all of these agents produce similar CNS effects. The term "cannabis" encompasses the various preparations derived from the Indian hemp plant *Cannabis sativa* and other Cannabis species. Marihuana and related drugs have some effects similar to those of the sedatives and, particularly in higher doses, to the hallucinogens.

ABUSE PATTERNS

The use of hallucinogens is most prevalent among educated, affluent young people who smoke marihuana more or less regularly. The usual pattern is an occasional "trip" separated from other episodes by several weeks or months. Physical dependence does not occur. A temporary tolerance to the effects of these drugs rapidly develops after a few daily doses. For most users, a feeling of satiety follows intoxication, resulting in longer intervals between doses than dictated by the tolerance phenomenon. In addition, there is a tendency toward diminished hallucinogen use with time, so that long term chronic abuse is rarely encountered.

Lysergic acid diethylamide (LSD) is the most potent hallucinogen known. The major effects of LSD ingestion are referrable to the CNS and are considerably influenced by the expectations of the user. The subjective experience is multifaceted and may include feelings of transcendence, hyperemotionality, novelty of perception, and a variety of ineffable alterations in consciousness. Most effects subside within eight to ten hours.

Marihuana smoking is extensively practiced in the United States. It is estimated that 26 million Americans have tried it, that 13 million smoke regularly, and that 2.5

TABLE 4 Commonly Abused Psychedelics

Indole Group
    Lysergic acid diethylamide (LSD)
    Psylocybin, psylocin
    Dimethyltryptamine (DMT)
    Diethyltryptamine (DET)
    Dipropyltryptamine (DPT)
    Iboga alkaloids
    Harmala alkaloids
    Myristicin compounds, Morning glory seeds.
Phenylethylamine Group
    Peyote, mescaline
    Dimethoxymethylamphetamine (DOM, STP)
    Methylene dioxyamphetamine (MDA)
    Methoxymethylene dioxyamphetamine (MMDA)
Miscellaneous
    Phencyclidine (PCP)
    Nutmeg
    Cannabis, Tetrahydrocannabinol (THC)

million do so daily. The use of more potent preparations such as hashish ("hash"), hashish oil, THC, and other cannabinoids, is less widespread. Smoking produces effects within a few minutes which persist for several hours. Oral ingestion has a longer onset and duration, and the intensity of intoxication is less controlled by the user. Cannabis intoxication produces mood changes, typically a mild euphoria; perceptual changes, particularly altered time sense; and various changes in thought processes. With higher doses disturbances of perception may be quite marked.

COMMON MEDICAL PROBLEMS

Hallucinogen abuse has been associated with severe depression, paranoia, and prolonged psychosis. Pre-existing psychiatric disorders may be of primary significance in these cases. It appears likely that for certain vulnerable individuals the intense drug experience is sufficient to disrupt psychologic equilibrium.

Information concerning the effects of long term marihuana use on health is accumulating rapidly. Habitual smokers are subject to an increased risk of developing bronchitis and other pulmonary diseases. There is conflicting evidence concerning other effects on physical and mental health. The possible psychologic consequences of chronic intoxication are the subject of much controversy.

Intoxication

Adverse reactions to hallucinogens are primarily psychologic and behavioral. A "bad trip" is characterized by diminished cognitive control, sensory overload, dysphoria, and panic. Fear of persistence of the reaction is common. Judgment is impaired and behavior is unpredictable. Somatic effects are sympathomimetic: pupillary dilatation; hyperthermia; tachycardia; hypertension; nausea; tremor; and hyperreflexia. "Flashbacks" are recurrences of elements of the drug-induced state subsequent to a period of known pharmacologic activity. The majority of these reactions occur within a few days of hallucinogen use and consist of transient episodes of subtle perceptual and affective alterations. In some cases the experience is an intense repetition of an unpleasant aspect of the acute state. Frequent "tripping" is associated with an increased frequency of flashbacks.

Adverse reactions to cannabis are rare in view of the extensive use of these preparations. Intoxication, especially with the more potent forms, can lead to toxic psychosis, paranoia, confusional states, and unpleasant emotional reactions. Perceptual distortions and hallucinations occur. Severe anxiety may be prominent. Physical findings are generally limited to conjunctival injection, tachycardia, hypertension, and dryness of the mouth. Deaths due to cannabis overdosage are virtually unknown. Toxicologic determinations are available for most of these substances, but are rarely necessary for diagnosis or treatment.

Most adverse reactions to hallucinogens and cannabis are handled uneventfully without medical assistance. Individuals who do seek treatment generally go to neighborhood facilities well known in the drug-using community. Those seen at conventional emergency services tend either to be experiencing more prolonged and intense emotional reactions or to be novices in drug abuse. Finding an understanding person in a serene environment will reassure most individuals on a "bad trip," "stoned," or having flashbacks. Characteristically, the user is in a highly suggestible state and will respond readily to "talk-down" techniques. Drug-induced panic can be dispelled by a therapist with a benevolent interest in the patient and a confident, deliberate manner. For patients who do not regain their composure, minor tranquilizers and sedatives have value as adjuncts to a supportive environment. Chemotherapy with phenothiazines carries the risk of anticholinergic reactions. Hospitalization is unnecessary except in extreme cases when psychosis or dysphoria persists.

Withdrawal

Withdrawal phenomena are not seen after discontinuation of hallucinogen use. Interruption of regular use of cannabis products can lead to irritability, sleeping difficulties, and disturbed gastrointestinal function. These symptoms are generally mild and subside rapidly without treatment.

INHALANTS

A variety of substances including anesthetics and solvents may be inhaled to produce brief episodes of intoxication. The use of volatile and gaseous anesthetics for such purposes actually antedates their medical applications. Organic solvents are mixtures of petroleum distillates and are found in household products such as varnishes, paint thinners, cleaning and lighter fluids, and glues. These chemicals enter the bloodstream through the pulmonary alveoli and rapidly induce alterations in consciousness.

ABUSE PATTERNS

Anesthetics are diverted for recreational use by health professionals and others who have access to these agents. Gases are administered from the tank, generally with the use of a facemask or other device. Volatile liquids are poured over a cloth which may be held up to the face or placed in the mouth. The intoxication is brief and inhalation is repeated periodically. Simultaneous intoxication with marihuana or other drugs is common.

Organic solvents are ubiquitous. Intentional sniffing of their vapors is primarily a phenomenon of childhood and adolescence. Youngsters who might have difficulty obtaining other mind-affecting substances find these to be readily available. Paraphernalia for solvent inhalation include moistened

TABLE 5 Commonly Abused Inhalants

Anesthetics
  Gases: Nitrous oxide, ethylene, cyclopropane, halothane
  Volatile liquids: Diethyl ether, chloroform, ethyl chloride
Organic Solvents
  Gasoline, kerosene, toluene, benzene, carbon tetrachloride
Miscellaneous
  Aerosols: Freon and other fluorocarbon propellants
  Amyl nitrite

cloths, bags, balloons, and atomizers. Aerosol abuse follows essentially the same pattern.

Inhalants induce a rapidly reversible organic brain syndrome which is similar in most respects to acute alcohol or sedative intoxication. A dreamy euphoria is typical. In some cases, hallucinations accompany the acute state. Drowsiness is a common aftermath. Tolerance and dependence usually are not seen with abuse of inhalants.

Amyl nitrite, which is administered by inhalation in the treatment of angina pectoris, occasionally is used for nonmedical purposes. Its reputation for enhancing the duration and intensity of sexual orgasm is responsible for perpetuation of its use in the drug culture. Hypotension is the major adverse effect.

COMMON MEDICAL PROBLEMS

The hazards of inhalation have not been firmly established. Damage to the brain, lungs, heart, liver, kidneys, and bone marrow occurs in some cases, although most of the evidence is drawn from studies of industrial exposure which may not be comparable to the occasional deliberate sniffing of vapors.

Intoxication

Inhalers infrequently receive emergency medical treatment, since the effects of these agents are generally quite short-lived. Adverse effects may include agitation, incoordination, confusion, disorientation, delirium, convulsions, and coma. Usually the inhaler stops before these symptoms emerge. Anoxia occurs with the use of hazardous inhalation techniques. In addition, some agents have direct respiratory depressant effects. Pulmonary edema may develop, further compromising oxygenation. Cardiac arrhythmias and hypotensive episodes are common. This cardiovascular toxicity may be aggravated by anoxia. Cases of sudden death after sniffing of aerosols have been reported and are believed to result from acute arrhythmias.

Removal of the causative agent and exposure of the patient to fresh air are often sufficient to reverse the toxic effects. For more severe reactions respiratory assistance and oxygen administration may be required. Hypotensive episodes should not be treated with sympathomimetics because of the dangers of precipitating an arrhythmia in a sensitized myocardium.

Supportive medical treatment usually leads to prompt recovery. Patients should be maintained under observation until cardiopulmonary functions have stabilized. Follow-up care in cases of severe poisoning should include assessment of hepatic and renal status. Psychiatric evaluation is indicated after acute symptoms have subsided, particularly for children.

Withdrawal

Withdrawal syndromes do not occur with most of these substances. Habitual use of ether can produce physical dependence and subject the user to a withdrawal syndrome similar to that seen with alcohol.

ALCOHOL ABUSE

Ethanol is a central nervous system depressant of the sedative–hypnotic class. Alcoholic beverages of all varieties have been employed extensively in Western cultures as socially-sanctioned intoxicants. Alcohol is also a foodstuff that supplies "empty" calories without essential vitamins and nutrients, distinguishing it from other psychotropic drugs and accounting for the chronic malnutrition of many heavy drinkers. The acute effects of alcohol ingestion on behavior and mood are familiar and do not require elaboration.

ABUSE PATTERNS

From a public health perspective, alcoholism is the most destructive of all drug dependencies. An estimated 10 million Americans are "problem drinkers" whose lives are characterized by a preoccupation with alcohol and a loss of control over its consumption. Drinking patterns vary, but chronic and recurrent abuse is found in all strata of society. Increasing use of alcohol by adolescents and increasing use of alcohol along with other drugs are recent trends of some concern. It is estimated that 20 per cent of all alcoholics habitually use other drugs as well.

The common terminology of alcoholism is imprecise. Consequently, no clear criteria mark the transitions from "social" drinking to "problem" drinking to alcohol addiction. As with other CNS depressants, continuous abuse produces both psychologic and physical dependence, cross-tolerance to sedatives, and vulnerability to severe abstinence phenomena.

COMMON MEDICAL PROBLEMS

Illnesses resulting from cumulative alcohol toxicity and accompanying chronic malnutrition affect all major organ systems and account for a disproportionate share of the morbidity and mortality encountered in medical practice. Alcoholics are subject to gastrointestinal bleeding, hepatic dysfunction, and pancreatitis. Chronic alcohol abuse is associated with Wernicke's encephalitis, Korsakov's psychosis, and other neuropsychiatric syndromes. The pathologic sequelae of alcoholism also include a number of cardiopulmonary, neuromuscular, hematologic, and metabolic disorders. Numerous injuries from automobile accidents, industrial accidents, and other causes are the indirect result of inebriation.

Intoxication

Acute alcohol intoxication may occur alone, may be superimposed upon a state of chronic intoxication, or may be complicated by other drug intoxications. Pathologic intoxication refers to an excited, combative, psychotic state following minimal alcohol intake by a susceptible individual. Mild to moderate intoxication ("simple drunkenness") is generally associated with less flagrant behavior.

As alcohol intoxication progresses in severity, clouded consciousness, slurred speech, ataxia, and hyporeflexia develop. Pupils become dilated and nystagmus is demonstrable. Gastric irritation may produce vomiting, which occasionally results in aspiration and pulmonary complications. Further CNS depression leads to stupor. In advanced stages hypoventilation, hypotension, and hypothermia are seen. A lapse into coma may be the prelude to respiratory failure; the margin between an anesthetic dose and a lethal dose of alcohol is narrow.

Blood alcohol levels can be roughly correlated with degree of intoxication, although tolerance and individual variability complicate interpretation of these data. Levels below 50 mg. per 100 ml. rarely produce significant effects. Increasing signs of intoxication are seen as blood levels rise from 100 to 200 mg. per 100 ml. At concentrations of 250 mg. per 100 ml. sedation is usually prominent; at 300 mg. per 100 ml. stupor may occur; and at 400 mg. per 100 ml. coma is likely. Higher levels are usually fatal. Chronic alcoholics require higher blood levels before similar physiologic effects are seen, although the lethal dose is not substantially altered. Blood alcohol determinations, or comparable analyses of urine, saliva, and expired air, are of value in confirming intoxication and gauging the contribution of alcohol ingestion to the over-all clinical condition of the patient. Other toxicologic tests, particularly barbiturate and other sedative levels, are indicated to detect polydrug toxicity. In addition to routine laboratory studies, a liver profile and serum amylase should be done. X-rays of the chest and skull are advisable.

Uncomplicated alcohol intoxication does not require treatment and should be followed by an uneventful recovery. In cases of pathologic intoxication, the patient must be prevented from harming himself or others. Parenteral sedatives can be used for this purpose, although physical restraint may be necessary until the crisis has passed. Alcoholic stupor is usually of brief duration, and if vital signs remain within normal limits specific therapeutic measures are unnecessary. Such patients should be kept under close observation for signs of advancing CNS depression. Injection of thiamine (100 mg.) is advisable in almost all cases.

Alcoholic coma is a life-threatening condition which requires supportive treatment and good nursing care. In the presence of compromised breathing and suppressed respiratory reflexes, a clear airway should be established, preferably by endotracheal intubation. Assisted ventilation with an oxygen-rich mixture is indicated for respiratory paralysis. Hypotension generally improves with adequate oxygenation and intravenous fluid administration. Additional treatments occasionally recommended include analeptic drugs, glucose and insulin solutions, and dialysis. Gastric lavage is unnecessary, unless recent ingestion of other drugs is suspected. The patient should be examined carefully to exclude other causes of coma and to detect concurrent illnesses or injuries. Attributing all findings to alcohol toxicity can delay accurate diagnosis and appropriate treatment.

Once the acute episode has resolved, patients should be evaluated to determine the need for medical aftercare and for treatment for alcoholism.

Withdrawal

Chronic alcohol ingestion produces physical dependence which becomes evident during a period of relative or absolute abstinence. The principal manifestations of the withdrawal syndrome are tremulousness, hallucinosis, convulsions, and delirium. The nature and intensity of the syndrome, which depend on the degree and duration of the preceding intoxication, range from a "hangover" to a full-blown case of delirium tremens.

Tremulousness may begin within a few hours after the last drink, along with flushed facies, hyperreflexia, irritability, anxiety, and insomnia. Typical gastrointestinal symptoms are anorexia, nausea, and vomiting. The coarse tremor may be quite striking after 24 hours of abstinence. Perceptual distortions dominate the clinical picture in some cases. Nightmares and misinterpretations of sensory input may be present. Alcoholic hallucinosis is characterized by frightening hallucinations occurring against a background of clear consciousness. This state may persist for several days, with a progressive loss of orientation and insight.

Grand mal type seizures ("rum fits") may occur within the first few days of abstinence, at times to the point of status epilepticus. Convulsions of a focal type should suggest the presence of another etiologic factor. A convulsive episode often ushers in the development of a delirious state.

Delirium tremens is the potentially lethal end-stage of alcohol withdrawal and is seen only in a small percentage of those undergoing the abstinence syndrome. In addition to the various combinations of symptoms described above, the patient displays profound confusion, disorientation, delusions, hallucinations, and extreme agitation. Signs of autonomic hyperactivity, such as fever, excessive sweating, and tachycardia usually are observed, and circulatory collapse may occur. Delirium can persist for several days. Ten to 20 per cent of such cases have a fatal outcome, particularly those complicated by infections, head injuries, or other disorders.

The milder forms of the abstinence syndrome require little treatment beyond modest doses of tranquilizers. Hospitalization is indicated in the presence of more severe or progressive symptoms. Examination for injuries and infections is essential. X-rays of the skull and chest should be obtained. Evaluation of liver functions also should be done.

Fluid administration to correct water and electrolyte imbalance is a vital component of the treatment regimen. Extreme dehydration is often encountered and may require up to 6 liters of intravenous fluids, one-quarter in the form of normal saline, in a 24-hour period. Serum electrolytes, including magnesium, should be monitored. Hypoglycemia develops occasionally and requires parenteral glucose administration. Thiamine and multivitamin supplements should be added to the parenteral fluids.

Vital signs should be followed closely for early detection of hyperthermia or shock, the most common lethal complications. Fever should be controlled with antipyretics, a cooling mattress, and treatment of intercurrent infections. Circulatory collapse requires blood or plasma transfusions, other intravenous fluids, and measures employed in treating shock from other causes.

A wide variety of sedative drugs have

been employed to ameliorate the alcohol abstinence syndrome. Benzodiazepines have become increasingly favored for this purpose, although some clinicians regard paraldehyde as the safest agent in view of the prevalence of liver disease among these patients. The use of phenothiazines in this setting is more controversial. Anticonvulsant medications are rarely necessary.

The value of a supportive emotional environment in moderating the course of withdrawal is remarkable and should not be neglected. Efforts to orient the patient to his surroundings and to explain procedures before they are undertaken generally are rewarded by an increase in cooperation. A well lighted room and contacts with familiar people help to allay anxieties and reduce agitation. Experience with "social model" detoxification techniques indicates that most episodes of alcohol withdrawal can be managed without any medical treatment.

The abstinence syndrome is self-limited, and recovery generally occurs within a week. These patients have major drinking problems to the point of alcohol addiction. Efforts to engage them in long term treatment are imperative if the pattern is to be broken.

References

Baselt, R. C., Wright, J. A., and Cravey, R. H.: Therapeutic and toxic concentrations of more than 100 toxicologically significant drugs in blood, plasma, or serum: a tabulation. Clin. Chem. 21(1):44, 1975.

Bourne, P. G., ed.: A Treatment Manual for Acute Drug Abuse Emergencies. Washington, D.C., National Clearing House for Drug Abuse Information, Publication No. 16, 1974.

Brecher, E. M. and the Editors of Consumers Reports: Licit and Illicit Drugs. Boston and Toronto, Little, Brown & Co., 1972.

Freed, E. F.: Drug abuse by alcoholics: a review. Int. J. Addictions 8(3):451, 1973.

Sapira, J. D.: The narcotic addict as a medical patient. Am. J. Med. 45(4):555, 1968.

Shearer, R. J., ed.: Manual on Alcoholism. Chicago, American Medical Association, 1968.

U.S. Department of Health, Education, and Welfare. First Special Report to the U.S. Congress on Alcohol and Health. Publication No. (HSM) 72–9099, Washington, D.C., 1971.

Wesson, D. R., and Smith, D. E.: A conceptual approach to detoxification. J. Psychedel. Drugs 2(2):161, 1974.

Chapter 56

DERMATOLOGIC EMERGENCIES

Howard M. Simons

INTRODUCTION

Considering the large area of the skin, the relative infrequency of cutaneous life-threatening emergencies may be surprising. Even in urticaria and erythema multiforme, both of which are seen fairly often, only a small percentage of cases require emergency treatment.

Although each emergency dermatologic condition is uncommon in its full-blown form, less severe variants occur often enough. More important, perhaps, is that only through a working knowledge of these entities can misdiagnoses be prevented, thus avoiding unnecessary laboratory studies and undue alarm to the patient and his family.

Much of the discussion in these sections is organized from the standpoint of major symptoms and signs. Classification by etiologic agent(s) would be theoretically more desirable, but in most instances etiology is obscure. Similarly, aside from cultures and microscopic examination for organisms, specific laboratory tests are rarely available and clinical impression remains the basis of diagnosis. A careful history and precise description of the skin lesion therefore assumes the greatest importance.

While few dermatologic conditions are life-threatening, patients with acute skin conditions frequently present at Emergency Departments. This probably reflects the suddenness of onset, the high visibility of the lesions, and the frequent severe pruritus. Reassurance of the patient and family is an important component of treatment.

RECOGNITION OF DERMATOLOGIC EMERGENCIES AND THEIR INITIAL MANAGEMENT

VESICULOBULLOUS ERUPTIONS

Toxic Epidermal Necrolysis

Toxic epidermal necrolysis is a cutaneous syndrome heralded by erythema, fever, bullae, and widespread exfoliation of the skin. This desquamation is probably its most characteristic feature and is similar in appearance to wet paper peeling off a wall (Fig. 1, A). The Nikolsky sign, where gentle pressure on normal skin causes bullae or further desquamation, is invariably present (Fig. 1, B). As the exfoliation progresses, the denuded surface appears moist, erythematous, and glistening, similar in appearance to a severe thermal burn—hence the alternative term for this condition, *scalded skin syndrome*. The process begins suddenly, and initial lesions usually appear around the eyes, oronasal area, and genitalia, with subsequent mucous membrane involvement.

The most common symptom, skin tenderness, is often severe. Even before clinical changes are seen in the skin, infants and younger children will remain very still because of the discomfort produced by movement. Other symptoms include anorexia, lethargy, diarrhea, and vomiting.

ETIOLOGY

The causes of toxic epidermal necrolysis fall into two main groups. In infants and children up to seven years of age, most cases are caused by epidermolytic toxin elaborated by staphylococci. In almost all cases of this milder form of the disease, the toxin is produced by group 2 staphylococci, usually phage type 71 or 55/71, but more recent reports have implicated group 1 as well. The mortality rate for infants is high, but drops to around 5 per cent in the one to six age group.

In adults, various drugs and chemicals cause a more severe form of toxic epidermal necrolysis characterized by more extensive mucous membrane involvement and a mortality rate of 30 to 40 per cent. The drugs most often cited are sulfonamides, phenylbutazone, salicylates, penicillins, and barbiturates, although a complete list of all drugs mentioned in the literature would exceed 100 preparations. One patient who developed the syndrome following the ingestion of gin and tonic was exquisitely sensitive to small quantities of quinine. Carbon monoxide and a fumigant containing acrylonitrile have been reported to produce toxic epidermal necrolysis following inhalation.

Although toxic epidermal necrolysis is reported in adult patients with a variety of diseases, it is not clear whether the skin changes are due to these diseases or to one of the many medications that these patients received.

RECOGNITION

In more severe forms of toxic epidermal necrolysis, the combination of widespread painful erythema and sheetlike exfoliation with flaccid bullae usually permits a rapid clinical diagnosis. Erythema multiforme also has peri-orificial involvement (Fig. 2), but often shows typical iris or target lesions (Fig. 3), a negative Nikolsky sign, and discrete lesions rather than widespread exfoliation. Erythema multiforme and toxic epidermal necrolysis are both reaction patterns to a variety of agents, and, in cases which cannot be separated clinically, both entities may be present at the same time.

Milder cases of toxic epidermal necrolysis that occur in children may be less easy to recognize clinically, and a high index of suspicion is essential. About 90 per cent of children are febrile and 50 per cent show leukocytosis, circumstances suggesting an infectious process but otherwise nonspecific. Although erythema may be absent, skin tenderness is an almost constant finding, resulting in an irritable, febrile child who appears afraid to move. There is usually a history of sore throat, ear ache, or rhinorrhea.

Division of toxic epidermal necrolysis into two major types should aid recognition. The milder staphylococcal type is seen mainly in children, whereas the more severe "drug" type shows more mucous membrane involvement and may be confused clinically with erythema miltiforme. It should be remembered, however, that the "drug" type may be seen in children as well as adults and that a few staphylococcal cases have been reported in adults.

Although the histology of the two types differs, frozen section techniques usually are unavailable, making this an impractical means of differentiating between the two.

MANAGEMENT

As soon as the presumptive diagnosis of toxic epidermal necrolysis is made, cultures should be obtained from the nasopharynx, blood, urine, unruptured bullae, skin, eyes, and ears. An intravenous drip should be started immediately to facilitate therapy and maintenance of fluid balance and nutrition. Although almost all patients will require hospitalization, patients 10 and under (and most older patients as well) should be started on treatment for penicillinase-producing Staphylococcus aureus infection while still in the Emergncy Department. Sodium nafcillin or sodium methicillin is the drug of choice, although the former has been used more widely in this condition. It is given intravenously in dosage of 50 mg. per kg. daily in divided doses every four hours for children, and in dosage of 0.5 to 1 gm. every four hours for adults. Erythromycin is also effective and should be used if the patient is allergic to penicillin. However, if parenteral medication is necessary cephalothin can be used cautiously.

In drug-induced cases, systemic steroids are clearly indicated, and moderate to high doses should be given, depending on the presence of relative contraindications to their use. The intravenous route should be used initially. One of the most challenging problems to confront the emergency physician is the severely ill child whose history and clinical appearance do not permit differentiation between toxic epidermal necrolysis and erythema multiforme, even though one or the other seems more likely. The child may be toxic, febrile, and dehydrated and have already received small doses of numerous medications. In such a patient, high-dose steroids should be combined with appropriate antibiotics, keeping in mind the possibility of a drug-induced syndrome. Systemic steroids do not appear to affect *Staphylococcus areus*-induced toxic epidermal necrolysis adversely, provided that an effective antibiotic is given simultaneously.

Local care of the skin may be life-saving in the seriously ill patient with the drug-induced variety and should be started in the Emergency Department if admission to the hospital will be delayed more than a few hours. Warmed silver nitrate, 0.5 per cent aqueous, should be applied as a compress to denuded areas in order to reduce the number of gram-negative organisms in these areas. Use of a rotating frame will aid compressing and also reduce trauma to the intact skin. Loss of heat can be reduced by placing the patient in a warm humidified room, and strict isolation procedures will reduce the chances of a life-threatening secondary infection. Fluids, electrolytes, and nutrition must be monitored and maintained, especially in infants.

Erythema Multiforme

Erythema multiforme (Figs. 2, 3), an acute disorder primarily affecting the skin and mucous membranes, has distinctive clinical lesions and multiple causes. Unfortunately, dermatologists, because of their tendency to describe in detail and to give adjectival names to minor variations of this entity, have encouraged nondermatologists to lump together under this heading a variety of conditions that do not belong there.

The lesions of erythema multiforme are well defined and quite characteristic. The multiforme appearance is related to the severity of the process and to the tendency for new crops of lesions to continue to appear.

ETIOLOGY

The causes of erythema multiforme are many, and each year several new "causes" are added to the list. Although little is known about the mechanisms of disease production, recent investigations suggest that small blood vessels in the skin become sensitized by bacterial, viral, or chemical products. A large number of recurrent cases are caused by, or at least are associated with, *Mycoplasma pneumoniae* and the virus of herpes simplex, and this may include the common "idiopathic" erythema multiforme that occurs in children and young adults during the winter and early spring. Other infections that may be related include histoplasmosis, trichomonas, influenza, ECHO and coxsackie viremias, orf, and fungal infections. Vaccinations with the viruses of vaccinia, mumps, and poliomyelitis have also been incriminated.

Although many drugs have been reported to produce erythema multiforme, those most often cited are the penicillins, sulfonamides, and barbiturates. Phenolphthalein, used as a laxative or as a dye in inexpensive red wines, produces a localized erythema multiforme reaction of the genitalia or lips. X-ray therapy, internal malignancies, and collagen diseases are other causes.

RECOGNITION

Erythema multiforme occurs most commonly in a mild form, but for unknown reasons it also may appear as a more severe toxic process often referred to as the Stevens-Johnson syndrome. Episodes of both forms resolve spontaneously in two to four weeks. However, rarely a fulminating course with secondary infection may lead to a fatal outcome.

The initial lesions of the mild form are bright red macules that typically appear suddenly on the hands and feet in symmetrical distribution. Other common sites are the forearms, elbows, and lower legs, and all these sites may be involved together. The lesions may coalesce and become general-

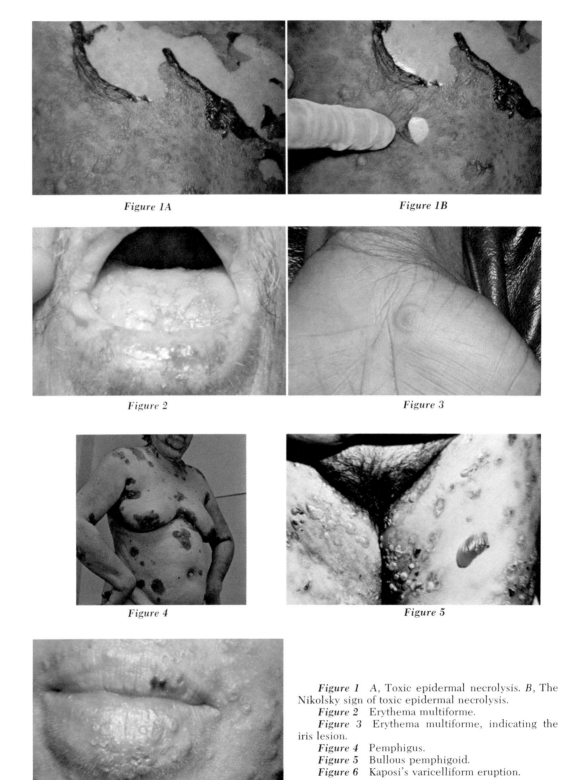

Figure 1A

Figure 1B

Figure 2

Figure 3

Figure 4

Figure 5

Figure 6

Figure 1 A, Toxic epidermal necrolysis. B, The Nikolsky sign of toxic epidermal necrolysis.
Figure 2 Erythema multiforme.
Figure 3 Erythema multiforme, indicating the iris lesion.
Figure 4 Pemphigus.
Figure 5 Bullous pemphigoid.
Figure 6 Kaposi's varicelliform eruption.

ized, but rarely is the trunk involved before the extremities. Mucosal lesions, present in about 30 per cent of cases, begin as vesicles or bullae that become eroded or crusted.

The red macules evolve to violaceous papular swellings or more frequently to the characteristic iris (or target) lesions. The latter are pathognomonic of erythema multiforme and show a thin peripheral red border, a middle pale zone, and a dusky center which may be vesicular. Iris lesions are edematous at first but later persist as macules until they fade, eight to 12 days after their initial appearance. Resolution occurs without scarring, but hyperpigmentation may persist for weeks to months. Pruritus is variable.

The Stevens-Johnson syndrome is characterized by severe mucosal involvement, especially of the mouth and eyes, although the vagina and urethra often show changes as well. The palate and oral mucosa show raw, tender surfaces covered by a sticky gray exudate; the lips may be swollen, bloody, crusted, and exquisitely tender. The patient cannot eat or drink or open his mouth to permit examination. The eyes are bilaterally involved with a purulent conjunctivitis; the lids are edematous, and crusting causes them to stick together. Corneal involvement with ulceration may occur, probably due to secondary bacterial infection. Genital lesions show a similar exudative clinical pattern, but the anal and nasal mucosae are rarely involved.

The skin may show the iris and maculoedematous lesions of the milder form or may display severe vesiculobullous lesions, frequently with hemorrhage. In other cases, severe mucosal involvement will occur without skin changes. Stevens-Johnson syndrome may be ushered in with fever, malaise, prostration, and a prodrome of flu-like symptoms; but these changes, along with pneumonitis, may be due to an underlying respiratory virus.

Recognition of erythema multiforme depends on the characteristic appearance of the eruption, and diagnosis is almost impossible during the prodromal period. If the patient is seen during the prodrome, an upper or lower respiratory infection may be suspected. On the other hand, erythema multiforme is often recurrent in children and young adults, and taking a thorough history may enable the astute emergency physician to predict the appearance of the eruption.

In sum, erythema multiforme is recognized by its characteristic symmetry, acral and mucosal distribution, and cutaneous iris or vesiculobullous lesions. With the use of rigorous clinical standards, false positive diagnosis may be avoided. There are no specific laboratory tests for erythema multiforme, and any abnormal findings usually reflect an underlying process or secondary infection. Recognition of erythema multiforme occasionally will require consideration of the following mucocutaneous disorders:

Pemphigus. In this more chronic and indolent process, the bullae are larger, break easily, and leave eroded lesions which tend to enlarge by detachment of the epidermis at the periphery. Involvement of the trunk is common, and erythema is rarely prominent. Mouth lesions are the first site of activity in more than one-half of cases; however, they are typically erosive and show little tendency toward crust formation. Nikolsky sign is present and may account for the localization of skin lesions to areas of the trunk that are exposed to friction or pressure (Fig. 4). If pemphigus is suspected, a Tzanck test performed on material scraped from the floor of a bulla will show *acantholytic* cells, swollen epidermal cells whose cytoplasm has condensed peripherally at the cell walls.

Behçet's Disease. This rare clinical entity reported most often from eastern Mediterranean countries is characterized by recurrent oral and external genital ulcerations in association with iritis and other destructive inflammatory changes of the eyes. The mouth lesions are quite similar to the erosions of recurrent aphthous stomatitis, and Behçet's disease is more easily confused with the latter than with erythema multiforme. Ocular involvement is usually progressive and severe, although it is initially unilateral in one-half of cases in contrast to erythema multiforme, where eye lesions are symmetrical. Behçet's disease may show varying multisystem involvement. Its other skin lesions are described as acneiform or pyodermatous when present.

Bullous Pemphigoid. In this skin disease of the elderly, large tense bullae appear in association with erythema in a wide distribution, although the axillae, groin regions, and flexor arm areas are more commonly involved (Fig. 5). Oral mucosal lesions occur in one-third of patients, but are few in number, rarely very painful, and never progress to severe stomatitis. Bullous pemphigoid may be further differentiated from erythema multiforme by: *(a)* its gradual onset and more chronic course; *(b)* the absence of iris lesions, although gyriform erythematous lesions are seen; *(c)* the sparing of acral areas; and *(d)* its rarity in patients under age 50, even though occasional childhood cases have been seen.

Toxic Epidermal Necrolysis. See page 1273. In most cases, the sheetlike exfoliation of this entity contrasts well with the more discrete vesiculobullous eruptions of erythema multiforme, and yet confusion between the two entities does occur. Favoring toxic epidermal necrolysis are a positive Nikolsky sign, exfoliation *around* the mouth rather than crusting of the lips, unilateral eye involvement, and the symptom of tender skin.

MANAGEMENT

The mild form of erythema multiforme usually requires little more than symptomatic treatment, reassurance about the benign prognosis, and an explanation to the patient about likely causes of this mucocutaneous disorder. In regard to the last, a thorough history and physical examination must aim at uncovering latent infections and must record all medications (including "over-the-counter" preparations) that the patient has taken. The patient should be asked specifically about fever sores, herpes infections, and cold sores present now or in the past and about any other cutaneous lesions he has noticed. A chest x-ray is indicated for even the mildest of respiratory symptoms associated with skin manifestations. Antibiotic treatment of *Mycoplasma pneumoniae* infection should be instituted if this underlying condition is found.

The discomfort of oral lesions may be reduced by warm saline gargles, aspirin, and viscous lidocaine. One tablespoon of lidocaine should be swished around in the mouth, held there for one minute, and then swallowed just before meals. Applications of Vaseline will soften superficial crusting around the eyes and lips.

In more severe cases of erythema multiforme, systemic steroids are indicated and should be started immediately as hydrocortisone 80 to 120 mg. every eight hours intravenously, or 60 to 90 mg. of oral prednisone daily in one stat dose if oral ingestion is tolerated. Since hospitalization is indicated in severe cases, antibiotics should be reserved for treatment of specific infections that may be uncovered later. All suitable cultures should be taken prior to institution of any antibiotic therapy.

Kaposi's Varicelliform Eruption

This somewhat cumbersome term refers to an infection by the viruses of either herpes simplex or vaccinia that occurs *only* in persons with a predisposing skin disease. The terms "eczema herpeticum" and "eczema vaccinatum" have the advantage of being more specific, but have not completely displaced the older term because (1) the two viral conditions are almost identical clinically and (2) a third agent, coxsackievirus A16, has also been shown to produce Kaposi's varicelliform eruption.

Although atopic dermatitis is by far the most common condition in which these infections occur, they are also known to infect patients with Darier's disease, seborrheic dermatitis, pemphigus, ichthyosis, and contact dermatitis on rare occasions.

RECOGNITION

The cutaneous eruption typically begins with the sudden appearance of massive crops of small vesicles that enlarge rapidly, develop characteristic central umbilications, and become pustular and crusted. Although abnormal skin usually shows the earliest involvement, later the process may become generalized. Crops of new lesions appear as the patient develops high fever, constitutional symptoms, and marked regional lymphadenopathy. The face frequently shows the most severe involvement and may be markedly edematous (Fig. 6).

Depending on the severity of the infection, the lesions may become confluent, severely erosive, or hemorrhagic. Secondary bacterial infection may obscure the primary lesions and occasionally contribute to mortality, although viremia and viral visceral involvement appear to be the main causes of death in this condition.

The most severe cases occur in infants and in other patients who have no antibodies against the causative viruses; therefore, recurrent attacks in the same individual are almost always milder. In eczema vaccinatum, a history of vaccination in the patient or a close family member usually will be obtained. On the other hand, the herpes simplex virus is more ubiquitous and thus more apt to cause recurrent attacks. Usually healing occurs in two to three weeks.

Since most patients (or their parents) assume that the skin problem is merely an exacerbation of atopic dermatitis, close examination of the clinical lesions and a high index of suspicion are required to recognize this occasionally fatal condition. The physician must steer away from the crusted or hemorrhagic confluent areas of the face and look for discrete lesions with characteristic central umbilications. The presence of fever and prostration also suggest that this is more than just an acute dermatitis.

The diagnosis of eczema vaccinatum is confirmed by a history of recent vaccination or exposure to a vaccinated person. Although eczema herpeticum also may have historical support, its diagnosis should be confirmed in the Emergency Department by examination of a smear (Tzanck test) taken from one of the lesions. The roof of an early vesicle or pustule is removed with a scalpel blade or fine iris scissors, and the residual fluid is gently removed with a small gauze sponge. The base of the vesicle or pustule is then scraped onto a glass slide with a scalpel blade and is stained with Giemsa's or Wright's stain. Finding multinucleated epithelial giant cells confirms the diagnosis of eczema herpeticum as these changes are absent in eczema vaccinatum or smallpox infections.

Differentiation of the latter two diseases may be difficult in geographic areas where smallpox occurs; here the emergency physician may have to base his working diagnosis on the absence of the rather severe prodromal symptoms and consistently centifugal distribution of the skin lesions of smallpox. Subsequent changes in antibody titers will make the distinction quite clear.

MANAGEMENT

Patients who have moderate to severe involvement with Kaposi's varicelliform eruption will always require hospitalization, and the nature and extent of initial management depend on the speed with which this is arranged. Bacterial cultures should be taken from the skin, especially from areas that appear to be secondarily infected. Intravenous penicillin should be used initially to treat the streptococcal and staphylococcal bacterial overgrowth always present in this condition. Cool compresses of a 1 to 40 solution of aluminum subacetate (Burow's solution) should be applied four times daily for 30-minute periods to facilitate crust removal, although localized pyodermatous areas will benefit more from warm aqueous compresses and gentamicin ointment.

Strict isolation technique should begin in the Emergency Department, and it is the responsibility of the emergency physician to insure its continuation during the patient's transferral to the hospital floor. The severely ill patient already has a viremia and overgrowth of resident bacteria on the skin; an additional pathogen may be more than he can handle. Also isolation separates the patient from medical personnel and other patients who may be susceptible to the viruses of Kaposi's varicelliform eruption.

The value of hyperimmune gamma globulin in the management of eczema vaccinatum is now well established, but is strongly disputed in eczema herpeticum in the doses that have been tried thus far. Preliminary reports indicate that intravenous use of adenine arabinoside is effective in most herpes infections, although dosages for its use have not yet been established. Although it has no known toxicity, its insolubility requires the administration of large intravenous fluid volumes, and it seems likely that more water-soluble adenine analogues will replace it in the future. Systemic steroids do not appear to be helpful, and may be dangerous in herpes conditions.

URTICARIA

Angioedema and urticaria may be discussed together, as they often occur together. Urticaria is an eruption of "hives" or welts, transient swellings of the skin which are well circumscribed, erythematous, and usually pruritic (Fig. 7). As they enlarge, their raised irregular borders surround paler centers. The term "angioedema" suggests a more severe form of urticaria with larger lesions and involvement of subcataneous or deeper structures. Although individual lesions rarely last longer than 36 hours, new crops of lesions may prolong the patient's discomfort indefinitely in the absence of treatment.

ETIOLOGY

The emergency physician will be confronted almost exclusively with acute episodes of the so-called immunologic (or allergic) form of urticaria, most often due to an antigen–antibody reaction in which histamine (and perhaps other substances) is released from mast cells. The production of immunologic urticaria requires the individual to form specific antibodies of the IgE class following exposure to an antigen. These specific antibodies become fixed to the surfaces of mast cells and, upon subsequent exposure to the antigen, act in some poorly understood manner to cause release of histamine from mast cell granules. Histamine, along with other chemical mediators, then either acts pharmacologically or activates other mediators or reflex actions that result in clinical urticaria.

Anaphylaxis and *serum sickness* are two urticaria-related conditions produced by variant immunologic mechanisms. Anaphylaxis is a symptom complex, potentially life-threatening, that involves the integumentary, respiratory, cardiovascular, and digestive systems, singly or in combination (for management of this life-threatening condition, see also Chapter 57). Angioedema, rather than urticaria, usually predominates, and typically is manifested in swollen eyelids, tongue, and lips. Edema of the larynx or lower bronchial tree can produce shortness of breath and a feeling of tightness in the chest. Wheezing may be severe. Cyanosis and more severe respiratory distress may be followed by asphyxiation. Hypotension occurs frequently in more severe cases, whereas gastrointestinal symptoms are seen less often. Anaphylaxis usually occurs immediately or within hours of antigenic exposure.

Serum sickness, on the other hand, usually begins seven to 14 days after antigenic exposure, and its usual symptoms of urticaria, arthralgia, fever, and lymphadenopathy begin insidiously. Serum sickness, which derived its name from its onset following injection of non-human serum, is now seen most frequently as a complication of drug therapy. When the antigenic substance has been injected, an intense reaction of urticaria or edema will often occur at the site of injection.

Although acute urticaria is easier to re-late to its precipitating agent than is chronic urticaria, the latter should be assumed to represent repeated episodes of acute urticaria occurring over a prolonged period. In both cases the antigenic substance is immediately present, and attempts to identify it must include consideration of the following possible causes:

Drugs. Urticarial drug eruptions are caused by an infinite variety of drug components. Penicillin heads the list because of the frequency and seriousness of its reactions, and even trace contamination by it in dairy products has caused urticaria. Aspirin, other over-the-counter products, nose and eye drops, diagnostic aids in radiology, and preservatives and dyes present in drugs and vitamins can cause urticaria. Reactions following intradermal skin tests are well known, but anaphylactoid and urticarial reactions may also follow *topical* applications of antibiotics and mechlorethamine in highly sensitive individuals.

Foods. Although many foods may cause urticaria, those most commonly cited are seafood, eggs, chocolate, berries, nuts, milk, and pork. A secondary group of frequent offenders includes oranges, wheat, chicken, corn, tomato products, and garlic. Foods are probably the most common cause of mild acute urticarial reactions that are recognized by the patient but require no medical treatment. Urticaria from foods is occasionally associated with gastrointestinal symptoms, fatigue, or headache. Urticaria from shellfish, nuts, and berries often appears within minutes of ingestion, whereas it may be delayed for several hours after intake of foods in which the antigen is formed by the digestive actions of proteolytic enzymes. Recent work has called attention to the role of food additives and dyes such as benzoic acid and azo dyes in the causation of urticaria, and the number of foods containing these materials is quite extensive.

Insects. (See also *Bites and Stings*, p. 804.) Urticarial reaction from insect stings results primarily from Hymenoptera (bees, wasps, hornets and yellow jackets) and should be differentiated from both the *normal reaction* to stings and the *delayed* or *localized reaction*. Most persons will experience swelling, redness, and burning pain at the site of the sting, occurring almost immediately and usually subsiding within several hours. The delayed or localized reaction is much less common, occurs from a few hours to a few days after the sting, and may be manifested by extension of the local swelling, increasing discomfort, varying distortions of the stung part, or vesicles. It does not result from an immunologic reaction but appears to depend instead on pharmacologic reactions of chemicals or toxins in the venom.

Wasps and hornets, in contrast to bees, are scavenger insects and can transmit infection when they sting. For this reason, a pyoderma or cellulitis may distort the clinical appearance of a normal or delayed reaction, making it unrecognizable. The infection itself may not be recognized before the local reaction has subsided.

Urticaria may occur independently of the preceding normal or localized reaction, in that a more severe localized reaction is not a forerunner of severe urticaria or anaphylaxis. Urticarial reaction may occur within minutes or not for many hours following the sting, and in milder cases the onset may be insidious.

In addition to stinging insects, generalized uriticarial reactions can be caused by biting insects on rare occasions. Mosquitoes lead the list of biting insects that produce these reactions, but urticaria has also been reported to follow bites by black flies, kissing bugs, fleas, deerflies, and horseflies.

RECOGNITION

The most valuable diagnostic tool is clinical evaluation with special emphasis on history taking. Since urticaria and angioedema may represent an early phase of anaphylaxis, specific questioning should be directed at detection of this potentially lethal condition. The patient should be asked about the presence of gastrointestinal symptoms, of lightheadedness or dizziness, of feelings of generalized warmth, and of soreness or tightness in the throat or chest. Although angioedema of the eyelids or oral cavity is easily detected (Fig. 8A and B), scrotal or vulvar edema is easily overlooked and often unnoticed by the patient who has pruritic urticarial lesions elsewhere. Mild hypotension or slight tachypnea may be early signs. Anaphylaxis is much more likely to occur following parenteral administration than following oral medication. Also the patient should be questioned about recent skin

tests and the possibility of an occult insect sting in which the normal reaction was inapparent.

Although the classic morphology of urticaria permits almost immediate recognition, difficulties may arise when the urticarial lesions are the early skin changes of another disease. Dermatitis herpetiformis, pemphigoid, lupus erythematosus, vasculitis, occult malignancies and lymphomas, and Loeffler's syndrome will occasionally present urticaria as an early sign. Atypical features or multiform lesions should arouse suspicion in the examining physician. Dermatitis herpetiformis and pemphigoid might show vesicular or crusted lesions, excoriations might suggest a malignancy or lymphoma, and in lupus erythematosus the urticaria may be accompanied or distorted by various erythematous lesions.

Although a large number of infections and infestations are associated with urticarial reactions, such cases usually present with longstanding (chronic) urticaria and are therefore less likely to challenge the emergency physician. Clinical evaluation, however, should consider such conditions as dermatophytosis, moniliasis, periodontal disease, amebiasis, helminth infestation, and other occult infections. The view that laboratory studies are *not* needed in acute urticaria and are *not* helpful in chronic urticaria is a little extreme, and some recourse to laboratory studies is indicated, especially if aimed at confirming a diagnosis rather than at groping for one. On the other hand, a routine blood count, urinalysis, and sedimentation rate might suggest the presence of an occult medical problem or infection. Further laboratory studies should be left for the follow-up physician unless the evaluation uncovers a specific clue.

The following conditions may be confused with immunologic (allergic) urticaria and must be considered in the differential diagnosis of urticarial reactions:

Cold Urticaria. At least two clinical forms exist. In the more common acquired cold urticaria, lesions usually appear within minutes of exposure to cold. Histamine appears to be the mediator of the reaction, but other agents almost certainly are involved. The production of a pruritic wheal following the application of an ice cube to normal skin for at least five minutes will confirm the diagnosis. Familial cold urticaria, a rare condition, appears to be a systemic reaction in which urticarial lesions are delayed in onset (with negative ice cube test), nonpruritic, and associated with arthralgias and a leukocytosis.

Cholinergic Urticaria. In this condition, sweating or exertion, emotional stress, and eating spicy foods produce characteristic 1- to 3-mm. wheals usually surrounded by a large red flare. The very small wheals and supporting history often are typical enough to suggest the diagnosis without recourse to administration of cholinergic drugs.

Hereditary Angioedema. This dominantly inherited condition is characterized by recurrent nonpruritic swellings of the skin and mucous membranes and is usually diagnosed in infancy or early childhood. No urticaria is present. Lesions often follow trauma, and many deaths occur from laryngeal obstruction.

Dermatographism. About one-third of the normal population shows the triple response of Lewis following firm stroking of the skin. The term dermatographism is applied when the triple response is persistent or exaggerated or produces a pruritic syndrome. Although dermatographism may be seen following emotional stress or drug reactions, the cause in most patients is not apparent. When a pruritic syndrome is present, scratching induces further dermatographism, and the appearance may mimic urticaria.

Papular Urticaria. Except in its name, this warm weather condition of children has almost no relationship to immunologic urticaria. Following some poorly understod sensitivity to biting insects, such as fleas or bedbugs, the patient develops papules, urticarial lesions, excoriations, and occasionally impetiginized crusted lesions. Although infants may show lesions on any skin surface, older children usually show the most activity on exposed parts of the arms and legs. In this condition, the urticarial lesions are small, round, and often excoriated or crusted; usually they are easily distinguished from the large transient lesions of other urticarias.

MANAGEMENT

Although the initial treatment of immunologic urticaria (and anaphylaxis) is epinephrine, its use depends to a great extent on the severity of the reaction. In the absence of hypotension, 0.3 ml. of 1:1000 epinephrine should be injected subcutaneously along with 50 mg. of diphenhydramine hydrochloride administered orally or intramuscularly. If the reaction is caused by medication injected into an extremity, proximal tourniquets and injection of epinephrine directly into the injection site should reduce absorption of the antigenic substance. Caution must be used if the patient is hypertensive or has cardiac disease. In such instances a much smaller initial dose of epinephrine is indicated.

Since hypotension may delay the absorption of epinephrine from a subcutaneous site, epinephrine should be given intramuscularly to these patients. An intravenous infusion should also be started so that antihistamines may be given by this route. Epinephrine may be repeated at five-minute intervals if no response is noted.

Since intravenously administered epinephrine increases the risk of cardiac arrhythmia, this route is reserved for life-threatening conditions, and only 1/100,000 epinephrine should be used. In patients receiving phenothiazine medications, epinephrine may produce a further paradoxic hypotension, and should be replaced by phenylephrine hydrochloride. Diphenhydramine hydrochloride should be given cautiously and never be repeated where bronchospasm is suspected, and in patients with asthma it should be replaced by another antihistamine such as promethazine hydrochloride.

When possible, a tourniquet should also be applied proximal to the site of a sting; and if the stinger remains, it should be scooped out carefully with a dull blade to avoid injection of more venom into the skin. All patients should be observed and treated until the symptoms have abated, and oral antihistamines should be continued for several days or until discontinued by the follow-up physician. Aspirin, but not other salicylates, is reported to aggravate urticarial reactions, and the patient should be warned of this.

PURPURA

Purpura is a change in color of the skin or mucous membranes or both resulting from extravasation of red blood cells. Although usually pink or red in color, various shades from orange-brown to blue-black are seen as the red cells break down to form various pigments. Smaller lesions, 3 mm. or less, are called *petechiae;* larger ones are known as *ecchymoses. Hematoma* refers to a palpable ecchymotic mass, often the result of trauma. In contrast, small purpuric lesions are almost always macular unless an associated inflammatory infiltrate makes them palpable.

Purpura is recognized by failure of a suspected lesion to blanch under application of firm pressure. Although finger pressure is most often used, diascopy, where the pressure is applied with a glass slide, provides better visualization of the lesion. Differentiating purpura from macular inflammatory lesions or telangiectasia may be especially difficult on the lower legs, and in such cases diascopy should always be used. In some cases purpura can be identified only with the help of a skin biopsy, but the latter usually is not considered an Emergency Department procedure.

Like pruritus or anemia, purpura is an indication of disease, not a disease per se. Although the diseases which cause purpura are quite numerous, only the small number which may present as an emergency condition will be discussed here. This number is further reduced by the omission of thrombocytopenic purpuras and coagulation defects, which are discussed in Chapter 49A.

Anaphylactoid Purpura (Henoch–Schönlein Purpura)

This syndrome (Fig. 9) results from acute or subacute inflammation of small blood vessels in the skin and, less commonly, in the gastrointestinal tract, joints, and kidneys. When purpura and gastrointestinal changes occur together, the term "Henoch's purpura" is often applied; "Schönlein's purpura" is used when joint changes are prominent. In recent years, however, this unnecessary splitting of the syndrome has been eliminated by using the term "Henoch-Schönlein purpura" synonymously with anaphylactoid purpura.

This is primarily a condition of children and young adults, with peak incidence in the four to seven age group. Twice as many males as females are affected. The syndrome is most common in early spring and follows upper respiratory infections in many pa-

tients. Despite the reported high incidence of preceding infections, no relationship between infection and this syndrome has been clearly established. Antistreptolysin 0 titers are not found to be elevated, and the renal involvement of anaphylactoid purpura differs qualitatively from the glomerulonephritis which follows streptococcal infections. Although numerous drugs have been incriminated as causative agents, the vast majority of cases have no drug history. The possibility that the syndrome results from hypersensitivity to an occult virus has been considered but never proved, although some experimental work suggests that an antigen–antibody reaction occurs in or near the small blood vessels.

Indeed, any mechanism that produces dilatation and altered permeability of the small vessels could account for the cutaneous hallmarks of anaphylactoid purpura: exudation and hemorrhage. Upon dilatation of the small vessels, the initial lesions are pink and macular, but within hours they become edematous or even urticarial. As hemorrhage occurs, their color darkens to red, then purple; the subsequent variable hues of resolving purpura are seen during the next several days.

Most cases of anaphylactoid purpura resolve spontaneously in three to five weeks although recurrences are seen in a small minority of patients.

RECOGNITION

The skin of patients with anaphylactoid purpura shows more than just purpura, although very few skin lesions will resolve without displaying at least some petechial component. The skin changes are polymorphous. Macules, papules, urticarial edematous lesions, palpable purpura, and, if the exudation is severe in the upper dermis, hemorrhagic bullae may be seen. Erosions, ulcers, and crusts are not common. Lesions are seen most commonly on the lower legs and ankles, but the buttocks, elbows, and forearms also are frequently involved. Localized edema of the face, hands, and feet often occurs in younger children and is apparently unrelated to any underlying renal involvement.

Gastrointestinal involvement usually produces colicky pain that is difficult to localize on abdominal examination. Vomiting, hematemesis, and melena also are frequently seen. The abdominal pain may be severe enough to cause confusion with an "acute abdomen," and this is especially likely if skin changes are minimal. On the other hand, intussusception does occur, requiring surgical correction.

The typical joint pain of anaphylactoid purpura is acute at onset, involves the knees and ankles most often, and occurs in the absence of joint swelling and redness. The pain may be transient and variable during the attack.

Recognition of anaphylactoid purpura is easy if the triad of palpable purpura, abdominal colic, and joint pain is present. Recognition also may be easy if purpuric lesions are present with involvement of only *one* of the other systems, provided the examining physician has an appreciation of the distribution and polymorphous appearance of the cutaneous changes. Since the syndrome recurs in some patients, a history of prior involvement may be obtained.

Laboratory tests are not especially helpful, although a normal platelet count rules out a thrombocytopenic cause for the purpura. The sedimentation rate is frequently elevated to a moderate degree. Although urinary abnormalities reflecting renal vascular involvement will be found in most patients, these are almost always absent in the early stages. Eventually, most of the patients will show microscopic hematuria, and approximately 40 per cent will have gross hematuria, proteinuria, or both. A small number of patients will develop severe renal involvement which may lead to permanent kidney damage. As with gastrointestinal involvement, the severity of the renal changes does not correlate with the severity of the cutaneous lesions.

Since noninflammatory diseases and coagulation defects usually cause purpura that is monomorphous and macular, confusion with anaphylactoid purpura is unlikely. In contrast, separation from conditions that produce inflammatory purpura or elevated lesions may be difficult, and one or more of the following conditions may have to be considered in the differential diagnosis.

Systemic Vasculitis. This entity, also known as leukocytoclastic angiitis because of its characteristic histologic features, may show skin lesions similar to those of anaphylactoid purpura but is a more chronic process and more variable in its clinical presentation. Although anaphylactoid purpura and systemic vasculitis appear to be related by their occasionally identical cutaneous changes and similar vascular pathologic processes, anaphylactoid purpura should be viewed as a well-defined, more acute clinical syndrome. In contrast, systemic vasculitis is seen more commonly in adults, has large vessel involvement resulting in cardiopulmonary and central nervous system changes, and causes fever in 75 per cent of cases. Skeletal involvement produces myalgia, stiffness, and weakness, in contrast to the transient joint pain of anaphylactoid purpura.

Gonococcemia. In a small percentage of gonococcal infections, the infecting organism will invade the blood stream and produce the triad of fever, arthritis, and skin lesions. The skin changes are typically either hemorrhagic or vesiculopustular on an erythematous base and usually are accompanied by an intermittent fever, chills, and mild to moderate prostration. The arthritis is mild and polyarticular at first, later becoming localized in one or two joints, and, unlike anaphylactoid purpura, may produce heat, tenderness, and swelling. The gonococcemic lesions are palpable, and most often involve the hand and fingers (Fig. 10), unusual sites for the skin lesions of anaphylactoid purpura. The latter condition is seen most commonly in youngsters, whereas gonococcemia is limited to persons, usually female, who are sexually active. Unfortunately, the gonococcus is difficult to demonstrate in the skin lesions, either by culture or by direct smear, although fluorescent antibody techniques have shown the organism to be present.

Meningococcemia. Although most patients with meningococcemia will be prostrate, febrile, and either obtunded or comatose, milder cases in which an alert patient complains of muscle aches, nausea, or cough may be difficult to separate from anaphylactoid purpura. As in the latter condition, the cutaneous changes of acute meningococcal diseases show purpura on a background of polymorphous lesions. The purpura is typically palpable, decidedly grayish in color, varies in size from a few millimeters to several centimeters, and is very irregular in outline—much like the coast of Maine. It has a more generalized distribution, but the buttocks and legs are predominantly involved. Except for epidemics

Figure 7   Urticaria.
Figure 8   *A,* Angiodema. *B,* Angiodema following therapy with systemic steroids.
Figure 9   Anaphylactoid (Henoch-Schön-lein) purpura.
Figure 10   Gonococcemia.
Figure 11   *A* and *B,* Progressive pigmentary purpura.

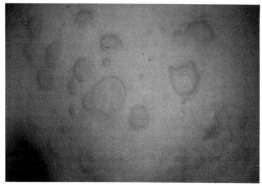

Figure 7

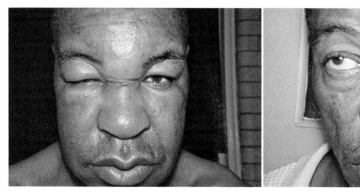

Figure 8A

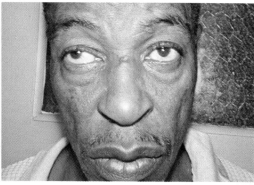

Figure 8B

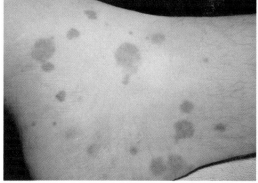

Figure 9

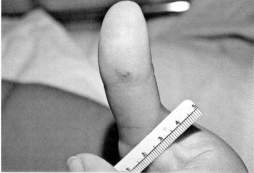

Figure 10

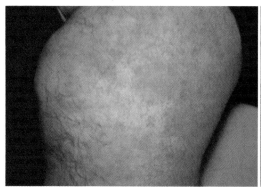

Figure 11A

Figure 11B

in the military, meningococcemia attacks the same age group subject to anaphylactoid purpura.

Any problems in differentiating anaphylactoid purpura from mild forms of acute meningococcemia are usually solved by laboratory tests. Leukocytosis is almost always present in acute meningococcemia, and spinal fluid examination may show a polymorphonuclear pleocytosis and gram-negative diplococci on culture or smear. Direct examination of material from a skin lesion is much less likely to demonstrate the organism.

Recurrent episodes of anaphylactoid purpura could be confused with chronic meningococcemia, a condition in which a transient bacteremia occurs every one to four days, resulting in distinct episodes of fever, chills, myalgias, anorexia, and skin lesions. The cutaneous changes appear in showers after the onset of the fever and evolve and fade as the fever and other signs of the bacteremia resolve, only to reappear with the next episode. The morphology of the skin lesions is much less regular. Poorly demarcated erythematous macules and papules are more common, but hemorrhagic lesions are also described, as well as a variety of vague intermediate lesions. Culturing the organism from the blood confirms the diagnosis.

Rheumatic Fever. Erythema marginatum occurs in 10 to 15 per cent of patients with acute rheumatic fever and may be confused with the skin changes of anaphylactoid purpura because of the associated joint involvement and its occurrence in a similar age group. Erythema marginatum begins as an erythematous macule or papule which enlarges peripherally, leaving a paler inactive center and producing an annular or polycyclic pattern. The advancing borders may be macular or elevated; their color may be pink, red, or dusky, but is *always* blanchable. Erythema marginatum typically enlarges rapidly, rarely lasts more than a few days, and leaves no residual marks. However, recurrent crops may prolong the skin changes for several weeks or longer. It is usually asymptomatic and is more common on the trunk and extremities than on the acra.

The evanescence, the rapid peripheral spread, and the immunologic relationship to streptococcal organisms suggest that erythema marginatum is probably a variant of urticaria. Occasionally, when the pale central part of the lesion is edematous, the similarity to a hive is striking. The lesion may be viewed as an inferior form of hive, a hive with scanty exudation and little or no pruritus.

The lesions of anaphylactoid purpura may be differentiated from erythema marginatum by the absence of peripheral spread and by the presence of purpura. Recognition of the former requires taking an adequate history; of the latter, a microscopic slide for diascopic examination.

Progressive Pigmentary Purpura. Although this chronic condition is seen almost exclusively in adults, it merits brief inclusion here more because of its importance to the diagnosis of purpura in general than because of its only superficial resemblance to anaphylactoid purpura. The use of the term *progressive pigmentary purpura* permits elimination of at least seven cumbersome eponymic designations, of which Schamberg's disease is probably the best known. The alternative term *capillaritis* stresses the microscopic changes. Its cause(s) is unknown.

Irregular orange-brown or yellow-brown patches typically begin on the lower legs or feet and spread proximally. The most characteristic clinical finding is the delicate pinpoint petechiae (cayenne pepper spots) seen within and at the periphery of older lesions (Fig. 11). Although pruritus is usually minimal or absent, some variants are pruritic and show a more generalized distribution. The process seems unrelated to other medical problems and may resolve spontaneously over many months or years.

Progressive pigmentary purpura is clinically differentiated from anaphylactoid purpura by the absence of ecchymoses, elevated lesions, and other epidermal changes; by its very chronic course without other system involvement; and by its frequency in middle-aged persons, especially males. Progressive pigmentary purpura could be confused more easily with a drug eruption, venous insufficiency, and Waldenström's hyperglobulinemic purpura.

Rocky Mountain Spotted Fever. Six or seven days after a tick bite, the infected patient usually develops grippelike symptoms (headache, myalgia, and malaise) and subsequently fever, chills, and joint symptoms. A blanchable erythema begins on the third or fourth day of fever on the wrists and ankles and spreads to the palms and soles as well as centrally to the arms, legs, trunk, and face. In time the erythema becomes dusky or bluish and, finally, petechial (Fig. 12).

Although the typical case of Rocky Mountain spotted fever is not easily confused with anaphylactoid purpura, a patient with a milder prodrome might be puzzling. In a more severely ill patient, meningococcemia may be difficult to rule out. Since routine laboratory tests are within or close to normal limits in Rocky Mountain spotted fever, its diagnosis must be clinical. The patient should be questioned carefully about recent tick bites, possible exposure to ticks, and the progression of the eruption and its relationship to early symptoms. The treatment of choice is tetracycline, 1 gm. every eight hours in adults, taken on an empty stomach.

MANAGEMENT

Although anaphylactoid purpura is an acute self-limited process, most patients are best treated in the hospital. Management generally centers around reassurance of the patient and his family, relief of the acute symptoms, and bed rest. Only in the mildest cases should this be attempted on an outpatient basis. Another reason for hospitalization is the uncertainty of the diagnosis: the possible confusion with rheumatic fever or sepsis.

Despite the large number of cases that appear to follow upper respiratory infections, antibiotics should not be given unless a specific infection is present or suspected. Joint pain is best treated by bed rest, as it allows the patient to assume the position that provides the most comfort. Since aspirin and phenacetin have gastrointestinal and renal side-effects, respectively, they should be strictly avoided. Acetaminophen or propoxyphene hydrochloride would be appropriate if analgesics are needed. The skin changes do not appear to be helped by topical corticosteroids.

Systemic corticosteroids are most valuable in treating painful arthritis, abdominal pain, and gastrointestinal hemorrhage. This last is the most dangerous acute problem in anaphylactoid purpura and should be treated with systemic corticosteroids as soon as the possibility of intussusception has been ruled out. Prednisone should be given in daily doses of 40 to 60 mg., depending on the age of the patient and the severity of the hemorrhage or pain. Localized soft tissue edema also responds rapidly to systemic corticosteroids although other cutaneous changes do not.

Intussusception occurs in about 3 per cent of affected children, and surgical consultation should be obtained if abdominal symptoms are severe. Renal changes in anaphylactoid purpura are slower to appear and are, therefore, usually not the concern of the emergency physician. The value of treating these changes with systemic corticosteroids or immunosuppressive agents has not yet been established.

Purpura Fulminans

This rare entity is characterized by the sudden appearance of large ecchymotic areas which often become necrotic or gangrenous (Fig. 13). These fulminating ecchymoses usually are on the extremities, although acral parts of the face may be involved. The skin changes are accompanied or soon followed by fever, chills, and vascular collapse, which may lead to death within one or two days. In patients who survive, gangrenous digits often will either self-amputate or require surgical amputation.

The etiology of purpura fulminans is better understood by its relationship to the syndrome of disseminated intravascular coagulation. Although purpura fulminans is most often described as occurring in children recovering from mild viral or bacterial infections, it is also seen in certain obstetric disorders, following pulmonary surgery, in prostatic carcinoma, and following certain snake bites. All of these conditions have been reported to show altered intravascular coagulation and increased fibrinolytic activity.

Apparently, clots form continuously in blood vessels as a normal occurrence, and this process may increase in various conditions, even without clinical thrombotic disease. In purpura fulminans and the diseases mentioned above, intravascular clotting is more extreme, more generalized, and results in the consumption of circulating fibrinogen.

Thus, coagulation in distal vessels and generalized defibrination explain the acral gangrene and large ecchymotic areas, respectively, that occur in purpura fulminans.

RECOGNITION

The combination of rapidly progressing hemorrhagic skin lesions with signs of prostration, fever, and shock is very suggestive of purpura fulminans. The ecchymoses are palpable and usually limited to the extremities initially, although they often spread centripetally, show some blistering necrosis, and may be joined by gangrene of the digits or of hemorrhagic areas. The typical patient is an otherwise healthy youngster who is convalescing from a minor infection.

Less severe forms of purpura fulminans merge with the syndrome of disseminated intravascular clotting, and it may be better to use the latter term in such cases, reserving purpura fulminans for the more explosive condition described above. The diagnosis of disseminated intravascular clotting is most often made on patients hospitalized with various ailments such as septicemias, leukemias, obstetric problems, and various carcinomas. As more sophisticated hematologic testing becomes available, it seems likely that all or most patients with these ailments will be shown to have increased clotting tendencies even in the absence of clinical bleeding.

On the other hand, patients with the intravascular coagulation syndrome come to the Emergency Department with signs of hemorrhage (purpura, hemoptysis, hematuria, etc.) or because of their underlying disease (septicemia, carcinoma, etc.); but without both present together, the correct diagnosis is difficult to make clinically. Any patient with *palpable* purpura should be questioned thoroughly about underlying cardiopulmonary conditions which could produce hypoxia, the presence of cancers especially of the prostate, recent treatment with chemotherapeutic agents, and infections of any kind. Acral and facial cyanosis are seen occasionally and are usually gun-metal or purplish and sharply outlined, and do not blanch with pressure.

The diagnosis of purpura fulminans or disseminated intravascular coagulation can almost always be confirmed by laboratory tests, which show a prolonged prothombin time and decreased fibrinogen and platelets. In patients with liver disease or in milder cases where tests may be equivocal, a skin biopsy is helpful.

MANAGEMENT

Although the intravascular coagulation syndrome usually is managed by treating the underlying disease, purpura fulminans produces such severe hemorrhage that it should be treated immediately with anticoagulation. Although the dose of intravenous heparin has not been clearly established for this condition, somewhere in the range of 80 to 100 units per kg. every four hours seems reasonable. The hemorrhage will continue for at least 18 to 24 hours before responding to heparin; treatment is usually continued for three or four days longer. Monitoring of the hemostatic factors usually shows a more rapid return to normal of fibrinogen than of platelets.

Supportive measures are essential, and acidosis and hypotension in particular should be treated vigorously in order to increase the already decompensated tissue perfusion. Blood transfusion may be indicated. Local skin care is aimed at preventing and treating infections which are expected to occur as the large ecchymotic areas become necrotic or gangrenous. Gentle compression with an antibacterial soap and applications of gentamicin ointment will be helpful.

Milder forms of disseminated intravascular coagulation rarely require heparin, since therapy for the primary process usually is available. The one exception is in acute leukemias where heparin may halt a hemorrhagic episode until the malignancy can be brought under effective long term control by chemotherapy.

NECROTIC ULCERATIONS

Pyoderma Gangrenosum

Pyoderma gangrenosum is an uncommon ulcerating inflammatory condition of the skin which starts as a painful acute process and then usually goes on to a chronic destructive course.

About 50 per cent of cases occur in association with ulcerative colitis, and although the pyoderma gangrenosum usually parallels the activity of the bowel disease, it may appear when the colitis is subsiding or may even precede the diagnosis of ulcerative colitis. Other patients with pyoderma gangrenosum have been reported to have regional ileitis, rheumatoid arthritis, cavitary or infectious lung disease, or a variety of other gastrointestinal lesions. Some patients appear to be in perfect health despite extensive search for one of the associated diseases. The finding of hypoproteinemias and paraproteins in some patients suggests that bacterial allergy may play a significant role in the production of pyoderma gangrenosum, and the appearance of new ulcers at the sites of bacterial skin tests supports this possibility.

Pyoderma gangrenosum occurs with equal frequency in males and females, and is much more common in adults than in children. In the latter, the skin changes are almost always associated with a gastrointestinal process. Healing occurs slowly, usually taking several months or longer. The resulting scars appear to be proportional to the size of the ulcerations.

RECOGNITION

The initial lesion is usually a small erythematous papulopustule that may become a tender or painful nodule before becoming necrotic. Generally, central ulceration occurs within several days and is followed by irregular peripheral enlargement or coalescence of other similar necrotic papulonodules to form multiple lesions of varying size and shape. The ulcers are most common on the legs and buttocks.

Surrounding the central partially crusted necrotic mass is a ragged overhanging edge which often displays a characteristic bluish-black hue. Peripheral to the edge is a bandlike area of erythema and edema which advances as the ulcer enlarges (Fig. 14).

Pyoderma gangrenosum is recognized by the combination of the above clinical features with a history of ulcerative colitis or other process known to be associated with necrotic skin changes. The patient should be asked specifically about symptoms of colitis and ileitis as well as about a history of such symptoms. Information about the initial appearance of the skin lesion(s) should be elicited, keeping in mind its fairly rapid

evolution. In rare cases, the initial papulopustule will wax and wane without ever showing central necrosis, merely persisting as a solitary lesion or more commonly a group of lesions which are tender or mildly painful.

Smear or culture of the necrotic mass for organisms is more apt to confuse than help, as a mixture of the resident flora and facultative transients is usually found. These organisms typically vary from lesion to lesion in the same patient. Other abnormal laboratory findings are difficult to evaluate and probably reflect the activity of an associated disease. Skin biopsy usually shows necrosis and acute inflammation of the upper dermis, with apparent secondary ulceration of the epidermis. Although this histology is nonspecific, the absence of vasculitis is helpful in diagnosis.

In cases where the clinical features are less typical or where an associated disease is not found, some of the following conditions may have to be considered in the differential diagnosis.

Factitious Dermatitis. In this condition, the patient consciously produces skin lesions in order to avoid work, to gain sympathy or narcotics, or for other selfish reasons. The lesions may be produced by a variety of agents, including the fingernails, sharp instruments, various chemicals, and heated metallic objects, and ulcerations suggestive of pyoderma gangrenosum may result. Factitious dermatitis is suspected much more often than it is proved, and observation of the patient and the skin changes over an extended period is almost always necessary to confirm this diagnosis. Helpful clues are the presence of pain which appears out of proportion to the amount of tissue destruction, sharp or angular edges to the lesion, and inappropriate response to treatment. Factitious lesions may spare the right hand and right arm of right-handed persons.

Iodermas or Bromodermas. These vegetating, often granulomatous lesions are apparently an allergic response to either one of the halides, and may follow ingestion of such drugs as potassium iodide, carbromal, or vitamin preparations. The lesions also may be seen in persons whose drinking water contains iodides or who have received an iodide preparation for a radiographic gallbladder study. The following features of iodermas and bromodermas are helpful in their differentiation from pyoderma gangrenosum: (1) their more exuberant and hyperkeratotic surface studded with small pustules; (2) their frequent occurrence on the face, a rare site for pyoderma gangrenosum; and (3) a history of exposure to halides. Oral administration of ammonium or sodium chloride facilitates removal of the halides from the body.

Sporotrichosis. This fungal disease is caused by *Sporotrichum schenckii* and most commonly occurs in gardeners, florists, or outdoor workers following trauma from a thorn or splinter. The initial lesion appears on the exposed surfaces as a nodule or pustule which ulcerates. Although painless, it has an appearance similar to pyoderma gangrenosum and at this stage would be difficult to differentiate from the latter. Although a few sporotrichotic ulcers will remain this localized, most are followed by lymphangitic spread, resulting in multiple painless subcutaneous lesions or indolent ulcers along the extremity. The fungus cannot be seen in potassium hydroxide smears, but is readily cultured on routine fungal media.

Vascular Ulcers. These usually occur on the lower legs, and will rarely approach the magnitude of pyoderma gangrenosum in the absence of well-established syndrome of venous or arterial insufficiency. Ischemia is more likely to produce gangrene than ulceration but not infrequently is the cause when venous or traumatic ulcerations heal slowly or fail to heal.

A special type of ischemic ulcer, the *hypertensive ulcer*, could be easily confused with pyoderma gangrenosum. This ulcer, occurring of course in hypertensive patients, usually involves the skin of the outer aspect of the lower leg just above the ankle. It begins as a dusky red, painful area which becomes purpuric and then ulcerates. The resulting ulcer is punched-out, has a necrotic center, and enlarges irregularly by peripheral spread, but rarely becomes larger than several centimeters. Pain is a persistent symptom and is unrelieved by bed rest. An erythematous halo, similar to that seen in pyoderma gangrenosum, may surround the ulcer if it is infected. Control of the infection and removal of the adherent eschar with enzymes and debridement are essential to the management of these indolent ulcerations.

Venous ulcers are a much more chronic condition, and almost always occur on a background of the chronic changes of stasis dermatitis. The latter consists of a variable combination of telangiectasia, petechiae, edema, atrophy, hemosiderin pigmentation, and secondary eczematous changes. The diagnosis is rarely in doubt when the full-blown picture is present, but may be more difficult when a trumatic ulcer fails to heal because of early stasis changes. In such cases, the presence of varicose veins or a history of venous surgery may be helpful.

MANAGEMENT

Most patients with pyoderma gangrenosum will require hospitalization, and the decision to initiate treatment in the Emergency Department is based on the activity of the skin lesions and the presence of an associated disease. The treatment of an underlying ulcerative colitis will facilitate healing of the skin, but the form of this treatment must be determined by the patient's previous response to therapy and the advice of the consultant gastroenterologist to whose service the patient will be admitted. Sulfapyridine or salicylazosulfapyridine is frequently effective, but may be combined with systemic corticosteroids if the bowel or skin lesions are especially destructive.

Relief of pain may be achieved with any of the usual analgesics, although aspirin should be avoided here, as its use is contraindicated in all conditions in which gastrointestinal bleeding may occur. Low dose narcotics occasionally are required.

Warm aqueous silver nitrate compresses (0.5 per cent) are advised for their antibacterial, debriding, and soothing effects. They should be applied for 20 minutes four times daily, followed by application of gentamicin ointment.

Intralesional injections of a corticosteroid suspension are reported to produce rapid healing of the necrotic ulcerations, and might be an ideal form of therapy in patients who have no underlying disorder or cannot tolerate systemic corticosteroids. Large amounts of an 8 mg./cc. concentration may be injected under and around the ulcerations without producing atrophy.

Coumarin Necrosis

This necrosis of the skin is an uncommon complication of treatment with coumarin congeners. It characteristically occurs three to ten days after initiation of anticoagulant therapy. Although the initial lesions are painful red areas, they evolve rapidly into purpuric swellings which ulcerate and form hemorrhagic eschars. The necrotic lesions, which occur almost exclusively in women, are strikingly asymmetric in distribution. They usually heal spontaneously in six to ten weeks, even if the coumarin derivative is continued.

Although these ulcerations usually are more benign than they appear clinically, occasional cases have shown deep extensions with considerable destruction and scarring. Amputation of a digit is a rare complication, but even milder forms may add considerably to the morbidity of patients who have other vascular diseases. Coumarin necrosis has contributed to death in several patients.

The cause of coumarin necrosis is unknown. Specific allergy to a coumarin congener has not been demonstrated in these patients, and vasculitic lesions are not seen histologically. A toxic endothelial change apparently occurs as an idiosyncratic reaction independent of the prothrombin level, and this is followed by localized intravascular coagulation.

RECOGNITION

The typical appearance of these multiple irregularly outlined infarcted lesions in a patient who was recently started on a coumarin anticoagulant usually affords immediate recognition. Pain is a consistent clinical finding. Although erythema is present at first, subsequently the infarcted skin is free of surrounding erythema. The affected skin usually overlies areas of increased body fat, such as the buttocks, thighs, breasts, or calves, although other areas may be involved less commonly.

These deep, bizarre ulcers are very suggestive of self-inflicted lesions, and if the history of coumarin anticoagulation is not obtained or is unavailable, the possibility of factitious dermatitis is difficult to rule out. Pyoderma gangrenosum and spider bites are discussed elsewhere in this section.

Less severe forms occasionally are seen in which the skin lesions persist as painful ecchymotic swellings without necrosis. These lesions may be difficult to differentiate from localized infection, but the absence of heat is a helpful diagnostic sign.

Since hemorrhage is the most common side-effect of coumarin therapy, the early changes of coumarin necrosis usually are assumed to be due to bleeding into the skin, and only a high index of suspicion will allow the correct diagnosis to be made in this early phase. It must be remembered that coumarin necrosis will always appear within three to ten days after the anticoagulant has been started and that over 90 per cent of reported cases appeared on days three to five. Although skin hemorrhage occurring during these early days could be confused with coumarin necrosis, hemorrhage is unlikely unless the prothrombin time is within or above the high therapeutic range. Hemorrhage into the skin is often accompanied by bleeding elsewhere, e.g., the gastrointestinal or genitourinary tracts.

MANAGEMENT

If coumarin necrosis is recognized early in its course, the *immediate* use of heparin may prevent subsequent infarction of the skin. One dosage schedule suggests immediate administration of 15,000 units of heparin intravenously, followed by 10,000 units every four to six hours until a total daily dose of 35,000 units has been given.

Although continuation of the coumarin congener does not adversely affect the healing of the necrosis that it produced, most authors recommend stopping the drug and administering vitamin K. On the other hand, this decision must be based on the possible risk to the patient of thrombosis and embolization, the processes the anticoagulant was initially given to control.

Once necrosis of skin has occurred, heparin is of no value, and treatment is merely symptomatic and supportive. Although most necrotic ulcers heal spontaneously with scar formation, surgical excision of larger areas followed by skin grafting has been recommended.

Loxoscelism

The bite of the brown house spider, *Loxosceles reclusa*, may produce a necrotic slough at the site of envenomation in association with systemic toxicity of variable severity. The spider is found in the southern and central parts of the U.S., where its natural habitat appears to be rocky or wooded areas. However, in colder regions it has moved indoors, where it lives unnoticed in closets, attics, and basements. Its tendency to live in old clothes and trunks no doubt accounts for sporadic cases in such nonendemic areas as Pennsylvania and California.

The brown spider is·8 or 9 mm. long and is fairly easily identified by the violin-shaped band on its cephalothorax.

RECOGNITION

The spider bite either is not felt or produces a slight stinging discomfort initially. However, pain may appear within two to ten hours, followed by erythema, tenderness, and occasionally blister formation. Subsequently an ischemic zone appears around the site, and the latter becomes indurated and hemorrhagic. An irregular, often stellate eschar slowly becomes demarcated over the next five to ten days, and with separation of the eschar an ulcer is seen.

Systemic toxic reactions occur in a small number of patients and are more severe in children. Chills, fever, weakness, nausea, vomiting, and restlessness have been described in association with a faint maculopapular erythematous eruption that is occasionally petechial. Hemolytic reactions are a rare complication that can be fatal in children.

Mild cutaneous changes with little or no systemic reactions may follow recluse spider bites and probably are much more common than the severe cases. If the spider is not observed, an itchy or mildly painful erythematous reaction that is not followed by necrosis might be ascribed to a hymenoptera sting. These milder forms are difficult to recognize, except in endemic areas.

The differential diagnosis of an early spider bite may include cellulitis, pyoderma, or hymenoptera sting. Severe pain that requires narcotics for control, a central vesicle or bleb, and a two-hour or longer delay in the onset of the local reaction favor recluse spider bites over stings. The general-

ized eruption after spider bites is usually morbilliform rather than urticarial. Although no laboratory tests are helpful early in the course, evidence for hemolysis may be found later: hemoglobinemia, thrombocytopenia, and bilirubin elevation. Subsequent necrotic ulceration is often *late* confirmatory evidence of the diagnosis.

MANAGEMENT

Pain, a delayed but common feature, is usually the reason for seeking medical treatment. The pain typically intensifies over several days before diminishing, and although non-narcotic analgesics should be tried initially, stronger preparations frequently are needed. The pain appears to be unrelated to the amount of tissue damage—to the degree that extremely painful spider bites may show no necrosis. Hydroxyzine hydrochloride 25 mg. three times daily should be prescribed for localized or generalized pruritus.

The value of systemic corticosteroids in preventing necrosis is disputed, and animal investigations have shown no benefit from this medication even when administered prior to envenomation. On the other hand, systemic corticosteroids appear to reduce the systemic reaction and hemolytic syndrome without altering the tell-tale eschar and slough.

Immediate or early excision with primary closure also has been suggested, but seems rather heroic when many recluse spider bites will resolve without necrosis. However, if elliptical excision of a small site is technically feasible it is probably a valuable form of therapy since it guarantees that a much larger, perhaps massive, necrotic slough will not occur. Surgical consultation should be sought.

Lymphangitis and cellulitis are occasional complications and should be treated with a suitable antibiotic.

COMMON DERMATOLOGIC PROBLEMS SEEN IN THE EMERGENCY DEPARTMENT

ECZEMATOUS DERMATITIS

Eczematous dermatitis should be viewed as a symptom complex resulting from inflammatory changes in the skin. Although divi-

sion of eczematous dermatitis into two types—acute and chronic—facilitates recognition and management, frequently both types occur together in the same patient.

Eczematous dermatitis is seen in association with many dermatologic conditions, and, taken together, these conditions account for disease in more than 30 per cent of all patients who seek dermatologic treatment. Since rubbing, scratching, or other irritation may cause "eczematization," almost any pruritic skin disorder may develop a superimposed eczematous dermatitis. Those most likely to be seen in the Emergency Department are discussed here.

RECOGNITION

Acute eczematous dermatitis is characterized by vesicles and bullae of variable size on an edematous and erythematous surface. As the vesiculobullae break, serum oozes forth, leading to crust formation. The involved area is warm, and the patient complains of burning discomfort or itch or both.

The best example of acute eczematous dermatitis is *contact dermatitis,* and perhaps the best known example of this is poison ivy dermatitis (Fig. 15). The contactant may be an allergic sensitizer, as in poison ivy, or a primary irritant. Recognition of contact dermatitis is based on the clinical changes of eczematous dermatitis localized to areas exposed to the suspected contactant.

Recognition of poison ivy or poison oak dermatitis is aided by a history of similar dermatitis in the past and of recent exposure to the oleoresin. Occasionally, skin changes may not appear until 10 to 12 days after exposure to the plant, although lesions usually appear from within a few hours to several days. The initial lesions usually are on the hands, arms, or fingers, but the oleoresin frequently is spread by the fingers to the eyes, genitalia, or elsewhere. Poison ivy may be carried to the patient indirectly by long-haired dogs or even by droplets on a windy day. Pruritus is prominent.

Skin involvement may be mild or severe depending on amount of exposure and degree of sensitivity of the individual. The eruption usually is asymmetric, often shows vesicles in a linear arrangement, and may show considerable edema, especially of the eyelids or face. A characteristic clinical finding is groups of fluid-filled lesions of varying sizes. Erythema multiforme (see page 1275) lacks this grouping and is much more symmetrical.

Autosensitization (id reaction) is an acute eczematous dermatitis which appears, often suddenly, in a patient who has a more localized eczematous condition elsewhere on the body. In the typical case, a patient's stasis dermatitis or tinea pedis will exacerbate, and an acute eczematous dermatitis will appear symmetrically on the arms, hands, upper trunk, or face. Autosensitization is not uncommon in infants who develop candidiasis of the diaper area. In most cases adequate therapy of the localized process produces rapid involution of the secondary skin lesions. Autosensitization is frequently misdiagnosed as a drug eruption, and only awareness of this condition will prevent discontinuance of valuable drugs.

Chronic eczematous dermatitis is characterized by dryness, scaling, and lichenification. Erythema is minimal or absent. Excoriations are an inconstant finding, depending upon whether the patient scratches or rubs the pruritic areas. In more severe cases, the skin may thicken, become hypertrophic or even nodular, and develop fissures.

Atopic dermatitis, defined by the presence of bronchial asthma or allergic rhinitis in the patient or his family, may show both acute and chronic eczematous dermatitis at different times in the same patient. In infants the process is more acute, appearing predominantly on the face as a diffuse erythema topped by tiny vesicles and crusts. In children and young adults, patchy chronic eczematous changes involve the trunk and limbs with some tendency toward localization in the flexural creases, although spasmodic episodes of acute lesions may appear from time to time. A localized form of atopic dermatitis known as *dyshidrotic dermatitis* occurs in children on the feet, and occasionally on the hands, as a mixture of acute and chronic eczematous changes. Deep-seated vesicles and bright erythema intermix with scaling, dryness, excoriations, and fissures, often in association with hyperhidrosis.

Lichen simplex chronicus (or neurodermatitis) is an excellent example of chronic eczematous dermatitis. In this localized variant of atopic dermatitis, sharply demarcated lichenified and scaling plaques occur typically on the hands, feet, neck, or vulvar skin (Fig. 16). Pruritus, always present to some degree in eczematous dermatitis, may be agonizing. As in other forms of atopic dermatitis, the etiology is unknown although a variable combination of constitutional, emotional, and environmental contactant factors appears to play a causative role. The elevated levels of serum IgE in persons with atopic dermatitis suggest that repeated subclinical whealing in the skin may induce the eczematous changes seen clinically. Since the severity of atopic dermatitis correlates with the levels of IgE, determination of this immunoglobulin might aid recognition.

Contact dermatitis and the various forms of atopic dermatitis may be difficult to tell apart, and occasionally the two conditions may occur together, as when a patient develops a contact dermatitis in response to a medication that has been applied to an area of atopic dermatitis. Other primary skin conditions—seborrheic dermatitis, lichen planus, and psoriasis, to name just a few—may develop superimposed contact dermatitis or secondary eczematization, and the primary process can be identified only by finding undisturbed lesions at other locations. On the other hand, although it is very helpful to be able to explain the process to the patient, most cases of eczematous dermatitis can be treated satisfactorily until reevaluation at a subsequent time gives more precise definition of the underlying problem.

MANAGEMENT

Poison ivy or poison oak dermatitis probably is the most common type of eczematous dermatitis requiring therapy in the Emergency Department, and its management will vary from reassurance to use of large doses of systemic corticosteroids in the more severe cases. Because poison ivy is a self-limited disorder (in the absence of additional contact), running its course over a period of several weeks, it presents classic conditions for the use of systemic corticosteroids. The latter are clearly indicated when the severity of the skin changes interferes with a vital function, causes severe discomfort, prevents employment, or produces or aggravates emotional or other disease. Systemic corticosteroids should not be used in mild cases or where they are contraindicated by other illnesses. Unfortunately, most cases fall somewhere between these two extremes, and the decision whether or not to use this potent medication must be based on consideration of the individual case.

The dosage of systemic corticosteroid is determined not only by the same considerations on which its use was determined, but also on the *phase* of the skin lesions. Since

an average case of poison ivy will reach peak severity after about three to five days, if a patient with poison ivy is started on systemic corticosteroids on day six, the required dose may be minimal. On the other hand, treatment of a patient on day one or two usually requires higher doses, and a less predictable course may be anticipated. Thorough questioning may reveal whether the patient is already improving and the course and severity of previous episodes of poison ivy, all of which may provide some predictive information.

Between five and 12 tablets of prednisone (5 mg.) are prescribed to be taken immediately and in a daily dose each morning thereafter. Usually this initial high dose must be maintained through day five or six, after which it is slowly reduced. The easiest way to reduce the corticosteroids is by means of telephone conversation with the patient every three to five days. No followup visits are needed since the patient usually is able to evaluate the skin's improvement for the physician. The patient even might be given the option of reducing the number of prednisone tablets on his own if improvement occurs sooner than expected. The medication should be continued until at least 14 to 18 days after the initial skin lesions appeared.

Ancillary measures include oral antihistamines for control of pruritus, avoidance of hot water and of overheating, which tend to increase itching, and frequent application of corticosteroid aerosol sprays.

Less severe or more localized forms of poison ivy are treated in the same way that other cases of acute eczematous dermatitis are treated: by drying the oozing vesiculobullous surfaces. Cool or cold compresses are applied three or four times daily for 30 minutes, and although water is effective, Burow's solution offers enough advantage to merit its routine use. Burow's solution is made in a 1:40 solution by dissolving a powder packet (provided by several pharmaceutical companies) into one pint of cold water. Between applications, the Burow's solution is refrigerated, thus insuring proper temperature of the compresses. This coldness reduces pruritus, removes heat from the inflamed surfaces, and provides topical anesthesia; and these values should be explained to the patient.

Topical corticosteroids are also of value in acute eczematous dermatitis and should be administered in lotion form. Small amounts are applied with the fingertips as frequently as possible.

Treatment of chronic eczematous dermatitis also centers around cold compresses, although the purpose here is to incorporate water into the dehydrated skin. To accomplish this, compressing is immediately followed by applications of corticosteroid ointments which reduce or prevent evaporation from wet surfaces. Explain to the patient that even without the preceding compresses topical corticosteroids are effective but require six to eight applications per day.

Relief of pruritus is essential to treatment of both forms of eczematous dermatitis, and management is rarely successful if pruritus continues. The patient should be given some insight into this situation and advised to use ice cubes or cold compresses in lieu of scratching. Antihistamines should be prescribed. Soap and bathing with warm water should be interdicted and the patient motivated to recognize and avoid environmental irritants.

Although acute eczematous dermatitis carries some risk of secondary bacterial infection, only grossly infected lesions require antibacterial therapy. Large numbers of resident and transient bacteria may be cultured from eczematized skin, but the addition of antibiotics to topical preparations has not been helpful and increases the likelihood of contact dermatitis from antimicrobial agents.

INFECTIONS

Bacterial Infections

IMPETIGO CONTAGIOSA

This very common superficial pyoderma is caused by either group A streptococci or *Staphylococcus aureus*, and frequently both bacteria are found together in skin lesions. Although investigators continue the debate over which organism causes the primary lesion and which is the secondary invader, there is little doubt that at least two clinical forms exist. Impetigo is much more common in children but may occur in any age group.

RECOGNITION

The characteristic lesion in the streptococcal form is an irregularly rounded cluster of tiny vesiculopustules that quickly rupture and become covered by heavy yellowish crusts. As these crusts enlarge on addition of new layers of dried seropurulent discharge, often the underlying erythema is obscured. Smaller lesions in an earlier phase of development may be found in adjacent skin areas. The face, hands, and arms are most commonly involved.

Although rheumatic fever does not follow group A streptococcal infection of the skin, many cases of acute glomerulonephritis have been preceded by streptococcal pyodermas. Lymphadenopathy may occur.

The staphylococcal form of impetigo typically shows flaccid bullous lesions, thin scalelike crusts, and circinate lesions with central healing. The lesions spread to other parts of the body, apparently by autoinoculation. Although these lesions bear a superficial resemblance to fungal infection, the latter is much more delicate and never so exudative. Satellite lesions frequently are present in staphylococcal impetigo.

Leukocytosis is present occasionally in streptococcal impetigo, but rarely in the staphylococcal form. Smear from moist lesions shows characteristic gram-positive cocci. Although cultures demonstrate the presence of one or both causative organisms, such procedures are economically impractical and rarely necessary. Nephritic changes seldom occur earlier than at least one week after streptococcal impetigo, but a baseline urinalysis is helpful.

Usually the two forms of impetigo are distinct enough clinically to permit differentiation, but milder forms may cause confusion. However, since treatment is similar in both, culturing and other efforts to tell them apart are not indicated.

MANAGEMENT

Although topical measures alone are adequate in early uncomplicated cases, there is an increasing tendency to use systemic antibiotics in all cases of impetigo. Perhaps systemic antibiotics are most valuable when the patient is unreliable in carrying out local care. Oral penicillin is effective in all streptococcal and most staphylococcal cases, but dicloxacillin should be used where a penicillinase-producing staphylococcus is suspected. Dosage is 250 mg. of either medication taken four times daily.

Topical measures should include warm water compresses or soaks two or three times

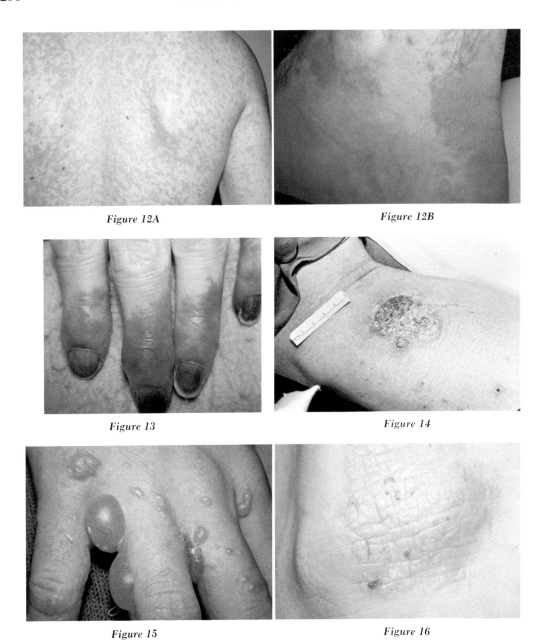

Figure 12A

Figure 12B

Figure 13

Figure 14

Figure 15

Figure 16

Figure 12 A and B, Rocky mountain spotted fever.
Figure 13 Purpura fulminans.
Figure 14 Pyoderma gangrenosum.
Figure 15 Acute eczematous dermatitis (poison ivy).
Figure 16 Lichen simplex chronicus (neurodermatitis).

daily to remove crusts, followed by application of gentamicin or another antibiotic ointment.

Although suppurative complications are decidedly rare in healthy patients with impetigo, persons with atopic dermatitis, diabetes, or other debilitating conditions are at greater risk. All patients should be evaluated at least superficially for upper respiratory infections, lymphangitis, and bacteremia, and reevaluated in three to five days to be certain that the pyoderma has responded to therapy. Since treatment with penicillin *does not* prevent nephritis, urinalysis four weeks after skin infection is indicated.

ECTHYMA AND ERYSIPELAS

These two skin infections are discussed together because both are caused by group A streptococci. Ecthyma can be considered a deeper form of impetigo whereas erysipelas is a superficial cellulitis characteristically seen on the face, scalp, or lower legs.

RECOGNITION

Ecthyma appears as superficial rounded erosions, often a centimeter or more in diameter, surrounded by indurated erythema. Very often multiple lesions are present on the involved area, which is usually on the lower legs. Children are commonly affected, and trauma appears to precede the infection.

In erysipelas, group A streptococci (and group G rarely) enter through a break in the skin and produce a now uncommon superficial cellulitis that is always hot, quite erythematous, and sharply demarcated from normal skin. Patients are usually febrile and at least mildly toxic. The fiery red lesion typically spreads peripherally but shows no central clearing. Erysipelas involves the lower legs in debilitated patients, apparently secondary to stasis dermatitis, chronic tinea pedis, or excoriations. In these patients repeated episodes may occur, resulting in chronic edema as lymph channels and nodes are replaced by fibrotic scar.

A moderate leukocytosis should be expected, and antistreptolysin 0 titer eventually rises. Like most streptococcal diseases elsewhere in the body, the lesion is nonexudative, making culture or smear of the organism difficult.

Erysipelas could be confused clinically with angioedema or acute contact dermatitis, and unilateral facial involvement might mimic herpes zoster. Angiodema does not show the deep erythema or heat of erysipelas, and contact dermatitis usually has more eczematous changes (see page 1293). The fever and leukocytosis of erysipelas are further differentiating features.

Streptococcal cellulitis may occur as a complication of erysipelas, or, more commonly, as a rapidly spreading erythema around a wound or other injury to the skin. Because subcutaneous tissues as well as skin may be involved, lymphangitis and septicemia are more likely complications. The process is tender, hot, and edematous, and associated with fever and systemic symptoms as may occur in erysipelas. Many cases *cannot* be distinguished from the latter although the advancing border of cellulitis is usually less distinct than the more superficial and less serious erysipelas. In cases that are clinically confusing, it seems prudent to diagnose the more dangerous condition and treat accordingly.

MANAGEMENT

The usual treatment for ecthyma and erysipelas is oral penicillin, although erythromycin is substituted if there is history of penicillin allergy. Antibiotic therapy should begin at once. Although ecthyma is treated on an outpatient basis, hospitalization for erysipelas may be indicated by severity of the process, by possibility of associated cellulitis, or by presence in the patient of other conditions that reduce defenses against infection.

Ecthyma usually benefits from application of warm water compresses two or three times daily to remove crusts, followed by topical gentamicin. On the other hand, the localizing effect of heat on infection is of little value in erysipelas and cellulitis when compared with the marked symptomatic relief afforded by cool compresses. Here, bed rest, elevation of the infected area, and protecting it from trauma are helpful. Because of their tendency to retain heat, ointments should be avoided; hydrating creams are beneficial in the scaly healing stages.

Systemic signs and symptoms usually improve within 48 hours of penicillin treatment, but the inflammatory changes of the skin resolve rather slowly. Both erysipelas and cellulitis recur frequently in patients with chronic lymphedema of the lower legs. In such cases, prophylactic penicillin therapy over long periods may be indicated.

FOLLICULAR INFECTIONS

Coagulase-positive staphylococci are the most common cause of infections that begin in the hair follicle. Young, active adults are involved typically. Irritation or inflammation of the skin may underlie folliculitis, as in dry skin, chemical exposures, scabies, or atopic dermatitis. Friction and maceration account for this condition after close shaving and in wrestlers or other athletes. A rather mysterious recurrent folliculitis occurs in children on the buttocks and thighs in the absence of predisposing causes such as malnutrition or hematologic disease.

RECOGNITION

Folliculitis is the term applied to a mild form of follicular infection that appears as erythema, slight tenderness and swelling, and perhaps pus formation at the follicular opening. Folliculitis is quite common but usually is trivial when only one or several lesions occur and frequently is left untreated.

A recurrent variant called *sycosis barbae* occurs in males in the beard area as perifollicular papules and pustules in association with scaling and erythema. This process slowly spreads to involve larger areas of skin and may affect the eyebrows and eyelashes, even producing blepharoconjunctivitis. *Tinea barbae*, fungal infection in the same general area, may be difficult to distinguish clinically from sycosis barbae, although scrapings from tinea barbae usually show fungal hyphae on potassium hydroxide examination.

Furuncles and *carbuncles* are deeper, more severe forms of follicular infection. The former is essentially a boil, a deep-seated perifollicular inflammation which usually follows folliculitis. It is indurated, always tender, and usually uncomfortable or frankly painful, especially when on the nose and ears where it is bound down against cartilage by overlying skin. The favored sites are hairy areas exposed to friction such as the neck, face, buttocks, and waistline.

Furuncles look like acne, but the latter appears in very limited distribution and usually is accompanied by comedones and a variety of inflammatory lesions In hidradenitis suppurativa, painful nodular lesions are sharply localized to the inguinal and axillary areas.

A carbuncle, infection of numerous contiguous hair follicles, begins as a very painful, firm erythematous lump. As suppuration occurs within it, pus appears from the numerous follicular orifices. The nape is the most common site. The patient is often febrile and appears ill. Although carbuncles are usually solitary, furuncles and folliculitis may be present in adjacent skin.

MANAGEMENT

The purpose of therapy in most follicular infections is to promote drainage of pus and necrotic material via the follicle itself. *Early lesions* must *never* be opened, picked, incised, or otherwise traumatized, as such procedures increase local inflammation and may lead to cellulitis or bacteremia. Therapy centers around warm (or hot) water compresses for 30 minutes three or four times daily to encourage "pointing" and subsequent drainage through follicular orifices. Thin applications of gentamicin ointment prolong effectiveness of the heat, and may also reduce bacteria in adjacent skin areas. As pointing occurs, a gentle incision through the follicular orifice with a No. 11 blade guarantees continuation of drainage.

Systemic antibiotics are used for deeper furuncles, for carbuncles, and for milder follicular infections in patients with diabetes, immunoglobulin deficiency states, and malnutrition. Although penicillin is surprisingly effective, in view of the large number of coagulase-positive staphylococci resistant to this medication it seems more prudent to use erythromycin or nafcillin. Furuncles around the nares and upper lip carry the additional risk of cavernous sinus thrombosis and meningitis, and should be treated with maximum antibiotic doses. Bed rest is helpful in severe cases.

Painful carbuncles of the nape are less responsive to therapy. The physician is best advised to avoid immediate incision, however, preferably relying upon local applications of heat, analgesics, and high doses of systemic antibiotics.

In recurrent furunculosis, a most baffling problem on occasion, local treatment must be thorough and persistent. Gentamicin ointment should be applied to the nares, fingernails, and perineum as well as to the sites of infection. Frequent use of antibacterial soaps is indicated, even at the risk of overdrying the skin, and dressings should be avoided except on actively discharging lesions. Since furuncles recur after cessation of systemic antibiotics, the latter are best avoided unless their prolonged use is acceptable.

Viral Infections

HERPES SIMPLEX

This worldwide viral infection, one of the most common infections of man, displays a variety of primary and secondary (or recurrent) forms. Although almost the entire population is infected with the virus, more than 98 per cent of all primary infections are either subclinical or so mild as to be unrecognized. Symptomatic primary infections are characterized by mild to moderate systemic reactions and localized lesions at the portal of entry of the virus.

RECOGNITION

The most common form of primary herpes simplex infection is *gingivostomatitis*, usually occurring in young children as painful widespread oral vesicles in association with fever and malaise. The gums are characteristically swollen, bloody, and erythematous, and eating and drinking produce severe discomfort. Tender submandibular lymphadenopathy commonly occurs. Other viral and bacterial infections usually involve only the posterior pharynx, and erythema multiforme is much more exudative. The triad of fetid breath, severe gingivitis, and anterior buccal involvement suggests the diagnosis of herpetic gingivostomatitis.

Herpetic *vulvovaginitis* produces similar constitutional symptoms, rapidly eroding vesicles on the vaginal mucosa and adjacent skin areas, pain, and inguinal lymphadenopathy. Dysuria and dyspareunia usually are present, and pruritus is a common complaint. In the male, multiple vesicles often center around the urethral meatus, and in the absence of fever would be difficult to differentiate from recurrent herpes simplex.

Herpetic *keratoconjunctivitis* is usually unilateral, may appear alarmingly severe and destructive, and displays swelling, exudation, and superficial ulceration of the cornea on occasion. *Kaposi's varicelliform eruption* may be either a primary or recurrent infection in a person with an underlying dermatitis. It is discussed on page 1278.

Inoculation herpes simplex is a primary infection that occurs in abraded or injured skin, and is an occupational hazard of physicians and nurses. It occurs most commonly on fingertips as clusters of tense papulovesicles that usually are painful. The patient is often febrile and more or less ill, and has regional lymphadenopathy. Careful clinical evaluation is required to differentiate this condition from bacterial infections, monilial paronychia, and recurrent herpes simplex infections.

Recurrent herpes simplex infections are many times more common than all of the primary forms taken together. They differ strikingly from the latter by their localized distribution and absence of fever and systemic symptoms. Recurrent infections frequently recur in the same general areas, but usually not at the exact sites. The most commonly involved areas are the lips and around the mouth, the face generally, and the genitalia, although the palms and buttocks are not uncommon sites.

Following a brief prodrome of burning or itching discomfort, one or several rounded clusters of tiny discrete vesicles appear on an erythematous base. The lesions become crusted in a day or two, almost always in the absence of a preceding oozing phase. With the one exception of palmar involvement, recurrent herpes infections are rarely complicated by secondary pyoderma or lymphangitis.

Whereas recurrent infections usually are recognized easily by their typical appearance and history, primary infections show less consistent changes and, being less common, are often misdiagnosed. On the other hand, the absence of a history of prior herpes lesions supports the diagnosis of primary infection, especially in older children and adults. Of the four clinical features of primary herpes infections (fever, lymphadenopathy, constitutional symptoms, and vesicular lesions), it is the cutaneous changes that most aid recognition. Oral and vulvar vesicles will often slough rapidly, producing whitish plaques or superficial erosions that are easily seen against the edematous and erythematous background mucosal surfaces. The fever of primary infections is almost always low-grade and often precedes by several days the onset of mucosal or cutaneous lesions.

The most helpful laboratory aid in the recognition of herpes infections is the Tzanck smear in which contents from an intact vesicle are examined microscopically. After removing the roof of the vesicle with a fine iris scissors, the fluid is blotted with gauze carefully so as not to disturb the cells below. Cloudy material from the floor of the lesion is then gently scraped with a dull No. 15 scalpel onto a glass slide as thinly as possible. After fixation in methyl alcohol the slide is treated with Giemsa stain according to the technique used for blood smears and is then examined under the microscope. Finding multinucleate giant epithelial cells confirms the diagnosis of herpes simplex, although similar bizarre viral cells also are characteristic of herpes zoster and varicella. In most primary herpes infections the patient's hemogram will show a low normal or decreased number of white blood cells and an increase in lymphocytes or monocytes.

MANAGEMENT

Most cases of primary herpes simplex infection produce enough discomfort and functional impairment to require hospitalization, although occasionally the patient or his family will delay seeking medical advice for four or five days so that the acute stage is already subsiding. Another notable exception is the inoculation type that typically occurs on the fingers of medical personnel. Patients with severe gingivostomatitis, almost always infants or young children, may require parenteral alimentation or fluid balance that should be initiated in the Emergency Department.

Although idoxuridine has proved valuable in the management of herpes simplex keratitis, it has been much less effective on skin lesions. On the assumption that this chemical is absorbed more readily on mucous membranes, it should be prescribed for the buccal and vaginal mucosae as a 0.1 per cent solution applied hourly during the waking hours and every three hours during the night. Keratoconjunctivitis should be managed by an ophthalmologic consultant.

Nonspecific symptomatic measures for primary infections include analgesics that often must be administered parenterally and intraoral lidocaine for patients old enough to hold this anesthetic in their mouths for several minutes before swallowing it. Use of lidocaine prior to meals may allow oral intake of food and liquid that would be otherwise intolerable. Cool or cold water compresses to the vulvar region are comforting, but, to avoid maceration, should not exceed 15 minutes four times daily. Spread-eagle positioning of the legs is also helpful.

The patient and/or his family should be reassured that the pain and discomfort of primary infections subside in five to eight days, although complete healing may require several weeks. On the other hand they must also be warned that herpes simplex lesions contain millions of viral particles that may infect susceptible persons, especially infants and children without prior exposure. Family members with eczematized or injured skin are especially at risk.

Management of *recurrent* herpetic infections is facilitated by dividing the course of infection into two phases: an early phase, the first 36 to 48 hours, in which the viruses are replicating and spreading; and a second phase in which viral activity is dormant and injured tissues are healing. Treatment during the early phase can shorten markedly the course of the recurrent infection, whereas second-phase therapy is much less spectacular, consisting of symptomatic measures. The emergency physician would appear to have the unique opportunity to initiate early-phase treatment in many cases.

Although initial reports indicated that early-phase herpetic lesions resolved more rapidly after application of a light-reactive dye and exposure to artificial light (a technique known as photoinactivation), other investigations have questioned both the efficacy and safety of this therapy.° It is hoped that agents such as idoxuridine and adenine arabinoside will be effective in recurrent skin lesions, but this must await the development of a more efficient delivery system. Hourly applications of alcohol or ether to early le-

---

°Recent reports have provided evidence that dye-light therapy may unmask the oncogenic potential of the virus. Also, treated cells may possibly become malignant through photodynamic mutagenesis. Accordingly, the FDA now considers this therapy to be controversial, and reports that further research is needed to resolve questions of efficacy and safety.

sions is reported to be helpful, but the tedium of such treatment probably produces inconsistent results. Because ether is volatile, it must be handled carefully. Flexible collodion, a mixture of ether and alcohol, usually is available in Emergency Departments and could easily be dispensed to patients.

Recurrent lesions more than 48 hours old usually are better treated by drying techniques: warm compresses followed by air drying and frequent applications of alcohol or witch hazel. Occlusive coverings should be avoided because they promote maceration and secondary infection. Topical steroids are of little help and seem no better than simple emollient creams in softening older lesions. It might be helpful to direct patients to begin treatment at the first indication of recurrent lesions, hopefully even before vesiculation has occurred.

HERPES ZOSTER

Both varicella and zoster are caused by the same virus, *Herpesvirus varicellae.* Whereas varicella occurs as a primary infection in patients without immunity to the virus, zoster represents activation of the virus in a person with partial immunity. Varicella-zoster infection may be compared superficially with herpes simplex infection in which distinctive primary infections may be followed by activation of the virus to produce localized herpes simplex lesions. Unlike herpes simplex, however, zoster almost never recurs.

The factors that cause activation of the varicella-zoster virus are basically unknown, although greater frequency of zoster in patients with Hodgkin's disease, lymphomas, leukemias and other cancers is well established. In patients who have received antimetabolites or x-ray therapy it is difficult to know if subsequent zoster is the result of therapy or of the disease under treatment.

RECOGNITION

The typical clusters of papulovesicles occurring in the skin of one or two contiguous dermatomes produce one of the most characteristic clinical pictures seen in dermatology. New lesions may appear over a period of several days' duration in a centripetal fashion such that the first cluster of lesions is often on the back somewhat lateral to the midline. The clusters are initially discrete and separated by normal skin but may become confluent in severe cases. Unilateral involvement with sharp cut-off at the midline is occasionally helpful in ruling out an acute eczematous dermatitis (like contact dermatitis) when the dermatomal distribution is not apparent.

When the ophthalmic branch of the trigeminal nerve is involved, ocular changes are likely These may vary from a mild keratoconjunctivitis to a deeper keratitis with ulceration or scarring. Since ocular changes may lag behind the skin lesions by several days, it is prudent to obtain early ophthalmologic consultation. Ocular involvement is supposedly more likely when the side of the nose shows vesicular lesions, indicating involvement of the nasociliary nerve. Involvement of the maxillary or mandibular divisions of the trigeminal nerve, although much less common, produces unilateral vesicles in the mouth.

Although motor system involvement in zoster is not common, partial paresis of an extremity occasionally is noted. Even though motor function returns, early recognition of the paralysis is crucial so that prompt physiotherapy can be used to prevent disuse atrophy of large muscle masses. A more characteristic example of motor involvement is the Ramsay-Hunt syndrome in which the geniculate ganglion is affected. This produces vesicles of the external auditory canal and ear lobe along with persistent earache and facial nerve paralysis that occasionally is permanent. Zoster in the sacral dermatomes (S2 to S4) may be accompanied by bladder dysfunction manifested either by acute urinary retention or by urinary frequency.

Pain is a prominent symptom in most older patients with zoster, and may be a diagnostic challenge when it precedes the skin lesions. Involvement of thoracic or lumbar dorsal roots may mimic myocardial infarction, peritonitis, or other painful syndromes although careful clinical evaluation usually will reveal the pain's superficial location. The finding of itching, paresthesias, hypesthesia, or hyperesthesia in a dermatomal distribution is very suggestive of zoster. Pain is almost always minimal or absent in young adults.

Zoster frequently is accompanied by regional lymphadenopathy and occasionally by mild constitutional symptoms. Although milder cases may heal uneventfully in two to four weeks, severe reactions with necrosis or hemorrhage may require several months and heal with scar formation. Elderly patients and those with reticuloendothelial diseases usually show more devastating skin changes, and the latter also may show disseminated or bilateral lesions.

Recognition of zoster rests almost totally on clinical findings, and rarely is recourse to laboratory aids indicated or helpful. The hemogram and sedimentation are normal unless secondary bacterial infection has occurred. The Tzanck smear (see page 1300) distinguishes zoster from erythema multiforme and dermatitis herpetiformis but not from herpes simplex occurring in a zosteriform distribution. The latter's history of recurrence, however, rules out zoster.

MANAGEMENT

Milder cases are managed by supportive outpatient treatment which centers around reassurance about anticipated duration and course of the viral illness, and symptomatic measures. Aspirin or propoxyphene hydrochloride should be tried first, although codeine compounds or stronger narcotics may be needed. Pruritus can be reduced by cool water compresses and oral antihistamines, along with calamine lotion which can be applied as often as needed to relieve itching. Topical steroids are of little value in either reducing pruritus or accelerating resolution of skin lesions. If compresses are prescribed, maceration is reduced by use of compresses for no longer than 15 minutes four times daily. Similarly, immersion of affected skin in bath water must be avoided in favor of short, coolish showers. It is doubtful that bed rest or other restrictions are necessary in these milder cases, although the patient should be warned of his contagion for children who have not had varicella.

Pain by itself is not necessarily an indication for hospitalization, although for a patient with other illnesses or debilitation, management may be aided by the hospital setting. Severe, hemorrhagic, or gangrenous skin changes require inpatient treatment and dermatologic consultation.

Systemic corticosteroids should be used in painful zoster to prevent postherpetic neuralgia, the most common complication of this infection. Postherpetic pain, although somewhat unpredictable, appears to be quite frequent following trigeminal involvement; it is uncommon in patients under 40 and increases in incidence and severity with age. The usual daily starting dose of prednisone is in the 40 to 60 mg. range; however, duration of treatment and dosage must be individualized according to severity of pain, response to treatment, and presence or absence of contraindications to the use of this medication. Skin lesions are not improved by systemic steroids. The help of an internist or dermatologist with prior experience in this area is essential.

Fungal Infections

DERMATOPHYTOSIS

Tinea, dermatophytosis, and "ringworm" refer to fungal infections caused by a related group of fungi which includes the three genera *Microsporum*, *Trichophyton*, and *Epidermophyton*. The term "ringworm," despite the clinical picture it evokes, has been a source of confusion for the nondermatologist, and preference should be given to the other two terms. By stressing the ringed morphology, this term has been misapplied all too often to erythema annulare, various eczematous lesions, and the herald patch of pityriasis rosea; and has slowed appreciation of the nonringed appearance of dermatophytosis of the hands, feet, and beard areas.

Dermatophytes, like bacteria, exist only as saprophytes or parasites, and, being essentially necrophilic, are found only in such dead tissue as hair, nails, and the stratum corneum. Although all dermatophytes invade the skin, some species appear to be excluded from hair and nails. Anthropophilic species of dermatophytes tend to produce milder and more chronic cutaneous lesions, whereas zoophilic fungi, which usually infect people from an animal source, evoke a more inflammatory skin lesion.

RECOGNITION

Enumeration of species and the clinical conditions they produce would be lengthy and inconsistent with the aims of this chapter. The following discussion by regions of the body should facilitate recognition of common dermatophyte infections while avoiding details and terms more valuable to mycologists or dermatologists. Additional information is available in mycology textbooks.

Recognition of fungal infections is aided immensely by *direct microscopic examination* of material from suspected lesions. The scales, subungual debris, or hairs are placed on a glass slide. Add one or two drops of 15 per cent potassium hydroxide and a coverslip, and heat the preparation gently for several seconds with a Bunsen burner. Although boiling should be avoided, any bubbles that appear can be removed by tapping the coverslip. Let the preparation stand, preferably on the microscope light, for 20 minutes to enhance clearing. Using reduced light, examine the slide under low power initially; switch to high power for details. The microscopic elements to look for are discussed below.

TINEA UNGUIUM

More common on the toenails than the fingernails, this infection typically begins at the distal edge of the nail as a whitish or yellow patch that slowly spreads proximally in irregular fashion. The nail plate thickens, becomes deformed, and is eventually lifted off the nail bed by the accumulation of subungual material, although many variations of the above changes are seen. The process is almost always asymptomatic.

Psoriasis is easily confused with tinea unguium, and it usually is necessary to examine all areas of skin in search of other lesions of psoriasis. The characteristic superficial pits of the nail plate in psoriasis are not found in fungal infection. Psoriasis is more symmetrical whereas tinea unguium frequently involves only one hand.

Identifying fungal elements on direct microscopy (see above) is more difficult here than in other regions of the body, and often repeated examinations are required. Using a sterile scalpel blade, obtain scrapings from the *undersurface* of the nail as proximally as possible. Try to avoid the usually abundant loose keratin debris present more distally. After heating, allow the slide to stand for at least 30 minutes before examining, as subungual debris is slow to clear. Finding translucent, branching linear filaments (hy-

phae), often segmented into anthrospores, confirms the diagnosis of dermatophyte infection. Hyphae must be carefully differentiated from the so-called mosaic artifact which is less translucent and follows the outlines of the keratinized cells.

TINEA CAPITIS

The most common form of dermatophytosis of the scalp is caused by *Microsporum audouini* and typically occurs as epidemics in prepubertal school children. These noninflammatory lesions are oval to round, are covered by a grayish scale, and contain hair that is uniformly broken off about 2 mm. from the scalp surface. The more inflammatory form of tinea capitis is contracted from young pets, is usually caused by *M. canis,* and often shows slight edema, vesiculation, and peripheral spread. In both forms, the lesions are asymmetric and variable in size. Kerion is an even more inflammatory reaction in the scalp that begins with follicular pustules that coalesce to produce a solitary boggy swelling ressembling an abscess.

The finding of several irregularly rounded areas of partial alopecia with broken off hairs (with or without scaling) is quite suggestive of tinea capitis. History of similar changes in siblings or schoolmates all but confirms the diagnosis. Sporadic cases and infections in adults are more easily mistaken for alopecia areata, although the latter is never scaly.

Examination of scalp lesions with Wood's light* will reveal bright green or yellow-green fluorescence of hairs in *Microsporum* infections but not in the much less common *Trichophyton* infections. In early infections where hyphae are still below the skin surface no fluorescence is seen. In such cases, epilate several hairs with a forceps and examine their roots under Wood's light. If this examination is still negative or equivocal, prepare a potassium hydroxide mount for microscopic examination. Select broken or lusterless hairs or hairs from the edges of

---

*Wood's light is an ultraviolet light fitted with a nickel oxide filter. It emits maximum radiation with wavelengths of about 3650 angstrom units and is useful in the diagnosis of erythrasma and tinea versicolor as well as tinea capitis. Always use Wood's light in a darkened room.

suspected lesions. In *Microsporum* infections, very small arthrospores form sheaths around hairs, and under low power these hairs appear to have a granular coating. With higher magnification, individual spores can be identified along the outside of the hairs in a so-called mosaic pattern. In *Trichophyton* infections, the arthrospores are larger and appear in parallel chains either outside the hair shafts or within the hairs.

TINEA CORPORIS

Dermatophytosis of the glabrous skin is more common in tropical areas and is a summertime disease in temperate climates. Its more common occurrence on exposed parts such as the face, hands, and arms supports the thesis that the disease is usually contracted from an animal or another human even though some lesions appear to result from self-inoculation. All known dermatophytes can produce tinea corporis, and the causative organisms appear to reflect prevailing fungi of the particular area.

The most common form begins as a mildly pruritic inflammatory papule that enlarges peripherally to produce a papulosquamous lesion with an elevated, vesicular, scaling border. With central clearing, an annular lesion is seen, although occasionally secondary areas of activity appear within the circle. Other lesions show a variable morphology, ranging from severely scaling eczematous patches to granulomatous nodules.

Most lesions of tinea corporis are solitary or few in number, totally asymmetric, round or oval, and discrete. These features aid differentiation from the other papulosquamous eruptions that usually are more widespread in their distribution. On the other hand, tinea corporis could be confused with the "herald patch" of pityriasis rosea, inpetigo, contact dermatitis, and even psoriasis on occasion. With few exceptions all solitary papulosquamous lesions should be examined for presence or absence of fungal elements.

TINEA CRURIS

Dermatophytosis of the crural or perineal folds is relatively common in men but quite rare in females. It displays the same peripheral spread as tinea corporis but has a more irregular often scalloped border and variable central clearing. Extension to the perianal skin or down the medial thighs occurs commonly. The process is usually bilateral.

Examination of scales treated with potassium hydroxide verifies the diagnosis. Erythrasma produces a brownish pink discoloration of intertriginous skin that fluoresces coral red with Wood's light. It never shows an active border or significant inflammation. In contrast to tinea cruris, candidiasis involves the vulvar and scrotal skin. It is fairly common in females. Intertrigo of the crural folds often shows striking similarities to tinea cruris, and the potassium hydroxide scraping may be the only way to make the correct diagnosis in such cases.

TINEA PEDIS

Only the acute form, consisting of vesiculation between the toes and/or on the plantar surfaces, is likely to challenge the emergency physician. It usually is caused by *Trichophyton mentagrophytes*. The process begins between or under the toes as a slight maceration and scaling that is invariably pruritic and is usually followed by fissuring and accumulation of hyperkeratotic debris. Acute episodes are marked by increased erythema, vesiculation, and extension of the vesiculobullous lesions to the plantar surfaces. Secondary bacterial infection may occur in the fissures or deep-seated buttonlike vesicles. If the patient tries to treat himself, the infected acute tinea pedis is likely to be further irritated by various antifungal medications (which are more or less irritating to start with). The clinical picture of tinea pedis thus varies from slight scaling of the fourth interspace (the most common site of initial involvement) to a crusted, oozing, edematous mess.

This acute process and its complications are more common in males and in persons who wear occlusive footwear and work on their feet. Plantar hyperhidrosis, warm weather, and poor bathing habits are contributing factors. Tinea pedis is exceedingly rare in prepubertal children.

Recognition of tinea pedis is aided by a history of recurrence in warm weather and improvement with antifungal preparations. The scaling hyperkeratotic and fissured phase displays a characteristic clinical picture, and its interdigital location is somewhat unique. In the vesiculobullous phase, microscopic examination of keratinous material is essential to recognition, and vesicle roofs are the best source of fungal elements. The roof should be removed with a fine scissors, thinned extensively before and after heating, and placed on the microscope light for 20 minutes for additional clearing.

Shoe contact dermatitis and dyshidrotic eczema rarely involve the intertoe spaces, typically involve the dorsal surfaces of the toes and feet, and usually produce more eczematous changes rather than discrete vesiculobullous lesions. Because pustular psoriasis is extremely difficult to differentiate from some cases of tinea pedis, the emergency physician should examine for the nail changes of psoriasis and psoriatic lesions elsewhere on the patient's body. Use Wood's light to detect the coral red fluorescence of erythrasma, a superficial bacterial infection found commonly in interdigital or other intertriginous areas.

In the acute form of tinea pedis with superimposed pyoderma or contact dermatitis, it is more essential to recognize and treat these complications than the underlying, often unrecognizable, fungus infection.

In marked contrast to this acute form is the chronic variety of tinea pedis most frequently caused by *T. rubrum*. This condition is recognized by its extreme chronicity, faint or absent erythema, and diffuse fine scaling that often involves the entire plantar surface and extends around the sides of the foot in the so-called "moccasin" distribution. It is usually bilateral and, unlike its acute counterpart, will occasionally produce a unilateral tinea manuum of similar appearance. Its increased incidence in patients with Cushing's disease or lymphomas suggests that reduced cell-mediated immunity may be an important underlying factor. Although patients rarely request therapy for it, *T. rubrum* infection is extremely common in adult males, should not go unrecognized, and will at least provide the emergency physician with an opportunity to practice and perfect his potassium hydroxide scraping technique.

MANAGEMENT

Griseofulvin is valuable in the treatment of dermatophytosis although its effectiveness in the different tineas is variable. It is most valuable in the treatment of *Tinea capitis* where the curative dose for children is 1 gm. four times daily for a total dose of 4 gm. Higher blood levels are obtained if griseofulvin is taken with a fatty meal. The patient and his parents should be warned of the contagiousness of this condition, and the patient should be advised not to share his hat, comb, brush, and towel with others. Mild shampooing two or three times weekly may help eliminate infectious scales and hairs. Siblings and other household children should be examined with Wood's light and reexamined along with the patient three weeks after treatment.

Griseofulvin is not without side-effects but appears to be especially well tolerated by children. Headache, gastrointestinal distress, and diarrhea are the most common complaints, but these can be eliminated by lowering the dosage or stopping and then starting the medication again. Although preliminary toxicologic studies had indicated that griseofulvin produced serious adverse hepatic and bone marrow reactions, no such side-effects have been experienced during almost 15 years of clinical use. Occasionally there will be a reduction in leukocyte counts; and even though this is transient and reversible, some caution is warranted in patients already receiving other bone marrow-depressing drugs. Because of its action on the liver enzyme system, griseofulvin reduces the effectiveness of coumarin anticoagulants; for the same reason, barbiturates reduce the antifungal activity of griseofulvin.

In *Tinea corporis* and *Tinea cruris* topical antifungal therapy is effective, usually making griseofulvin unnecessary. Tolnaftate, haloprogin, and miconazole nitrate are valuable in these conditions, and the latter two agents appear to be effective in candidiasis as well. The cream form should be applied three times daily to lesions of the glabrous skin, whereas lotion is preferable in intertriginous infections in order to reduce maceration. Crural lesions are additionally benefited by cool water compresses to remove sweat and debris and by avoidance of tight-fitting or occlusive underclothing. The patient should be seen for follow-up two weeks after treatment is begun.

In the vesicular type of *Tinea pedis*, emergency treatment centers around warm water soaks three times daily to soften the skin and remove debris, followed by applications of either tolnaftate, haloprogin, or miconazole nitrate cream. The cream should be spread thinly over the entire plantar surface and usually between and under the toes as well. If excessive hyperkeratosis or deep-seated vesiculobullae are present, a thin layer of Whitfield's ointment should be applied over the antifungal cream. Whitfield's ointment, a keratolytic containing 3 per cent salicylic acid and 6 per cent benzoic acid, should not be used in ambulatory patients as it may increase maceration. It should also be avoided if secondary contact dermatitis or bacterial infection is present.

CANDIDIASIS

This fungal infection principally involves skin and mucous membranes and only rarely produces systemic disease. The causative organism is almost always *Candida albicans* although other Candida species are implicated occasionally. Since *C. albicans* (as well as other Candida species) is a harmless resident of normal skin, mucous membranes, and the gastrointestinal tract, its isolation from pathologic conditions in these areas is difficult to evaluate.

The virulence of *all* Candida species seems quite low, and it is generally assumed that in all cases of candidiasis local or systemic factors predispose the patient to this fungal disease. Diabetes mellitus, antibiotic or corticosteroid therapy, use of oral contraceptives, obesity, and lymphoreticular disease are some of the better known processes that are associated with candidal infection. Infancy, pregnancy, and old age produce certain physiologic changes that also allow the yeast to assume a pathogenic role.

RECOGNITION

Oral candidiasis (thrush) shows well defined, creamy white patches on any portion of the oral mucous membranes. This creamy material, often compared to curds of milk, appears crumbly when disturbed, and its removal reveals an erythematous base. Its incidence in infants has decreased greatly, and it is now more a problem of premature infants and of adults with debilitating disease or following antibiotic therapy.

A similar reaction occurs in *Candidal vaginitis*, but here the process is exudative and more inflammatory. A yellowish-white milky discharge that may contain curd-like material dominates the clinical picture. The vaginal mucosa, and usually the vulvar skin as well, is erythematous, swollen, and extremely pruritic. Scratching may cause excoriations, erosions, and additional inflammation, often with extension of the process over the perineum and into the crural areas.

Candidal intertrigo is the most common *skin* infection, usually seen in inguinal, axillary, and inframammary folds. The intergluteal cleft and the spaces between the fingers and toes show occasional involvement. Candidiasis in these areas is almost always superimposed on intertrigo or seborrheic dermatitis, and frequently is difficult to separate clinically from these two underlying conditions. Clues to its presence are (a) an *intense erythema* that is surprisingly non-tender and non-edematous, (b) sharply demarcated, peripherally spreading *scalloped* borders, and (c) *satellite vesiculopustules*. Interdigital candidiasis shows a moist red macerative lesion surrounded by scaling overhanging borders, and because of this eroded appearance has been given the name of "erosio interdigitalis blastomycetica."

Candidal paronychia produces erythema, fusiform swelling, and tenderness in the paronychial tissues. Although slight pus formation usually occurs, it is not clear whether this is due to the yeast infection or to an associated bacterial overgrowth. Widening and/or deepening of the nail groove is almost pathognomonic of candidal infection in this area. These paronychial changes are chronic, interrupted by more acute intermittent episodes, and usually produce secondary dystrophic changes in the nail plate.

Paronychial infection *always* precedes the nail changes of candidiasis, and a diagnosis of the latter is untenable without at least some history of paronychial inflammation. These nail changes are directly proportional to the amount of nail matrix injury resulting from paronychial activity, and can be differentiated from tinea unguium (see page 1303) by their proximal location and absence of subungual debris. One or several fingers may be involved. Candidal paronychia is almost totally confined to persons whose hands are frequently wet, such as bartenders, housewives, and waitresses.

In the presence of clinical changes suggestive of candidiasis, the diagnosis should be confirmed by demonstration of large numbers of fungal elements in material from mucosal or skin lesions. Scrapings may be examined microscopically with the potassium hydroxide technique (see page 1303), but use of either Gram's or Giemsa stain facilitates identification of the small (2 to 4 μ), oval thin-walled cells. Pseudohyphae* and budding yeast cells are usually also present. It should be stressed that since *C. albicans* may be found normally in the vagina and gastrointestinal tract and may colonize intertriginous areas under special circumstances, demonstration of this organism in clinical lesions is significant *only* if these lesions are consistent with clinical changes generally accepted as being produced by the organism.

Recognition of candidiasis is further aided by the presence of one or more underlying conditions known to predispose the patient to this infection. Inquire about immunosuppressive drugs, systemic corticosteroids, and antibiotics. History and physical examination may reveal a tendency toward excessive sweating, obesity, or intertrigo. Candidiasis could be the first sign of pregnancy, diabetes, or immune deficiency. Although it seems unreasonable to expect the emergency physician to investigate all these possibilities, a blood glucose determination usually is indicated.

MANAGEMENT

Specific anticandidal *topical* agents have generally replaced Castellani's paint and gentian violet in the management of this fungal infection, although safe and effective *systemic* agents are still not available. Griseofulvin is ineffective.

For oral lesions, direct the patient to suck on one nystatin oral tablet three times daily until it completely dissolves in his mouth. In infants and children, 1 cc. of nystatin oral suspension is placed in the mouth four times daily. For candidal vaginitis, prescribe nystatin vaginal tablets twice daily for two weeks, inserted into the vagina with an applicator that comes with this product.

Amphotericin B or haloprogin should be prescribed in lotion form for candidal inter-

trigo or other skin lesions. Sweating and maceration can be reduced by avoiding hot water, tight-fitting clothing, and excessive physical activity. Cool water compresses will provide cleanliness, remove debris and perspiration, reduce pruritus, and soothe inflamed skin at the same time, but should be used only two or three times daily for no longer than ten minutes. Candidal paronychia requires scrupulous avoidance of moisture, and a simple way to achieve this is by application of clear nail lacquer on top of the antifungal lotion. Suggest finger cots for unavoidable wet work.

References

Ackerman, A. B., Miller, R. C., and Shapiro, L.: Gonococcemia and its cutaneous manifestations. Arch. Derm. *91*:227, 1965.

Allen, D. M., Diamond, L. K., and Howell, D. A.: Anaphylactoid purpura in children (Schönlein-Henoch syndrome). Am. J. Dis. Child. 99:833, 1960.

Ansell, B. M.: Henoch-Schönlein purpura with particular reference to the prognosis of the renal lesion. Br. J. Dermatol. 82:211–215, 1970.

Ashton, H., Frenk, E., and Stevenson, C. J.: The management of Henoch-Schönlein purpura. Br. J. Dermatol. 85:199–203, 1971.

Baker, H., and Levene, G. M.: Cutaneous reactions to anticoagulants. Brit. J. Dermatol. *81*:236–237, 1969.

Benoit, F. L.: Chronic meningococcemia. Am. J. Med. 35:103–112, 1963.

Berger, R. S.: A critical look at therapy for the Brown Recluse spider bite. Arch. Dermatol. *107*:298, 1973.

Callaway, J. L., and Tate, W. E.: Toxic epidermal necrolysis caused by "gin and tonic." Arch. Dermatol. *109*:909, 1974.

Champion, R. H., et al.: Urticaria and angio-edema. Brit. J. Dermatol. *81*:588–597, 1969.

Daughters, D., Zackheim, H., and Maibach, H.: Urticaria and anaphylactoid reactions after topical application of mechlorethamine. Arch. Dermatol. *107*:429–430, 1973.

Deykin, D.: The clinical challenge of disseminated intravascular coagulation. N. Engl. J. Med. 283:636–644, 1970.

Dillaha, C. J., et al.: North American loxoscelism. J.A.M.A. *188*:33–36, 1964.

Everett, E. D., and Overholt, E. L.: Hemorrhagic skin infarction secondary to oral anticoagulants. Arch. Dermatol. *100*:588–591, 1969.

Fardon, D. W., et al.: The treatment of Brown spider bite. Plast. Reconstr. Surg. *40*:482–488, 1967.

Gardner, L. W., and Acker, D. W.: Triamcinolone and pyoderma gangrenosum. Arch. Dermatol. *106*:599–600, 1972.

Higgins, P. G., and Crow, K. D.: Recurrent Kaposi's varicelliform eruption in Darier's disease. Br. J. Dermatol. 88:391–394, 1973.

Juel-Jensen, B. E.: Severe generalized primary herpes treated with cytarabine. Br. Med. J. 2:154–155, 1970.

Kahn, G., and Danielsson, D.: Septic gonococcal dermatitis. Arch. Dermatol. 99:421–425, 1969.

---

*Pseudohyphae are filaments composed of elongated budding cells that have failed to detach. Unlike true hyphae, they have unequal diameters along their length.

Kahn, S., Stern, H. D., and Rhodes, G. A.: Cutaneous and subcutaneous necrosis as a complication of coumarin-congener therapy. Plast. & Reconstr. Surg. 48:160–166, 1971.

Kazmier, F. J., et al.: Treatment of intravascular coagulation and fibrinolysis (ICF) syndromes. Mayo Clin. Proc. 49:665–672, 1974.

Kelly, J. F., and Patterson, R.: Anaphylaxis. Course, mechanisms and treatment. J.A.M.A. 227:1431–1436, 1974.

Koch-Weser, J.: Coumarin necrosis (Editorial) Ann. Intern. Med. 68:1365–1367, 1968.

Lowney, E. D., et al.: The scalded skin syndrome in small children. Arch. Dermatol. 95:359–369, 1967.

Lyell, A.: A review of toxic epidermal necrolysis in Britain. Br. J. Dermatol. 79:662–671, 1967.

Moschella, S. L.: Pyoderma gangrenosum. Arch. Dermatol. 95:121–123, 1967.

Nalbandian, R. M., et al.: Petechiae, ecchymosis and necrosis of skin induced by coumarin congeners. J.A.M.A. 192:603–608, 1965.

Nalbandian, R. M., et al.: Coumarin necrosis of skin treated successfully with heparin. Obstet. Gynecol. 38:395–399, 1971.

Nielsen, L. T.: Chronic meningococcemia. Arch. Dermatol. 102:97–101, 1970.

Perry, H. O.: Pyoderma gangrenosum. South. Med. J. 62:899–908, 1969.

Radimer, G. F., Davis, J. H., and Ackerman, A. B.: Fumigant-induced toxic epidermal necrolysis. Arch. Dermatol. 110:103–104, 1974.

Robboy, S. J., et al.: The skin in disseminated intravascular coagulation. Br. J. Dermatol. 88:221–229, 1973.

Ross, C. M.: The acute defibrination syndrome. Arch. Dermatol. 87:213–218, 1963.

Sahn, D. J., and Schwartz, A. D.: Schönlein-Henoch syndrome. Pediatrics 49:614, 1972.

Shelley, W. B.: Consultations in Dermatology II. Philadelphia, W. B. Saunders Co., 1974, pp. 250–255.

Shelley, W. B.: Consultations in Dermatology. Philadelphia, W. B. Saunders Co., 1972, pp. 166–170.

Wheeler, C. E., and Abele, D. C.: Eczema herpeticum, primary and recurrent. Arch. Dermatol. 93:162–173, 1966.

Chapter 57 DRUG REACTIONS

George J. Caranasos

An adverse drug reaction (ADR) is an unintended and undesired effect of a drug used for prophylactic, therapeutic, or diagnostic purposes. The incidence of ADR's in ambulatory patients is unknown, but ADR's are the reason for admission of about 3 per cent of medical patients and in medical patients hospitalized for other causes a 10 to 18 per cent incidence of ADR's is found. Although most ADR's are of minor severity, serious and fatal reactions do occur. About 85 per cent of ADR's are due to pharmacologic effects, and the remainder are mediated by immunologic mechanisms. Drug factors predisposing to adverse effects include excessive drug dose, use of many drugs simultaneously, inherent propensity of a given drug to cause adverse effects, and drug interactions. Patient factors that may lead to ADR's include age (higher incidence in the very young and the old), genetic factors (e.g., glucose-6-phosphate dehydrogenase deficiency), underlying disease (e.g., renal insufficiency), and a history of a previous ADR (ADR's are more frequent in individuals with a prior ADR to any drug).

Detection of ADR's necessitates a high level of suspicion, a knowledge of the common adverse effects of drugs prescribed, and a careful history of drugs used, including both prescription and over-the-counter preparations. The incidence of ADR's can be diminished by prescribing drugs in appropriate doses and with clear instructions to the patient for proper administration, by avoiding unnecessary drug exposure, and by using drugs less likely to produce adverse effects. Drugs, and their congeners, to which an individual is allergic obviously should not be administered. One must also be aware of any underlying diseases in a patient and what medicines are being taken or are likely to be taken before prescribing new drugs.

ANAPHYLAXIS

Anaphylaxis is an acute, potentially fatal allergic reaction most often due to parenteral, rarely to oral, drug administration (Table 1). Penicillins, iodinated contrast media, and BSP are the drugs most frequently implicated. Atopic individuals are predisposed to anaphylaxis. A negative history of an ADR to a drug does not preclude the occurrence of anaphylaxis. Symptoms

TABLE 1 *Causes of Anaphylaxis*

Drugs	
Antimicrobials	penicillins, cephalosporins, sulfonamides, streptomycin tetracyclines, nitrofurantoin (Furadantin)
Iodinated contrast media	
Local anesthetics	procaine (Novocain), lidocaine (Xylocaine)
Analgesics	salicylates, aminopyrine, phenylbutazone (Butazolidin), indomethacin (Indocin)
Hormones	insulin, ACTH
Enzymes	trypsin, chymotrypsin, penicillinase (Neutrapen)
Heterologous antisera Antilymphocyte globulin Pollen extracts Vaccines	
Other drugs	sulfobromophthalein (BSP) sodium dehydrocholate (Decholin), dextrans, iron-dextran (Imferon), probenecid (Benemid), tripelennamine (Pyribenzamine), heparin, meprobamate, thiamine, folic acid
Other Agents	Hymenoptera stings (bee, wasp, hornet), snake venom, foods (shellfish, egg albumin, nuts)

begin between five and 60 minutes after parenteral drug administration. Laryngeal edema and hypotension are most often associated with a fatal outcome. Symptoms may respond rapidly to therapy or may last for a day or more.

Cutaneous and respiratory manifestations are the most common, but cardiovascular dysfunction may supervene. Skin lesions include a generalized sensation of warmth or burning, diffuse urticaria, and angioedema, especially of the face and tongue. Respiratory distress results from either laryngeal edema with stridor and airway obstruction or from bronchospasm, which leads to tightness in the chest, tachypnea, cough, wheezes, and occasionally rales. Hypotension leads to tachycardia, dizziness, and syncope. Anoxia due to respiratory tract involvement can potentiate vascular collapse and lead to cardiac arrhythmias and cardiac arrest. Occasionally nausea, vomiting, abdominal cramps, and diarrhea may be present. Respiratory or cardiovascular patterns can occur without skin lesions.

Early diagnosis and treatment are mandatory to avert death, which can occur within 15 minutes. There must be constant attention to an adequate airway and perfusion. Any agent known to cause anaphylaxis should be injected below the deltoid area in the arm, if possible, and emergency equipment should be available. The following measures should be taken:

(1) Aqueous epinephrine, 1:1000, 0.3 to 0.5 ml. IM. Urticaria, bronchospasm, and hypotension usually improve. Epinephrine may be repeated in five to 15 minutes if necessary. In profound hypotension the aqueous epinephrine dose can be diluted in 10 ml. saline and can be given *slowly* intravenously, but this method may precipitate cardiac arrhythmias.

(2) To retard absorption of an injected drug place a tourniquet proximal to the injection site and infiltrate the area with aqueous epinephrine, 1:1000, 0.3 ml.

(3) If laryngeal edema progresses, a tracheostomy is necessary. An endotracheal tube may not pass through an edematous larynx.

(4) Start an intravenous infusion of saline.

(5) Persistent bronchospasm after epinephrine therapy should be treated with the administration of aminophylline, 500 mg. I.V. *slowly.* Aminophylline may increase

hypotension and should not be used in patients responding to epinephrine.

(6) Oxygen and assisted ventilation are helpful. A positive pressure breathing apparatus with nebulized isoproterenol (Isuprel) 1:200 (0.5 ml. in 1.5 ml. saline) often helps relieve bronchospasm.

(7) Prolonged hypotension may respond to intravenously administered plasma or colloids (e.g., dextran). Vasoconstrictors such as metraminol bitartrate (Aramine) or levarterenol bitartrate (Levophed) may be needed. Normovolemic hypotension due to a reduced cardiac output responds to an infusion of isoproterenol. Hypotension can lead to metabolic acidosis, which should be treated with intravenously administered sodium bicarbonate. Cardiac arrhythmias are treated with appropriate antiarrhythmic drugs and the dose of catecholamines reduced.

(8) Antihistamines are usually administered to block further histamine binding at target cells. Diphenhydramine (Benadryl), 50 mg. I.M., should be given early in the course of treatment.

(9) Corticosteroids do not act rapidly enough to reverse acute anaphylaxis. Prolonged anaphylaxis and persistent hypotension or bronchospasm, however, should be treated with hydrocortisone succinate (Solu-Cortef), 100 to 500 mg. I.V., every six hours.

(10) Cardiorespiratory arrest is managed with external cardiac massage and assisted ventilation.

SERUM SICKNESS

Serum sickness is an allergic disorder characterized by skin lesions, fever, arthralgias, and lymphadenopathy that appear seven to 12 days after initial drug exposure, but in a shorter period of time in a sensitized person. Although the reaction originally was described as due to horse serum, drugs are now the most common cause (Table 2), notably penicillin.

Skin lesions are the most frequent findings. Edema and urticaria at a drug injection site may be the initial manifestations. Urticaria are the most frequent cutaneous lesions, but morbilliform and scarlatiniform rashes occur, and rare instances of erythema nodosum, erythema multiforme, and vasculitic purpura have been observed. Angioedema usually involves the face but may af-

TABLE 2 Drugs That Cause Serum Sickness

Drugs that Commonly Cause Serum Sickness

antimicrobials	penicillin
	sulfonamides
	streptomycin
hydantoin anticonvulsants	
thiouracils	
heterologous serums and vaccines	

Drugs that Uncommonly Cause Serum Sickness

ACTH	isoniazid
arsenicals	mercurials
barbiturates	tetracyclines
bismuth compounds	phenolphthalein
erythromycin	phenylbutazone
griseofulvin	(Butazolidin)
heparin	probenecid (Benemid)
hydralazine (Apresoline)	quinidine
iron-dextran (Imferon)	quinine
insulin	salicylates
iodides	tripelennamine
iodinated contrast media	(Pyribenzamine)

fect the glottis and external genitalia. Low grade fever usually is present but may be more markedly elevated in severe cases. Arthritis and arthralgias, usually migratory polyarthritis of large joints, are common. Lymphadenopathy occurs in most patients, but may be mild or restricted to the lymph nodes draining the site of drug injection. Often there is malaise, anorexia, headache, and myalgias. Although neurologic and cardiac involvement are rare, they are potentially lethal. There may be peripheral neuritis, polyneuritis, or meningoencephalitis with residua in a minority of patients so affected. Angina pectoris and acute myocardial infarction from involvement of the coronary arteries are rare sequelae.

Laboratory findings are sparse. A mild leukocytosis occurs with the acute illness, and eosinophilia may appear during recovery. The urine may show small amounts of protein and occasionally red blood cells and white blood cells, but renal function is maintained.

The illness is self-limited and subsides in two to three weeks. Residua or death may follow the infrequent involvement of the nervous system and heart.

Treatment is mainly directed at alleviating symptoms.

(1) Urticaria and angioedema are quickly alleviated by subcutaneous injection of 0.2 to 0.3 ml. of aqueous epinephrine 1:1000. Epinephrine also is effective in managing glottal edema, which, however, may be severe enough to require tracheostomy. Antihistamines such as diphenhydramine hydrocholoride (Benadryl), 25 to 50 mg. orally every four to six hours, provide more prolonged relief of urticaria and angioedema.

(2) Fever, discomfort, and joint pains are alleviated by aspirin 300 to 600 mg. every four hours.

(3) Parenteral fluids may be needed to treat dehydration.

(4) In severe cases, when symptoms are not relieved by the above measures, or if there is either nervous system or coronary artery involvement, corticosteroids (e.g., prednisone, 60 mg. daily) should be used.

ASPIRIN-INDUCED ASTHMA

Aspirin can cause severe wheezing in up to 10 per cent of asthmatic patients by a poorly understood nonimmunologic mechanism. These individuals usually have a family history of asthma, rhinorrhea, nasal polyps, and chronic sinusitis that antedates the onset of aspirin sensitivity. Most of these patients have perennial (intrinsic) asthma and wheeze when aspirin is not given. A low incidence of atopy and negative skin tests are characteristic.

Salicylates other than aspirin do not precipitate wheezing, but sensitivity to the following structurally dissimilar drugs also exists: indomethacin (Indocin), aminopyrine, mefenamic acid (Ponstel), and tartrazine, a yellow food dye.

In a few minutes to two hours after ingestion of aspirin or the other drugs listed, severe, potentially fatal bronchospasm occurs. There may be accompanying rhinorrhea, flushing, pruritus, urticaria, or hypotension.

In order to prevent this reaction, a sensitive individual should be warned against taking all precipitating drugs and over-the-counter preparations that may contain aspirin.

Treatment is the same as for any asthmatic attack, except that wheezing is characteristically severe and often does not respond to the usual measures but requires corticosteroid therapy. Initial measures include:

(1) Aqueous epinephrine 1:1000, 0.3 to 0.5 ml. subcutaneously, which may be repeated in 15 minutes if necessary.

(2) Aminophylline, 250 to 500 mg. I.V. *slowly* over five to ten minutes.

(3) Adequate hydration, which may require intravenous administration to loosen secretions.

(4) If carbon dioxide retention and respiratory acidosis occur, these should be corrected with intravenously administered sodium bicarbonate, since a normal blood pH facilitates the effectiveness of drug therapy.

(5) Corticosteroids usually should be employed in conjunction with the above measures. If the patient is unable to take oral medicines, hydrocortisone succinate (Solu-Cortef), 100 mg. I.V. should be given every six hours. When or if oral medicines can be taken, prednisone, 15 mg. every six hours, should be used. Corticosteroids should be tapered over a week as the attack subsides.

AGRANULOCYTOSIS

Agranulocytosis is a drug-induced marked decrease or absence of polymorphonuclear leukocytes (PMN) accompanied by a decreased total white blood cell count. The absolute number of PMN's may fall between 0 and 500 per cu. mm. There are two causative mechanisms: (a) an immunologically mediated type in which PMN's are rapidly destroyed in the blood after drug ingestion in a sensitized individual; and (b) a more slowly developing toxic type that suppresses bone marrow granulocyte production after several weeks of continuous drug therapy (Table 3).

The immunologic type is ushered in by chills, fever, malaise, sore throat, and hypotension coincident with the peripheral destruction of PMN's. There are no specific symptoms of the toxic form, but chills and

TABLE 3   *Drugs Causing Agranulocytosis*

Immunologic type	aminopyrine, dipyrone, phenylbutazone (Butazolidin), thiouracils, sulfonamides (and many others less frequently)
Toxic type	antineoplastic drugs (dose-related)
	all phenothiazines except promethazine (Phenergan) and methdilazine (Tacaryl)

fever appear if bacterial infection supervenes. The great danger in both forms is bacterial infection, which is associated with a mortality rate of about 20 per cent.

The hematologic findings are the same in both forms and consist of an absence or near absence of PMN's and a depressed white blood cell count. In the immunologic type, PMN's may return rapidly or after a week or so, and in the toxic type PMN's return more gradually during about a two-week period after stopping the causative drug.

As part of the treatment, (1) patients should be hospitalized and all suspected causative drugs discontinued.

(2) Protective isolation may be employed in an attempt to prevent bacterial infections, but its efficacy is unproved.

(3) Prophylactic antibiotics do not prevent infections, but are associated with the development of infections due to bacteria resistant to the antibiotics used.

(4) When fever is present, blood cultures should be performed as well as cultures of other sites clinically indicated.

(5) If bacterial infections do occur, they should be treated promptly with appropriate antimicrobial agents.

THROMBOCYTOPENIA

Thrombocytopenia is so frequently drug-induced that drugs should always be considered as a possible cause. Drug-induced thrombocytopenia is often due to immunologic mechanisms. In such instances, platelet counts can fall to very low levels in minutes or hours after drug exposure in a sensitized individual. Almost any drug can cause thrombocytopenia. Antineoplastic agents produce a dose related fall in platelets and other blood elements.

Clinical manifestations of thrombocytopenia include petechiae, ecchymoses, bleeding gums, epistaxis, gastrointestinal bleeding, or hemorrhage from other sites. Intracranial hemorrhage is uncommon.

Platelet counts can be depressed to levels of 500 per cu. mm. Bone marrow aspiration usually shows normal numbers of megakaryocytes. Some drugs (e.g., antineoplastic agents) damage megakaryocytes, leading to a diminished number of megakaryocytes, which may contain vacuoles.

The initial step in treatment is to (1) discontinue all drugs. If clinically necessary, structurally unrelated compounds with similar pharmacologic effects can be substituted. If thrombocytopenia is drug-induced, normal numbers of platelets should be present in about two weeks. In thrombycotopenia induced by gold salts, which are retained in the body for prolonged periods, a fall in platelets may not occur for up to a month after the last injection and may persist for a protracted period.

(2) Bed rest is advisable to decrease the risk of trauma and bleeding.

(3) Prednisone in doses of 60 mg. daily should be given if the platelet count is lower than 10,000 per cu. mm. and probably if the platelet count is below 25,000 per cu. mm.

(4) If hemorrhage occurs, platelet transfusions should be given. Greatest benefit accrues if the causative drug has been cleared.

UPPER GASTROINTESTINAL BLEEDING

Of the many drugs implicated in producing upper gastrointestinal bleeding (Table 4), aspirin has been incriminated most often. A possible link to aspirin ingestion has been found in 5 per cent of patients presenting with upper gastrointestinal bleeding. Salicylates can cause hemorrhagic gastritis and peptic erosion or ulceration with bleeding. Uncommonly, a previous peptic ulcer may be reactivated. Phenylbutazone (Butazolidin), oxyphenbutazone (Tandearil), and indomethacin (Indocin) can produce similar effects. About 60 per cent of corticosteroid-induced peptic ulcerations occur in the stomach and usually follow high-dose, prolonged therapy, but ulcerations may develop rapidly with relatively small doses. Often, there are no symptoms until bleeding or perforation occurs. Corticosteroid-induced ulcers may heal with multi-

ple feeding and antacid treatment, even though corticosteroids are continued. The small doses of reserpine and its congeners used to treat hypertension rarely cause peptic ulceration. Anticoagulant therapy increases the hazard of gastrointestinal bleeding if ulcerogenic drugs are taken concomitantly or if a peptic ulcer is present.

Clinically there may be indigestion or epigastric distress. With slow bleeding the stools become positive for occult blood, and iron deficiency anemia may appear. In more acute bleeding, hematemesis, melena, hypotension, and syncope may occur.

Treatment is directed at stopping bleeding and maintaining intravascular volume as with bleeding from any other cause.

(1) Ulcerogenic drugs should be discontinued. If corticosteroids are the cause, the drug should be tapered slowly, if this is possible, but healing may occur with antacids and diet therapy while the drug is still being administered.

(2) If ulceration is demonstrated radiographically or endoscopically, or if symptoms are troublesome, multiple feedings and antacids between feedings should be used.

(3) If continued salicylate therapy is deemed necessary, as in patients with rheumatoid arthritis, enteric coated preparations may be used, but their absorption tends to be erratic and symptoms may recur.

(4) If anticoagulants are the cause of bleeding, the clotting defect produced by heparin is counteracted by protamine and that of the coumarin derivatives by vitamin K analogues.

(5) Iron deficiency anemia following slow bleeding should be treated with iron therapy (e.g., ferrous sulfate 300 mg. three times a day) best given with meals and at least an hour before antacids are taken to avoid binding and diminished iron absorption. Iron therapy should continue for three months after blood values have returned to normal in order to replenish iron stores.

TABLE 4. Drugs Causing Upper Gastrointestinal Bleeding

anticoagulants
salicylates
phenylbutazone (Butazolidin)
oxyphenbutazone (Tandearil)
indomethacin (Indocin)
reserpine
mefenamic acid (Ponstel)
ethacrynic acid (Edecrin)

EXFOLIATIVE DERMATITIS*

Exfoliative dermatitis is a more or less generalized scaly, inflammatory skin disorder due to drugs (Table 5), other skin diseases, hematologic or other malignancies, or unknown causes. Most of the skin, includ-

*See also Chapter 56.

TABLE 5   Drugs Known to Cause Exfoliative Dermatitis

Antimicrobials	penicillin°, sulfonamides°, tetracyclines, streptomycin, isoniazid, PASA
Barbiturates°	
Hydantoin anti-convulsants°	
Analgesics	phenylbutazone (Butazolidin)°, salicylates
Heavy metals	arsenicals°, gold salts, mercurial diuretics, antimony compounds
Other drugs	actinomycin D, allopurinol (Zyloprim), BAL, chloroquine (Aralen), chlorpropamide (Diabinese), codeine, griseofulvin, iodides, phenothiazines, quinacrine (Atabrine), quinidine, quinine, thiouracils, vitamin A

° Common cause of disorder.

ing the scalp, palms, and soles, becomes erythematous, dry, and scaly, but some areas may be moist. Itching is common. The hair and nails may be secondarily damaged or lost. Lymphadenopathy occurs often, even in the absence of leukemia or lymphoma. About 20 per cent of patients have hepatomegaly.

Continuous exfoliation of the skin leads to a negative nitrogen balance, hypoalbuminemia, edema, and loss of muscle mass. A diminished protective skin barrier results in external water loss. Defects in temperature regulation occur, with chilly feelings and fever in about 40 per cent of patients and hypothermia in some. Patients are prone to develop bacterial infections.

The course depends on the etiology, with the best prognosis in the drug-induced group.

The first principle of therapy in drug-induced exfoliative dermatitis is (1) to discontinue the causative drug. This alone often leads to rapid clearing.

(2) Chilliness from increased heat loss through the damaged skin is treated by insuring a warm ambient temperature, adequate bed clothes, and a heat cradle if necessary.

(3) Skin care should include warm tub baths, with care to avoid chilling, and lubri-cation of the skin, best accomplished with solid Crisco.

(4) Corticosteroids ameliorate symptoms and shorten the course of illness. Prednisone, 60 mg. daily in divided doses, should be started and tapered as the skin lesions heal.

(5) A careful record of intake and output and serum electrolyte values must be maintained. Fluid and electrolyte disturbances usually require parenteral fluid therapy.

(6) Infections should be cultured and promptly treated with appropriate antimicrobial agents.

STEVENS-JOHNSON SYNDROME

The Stevens-Johnson syndrome is an acute, severe form of erythema multiforme with skin and mucous membrane lesions. About 35 per cent of cases are due to drugs, the most frequently implicated being penicillin, phenolphthalein, sulfonamides, barbiturates, and hydantoin anticonvulsants. Other causes include herpes and mycoplasma infections, vaccines, deep x-ray therapy, malignancies, pregnancy, and foods.

Skin lesions tend to be symmetrical, are most numerous on the extensor areas of the distal parts of arms and legs, and often involve the palms and soles. The typical lesion begins as a red spot. Small bullae may develop in the center; these then become surrounded by concentric circles of deeper color, the so-called "iris" or target lesions. Although the iris lesion is characteristic, it is not always present. Vesicular and erosive lesions frequently occur in the mouth and on the gums and tongue. The lips are often swollen and encrusted. Conjunctival and genital lesions occur in most patients. Other frequent findings are fever, toxemia, myalgias, arthralgias, and less often cough with patchy pulmonary infiltrates.

Laboratory abnormalities are few. Mild anemia occurs in severe cases and there may be leukocytosis, usually due to secondary infection.

Most cases abate in two weeks but severe forms may last up to six weeks. Skin lesions heal without scarring. Blindness may result from scarring of ocular lesions. There is a low mortality rate.

Treatment consists of: (1) discontinuing all suspected drugs.

(2) Corticosteroids are beneficial in severe cases. If the patient is able to swallow, prednisone in divided daily doses of 60 to 100 mg. is given until improvement occurs and the dose is then tapered. If mouth lesions prevent swallowing, hydrocortisone succinate (Solu-Cortef), 100 mg. I.V. every six to eight hours may be used.

(3) Fluid and electrolyte imbalances can occur in patients unable to take oral sustenance. This should be corrected with intravenous fluid administration.

(4) Mouth care is important for oral lesions. Raw areas should be cleaned with saline soaks and then covered with glycerine, propylene glycol, or triamcinolone acetonide in emollient dental paste (Kenalog in Orabase).

(5) Patients with eye involvement must receive care from an ophthalmologist. Conjunctival involvement plus drying and turning in of the lashes can lead to corneal abrasion with infection and later corneal opacification and, rarely, rupture of the globe.

TOXIC EPIDERMAL NECROLYSIS*

Toxic epidermal necrolysis resembles a burn and is also termed the "scalded skin syndrome." In adults the disease usually is due to drug reactions, but in children staphylococcal infections are the commonest cause. Cases also have been associated with smallpox vaccination, leukemias, lymphomas, and no ostensible cause. The drugs most commonly implicated are phenylbutazone (Butazolidin), hydantoin anticonvulsants, sulfonamides, and tetracyclines.

Clinically, skin lesions resemble a burn, with tender, red areas over which the epidermis easily strips off. Elements of the Stevens-Johnson syndrome may occur concomitantly with iris lesions and oral and conjunctival involvement.

Few laboratory abnormalities occur.

---

*See also Chapter 56.

The white blood cell count and erythrocyte sedimentation rate usually are normal. Occasionally there is transient albuminuria and modest urea nitrogen retention.

Milder cases recover without incident. If half the area of skin is involved, the mortality may be as high as 40 per cent. Death occurs from shock due to fluid losses from the injured skin, secondary bacterial infection, and, rarely, from disseminated intravascular coagulation.

Treatment begins by: (1) discontinuing all drugs.

(2) Fluid and electrolyte balance must be maintained.

(3) A turning frame facilitates moving the patient to avoid prolonged pressure on involved areas of skin.

(4) The role of corticosteroid therapy is not clear. In severe cases, large doses of prednisone, 100 to 150 mg. daily, may be beneficial if given early in the course of illness and tapered as skin lesions clear.

(5) Isolation is not necessary, but hand washing and aseptic techniques should be used to try to prevent infection.

(6) Prophylactic antibiotics do not prevent infection but allow growth of resistant organisms. If bacterial infections occur, however, they should be appropriately treated.

References

Abrahams, I., McCarthy, J. T., and Saunders, S. L.: One hundred and one cases of exfoliative dermatitis. Arch. Dermatol. 87:96, 1963.

Bianchine, J. R., et al.: Drugs as etiologic factors in the Stevens-Johnson syndrome. Am. J. Med. 44:390, 1968.

Chodirker, W. B. and Vaughan, J. H.: Serum Sickness. In Fitzpatrick, T. B., et al.: Dermatology in General Medicine. New York, McGraw-Hill, 1971, p. 1274.

Kelly, J. F., and Patterson, R.: Anaphylaxis: course, mechanism and treatment. J.A.M.A. 227:1431, 1974.

Lancet (editorial): Aspirin and gastrointestinal bleeding. Lancet 2:460, 1967.

Lockey, R. F., Rucknagel, D. L., and Vanselow, N. A.: Familial occurrence of asthma, nasal polyps, and aspirin intolerance. Ann. Intern. Med. 78:57, 1973.

Lyell, A.: A review of toxic epidermal necrolysis in Britain. Br. J. Dermatol. 79:662, 1967.

Miescher, P. A.: Drug-induced thrombocytopenia. Semin. Hematol. 10:311, 1973.

Pisciotta, A. V.: Immune and toxic mechanisms in drug-induced agranulocytosis. Semin. Hematol. 10:279, 1973.

Chapter 58   POISONINGS

A. Emergency Toxicology and General Principles of Medical Management of the Poisoned Patient
B. Management of Specific Poisonings.
C. Intoxication and the Alcohol Abstinence Syndrome

A. EMERGENCY TOXICOLOGY AND GENERAL PRINCIPLES OF MEDICAL MANAGEMENT OF THE POISONED PATIENT

George R. Schwartz

CHAPTER OVERVIEW

The range of possible substances that can cause poisoning is vast. In fact, every substance is a potential poison if it is admitted into the body in large enough quantities. To provide a compendium of all possible poisons is therefore impossible for practical purposes. Chapter 58B does list 172 substances commonly involved in poisonings and includes a synopsis of medical management in such cases. Moreover, throughout this book, the diagnosis and treatment of poisonings and drug overdoses are discussed in some detail. The index has been designed to allow ready reference to these discussions, which are listed under the general heading of "Poisonings."

The principal thrust of this chapter is the following:

1. To provide a brief historical introduction and review the basics of emergency toxicology.

2. To detail the method of evaluation of a poisoned patient or one in whom poisoning is suspected.

3. To describe the sequence of good general medical management in cases of poisonings.

4. To describe the role of the laboratory in the poisoned patient.

5. To describe techniques involved in the management of poisonings; their indications and contraindications (e.g., emesis, lavage, dialysis).

6. To present an approach to symptom and sign analysis when poisoning is present or suspected but the actual substance involved is not known.

7. To present some of the controversies that exist among experts in poisoning management and the reasons for the differences of opinion (for example, the management of

ingestion of petroleum distillates, the efficacy of dialysis and other techniques).

8. To review common food poisonings and their management.

Commercial Information Services

Every emergency department should have a special area in which information about poisonings is collected. This includes books, standard protocols, telephone numbers, and microfilm information equipment when available. Over the past decade some cities have seen development of area-wide poison control centers where information is readily available by experts. More commonly, however, the expansion of such centers has not kept pace with the new information, and funds have been insufficient for 24-hour coverage by highly skilled toxicology experts. As a result, several commercial services have been established which offer subscribing hospitals information on microfilm as well as a microfilm projector. The commercial service updates the information on a regular basis. Personal experience has demonstrated that these services can be very useful. However, the appropriate use of such services requires training of the personnel in asking suitable questions of the patient or those accompanying the patient. Of course, the microfilm units are not portable, and this limits their use outside the hospital or poison control center.

Historical Survey

The history of poisonings is as old as man. Earliest man had to contend with animal venoms and poisonous plants. In some instances this knowledge of poisons (for example, curare) was used for hunting. Hippocrates mentions poisons in some detail, and the well-known draught of Socrates was hemlock, the state poison of the Greeks. Aristotle included information about poisonings in his writings; and Dioscorides, a Greek physician in the court of Nero, classified poisons. In fact, Dioscorides' classification into plant, mineral and animal poisons is still a convenient format.

The early Romans developed deliberate poisoning into a profession, and a cadre of experts emerged who sold their services, primarily for political assassination. However, like the "contract killers" or "hit men" of our current day, their knowledge of poisons and methods of poisoning could be sold to the highest bidder.

Most early poisons were of plant origin, but there is evidence that heavy metal poisoning and arsenic poisoning was known. Arsenic was the likely agent used in the murder of Claudius which resulted in Nero becoming emperor of Rome.

In the Middle Ages deliberate poisonings continued, and in the Renaissance such well-known families of poisoners as the Borgias became prominent in Italy.

The most powerful historical influence on the development of a science of toxicology was probably Phillipus Aureolus Paracelsus. Born Theophrastus Bombastus von Hohenheim, he assumed the name Paracelsus and throughout the 16th century lived in a peripatetic manner. Many of his ideas were new to his time, and he was often viewed as a maverick physician and sometimes ridiculed. His major contribution in the field of poisonings was his visionary realization that poisoning is often a matter of dose and that the difference between the therapeutic and highly toxic effects of a substance is usually dose-related.

Until the 20th century, the major focus was on detection and description of poisonings rather than on treatment and antidotes. The tremendous advances in pharmaceuticals, new technology and enhanced knowledge of the chemical nature and action of substances have given impetus to more effective treatment. The growth of Emergency Medicine has served to focus more attention on applied toxicology, since facilities are more advanced and time delays from the time of poisoning to that of treatment have been reduced. Skilled Emergency Physicians are extremely important in rapidly diagnosing and initiating suitable treatment.

EMERGENCY TOXICOLOGY

The field of toxicology (the science of poisons) is broad and multidisciplinary. *Emergency toxicology is the application of toxicologic knowledge within a limited time frame and often limited data base in order to formulate the most effective treatment plan.*

To formulate such a plan clinical information must be integrated with knowledge of the physiologic dynamics of the poisonous substance. Symptom and sign analysis (Table 1) may enable possible or presumptive identification of the poison when information is inadequate or the patient is unable or unwilling to provide it.

When dealing with the emergency situation, first and foremost is attention to supporting vital functions. The basic medical management will be reviewed in the next section. The following is an outline of the questions which should be kept in mind when evaluating a poisoned patient.

1. *Nature of poison and route of entry*
   a. What is the chemical nature of the poison?
   b. Is the dose potentially lethal?
   c. Was the substance taken orally, parenterally, or through the skin, lungs, GI tract, or rectum?
   d. Can the substance be rapidly eliminated (e.g., via emesis), counteracted, or neutralized?
2. *Absorption dynamics and distribution in body*
   a. What is the time course of absorption and/or effect? Is emesis or lavage likely to be effective? If delays have occurred or if the route of entry was other than oral, can the substance be counteracted or bound? (In this context consider antidotes, antibodies, binding agents, etc.)
   b. Will activated charcoal be of value?
   c. What is the target organ of the poison? Where is the storage site in the body (e.g., fat storage, bound to plasma protein)? Which system will be compromised or injured by

TABLE 1 *Symptom and Sign Analysis to Assist in Identification of Chemical Agent or Class of Agent When Type of Poisoning Is Not Known*

AGENT	STATE OF CNS	CONVULSIONS	PUPILS	SALIVARY ACTIVITY	RESPIRATIONS	HEART RHYTHM AND RATE	BLOOD PRESSURE	DIARRHEA	SKIN CHANGE
Atropine-like or anticholinergic syndrome	Excitability, coma if severe	Possible	Dilated,	Dry	Usually ↑ ↓ if severe	Tachycardia	↑ Slightly ↓ in severe	No	Flushed
Cholinergic type	Excitability, coma if very severe	Usually not	Constricted	Secretions increased markedly	Possible wheezes; ↓ respirations in severe cases	Bradycardia	→	Yes	Flushed; may be in shock if severe
CNS tranquilizers, barbiturate type	Depressed	Not usual	Nystagmus, midpoint unless hypoxic, and then dilated	No marked change	↓ ↓ possible pulm. edema	Tachycardia	→	Possible	May be in shock state
CNS tranquilizers, nonbarbiturate (minor type)	Depressed	Not usual	Not changed unless very severe—then dilated	No marked change	→	Tachycardia	→	No	VS usually maintained unless very severe
CNS tranquilizer, phenothetazine type	Depressed	Possible	Either slightly constricted or no marked change	Dry	Slightly depressed unless very severe	Tachycardia	→	No	Flushed
Aspirin	Usually depressed	Possible	No marked change	No marked change	↑ ↑	Tachycardia	↓ in severe	Possible	Not marked
Narcotic	Depressed	Not usual	Constricted	Tend to dry	↓ ↓ Possible pulm. edema	Tachycardia	→	No	Not marked
Carbon monoxide	Depressed	Possible if severe	No marked change	No marked change	↑	↑	→	Possible	Red color
Neuromuscular blocking agent	No change until hypoxic	No	No change	No significant change	→ →	↑	→	Possible	Not marked
Cardiovascular—digitalis	Slightly depressed	If severe	No marked change	No marked change	No marked change	Slow rate arrhythmias	→	Yes	Not marked
Adrenergic—e.g., amphetamine	Excited	No	Dilated	Dry	Increased	Tachycardia, possible arrhythmias	↑	No	Flushed
Alcohol	Depressed if severe	No	No marked change	Slightly increased	→	Tachycardia	→	Possible	Flushed
Cyanide	Depressed	Frequent	Not much change unless severely hypoxic; then dilated	Not much change	↓ ↓	Tachycardia and arrhythmias	→	Possible	Cyanosis

the poison? Can this organ injury be reduced or prevented?

    d. Will metabolism produce other products which might be hazardous?

  3. *Excretion dynamics*

    a. How is the substance excreted? Is it excreted in the urine or stool, through the lungs, via liver and biliary system, or other routes?

    b. Can excretion be hastened (e.g., with purgatives, with diuresis, through acidification or alkalinization of the urine, using dialysis or ion-exchange resins, through blood exchange)?

  4. *The role of the laboratory*

    a. Are there specific tests of poison level (e.g., serum alcohol, barbiturate)?

    b. What tests will be useful in evaluating the clinical status of the patient? Which tests will allow determination of any baseline values as well as allowing the course of organ injury to be followed?

Metabolism of Toxic Substances

Metabolic reactions within the body have evolved so as to be able to cope with limited quantities of almost any chemical substance. The metabolic reactions, however, are not basically programmed for detoxification so that when acting on a poison some metabolic products may be as active chemically or even more dangerous than the original poison. It is worthwhile to remember also that metabolic systems are often less developed in the young so that in infants and children some toxicants may be active at lower dose ranges and may remain active for a longer period of time. For example, some barbiturates depend on liver metabolism—primarily, hexabarbital and secobarbital (phenobarbital less than the others).

There are four major types of enzymatic metabolic reactions: hydrolysis, oxidation, reduction, and conjugation. The precise metabolic fate of most poisons has not been described, and medical science has not progressed to such a point that any of these processes can be substantially hastened. As a result, metabolic treatment of poisoning is rudimentary at best, and technologic ad-

vances have been made in the direction of enhancing elimination by use of such devices as dialysis machines.

BASIC MEDICAL MANAGEMENT OF POISONINGS

The basic elements of the medical management of poisonings are as follows:

  1. Support vital functions

  2. Identify agent (when possible)

  3. Remove, neutralize, or reverse effects

  4. Hasten excretion

  5. Treat damaged or poisoned organs or systems

INITIAL MANAGEMENT

When a patient has been poisoned the immediate view must be to maintain life. The vital functions must be evaluated and supported as necessary. Most commonly this refers to the respiratory system since many drugs and poisons act to depress the respiratory center. At times, however, maintenance of blood pressure and treatment of shock-like states are necessary. Any cardiac irregularity must be identified and monitored.

During the initial evaluation and support of vital functions a member of the emergency department team should make efforts to identify the poison. If the patient cannot or will not provide this information, all sources of history should be rapidly explored. Information from friends, knowledge of available drugs and poisons, empty bottles, and previous treatments or physicians must be assessed. Table 1 illustrates a symptom and sign analysis. Using nine easily observed signs, one may possibly place an unknown poison in one of the drug categories shown. Such categorization is particularly important when large doses have been taken, and reversal should be undertaken when such treatment is possible. For example, the so-called "anticholinergic syndrome" can be produced by a large number of drugs, and physostigmine has demonstrated value in reversing some of the abnormalities. Table 2 indicates some compounds involved in the "anticholinergic syndrome", and the use of physostigmine in such instances Identification as to class or type of drug may be extremely useful when dialysis is considered.

Although identification or probable

***TABLE 2 Common Drugs That Produce the "Anticholinergic Syndrome"
and the Use of Physostigmine in Such Cases***

DRUGS	TREATMENT
Elavil Atropine Ornade Benadryl Bentyl Sinequan (doxepin) Homatropine Scopolamine Tofranil and other tricyclic antidepressants Probanthine Sominex (methapyrilene)	Use physostigmine (side effects are those of cholinergic stimulation and can be reversed with atropine). If atropine reversal is necessary, use a dose half that of physostigmine. *Children:* 0.5 mg. I.V. slowly. The dose may be slowly raised to 2.0 mg. or stopped prior to that if cholinergic symptoms (e.g., salivary glandular activity, diarrhea) become prominent. *Adults:* Begin with 2.0 mg. slowly I.V.—raise to 4.0 mg. if no effect. Repeat if anticholinergic symptoms again become prominent. The anticholinergic poisoning symptoms include CNS hyperactivity and seizures initially; but with marked overdosage, coma and medullary paralysis may occur. Tachycardia, mydriasis, and decrease in secretions are also prominent.

identification of the poison is important, excessive time must not be expended at this point on specific or class delineation. Frequently overdoses with suicidal intent involve more than one drug and the clinical picture can be confusing. The higher priority is to support vital functions and remove the agent or reverse its action. If there is a possibility of a narcotic or opiate-like substance being involved, a trial of naloxone (Narcan) can be undertaken with little risk. Similarly, if insulin or an insulin-like substance is possibly involved, a solution of 50 per cent dextrose can be infused after blood has been taken for glucose determination. The use of the paper sticks for rapid glucose determination can be helpful as well, although they deteriorate with age.

REMOVAL OF ORALLY INGESTED POISONS

Most poisonings occur through oral ingestion, and the most effective means of removal is by induction of emesis. Although

TABLE 3 Contraindications to Emesis

1. The ingested substance is nontoxic in the existent dose range.
2. The ingested substance is a caustic alkali or acid.
3. In petroleum distillate ingestion. (There is controversy if the amount taken is large, since the dangers of systemic absorption may outweigh the risk of aspiration.)
4. If the patient is comatose or has a substantially depressed gag reflex.
5. If the substance ingested has strong antiemetic properties, emesis induction, while not contraindicated, might not be successful.

this procedure is usually safe, there are situations in which emesis induction (usually through use of ipecac syrup) should not be undertaken. Table 3 lists such contraindications. In the presence of an impaired state of consciousness and a depressed gag reflex, chances of aspiration are increased. To avoid this potentially disastrous complication such patients require gastric lavage with a cuffed endotracheal tube in place.

PETROLEUM DISTILLATE INGESTION

There has been considerable controversy as to the proper management in cases of petroleum distillate ingestion. Certainly, in the presence of a depressed gag reflex experts are in accord that emesis should not be induced. Some physicians feel that if the ingestion is large (for example, greater than 30 cc.), lavage should be undertaken with an endotracheal tube in place. If the patient is alert and the gag reflex is intact, some authorities feel that there is sufficient data supporting the safety of ipecac use (HEW, 1976). On the other hand, Arena (1976) has pointed to the low death and complication rate from petroleum distillate ingestion, with almost all deaths resulting from aspiration and pulmonary complications. He concludes that emesis is to be generally avoided in such ingestions. Some physicians have adopted a middle-of-the-road position that with large petroleum distillate ingestions lavage should be instituted with a cuffed endotracheal tube in place. The American Academy of Pediatrics, through HEW, released *The Handbook of Common Poisonings in Children* in 1976, which advised emesis in an alert patient who has ingested large amounts of kerosene or related petroleum distillates. The emesis should be performed with the patient in an upright position; "This recommendation is made on the basis of newer information which shows the safety of Ipecac syrup–induced emesis following hydrocarbon ingestion." Particularly dangerous hydrocarbons (such as those containing camphor, pesticides, heavy metals or halogenated solvents) are hazardous at lower dosages.

USE OF LAVAGE OR EMESIS

How long after oral ingestion should lavage be undertaken or emesis induced? This is a frequent and highly relevant question posed daily in most large emergency facilities. There is no set answer, but review of some physiology is a good evaluative approach to this dilemma. While the average time to empty half of the stomach contents through the pyloris depends on many factors, the figure of one-half to one hour is often used. Certainly the exact time is related to the nature of the ingested material and the quantity. There is also a good deal of individual variation. Factors that should be considered include the following:

1. The ingested poison may slow gastric motility and emptying. Also, it may be ingested while there is food within the stomach, and the time for passage into the intestine can be very different if the stomach is full.

2. Deliberate or accidental overdosage or poisoning can be accompanied by a marked sympathetic nervous system response, which can cause a delay of hours of gastric emptying. Also, the ingested poison may itself have the pharmacologic action of slowing gastric emptying.

3. Some ingested substances (for example, methyl salicylate) can be re-excreted into the stomach.

Because of the above, emesis or lavage can result in substantial returns of the poison, in some instances four, six and even eight hours after ingestion. Occasionally, ingested drugs can remain in the stomach for days. If the amount ingested is dangerous, emesis should be induced, therefore, even if a substantial time delay is involved. In my personal experience, a 30-year-old woman ingested 100 tablets of aspirin soon after eating a large meal. Ten hours later gastric lavage returned a portion of the meal and the aspirin.

Gastric Lavage. Gastric lavage should be used when emesis is contraindicated and emptying of the stomach is necessary. A tube can readily be passed via the oral route in children. In adults a nasal route can be used, but the size of the tube is therefore limited, and the oral route with at least a size 28 Fr. is preferable. The usual NG tube can be used for liquids, but gets obstructed if aspiration of tablets is necessary. The double lumen tube allowing lavage solution to be infused while the tube is connected to suction is a useful innovation. If the state of consciousness is diminished or a depressed gag reflex is present, lavage should be performed with a cuffed endotracheal tube in place to avoid aspiration. Remove all foreign bodies (e.g., false teeth) from the mouth prior to lavage.

Position the patient in such a way that his left side is down (to allow pooling of gastric contents and limit passage into the duodenum), and the head should be lowered. Such precautions are essential to minimize chances of aspiration. Upon beginning lavage, material should be saved for visual inspection and laboratory analysis when indicated.

Lavage fluid should be normal saline in children to avoid the possibility of water intoxication, but in adults ordinary tap water or half normal saline is satisfactory. Lavage with smaller aliquots (50 cc. in children, 200 to 300 cc. in adults) and continue until

TABLE 4   Induction of Emesis

INDUCER	DOSE/ADMINISTRATION	DANGERS	REASONS FOR FAILURE
Ipecac syrup	Child: 10–15 cc. po Adult: 20–30 cc. po Follow with glasses of water; may repeat dose once after 20 min.	If emesis does not occur, must lavage due to possible cardiovascular irritation.	1. Ingested substance antiemetic 2. Inadequate water 3. Decreased state of consciousness
Apomorphine	Child: 0.03 mg./lb. BW I.V. Adult: 6.0 mg. I.V. Stomach should be full (give water).	Respiratory depression may occur. Narcan must be immediately available to reverse.	Depressed consciousness

TABLE 5 *Antidotes That Chemically Counteract Effects or Serve as Binding Agents°*

NATURE OF POISON	TREATMENT AGENT
Cholinergic compounds (e.g., organophosphates, DDT)	Atropine: begin with 1.0 mg. I.V. in adults Children's dose dependent on weight, (.05 mg./kg.)
cyanide poisoning	Amyl nitrate
nitrates and nitrites	Methylene blue (0.2 ml./kg. I.V. given over 5 minutes in saline
carbon monoxide	Oxygen
Narcotics (e.g., morphine, heroin, methadone, Demerol, and to lesser extent, propoxyphene [Darvon], Talwin, Percodan	Naloxone (Narcan): begin with 0.4 mg. I.V. in adults 0.01 mg./kg. BW in children
Anticholinergic compounds (see Table 58-2)	Treat with physostigmine (see Table 58-2 for dose)
Iron overdose	Use Desferal: Adult, 1–2 gm. I.V. or I.M. Child, 90 mg./kg. BW I.V. or I.M. *Note:* Dangerous in renal disease
Heparin	Protamine sulfate – give as 1% solution in equal dosage to the heparin
Coumadin	Vitamin K: Give up to 10 mg./minute to maximum of 100 mg. (depending upon amount ingested)
Metal poisonings: Cadmium, cobalt, copper, lead, nickel	Use calcium EDTA (Versene)
Antimony, arsenic, gold, nickel, lead	Bind with dimercaprol (BAL)
Mercury	Bind with penicillamine

°Most poison antidotes are nonspecific, but those that chemically counteract or bind poisons tend to be more effective. Delays prior to their use should be minimized.

the return is clear. Use of larger aliquots of lavage fluid should be avoided, since distending the stomach tends to force gastric contents through the pylorus.

USE OF ACTIVATED CHARCOAL (PHYSICAL BINDING)

Activated charcoal slurry (1 or 2 tbsp. per glass of water) should be given after emesis or lavage is concluded. Its effectiveness is widespread and its use is limited only in cyanide poisoning. If the patient cannot swallow, the slurry can be instilled via a lavage tube.

While it is common practice to prepare the slurry freshly for each patient, using an aqueous suspension of activated charcoal offers much in convenience and has been shown to be as effective as that prepared freshly even after a year (Chin et al., 1970).

CHEMICAL REVERSAL OF ACTIONS OF POISONS

Table 2 indicates the use of physostigmine in poisoning by anticholinergic agents. Table 5 reviews some antidotes that act in a relatively specific manner either by stimulating opposing systems (e.g., use of atropine to counteract cholinergic poisons), by employing principles of competition for receptor sites (e.g., Narcan in opiate overdoses), by supplementing depleted substances (e.g., vitamin K in Coumadin overdose) or through chemical binding actions (e.g., calcium EDTA, BAL, or penicillamine in heavy metal overdosages).

This listing is not complete and does not include the use of antivenins (covered in the sections dealing with snake bites and insect bites) or specific antibodies (such as the use of antibodies in digoxin intoxication (Smith, 1976).

TECHNIQUES TO SPEED EXCRETION

Speeding Intestinal Excretion. The three most commonly used cathartics are sodium sulfate, 10 to 30 gm. in 8 oz. of water, castor oil, 30 cc., given orally, and magnesium sulfate (Epsom salts) 15–30 gm. in water (for adults) and 250 mg./kg. in children. Castor oil should certainly be avoided if there is vomiting or a depressed gag reflex. Because of the possible hazards associated

TABLE 6　Common Drugs in Which Forced Diuresis Will Not Be Effective in Speeding Excretion*

Short- and medium-acting barbiturates
Glutethimide
Methaqualone
Phenothiazines
Tricyclic antidepressants
Ethchlorvynol
Paracetamal
Phenytoin

*These drugs are listed because of their frequent involvement in overdoses and because of the possible complications of such diuresis coupled with its ineffectiveness, the procedure should be avoided.

with use of castor oil, it should rarely, if ever, be used.

Forced Diuresis. Forced diuresis can be useful when the drug or active metabolites of the drug are excreted in the urine and when diuresis increases such excretion. Because diuresis will reduce reabsorption, drugs which are not resorbed will not have hastening of elimination with diuresis. Thus, it is important to recognize that merely increasing urine flow may have no effect at all in speeding excretion. Table 6 indicates some common drugs which are not excreted in increased amounts with increased urine flow (Prescott, 1975).

On the other hand, increased flow will speed excretion of a substance such as phenobarbital.

Forced diuresis is not a benign procedure and dangers or complications that may occur include (1) pulmonary edema, (2) electrolyte and acid-base disturbance, (3) water intoxication, and (4) cerebral edema. Whenever forced diuresis is performed, the patient's renal status must first be known as well as acid-base balance, electrolytes, and cardiopulmonary status. Weight changes should be closely monitored. Precautions are of particular importance in an older population.

The use of forced diuresis (generally mannitol-induced, but a diuretic such as furosemide can be used) remains of limited benefit. Beckett (1974) points out that at most the rate of elimination can only be increased twofold. Of more utility is diuresis coupled with pH control. For example, amphetamine, quinine, and other basic drugs will be more rapidly excreted in a more acid urine because of increased ionization. On the other hand, phenobarbital excretion by renal means can be increased as much as sevenfold with forced alkaline diuresis (Prescott, 1975). Forced alkaline diuresis is also effective in salicylate and butabarbital overdose. Alkaline diuresis is usually accomplished with bicarbonate, 1–2 mEq./kg. given I.V. Potassium depletion is a danger and must be monitored. Acid diuresis can be well accomplished with ascorbic acid given orally or I.V. (500 mg. to 2 gm.). The urine pH should be about 5.

USE OF HEMODIALYSIS

According to Prescott (1975), "Poisoned patients are often subjected to unnecessary and potentially harmful hemodialysis and forced diuresis." Experience from a large poison treatment center clearly shows that the great majority of patients recover with supportive therapy and good nursing care (Matthew and Lawson, 1970). Prescott calls for a minimum of "meddlesome medical interference." As technologic advances provide simpler hemodialysis units they will become available for use in emergency departments to a vastly greater extent. It is therefore of importance to understand some of the physicochemical and pharmacologic principles involved in hemodialysis of an ingested drug.

Firstly, the basic principle underlying hemodialysis is that blood containing circulating drugs or metabolites of those drugs will be cleared of the poisonous chemicals through their passage via a semipermeable membrane into fluid containing none of the drug. Thus, effective dialysis requires a plasma concentration of the drug high enough to ensure that enough is removed to favorably influence the clinical course. If the poison has wide distribution in the body and toxic effects are related to tissue concentration, then the amount in plasma would tend to be only a small fraction of the total, and lowering of plasma level might have no significance. Even if the substance is highly dialyzable, supportive treatment would be indicated in the type of situation cited. For example, after distribution of the drug haloperidol, the plasma contains only 0.25 per cent of the total amount of drug in the body (Prescott, 1975). On the other hand, if the drug is being actively absorbed from the small intestine and distribution has not occurred, dialysis during this period of time might be of much greater value. The next factor of importance is the molecular weight of the drug (which is generally assumed to bear directly on molecular size). Clearance through a dialysis membrane is directly proportional to the blood concentration and is related to the molecular weight. In fact, the relationship between molecular weight and clearance is such that doubling the molecular weight reduces clearance by greater than twofold. As the molecular weight approaches 350, and using the currently available membranes, the rate of drug permeation is reduced to such a low level that dialysis is unlikely to make any significant difference (Schreiner and Teehan, 1972). Also, if the drugs are of low molecular weight but are bound to a carrier (e.g., plasma protein), dialysis efficacy is markedly reduced.

The use of hemodialysis is another area of substantial controversy in poison management. While Prescott (1975) is negative in his views toward hemodialysis, other investigators (e.g., Schreiner and Teehan, 1972) advise its use in many more instances. The diverging opinions probably reflect the lack of large-scale, controlled studies, which are very difficult to perform in the clinical practice of medicine, particularly for those advocates of dialysis who face an ethical problem if they withhold the very procedure they believe will help the patient.

The following principles regarding hemodialysis in the management of poisonings are those generally acceptable at the current time:

General guidelines for hemodialysis in management of poisonings:

1. Dialysis should be considered when the drug is largely confined to the blood and is dialyzable. For example, some common agents in which dialysis has been employed include salicylates, phenylbutazone, phenobarbital, sulfonamides, sulfonylureas, methanol, and ethylene glycol.

2. Dialysis is of no use with irreversibly acting drugs once they have entered the body (e.g., cyanide, organophosphate cholinesterase inhibitors).

3. Dialysis should not be used if effective pharmacologic or biochemical antagonists are available (for example, Narcan for narcotics).

4. Dialysis is of increasingly limited value as the molecular weight of the chemical substance approaches 350. This is due to the slowness of dialysis through available membranes.

5. Hemodialysis should be considered only when the amount ingested is dangerous to life and when the speed of elimination via hemodialysis is substantially greater than elimination through usual metabolic and excretory pathways.

6. Hemodialysis may be of value in severely intoxicated patients who have impairment of the usual routes of elimination (for example, renal impairment, liver disease, or cardiac disease resulting in impaired excretion).

7. Hemodialysis should be used only when the dangers have been assessed and benefits outweigh the dangers. The major dangers include hemorrhage, air embolism, infection, electrolyte abnormality, and circulatory overload.

Peritoneal dialysis may be employed when hemodialysis is not available. Although generally less desirable, peritoneal dialysis and exchange transfusion may be more useful in small children. The newest innovation is a charcoal perfusion device. Further testing is needed to clearly define its use.

ROLE OF THE CLINICAL LABORATORY IN ACUTE POISONING

The current role of the clinical laboratory in the medical management of acute poisoning is primarily that of providing data on electrolytes, acid-base status, blood gas and respiratory status, and organ function tests (tests of liver and kidney function, tests of the hematologic system, and generally nonspecific tests).

While determination of salicylate level, barbiturate level, carboxyhemoglobin, alcohol, iron, lead, and digoxin are often performed in hospital laboratories, the delays often render the results of little use for the immediate treatment. Qualitative testing can be helpful when the agent causing the poisoning is unknown, but this is currently unavailable except in advanced poison treatment centers. For example, Widdop (1975) describes a capability at his poison unit in England of rapidly measuring at least 25 drugs through use of chromatography, spectrophotofluorometry, and other techniques. Such laboratory capability is extremely rare in the United States.

Although at present specific testing, either qualitative or quantitative, is rudimentary (even at advanced centers), projection of technologic advances in this area is reasonable. Table 7, prepared by Done (1975), lists the therapeutic, toxic, and lethal levels of well over 100 drugs. As techniques of

TABLE 7   *Compendium of Therapeutic, Toxic, and Lethal Blood Levels of Pharmacologic Agents*

The significance of a blood level

Compound	Therapeutic or normal	Toxic	Lethal
Acetaminophen	3 mg.%	4 hr.: 12 mg.% 12 hr.: 5 mg.% or half-life in serum > 4 hr.	30 mg.% 12 mg.%
Acetazolamide	1-1.5 mg.%	—	—
Acetohexamide	2.1-5.6 mg.%	—	—
Acetone	—	20-30 mg.%	55 mg.%
Acetylsalicylic acid	see Salicylate		
Aluminum	0.03 mg.%	—	—
Aminophylline	1-2 mg.%	2-4 mg.%	—
Amitriptyline	8-20 μg.%	40 μg.%	0.5-2.0 mg.%
Ammonia	50-170 μg.%	—	—
Amphetamine	2-3 μg.%	> 10 μg.%	0.05-0.2 mg.%*
Arsenic	7 μg.%	0.1 mg.%	0.1-1.5 mg.%
Aspirin	see Salicylate		
Aventyl	see Nortriptyline		
Barbiturates			
short-acting	0.2-0.4 mg.%	0.7 mg.%	1-3 mg.%†
intermediate	0.1-0.5 mg.%	1-3 mg.%	3-5 mg.%†
phenobarbital	1-2.5 mg.%	4-6 mg.%	8-15 mg.%†
barbital	ca. 3 mg.%	6-8 mg.%	10 mg.%
Benadryl	see Diphenhydramine		
Benemid	see Probenecid		
Benzedrex	see Propylhexedrine		
Benzene	—	any measurable amount	.094 mg.%
Boric acid	0.08 mg.%	4 mg.%	5 mg.%
Bromide	5 mg.%	50 mg.%	100-200 mg.%
Brompheniramine	0.8-1.5 μg.%	—	—
Butazolidin	see Phenylbutazone		
Cadmium	—	0.005 mg.%	—
Caffeine	—	0.5 mg.%	10-15 mg.%
Carbamazepine	0.2 mg.%	0.8-1 mg.%	—
Carbon monoxide	7-13% carboxyhemoglobin	25-35%	60%
Carbon tetrachloride	—	2-5 mg.%	—
Carisoprodol	1-4 mg.%	—	—
Celontin	see Methsuximide		
Chloral hydrate	1 mg.%	10 mg.%	10-25 mg.%†
Chlordiazepoxide	0.1-0.3 mg.%	0.55 mg.%	2-3 mg.%
Chloroform	—	7-25 mg.%	39 mg.%
Chloroquine	0.15 mg.%	—	1 mg.%
Chlorpheniramine	—	2-3 mg.%	—
Chlorpromazine	0.05-0.1 mg.%	0.1-0.2 mg.%	0.3-1.2 mg.%
Chlorpropamide	3-14 mg.%	—	—
Chlorprothixene	0.004-0.03 mg.%	—	—
Chlorzoxazone	1-2 mg.%	—	—
Codeine	2.5 μg.%	—	0.2 mg.%
Copper	100-150 μg.%	540 μg.%	—
Compazine	see Prochlorperazine		
Cyanide	0.015 mg.%	—	0.5 mg.%
Darvon	see Propoxyphene		
DDT	1.3 μg.%	—	—
Demerol	see Meperidine		
Desipramine	.059-0.14 mg.%	—	0.3-2 mg.%
Dextropropoxyphene	see Propoxyphene		
Diabinese	see Chlorpropamide		
Diamox	see Acetazolamide		
Diazepam	0.1-0.25 mg.%	0.5-2 mg.%	2 mg.%
Dieldrin	0.15 μg.%	—	—
Digitoxin	1-3 μg.%	—	3 μg.%
Digoxin	0.07-0.2 μg.%	0.2 μg.%	0.4 μg.%
Dilantin	see Diphenylhydantoin		
Dilaudid	see Hydromorphone		
Dimetane	see Brompheniramine		

Note: Very few of these determinations can now be done by hospital laboratories, but with technologic advances in the future, such laboratory results may be available for physicians treating poisoned patients. Knowledge of the blood levels can be currently useful for clinical research.

TABLE 7 *Compendium of Therapeutic, Toxic, and Lethal Blood Levels of Pharmacologic Agents* (Continued)

The significance of a blood level

Compound	Therapeutic or normal	Toxic	Lethal
Dinitro-o-cresol	—	3-4 mg.%	7.5 mg.%
Diphenhydramine	0.1-0.5 mg.%	—	1 mg.%
Diphenylhydantoin	0.5-2.2 mg.%	1-5 mg.%	5-10 mg.%
Divinyl oxide	—	—	70 mg.%
Doriden	see Glutethimide		
Doxepin	—	—	1 mg.%
Dymelor	see Acetohexamide		
Elavil	see Amitriptyline		
Ethanol	50 mg.%	150 mg.%	400 mg.%
Ethchlorvynol	0.2-1.5 mg.%	2 mg.%	10-15 mg.%
Ethinamate	0.5-1 mg.%	—	—
Ethosuximide	2.5-7.5 mg.%	—	—
Ethyl chloride	—	—	40 mg.%
Ethyl ether	90-100 mg.%	—	140-189 mg.%
Ethylene glycol	—	150 mg.%	200-400 mg.%
Flexin	see Zoxazolamine		
Fluoride	0-0.05 mg.%	—	0.2-0.3 mg.%
Fluothane	see Halothane		
Furadantin	see Nitrofurantoin		
Gantrisin	see Sulfisoxazole		
Gold	300-600 μg.%	—	—
Glutethimide	0.02-0.75 mg.%	1-8 mg.%	3-10 mg.%*
Halothane	15 mg.%	—	20 mg.%
Heroin	see Morphine		
Hexachlorophene	—	—	1 mg.%
Hydrogen sulfide	—	—	0.092 mg.%
Hydromorphone	—	—	0.01-0.03 mg.%
Imipramine	0.005-0.016 mg.%	0.06 mg.%	0.2-0.4 mg.%
Inderal	see Propranolol		
Isopropanol	—	—	80 mg.%
Iron (serum)	0.04-0.2 mg.%	0.6 mg.%	1 mg.%
Lactate	10-20 mg.%	—	75 mg.%
Lead	0.005-0.06 mg.%	0.1 mg.%	0.2 mg.%
Librium	see Chlordiazepoxide		
Lidocaine	0.2 mg.%	0.6-1 mg.%	—
Liquiprin	see Acetaminophen		
Lithium	0.42-0.83 mg.%	1.39 mg.%	1.39-3.47 mg.%
LSD	—	0.1-0.4 μg.%	—
Madribon	see Sulfadimethoxine		
Magnesium	1.5-2.5 mEq./liter	—	5 mEq./liter
Manganese	0.015 mg.%	0.46 mg.%	—
Marijuana (as THC)	7 μg.%	—	—
Mellaril	see Thioridazine		
Meperidine	60-65 μg.%	0.2 mg.%	0.5-3 mg.%*
Meprobamate	0.5-1.5 mg.%	—	5-20 mg.%†
Mercury	0.006-0.012 mg.%	—	0.3 mg.%
Methadone	48-86 μg.%	—	0.1-0.4 mg.%
Methamphetamine	—	0.01-0.5 mg.%	0.1-4 mg.%*
Methanol	—	20 mg.%	89 mg.%
Methapyrilene	0.2-0.4 mg.%	3-5 mg.%	5 mg.%
Methaqualone	0.5 mg.%	1-3 mg.%	2-3 mg.%
Methsuximide	0.25-0.75 mg.%	—	—
Methylene chloride	—	—	28 mg.%
Methylene dioxyamphetamine	—	—	0.4-1 mg.%
Methyprylon	1 mg.%	3-6 mg.%	3-10 mg.%
Milontin	see Phensuximide		
Morphine	0.01 mg.%	—	0.05-0.4 mg.%*
Mysoline	see Primidone		
Nebs	see Acetaminophen		
Nickel	0.041 mg.%	—	—
Nicotine	0.03 mg.%	0.5-1 mg.%	0.5-5.2 mg.%
Nitrofurantoin	0.18 mg.%	—	—
Noctec	see Chloral hydrate		
Noludar	see Methyprylon		
Norpramin	see Desipramine		
Nortriptyline	10-16 μg.%	0.5 mg.%	1 mg.%

TABLE 7   Compendium of Therapeutic, Toxic, and Lethal Blood Levels of Pharmacologic Agents (Continued)

The significance of a blood level

Compound	Therapeutic or normal	Toxic	Lethal
Orinase	see Tolbutamide		
Orphenadrine	—	0.2 mg.%	0.4-0.8 mg.%
Oxalate	0.2 mg.%	—	1 mg.%
Papaverine	0.1 mg.%	—	—
Para-methoxyamphetamine	—	—	0.2-0.4 mg.%
Paraldehyde	5-8 mg.%	20-40 mg.%	50 mg.%
Pentazocine	0.05 mg.%	0.2-0.5 mg.%	0.3-2 mg.%*
Perphenazine	—	0.1 mg.%	—
Phencyclidine	—	—	0.1 mg.%
Phenmetrazine	—	—	0.4 mg.%
Phensuximide	1-1.9 mg.%	—	—
Phenylbutazone	5-15 mg.%	—	—
Placidyl	see Ethchlorvynol		
Potassium (serum)	4-6 mEq./liter	6-8 mEq./liter	8 mEq./liter
Primidone	1-2 mg.%	5-8 mg.%	ca. 10 mg.%
Probenecid	10-20 mg.%	—	—
Procainamide	0.6 mg.%	1 mg.%	1.2 mg.%
Prochlorperazine	—	0.1 mg.%	—
Promazine	—	0.1 mg.%	—
Propoxyphene	5-20 µg.%	0.1 mg.%	0.1-3 mg.%†
Propranolol	0.0025-0.02 mg.%	—	0.8-1.2 mg.%
Propylhexedrine	—	—	0.2-0.3 mg.%
Quaalude	see Methaqualone		
Quinidine	0.3-0.6 mg.%	ca. 1 mg.%	3-5 mg.%
Quinine	—	0.2 mg.%	1 mg.%
Rela	see Carisoprodol		
Salicylate	2-10 mg.%	6 hr.‡: 50 mg.%	90-120 mg.%
	30 mg.% for rheumatics	12 hr.‡: 40 mg.%	70-100 mg.%§
		24 hr.‡: 25 mg.%	50-65 mg.%§
		48 hr.‡: 10 mg.%	20-30 mg.%§
Sinequan	see Doxepin		
Sodium	135-145 mEq./liter	160 mEq./liter	200 mEq./liter
Soma	see Carisoprodol		
Sparine	see Promazine		
Strychnine	—	0.2 mg.%	0.9-1.2 mg.%
Sulfadiazine	8-15 mg.%	—	—
Sulfadimethoxine	8-10 mg.%	—	—
Sulfaguanidine	3-5 mg.%	—	—
Sulfanilamide	10-15 mg.%	—	—
Sulfisoxazole	9-10 mg.%	—	—
Talwin	see Pentazocine		
Taractan	see Chlorprothixene		
Tegretol	see Carbamazepine		
Theophylline	1-2 mg.%	2-4 mg.%	—
Thiocyanate	—	—	20 mg.%
Thioridazine	0.10-0.20 mg.%	—	0.5-2 mg.%
Thorazine	see Chlorpromazine		
Tigan	see Trimethobenzamide		
Tin	0.012 mg.%	—	—
Tofranil	see Imipramine		
Tolbutamide	5.3-9.6 mg.%	—	—
Toluene	—	—	1 mg.%
Tribromoethanol	—	—	9 mg.%
Trichloroethane	—	—	10-100 mg.%
Trilafon	see Perphenazine		
Trimethobenzamide	0.1-0.2 mg.%	—	—
Tylenol	see Acetaminophen		
Uric acid	3-7 mg.%	—	20 mg.%
Valium	see Diazepam		
Valmid	see Ethinamate		
Warfarin	0.1-1 mg.%	—	—
Xylocaine	see Lidocaine		
Zarontin	see Ethosuximide		
Zinc	68-136 µg.%	—	—
Zoxazolamine	0.3-1.3 mg.%	—	—

*Higher level is for tolerant users. †Lower level applies in presence of alcohol. ‡After single acute ingestion only. §Lower figure indicates severe poisoning and death is possible; higher figure almost certain lethality.

measurement improve, more of such specific tests will be performed, allowing better correlations of clinical state with serum level dynamics.

FOOD POISONING

Food poisonings occur most commonly when previously prepared food contaminated by bacteria is allowed to remain without refrigeration for several hours. These poisons are usually staphylococcal in origin. Improperly canned food in sealed containers can allow growth of anaerobic organisms.

Poisoning Caused by Bacterial Enterotoxins

The enterotoxins are produced by bacteria growing in the food, most commonly *Staphylococcus aureus*, but also *Clostridium perfringens*, *Bacillus cereus*, and *Vibrio parahemolyticus*. *Clostridium botulinum* is a rare but deadly cause, and disease is caused by its exotoxin.

CLINICAL PRESENTATION

Staphylococcal Food Poisoning. Generally symptoms begin within six hours and are heralded by violent vomiting and abdominal cramps. The onset is usually sudden. History is extremely important in diagnosis. The usual absence of diarrhea is a helpful differential point. Characteristically associated with creamy foods and casseroles, the vomiting may lead to rapid dehydration and electrolyte imbalance.

Other Bacterial Food Poisoning Symptoms appear within 6 to 24 hours and consist of profuse diarrhea, tenesmus and lower abdominal cramps. Vomiting is not usually a prominent symptom. This presentation is characteristic of *Clostridium perfringens* food poisoning.

TREATMENT

Treatment is supportive, with I.V. solutions, antinauseants, and anticholinergics. Initially the patient should have nothing by mouth (npo) and progress to clear liquids.

Botulism

CLINICAL PRESENTATION

Patients will usually present 12 to 48 hours after ingestion, although longer delays have been reported. The symptoms are to some extent dependent on type of toxin, of which three account for almost all cases: type A, B, or E.

Improperly canned food accounts for the main problem, as it allows an anaerobic environment in which the organism can grow.

While abdominal symptoms, nausea and vomiting are usually considered to be associated with botulism, they are not found in more than half of those persons with type A and B poisoning, whereas intestinal symptoms are the rule in type E poisoning. Weakness and malaise are nonspecific but common findings. The best clues to diagnosis come from the neurologic findings, which include vertigo, failure of accommodation, blurred vision, difficulty with speaking or swallowing, and progressive paralysis. The most dangerous development is paralysis of the respiratory muscles. As a rule, patients, despite their neurologic symptoms, remain alert and oriented. Fever is rare. Botulinum toxin type A causes interference with neuromuscular transmission leading to respiratory paralysis.

TREATMENT

1. Maintain vital signs, particularly respiration. A tracheostomy and ventilator may be needed. I.V. feeding is necessary.

Since botulism is so rare, it is important to have a high index of suspicion when patients present with vague neurologic symptoms of a widespread nature without any apparent cause.

2. Get antitoxin (call CDC 404-633-3311, day; or 404-633-2176, night). (Equine antitoxin can be given with steroids to reduce allergic response.)

3. Eliminate unabsorbed toxin with gastric lavage and cleansing enemas.

4. Guanidine (still experimental but has shown promise) must be given, 15 to 50 mg./kg. B.W. per day, in four or six divided doses, through a nasogastric tube. Excess dosage causes tremors and muscle twitches.

Common "Food" Poisoning Caused by Organisms

"Traveler's diarrhea": This common condition is a syndrome of acute watery diarrhea resulting from infection by an enteropathogen (usually enterotoxigenic *E. coli*). The condition is often acquired while traveling through developing countries. Prophylactic treatment with antibiotics will decrease attack rates with doxycycline (100 mg. daily) appearing to be the most effective protective agent.

Salmonella: Diarrhea 8 to 24 hours after ingestion. Nausea and vomiting present but less prominent. Severe chills and fever occur. Treatment is symptomatic. There is no evidence that antibiotics are of benefit as long as the condition is gastroenteritis and not an enteric fever with salmonella bacteremia.

Shigella (Shigellosis): Symptoms may begin within hours or after weeks. Generally, diarrhea is predominant, with mucus, bloody feces, and severe cramps. Abdominal tenderness and fever are common. There is controversy regarding efficacy of antibiotic treatment. Ampicillin is often used in such cases unless culture reports suggest another antibiotic.

Amebic colitis demands antimicrobial therapy, usually metronidazole, followed in 1 week by diiodohydroxyquin (to eradicate cysts).

Food Poisonings Caused by Chemicals Naturally Present

INTRODUCTION

As has been previously discussed, the difference between what is therapeutic and what is toxic may just be a question of dosage. Foods are composed of many chemical substances that are essential for life, such as carbohydrates, proteins, minerals, and vitamins. However, many foods contain chemical substances that are part of their nature but do not appear to be involved in nutritional processes. In many cases, the chemicals exert modest effects, and even ingestion of large quantities will not exert apparent toxic effects. For example, lettuce contains the chemical lactucin, which exerts sedative effects when it is concentrated. Another example is spinach, which has a high oxalic acid content; but even with larger ingestions, which might produce feelings of malaise and bloating, a spinach overdose would only rarely present as a clinical problem. On the other hand, there are common foods that can cause severe poisoning because of their being underripe, or because too much has been taken, or because the patient has been taking a pharmacologic agent that interacts in some way with a chemical or chemicals in a food. For example, the "vomiting sickness" of Jamaica has been traced to eating the unripe akee fruit.

The toxic substance has been termed "hypoglycin" because it acts to rapidly lower blood sugar.

The common potato plant ordinarily has leaves that contain belladonna-type actions. When some potatoes are unripe, belladonna poisoning can occur. In fact, deaths have been linked to eating potatoes.

Alcohol is an example of toxicity of a common food in which overdosage may be lethal. However, there are many more. Severe toxicity with sympathomimetic effects can come from overdose of nutmeg due to the content of myristin, and a prized fish of Japan called "fugu" contains a toxin that exerts cholinergic effects. Overdose can cause cholinergic poisoning.

As an example of food-drug interactions, the presence of tyramine in aged cheese, pickled herring, chianti wine, and some other aged foods can cause hypertensive crises in patients who are taking monoamine oxidase inhibitors for treatment of depression.

MUSHROOM POISONING

While the *Psilocybe* mushroom has gained notoriety, poisoning from ingestion of these mushrooms can induce severe vomiting, abdominal cramps, and marked hallucinations but is relatively benign due to a large tolerance of the body to psilocybin. The mushroom *Amanita muscaria* has also been eaten for its hallucinatory effects, and the vikings were said to have consumed them prior to going into battle because of the rage-like reaction induced. With overdose, muscarine causes parasympathomimetic symptoms that occur usually within one half hour after ingestion and cause profuse salivation, lacrimation, bradycardia, and other cholinergic responses. Treatment involves atropine, which can be given at a dosage of 0.5 to 1.0 mg. I.M. or I.V. (when symptoms warrant). This dosage can be repeated every 30 minutes.

The most severe mushroom poisoning comes from those containing peptide toxins (phallotoxins or amatoxins). These can be deadly at low doses. Symptoms may be delayed from several hours to as long as 24 hours after ingestion. Severe abdominal pain, diarrhea, and vomiting are present. Amatoxins cause liver, brain, and renal tubule cell injury, which may lead to death. Early treatment consists of the following:

1. Supportive treatment, with monitoring of vital signs and urine output. Renal

TABLE 8   Other Food Poisonings and Their Treatment°

NAME	FOOD INVOLVED	SYMPTOMS/SIGNS	TREATMENT
Favism	Fava bean	Glucose-6-phosphate dehydrogenase deficiency (inherited) produces hemolysis, severe anemia	*Supportive:* monitor urinary output, transfusions as needed
Fish poisoning (ichthyosarcotoxism)	Ciquatera (sea bass snapper, barracuda)	For unknown reasons fish usually good as food contain a toxin that causes weakness, paresthesia, GI symptoms, and in fatal cases, respiratory paralysis	Gastric lavage, respiratory support as needed
	Puffer fish	Far Eastern locality contains a neurotoxin that can cause paralysis	
	Tuna, mackeral	Bacteria act on histidine in flesh producing a toxin with GI symptoms; headache and allergic manifestation	
Shellfish poisoning	Mussels and clams usually along Pacific coast— June to October	Paresthesias, neurologic symptoms, respiratory paralysis	Supportive, particular attention to respiratory function
Ergotism	Grain with ergot fungus	Hypertension, vasoconstriction, CNS symptoms	Vasodilatation by amyl nitrate inhalation or papaverine infusion
Chinese restaurant syndrome	Monosodium glutamate	Flushing, diaphoresis, weakness, headaches, pruritus	No specific treatment
Diascorism	Toxic yam with diascorine	Convulsions, deaths have occurred	Anticonvulsants
Cyanide poisoning	Pits from apricots, cherries, cassava, unripe millet, bitter almonds	Metabolic poisoning, loss of consciousness, cyanosis, convulsions	Amyl nitrate, oxygen
Hemagglutination	Castor bean, partially cooked bean flakes, kidney bean flour, legume seeds	Nausea, vomiting, respiratory impairment, anemia; deaths reported from castor beans	No specific treatment
Cycad poisoning	Cycad starch and leaves (eaten in Philippines, Malay)	Neurologic symptoms, weakness, paresthesias	No specific treatment
Lathyrism	Some beans, peas	Muscular weakness, partial paralysis, spinal cord impairments	No specific treatment

°Of the food poisonings listed the fish and shellfish contain poisons generally not present in a dangerous amount (the puffer fish is an exception). Ergotism is due to a fungus contaminant. On the other hand, yam poisoning, cyanide poisoning, hemagglutination reaction, cycad poisoning, lathyrism, and favism result from chemicals that are natural constituents of the foods.

TABLE 9 *Poisonous Plants and Their Chemical Actions in the Body*

PLANT	CHEMICAL ACTIONS
Jimson weed Larkspur Tomato and potato leaves	Atropine-like actions

Morning glory
    seeds
	LSD (lysergic acid
	    diethylamide)

Crocus	Colchicine-like effects
Foxglove Nightshade Lily-of-the-valley Christmas rose	Cardiac glycosides (digitalis-like)
Mistletoe	Sympathomimetic amines
Poinsettia	Parasympathomimetic (cholinergic effects)
Hemlock	Strychnine-like
Mountain laurel	Curare-like
May apple Wisteria	Irritating resin-like podophyllin

failure may occur. Urine output must remain high. Early diuresis may be necessary.

2. Large doses of steroids have been used empirically.

3. Hemodialysis or peritoneal dialysis to be used early, where available, because of the small molecular size of the peptide toxins. This may have substantial benefit if used early.

4. Penicillin, chloramphenicol, and sulfamethoxazole have been used in animals to decrease binding of the toxin to albumin. This might aid if dialysis is used subsequently.

If severe poisoning has occurred, all the above measures should be instituted as early as possible.

MISCELLANEOUS FOOD POISONS

Table 8 summarizes some other food poisonings and their treatment.

PLANT POISONINGS

The number of plants that can exert toxic actions is vast. For purposes of emergency treatment it is useful to identify the major type of chemical actions caused by the poisoning. Table 9 identifies common plants and their chemical actions.

Bibliography

American Academy of Pediatrics: Handbook of Common Poisonings in Children. Department of Health, Education, and Welfare, Publication FDA 76-7004, 1976.

Arena, J.: Poisoning. J.A.M.A. 232:1272, 1975.

Arena, J.: Treatment of Poisoning. Springfield, Ill., Charles C Thomas, Publisher, 1976.

Beckett, R.: Comments on article by Prescott, L.F.: Limitations of hemodialysis and enforced diuresis. *In* The Ciba Foundation: The Poisoned Patient: The Role of the Laboratory. New York, Excerpta Medica, 1974.

Casarett, L., and Doull, J.: Toxicology. New York, Macmillan, 1975.

Chin, L., Picchioni, A. L., and Duplisse, B. R.: The action of activated charcoal on poisons in the digestive tract. Toxicol. Appl. Pharmacol. 16:799, 1970.

Decker, W. J., et al.: Inhibition of aspirin absorption by activated charcoal. Clin. Pharm. Ther. 10:710, 1969.

Der Marderosion, A.: Poisonous plants in and around the house. Am. J. Pharm. Ed. 30:1, 1966.

Done, A.K.: The toxic emergency. Emerg. Med. 7:242–251, Oct. 1975.

Gleason, M. N., and Gosselin, R. E.: Clinical Toxicology of Commercial Products. Baltimore, The Williams & Wilkins Co., 1969.

Levy, G., and Tsuchiya, T.: Effect of activated charcoal on aspirin absorption. Pharmacology 11:292, 1969.

Matthew, H., and Lawson, A.: Treatment of Some Acute Poisonings. Edinburgh, Churchill-Livingstone, 1970.

Prescott, L.F.: Limitations of hemodialysis and forced diuresis in the poisoned patient. *In* The Ciba Foundation: The Poisoned Patient: The Role of the Laboratory. New York, Excerpta Medica, 1974.

Schreiner, G. E., and Teehan, B. P.: Dialysis of poisons and drugs. Trans. Am. Soc. Artif. Organs 18:563, 1972.

Smith, T. W.: Reversal of digoxin intoxication with digoxin-specific antibodies. N. Engl. J. Med. 294: 797, 1976.

Thienes, C. H., and Haley, T. J.: Clinical Toxicology. Philadelphia, Lea & Febiger, 1972.

Widdop, B.: Drug analysis in the overdosed patient. *In* The Ciba Foundation: The Poisoned Patient: The Role of the Laboratory. New York, Excerpta Medica, 1974.

B. MANAGEMENT OF SPECIFIC POISONINGS*

Jay Arena

1. Acetaldehyde
See Metaldehyde.

1a. Acetaminophen
This compound (half-life, 1 to 2 hr.) does not produce the GI hemorrhagic or acid-base disturbance of aspirin but has a more subtle form of hepatic toxicity which can be serious. Treatment is symptomatic and supportive. Oral methionine (Pedameth), 2.5 gm. every 4 hr. up to 10 gm., has recently been found effective in reducing the frequency and severity of acetaminophen-induced liver damage. (This use of methionine is not listed in the manufacturer's official directive.) Although this compound has few side effects and is of low toxicity, it has the potential to aggravate pre-existing hepatic disease, and thus should only be given early (before 12 hr.) after ingestion, before the likely acetaminophen hepatic effects take place. N-acetylcysteine (Mucomyst) appears to act as a glutathione substitute and to directly combine with the toxic acetaminophen metabolite. It is presently being recommended as the oral drug of choice (loading dose of 140 mg. per kg., followed by 70 mg. per kg. every 4 hr., for a total of 18 doses), if given within 12 hrs. after ingestion. (This use of N-acetylcysteine is not listed in the manufacturer's official directive.)

2. Acetanilid
Gastric lavage or emesis. Saline cathartic. Methylene blue for methemoglobinemia. Discontinue drugs in chronic poisoning or idiosyncrasies.

3. Acetic Acid (Glacial)
Magnesium oxide. Demulcents. For inhalation, treat pulmonary edema. Shock therapy.

4. Acetone
Gastric lavage or emesis. Analeptics and respiratory stimulants if necessary. Artificial respiration and oxygen.

5. Acetylsalicylic Acid (Aspirin)
See Salicylates.

6. Alkalis
Give milk and force water, followed by diluted vinegar or fruit juices by mouth. Do not use strong acids. Demulcents. Cortico-steroids to prevent stricture. Esophageal dilatation after fourth day. Broad-spectrum antibiotics.

7. Aminophylline See Xanthines.

8. Ammonia (Ammonium Hydroxide)
See Alkalis. Do not dilute with water, because heat may be generated.

9. Amphetamine
Gastric lavage or emesis. Activated charcoal. Sedation or short-acting barbiturates with caution. Chlorpromazine (Thorazine), 1 to 2 mg. per kg. intramuscularly and repeat if necessary, is treatment of choice.

10. Amyl Acetate (Banana Oil, Pear Oil)
See Acetone.

11. Aniline and Derivatives (Dimethylaniline, Nitroaniline, Toluidine)
Gastric lavage or emesis. Artificial respiration and oxygen. For skin contact, thorough cleansing. Methylene blue for methemoglobinemia.

12. Antihistaminics
Gastric lavage or emesis. Activated charcoal. Saline cathartic. Do not use stimulants. Levarterenol for hypotension. Short-acting barbiturates with caution.

13. Antimony
Gastric lavage with 1 per cent sodium bicarbonate solution. Demulcents. BAL. Maintain fluid and electrolyte balance.

14. Antipyrine (Phenazone)
See Acetanilid.

15. ANTU (Alphanaphthylthiourea)
Gastric lavage or emesis. Saline cathartic. Oxygen. Avoid oils (more readily soluble).

16. Arsenic Trioxide (White Arsenic)
Gastric lavage or emesis. 30 ml. tincture of ferric chloride and 30 gm. of sodium carbonate in 120 ml. of water as antidote in lavage (remove precipitant). BAL. Shock therapy.

17. Arsine Gas
Move from environment. Exchange transfusion. BAL (ineffective). Industrial prevention with education, ventilation, etc.

18. Aspidium (Male Fern) Oleoresin
Gastric lavage or emesis. Activated charcoal. Saline cathartic. Demulcents. Short-acting barbiturates. Artificial respiration and oxygen. Avoid fats and oils.

---

*Modified from Arena: *Poisoning: Toxicology, Symptoms, Treatment*, 4th ed. Springfield, Ill., Charles C Thomas, Publisher; and *Davison's Compleat Pediatrician*, 9th ed., Lea & Febiger.

19. Atropine

Gastric lavage with 4 per cent tannic acid solution or emesis. Pilocarpine or physostigmine for parasympathomimetic effects. Miotic for eyes. Oxygen. Small doses of barbiturates, chloral hydrate, or paraldehyde for delirium or convulsions. Cold packs or alcohol sponging. Indwelling catheter.

20. Barbiturates

Adequate pulmonary ventilation and control of shock are of prime importance; analeptics are considered secondary, if not actually contraindicated.

Immediate gastric lavage with a solution of saline and activated charcoal. Continue lavage with isotonic saline until the return is clear. Use castor oil for instillation and withdrawal to increase solubility of sedatives and dissolve concretions. Ensure clear airway. Respiratory stimulants such as picrotoxin or pentylenetetrazol (Metrazol), administered in subconvulsive doses (therapy equivocal): bemegride (Megimide) and ethamivan (Emivan). Artificial respiration. Administration of 100 per cent oxygen. For circulatory depression and shock caused by depression of vasomotor center, as well as direct action on smooth muscle in blood vessel wall: pressor amines such as levarterenol (which acts directly on vascular smooth muscle). Intravenous hydrocortisone. Blood transfusions. Trendelenburg position. For water loss from skin and lungs, decrease in urine, electrolytes variable: adequate hydration with 5 to 10 per cent glucose in water to facilitate renal elimination of barbiturates. Use of electrolytes based on analysis of plasma. After the vital signs have been stabilized and adequate renal function has been ascertained, urea or Diamox-induced (forced) osmotic diuresis with alkalization of urine has proved to be effective and successful therapy in reducing mortality, severity of intoxication, and duration of treatment and hospital stay, and is now the treatment of choice in most centers. For hypostatic pneumonia resulting from hypotension and hypoventilation: prophylactic antibiotics. For depression of kidney function resulting from hypotension and central antidiuretic action of barbiturates: exchange transfusions (children). Intermittent peritoneal dialysis. Artificial kidney (lipid dialysis). For cerebral edema: mannitol or urea.

21. Barium (Soluble Salts)

Gastric lavage with 3 or 5 per cent solution of either magnesium or sodium sulfate. 10 ml. of 10 per cent sodium sulfate intravenously, repeated in 30 minutes for serious symptoms. Artificial respiration and oxygen. Procainamide for ventricular arrhythmias. Potassium.

22. Benadryl (Diphenhydramine HCl)
See Antihistaminics.

23. Benzene (Benzol)

Gastric lavage or emesis. Artificial respiration and oxygen. Shock therapy. Blood transfusion if necessary. Avoid fats, oils, alcohol, and epinephrine or related drugs (induces ventricular fibrillation).

24. Benzene Hexachloride (BHC)

Gastric lavage or emesis. Wash skin thoroughly. Short-acting barbiturates. Avoid fats, oils, and epinephrine.

25. Benzine (Petroleum Ether, Naphtha)
See Kerosene.

26. Beryllium

Calcium disodium edetate (edathamil). Corticosteroids for chemical pneumonitis. Excision of skin granulomas and ulcers. Prevention with education of berylliumusing workers or operators.

27. Bismuth (Soluble Compounds)

Gastric lavage or emesis. Activated charcoal. Saline cathartic. BAL. Discontinue medication at first sign of toxicity. Methylene blue for methemoglobinemia.

28. Boric Acid (Boracic Acid)

Gastric lavage or emesis. Saline cathartic. Shock and convulsive therapy. Peritoneal dialysis or exchange transfusion.

29. Botulism   See Chapter 38A.

30. Bromides

Discontinue all sources of bromides. 6 to 12 gm. of sodium chloride in divided doses with 4 liters of water daily for 1 to 4 weeks (adult dose). Isotonic salt solution or ammonium chloride IV in more serious cases. Hemodialysis with artificial kidney.

31. Cadmium

Gastric lavage or emesis. Move patient from exposure. Saline cathartic. Calcium disodium edetate (edathamil). BAL contraindicated (BAL and cadmium combination is nephrotoxic). Artificial respiration and oxygen. Antibiotics and corticosteroids for chemical pneumonitis and pulmonary edema.

32. Caffeine   See Xanthines.

33. Camphor

Gastric lavage or emesis. Demulcents.

Short-acting barbiturates. Artificial respiration and oxygen. Shock therapy. Avoid fats, oils, alcohol, and opiates.

34. Cantharidin (Spanish Fly, Russian Fly)

Gastric lavage (cautiously because of corrosive effects) or emesis. Demulcents. Therapy for shock. Short-acting barbiturates. Adequate fluids for diuresis. Avoid morphine because of respiratory depression.

35. Carbon Dioxide

Terminate exposure; move patient to fresh air. Artificial respiration and oxygen. Respiratory and blood pressure stimulants.

36. Carbon Disulfide

Gastric lavage or emesis, if ingested. Move from exposure. Artificial respiration and oxygen. Pulmonary edema and therapy for shock. Short-acting barbiturates. Prevention: maximum allowable concentration (MAC) must be observed at all times. For skin contact, wash thoroughly.

37. Carbon Monoxide

Move patient from exposure immediately. Artificial respiration and oxygen. Administration of 100 per cent oxygen in a pressure chamber, if available. Hypothermia. Blood transfusion or washed red blood cells given early. Chronic carbon monoxide poisoning and therapy are questionable.

38. Carbon Tetrachloride

Gastric lavage or emesis, if ingested. Move from source of exposure. Remove contaminated clothes. Artificial respiration and oxygen. Shock therapy with special emphasis on fluid and electrolytes in face of oliguria or anuria. Avoid fats, oils, alcohol, epinephrine, and related compounds. Prevention: use of less toxic chemicals such as methyl chloroform.

39. Chloral Hydrate

See Barbiturates.

40. Chlorates

Gastric lavage with care, or emesis. Demulcents. Shock therapy. Methylene blue for methemoglobinemia.

41. Chlordane

Gastric lavage or emesis. Short-acting barbiturates. For skin contamination, thorough washing of skin and removal of contaminated clothing. Avoid fats, oils, demulcents, and epinephrine, which should never be used for any halogenated insecticides.

42. Chlorinated Alkalis (Hypochlorites, Chlorine)

Gastric lavage or emesis for large amounts only. Demulcents. Move from exposure; wash skin thoroughly. Antibiotics and corticosteroids for pulmonary edema and pneumonitis from chlorine inhalation. Oral magnesium oxide (paradoxic as it may sound) to prevent formation of irritating hypochlorous acid.

43. Chloroform

Gastric lavage or emesis. Demulcents. Artificial respiration and oxygen. Respiratory and cardiac stimulants. 10 per cent calcium gluconate intravenously (slowly).

44. Chlorothiazide (Diuril)

Discontinue use of drug. Correct fluid and electrolyte imbalance.

45. Chromium (Potassium Salt, Chromic Oxide)

Gastric lavage or emesis. Demulcents. 1 per cent aluminum acetate wet dressings for skin contamination. 10 per cent edetate (edathamil) ointment for skin ulcers. Remove from source of exposure whether it be from inhalation or skin contact.

46. Cocaine

Gastric lavage or emesis. Remove drug from skin or mucous membranes. Short-acting barbiturates. Artificial respiration and oxygen.

47. Codeine

Gastric lavage or emesis. Saline cathartic. Nalorphine (Nalline), levallorphan (Lorfan) or preferably naloxone (Narcan). Artificial respiration and oxygen. Maintain body heat and fluid balance.

48. Colchicine

Gastric lavage or emesis. Saline cathartic. Artificial respiration and oxygen. Shock therapy. Discontinue or reduce dosages of drug at first sign of toxicity.

49. Copper

Gastric lavage or emesis if vomiting has not occurred. Demulcents. Shock therapy. Calcium disodium edetate (edathamil). Penicillamine derivatives.

50. Cosmetics

Deodorants (aluminum salts, titanium dioxide, antibacterial agents); depilatories (soluble sulfides or calcium thioglycolate): gastric lavage or emesis, if large amount ingested. Hair dyes: discontinue use if allergy develops.

51. Curare

Discontinue drug immediately. Endotracheal catheter and use a positive pressure artificial respirator with oxygen until muscle function returns. Neostigmine or edrophonium chloride. Cold packs or alcohol sponging for temperature elevation.

52. Cyanides (Hydrogen, Potassium, Sodium)

Gastric lavage or emesis, if ingested. Artificial respiration and oxygen. Remove contaminated clothing and wash skin thoroughly. Use cyanide poison kit with directions.

53. DDT (Chlorobenzene Insecticide, TDE, DFDT, DMC, Methoxychlor, Neotrane, Ovotran, Dilan, Dimite)

Gastric lavage or emesis. Saline cathartic. Short-acting barbiturates. Artificial respiration and oxygen. Remove contaminated clothing and wash skin thoroughly. Avoid fats, oils, demulcents, epinephrine, and related compounds.

54. Demerol HCl (Meperidine HCl)

See Morphine.

55. Detergents (Anionic and Nonionic Surfactants, Phosphate Salts, Sodium Sulfate and Carbonate, Fatty Acid Amides)

Unless taken in large quantities, no serious toxic symptoms other than gastrointestinal symptoms; at present causing havoc with public water supplies.

56. Diamethazole (Asterol)*

Use as directed only or discontinue use. Should not be used in children under 6 years of age. Short-acting barbiturates.

57. Dichlorohydrin

See Carbon Tetrachloride.

58. Dichlorophenoxyacetic Acid (2,4-D; 2,4,5-T Esters or Salts)

Gastric lavage or emesis. Quinidine sulfate to relieve myotonia and suppress ventricular arrhythmias. Antipyretic for hyperpyrexia.

59. Dieldrin

See Chlordane (Indane Derivatives).

60. Diethyltoluamide (Dimethylphthalate, Indalone)

Gastric lavage or emesis. Demulcents. Short-acting barbiturates.

61. Digitalis (Purple Foxglove) (Digitoxin)

Discontinue use. Gastric lavage or emesis for accidental or suicidal ingestion.

Disodium or dipotassium edetate. Potassium chloride, orally or intravenously, under electrocardiographic observation. Procainamide, quinidine, phenytoin (Dilantin), propranolol hydrochloride, lidocaine, or atropine.

62. Dilantin Sodium

See Diphenylhydantoin Sodium.

63. Dimethyl Sulfate

Move to fresh air; eyes, skin, and mucous membranes should be washed thoroughly with water. Weak alkali wet dressings for skin burns. Antibiotics and corticosteroids for pneumonitis. In contaminated areas deactivate by spraying with water or 5 per cent sodium hydroxide solution.

64. Dinitro-ortho-cresol (Dinitrophenol Derivatives)

Gastric lavage with sodium bicarbonate solution or emesis. For skin contamination wash thoroughly with weak alkaline solution. Oxygen and circulatory stimulants. Reduce temperature with cold packs or alcohol sponging. Maintain fluid and electrolyte balance.

65. Dioxane

See Acetone.

66. Diphenhydramine HCl (Benadryl HCl)

See Antihistaminics.

67. Diphenylhydantoin Sodium (Dilantin Sodium)

Gastric lavage or emesis for ingestion. Discontinue use or reduce dosage.

68. Dithiocarbamate (Ferbam)

Discontinue use of spray. Avoid alcohol.

69. Doriden

See Barbiturates.

70. Emetine (Alkaloid of Ipecac)

Gastric lavage if emesis has not taken place. Maintain fluid and electrolyte balance. Cautious digitalization. Cardiac pacemaker until EKG is normal and pulse is regular.

71. Ephedrine

Gastric lavage or emesis. Activated charcoal. Short-acting barbiturates. Phentolamine (Regitine) early, to block hypertensive effects.

72. Epinephrine (Adrenalin)

See Ephedrine.

73. Ergot Derivatives

Gastric lavage or emesis. Activated charcoal, 1 to 2 tbsp. in water. Saline cathartic.

---

*This product was discontinued in the United States in 1966 but is still available in Europe.

Atropine sulfate for abdominal pain and spasm, 10 per cent solution of calcium gluconate for myalgia, and papaverine HCl or mecholyl as vascular antispasmodic. Short-acting barbiturates and artificial respiration and oxygen, if necessary.

74. Essential (Volatile Oils)
100 ml. of castor oil, then remove by gastric lavage. Saline cathartic. Demulcents. Short-acting barbiturates. Artificial respiration and oxygen. Maintain fluid and electrolyte balance.

75. Ether
Artificial respiration and oxygen. Maintain adequate airway, blood pressure, and body temperature.

76. Ethyl Alcohol (Pure) (Whiskey = 40 to 50 per cent alcohol; wines = 10 to 20 per cent alcohol; beers = 2 to 6 per cent alcohol)
Gastric lavage or emesis. Sodium bicarbonate, 1 tsp. to 1 pt. water, every 1 to 2 hours to prevent acidosis. Intravenous bicarbonate for acidosis. Caffeine and sodium benzoate or strong coffee. Hypertonic glucose or urea for cerebral edema. Intravenous glucose for hypoglycemia. Avoid depressant drugs (barbiturates interfere with enzymatic action of alcohol dehydrogenase) and potent respiratory stimulants.

77. Ethylene Chlorohydrin (Ethylene Dichloride)
Gastric lavage or emesis. Move from exposure. Artificial respiration and oxygen. Thorough washing for skin contact. Epinephrine or levarterenol for maintaining blood pressure.

78. Ethylene Glycol (Diethylene Glycol, Propylene Glycol)
Gastric lavage or emesis. Artificial respiration and oxygen. Ten per cent calcium gluconate intravenously to precipitate metabolic product, oxalic acid and oxalates. Maintain body temperature, fluids, and electrolytes. Short-acting barbiturates. Dialysis. Oral and intravenous ethyl alcohol (see Methyl Alcohol).

79. Ferrous Sulfate (Copperas, Green Vitriol; approximately 20 per cent elemental iron)
Clearance with suction and maintenance of open airways. Control of shock with available intravenous fluids, blood, plasma, and oxygen. Gastric lavage with concentrated solution of sodium bicarbonate, 5 per cent disodium phosphate, or milk until returning fluid is clear. Critically ill patients should receive calcium disodium edetate (edathamil) intravenously; if none given orally, intravenous dose should be 70 to 80 mg. per kg. BW per 24 hours in dextrose or isotonic saline solution in 0.5 to 2 per cent concentration; if used orally (and rate of its absorption through a gut wall damaged by iron is not known), only half the aforementioned dose should be used intravenously, 35 to 40 mg. per kg. BW per 24 hours. Guided by the clinical picture and daily iron levels in serum and, if measurements are available, by the urinary output of calcium disodium edetate (edathamil) and iron, intravenous and/or oral calcium disodium edetate (edathamil) is continued in a total daily dose of no more than 70 to 80 mg. per kg. BW; duration of treatment with this drug should not be, and need not be, longer than 5 days. Deferoxamine (Desferal), a chelating agent, has been demonstrated to be effective in the treatment of acute iron poisoning. Dosage recommended is 5 to 10 gm. by mouth or nasogastric tube and 1 to 2 gm. intravenously (slowly to avoid hypotensive effects) or intramuscularly. Parenteral therapy can be repeated if serum iron levels remain high. Follow-up liver function tests and study of gastrointestinal tract with a radiopaque medium for strictures.

80. Fluorides (Fluorine, Hydrogen Fluoride, Fluorosilicates [insoluble])
Gastric lavage or emesis with lime water (0.15 per cent calcium hydroxide), calcium chloride solution (1 tsp. per 1000 ml. water), or milk. 10 per cent calcium gluconate intravenously or intramuscularly. Demulcents. For inhalation move to fresh air. Artificial respiration and oxygen. Prophylactic antibiotics and corticosteroids for pulmonary irritation and edema. Wash skin immediately and thoroughly with water and apply magnesium oxide paste with 20 per cent glycerin.

81. Fluoroacetate Sodium
Gastric lavage or emesis. Saline cathartic. 10 per cent calcium gluconate or sodium glycerol monoacetate (Monacetin). Short-acting barbiturates. Procainamide for arrhythmia. For skin contact, wash thoroughly.

82. Food Poisoning (Botulism)
Types A and B polyvalent antitoxin (inadequately processed vegetables and

meats) or Type E antitoxin (fish and marine products). Trivalent (A, B, E) antitoxin now available.* Maintain an airway. Parenteral fluids.

83. Formaldehyde (Formalin)
Gastric lavage with 0.1 per cent ammonia or 1 per cent ammonium carbonate solution. Saline cathartic. Combat shock or collapse; levarterenol if necessary.

84. Glutethimide (Doriden)
See Barbiturates.

85. Gold
Discontinue use of parenteral therapy. Dimercaprol (BAL). Antihistaminic therapy. Supportive therapy for renal and hematologic effects.

86. Hydralazine (Apresoline, Phthalazine Derivatives)
Gastric lavage or emesis. Discontinue use or reduce dosage. Maintain blood pressure.

87. Hydrochloric Acid (Muriatic Acid)
Do not use gastric lavage after 1 hour of ingestion. Neutralize acid with magnesium oxide, milk of magnesia, or lime water. Give demulcents. Maintain blood pressure, fluids, and electrolytes. Antibiotics and corticosteroids to prevent infection and strictures. Thorough washing of skin and application of magnesium oxide paste. Gastroscopy for determining corrosive injury to the stomach.

88. Hydroquinone
Gastric lavage or emesis. Saline cathartic. Methylene blue for methemoglobinemia.

89. Hypochlorites (Clorox, etc.)
See Chlorinated Alkalis.

90. Iodine (Iodoform, Iodides)
Give suspension of starch or flour or 1 to 5 per cent solution of sodium thiosulfate. If not available, use milk or egg white. Follow by gastric lavage. Regulate fluids and electrolytes, depending on degree of renal involvement. Epinephrine, diphenhydramine (Benadryl), or hydrocortisone for anaphylactoid reaction.

91. Isoniazid
Prompt gastric lavage or emesis (symptoms appear within 30 minutes). Discontinue drug or reduce dosage. Pyridoxine, 200 to 400 mg. intravenously. Short-acting barbiturates intravenously for convulsions. Parenteral sodium bicarbonate for acidosis. Hemodialysis. Osmotic diuresis (mannitol, urea, furosemide, or ethacrynic acid) hastens excretion.

92. Isopropyl Alcohol (Rubbing Alcohol)
See Ethyl Alcohol.

93. Kerosene (Petroleum Distillates: Benzine, Gasoline, Naphtha, Mineral Seal Oil, etc.)
Prevent aspiration. Gastric lavage or emesis to be avoided. 50 ml. of mineral or vegetable oil by mouth (if not forced). Oxygen and antibiotics. Corticosteroids for pulmonary edema and chemical or lipoid pneumonitis (particularly for mineral seal oil aspiration). Results are equivocal, yet since therapy is short range, it may benefit those with severe pulmonary distress.

94. Lead
Gastric lavage with 1 per cent sodium sulfate solution, followed by saline cathartic for immediate ingestion. Calcium disodium edetate (edathamil) intravenously or intramuscularly for 5 days and repeat if necessary. 4 per cent urea (30 per cent in severe cases) intravenously for encephalopathy with increased intracranial pressure; craniectomy may be necessary. Mannitol and/or adrenal corticosteroids are also used for this purpose and often preferred. 10 per cent solution of calcium gluconate or morphine for severe abdominal pain (colic). Early diagnosis and treatment are paramount in preventing death or serious sequelae in children. BAL combined with calcium disodium edetate (edathamil) therapy is more effective in lead encephalitis than use of edetate (edathamil) alone. Penicillamine (Cuprimine) as an oral chelating agent has recently been reported to be effective and should be used as adjunctive therapy.

95. Mace (Anti-Riot Gas)
See Tear Gases.

96. Manganese
Remove from further exposure. Antibiotics and corticosteroids for pneumonitis. Calcium disodium edetate (edathamil) may be beneficial if given early. Antiparkinsonian

---

*U.S. Communicable Disease Center, Atlanta, Georgia. Telephone number for day coverage is (404) 633-3753 (-4, -5, -6); for nights and weekends, (404) 633-2176.

drugs. Diphenylhydramine (Benadryl), biperiden hydrochloride (Akineton), or methylphenidate hydrochloride (Ritalin).

97. Marijuana
Removal of drug exposure (characteristic "burnt rope" acrid odor on clothes and body). There are no withdrawal symptoms except with extreme cases of habituation.

98. Meperidine HCl (Demerol HCl)
See Morphine.

99. Meprobamate (Equanil, Miltown, etc.)
Gastric lavage or emesis. Saline cathartic. Artificial respiration and oxygen. Maintain blood pressure with methoxamine hydrochloride.

100. Menthol
See Phenol.

101. Mercury Compounds
Gastric lavage immediately with egg white solution or with 5 per cent sodium formaldehyde sulfoxylate; if unavailable, a 2 to 5 per cent solution of sodium bicarbonate may be used. Magnesium sulfate as cathartic (early only). BAL. Penicillamine derivatives (oral antidote). Maintain fluid and electrolyte balance and nutrition. Spironolactone (Aldactone) has prevented renal tubular necrosis in experimental animals (rats).

102. Metaldehyde (Changes to Acetaldehyde)
Gastric lavage or emesis. Demulcents. Short-acting barbiturates. Artificial respiration, oxygen, and antibiotics. Parenteral chlorpromazine and calcium gluconate.

103. Methadone (Dolophine)
See Morphine.

104. Methyl Alcohol
To prevent the formation of formic acid and formates, 10 ml. ethyl alcohol per hour can suppress the metabolism of methyl alcohol. In severe poisoning ethyl alcohol can be given intravenously in 5 per cent concentration in bicarbonate or saline solution and 3 to 4 oz. of whiskey (45 per cent alcohol) orally every 4 to 6 hours for 1 to 3 days. Combat acidosis. Hemodialysis.

105. Methyl Bromide (Chloride, Iodide)
Move from exposure. Artificial respiration and oxygen. Epinephrine for bronchospasm; antibiotics and corticosteroids for pneumonitis. Prevention: safety dispensers for fumigant use.

106. Methyl Salicylate (Oil of Wintergreen)
See Salicylates. Gastric lavage, however, may be worthwhile, even several hours after ingestion, because methyl salicylate is poorly absorbed.

107. Metrazol
See Pentylenetetrazol.

108. Morphine (Codeine, Heroin, Propoxyphene [Darvon], Meperidine [Demerol], Dihydromorphinone [Dilaudid], Opium Alkaloids [Pantopon])
Gastric lavage (before loss of consciousness). Do not use syrup of ipecac or apomorphine. Activated charcoal. Saline cathartic. Delay absorption of intramuscular drug with tourniquet and cryotherapy. Maintain adequate airway, body temperature, fluids, and electrolytes. Give narcotic antagonists Nalline or Lorfan. Naloxone hydrochloride (Narcan) is preferable. Ephedrine for hypotension and bradycardia—methoxamine or phenylephrine if pulse is rapid. Doxapram hydrochloride (Dopram), 3 to 5 ml. intravenously, is the respiratory stimulant of choice, but it has short-lasting effects (3 to 5 minutes).

109. Muscarine (Some Mushrooms)
Artificial respiration with oxygen. Atropine, 1 to 2 mg. every hour until free of respiratory effects. PAM or Protopam chloride may be useful adjunct therapy. Gastric lavage or emesis if vomiting has not occurred.

110. Naphthalene (Mothballs, Repellents, etc., Paradichlorobenzene, Camphor)
Gastric lavage or emesis for ingestion. Give sodium bicarbonate every 4 hours to maintain alkaline urine and prevent renal blockage with acid hematin crystals. Blood transfusions as necessary. Short-acting barbiturates. Avoid use of milk, oils, or fatty foods. In prevention, these products should be kept away from hands and clothes of children (symptoms produced not only by ingestion but also by inhalation and transcutaneous absorption).

111. Naphthol
See Phenol.

112. Nickel (Nickel Carbonyl)
Remove from skin by thorough washing. Artificial respiration and oxygen. BAL. Antibiotics and corticosteroids for pneumonitis.

113. Nicotine
Gastric lavage or emesis. Activated char-

coal. Short-acting barbiturates. Artificial respiration and oxygen; use of positive pressure resuscitator through period of respiratory failure may prevent death. Thorough washing of skin and removal of clothing will be necessary for skin contamination.

114. Nitrates, Nitrites
Gastric lavage or emesis. Saline cathartic. Methylene blue for methemoglobinemia. Maintain blood pressure with levarterenol. Short-acting barbiturates for convulsions.

115. Nitric Acid
Give large amounts of water. Neutralize with lime water, magnesia, etc. Gastric lavage cautiously if seen within the first half hour. Gastroscopy to detect caustic burns of the stomach. Demulcents. Morphine for pain, but avoid large doses and possible depression. Shock therapy. Corticosteroids to prevent stricture formation. For eye and skin contact wash thoroughly with water: *do not use chemical antidotes.*

116. Nitrobenzene
Gastric lavage or emesis. Artificial respiration and oxygen. Methylene blue, 1 per cent solution, for methemoglobinemia. Avoid fats and oils.

117. Opium
See Morphine.

118. Oxalates
Gastric lavage with calcium lactate solution, 10 gm. (2 tsp.) per 100 ml. 10 per cent calcium gluconate intravenously. Give milk and demulcents.

119. Paraldehyde
Gastric lavage or emesis. Artificial respiration and oxygen. Maintain body temperature, fluids, and electrolytes.

120. Parathion (Phosphate Ester Insecticides) (Malathion, Systox, EPN, Diazinon, Guthion, Trithion, TEPP, OMPA, Co-Ral, Phosdrin)
Prompt induction of emesis or gastric lavage with 5 per cent $NaHCO_3$ for ingestion only. Decontaminate by removal of all soiled clothes and thorough washing of skin. Maintain clear airway and respirations with laryngeal intubation and artificial respirations and oxygen. Atropine, 1 to 2 mg. intramuscularly or intravenously and repeat at 20 to 30 minute intervals, as soon as cyanosis has cleared (chance of ventricular fibrillation).

Continue atropine until definite improvement occurs and is maintained (sometimes 2 or more days). The total dosage (required may be phenomenal (over 300 mg.). PAM (pralidoxime chloride), a cholinesterase reactivator as 5 per cent solution intravenously. Avoid narcotics, barbiturates, epinephrine, aminophylline, ether, and phenothiazine derivatives because they further reduce cholinesterase activity and some are respiratory depressants.

121. Pentachlorophenol
Gastric lavage or emesis. Removal of contaminated clothing and thorough washing of skin. Short-acting barbiturates.

122. Pentylenetetrazol (Metrazol)
Delay absorption of intramuscular drug with tourniquet and cryotherapy. Gastric lavage or emesis for ingestion. Short-acting barbiturate for convulsions. Cold packs and alcohol sponging for hyperthermia.

123. Permanganate, Potassium
Thorough lavage of stomach with 3 per cent hydrogen peroxide (10 ml. in 100 ml. of water). Milk or demulcents. Combat collapse and shock.

124. Phenacetin Acetophenetidin)
See Acetanilid.

125. Phenol (Derivatives) (Creosote, Guaiacol, Resorcincol, Thymol)
Careful gastric lavage, followed by 60 ml. of castor oil which dissolves phenol and hastens its removal. Activated charcoal. Maintain body temperature, fluids, electrolytes. For skin and mucous membranes, wash thoroughly and follow by application of castor oil or 10 per cent ethyl alcohol. Short-acting barbiturates for convulsions and antibiotics as prophylaxis in pulmonary edema.

126. Phenolphthalein
Gastric lavage or emesis. Activated charcoal. Castor oil if given early to hasten the drug through the intestinal tract, but no other solvents because they increase laxative action.

127. Phenothiazine Derivatives
Discontinue drug or reduce dosage. In blood dyscrasias or jaundice do not change to another derivative. Gastric lavage for ingestion of large doses. Antiparkinsonian drugs are rarely necessary. Injectable diphenhy-

dramine hydrochloride (Benadryl) is effective in treatment of extrapyramidal symptoms. Biperiden (Akineton) parenterally or orally. Methylphenidate (Ritalin).

128. Phosphoric Acid
See Acetic Acid.

129. Phosphorus (Red [Nonabsorbed, Nontoxic], Yellow [Volatile and Highly Toxic], Phosphine)
Thorough gastric lavage with potassium permanganate (1:5000) or 3 per cent hydrogen peroxide. Copper sulfate, 0.25 gm. in glass of water, forms insoluble copper phosphide. 100 ml. of mineral oil as a solvent (to prevent absorption and hasten elimination) and repeat in 2 hours. Maintain body temperature, fluids, and electrolytes. Give glucose, vitamin K, and 10 per cent calcium gluconate, if indicated. Exposure to phosphine must be terminated at once, and use of contaminated water for drinking or bathing should be forbidden.

130. Physostigmine (Eserine) (Pilocarpine, Neostigmine, Methacholine [Mecholyl], Muscarine)
Gastric lavage or emesis. Maintain artificial respiration until antidote (atropine) can be given. Keep patient fully atropinized (1 to 23 mg. per hour intramuscularly) throughout entire crisis. Maintain airway and remove pulmonary secretion (postural drainage).

131. Picrotoxin
Gastric lavage or emesis. Slow absorption of injected drug by application of cold and/or tourniquet. Short-acting barbiturate. Cold packs or alcohol sponging for hyperthermia.

132. Procaine
See Cocaine. (Procaine is much less toxic.)

133. Pyrethrum (Insect Flowers)
Gastric lavage or emesis unless kerosene is more suspected than pyrethrum. Demulcents. Short-acting barbiturates for convulsions.

134. Pyribenzamine (Tripelennamine)
See Antihistaminics.

135. Quaternary Ammonium Compounds (Cationic Detergents)
Gastric lavage with soapy water, milk or gelatin solution, or emesis. Demulcents or soapy solution. Maintain clear airway; artificial respiration and oxygen. Short-acting barbiturates for convulsions. Atropine recommended without good basis for its use. Avoid alcohol. Thoroughly wash with soap and water for excessive skin contacts.

136. Quinine and Cinchona-like Compounds (Quinidine, Synthetic Hydrocupreine Compounds [Optochin, Numoquin], Plasmochin, Chloroquine [Aralen], Quinacrine [Atabrine])
Gastric lavage or emesis. Discontinue use of drug. Activated charcoal. Levarterenol for hypotension. Artificial respiration and oxygen.

137. Radiation Syndrome
Remove external clothing and wash clothing and entire body with soap and water. Fresh blood or platelet-enriched plasma. Bone marrow replacement. Antibiotics as prophylaxis for infections.

138. Rotenone
Gastric lavage or emesis if vomiting has not already occurred. Wash thoroughly for skin contact. Short-acting barbiturates. Avoid fats and oils.

139. Ryania
See Rotenone.

140. Sabadilla (Cevadilla)
Demulcents. Activated charcoal. Gastric lavage is usually unnecessary because vomiting occurs early.

141. Salicylate
I. Immediate (emesis or gastric lavage)
  A. Evaluation method of severity of intoxication (extrapolation method of Done)
  B. Appraisal of status of dehydration
  C. Determination of acid-base imbalance. Test urine with Phenistix paper and Nitrazene paper.
  D. Determination of electrolyte imbalance
  E. Draw blood for the following laboratory tests:
    1. Salicylate level
    2. CO_2-combining content
    3. Plasma CO_2 content
    4. pH
    5. Serum electrolytes
II. Pending laboratory report
  A. Start intravenous fluids (5 per cent glucose in 1/3 isotonic saline)
  B. If dehydration is severe, hydrating solutions should be given at the rate

of 8 ml. per sq. m. body surface per minute for 30 to 45 minutes.

C. After that time, slow down hydrating solution to 2 ml. per sq. m per minute

D. Correct bicarbonate and potassium deficits as indicated (average requirement: 5 mEq. $NaHCO_3$ per kg. BW and 2 mEq. K per kg. BN for 12 hours)

E. In presence of clinical acidosis and acid urine, $NaHCO_3$ should be given in initial hydrating solution

F. Cool water body sponging for pyrexia

III. In life-threatening intoxication, consider exchange transfusion in small infants, peritoneal dialysis with 5 per cent albumin solution (Albumisol), or dialysis with artificial kidney

IV. Administer vitamin K and B complex, the route of administration depending on the condition of the patient

V. Maintenance management

A. Test each urine voided with Nitrazine paper

B. Periodic (frequent) determination of:

1. Blood CO_2-combining power
2. Blood CO_2 content
3. Blood pH

142. Santonin

Gastric lavage or emesis. Saline cathartic. Short-acting barbiturates. Avoid opiates.

143. Sea Nettle (Portuguese Man-of-War)

The following procedures are recommended: (1) Remove adhering tentacles with the use of gloves, bathing towel, seaweed, gunny sack, dry sand, salt, sugar, or any dry powder. This should be done immediately. (2) Pour alcohol over the wounded areas as soon as possible. Rinse the skin off with salt water after at least 2 minutes have elapsed. Do not rub the wounded area with sand. (3) Apply a corticosteroid-analgesic balm, preferably by aerosol.

144. Selenium

Move from occupational environment. Eliminate from diet. Bromobenzene solution, 0.25 to 1 gm. in lavage.

145. Silver Nitrate

Dilute with isotonic saline solution (0.9 per cent = 1 tsp. salt per 1 pt. water) and thorough lavage of stomach; a relatively insoluble and noncorrosive silver chloride is formed in this reaction. Sodium sulfate cathartic (1 oz. per cup of water). Milk or demulcents. Shock therapy. Meperidine (Demerol) or codeine for pain.

146. Solanine

Gastric lavage or emesis. Activated charcoal. Pilocarpine. Artificial respiration and circulatory stimulants as necessary.

147. Squill (Red, White)

See Digitalis. Gastric lavage or emesis. Demulcents. Quinidine sulfate. Avoid epinephrine or other stimulants.

148. Strychnine

If symptoms have begun, avoid gastric lavage or emesis. Activated charcoal, followed by gastric lavage if asymptomatic. Short-acting barbiturates. Avoid stimuli and opiates. Artificial respiration and oxygen. Muscle relaxants; diazepam (Valium) is particularly effective.

149. Sulfides (Carbon Disulfide, Soluble Sulfides, Hydrogen Sulfide)

Move from exposure. Artificial respiration and oxygen. Remove swallowed poison by gastric lavage or emesis. Wash skin thoroughly for skin contact and use burn therapy. Antibiotics prevent secondary infection.

150. Sulfonamides

Gastric lavage or emesis for overdosage. Discontinue drug. Alkali and large intake of fluid if renal function is normal. Hemodialysis in severe poisoning.

151. Sulfur Dioxide

Move to fresh air. Artificial respiration and oxygen. Antibiotics and corticosteroids for pneumonitis.

152. Sulfuric Acid

See Hydrochloric Acid.

153. Tear Gases

The most frequently used preparations are chloracetophenone, ethylbromoacetate, bromoacetone, bromobenzyl cyanide, and bromomethylethylketone. *Alpha-chloroacetophenone*, even though called a "gas," is actually a fine powder. In commercial blast-dispersion cartridges, it is mixed half and half with silica anhydride, and a standard shotgun primer is used as a propellant. The mixture is an effective lacrimator in concentrations as low as 2 ppm. of air. It can cause extreme irritation and edema of the mucous membranes of the nose and eyes if discharged into the face and temporary blindness may result. *Mace* contains recrystallized 2-chloroacetophenone (0.9 per cent 1,1,1-trichloroethane), solvents and propellants—Freon, kerosene, methylchloroform, 4.0 per cent.

The eyes should be irrigated for 15 minutes with isotonic saline solution of water, followed by an anti-flammatory eye ointment. For clothing and skin contamination the clothes should be removed and a thorough shower taken.

154. Tetrachloroethane
See Carbon Tetrachloride.

155. Thallium
Gastric lavage or emesis. For skin contamination, wash thoroughly. Activated charcoal twice a day, 1 to 2 tbsp., and potassium chloride, 3 to 5 gm. daily for 5 to 7 days. BAL. Dithizon (no preparations marketed for therapeutic use), 10 mg. per kg. BW twice a day for 5 days. Maintain body temperature, blood pressure, fluids, and electrolytes. Antibiotics for pneumonitis. Artane for tremors and ataxia.

156. Thiocyanates
Inorganic: Gastric lavage or emesis. Saline cathartic. Give 2 to 4 liters of fluid daily if renal function is normal. Hemodialysis or peritoneal dialysis, if necessary.

Organic (lauryl, ethyl, and methyl thiocyanate, lethane 60): See Cyanides.

157. Thiourea
Discontinue use of drug. Antibiotics and corticosteroids for bone marrow depression.

158. Thiram (Tetramethylthiuram Disulfide)
Gastric lavage or emesis. Wash thoroughly for skin contact and remove contaminated clothing. Avoid fats, oils, lipid solvents, and especially alcohol. Artificial respiration and oxygen.

159. Toxaphene
See DDT.

160. Trichloroethylene
See Carbon Tetrachloride.

161. Tricyclic (Dibenzazepine) Compounds
Treatment of intoxication from tricyclic antidepressant tranquilizers is supportive and symptomatic, with particular attention to the correction of cardiac arrhythmias and maintenance of blood pressure and respiration. Vital signs should be monitored continuously. EKG monitoring is advisable, and severely intoxicated cases should be treated in an intensive care unit. Cardiac arrhythmias

may progress to cardiac arrest owing to ventricular fibrillation or asystole. Death may occur rapidly after a sudden drop of blood pressure and pulse rate. The use of defibrillators and internal or external pacemakers has been advocated. However, in one nonfatal case, an external DC defibrillator produced no alleviation of arrhythmias, and in a fatal case an external pacemaker was tried unsuccessfully. Although documentation is limited, some arrhythmias were controlled in individual patients by use of the parasympathomimetic drugs; physostigmine, drug of choice (readily crosses the blood-brain barrier, 1 mg. intravenously); pyridostigmine (Mestinon) and neostigmine (Prostigmin) or by the beta-adrenergic blocking agent, propranolol (Inderal). Since it is not possible to predict which patient will respond, it may be necessary to try more than one antiarrhythmic drug. Intravenous sodium diphenylhydantoin has had dramatic antiarrhythmic properties and may also be of value in preventing convulsions which occur frequently. Congestive heart failure is treated by digitalization. However, rapid digitalization should be avoided in a situation in which multiple ventricular ectopic beats are likely to occur. The administration of sodium bicarbonate and potassium may aid in treating the cardiovascular effect.* Convulsions may cause a dangerous increase in the cardiac workload. Agitation, tremors, and convulsions have been successfully treated with parenteral barbiturates. However, use of barbiturates is questionable if drugs that inhibit monoamine oxidase have also been taken by the patient in overdosage or in recent therapy. Also, barbiturates may increase respiratory depression, particularly in children. It is advisable to have equipment available for artificial ventilation and resuscitation. Diazepam (Valium) has been used as an alternative to barbiturates for controlling convulsions, and is considered the drug of choice by some. Hypotension and shock may be treated by intravenous fluids of glucose, saline solution, or plasma, and cautious administration of vasopressor agents such as levarterenol (*l*-norepinephine; Levophed), phenylephrine, or metaraminol which will increase blood pressure without increasing heart rate. Any of these sympathomimetic drugs may induce cardiac arrhythmias and must therefore be

---

*In one series sodium bicarbonate was the most clinically effective method of treatment of arrhythmias in children; experimental studies support this view.

used with caution. Other sympathomimetic drugs such as epinephrine and isoproterenol which stimulate the beta receptor sites of the heart should be avoided, because they cause additional increases in the heart rate and may lead to fatal ventricular fibrillation. Respiration must be maintained. Intratracheal artificial respiration is effective and the need for it should be anticipated. Patients should be observed for possible recurrence of respiratory distress following resumption of spontaneous breathing. Various methods have been attempted to hasten excretion of these drugs. They are absorbed quickly from the gastrointestinal tract and are largely bound to plasma proteins. In addition, they are rapidly accumulated in the body tissues, so that high serum concentrations do not occur. They are exreted in the urine largely as glucuronides of the demethylated and hydroxylated metabolites. They are also reportedly secreted into the stomach after absorption. Beneficial effects have been reported from use of exchange transfusion, repeated gastric lavage, and osmotic diuresis. Although evidence is equivocal as to the effectiveness of osmotic diuresis in removing significant amounts of these drugs, it is the general belief that diuresis is beneficial. Osmotic diuresis with mannitol has been employed in the treatment of a number of cases of intoxication with tricyclic antidepressant drugs. In one adult, only 5 per cent of the ingested dose of amitriptyline was recovered in the urine (as amitriptyline and its principal metabolites) after a 10 hour period of forced diuresis with mannitol. Since these drugs also promote urinary retention, catheterization should be considered if diuresis is attempted. Care must also be used to prevent overhydration leading to increased cardiac workload. Continuous or repeated gastric lavage has also been recommended to speed excretion. Although continuous gastric lavage was effectively employed in a child intoxicated with imipramine who exhibited coma, convulsions, and cardiac disturbances, it may be unwise to attempt during convulsive stages. Hemodialysis and peritoneal dialysis are not effective in removing significant amounts of these drugs.

162. Tridione (Trimethadione)
Gastric lavage or emesis. Saline cathartic. Methylene blue for methemoglobinemia. Remove contaminated clothing and wash skin thoroughly. Short-acting barbiturates.

163. Trinitrotoluene (TNT)
Gastric lavage or emesis. Saline cathar-

tic. Methylene blue for methemoglobinemia. Remove contaminated clothing and wash skin thoroughly. Short-acting barbiturates.

164. Tri-ortho-cresyl Phosphate ("Machine Oil")
Gastric lavage or emesis. Treat as for paralysis poliomyelitis with hydrotherapy, massage, and orthopedic care. Respirators or rocking bed until sufficient recovery occurs.

165. Tripelennamine (Pyribenzamine)
See Antihistaminics.

166. Turpentine
Gastric lavage or emesis. Demulcents. Saline cathartic. Stimulants for depression. Artificial respiration and oxygen if necessary.

167. Veratrum (Hellebore)
Gastric lavage or emesis. Activated charcoal. Saline cathartic. Atropine every hour to block reflex fall of blood pressure. Phentolamine hydrochloride or other sympathetic blocking agents should be given if hypertension present.

168. Vitamins (Vitamin A, Vitamin D, Vitamin K)
Discontinue use or reduce dosage. Symptomatic and supportive therapy as indicated.

169. Warfarin (Coumadin, Panwarfin)
Gastric lavage or emesis. Vitamin K in adequate dosage. Transfusion of fresh blood if hemorrhage is severe.

170. Xanthines (Aminophylline, Theophylline, Theobromine, Caffeine)
Gastric lavage or emesis. Antacids or demulcents. If suppository, remove by enema. Short-acting barbiturates. Oxygen.

171. Xylene (Benzene, Toluene, Cumene, Mesitylene)
Cautious gastric lavage. 50 ml. of mineral oil left in stomach. Saline cathartic. Artificial respiration and oxygen. Avoid digestible fats, oils, and epinephrine. Wash thoroughly for skin contact.

172. Zinc (Sulfate, Oxide, Phosphide [Releases Phosphine on contact with water; See Phosphine under Phosphorus])
Gastric lavage or emesis for ingestion. Move patient from source of inhalation. Artificial respiration and oxygen. Antibiotics and corticosteroids for "metal fume fever" and pneumonitis.

C. INTOXICATION AND THE ALCOHOL ABSTINENCE SYNDROME

David H. Knott, Robert D. Fink, and Jack C. Morgan

Changing attitudes and laws concerning the responsibility of the institutional health care system toward alcohol-related disorders have created confusion, ambivalence, and apprehension among members of the medical profession. Legislative trends are dictating a more health-oriented, nonpunitive approach to acute alcohol problems. Although a legislative mandate employing the "disease aspect" of acute alcohol problems may be appropriately altruistic, it nevertheless is creating confusion, particularly for the emergency medical system, concerning the most effective and realistic approach to be taken.

The question of how to treat alcohol intoxication and withdrawal has plagued man for thousands of years. Presently, the fundamental problem is twofold: (*a*) how to recognize and properly manage medical-surgical-psychiatric emergencies that are complicated by the effects of alcohol intoxication or abstinence; and (*b*) how to triage patients so that only those most seriously affected utilize emergency care facilities. Emergency Departments should not serve as detoxification centers but rather as a back-up service to handle severe cases. Historically, however, the effectiveness of detoxification centers has not been particularly promising. One should anticipate that emergency medical service facilities will be given a gradually increasing responsibility in this area until more effective detoxification programs are developed.

Skillful diagnosis is essential for proper management. Although this maxim is obvious, frequent errors in management result from inadequacies in differential diagnosis. The use of the term "acute alcoholism" is overly simplistic and fails to provide the exactness and detail necessary for accurate diagnosis and treatment, which must be individualized. The following discussion will focus on the diagnosis and treatment of the medical-psychiatric problems associated with and usually caused by the use of alcohol as they might present to an emergency health care facility. The acute phase of alcohol abuse can be divided into:

A. Alcohol Intoxication
B. Alcohol Abstinence Syndrome
C. Alcohol-related Toxic Psychoses
   1. Pathologic Intoxication
   2. Alcoholic Hallucinosis
   3. Alcoholic Paranoid State
D. Combined Alcohol-Drug Abstinence Syndrome

ALCOHOL INTOXICATION

DIAGNOSIS

Some of the well-known signs and symptoms of alcohol intoxication include dilated pupils that react slowly to light, nystagmus, dysarthria, dysmetria, ataxia, and emotional lability—including paranoia, combativeness, and a marked impairment in judgment. The severity of the clinical condition depends on the blood alcohol level and on the biologic tolerance of the individual to alcohol. It is important to relate the severity of the clinical condition with the blood alcohol level. The odor of alcohol on a patient's breath cannot be taken as evidence in this regard: either direct measurement or an estimation of the blood alcohol concentration (BAC) is necessary.

A useful and easily determined estimation of BAC is the plasma osmolality (Beard, et al., 1974). The increment in plasma osmolality caused by a unit increase in plasma alcohol is linear—i.e., a rise in plasma osmolality of approximately 22 milliosmoles/kg. H_2O (acutal figure is 21.7) reflects a 100 mg. per cent increase in plasma alcohol. For example, if one assumes an average normal plasma osmolality of 290 (275 to 295) and the measured plasma osmolality of the intoxicated patient is 356, then the estimate of the BAC is 300 mg per cent or 0.3 per cent. One must always be aware that concomitant conditions (trauma, infection, multiple drug use, etc.) can complicate the clinical picture; therefore, correlating the signs and symptoms with the BAC is necessary for an effective treatment regimen.

MANAGEMENT

The lethal effects of alcohol are primarily due to suppression of the medullary respiratory center. Unless vital functions (particularly respiration) are threatened, treatment of alcohol intoxication should be supportive and conservative. Psychotropic agents should be withheld unless a definite and clinically significant abstinence syndrome occurs (see below). Commonly associated disorders, such as hemorrhage, infection, trauma, etc., should be searched for and treated appropriately.

There have been many attempts in the past to mitigate the effects of alcohol intoxication by increasing the rate of alcohol metabolism and elimination. Such efforts as the use of glucose and insulin, steroids, thyroid hormones, oxygen inhalation, and analeptic drugs have produced equivocal results at best and frequently complicate the picture. There is some evidence that intravenous fructose (1,000 cc. of 10 per cent frucose) will decrease the morbidity of alcohol intoxication, although the mechanism is not yet well-understood (Merry and Marks, 1967). Since it is known that the signs and symptoms of alcohol intoxication (especially the neurologic and affective ones) are exacerbated by actual and relative hypoglycemia, any measure (oral fruit juices, etc.) that will increase and possibly stablize blood glucose should exert a salutary effect. Because of the depressant effect of alcohol on the central nervous and cardiovascular systems, any emergency invasive technique must be performed with caution in the intoxicated patient.

ALCOHOL ABSTINENCE SYNDROME

DIAGNOSIS

Although delirium tremens (loosely defined) is the type of alcohol abstinence syndrome most frequently encountered, the diagnostic criteria and etiologic factors pertaining to the syndrome of delirium tremens have been subjected to extensive interpretation and controversy. The severity of the abstinence syndrome depends on many factors, such as the amount of alcohol consumed (and how rapidly it was consumed), the height and duration of the blood alcohol level, the age of the individual, the degree of tissue tolerance to alcohol, and the general physical and psychologic condition of the patient. Rather than simply using the terms "impending delirium tremens" or "delirium tremens," these authors have found it more useful clinically to describe the alcohol abstinence syndrome according to four stages (Knott, et al., 1974). This approach allows more individualized and effective treatment.

These stages are:

Stage I. Psychomotor agitation, autonomic hyperactivity, tachycardia, hypertension, diaphoresis, anorexia, insomnia, occasional auditory and visual illusions.

Stage II. Symptoms and signs of Stage I plus hallucinations, which can be auditory, visual, tactile or olfactory. The hallucinations are usually of a mixed type. They are frequently threatening. They can be intermittent and transient and usually are followed by total or partial amnesia of the hallucinatory experience.

Stage III. Signs and symptoms of Stages I and II plus delusions, disorientation and delirium. These states can be intermittent and transient and usually involve some amnesia of the experience. In the authors' experience, if Stage III exists, there are frequently coexistent medical-surgical problems, prominent among which are trauma, hemorrhage, infection, multiple drug misuse and severe fluid and electrolyte derangements.

Stage IV. Signs and symptoms of Stages I, II, and III, plus seizure activity—typically of the grand mal variety. There are reports that not infrequently a seizure can precede the development of Stages I, II, and III (Victor, 1973). Within the first 96 hours of the abstinence syndrome, seizure activity can occur exclusive of other symptomatology. Such seizures have been termed "rum fits" or "alcoholic epilepsy" and usually are due to alcohol withdrawal, not to underlying chronic CNS pathology.

These four stages are unpredictably progressive and frequently overlap. This syndrome can occur at any time after the blood alcohol level begins to decrease until as long as 72–96 hours after the last drink. Characteristically the most dramatic symptoms will occur within a 12- to 48-hour period after the cessation of alcohol ingestion.

MANAGEMENT

The abstinence syndrome involves a state of neurophysiologic hyperarousal complicated by some specific pathophysiologic states associated with the pharmacology of alcohol. Treatment is directed toward amelioration of both the hyperarousal state (psychopharmacologic approach) and the generalized pathophysiologic disturbances (medical management).

PSYCHOPHARMACOLOGIC APPROACH

The use of psychotropics in the emergency situation should be dictated by the severity of the abstinence syndrome. Avoid oversedation and polypharmacy; signs and symptoms should be "titrated." Repeated drug administration should be determined by clinical response rather than by routine "standing orders." The authors' experience is that, for Stage I, the milder psychosedatives are most useful—an example would be hydroxyzine (Vistaril), 50 to 100 mg. orally or I.M. every two to three hours as needed to control symptoms. This approach avoids the potential development of oversedation and CNS depression, which may complicate the clinical picture if more potent sedatives are used routinely. If hydroxyzine is ineffective, or if the patient has a history of alcohol withdrawal seizures, diazepam (Valium) 10 to 20 mg. I.M. (I.V. for the severely agitated patient) may be given every two to four hours as needed for symptom control.

The hallucinations of Stage II can be effectively aborted by administration of haloperidol (Haldol), 2.5 to 5 mg. I.M. every two to four hours as needed, while the patient is maintained on psychosedatives. In Stage III, haloperidol may be useful, but adequate sedation is more often effected by administering parenteral phenobarbital. Seizure activity can be controlled and prevented with diazepam.

No drug is unique and specific for the abstinence syndrome, and prescribing practices should be based on a thorough understanding of the pharmacology of the psychotropic agent, its actions, side-effects, and any predictable idiosyncrasies in the reaction of the alcohol-abusing individual to that particular compound. Symptom control can be ascertained by measuring vital signs. A decrease in blood pressure, pulse, and psychomotor agitation and no progression to psychotic symptoms (hallucinations, delusions, etc.) indicate proper management of the hyperarousal state.

MEDICAL MANAGEMENT

Some of the pathophysiologic states consequent to alcohol abuse affect the course of the abstinence syndrome. Mismanagement or neglect of these states increases the morbidity of this condition. Specific attention in the emergency situation to fluid and electrolyte disturbances, abnormalities in carbohydrate metabolism, gastrointestinal dysfunction, infection, and trauma can expedite recovery.

Fluid and Electrolyte Metabolism. Recent basic and clinical investigations have shown that alcohol has a biphasic action on fluid balance (Beard and Knott, 1968). As long as the blood alcohol concentration is increasing, it promotes a diuresis. The increased urine formation is a result of an increase in the free-water clearance. This is effected by an inhibition of antidiuretic hormone by rising levels of blood alcohol. During the diuretic phase, Na^+, K^+, and Cl^- are retained. By contrast, stable or decreasing blood alcohol levels are associated with an antidiuresis, and with continued fluid (or food) ingestion positive water balance frequently results.

The over-all result of this biphasic action is the accumulation of electrolytes (Na^+, K^+, Cl^-) and water. This creates an isosmotic expansion of total body water, which is distributed proportionately throughout all fluid compartments and particularly—and more importantly—throughout the intracellular space of the central nervous system. Serum electrolyte levels in such instances will be in the normal range.

A state of *dehydration*, occasionally in association with hyponatremia, hypokalemia, and hypochloremia usually prevails only when protracted vomiting, diarrhea, malnutrition, or a combination of these are prominent concomitants of the abstinence syndrome. Low serum K^+ values may be due to hyperventilation, which is encountered frequently in acute withdrawal. The respiratory alkalosis and the associated extracellular to intracellular shift of K^+ are physiologic consequences of hyperventilation. Replacement of K^+ is not needed in this situation, unless cardiovascular or neuromuscular symptoms of hypokalemia are noted.

In contrast to the empiric use of intravenous fluids, the use of diuretics in the acutely withdrawing patient who is overhydrated is an effective treatment adjunct (Knott and Beard, 1969). In the authors' experience, a single oral or parenteral dose of furosemide (Lasix, 40 to 80 mg.) will effect a safe, rapid diuresis and often will shorten the period of detoxification.

In addition to a retention of Na^+, alcohol causes an intracellular shift of sodium. This alters transcellular membrane potential and could possibly lead to commonly encountered abnormalities such as cardiac arrhythmias, generalized myalgias, and seizure diathesis. Many of the traditional anticonvulsant drugs, such as diphenylhydantoin (Dilantin), decrease intracellular Na^+. In some instances Dilantin is administered (400 mg. daily for three to four days) to reverse this disorder of Na^+ partition. It is important to indicate that Dilantin per se in the seizure-prone individual will *not* necessarily prevent convulsions in the initial 72- to 96-hour period of the abstinence syndrome; in these individuals additional drugs such as diazepam or phenobarbital may be necessary for prophylaxis and control.

The empiric use of magnesium (Mg^{++}), usually as $MgSO_4$, in acute alcohol withdrawal is a controversial issue. Experimental and clinical impressions with regard to this agent are somewhat equivocal, but some evidence strongly suggests that excessive alcohol ingestion is associated with a decrease in total exchangeable Mg^{++} (Victor, 1973). In the authors' experience, a replacement (not therapeutic) dosage of $MgSO_4$ (2 cc. of 50 per cent $MgSO_4$) intramuscularly every four to six hours for a total of six to eight doses is useful in returning magnesium stores to normal and theoretically reduces the hyperirritability of neural tissue.

Abnormalities in Carbohydrate Metabolism. Hypoglycemia has been associated with the acute withdrawal syndrome primarily in those suffering from malnutrition

(Field, et al., 1963). It is important to recognize the lability of blood glucose during the withdrawal period. Chronic alcohol ingestion partially depletes hepatic glycogen stores and impairs gluconeogenesis.

Catecholamines, which increase in association with early withdrawal, have a glycogenolytic effect that may lead to normal or even elevated blood sugar levels. As the patient becomes calmer and as catecholamine release decreases, the blood glucose can fall rapidly without the protective effect of adequate glycogen stores in the liver. This leads to increased agitation and may precipitate seizure activity. Oral sustenance during the period of the abstinence syndrome is essential. Intravenous dextrose and water may be necessary for those patients unable to tolerate oral nutrition. Thiamine (100 mg. daily) should be administered parenterally in conjunction with parenteral fluids.

Gastrointestinal Dysfunction. Gastritis and toxic hepatitis are frequently found in this patient population and should be treated accordingly. Subacute pancreatitis occurs more often than previously suspected. Urinary amylase levels are frequently necessary to confirm the presence of this condition as serum amylase may be in the normal range. A regimen should include, where appropriate, antacids, anticholinergics, and proper dietary restrictions.

Infection. Alcohol suppresses leukopoiesis, decreases leukocytic reserves and can decrease gamma-globulin levels (Beard and Knott, 1966). The patient suffering the acute abstinence syndrome is susceptible to infection, particularly of the respiratory tract. Any infectious or inflammatory process associated with trauma has a more serious course in the patient whose immune mechanism has been impaired by alcohol. Aggressive management, preferably using bactericidal drugs, decreases morbidity.

Alcohol impairs motor function. As a result, trauma is a frequent complication of alcohol intoxication and withdrawal, and should certainly be suspected while the patient is being evaluated.

Any undiagnosed and untreated medical-surgical condition exacerbates the abstinence syndrome and can result in the progression from mild forms of Stage I to the severe condition of Stage IV.

The *primary responsibility of emergency medicine in this regard is to:* (a) not overtreat or iatrogenically complicate the condition, e.g., by oversedating the patient or overzealously using intravenous fluids; (b) ameliorate the hyperarousal state and the pathophysiology associated with the abstinence syndrome through total medical management; and (c) recognize that acute care is only a precedent to longer range rehabilitative efforts which obviously exist outside of the Emergency medical system.

ALCOHOL-RELATED TOXIC PSYCHOSES

Some variants of the abstinence syndrome present as emergency situations, yet only remotely resemble the classic picture described above. The complication of alcohol abuse in the functional psychiatric disorders, such as latent or borderline schizophrenia, and in the more disturbed premorbid personalities, such as paranoid or explosive types, can frequently produce a toxic psychotic state (Chafetz, 1967). Important points for consideration in differentiating the alcohol abstinence syndrome of the delirium tremens variety and the other alcohol-related toxic psychoses are:

(a) Extent or absence of psychomotor agitation and autonomic hyperactivity.

(b) Type and nature of hallucinations (mixed or pure—auditory, visual, tactile, pleasant, or threatening).

(c) State of sensorium—is there a coexistent disorientation in one or more spheres?

(d) Extent of amnesia of the psychotic episode.

(e) Presence of coexistent disorders—especially infectious or traumatic.

(f) Onset in regard to drinking pattern and duration of the psychotic episode.

While many variants have been described, there is frequently an overlapping of symptomatology. Some of the more common, yet still infrequent toxic psychoses are described below.

PATHOLOGIC INTOXICATION

This psychosis is actually associated with alcohol intoxication rather than abstinence. It is characterized by a markedly impaired sensorium with confusion and disorientation developing after consumption of small quantities of alcohol. There is frequently a sudden onset of markedly aggressive and hostile behavior. Impulse control is generally lacking, and destructive behavior is not uncommon. This often necessitates intervention by law enforcement personnel. There may be superimposition of psychotic symptomatology, including hallucinations, usually of a visual type, and delusions. There is a definite paranoid trend in some cases. Total amnesia of the psychotic episode is frequently observed. The etiology of pathologic intoxication is poorly understood. In some cases there is a question as to whether this represents an alcohol-induced temporal lobe dysrhythmia (Bach, et al., 1970). Treatment for the agitated phase can be accomplished with phenobarbital in doses sufficient to produce a sedative effect. Halperidol (Haldol) can be used to control psychotic symptoms.

ALCOHOLIC HALLUCINOSIS

This syndrome can occur as early as 72 to 96 hours after blood alcohol levels begin to decline. However, it may present with onset as late as four to seven days after the last drink. It is characterized by auditory hallucinations (rarely accompanied by visual hallucinations), delusions, and paranoid ideation. The sensorium can be clear (the patient is oriented in all spheres) and autonomic hyperactivity and psychomotor agitation are frequently absent. There is little or no amnesia of the psychotic period. This point should be considered when taking a history of previous episodes. A concomitant systemic infection is frequently present. Adequate treatment consists of aggressive use of a neuroleptic—e.g., haloperidol (Haldol) or chlorpromazine (Thorazine)—in conjunction with diagnosis and treatment of any associated medical disorders.

ALCOHOLIC PARANOID STATE

At times the alcoholic paranoid state is confused with paranoid schizophrenia. It can occur days after the last drink and can last from days to weeks. It may be insidious in onset and is related to both the amount of alcohol consumed and the duration of drinking. Frequently it is characterized by suspicion, distrust, jealousy, paranoid delusions (especially of marital infidelity), and amnesia of the psychotic episode. While this condition responds well to neuroleptic medication (chlorpromazine or haloperidol), recurrence is unpredictably associated with a resumption of alcohol ingestion.

These toxic psychoses must be differentiated from the alcohol abstinence syndrome because they demand aggressive administration of neuroleptics (such as a phenothiazine or haloperidol) rather than psychosedatives. A more disturbed premorbid personality and functional psychiatric disorder frequently is involved, thus necessitating more careful attention to psychiatric referral and follow-up.

COMBINED ALCOHOL–DRUG ABSTINENCE SYNDROME

Emergency services will be confronted with patients who are misusing a variety of drugs including alcohol. An increasing problem is the combination of alcohol plus sedative-hypnotics (minor tranquilizers, such as diazepam, chlordiazepoxide, barbiturates, and various soporifics). Depending on the rate of metabolism of the drugs involved, the abstinence syndrome can occur in two or more stages (e.g., alcohol abstinence in the first 12 to 48 hours and sedative hypnotic abstinence four to seven days after cessation of drug ingestion). A careful drug history obviously is necessary for proper management and referral to the aftercare system (Fink, et al., 1974).

Emergency medical services should be prepared to diagnose and treat the seriously disturbed patient suffering alcohol intoxication and abstinence. These services can function best if they (a) concentrate on meeting only the medical-surgical-psychiatric needs of the patient, (b) do not allow expenditure of health manpower for the treatment of simple, uncomplicated drunkenness, and (c) insist that a referral system be established so that once detoxification is initiated or accomplished the patient has access to an aftercare system designed to ascertain and manage his psychosocial needs.

References

Bachy, R. G., Lion, J. R., and Ervin, F. R.: Pathologic intoxication – clinical and electroencephalographic studies. Am. J. Psychiat. 127:698, 1970.

Beard, J. D., and Knott, D. H.: Hematopoietic response to experimental chronic alcoholism. Am. J. Med. Sci. 252:260, 1966.

Beard, J. D., and Knott, D. H.: Fluid and electrolyte balance during acute withdrawal in chronic alcoholic patients. J.A.M.A. 204:135, 1968.

Beard, J. D., Knott, D. H., and Fink, R. D.: The use of plasma and urine osmolality in evaluating the acute phase of alcohol abuse. South. Med. J. 67:3, 271, 1974.

Chafetz, M.: Personality Disorders. III: Sociopathic Type: The Addictions: Alcoholism. In Freedman, A. M., and Kaplan, A. L. (eds.): Comprehensive Textbook of Psychiatry. Baltimore, Williams & Wilkins Co., 1967, p. 1011.

Field, J. B., Williams, H. E., and Mortimore, G. D.: Studies on the mechanism of alcohol induced hypoglycemia. J. Clin. Invest. 42:497, 1963.

Fink, R. D., Knott, D. H., and Beard, J. D.: Sedative-hypnotic dependence. Am. Fam. Physician 10:3, 116, 1974.

Israel-Jacard, Y., and Kalant, H.: Effect of ethanol on electrolyte transport and electrogenesis in animal tissues. J. Cell Comp. Physiol. 65:127, 1965.

Knott, D. H., Beard, J. D., and Wallace, J. A.: Acute withdrawal from alcohol: a diagnostic and therapeutic problem. Postgrad. Med. 42:109, 1967.

Knott, D. H., and Beard, J. D.: A diuretic approach to acute withdrawal from alcohol. South. Med. J. 62:485, 1969.

Knott, D. H., Beard, J. D., and Fink, R. D.: Acute withdrawal from alcohol. Emerg. Med. 6:No. 2, 87, 1974.

Marinacci, A., and Von Hagen, K.: Alcohol and temporal lobe dysfunction. Behav. Neuropsychiat. 3:2, 1972.

May, P. R. A., and Ebaugh, F. G.: Pathological intoxication, alcoholic hallucinosis and other reactions to alcohol. Q. J. Stud. Alcohol 14:200, 1953.

Merry, J., and Marks, V.: Effect on performance of reducing blood alcohol with oral fructose. Lancet 2:1328, 1967.

Stokes, P. E., and Lasley, B.: Further Studies on Blood Alcohol Kinetics in Man as Affected by Thyroid Hormones, Insulin and d-Glucose. In Maickel, R. P. (ed.): Biochemical Factors in Alcoholism. Oxford, Pergamon Press, 1967, p. 101.

Sullivan, L. W., and Herbert, F.: Suppression of hematopoiesis by ethanol. J. Clin. Invest. 43:2048, 1964.

Victor, M., and Adams, R. D.: Effects of Alcohol on the Nervous System. In Merritt, H. H., and Hare, C. C. (eds.): Metabolic and Toxic Diseases of the Nervous System. Baltimore, Williams & Wilkins Co., 1953, p. 526.

Victor, M.: The role of hypomagnesemia and respiratory alkalosis in the genesis of alcohol withdrawal symptoms. Ann. N.Y. Acad. Sci. 215:235, 1973.

Wolfe, S. M., and Victor, M.: The relationship of hypomagnesemia and alkalosis to alcohol withdrawal symptoms. Ann. N.Y. Acad. Sci. 162:973, 1969.

Chapter 59   PEDIATRIC EMERGENCIES

Garrett E. Bergman

GENERAL

Although basic physiologic responses to trauma, infection, metabolic stresses, and drugs are similar in patients of all ages, clinically, children often react differently from adults. In children the spectrum of responses to various stresses may be different, or if similar reactions do occur, they may progress at a different rate, with very different consequences.

For example, the young child with salicylate intoxication will often present with a metabolic acidosis, having rapidly progressed through the initial stage of respiratory alkalosis that is usually seen when older children and adults present. On the other hand, peritoneal localizing signs appear later in the course of appendicitis in young children, and the diagnosis must be suspected from less specific findings. For this reason, the physician dealing with children in an emergency situation must become familiar with the patterns of normal and expected responses to various childhood stresses of illness and trauma. With experience, it is usually possible to distinguish the distress of a child with a minor illness from that of a child who is seriously ill.

Elsewhere in this text the assessment of conditions that may affect children as well as adults is presented. This chapter will focus on particular emergencies and conditions characteristic of or restricted to children. Additionally, common problems that present differently or need to be assessed differently in children will be covered.

INITIAL ASSESSMENT

Most historical information concerning the child will be provided by the parent or guardian, who may recognize and report subtle alterations early in the course of a disease. In situations of obvious gravity, as might be encountered in an emergency unit setting, it is prudent to elicit historical material while assessing the patient objectively by examination. Information to be elicited early in evaluation includes the following:

1. The chief symptom and its consequences
2. How and when the problem began and how it has progressed
3. Associated symptoms such as fever, pain, lethargy, or anorexia
4. The presence of any congenital or chronic disease state
5. Means and results of treatment that had been employed prior to arrival

Frequently, the emergency setting is the first encounter between the physician and patient. Although a child is often very frightened and upset, a reassuring, gentle approach will often ensure the child's cooperation so that the physician can achieve a more complete and accurate evaluation. To lessen their apprehension, it is important to fully explain all procedures to children over two or three years of age before performing them. When possible, the child should be examined while in the parent's lap or with the parent standing close or even directly in contact with the patient or the examining bed; this security will often decrease the crying and struggling. For the younger child in whom cooperation is impossible, the judicious use of restraints is warranted, as necessary, for evaluative procedures such as adequate examination of the ears, diagnostic procedures such as venesection and lumbar punctures, and therapeutic measures such as suturing and other surgical procedures. One can use commercially available restraint boards ("papoose boards"), but frequently, a folded bedsheet and an experienced assistant can provide effective immobilization.

In the physical examination of a child, one looks for essentially the same alterations as in an adult. To determine objectively the state of consciousness, the responses to stimuli, the state of cardiac and respiratory functioning, and so on calls for the same precise methods and skills of observation.

In addition to the usual sites of diagnostic venesection, children have additional superficial veins that can be used when hand and arm veins are no longer available. In infants, the veins of the scalp can be used for diagnostic sampling and therapeutic infusions. The familiar "butterfly" infusion needles are as useful for drawing blood samples from superficial veins as for infusing fluids for therapy. The external jugular veins are fairly easy to puncture for blood sampling, but should rarely be used to infuse fluids because of the risk of extravasation into the neck and pleural space. The internal jugular vein should be used only as a last resort, perhaps for emergency administration of drugs or fluids, and insertion of a central venous pressure catheter. Many hospital laboratories are now equipped to determine blood values on small quantities of blood by microtechniques; for some, venous blood is not required, and capillary samples can be used.

LIFE-THREATENING EMERGENCIES

Severe dysfunction or failure of the *cardiovascular, respiratory,* or *central nervous system* can acutely jeopardize life. The basic life support measures that must be provided are the same as for adults—establishment of an airway, ventilation, cardiac support, and drugs as necessary—and are all designed to re-establish effective oxygenation of the central nervous system and other vital organs. The specific procedures to be followed are outlined in Chapter 8. There are some differences in recommended techniques in children, as follows:

Establishing an Airway. The trachea of an infant is very pliable; exaggerated neck extension can cause buckling of the trachea and occlusion of the airway. Often a problem arises as to the appropriate size of endotracheal tube to use for intubation. The "rule of thumb" is to use an endotracheal tube that is the same size as the child's thumbnail, as his thumbnail has about the same diameter as his trachea.

Cardiac Compression. To apply pressure to the child's more compliant thorax, and thereby effect cardiac compression, less force is required than would be for an adult. For infants and young children, only one hand may be used (see also procedure, p. 291).

Infant: Circle the thorax with both hands, thumbs meeting over the mid-sternum, and fingertips meeting posteriorly; depress the sternum $1/2$ to $3/4$ inch about 100 times per minute.

Young Child: Place three fingers or the heel of one hand over the mid-sternum and compress with immediate force from the elbow to depress the sternum $3/4$ to $1^1/2$ inches at a rate of 80 to 100 times per minute.

Older Child: Use technique described for adults but with elbows bent to absorb some of the force, at a rate of 60 to 80 times per minute.

Drugs. Drugs with recommended dosage schedules for use in support of resuscitation measures are listed in Table 1.

By developing a dynamic approach to the evaluation of a child in an emergency setting, the physician can accurately and efficiently assess the severity of the illness or trauma and institute the necessary therapeutic measures simultaneously. From the history, he can determine how the problem has evolved and how previous treatments have altered its course. By observation and physical examination, he can determine how the problem is affecting the child at present. In a life-threatening situation, he can provide life support measures as necessary. Because most children have been essentially healthy prior to the acute episode, they are likely to respond favorably, with excellent long-term prognosis, to therapeutic interventions. It can be a very rewarding experience to treat children and observe their rapid recovery.

PROBLEMS IN THE FIRST THREE MONTHS OF LIFE

Problems for which young infants are brought to the emergency unit range from extremely trivial matters to situations of serious morbidity. Inexperienced parents may interpret variations in the infant's normal activity as an emergency and may anxiously seek

TABLE 1 *Use of Drugs for Resuscitation Support*

DRUG	CONCENTRATION	DOSE	ROUTE	COMMENTS
Epinephrine	1:10,000 (0.1 mg./ml.)	0.01 mg./kg. up to 0.5 mg. (0.1 ml./kg. of 1:10,000)	Intravenous, intracardiac	
Atropine		0.4 mg. as bolus	Intravenous	May repeat, up to 2 mg.
Sodium bi-carbonate	Approx. 1 mEq./ml.	1.0 to 4.0 mEq./kg. (1.0 to 2.0 mEq./kg. per 5 minutes of arrest)	I.V. slow push	Repeat every 5 to 10 minutes
Calcium gluconate	10% (100 mg./ml.)	1 to 2 ml./kg.	I.V. slow push	Repeat every 10 minutes as necessary
Isuprel	0.2 mg./ml.	1 mg./100 ml. D5/0.25 normal saline	I.V. drip	Titrate to desired effect

advice. Eliciting a background family history of serious illness or death in a previous child may give the physician a more empathic understanding of the parents' seeming over-concern. Nevertheless, it is imperative that the physician recognize those clinical signs indicating a serious alteration in the health of the infant.

The general responses of an infant to external or internal stimuli are global rather than specific to the body part or system affected. A healthy infant has a fairly predictable range of activity, which includes visual exploration of his environment, nondirected spontaneous movements of his extremities, vocalizations and facial expressions in response to internal or social stimuli, and crying as a means of communicating his various needs, such as relief of hunger or physical discomfort or the desire for more social stimulation. In as early a setting as the newborn nursery, one can recognize distinct differences in temperament; some children being much more demanding, much more active, or more easily prone to crying than others. Infants may want to eat six to ten times a day, may urinate up to 16 to 20 times a day, and may have a bowel movement after each feeding. They usually sleep after each feeding, but may desire play and stimulation between feedings by one month of age. A healthy baby whose needs are being met appears contented. An infant stressed by physical or emotional trauma may be irritable, usually does not feed or sleep according to a predictable schedule, is rarely interested in his surroundings, and may make it difficult

for his guardian to relieve his distress by previously effective measures; a few or all of his observable behaviors may differ from his established pattern.

INFECTION

Early in life, the infant is protected against many infections by the transplacentally transported maternal immunoglobulins, primarily IgG. An established infection in an infant, however, is poorly localized by his incomplete host defenses, and as result, clinical signs and symptoms may not specifically indicate the site of infection. White blood cell functions, opsonins, components of the complement and properdin systems, and cellular immune mechanisms may all contribute to host deficiency to some degree early in life. Blood cultures frequently are positive when obtained in the presence of otitis media, urinary tract infection, or staphylococcal pyoderma, with secondary infection sites from septic emboli not uncommon, even up to two years of age.

Fever in the first three months of life must be recognized as a serious symptom, and its cause must be fully determined. The body temperature of a healthy infant can fluctuate by 1.5° F. daily, up to perhaps 100.5° F. rectally. Any elevated temperature should be considered abnormal, possibly a sign of sepsis, and appropriate diagnostic measures (blood cultures, lumbar puncture, chest x-ray, urine culture) must be taken, even if clinical examination reveals a seemingly benign infection. The decision to treat with intravenous antibiotics pending culture results must be individualized, based upon all the clinical information and laboratory findings together.

Respiratory Infections. The gamut of respiratory infections ranges from simple rhinitis to pertussis to bronchiolitis to staphylococcal pneumonia. All may be characterized by tachypnea, cough, and fever but can be distinguished by characteristic presentations, primarily related to degree of toxicity and respiratory embarrassment produced. With coryza, nasal congestion may cause mild to moderate intermittent respiratory distress in the young, obligate nose-breathing infant, even with occasional use of accessory muscles or respiration. The usual pattern of the child's behavior is not disrupted significantly. Simple measures such as humidification (cool mist vaporizer) and saline nose drops ($1/4$ teaspoon of table salt to 8 oz. of boiled water) are usually sufficient treatment. Proprietary oral decongestants are rarely helpful in this age group, and with excessive administration, the undesirable side effects are hard to avoid.

Intercostal, subcostal, and suprasternal retractions; paradoxical breathing; and grunting with expiration suggest serious impairment of ventilation. If sudden in onset and in the absence of signs of infection, upper airway obstruction or aspiration of foreign material should be suspected, and immediate diagnostic and therapeutic steps should be taken. If fever is present, or the distress has been increasing in severity over six to 18 hours, or if generalized toxicity is present, a serious pneumonitic process is likely. Particularly, if the child or his caretaker has any presumed or known staphylococcal infection, treatment of staphylococcal pneumonia should be instituted with a semisynthetic, penicillinase-resistant antibiotic on clinical grounds because of its rapidly progressing course and attendant mortality. Any significant respiratory embarrassment in the infant calls for hospitalization, careful assessment, and aggressive treatment. It is common for salicylate intoxication to present with respiratory symptoms, sometimes severe hyperpnea, in the infant.

Wheezing is the hallmark of *bronchiolitis.* Most cases are caused by respiratory syncytial virus, but bronchospasm can occur both in bacterial and viral infections. Beginning with a coryzal picture, bronchiolitis progresses over three to seven days to varying degrees of severity. Most infants handle this infection well, and cool air humidification alone is sufficient therapy. Mild oral bronchodilators may relieve some distress if there is reversible reflex bronchospasm. Steroids and antibiotics do not seem to alter the course of viral bronchiolitis (Wright and Beem, 1965). There is still a small number of children who will require ventilatory assistance during the height of their illness. The degree of respiratory distress can be determined by assessing heart rate, respiratory rate, and how tired the child is becoming from the work of breathing. Determination of arterial blood gases, which is an objective measurement of how well the patient is able to handle the respiratory embarrassment, should be done whenever there is a question of respiratory decompensation. In a small number of children, particularly those with underlying cardiac or pulmonary disease, bronchiolitis can become life-threatening, particularly if bacterial infection develops secondarily. Recurrent episodes of "bronchiolitis" may actually be recurrent asthma, acute exacerbations of chronic pulmonary disease, the results of anatomic abnormalities of the intrathoracic structures, or the recurring effects of an aspirated foreign body.

Interstitial pneumonia can present as bronchiolitis, with wheezing, or as a mild pneumonia, with dyspnea. Most often, it is viral in etiology and is self-limited, but because of the difficulty in predicting the severity of respiratory embarrassment and the likelihood of bacterial superinfection in this age group, careful repeated evaluations are necessary. Occasional cases will progress to obliterative bronchiolitis. Viral pneumonia can also become potentially life-threatening for children with underlying cardiac or pulmonary disease.

Radiographic examination of the respiratory tract in young children often yields results that will not alter the management of their illness, but the typical findings of various conditions should be well recognized. Early in a pneumonitic process, no infiltration of consolidation may be seen but significant hyperexpansion of the lungs will be present. By observing the flattening of the diaphragms (up to 10 or 11 ribs visible above the diaphragm posteriorly) and a decrease in the cardiothoracic ratio, the diagnosis of bronchiolitis, asthma, or pneumonia could be supported. Later in the course of each of these entities, interstitial infiltrates, atelectasis, lobar consolidation, or fluid in the fissures or pleural space may be seen. Many infants with pneumonia will become dehydrated early in their illness from increased insensible water losses; only when they are rehydrated will their pulmonary infiltrate be visible on the x-ray films. When one observes signs of upper airway obstruction, AP and lateral views on neck x-ray, barium swallow x-ray, and laryngoscopy or bronchoscopy may be indicated to look for intraluminal foreign bodies or narrowing of the upper airway due to retropharyngeal abscess, epiglottitis, or other inflammatory disease processes. These studies could also demonstrate a structural (congenital) defect such as vascular ring from aberrant vessels or segmental bronchial stenosis, both of which could cause recurrent respiratory difficulties.

Urinary Tract Infections. Urinary tract infections are common and are frequently overlooked in infants. Aspiration of the urinary bladder for urinalysis and culture is an established and safe procedure; after cleansing the skin with an antiseptic of choice, insert a 22 gauge 1½ inch needle connected to a 6 cc. to 12 cc. syringe 1 cm. above the symphysis in the midline to a depth of 1 to 2 cm. and aspirate the urine. With ultrasonography, one can determine whether urine is present in the bladder. Bacteria and white blood cells in the urine obtained this way could not be from contamination, and their presence, even in small numbers, is significant.

Frequently, infants with urinary tract infections have no symptoms or signs except fever. There may be clinical jaundice, hyperbilirubinemia (both direct and indirect), poor weight gain, poor feeding, vomiting, and irritability. Many infants with urinary tract infections do not have anatomic abnormalities of the urinary collecting system, but all infants with urinary tract infections should be evaluated with intravenous pyelography and other indicated studies when the infection has subsided.

Gastrointestinal Infections. Gastrointestinal infections can cause more serious consequences to the infant earlier in the course of the disease than is the case in older children. Excessive fluid losses due to diarrhea, vomiting or intestinal pooling will compromise the small infant's intracellular and intravascular volumes sooner than in the older child or adult because of the following:

1. Insensible water losses are greater because of a greater surface area/body weight ratio in the infant.

2. The usual renal homeostatic mechanisms of acidifying and concentrating the urine are not yet fully developed, so there is less ability to compensate for alterations in fluid and electrolyte balance.

3. Relatively small volumes of fluid loss, which may actually represent a significant percentage of loss in the small infant, may be considered insignificant by the parent. In addition, home remedies for diarrhea and vomiting, such as giving improper electrolyte solutions (boiled milk, solutions of salt and sugar) or enemas (iced tea, milk, magnesium sulfate), may accelerate the pathologic process.

Most gastroenteritis in children is viral. In infants, however, enteric pathogens, including enteropathogenic strains of *E. coli,* cause many serious gastrointestinal disturbances. Clinical staging and treatment of dehydration will be covered later in this chapter. For simple diarrhea and vomiting, restricting oral intake to frequent small feedings of clear liquids will usually reverse the problem in 24 to 36 hours. "Starvation stools," which are green in color and watery in consistency, can develop after several days of restricted oral intake; solid foods such as rice, bananas, and apple sauce could then be given to reverse the diarrhea.

FAILURE TO THRIVE

The pivotal role of the Emergency Physician is to recognize when this condition is present. Thus, suitable charts of height and weight percentiles must be available. A place on the record for recording these percentiles may simplify such recognition.

Beyond the immediate postnatal period, healthy, full-term infants fed a sufficient number of calories in a balanced nutritional diet will gain weight at the rate of about ¾ ounce per day. Although it is not advisable for parents to weigh their child frequently, this figure is a useful guideline with which the physician can assess the general growth of the infant in the first three months. It is well to remember that scales may not be comparable. Some daily weight fluctuations (variable oral intake from illness, a greater number of bowel movements) should be expected. Weight should be measured and recorded on every visit for any child under six months of age, any child who appears small for his age, and any child with a subacute or chronic illness. Frequently, a child brought to the emergency physician for an acute episodic illness is found to have suboptimal weight gain. Evaluating and treatment of such an infant who "fails to thrive" usually presents a challenge, and referral should be made for detailed evaluation and treatment.

Recognition of Failure to Thrive. There are two broad categories of problems leading to poor growth in infancy: environmental and organic. Often, upon initial evaluation by history and physical examination, it becomes evident that the infant is not receiving a sufficient nutritional base on which to gain weight adequately; this deprivation can be due to parental ignorance or a disordered parent-child relationship (child abuse or neglect). Even when an adequate diet is present, however, a disturbed emotional environment can result in inadequate intake and absorption of food. Certain characteristics of the child may contribute to the abnormal relationship; a child with a physical handicap or a neurologic disease may evoke feelings of rejection, anger, and guilt in his parents.

When a complete history and physical examination do not suggest an obvious cause or the course of treatment for poor weight gain, hospitalization can provide a milieu in which diagnostic and therapeutic procedures can be performed simultaneously. Some causes for failure to thrive and the tests for them are listed in Table 2.

Although a large number of organic conditions can cause failure to thrive, most situations of unexpected poor growth are due to a pathologic psychosocial environment. An intensive multidisciplinary approach can help, in some cases, to establish patterns of parenting behavior conducive to the infant's better health.

TABLE 2　Causes of Failure to Thrive and Tests for Assessment

CAUSE	SCREENING TESTS
ENVIRONMENTAL	
Inadequate intake of food	History, observation in hospital
Emotional deprivation	History, observation in hospital
Environmental disruptions	History, observation in hospital
Rumination	Observation in hospital
ORGANIC	
Central nervous system abnormalities	Neurologic examination, developmental assessment, transillumination of skull, brain scan
Intestinal malabsorption	Observation in hospital, stool fat
Cystic fibrosis of the pancreas	Sweat test
Intestinal parasites (rarely a cause in temperate climates)	Stool examination for ova and parasites
Partial cleft palate	Physical examination, observation of feeding
Chronic heart failure	Physical examination, roentgenogram of chest
Endocrine disorders	Construction of growth chart, blood test for thyroid reaction, films for bone age
Idiopathic hypercalcemia	Serum calcium
Turner syndrome (females), other chromosomal disorders	Chromosomal analysis, in particular with peculiar facies
Renal insufficiency	Urinalysis, blood urea nitrogen
Renal tubular disorders	Urinalysis, urinary amino acid
Chronic infection (usually tuberculous or mycotic)	Tuberculin test, chest roentgenogram, temperature pattern in hospital
Chronic inflammation (e.g., rheumatoid arthritis)	Physical examination
Malignancies (especially of kidney, adrenal glands, brain)	Roentgenograms of abdomen and chest, intravenous urography, brain scan

Source: Vaughan, V. C., and McKay, R. J. (eds.): Textbook of Pediatrics, 10th ed. Philadelphia, W. B. Saunders Co., 1975, p. 1653.

Excessive vomiting, causing poor weight gain or a weight loss in the infant, can be the result of overfeeding or organic disease. The overfed, usually overweight, baby will regurgitate undigested food shortly after feeding. This, the "wet burping" of small amounts of food must be differentiated from the forceful vomiting of a child with malrotation of the bowel or pyloric stenosis. Renal tubular defects, adrenogenital syndrome, various infections, and some neurologic diseases can also be associated with vomiting.

Numerous organic conditions can cause an abnormal character to the stools and malabsorption. In carbohydrate malabsorption, either primary (due to congenital enzyme deficiency) or secondary to a diarrheal state, the stool pH will be less than 6.0 and will show evidence of reducing substances with Clinitest tablets. Cystic fibrosis and celiac sprue often cause malabsorption and "failure to thrive" in infancy. Enteric pathogens can cause diarrhea, malabsorption, and weight loss for up to several weeks. The presence of mucus or blood, or a green color and watery consistency to the stool, with or without the presence of numerous neutrophils on a stained smear of stool, should raise the suspicion of bacterial disease.

TRAUMA

Beyond the first year of life, accidents account for the single most common cause of death in children. As advances are made in the prevention and treatment of infections and congenital anomalies, the importance of trauma as a cause of morbidity and mortality in children increases. The differences in the recognition and treatment of trauma in children relate to specific physiologic characteristics. The bones of a child can often withstand a greater stress before a fracture occurs; there is a greater ratio of cartilaginous matrix to mineral in growing bone. Only in a growing child, obviously, could a fracture interrupt the epiphyseal growth plate of a long bone; if not recognized and treated, an epiphyseal fracture could cause disordered longitudinal growth of bone after healing, resulting in a permanent deformity. As a rule, the growing bones and tissues of children will heal better with fewer complications than adults because children have a greater capability to repair, replace, and remold diseased or injured tissue. On the other hand, a less than extensive burn on a child may quickly precipitate shock from a decreased vascular space; a smaller blood volume and greater ratio of surface area to blood volume make burns a more serious form of trauma in children.

BURNS

Among children aged one to four years, burns represent the leading cause of accidental death in the home. Burns can be caused by hot liquids, space heaters, electricity, chemicals, or combustion of flammable liquids or materials such as clothing. Hot liquids, usually foodstuffs, cause scalding burns. Electrical burns from household appliances, wires, or outlets can cause extensive local tissue necrosis; except for the severe bleeding that can result from electrical burns of the mouth, few complications usually result. Chemical burns encountered in the home are usually limited to esophageal burns from ingestion of caustic material such as lye or a drain-cleaning agent, which can result in severe long-term morbidity for the victim.

A good history is important in evaluating the likely severity of a burn, as often the degree as well as extent of a burn cannot be readily estimated initially. Burns from hot liquids spilled on clothing may be worse if the clothing was not immediately removed; steam burns may be more extensive than initially recognized. In estimating the severity of a thermal burn in terms of the percentage of surface area involved, the "rule of nines" employed in adult burn victims is not directly applicable to children because their body surface area proportions differ. Above age six to eight years, the differences are minor enough to be disregarded; the main difference is the larger percentage area of the head in proportion to the trunk. Under age five years, the head should be considered 15 to 20 per cent of the surface area, the trunk 30 to 35 per cent, and the legs each about 15 per cent. Criteria for admission to the hospital vary. In general, burns involving over 15 per cent of surface area; the neck, hands, feet, perineum, or face; or children under two years of age require in-hospital management. Under other conditions, in the absence of respiratory embarrassment or smoke inhalation, and in the presence of a favorable home situation and assured follow-up, partial thickness burns in nonvital areas of less than 15 per cent can be managed outside the hospital.

In the management of a thermal burn, the seriousness of the burn and associated injuries must be ascertained early. The airway is evaluated, the need for ventilatory assistance is determined, the need for nasogastric intubation for gastric decompression is assessed, blood is drawn for baseline studies, and fluid therapy is begun via intravenous catheter. The calculation of fluid requirement by various methods is available in Chapter 39A. In cases of serious burns, urinary output is monitored by urethral catheter. Antibiotics are not routinely administered.

Chemical esophagitis from caustic ingestion is one of the few instances of accidental ingestion in which emesis is contraindicated. Nothing should be given by mouth for 6 to 18 hours, at which time an examination by esophagoscopy may delineate the extent of mucosal burn. Steroids and antibiotics are often given if significant inflammation is seen; the full degree of morbidity may not be evident for several days or weeks as the healing tissues sclerose, requiring esophageal dilatations.

CHILD ABUSE

It is imperative to remember that trauma of almost any form, even the more bizarre, may be willfully and intentionally inflicted upon a child by an adult, including a parent, relative, or other caretaker. The combination of multiple fractures of the extremities and subdural hematoma was recognized as an entity in 1942 by John Caffey. In 1962 the term "battered child syndrome" was given by Henry Kempe to the entity of trauma inflicted purposely on a child. It is clear today that the incidence of child abuse is closely related to the physician's ability to recognize the possibility of nonaccidental trauma. Specific clinical observations that should raise suspicion of child abuse are as follows:

1. Episode of injury not explained fully by history

2. Recurrent injury (fractures, burns) to a young child

3. Presence of more than one fracture, especially if in separate stages of healing

4. Advanced underlying disease, such as malnutrition, advanced stage of infection, or delay in seeking medical advice

Certain injuries should be considered more likely to be secondary to abuse:

1. Subdural hematoma

2. Multiple fractures

3. Trauma involving perianal or genital areas

4. Clear marks of cigarette burns, heater elements, human bite, belt buckles

5. Any burn or fracture in an infant

The goals of recognizing and dealing with child abuse and neglect and potential child abuse are primarily to protect the child from further injury or death and to remedy the disordered family relations that have led to abuse. Statistics show that greater than 50 per cent of children recognized to have been abused have been purposefully injured previously. It has been estimated that the mortality rate may be 3 to 4 per cent, with a 30 per cent permanent physical disability rate.

To be effective in dealing with the parents in such a situation, one should keep in mind that such people often have certain characteristics that may set them aside from most adults. They have, as a rule, a low self-esteem and a constant fear of criticism and punishment; they will be easily threatened by any suggestion that they were guilty or responsible for the injury. They may feel that they have an obligation to punish the child. They generally have not learned to have trust and confidence in other people. Characteristically, such parents frequently had been abused as children. They will be suspicious of the physician's motives in offering help by suggesting hospitalization.

To deal effectively with such a family demands a long-term multidisciplinary approach; one cannot expect much to be accomplished therapeutically in the acute setting. By approaching the family in an empathic fashion, displaying genuine concern for the child and for the parents, one may achieve sufficient rapport to allow for the hospitalization of the child. Hospitalization is imperative in order to coordinate the diagnostic and therapeutic plans. For children under five to six years, hospitalization also provides the protection of separation and "defuses" a tense situation. The physician's approach to the parents in the initial contact might be as follows: "I'm not sure how your child could have gotten such an injury from the accident you describe. I feel we need to hospitalize him to do the necessary tests and find out how we can best help him. This must be upsetting to you, I realize, but I feel that with your help we can find out how your child was injured and work out a good plan which will be helpful."

ACUTE OBSTRUCTIVE RESPIRATORY DISEASE

In the conscious child, sudden obstruction to normal ventilation leads with variable rapidity to apprehension, agitation, delirium, and unconsciousness. If the obstruction is not quickly relieved and ventilation re-established, death is likely to result. The airway of a child can become obstructed at any point, from the nose to the alveoli, with significant consequences. In the unconscious patient, the tongue can block the oropharynx and cause a potentially preventable death.

At birth, the neonate begins to supply his oxygen needs independently. Except when crying, many infants can breathe only through their nostrils. (Occasionally, an infant may become irritable and agitated when nasal secretions from an upper respiratory infection partially obstruct the nostrils.) Complete bilateral choanal atresia can produce a respiratory emergency, particularly at times of feeding or earlier, if the infant cannot breathe through his mouth at all. He will then make vigorous attempts to breathe but will become more cyanotic. Since the obstruction may consist of only membranous tissue, the passage of a rubber catheter through both nares to the posterior nasopharynx may be curative. In any case, an oral airway should be inserted and the baby fed by endogastric tube until he learns to breathe through his mouth or surgical correction of the congenital anomaly can be undertaken.

Respiratory tract obstruction at the laryngeal level most often is due to laryngeal edema (anaphylaxis, infection, or foreign body), laryngospasm, or direct trauma to the larynx. Any foreign matter in the larynx could precipitate reflex laryngospasm, including an aspirated foreign body, inhalation of irritant fumes, or water in a near-drowning; the protective nature of this mechanism is obvious. Congenital malformations, laryngeal web, laryngomalacia and papillomas rarely cause respiratory embarrassment.

"Croup" syndrome is the clinical presentation of upper airway obstruction at the laryngotracheal level and includes several entities. Acute spasmodic croup is thought to be an allergy-equivalent condition seen in young children aged one to three years. After a day or two of mild coryzal symptoms, the child awakens in the middle of the night with severe apprehension, inspiratory dyspnea, and on expiration a metallic, barking cough characteristic of laryngeotracheitis. Often the cool night air encountered on the hectic ride to the hospital relieves most of the distress from respiratory embarrassment. As this is often a recurrent problem, the parents should be advised that a quiet walk with the child in the cool moist outside air or 15 minutes in a bathroom in which the steaming hot shower is running may be sufficient treatment.

Spasmodic croup must be differentiated from infectious croup (laryngeotracheobronchitis), which is usually due to parainfluenza virus types 1, 2, and 3. Differentiating characteristics of the latter include fever and other signs of systemic toxicity, the usually more significant prodromal period, and the more prolonged course of up to a week's duration. On physical examination there are signs of upper respiratory tract infection with rhinitis, pharyngitis, and bronchitis/bronchiolitis. Treatment consists primarily of humidification, especially at night.

Epiglottitis is an acute life-threatening emergency which can present with similar symptoms of upper respiratory obstruction. Usually seen in children three to seven years of age, but occasionally seen in older children and even adults, epiglottitis is most often due to *Hemophilus influenzae* type B. After a short period of mild prodrome in some children, there is the sudden onset of high fever, sore throat, and dyspnea, rapidly increasing in severity over a few hours or even minutes. Typically, the child sits forward, drooling and showing the effects of respiratory embarrassment, specifically inspiratory stridor, hoarseness (but not aphonia), a brassy cough, dysphagia, and when hypoxia occurs, irritability, agitation, and restlessness. It must be emphasized that any stimulation of the pharynx, such as by a tongue depressor or by an examining finger, may precipitate acute laryngospasm and sudden cardiorespiratory arrest in a hypoxic child. Pharyngeal examination in such an instance should be performed only when the means for immediate

TABLE 3 Drug Dosages in Asthma

DRUG	DOSE	ROUTE	COMMENT
Epinephrine	0.01 ml./kg. of 1:1000	Subcutaneously	May repeat up to three injections 15 minutes apart
Ethylnorepinephrine	0.02 ml./kg.	Subcutaneously	Very little cardiovascular effect, only bronchodilatation
Susphrine	0.005 ml./kg.	Subcutaneously	Immediate as well as prolonged effect
Aminophylline°	4 mg./kg. diluted in 50 to 100 cc. fluid	Intravenously	Bolus injection over 15 to 20 minutes; repeat in 6 hours
	4 to 6 mg./kg.	Orally	Effective orally in mild attacks; repeat every 4 to 6 hours
Sodium bicarbonate	2 to 4 mg./kg.	Intravenously	Initial bolus empiric; further doses determined by blood gas determinations

°Rectal administration not advised in children because of unpredictable absorption rate.

endotracheal intubation, oxygen administration, and intensive monitoring are available. Often, tracheotomy is required. Some recommend elective tracheotomy whenever the diagnosis is made unequivocally. Others suggest that nasotracheal intubation is an effective and safe alternative, with perhaps fewer complications when used for only two or three days. Blood cultures are positive in 75 to 90 per cent of cases; antibiotics for ampicillin-resistant *H. influenzae* should be given intravenously in large doses.

Bronchial and bronchiolar airway obstruction is due to a combination of contraction of the smooth muscle, edema of the mucous membrane, and increased secretions in the airway from the lining mucous membranes. The "final common pathway," leading to a decreased FEV_1 and wheezing, can be precipitated by infection, a foreign body, or the clinical syndrome asthma. In bronchiolitis, the signs of infection are present from at least the onset of respiratory symptoms; fever, rhinitis, and an age under two years suggest the diagnosis of viral bronchiolitis. The asthmatic child usually presents with the typical picture of wheezing, cough, air hunger, fatigue, and apprehension. The onset is usually abrupt, occasionally triggered by a recognized environmental (odors or fumes) or emotional (school exam, misdirected anger) stress, or certain viral upper respiratory tract diseases (see also Chapters 3 and 40).

ABNORMAL CARDIAC FUNCTION

In children cardiac disease is more often congenital rather than acquired. Congenital defects and complications or prematurity and immaturity account for most deaths in the first three months of life. One-half of the deaths due to congenital defects are due to cardiovascular defects; the incidence of such defects is approximately 0.8 per cent of live births. During the immediate postnatal period, significant changes in circulation takes place, completing the transition from a fetal to an adult functional pattern in the first few days of life. Almost immediately after birth, pulmonary vascular resistance begins to decrease markedly in response to an increase in PO_2 in the pulmonary arteries. As the ductus arteriosus and foramen ovale close functionally (anatomic closure may not occur until two to three months of life), there is less shunting of blood away from the lungs. It is during this time that specific cardiovascular defects dependent on the fetal pattern of blood shunting can precipitate problems in the infant.

HEART FAILURE

Heart failure in infants can produce symptoms and signs which superficially mimic other conditions. Weight loss, lethargy, and tachypnea may suggest an infectious process (bronchiolitis, meningitis) or a systemic metabolic problem (salicylism, renal tubular acidosis, chronic renal disease). Rales and low-grade fever could further support a pneumonitic process. Often an enlarged liver is overlooked in examination, or is attributed to depression of the diaphragms from primary respiratory disease. The combination of these findings with lethargy, poor feeding and poor weight gain, an ashen gray color or cyanosis, tachypnea and tachycardia, a gallop rhythm and enlarged heart on physical examination, and a chest x-ray demonstrating cardiomegaly support the diagnosis of heart failure. The pulmonary vasculature can be increased (patent ductus, transposition of the great vessels), normal (cardiomyopathy, coarctations of the aorta), or decreased (pulmonary atresia or stenosis, tetralogy of Fallot, pulmonary hypoplasia).

Physical examination, electrocardiogram, and a cardiac series x-ray examination are usually sufficient for the experienced clinician to make a probable diagnosis and institute appropriate therapy: oxygen, diuretics, morphine, and digitalis are the mainstays of therapy for heart failure due to any cause. Certain congenital cardiac defects demand immediate surgical intervention with the creation of a palliative shunt to prolong life (transposition of the great vessels, pulmonary atresia, tricuspid atresia).

ACUTE RHEUMATIC FEVER

The incidence of acute rheumatic fever is decreasing, but rheumatic heart disease is still by far the most common form of acquired heart disease in children. Sufficient numbers of studies demonstrating poor patient compliance in penicillin treatment of streptococcal infections would suggest that other factors, possibly better nutrition or alterations in the pathogenicity of the streptococcus, are responsible. Recommended treatment schedules for the prevention of acute rheumatic fever following streptococcal pharyngitis are as follows:

1. Benzathine penicillin G, 1,200,000 units intramuscularly.

2. Penicillin G, 200,000 units orally, three to four times a day for ten days. Attack rate of acute rheumatic fever after streptococcal infection is about 0.3 per cent in nonepidemic infections and up to 3 per cent in epidemics; after adequate treatment, the attack rate is approximately one-tenth these rates.

Presenting signs and symptoms of acute rheumatic fever are age-dependent. In young children, carditis with heart failure may be the initial manifestation; in school age children, migratory arthralgias or choreiform movements bring the patient to the physician's attention. The major and minor Jones' criteria for the diagnosis of acute rheumatic fever are listed in Table 4.

The physician's high index of suspicion for rheumatic fever when confronted with a child presenting with even minimally suggestive symptoms is the most important factor in making the diagnosis. Treatment consists of hospitalization, bed rest, sedatives, digitalis for heart failure, aspirin for the arthritis and fever, corticosteroids for the pancarditis, and penicillin at therapeutic levels for ten days followed by long-term daily prophylaxis.

A suggested schedule for digitalization of

TABLE 4 *Diagnostic Criteria for Acute Rheumatic Fever*

MAJOR MANIFESTATIONS	MINOR MANIFESTATIONS	SUPPORTING EVIDENCE OF STREPTOCOCCAL INFECTION	OTHER FINDINGS
Carditis	Fever	Recent scarlet fever	History of recent sore throat
Polyarthritis	Arthralgia*	Throat culture positive for group A streptococci	Family history of rheumatic fever
Chorea	Previous rheumatic fever or rheumatic heart disease	Increased ASO or other streptococcal antibodies	Abdominal pain Epistaxis
Erythema marginatum Subcutaneous nodules	Positive acute phase reactants: Increased erythrocyte sedimentation rate C-reactive protein Leukocytosis Prolonged P–R interval†		Tachycardia Rheumatic pneumonia Pallor and anemia Precordial pain Weight loss Malaise

*Should not be considered as a minor manifestation in patients in whom polyarthritis is the major manifestation.
†Should not be considered as a minor manifestation in patients in whom carditis is a major manifestation.
Source: Vaughan, V. C., and McKay, R. J. (eds.): Textbook of Pediatrics, 10th ed. Philadelphia, W. B. Saunders Co., 1975, p. 552.

TABLE 5   *Digitalization Schedule for Children*°

GROUP	TOTAL DOSE OF DIGOXIN (mg./kg.)	MAINTENANCE DOSE AS FRACTION OF DIGITALIZING DOSE
I Premature infants, neonates up to 2 weeks of age, infants with renal impairment or myocarditis	0.05 to 0.06	1/4
II Infants 2 weeks to 2 years of age	0.075	1/3
III Children 30 to 75 lb.	0.05–0.06	1/4 to 1/5
IV Children over 75 lb.	0.03–0.05	1/5

°Digitalization is accomplished after a baseline EKG by giving the total 24-hour dose in increments every 6 to 8 hours (1/2, 1/4, 1/4). Maintenance is given as one-half the total dose every 12 hours. Digoxin is available as an elixir in 50 ml. bottles containing 0.05 mg./ml.

children is given in Table 5. A summary of arrhythmias seen in children and their management is given in Table 6.

HEMATOLOGIC DISEASE

Anemia, neutropenia, and a bleeding diathesis due to thrombocytopenia or to a coagulation factor deficiency can all cause a life-threatening emergency. Neutropenia in children is rare except in those receiving antimetabolite chemotherapy for malignant disease. The risk of overwhelming septicemia increases dramatically as the total neutrophil count falls below 1000 per cu. mm.; in such a child, fever of any degree should be taken as a sign of sepsis and appropriate measures should be taken. Aplastic anemia, immune neutropenia, viral infections, leukemia, or drug exposure can all cause neutropenia. A particular form of superficial necrotic spreading skin ulcer called *ecthyma gangrenosum* is due to *Pseudo-monas* species and can occur in neutropenia patients.

ANEMIA

Life-threatening anemia is encountered rarely. Acute hemorrhage usually causes circulatory collapse from volume loss rather than there being any specific effects of anemia. The subacute development of anemia such as autoimmune hemolytic anemia, acute hemolysis in a G-6-PD–deficient patient or an aregenerative crisis in a child with any chronic hemolytic anemia (see discussion of sickle cell anemia later in this chapter) usually causes symptoms for a few days before high output heart failure develops. With a more indolent progression of anemia, as can be seen in children who develop severe iron deficiency anemia, no change in activity level or physical condition may be noted until the child presents with heart failure, develops pneumonia, or his hemoglobin level falls below 3 to 4 gm./dl.

TABLE 6   *Causes and Treatment of Arrhythmias Most Often Seen in Children*

ARRHYTHMIA	CAUSE	TREATMENT
Sinus arrhythmia	Physiologic	None; may require EKG to verify diagnosis
Extrasystoles	Drugs (digitalis, sympathomimetics, xanthines)	Change drug dosage
Paroxysmal atrial tachycardia	? infection; may *cause* chronic heart failure	Vagal stimulation (carotid or eyeball pressure), digitalis
Ventricular tachycardia (rare)	Myocarditis, post cardiac surgery	Electroconversion; lidocaine, quinidine
Atrial flutter	Myocarditis, infections, post cardiac surgery	Digitalis; then quinidine
Atrial fibrillation	Rheumatic heart disease, congenital heart disease	Digitalis, then quinidine

Rapid correction of severe anemia in a child can also precipitate heart failure, from fluid overload; partial exchange transfusion, administration of rapid acting diuretics intravenously just prior to transfusion (furosemide, 1 mg./kg.) and correcting anemia in step-wise fashion (up to 5 or 6 gm./dl. first day, 8 gm./dl. second day, 11 gm./dl. if necessary on the third day) may prevent this complication. Except for volume replacement in acute hemorrhage, cross-matched and fully prepared packed red blood cells only are proper to treat anemia when transfusion is indicated. The volume of packed red blood cells to give should be calculated by the formula: 4 × patient's weight (kg.) × desired change in hemoglobin concentration. Generally, a transfusion is indicated in a self-limited anemia correctable only to treat frank or incipient heart failure; it is rarely indicated in nondeficiency anemia. In the presence of any anemia, an assessment of responsive reticulocytosis and a platelet and white blood cell count are indicated to rule out aplastic anemia of the bone marrow.

Except following trauma or surgery, children with a congenital or acquired bleeding diathesis do not exhibit life-threatening symptoms. Children with a rare severe coagulation factor deficiency or abnormal platelet count or function can suffer serious hemorrhage with trauma. A carefully taken family and personal history will be indicative of a bleeding problem in over half the cases; a prothrombin time, partial thromboplastin time, and Ivy bleeding time (a physiologic test for adequate platelet count and function) will screen for almost every hemorrhagic disorder likely to cause a problem.

In dealing with uncontrollable hemorrhage, local factors causing prolonged bleeding must be recognized and treated first. After volume replacement, if necessary, to prevent or delay shock has been given, 7 ml./kg. of fresh, frozen, type-specific plasma can be given in an unknown bleeding diathesis to correct any deficit or coagulation factors to above symptomatic levels. For less serious bleeding, such as soft tissue hematomas and hemarthroses in children with known deficiency, specific preparations can be given according to the recommended schedules of administration.

THROMBOCYTOPENIA

Idiopathic (autoimmune) thrombocytopenic purpura is the most common cause of symptomatic thrombocytopenia seen in children. It is generally a well-tolerated, self-limited disease; most children recover spontaneously in a few months. The presentation is usually the acute development of cutaneous bleeding, petechiae and ecchymosis, often mucous membrane bleeding and epistaxis in an otherwise well child. Diagnosis is made by excluding other causes of thrombocytopenia, specifically drug or live virus vaccine exposure and marrow failure or replacement.

Most serious bleeding normally occurs in the first few days of the disease; corticosteroids may have a therapeutic role in the treatment of serious bleeding manifestations but are not indicated on a routine basis. Platelet transfusions are not very effective because they too are affected by the circulating antibodies that cause the thrombocytopenia. Life-threatening hemorrhage, such as intracranial bleeding, is an indication for immediate splenectomy which removes a major site of antibody production and the site where "sensitized" platelets are removed from circulation. Most children will demonstrate an immediate rise in platelet count postoperatively. Other forms of thrombocytopenia may respond well to platelet transfusions, one unit of platelet concentrate per 5 kg. of body weight.

SICKLE CELL ANEMIA

The patient with *sickle cell anemia*, whether homozygous (SS), hemoglobin S-C, or hemoglobin S-thalassemia, can present a life-threatening emergency in several ways. Specific organ involvement, such as pulmonary infection or infarction, or sudden large vessel cerebrovascular occlusion can create problems of significant consequence. An unusual complication seen in young children and in pregnant women with sickle cell anemia is a sequestration crisis. For unknown reasons, the red blood cells suddenly become sequestered in the spleen or liver, causing severe anemia, massive splenomegaly (or hepatomegaly), and shock within minutes or a few hours. Immediate simple transfusion or exchange transfusion with nonsickling packed red blood cells is required.

Splenic hypofunction, even in the presence of palpable splenomegaly, can predispose a patient with sickle cell anemia to sudden overwhelming sepsis, with all the associated complications. *Streptococcus pneumoniae* is most often involved; staphylococcus, *Hemophilus influenzae*, and *Salmonella* may also be responsible. Fever and signs of infection in a child with sickle cell anemia must be considered potentially lethal, and antibiotics should be used with perhaps less restraint than in immunologically competent patients.

Sudden severe anemia with impending high output heart failure can occur in patients with sickle cell disease from a hyperhemolytic crisis and from an aregenerative crisis; transient marrow failure can be associated with drugs, infection, or platelet deficiency. These complications usually are short-lived and correctable; transfusion may be required.

SEIZURES

Although the causes of generalized seizures in children are varied, the commonest cause by far is the simple febrile convulsion due to elevated body temperature. Characteristics of such benign generalized seizures are their association with extracranial febrile illness, occasionally familial incidence, peak occurrence between ages six months and four years (although children up to age five or six can develop such a seizure), and a short duration generally of less than five minutes. It is necessary to determine that the site of infection is not the central nervous system; many advocate routine examination of the cerebrospinal fluid in all children presenting with their first febrile convulsion. Treatment, after the convulsion stops, consists of simply treating the underlying cause of fever, lowering the body temperature (salicylates, acetaminophen, and sponging with tepid water), and one intramuscular dose of phenobarbital, 3 to 5 mg/kg. Occasionally, children will have a second short convulsion within 12 to 24 hours. An underlying convulsive disorder, precipitated by fever, should be suspected if the seizure lasts longer than 10 minutes, has any atypical features such as lateralizing signs, or is the third or fourth such episode. An electroencephalogram should be obtained in all children who have a febrile convulsion at least one week after the seizure. On the basis of these evaluations, daily maintenance anticonvulsant therapy may be necessary. Intermittent oral phenobarbital given to prevent a seizure concomitant with subsequent episodes of fever should not be effective, since therapeutic serum concentrations (10 to 20 mg./liter) are achieved only after several days or weeks of administration. It is important to stress that the normal child with an uncomplicated febrile convulsion has little likelihood of developing recurrent nonfebrile seizures or brain damage, as parents may anticipate the worst.

Recurrent and nonfebrile seizures rarely present any life-threatening risk as long as certain precautions are observed. During the acute convulsive episode, an adequate airway must be maintained. Loosen the clothing around the child's neck, turn him on his side so that oral secretions can drain, minimize unnecessary stimulation and give oxygen by mask if the convulsion is of long duration. Do not attempt to place any object in his mouth, even a plastic airway, as these may cause more local trauma and may obstruct the patient's breathing. The only other precaution necessary is to protect the patient from harming himself, as he might if he fell off the examining bed or litter. Oxygen administration by mask may be required in prolonged seizures.

A drug regimen recommended to treat status epilepticus consists of up to three intramuscular injections of phenobarbital, 5 to 6 mg./kg. (up to 200 mg. per dose), separated by 15 minute periods. The endpoint of treatment is a cessation of generalized convulsion; twitching or intermittent contractions of one or two muscle groups after a severe convulsion does not require further therapy. If a total of 15 mg./kg. over 45 to 60 minutes is ineffective, diazepam can be given by slow intravenous titration (no faster than 1 mg. per minute by use of a 2 to 3 cc. syringe). Usually, less than 5 mg. (2.5 cc.) is required. The major hazard is that intravenous diazepam can precipitate sudden respiratory arrest, especially in combination with phenobarbital.

In an occasional child, hypocalcemia, hypoglycemia, pyridoxine dependency, uremia, hypertension, or metabolic encephalopathy (Reye's syndrome, lead intoxication, electrolyte disturbance) can precipitate a generalized convulsion. These conditions may or may not be suggested by the clinical evaluation, and appropriate evaluations would be indicated.

DEHYDRATION

In the normal state of homeostasis, there is a balance between intake and loss of water and electrolytes maintained by specific regulatory mechanisms. When losses exceed intake and exceed the ability of the body to compensate for these losses, the deficit which develops can produce serious consequences. Children are more prone to dehydration than adults for many reasons. Their ratio of surface area to body weight is greater, leading to greater irreversible losses through the skin. They are more susceptible to viral illnesses, many of which cause increased losses through diarrhea and vomiting. The compensatory mechanisms of adults, primarily pulmonary and renal, can handle a wider range of variation in volumes of fluids and amounts of electrolytes. The more rapid development and progression of dehydration in children makes its recognition and treatment critical, as it is potentially a life-threatening emergency.

Most increased losses consist of hypotonic fluids; a relative excess deficit of water over electrolytes develops in the patient. However, the resulting state is dependent not only on the quantity and quality of the losses but also on the nature of the concomitant intake. Boiled milk formula given to a baby with diarrhea is likely to cause a hypernatremic dehydration, whereas plain water (or other nonelectrolyte solution) re-placement is likely to cause a hyponatremic dehydration. The three types of dehydration differ in their pathogenesis, in the physical findings in the patient, and in the recommended treatment: by definition, isotonic dehydration is isonatremic, with serum sodium between 130 and 150 mEq./liter; hypotonic (hyponatremic) if serum sodium is lower; and hypertonic (hypernatremic) if serum sodium is higher than 150 mEq./liter.

To determine the magnitude and type of deficit a patient is suffering, it is necessary to know the duration of illness, the kind and amount of intake during this period, the nature and amount of his abnormal losses, his weight changes, the presence of any underlying renal, pulmonary, or central nervous system disease, and any drugs that were taken during this time. The amount of body weight loss acutely is the best indication of the magnitude of the water losses. Out of the infancy age period, a 3 per cent weight loss represents mild dehydration, 6 per cent loss is considered moderate, and 9 per cent or more severe. In infants, a larger percentage of the body weight is extracellular fluid, so a 5 per cent weight loss would represent mild dehydration, 5 to 10 per cent moderate dehydration, and above 10 per cent severe dehydration.

In *isotonic* dehydration, losses of water are almost exclusively from the extracellular compartment with fairly well maintained intracellular water. In *hypertonic* dehydra-

TABLE 7   Clinical Findings of Dehydration

	ISONATREMIC DEHYDRATION (PROPORTIONATE LOSS OF WATER AND SODIUM)	HYPONATREMIC DEHYDRATION (LOSS OF SODIUM IN EXCESS OF WATER)	HYPERNATREMIC DEHYDRATION (LOSS OF WATER IN EXCESS OF SODIUM)
ECF volume	Marked decrease	Severely decreased	Decreased
ICF volume	Maintained	Increased	Decreased
Skin			
Color	Gray	Gray	Gray
Temperature	Cold	Cold	Cold or hot
Turgor°	Poor	Very poor	Fair
Feel	Dry	Clammy	Thickened
Mucous membrane	Dry	Slightly moist	Parched†
Eyeball	Sunken and soft	Sunken and soft	Sunken
Fontanel	Sunken	Sunken	Sunken
Psyche	Lethargic	Coma	Hyperirritable
Pulse	Rapid	Rapid	Moderately rapid
Blood pressure°°	Low	Very low	Moderately low

°Reflects magnitude of fluid loss from ECF.
†Tongue often has shriveled appearance due to loss of cellular fluid.
°°Signs of shock rather than of dehydration itself.
Source: Vaughan, V. C., and McKay, R. J. (eds.): Textbook of Pediatrics, 10th ed. Philadelphia, W. B. Saunders Co., 1975, p. 255.

tion, there are approximately equal losses from both compartments; intracellular fluid shifts out of the cells to maintain the intravascular volume. In *hypotonic* dehydration, fluid shifts from the extracellular (intravascular space) compartment to the intracellular compartment, leading to poor maintenance of intravascular volume and the *earlier onset of shock*. Documentation of weight loss gives the most accurate assessment of degree of water deficit; Table 7 lists clinical findings of dehydration.

Therapy for dehydration consists of supplying the required maintenance fluids and electrolytes and correcting the deficits. Because of impending shock from volume depletion, it is often necessary to begin fluid replacement before the initial blood electrolyte determinations are completed. A solution containing 5 per cent dextrose and 0.9 per cent sodium chloride can be given as a bolus of 20 ml./kg. over 15 minutes to reverse impending circulatory collapse. In all forms of dehydration, the fluid given should contain sodium in a concentration between 0.3 and 0.9 per cent; regardless of the patient's serum sodium, such a fluid will begin to correct the abnormality toward isonatremia. Under no circumstances should a child beyond infancy be given intravenous fluids that do not have sodium, as seizures from water intoxication can quickly result. Various balanced salt solutions containing lactate, bicarbonate, and other electrolytes in addition to sodium chloride have been used effectively as initial therapy; potassium supplements should be withheld until renal function is demonstrated. Hyponatremic and isotonic dehydration can be easily corrected within 24 to 36 hours; hypernatremic dehydration is treated over a two- to three-day period because of the risk of convulsions if the serum sodium is decreased rapidly.

INFECTIONS

Beyond early infancy, except in unusual cases of immune deficit, the biology of infectious agents in children is essentially the same as that in adults. Infections can, however, cause greater morbidity and mortality in children for several reasons. The spectrum of potentially infectious agents in children is broader than in adults; organisms responsible for many of the viral and bacterial diseases experienced in childhood elicit

TABLE 8   Common Infectious Agents

INFECTION	AGE	PREDOMINANT ORGANISM
Pneumonia	<2 years	Respiratory syncytial virus *Hemophilus influenzae* (*Staphylococcus aureus*)
	>2 years	Pneumococcus *Mycoplasma pneumoniae* Viruses
Bacterial meningitis	Neonatal	Enteric organisms
	>8 years	*Hemophilus influenzae* Pneumococcus (*Neisseria meningitidis*)
	8 years to adult	*Neisseria meningitidis* Pneumococcus
Otitis media	<8 years	Respiratory virus Pneumococcus *Hemophilus influenzae*
	>8 years	Pneumococcus Respiratory virus
Enteritis	<2 years	Virus Enteropathogenic *E. coli*
	>2 years	Virus *Salmonella* sp. *Shigella* sp.

the production of protective antibodies so that only the first encounter with that organism is likely to cause illness. For this and other not fully understood reasons, organisms likely to cause a particular disease differ at different ages (see Table 8).

PNEUMONIA

Pneumonia in young children generally causes more significant respiratory embarrassment than it does in adults. In many cases, pneumonia in a child under four years of age can be diagnosed with fair accuracy by inspection: tachypnea, intercostal and subcostal retractions, use of accessory muscles of respiration, a thick nasal discharge, vomiting, fever, irritability, and prolonged expiration with wheezing may be observed before physical examination and x-rays verify the diagnosis. In older children, the symptoms and signs are likely to be more specifically referrable to the lower respiratory tract, although children often complain primarily of abdominal pain in pneumonia. The response of a child to this infection varies mainly with the organism involved but also with numerous environmental and constitutional factors—acute and chronic nutritional state, age, associated disease, ambient temperature, and how quickly the parent recognizes illness and seeks medical attention. "Pneumonia" is a clinical diagnosis in children, not an x-ray diagnosis, as the typical progression of roentgenographic changes may lag behind the progression of the disease by several days: often, only overexpansion of the lung fields is appreciated on x-ray when the diagnosis of pneumonia is made.

Whether a child requires hospitalization for pneumonia should be determined on an individual clinical basis rather than by rigid guidelines. The following criteria could be used:

1. What degree of respiratory embarrassment exists now or is likely to develop? The presence of any complication such as pneumothorax or significant pleural fluid, or the question of blood gas determinations being necessary implies hospital care is required.

2. What is the likely etiologic agent and what is the course of pneumonia due to that organism? Rapid defervescence of fever and symptoms is expected following penicillin treatment of streptococcal pneumonia infection, but interstitial pneumonia due to respiratory syncytial virus is likely to run a 5- to 10-day course.

3. How well can the child maintain a state of good hydration in view of the expected increased insensible losses from hyperpnea and tachypnea and decreased intake? Will vomiting, anorexia, or just the ventilatory effort interfere with adequate fluid intake?

4. Are there any underlying diseases present which might increase the morbidity or consequences of pneumonia, such as anemia or heart disease?

5. How reliable and capable will the parents be in carrying out the recommended therapies? How well are the parents able to accept this responsibility?

Pneumonia in infants and young children is often viral in etiology, with respiratory syncytial virus playing a predominant role in bronchitis and bronchiolitis as well as pneumonia. Influenza virus, during epidemics in a community, can cause a pneumonic process in young children which may develop into obliterative bronchiolitis and chronic pulmonary disease. Staphylococcal pneumonia is a serious form of pneumonia that can occur in infants as a primary infection, secondary to staphylococcal abscesses elsewhere, or secondary to measles, varicella, or other types of viral pneumonia. Symptoms usually are severe and progress rapidly with marked respiratory embarrassment. Pneumatocele formation occurs with progression of the disease, and complications such as empyema, abscess formation, and pneumothorax may delay the resolution of the disease for several months. Measurement of the white blood cell count and differential blood cell count may help determine the etiology of pneumonia; if the total white blood cell count is more than 10,000 per cu. mm. or if the total number of immature polymorphonuclear leukocytes is greater than 500 per cu. mm., bacterial disease is more likely.

Treatment of pneumonia in children may include appropriate antibiotics, adequate fluid administration, antipyretics, postural drainage, and respiratory support when necessary.

MENINGITIS

Meningitis can be a rapidly progressing infection, causing death within hours of onset. Although there is usually a prodrome of a respiratory illness, signs of meningeal irritation (convulsion, irritability, vomiting, headache, stiff neck) frequently develop suddenly and progress rapidly to stupor, coma, shock, and death. The classical physical signs of meningeal irritation are not sensitive enough to be reliable in young children; the younger the child, the more liberal must be the criteria for performing a diagnostic lumbar puncture. Examination of the cerebrospinal fluid must include cell count and differential, Gram stain of centrifuged sediment, and determination of sugar and protein content. *Diplococcus pneumoniae* particularly may be present in the spinal fluid in large numbers before the expected neutrophil response occurs.

ACUTE OTITIS MEDIA

Criteria for diagnosing acute purulent otitis media lack selectivity and reliability. When one sees a bright red, bulging, painful tympanic membrane in a febrile child, there is rarely a doubt of otitis media. When one sees distortion of the normal landmarks or some injection of the tympanic membrane, pneumatoscopy may help verify the presence of fluid in the middle ear. Pain in the ear is not a reliable sign of purulent otitis; con-

TABLE 9   *Etiology of Acute Otitis Media—Based on Culture of Middle Ear Aspirates*

NEONATAL PERIOD	UNDER EIGHT YEARS OF AGE	OVER EIGHT YEARS OF AGE

E. coli
Other gram-negative
   organisms
Staphylococcus aureus
	Viral?
	Diplococcus pneumoniae,
	   25–50%
	Hemophilus influenzae,
	   15–25%
	Streptococcus, 5%
	Others—*Neisseria catarrhalis*,
	   Mycoplasma pneumoniae,
	   Staphylococcus sp.
		Viral?
		Diplococcus pneumoniae,
		   50–75%
		Hemophilus influenzae,
		   5%
		Streptococcus, 25%
		Others

versely, perhaps one-third to one-half of children with otitis do not have significant fever. The color of the tympanic membrane does not correlate well with the presence or absence of infection; gray or yellow-white eardrums often are associated with infection. The most sensitive sign may be distortion of the tympanic membrane, but even this is not highly specific. Unless tympanocentesis is performed, one must use clinical experience as the basis for judging whether acute otitis media is present, the most likely organism, and the antibiotic that is indicated (see Table 9).

Oral sympathomimetic decongestants may offer symptomatic relief, but the incidence of a persistent mucoid or serous middle ear fluid collection probably is not changed by adding a decongestant to the treatment. Antihistamines are not effective in the acute episode. Since severe pain in the ear is often the chief complaint, a strong analgesic such as codeine (0.5 to 1.0 mg./kg.) up to 15 mg. every six hours may be helpful for 24 to 48 hours.

References

Eichenwald, H. F.: Pneumonia syndromes in children. Hosp. Pract. Vol. 89, May 1976.

Graef, J. W., and Cone, T. E. (eds.): Manual of Pediatric Therapeutics. Boston, Little, Brown and Co., 1974.

Grosfeld, J. L. (ed.): Symposium on childhood trauma. Pediatr. Clin. North Am. 22(2): 267–514, May 1975.

Gruskin, A. B.: Fluid therapy in children. Urol. Clin. North Am. 3(2):277, 1976.

McCarthy, P. L., Jekel, J. F., and Dolan, T. F.: Temperature greater than or equal to 40° C. in children less than 24 months of age: a prospective study. Pediatrics 59:663, 1977.

McMillan, J. A., Nieburg, P. I., and Oski, F. A.: The Whole Pediatrician Catalog. Philadelphia, W. B. Saunders Co., 1977.

Rowe, D. S.: Acute suppurative otitis media. Pediatrics 56:285, 1975.

Smith, Clement A. (ed.): The Critically Ill Child—Diagnosis and Management, 2nd ed. Philadelphia, W. B. Saunders Co., 1977.

Vaughan, V. C., and McKay, R. J. (eds.): Nelson Textbook of Pediatrics, 10th ed. Philadelphia, W. B. Saunders Co., 1975.

Wolf, S. M., et al.: The value of phenobarbital in the child who has had a single febrile seizure: a controlled prospective study. Pediatrics 59:378, 1977.

Wright, F. H., and Beem, M. O.: Diagnosis and treatment: management of acute viral bronchiolitis in infancy. Pediatrics 35:334, 1965.

Part IV

EMERGENCY
MEDICAL SYSTEMS

Chapter 60   EMS IN PERSPECTIVE

Blair L. Sadler, Alfred M. Sadler, Jr.,
and Samuel B. Webb, Jr.

THE PAST DECADE

As recently as ten years ago, emergency medical services (EMS) was a neglected area of health care. Many ambulance services were run by funeral homes and most services were staffed by inadequately trained personnel. Hospital emergency rooms were often understaffed, poorly organized, and often committed to a substitutive function of providing general medical care in the community.

And yet, EMS is one of the most widely discussed health topics in the United States today. This is not surprising, since heart attacks and accidents are two of the country's major killers, and it is widely believed that prompt quality emergency medical care could save many lives and reduce the severity of many injuries.

More fundamentally, in most parts of the country, no one had assumed clear-cut responsibility for EMS as such. Unlike police and fire services with high visibility, strong national organizations, and a position of prominence at state and local levels, ambulance services were often neglected and ignored. Unlike the development of sophisticated techniques and systems of managing certain specialized health care problems, emergency medicine was not given a priority by the nation's medical schools. Little research was being done, and many young Americans were receiving an M.D. degree without having been taught the basics of

emergency medicine. Small wonder that many physicians felt ill equipped to respond to emergencies in such common instances as the roadside accident.

THE MAGNITUDE OF THE PROBLEM

U.S. national statistics underscore the magnitude of EMS needs. For example, accidents are the leading cause of death between the ages of 1 and 37 and the fourth leading cause of death at all ages. Among accidental deaths, those due to motor vehicles constitute the leading cause for all age groups under 75 (U.S. Department of Health, Education and Welfare). Trauma patients use more hospital days than all heart patients or obstetrical patients and more than four times as many hospital days as all cancer patients. Studies suggest that mortality from vehicular accidents alone could be reduced by 15 to 20 per cent by proper medical care at the scene of the accident or en route to an emergency facility—a saving nationally of approximately 11,000 lives (Frey et al., 1969).

It is also estimated that from 5 to 20 per cent of the 700,000 deaths resulting annually from heart disease—the leading cause of death at all ages—might be prevented if the public were educated to recognize the symptoms of heart attacks and if comprehensive EMS systems were available throughout the nation (Cretin, 1974). Similarly, 5000 deaths each year from other causes such as poisoning, drownings, and drug overdoses might be prevented by immediate medical attention. These are merely some of the major problems that require effective emergency medical response and illustrate the potential value of a good EMS system.

The content of this chapter is developed in greater detail in *Emergency Medical Care: The Neglected Public Service*, by A. M. Sadler, B. L. Sadler, and S. B. Webb, Jr., published by the Ballinger Publishing Co., 1977.

THE EMERGING NATIONAL INTEREST IN EMS

During the past five years a number of well-established organizations have intensified their efforts in the area of emergency services as professional and public interest in emergency care has increased. These organizations include the American College of Surgeons, the American Health Association, the National Safety Council, the American Academy of Orthopedic Surgeons, the American Medical Association, and the American Hospital Association. The Joint Commission on Accreditation of Hospitals has established new standards for emergency department accreditation. Many community colleges and junior colleges have become involved in the training of emergency medical technicians and other emergency medical personnel. Medical and nursing schools are giving greater attention to clinical emergency care problems, while emergency care organization, financing, and evaluation issues are receiving increasing recognition as legitimate topics for health services research.

Several new organizations have been formed to address the emergency care problem. These include the American Trauma Society, the Emergency Department Nurses' Association, the American College of Emergency Physicians, the Society for Critical Care Medicine, the University Association for Emergency Medical Services, and the Society for Total Emergency Preparedness. Although each organization is concerned with different phases of emergency care, each has helped to raise the level of public awareness and concern about EMS—which is being translated into local action. Communities are establishing emergency medical councils and in some places are recognizing emergency medical care as the third public emergency service (along with police and fire services), deserving of public support and standards of quality control.

THE INITIAL FEDERAL ROLE AND THE U.S. DEPARTMENT OF TRANSPORTATION INITIATIVE

With one exception, federal and state governmental agencies did not keep pace with the efforts of professional and lay organizations to improve emergency medical

services. Throughout most of the 1960s, the Division of Emergency Health Services was the only office within the Department of Health, Education, and Welfare (DHEW) that was identified as having responsibility for improving emergency health services. This office operated with limited funding and authority. Through economic necessity, and no doubt under direction from higher governmental echelons, it focused its attention mostly on disaster preparedness and information dissemination.

The first significant evidence of congressional concern about EMS was the enactment of the National Highway Safety Act of 1966. This act authorized the U.S. Department of Transportation (DOT) to set guidelines for EMS. Under standard 11 of the law, DOT has provided funds for the purchase of ambulances and equipment, the installation of communications systems, the development and widespread support of emergency medical technician training programs, and the development of statewide EMS plans.

Under this law, federal funds have been allocated to each state on a block-grant basis and are matched by state resources. Funds are distributed through each governor's "highway safety representative" (on a largely unpublished basis) for each of 16 approved highway safety standards. Since, in some states, other standards have received greater priority than the EMS standard 11, few DOT dollars went into improved EMS. In other states, however, EMS has been given priority and sizable DOT funds have been allocated to this area.

Undoubtedly, the most widely known result of the DOT programs has been the development of a new health professional—the emergency medical technician–ambulance (EMT). With contributions of several national organizations, including the National Academy of Sciences (NAS), a specially designed 81-hour course was developed to teach emergency care fundamentals. A graduate of the course is designated an EMT-1, and in recent years, this has become widely accepted as the minimum level of training for persons treating patients at the emergency scene or en route to a hosptial via ambulance (NRC report, 1972).

The growth of the EMT training has been impressive. As of 1976, DOT estimates that 146,500 individuals have been trained as EMTs in all states. This now constitutes 60 per cent of the 258,000 ambulance attendants that need training.* A 20-hour refresher course has also been developed and is now used widely. DOT standards suggest that EMTs take the refresher course at least every two years.

DOT continues to support training programs as well as the purchase of vehicles and equipment, although their total EMS funds have decreased as HEW's role has increased. DOT has supported the NAS in developing national standards for the EMT through a national registry that is giving a certification examination, and in developing training guidelines for the advanced EMT (EMT-II). The EMT-II is trained to perform cardiac defibrillation, read electrocardiograms at the emergency scene, administer certain drugs, and perform other advanced life-saving procedures under the remote supervision of a physician. DOT estimates that between 8,000 and 10,000 individuals have completed some type of EMT-II (paramedic) training. DOT also continues to support the Military Assistance in Safety and Traffic (MAST) program designed to use helicopters in EMS settings.

THE INITIAL DHEW EFFORT — FIVE "DEMONSTRATION" PROJECTS

In 1972 the Health Services and Mental Health Administration (HSMHA) was designated the lead agency for EMS within DHEW and a program to develop five "total EMS systems" was launched. In June 1972, contracts totaling $16 million were awarded to five areas: the State of Arkansas, a three-county area of southern California (San Diego), a seven-county area of northeastern Florida (Jacksonville), the State of Illinois, and a seven-county area in southeastern Ohio (Athens).

As stated by DHEW official John S. Zapp, the "purpose of the EMS demonstration projects is not primarily to provide improved emergency services to the citizens of the respective areas, although this may be an important ancillary effect. The primary purpose is to develop and demonstrate various approaches to providing emergency

medical care in a systematic and comprehensive manner so that other states and communities can look to these experiences in developing EMS systems for their citizens."

One common thread running through these demonstration efforts was the emphasis on a regional approach to improving emergency medical care. It was becoming increasingly accepted that all communities and hospitals could not provide comprehensive EMS, and that our society could not afford unnecessary competition and duplication of effort. The emphasis on shared resources and a regional approach to emergency care provided the basis upon which two recent national efforts in emergency care have been launched: The Robert Wood Johnson Foundation Program and the Emergency Medical Services Systems Act of 1973.

REGIONALIZATION — THE ROBERT WOOD JOHNSON FOUNDATION PROGRAM

Based on the experiences of the demonstration projects and being cognizant of the growing national interest in EMS, the Robert Wood Johnson Foundation decided to make a major commitment to the field of EMS in the summer of 1972. The foundation's focus was on the point of public access to emergency medical care. The foundation recognized that in most parts of the country citizens had no easily identifiable place to call when they needed emergency medical assistance. Furthermore, in those few places where a well-publicized emergency medical number existed, the person receiving the call seldom was trained to deal directly with a request for such help. Even with trained dispatch personnel, the necessary assistance was often not readily mobilized because of ineffectual communication among the available emergency response agencies (ambulance, police, fire department, and hospitals).

It was further evident that in areas where communications systems did exist, many were hampered by political struggles and jurisdictional boundaries that prevented a patient from being taken to the most appropriate center for care. The foundation concluded that emergency medical care could be strengthened through regionally based communications systems that integrated an area's emergency care resources into a comprehensive network of services.

---

*Robert Motley, National Highway Traffic Safety Program, Department of Transportation, June 1976 (personal communication).

Thus, on April 9, 1973, $15 million was authorized for a nationwide program to encourage communities to develop regional emergency medical response systems based around easily identified, visible access points.* Forty-four regions were designated for grant support of up to $400,000 each in 32 states and Puerto Rico.

The grant program, which ended in late 1977, should yield considerable information concerning the problems of organizing regional systems of emergency care. This information should be relevant to the implementation of the national planning legislation and other health planning. Certain aspects of the program, particularly those related to regionalization, have been analyzed by the Rand Corporation, which will publish the conclusions of its independent analysis in 1978.

REGIONALIZATION – THE EMERGENCY MEDICAL SERVICES SYSTEMS ACT OF 1973

Public Law 93-154 was signed by the President on November 4, 1973. The purpose of the legislation is to provide incentives to appropriate units of government to inventory their resources for providing comprehensive EMS, to identify the gaps in such services, to remedy these deficiencies through better coordination and utilization of existing resources, and to develop the new components essential to the achievement of an integrated, comprehensive area EMS system.

The Law, which authorized $185 million over three years, provides funds for "feasibility projects" (Section 1202), "establishment and initial operations of systems" (Section 1203), and "expansion and improvement" of systems (Section 1204). The Law requires that 314 (a) and (b) agencies (Comprehensive Health Planning) have an opportunity to review and comment on all applications.

The legislation seeks to integrate the following 15 elements into regional EMS systems: manpower, training, communications, transportation, facilities, critical care units, public safety agencies, consumer participation, accessibility to care, transfer of

patients, standardized patient record keeping, public information and education, independent review and evaluation, disaster linkages, and mutual aid agreements. The Division of Emergency Medical Services in HEW has divided the country into approximately 300 EMS regions. Over a quarter of the country has received federal support under the Law for developing basic life support regional EMS systems.

THE INCREASING STATE ROLE IN EMS

Concurrent with the major foundation and federal efforts in emergency care has been the growth of interest and commitment at the state level. In no area is this more dramatically demonstrated than in the widespread enactment of state legislation relating to EMS during the past several years.

According to the National Emergency Medical Services Information Clearinghouse (NEMSIC) at the University of Pennsylvania, 21 states have adopted "comprehensive" emergency medical services legislation in the past five years. Typically, these laws include the creation or expansion of a state division of EMS (usually under its department of health), with licensing and standard-setting authority, and authorization for state or regional EMS councils to develop EMS plans and provide continuing advice. Many also include development of a state EMS communications plan, authorization for incorporated cities or counties to contract for or operate ambulance services, and authority to categorize hospital emergency departments.

Several other states have limited their legislation to ambulance services. These usually include minimum standards relating to training of ambulance personnel, types of equipment and vehicles, and some requirements regarding licensure of ambulance providers. Other laws provide exemption for physicians, nurses and EMTs from civil liability, and modify licensure provisions to permit advanced EMTs to function up to their level of training at the emergency scene if they are acting under physician supervision and control.* In addition to increased

---

*Dr. David Rogers, president of the foundation, and Dr. Philip Handler, president of the NAS, jointly announced the program.

*Other states have passed laws to implement Standard 11 of the Highway Safety Act of 1966. Understandably, this legislation tends to focus less on comprehensive EMS systems and more on driver education, alcohol abuse education and prevention, elimination of road hazards, and other highway-related programs.

legislative activity, several states have begun to appropriate more funds for EMS.

REGIONALIZED EMS COMMUNICATIONS AND FCC DOCKET #19880

The importance of communications as the link to bring all the various components of an EMS system together has long been recognized, but until recently, the nation's communications capability was not up to the task. In 1967 the President's Commission on Law Enforcement and Administration of Justice recommended that a single number be established for reporting police emergencies, and in 1968, the American Telephone and Telegraph Company announced that it would make the digits 911 available for national implementation. As interest in 911 developed, it became clear that the number could be used for fire and medical emergencies as well. In March 1973, Clay T. Whitehead, Director of the Office of Telecommunications Policy in the Executive Office of the President, issued a national policy statement, (Bulletin 73-1) which recognized the benefits of 911 and encouraged its nationwide adoption.

In November 1973, the Office of Telecommunications Policy submitted a detailed study of emergency medical communications to the FCC. The report ("Communications in Support of Emergency Medical Services") contained many detailed recommendations for changing the FCC rules. The most fundamental recommendation was that the FCC establish a medical services category in the "special emergency radio service." The study, which was carried out by the Interdepartment Radio Advisory Committee, became known as the IRAC Report.

The OTP report and comments on it from over 200 sources led to the adoption of Docket #19880 by the FCC in July 1974. New FCC rules provide for a medical services category, expand the licensure eligibility provisions, make available several additional UHF frequencies (both for dispatch and telemetry), and augment VHF capability. The rules support the development of coordinated, "area-wide" EMS communications systems and the establishment of central dispatch and control centers.

The DHEW program guidelines issued in support of the Emergency Medical Services Systems Act of 1973 support the position taken in Docket #19880. The DHEW regulations state:

the system should include a system command and control center which would be responsible for establishing those communication channels and allocating those public resources essential to the most effective and efficient EMS management of the immediate problem.... The essentials of such a command and control center are that (a) all requests for system response are directed to the center; (b) all system resource response is directed from the center; and (c) all system liaison with other public safety and emergency response systems is coordinated from the center.

Thus, not only has FCC Docket #19880 made available the needed additional UHF and VHF frequencies, but it enhances the development of regional emergency medical response systems as advocated in the Robert Wood Johnson Foundation and DHEW programs.

PHYSICIANS SPECIALIZATION

There has also been growing physician interest in emergency medical care. This is evidenced in the increasing leadership of many physicians in organizing and developing EMS systems, and by others in the full-time practice of emergency medicine. It is reflected by the growth of the American College of Emergency Physicians established in 1968 and by the recent development of residency programs in emergency medicine.

In 1975, the American Medical Association's House of Delegates recommended to their Council on Medical Education (CME) that emergency medicine emerge as a new specialty with accreditation and certification comparable to other specialty areas. In 1976, the American College of Emergency Physicians and the University Association of Emergency Medical Services jointly filed a formal request to the AMA's CME and the American Board of Medical Specialties (ABMS) for such recognition, and this is being considered by the Liaison Committee on Specialty Boards (a joint committee of the AMA's CME and the ABMS). As of 1978 the issue of Emergency Medicine as a specialty is still unresolved.

EMS: ITS FUTURE

The importance of EMS as a national health issue received a visible boost at a

White House conference held on January 6, 1976, during which many recent developments in the field were reviewed. At the conference, President Ford described the recent HEW EMS initiative as an "excellent program" and concluded that the "federal demonstration projects had proven their worthiness" in saving lives. He called it "a program that is totally justified" and stated that "it illustrates that people at the local level are best able to decide how federal monies should be spent." However, the President indicated his opposition to continuing categorical federal programs and his preference for bloc grants to states. This strategy, termed the Financial Assistance for Health Care Act, was announced by the President a few weeks later in his State of the Union Address.

Later in January 1976, hearings were held before the Senate's Subcommittee on Health of the Committee on Labor and Public Welfare to consider extending the Emergency Medical Services Systems Act of 1973 which was scheduled to expire in 1976. Testifying for the administration, Dr. Theodore Cooper, assistant secretary for health, stated that the EMS Act had "successfully demonstrated emergency medical services techniques to local communities" and had "resulted in substantial numbers of lives saved." After concluding that "a great deal has been accomplished to improve the awareness and the delivery" of EMS systems, Dr. Cooper asserted that continuation of the existing legislation was "no longer necessary." Instead he urged the adoption of the President's bloc grant approach while assuring that existing federal EMS grantees would be guaranteed phase-out support over three years.

In contrast, all public testimony and statements from committee members strongly favored continuing the EMS legislation. For example, Senator Alan Cranston warned that the "systematic regional approach" which was "the basic justification" for the legislation would probably be lost under the bloc grant strategy.

In the fall of 1975, the U.S. General Accounting Office conducted a preliminary assessment of EMS activity under the 1973 Act based on a review of 12 HEW grantees. In support of the program, the GAO concluded that sufficient data were available to show that communities had been able to up-grade their EMS resources and that it was "fair to assume" this had "resulted in some decrease in mortality and morbidity." However, the GAO noted that truly integrated regional EMS systems were being established with difficulty because regional management entities often lacked control over their system's resources. This was causing delays in obtaining local commitments to provide operating funds after the grant period, and in obtaining agreements concerning the optimal number and location of ambulances, categorization of emergency facilities, operation of regional communications systems (with central command and control authority), and the use of standardized patient record-keeping forms. The GAO concluded that changes in the proposed legislation might overcome these barriers and urged HEW to better coordinate its efforts with other federal agencies who were also involved in EMS (Ahart, 1976).

Subsequently, on February 12, 1976, the Office of Management and Budget reaffirmed the HEW position opposing enactment of the extension legislation. Instead, they urged the adoption of President Ford's Financial Assistance for Health Care Act, which they believed would give states "the flexibility necessary to support . . . projects tailored to the particular needs of the State and its subdivisions."

However, as expected, the Congress voted favorably on the extension bill titled the Emergency Medical Services Amendents of 1976. Although the new act makes numerous changes in the 1973 Act (including several recommended by the GAO), the basic approach of developing regional EMS systems containing 15 components remains intact. During 1977 through 1979, the bill authorizes $200 million for training, and $14 million for a new burn injury program. Undoubtedly with some ambivalence, President Ford signed the bill into law on October 21, 1976.

During the past decade, EMS has emerged from a minor and obscure position to one of high visibility and activity. The recognition at national, state, and local levels of the importance of improved emergency medical services and the role of emergency ambulance care as a third public service is both striking and encouraging. Whether the regional systems now under development throughout the country will ever become self-sufficient once federal funding ends is far from clear. This will depend in large measure on whether local governments are convinced that quality emergency medical care is an essential public service that is worthy of continued financial support. It will probably be close to another decade before we know the answer.

References

G. J. Ahart, Director, Manpower and Welfare Division, U.S. General Accounting Office, "Statement on Emergency Medical Services Systems Act of 1973," given before Subcommittee on Health, Committee on Labor and Public Welfare, Washington, D.C., January 23, 1976. For the complete report which reaches the same basic conclusions, see "Progress, But Problems in Developing Emergency Medical Services Systems," Report to the Congress by the Comptroller General of the United States, July 13, 1976.

S. Cretin: A Model of the Risk of Death from Myocardial Infarction. Technical Report 09–74. Cambridge, Mass., Operations Research Center, Massachusetts Institute of Technology, 1974.

Federal Communications Commission, "Medical Communications Services," Federal Register 39, 137, Part III (July 16, 1974): 26116–126.

Frey, C. F., Huelke, D. F., and Gikas, P. W.: Resuscitation and survival in motor vehicle accidents. J. Trauma 9(4):292–310, 1969.

Hearings Before the Sub-Committee on Public Health and the Environment of the Committee on Interstate and Foreign Commerce, House of Representatives, Highway Safety Programs Manual, Vol. 11, "Emergency Medical Services," U.S. Department of Transportation (January 1969), Appendix A to the Emergency Medical Services Act of 1972 (Part II), Serial No. 92-84, Washington, D.C., June 13–15, 1972.

Hearings Before the Sub-Committee on Public Health and the Environment of the Committee on Interstate and Foreign Commerce, House of Representatives, Military Assistance to Safety and Traffic Program (MAST), "Report of Test Program by the Interagency Study Group," U.S. Department of Defense, Department of Transportation, Department of Health, Education and Welfare (1970), Appendix A to the Emergency Medical Services Act of 1972 (Part I), Serial No. 92-84, Washington, D.C., June 13–15, 1972, pp. 146-150. For additional analyses of the MAST program see M. D. Keller and W. R. Gemma: "A Study of Military Assistance in Safety and Traffic (MAST); San Antonio, Texas," Ohio State University, Department of Preventive Medicine, Columbus, Ohio (July 1971) and Stanford Research Institute, "Evaluation of Operations and Marginal Costs of MAST Alternatives," U.S. Army, Office of the Chief of Staff, Washington, D.C., October 1971.

National Academy of Sciences, National Research Council, Division of Medical Sciences: Advanced Training for Emergency Medical Technician–Ambulance. Washington, D.C., September 1970.

National Academy of Sciences, National Research Council, Division of Medical Sciences, Committee on Emergency Medical Services: Roles and Resources of Federal Agencies in Support of Comprehensive Emergency Systems. Washington, D.C., National Research Council, March 1972.

National Emergency Medical Services Information Clearinghouse, Report, "Evaluation of Emergency Medical Services: Basic Guidelines," Department of Community Medicine, University of Pennsylvania, Philadelphia, Pennsylvania, 1975.

U.S. Department of Health, Education and Welfare, National Center for Health Statistics, Public Health Service, Health Resources Administration: Vital Statistics of the United States. 2:441–443, 1973.

Chapter 61

EMERGENCY MEDICAL SERVICES PLANNING AND EVALUATION

J. William Thomas and C. Gene Cayten

Programs that are designed to improve emergency medical services are growing in number and scope. An increasing awareness of the need for better emergency care has led many organizations, governmental and private, to provide financial support for upgrading EMS communications, ambulance, and hospital services. To utilize these resources effectively, new EMS programs should be preceded by careful planning efforts and should involve continuing evaluation of the quality of services rendered.

The first section of this chapter presents a step-by-step approach for EMS system planning. The second section, dealing with performance evaluation, examines techniques for appraisals of quality of care. In the final section, approaches for obtaining planning and evaluation data are given, and an information system for routinely collecting and reporting such data is described.

EMERGENCY MEDICAL SERVICES PLANNING

More than any other aspect of medical care, the handling of emergency cases depends on a close coordination of community resources. Because of past neglect, however, emergency care in many communities still relies on a fragmented assortment of transportation, communication, hospital, and phy-

sician services. Hospitals not infrequently have been concerned only with the operation of their own Emergency Departments. Ambulance organizations and police and fire departments have set up their own procedures for responding to requests for emergency assistance with little emphasis on coordination among themselves or between emergency transportation services and hospital Emergency Departments.

Potential benefits of better planning are impressive. Although the exact figure is open to some question, it has been estimated that up to 20 per cent of accidental highway deaths and prehospital coronary deaths could be avoided if prompt, effective emergency medical care were available (Hanlon, 1973). In addition to the approximately 35,000 deaths from myocardial infarction and 12,000 deaths from vehicular accidents that might be prevented each year, properly organized and equipped emergency medical services systems might annually save the lives of 13,000 who die from nonvehicular trauma, stroke, poisoning, drowning, and other accidents (Huntley, 1971). A significant reduction in the pain, suffering, and permanent disabilities related to nearly 12 million nonfatal injuries that occur each year could also be achieved by providing better emergency care.

While the benefits of improved EMS planning are great, so are the problems that must be addressed. Visits to hospital Emergency Departments now exceed 50 million and are rising at 10 per cent per year, a rate greater than any other measure of hospital utilization (American Hospital Association, 1972). Yet only 10 per cent of the nation's 5000 Emergency Departments are equipped and staffed to handle both medical and surgical emergencies, and less than 17 per cent have 24-hour physician coverage (Hanlon, 1973). In the area of prehospital emergency care, ambulances are underequipped and ambulance personnel undertrained. Although an increasing number of ambulance personnel are being trained to the emergency medical technician (EMT) level, many others still do not have even basic first aid training.

The Scope of Emergency Medical Services

Figure 1 illustrates the diverse aspects of a system for accidents and medical emergencies. Effective planning must accompany each step of this sequence.

Demand for emergency medical services is shown to be influenced by a number of population and environmental factors. These include the age and general health status of the population, geographic and meteorologic characteristics, and the employment and industrial composition of the area. Prevention programs tend to mitigate the ef-

fect of these factors, reducing both the number of accidents and medical emergencies and the severity of those incidents that do occur. Such programs are based on legislation (e.g., speed limits, automobile seatbelt laws) and/or public education (e.g., public first-aid training, information on how to recognize a heart attack and how to summon an ambulance quickly).

The speed with which medical assistance can be summoned in an emergency situation depends on the community's emergency communication system. If several different telephone numbers must be called before an ambulance can be located, it will generally take longer to get stabilizing care to the patient. The quality of care delivered once the ambulance arrives depends on the community's emergency medical transportation system, which should consist of appropriately designed and equipped vehicles and well-trained ambulance personnel.

Once at the hospital, the patient relies upon the resources available to the Emergency Department. The quality of emergency care provided by the hospital is a function of Emergency Department equipment, emergency physicians and nurses, other physician specialists in the hospital, and the availability of supporting hospital services such as laboratory, x-ray, and blood bank. While the "EMS system" is frequently considered to stop at the Emergency Department, the statisfactory outcome of emergency incidents depends to a great ex-

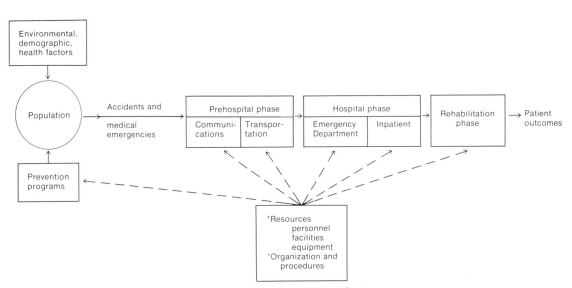

Figure 1. Aspects of EMS planning.

tent on the medical care provided in the hospital to patients admitted through the Emergency Department and the rehabilitation care provided both in the hospital and subsequent to hospital discharge.

The American Hospital Association says of EMS Planning (AHA, 1972):

The objective of community planning for emergencies is to devise a system that will get the patient to the right place in the appropriate time for the right treatment of the emergency condition he represents ... Coordinated joint action is essential.

In developing and carrying out community EMS programs, planners must appropriately balance the resources—pesonnel, facilities, equipment—allocated to each aspect of emergency health care, and they must determine the manner in which these resources are to be organized and operated so as to achieve the necessary coordination between the various EMS system elements.

Steps of the Planning Process

Emergency medical services system planning is comprised of activities similar to those of planning for general health services or for any public or private organization. Planning, the process of making coordinated decisions that individually and collectively have consequences far into the future, normally involves two key concepts:

(1) Goals orientation. A set of general goals for the system must be agreed upon, and priorities among goals established.

(2) An on-going process. As old goals are achieved, new goals are set. As experience indicates needed modifications, goals and/or programs should be changed.

As illustrated in Figure 2, the general planning process involves the following activities (Hamilton and Thomas, 1973):

(1) Setting general goals.

(2) Describing the status of the system being planned for.

(3) Developing specific objectives consonant with the general goals.

(4) Devising alternative approaches for achieving objectives.

(5) Selecting alternatives and structuring activity programs.

(6) Implementing the program.

(7) Evaluating progress with consequent modification of goals and alternative approaches.

Planning, as presented in these steps, is not an isolated or one-time activity. It is an integral part of system management and control, providing the objectives to be pursued for the system and feedback information on the effectiveness of programs undertaken. Like management, planning must be a continuous process.

SETTING GENERAL GOALS

It is generally agreed that the over-all goal of the EMS system is to diminish the death and disability resulting from medical emergencies. Some would qualify this goal by requiring emergency care to be rendered in a humane fashion conducive to patient satisfaction. However, a single over-all goal will not suffice for planning. Several general goals must be formulated to serve as broad statements of intentions for the future status of the system. These should be long-range and achievable only after successful comple-

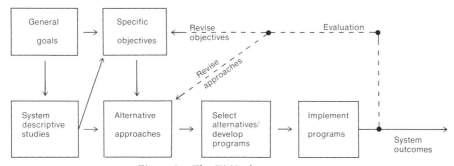

Figure 2. The EMS planning process.

tion of several coordinated programs. Since a system (e.g., emergency medical services system) consists of many separate though interacting elements, at least one general goal for each system element should be expressed. Examples of general goals that might be considered appropriate for an emergency medical services system include the following:

Reduce the severity of injuries associated with highway accidents.

Improve access to the emergency medical transportation system.

Improve the appropriateness of care provided in hospital Emergency Departments.

Improve the quality of prehospital medical care.

Improve the financial viability of hospitals maintaining Emergency Departments.

It may be noted that in defining the goals to be pursued, the planner is also defining the limits of the system. Thus, with the set of goals listed above, hospital inpatient care and rehabilitation care are not considered part of emergency medical services. In this case, the descriptive studies, specific objectives, and alternatives formulated will focus on prevention, communications, transportation, and Emergency Department operations only.

Constraints on the narrowness of EMS system goals are included in the Emergency Medical Services Act of 1973 (P.L. 93–154). Under this act, communities requesting federal funds for EMS system feasibility studies, system development, or expansion or improvement of an existing EMS system must present a plan which addresses the following:

Health and allied professionals.

Training/continuing education.

Central communications system.

Ground, air, and water vehicles.

Easily accessible EMS facilities.

Access to specialized critical medical care units.

Coordination with public safety agencies.

Consumer participation.

EMS services to those unable to pay.

Patient transfers.

Standardized records.

Public education including medical self help and first aid.

Periodic review and evaluation.

Disaster plan.

Reciprocal services with neighboring areas.

DESCRIBING THE STATUS OF THE SYSTEM

With the general goals providing a framework, studies are then performed to determine:

(1) Current demand and the nature of services provided by the system.

(2) The resources currently employed within the system and any constraints on their use.

Together, these studies indicate where improvements are needed, and they provide a yardstick against which future progress can be measured. Boyd (1974) has suggested that a system narrative, a chronologic listing of actions taken on behalf of a typical emergency patient, is also a valuable part of the system description.

Some of the factors to consider in surveying the status of an emergency medical service system are listed below.

(1) Factors Describing the Need for Emergency Care

Population distribution and trends, including changes in demographic characteristics, such as the proportion of elderly or the proportion of young children.

Socioeconomic, occupational, educational, and cultural mix.

Industrial-residential balance.

Hazard areas, such as large highways, industrial plants, and recreation areas.

Number of persons actually using emergency transportation and hospital Emergency Department services, by types of problem (trauma, heart attack, etc.), age (pediatric, adult), time of day and day of week.

(2) Factors Describing EMS Resources and Constraints

Accessibility of transportation facilities.

Capabilities of hospital Emergency Departments: personnel, equipment, support services.

Capabilities of emergency communications system.

Characteristics of ambulance services: number and type of vehicles, equipment, personnel training.

Availability of first aid training programs and the extent to which they are used.

Patterns of third-party payment.

Legal and regulatory barriers to facility

categorization and the use of paramedics on ambulances.

SPECIFYING OBJECTIVES AND DEVISING ALTERNATIVES

In planning for the achievement of a broad, long range goal, the required activities are segmented and described in a group of specific, shorter range objectives. At any time, one or more specific objectives related to each of the system's general goals will be pursued. As one specific objective is met, it is replaced by another objective associated with the same general goal.

Specific objectives are concerned with closing gaps in indicators of system performance. Comparison of system structure and performance to available standards and/or to EMS systems developed in other communities may aid in identifying gaps and defining objectives. If the descriptive studies indicate that 20 per cent of ambulance responses take longer than 15 minutes, an objective might be to reduce this proportion to 5 per cent. If only 30 per cent of myocardial infarctions are seen by specialists in the Emergency Department, an objective might be to increase this to 75 per cent. The gap with which each objective is concerned is the difference between the current value of the system performance measure and its desired value (Palmer and Sisson, 1972). Objectives should also include a time period in which the gap is to be closed. Thus, one year might be allowed for decreasing to less than 5 per cent the proportion of ambulance responses taking longer than 15 minutes.

Associated with each specific objective will be several courses of action that could be taken. These alternatives may be devised by local system managers or planning experts, or they may be suggested from the experiences of other communities. Several specific objectives with related courses of action for an EMS system are listed below.

OBJECTIVE: Increase the proportion of emergency patients transported by ambulances to 80 per cent by the end of the current year.

Possible Alternatives:

Buy four new ambulances.

Undertake a public education program on how to call an ambulance.

Install a central ambulance access system, such as the 911 telephone number.

Coordinate emergency transportation providers so that if one is called and no ambulances are available there, the call can be transferred to a provider that can respond.

OBJECTIVE: Increase the proportion of ambulance users who are transported in vehicles meeting American College of Surgeons standards to 95 per cent in six months' time.

Possible Alternatives:

Equip all current ambulances to American College of Surgeons standards.

Purchase new ambulances meeting standards.

Have central ambulance dispatchers send, whenever possible, ambulances which already meet standards.

OBJECTIVE:' In 18 months' time have at least 80 per cent of emergency patients treated at hospital Emergency Departments which meet AMA guidelines for comprehensive emergency centers.

Possible Alternatives:

Phase out nonconforming Emergency Departments.

Upgrade all Emergency Departments to comprehensive center standards.

Categorize Emergency Departments according to capability, and train ambulance personnel to select the appropriate facility.

Undertake a public education program dealing with selecting Emergency Departments appropriate to the patient's illness or injury.

OBJECTIVE: By December of next year have all rescue requests for cardiac emergencies serviced by ambulance personnel trained to the advanced emergency medical technician (EMT II) level.

Possible Alternatives:

Have the State Legislature enact enabling legislation to allow paramedics to give injections and provide other necessary treatment.

Train all ambulance personnel to the EMT-II level and equip all ambulances accordingly.

Have dispatchers elicit information from callers on the nature of the emergency condition, and send only specially staffed and equipped mobile coronary units for all cardiac emergencies.

Experience indicates that the *process* of setting objectives is often an important determinant of whether the objectives will eventually be achieved. Since EMS system improvements affect numerous organizations and agencies and available resources typically are limited, the economic, political, and social feasibility of accomplishing individual objectives must be weighed carefully. Such considerations argue strongly for involving representatives from the various sectors concerned—politicians, payers, providers, consumers—when specific objectives are being determined. If each group is represented during the objective-setting process, support for programs aimed at accomplishing the objectives is more likely.

SELECTING APPROACHES AND IMPLEMENTING PROGRAMS

For each of the objectives specified, one or more courses of action would be selected. For instance, to increase the proportion of emergency patients treated at comprehensive emergency centers, the alternative chosen might be to phase out nonconforming Emergency Departments. However, to have all cardiac emergency rescue requests served by trained EMT-II's, it might be decided both to pass enabling legislation and to train all ambulance personnel to the EMT-II level.

Techniques appropriate for selecting among alternatives differ with the type of decision being made. In some cases, a simple cost analysis may be used. In others, sophisticated statistical and operations research methods such as a queuing analysis, simulation, or various optimization techniques may be employed. Where the needed resources or the expected outcomes are difficult to quantify, subjective assessments by local experts or trained consultants may be the basis of decisions.

In selecting particular approaches for accomplishing objectives, EMS planners will first specify the criteria by which alternatives will be compared. Cost is one factor that usually must be considered; the time period required before results will be observed is another. Also to be evaluated are problems which may be encountered when implementing a prospective approach. Is the approach politically feasible in view of the strongly parochial interests of many of those concerned? Is it economically feasible; i.e., can the development and operating costs be covered by present and anticipated sources of funds? Is the approach likely to stimulate undesirable behavior on the part of providers or users of the system (e.g., cessation of certain services, overutilization of services)? It sometimes may prove necessary to give extra weight to certain less cost-effective approaches because of their potential for securing political and/or public support for future programs. For example, expensive telemetry may be used on a temporary basis

in order to facilitate public and professional acceptance of medical care (e.g., administering drugs) provided by EMT's. Some communities have learned that properly trained EMT-II's can effectively read an EKG and administer medications without telemetry and physician consultation. However, as an implementation strategy, these communities have gone through a phase utilizing telemetry in order to build up the necessary public and professional acceptance.

Program implementation is a particularly difficult aspect of the EMS planning process. Police departments, fire departments, private and volunteer ambulance organizations, and numerous hospitals may all be involved in different phases of providing emergency medical services in a defined region. Each of these groups functions independently, and implementation of the EMS programs must rely heavily on their general goodwill and cooperative efforts. An EMS system administrator may plan, evaluate, and recommend, but usually he cannot manage the system. Because of his lack of authority, determining which changes are appropriate is often far less difficult than directing their implementation.

PROGRAM EVALUATION AND INFORMATION FEEDBACK

Continual performance evaluation is a key aspect of system management and planning, but it also serves several other very important functions. With a wide variety of individuals and agencies concerned about the nature of emergency medical services provided to the community, information on system performance helps answer questions such as the following:

Consumer: Is prompt and courteous service being provided?

Educator: Do the rescue men I have trained know what they need to know to handle the problems they actually encounter?

Politician: Does the EMS system reflect favorably on my administration?

Federal Agency: Does the EMS system fulfull the federal guidelines for refunding?

Researcher: Which components of this system provide the most impact for the least cost?

Health Department: Are deaths and disabilities being reduced?

In an ongoing planning process, the values of system performance measures are monitored continually in order to evaluate the effectiveness of programs already implemented and to determine if, and when, specific objectives have been achieved. If one objective was to have 80 EMT-I's trained by 1977, was this accomplished? If, according to plan, patients with multiple trauma are to be transported only to hospitals categorized as Type A, what percentage of these patients are actually brought to such hospitals? Based upon this feedback information, objectives may be revised or replaced, and new approaches to achieving current objectives may be developed.

EMERGENCY MEDICAL CARE EVALUATION

Because of the peculiarly complex medical issues and interrelationships involved, quality of emergency medical care is often considered separately from program appraisal. The difficult problems can be characterized as follows:

(1) There is little agreement on what constitutes "appropriate outcomes." Simple death rates are too insensitive, and if morbidity is considered as well, reductions in death rates often lead to increased morbidity.

(2) Adequate scales or measures are difficult to obtain. Unlike dollar costs, specific values of morbidity are difficult to assign. While much effort has been put into developing health indices or indices of function, the state of the art is not sufficiently advanced to make these measures generally usable.

(3) Data on health system outcomes are difficult and often expensive to obtain.

General EMS Evaluation Methods

The last ten years have witnessed progress toward relative sophistication in evaluation of medical care. Avedis Donabedian's (1969) work stands out as a significant milestone, setting forth a basic framework of structure, process, and outcome modes of medical care evaluation. *Structure*, or input, evaluation measures the credentials and level of training of personnel, the adequacy of facilities and equipment, and the method of organizing resources in the EMS system. Although inputs may be measured easily and relatively unambiguously, the validity of structural standards remains uncertain. No research has yet been able to demonstrate that fulfilling the input standards of a "model" EMS system (one meeting all available standards for facilities, equipment, and personnel) has any impact on patient health.

Process evaluation assesses elements in the performance of medical care. Process assessment techniques include certification as to the appropriateness of care, statistical display, analysis of patterns of care, case review with implicit or explicit criteria, and appraisal of the data used for clinical decision making. Currently, most process evaluation methods consist of direct observation and record audits seeking the presence or absence of certain information. Though research findings have indicated somewhat stronger correlations between process indicators and patient outcome measures than between input factors and patient outcome measures, even these relationships are considered weak. Particular validity and reliability problems have been noted when employing explicit process criteria in medical record audits.

Outcome measures for medical care appraisal include assessment of mortality and morbidity, days of hospitalization, days of disability, indices of function and activity-of-daily-living, degrees of disability, etc. Although these indicators can give an over-all picture of a population's health status, they cannot accurately portray the effects of medical care within a particular phase of the system. As shown in Figure 2, the primary reason for evaluating emergency medical services is to indicate where changes in system structure or in medical procedures are most needed. Monitoring outcome measures and comparing observed values to standards or to results observed in other communities may indicate that problems exist and improvements are warranted; however, taken alone, they fail to provide adequate guidance as to where changes should be made and which objectives and current programs should be modified.

USING EVALUATION MEASURES

Since outcome measures are the most important indicators of over-all system success, they should be considered a part of any evaluation program. However, because patient outcome measures are not sensitive to the individual phases of emergency care,

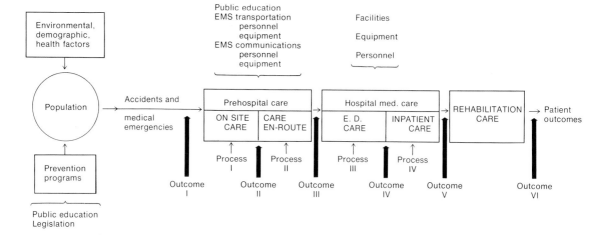

Figure 3. Aspects of EMS evaluation.

other types of indicators must be employed as well. Rules appropriate when selecting and applying EMS evaluation criteria include the following:

(1) Use intermediate outcome measures, i.e., outcome measures that reflect care given at each phase along the EMS system continuum. Make the intermediate outcome measures such as age and sex, as diagnostically specific as possible.

(2) Use structural (or input) evaluation to supplement the intermediate outcome measures.

(3) Use process type evaluation to supplement the intermediate outcome measures.

Figure 3 indicates points where intermediate outcome measures may prove useful. For each phase of the emergency medical services program, measures selected should reflect, as directly as possible, the specific objectives being pursued. The number of accidents per 100,000 population and the number of accidents per mile traveled might indicate the general results of a total prevention program for automotive accidents. However, the percentage of alcohol-induced accidents should reflect more directly the impact of programs designed to curb drinking and driving. To monitor the effectiveness of care provided at the accident scene, intermediate outcome measures might include the proportion of patients with cardiac arrest who are successfully resuscitated and the proportion of patients with massive external hemorrhage in whom shock is prevented or reversed. The percentage of patients, found alive, who are dead on arrival at the hospital can be used as a crude

intermediate outcome measure of the entire prehospital phase.

During the early stages of a general EMS system improvement program, particular emphasis may be placed on structural evaluation. Structural appraisal (surveys) frequently can be useful in comparing the adequacy of a given EMS system to standards or to a system operating in another community. For example, the objective of saving patients with cardiac arrest often may be served most effectively by obtaining properly designed ambulances with defibrillators and trained paramedics. The validity of structural accomplishments should not be assumed blindly, however. Gibson (1974) has posed the haunting notion that "the emergency system is dealing with a finite set of patients who are going to die or survive solely as a function of their condition and that the only effect of EMS expenditures is in influencing when and where the death takes place." While structural assessments may temporarily be emphasized, they should be supported by ongoing outcome evaluations designed to reflect the ultimate impact of system improvements.

Complementing the use of outcome and structural types of appraisal, a program to evaluate the process of medical care should be developed. Areas where system structure appears appropriate and yet crude outcome data show poor results should be of particular interest. For example, if a community maintains (by structural standards) a good public education program, good communication system, well-equipped vehicles, and well-trained personnel, and still shows a high number of prehospital coronary deaths, then evaluation of the process of the prehospital medical care may be expected to yield useful data.

Prehospital care process appraisal can focus on review of ambulance forms completed by the EMT's. These records may be checked to determine whether clinical findings indicated correlate with therapy provided. EMT practical skills, such as application of splints, insertion of an intravenous line, bandaging and positioning, can be checked readily by physicians and nurses on patients delivered to the Emergency Department. Also appropriate for review are evaluations made by emergency physicians and nurses concerning the techniques used by an EMT in rendering care within the Emergency Department to newly delivered patients.

INFORMATION SYSTEMS FOR EMS PLANNING AND EVALUATION

A comprehensive program of emergency medical services evaluation will require detailed data on intermediate patient outcomes, system structural characteristics, and medical care processes. A few sources, such as the ambulance record for prehospital process review, have already been mentioned. Data for system evaluation and planning typically must be obtained from a variety of such sources, and several alternative approaches to gathering these data are often required. One method, the periodic survey, is appropriate for data that are relatively stable and unchanging over time. Examples of such data include population size and demographic characteristics, geographic area size, road and terrain characteristics, number of ambulances and their locations, hospital locations, and Emergency Department capacities. The special data study, a second method, provides information on questions of momentary interest or questions that, once answered, only infrequently need to be addressed again. The size and socioeconomic composition of particular Emergency Department service districts, the total financial impact of an Emergency Department on its hospital and the relative effectiveness of alternative clinical treatments for a particular class of trauma are questions most appropriately answered through specially designed data studies.

The third approach to obtaining EMS information involves routine and continuing collection of certain predetermined data items. To be monitored on such a basis, data items should be related to questions of continuing concern and susceptible to change over short time intervals. Included in this category might be ambulance response time for each emergency incident, the severity and nature of emergencies occurring during various daily time periods, and the magnitude and nature of emergency department utilization at specified hospitals. While surveys and special data studies are important elements of the emergency medical services planning and evaluation process, establishing and maintaining systems and procedures for ongoing monitoring and data collection represent the greater challenge to EMS planners and administrators.

EMS Information System Overview

An EMS information system is a system, usually computer-based, for collecting, storing and analyzing incident-specific data on each medical emergency occurrence in order to support specified management planning decisions. Figure 4 illustrates the data flow and principal elements of such a system.

Typically, the emergency patient's first contact with the emergency medical services system is the central medical emergency dispatcher. Trained to elicit certan vital information from the caller, the dispatcher follows a questioning protocol in order to determine: (a) geographic location of the emergency; (b) nature of the emergency; (c) number of persons involved; (d) medical severity of the patient(s); (e) time of emergency occurrence.

Knowing the availability of ambulances under his control, he may then dispatch an appropriately staffed and equipped vehicle to the emergency site. The dispatcher's record is subsequently updated to reflect the information on which his decision was based and the identification of the ambulance he selected.

The next source of data on the patient encounter is the ambulance record. This document includes a summary description of

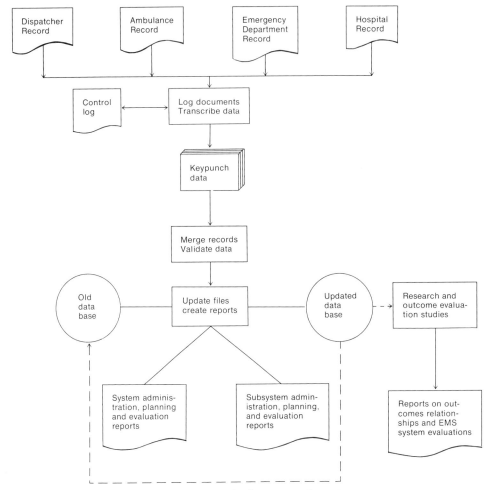

Figure 4. Emergency medical services information system.

the patient's condition over time — vital signs, type of illness/injury, medical severity — and the steps taken to provide stabilizing medical care at the scene and in transit to a hospital emergency department.

Within the Emergency Department, the patient's medical record constitutes the primary source of data. It includes: *(a)* demographic characteristics (age, sex, race, etc.); *(b)* vital signs and examination findings; *(c)* diagnoses/nature and bodily location of injuries; *(d)* ancillary services utilized, and results of tests; *(e)* identification of attending physician(s); *(f)* disposition of the patient (treated and released, admitted in severe condition, expired, etc.); *(g)* insurance coverage and billing information.

For patients admitted to the hospital, hospital record data — complications, length of stay, charges, etc. — also may be needed.

From such data, a variety of routine analyses and reports may be prepared by the EMS information system. These will normally deal with the utilization of various services and the performance of the many elements of the emergency medical services system in responding to patient needs.

Hospital Emergency Department utilization reports may indicate the number of encounters in the latest time period broken down by such variables as day of week, time, diagnosis, financial coverage, age, sex, and geographic origin. Statistics on physician and nurse utilization may be described in similar detail, and ancillary service usage patterns may be shown.

Ambulance reports may indicate the proportion of time each vehicle was in use, the number of runs (cumulative and by vehicle) by day of week, time, nature and severity of emergency, geographic location, etc. Utilization of equipment and supplies may be provided as well. For the emergency communications subsystem, reports may show the number of calls received by day of week and time of day. Information on false alarms provided in EMS information system reports is useful in restricting abuse of emergency telephone numbers.

Operating performance of the EMS system may be reported through a variety of process and outcome measures. Possible examples include average and maximum ambulance response times, proportion of severely ill/injured patients first seen by trained paramedics, proportion of severely ill/injured patients seen by physician specialists in Emergency Departments, change in patient vital signs from initial contact to Emergency Department discharge, patient disposition when leaving Emergency Department, and length of hospital stay.

Information System Functions and Characteristics

Specific data elements to be monitored on a routine basis and the statistics to be reported periodically will be selected by local EMS planners and administrators on the basis of questions and decisions of greatest concern to them. Data elements which serve as input to an EMS information system should be (Rosenfeld, et al., 1974):

(1) *Relevant* to the specific objectives of the overall EMS system and its component subsystems.

(2) *Valid* as important indicators of performance.

(3) *Reliable* when recorded by different individuals at different times.

(4) *Comprehensive* in the sense that, taken together, the data elements provide an understanding of the total operation and of relationships between components of the system.

(5) *Parsimonious* in that only data items essential to questions of continuing interest are included. Collecting and reporting interesting but nonessential data may greatly increase information system costs and also may impair the usefulness of the system by hiding essential information in lengthy tables of unwanted statistics.

The functions that an EMS information system is designed to serve should be consistent with the general goals and specific objectives of the EMS system itself. In selecting the data elements that make up the information system, the above attributes help ensure that the information reported serves the appropriate objectives and is of sufficient quality to remain useful on an ongoing basis. Although the particular functions desired will vary from community to community and, for a single EMS information system, will vary over time, the list below describes areas in which useful information may be routinely provided:

Ambulance service management – e.g., identifies where ambulances should be stationed at different periods of the day, how individual vehicle service districts should be defined, etc.

Emergency Department management – e.g., evaluates the adequacy of physician and nurse staffing for each Emergency Department, identifies indigent patients who qualify for Medicaid or other assistance programs, provides information on patient origin and financial and demographic characteristics.

EMS system resource need projections – e.g., identifies trends for planning ambulance needs, personnel requirements, communication system capacity, and hospital utilization.

Public education – e.g., provides input to programs for improving community knowledge of how to procure emergency medical service, and identifies needs for general first aid training.

Improved paramedic training – provides information on nature of emergency problems encountered by paramedics and feedback on adequacy of past training programs.

SUMMARY

EMS planning should be viewed as an active, continuing process. General goals for the system and each of its components provide the framework for ongoing planning and management. At the inception of the planning effort, data studies must be performed for assessing the adequacy of the various components of the EMS system and for formulating objectives for their improvement. Each objective gives rise to several courses of action, and from these, specific programs are selected for implementation. Thereafter, system and subsystem performance are monitored continually to evaluate effectiveness of programs and to determine whether objectives have been achieved. As early objectives are met, new ones are selected.

Evaluation is a key aspect of the EMS

planning process. Its purposes are to indicate whether emergency medical services are effective in saving lives and reducing disability, and, more importantly, to show *where* − prevention, prehospital care, Emergency Department care, hospital and rehabilitation care − improvements are needed. Techniques available for evaluating emergency medical services include assessments of system structure, medical care process, and patient outcomes. Because none of these techniques alone is wholly adequate, an evaluation program should provide for all three approaches.

Effective EMS planning and evaluation at both the system and subsystem levels rely on accurate, up-to-date information. Methods of obtaining data include periodic survey, special data study, and use of a computer-based information system. Drawing upon records from dispatchers, ambulances, Emergency Departments, and hospitals, the information system provides for routine reporting of numerous utilization and performance measures. With such information regularly available, EMS providers and planners are better able to identify areas where new resources can be productively employed and improvements achieved.

References

American Hospital Association: Emergency Services. Chicago, 1972.

American Medical Association: Developing Emergency Medical Services. Chicago, 1971.

Baker, S. P., et al.: The injury severity score: a method for describing patients with multiple injuries and evaluating medical care. J. Trauma *14*:3, 187, 1974.

Boyd, D. R.: Emergency Medical Service Response Systems Workshop. Sponsored by the AMA and the Robert Wood Johnson Foundation, Atlanta, Ga., August 22–23, 1974.

Brook, R. H.: Critical issues in the assessment of quality of care and their relationship to HMO's. J. Med. Ed. *48*:April, 1973.

Brook, R. H., and Appel, F. A.: Quality of care assessment: choosing a method for peer review. N. Engl. J. Med. 288:25, 1323, 1973.

Donabedian, A.: A Guide to Medical Care Administration. Vol. 2, Medical Care Appraisal − Quality and Utilization. New York, American Public Health Association, 1969.

Gibson, G.: Guidelines for research and evaluation of emergency medical services. Health Services Reports 89:2, 99, 1974.

Hamilton, W. F., and Thomas, J. W.: Emergency Health System Planning: An Annotated Bibliography. Leonard Davis Institute of Health Economics, University of Pennsylvania, Philadelphia, August, 1973.

Hanlon, J.: Emergency medical care as a comprehensive system. Health Services Reports 88, 579, 1973.

Huntley, H. C.: National status of emergency health services. Proceedings of the 2nd National Conference on Emergency Health Services, Dec. 2–4, 1971. Publication no. DEHS-16. Washington, U.S. Government Printing Office, 1966.

National Academy of Sciences-National Research Council: Accidental Death and Disability: The Neglected Disease of Modern Society. Washington, 1966.

National Safety Council: Accident Facts. Chicago, 1972.

Palmer, B. Z., and Sisson, R. L.: An Advanced Health Planning System. Government Studies and Systems, Inc., University City Science Center, Philadelphia, 1972.

Rosenfeld, L. S., Rodak, J., and Coulter, E.: Regional Emergency Medical Services in North Carolina: Monitoring and Evaluation. University of North Carolina, Chapel Hill, 1974.

Skudder, P. A., et al.: Hospital emergency facilities and services: a survey. Bull. Am. Coll. Surgeons *46*:2, 44, 1962.

Willamain, T. R.: The Status of Performance Measures for Emergency Medical Services. Technical Report, TR-06-74, Operations Research Center, M.I.T., Cambridge, Mass., July, 1974.

Williamson, J. W.: Evaluating quality of patient care: a strategy relating outcome and process assessment. J.A.M.A. *218*:4, 564, 1971.

Selected Annotated Bibliography

Brook, R. H.: Critical issues in the assessment of quality of care and their relationship to HMO's. J. Med. Ed. 48:April, 1973.

The purpose of this paper is to examine the relevant components of the quality of care issue, especially as they pertain to the medical care received by the enrollees of prepaid group practices. Brook discusses the problems with the definition of "quality of care," and he assesses the strengths and weaknesses of various methods of assessment using Donabedian's categorization as a guide. Most of this article consists of an extensive literature review of the state of medical care appraisal. The review reveals that nearly every study published demonstrates large deficiencies in quality of care.

Boyd, D., and Flashner, B.: The Critically Injured Patient: Concept and the Illinois Statewide Plan for Trauma Centers. Illinois Department of Public Health, Division of Emergency Medical Services, May 1972.

This is a detailed description of the planning and implementation process for the EMS system for the State of Illinois. Included are chapters on: regionalization and categorization, planning, transportation and communications, education and training, epidemiology, trauma registry, physical rehabilitation, and accident prevention. Also included are the legal statutes used in the implementation of the system.

Donabedian, A.: A Guide to Medical Care Administration, Vol. 2. Medical Care Appraisal—Quality and Utilization. New York, American Public Health Association, 1969.

This volume is based on a series of papers prepared by the Program Area Committee on Medical Care Administration of the American Public Health Association and is intended to serve as a guide for the administrator. It represents the "classic" work in medical care appraisal; Donabedian lays out his trichotomy of structure, process, and outcome and uses it as a frame of reference for discussing techniques, issues, and implementation. An extensive annotated bibliography is included.

Gibson, G.: Guidelines for research and evaluation of emergency medical services. Health Services Reports 89:2, 1974.

With the EMSS Act of 1973 research and evaluation is no longer a desirable by-product of Federal funding, but rather a major precondition for initial awards and subsequent renewal. This paper outlines methodologies for baseline and ongoing evaluation and commends their use by program applicants under the 1973 EMSS Act. Gibson's model for baseline evaluation includes: resources (hospital and ambulance), patient need data (as well as patient demand), and resource utilization. He suggests methodologies for collecting data and criteria for evaluating it. Outcome measures have been ignored; Gibson discusses the difficulties in doing outcome assessment, yet strongly recommends their inclusion and suggests several measures. Ongoing evaluation should employ experimental designs: to assess pre- to post-intervention changes in a project and control area; to assess effects of specific interventions (e.g., training); to assess exogenous goals set by the funding agency.

Keller, M., and Gemma, W.: Emergency medical services: status and opportunities in federal, state and local interaction. J. Am. Coll. Emergency Physicians, Fall, 1972.

A review of Federal agencies concerned with various aspects of emergency health services is provided by this paper. Also shown are the incentives for special concern for emergency health services. The importance of directing many new activities in emergency medical service through agencies at state and sub-state levels is stressed.

Rosenfeld, L. S., et al.: Regional Emergency Medical Services in North Carolina: Monitoring and Evaluation. University Program in Health Services Evaluation, University of North Carolina at Chapel Hill, 1974.

This report, produced by the Program in Health Services Evaluation of the University of North Carolina under contract with H.E.W., explores strategies that may be useful in EMS evaluation. It is aimed at those responsible for program planning and organization to aid them in clarifying the value of accumulation and analysis of data. The theme is adaptation of the principle of regional organization of health services to EMS.

Chapter 62

FINANCING THE EMERGENCY MEDICAL SYSTEM

William F. Hamilton

INTRODUCTION

The financial aspects of out-of-hospital emergency services are central to an understanding of the problems and opportunities facing regional EMS systems. This chapter reviews those factors which influence the cost and financing of pre-hospital care and raises several economic issues that require careful consideration in both developing and established EMS programs.

The availability of financial support from both public and private sources has stimulated widespread interest and considerable progress in the development of regional EMS systems in recent years. A primary thrust of these developmental efforts has been toward improved out-of-hospital services. Experiences gained through such projects have provided useful insights into how emergency medical services can best be organized and operated in a variety of settings.

Recent experiences with regional EMS programs also suggest that many communities have not adequately assessed the cost and revenue implications of proposed EMS system improvements. Accurate economic information is an essential input to responsible EMS system planning and development decisions. Not surprisingly, the two questions most commonly asked by local decision makers are (1) What will it cost? and (2) How can it be financed? These key questions and the factors which determine the answers will be considered in the following sections.

EMS SYSTEM COSTS

For the purposes of this discussion, out-of-hospital EMS costs can be related to

three major system functions: transportation, communications, and management. While detailed discussion of cost categories for an EMS system is beyond the limits of this chapter, a suggested breakdown is presented in Table 1.

The costs of out-of-hospital emergency medical services are influenced by many factors and can vary significantly from community to community. System structure, size, and sophistication as well as community characteristics are important cost determinants in most cases. A recent study of selected EMS systems in varying stages of development revealed over-all EMS operating costs (including hospital costs) ranging from $7 to $15 per capita. Of this total, between $2 and $4 per capita went for out-of-hospital services. Current HEW estimates of operating costs for fully developed EMS systems range between $4 and $7.50, depending upon the degree of sophistication achieved (i.e., basic vs. advanced life support).

TRANSPORTATION COSTS

The costs of operating ambulance services typically range between 20 and 30 per cent of total EMS system costs. Personnel costs account for the largest portion of ambulance service costs, often as high as 75 per cent, but may vary significantly with staffing arrangements (e.g., full-time vs. volunteer personnel) and qualifications. Administrative costs average about 10 per cent but vary with the nature of both the organization and the management activities undertaken (e.g., data processing, evaluation). The costs of equipment, training, and space depend largely on the type and sophistication of the services provided.

TABLE 1   Pre-Hospital EMS Cost Categories

TRANSPORTATION

a. Personnel expense: salaries and benefits to all those included in the organization who carry out the primary function of the service, i.e., ambulance drivers, telephone operators, EMTs.
b. Administrative expense: salaries and benefits of all supervisory and clerical staff (or those supportive of the primary care personnel), and insurance expense for personnel, vehicles, equipment and all other property.
c. Medical supplies: all medical items used while delivering emergency health care, i.e., oxygen, bandages, syringes, drugs, etc.
d. Vehicle operating and maintenance expense: all nonmedical items which are used to operate and maintain ambulance vehicles, i.e., tires, batteries, oil, gasoline, state inspections, and all maintenance charges.
e. Garage and office expense: all expenses incurred for housing ambulances, ambulance crews, administrative and clerical staff.
f. Vehicle and equipment depreciation: depreciation of all ambulances and their equipment (other than communication equipment).

COMMUNICATIONS

a. Dispatcher personnel expense: the salaries and benefits to all those included in providing EMS communication. Supervisory and clerical expenses are included in transportation costs and do not appear here.
b. Equipment maintenance: the periodic maintenance (whether preventive or repairs) of all communication equipment. Maintenance is often included in the equipment purchase contract.
c. Telephone service: all telephone utility expenses of telephone, line, and equipment rental or leasing, whether an 800 number, 7-digit number, or 911 number is used.
d. Equipment depreciation: depreciation of all communication equipment. Depreciated once a 10-year period, with no salvage value on a straight line basis.

SYSTEM MANAGEMENT

a. Personnel expense: salaries, wages and benefits of all clerical and administrative personnel involved in the management of the total system. Consultants are excluded.
b. Office expense: rental, lease or purchase of all office equipment and supplies.
c. Travel expense: any expenses incurred for travel of EMS officials.
d. Consultant services: the payment of all contracted consultants whether for communication, transportation, or hospital ED purposes.
e. Data processing services: the payment for computer time, terminal rental and manual labor attributed to data processing.

The burden of fixed costs (those incurred regardless of the number of runs made) and the resulting impact of underutilization are most apparent in EMS transportation services, especially in rural regions. Substantial fixed costs result in a high cost of maintaining an adequate ambulance response capability in sparsely populated areas. Thus, per capita costs generally reflect a strong inverse relationship to population density (i.e., per capita costs increase significantly as distance increases and the number of runs decreases).

COMMUNICATIONS COSTS

The communications costs associated with EMS may range from as little as 2 per cent of total EMS costs where costs are shared with other public services to as much as 35 per cent in rural areas where extensive communications networks are maintained solely for EMS purposes. Significant economies can be achieved where police, fire, and ambulance communications are combined. Factors influencing communications costs include the sophistication of the equipment in use and the degree to which dispatching is centralized to permit most efficient use of both personnel and equipment.

SYSTEM MANAGEMENT COSTS

The costs associated with system management vary with the range of management functions performed. Public information programs, system planning and evaluation, legislative liaison, and fund-raising are a few of the activities which might be included in system management. In carrying out these functions, costs may be incurred for a regional coordinator or EMS Council staff, for consultation, and for office, travel, and data processing services. Management costs are generally only 1 or 2 per cent of total EMS costs, with a tendency toward higher costs in early stages of EMS system development.

FUNDING SOURCES

It is often useful to distinguish between two types of funding for EMS systems. *Developmental* or grant funds have been made available by the federal government (principally HEW and DOT), by state governments, and by private foundations (especially the Robert Wood Johnson Foundation) for such "start-up" activities as system planning and organization, equipment purchases, and personnel training. *Operational* funding, on the other hand, is directed toward the expenses of system operation which continue long after developmental funds have been expended to get an EMS program started.

There can be little doubt that developmental funding programs over the past five years have led directly to the creation of regional EMS systems across the country. In many cases, however, there have been serious problems in obtaining permanent financing for ongoing system operations that were supported initially by grant funds. This is due at least in part to the fragmented nature of EMS financing and to the complex set of revenue sources through which EMS operating costs must be supported. These sources include patient service revenues (user fees and insurance reimbursements), family subscriptions, general taxes, special purpose taxes, and contributions.

Service charges and subscriptions are major sources of operating funds for emergency transportation. Ambulance services typically charge a base fee with additional mileage charges and supplementary charges for special services. Ambulance charges vary widely, but tend to be higher in urban areas than in rural areas. In urban areas, a fixed fee is quite common; rural ambulance services more frequently add a mileage charge. Collection rates are poor for many ambulance services, ranging between 30 and 50 per cent of charges. However, several groups have achieved collection rates above 80 per cent through the persistent pursuit of delinquent accounts and threats of legal action. In many areas, local governments subsidize at least a portion of ambulance operating costs. The methods for determining subsidies vary, with some set in proportion to the population served, some in relation to the number of ambulance runs actually made, and others set at what appear to be arbitrary fixed levels.

As a rule, the costs of EMS communications and system management are borne by local taxpayers or by developmental funds where grant support is available. Patient payments can be charged in most systems only by the units which contact the patient directly (i.e., the ambulance and the hospital emergency room). It will, therefore, often be necessary to develop new organizational mechanisms in most communities before such revenues can be utilized to support "overhead" activities like communications and system management.

FINANCING APPROACHES

Several innovative tax-based approaches to financing the over-all costs of EMS systems have been developed. Some states have enacted laws permitting single or multi-county EMS districts to levy property taxes for funds to support emergency medical services. In Atlanta, for example, counties participating in the regional system contribute on a per capita basis to support system management and operation of a central communications system. The Pennsylvania no-fault automobile insurance law specifically includes EMS communications cost as a reimbursable expense along with ambulance charges. A multi-parish private ambulance service in southwestern Louisiana operates much like a regulated monopoly, with costs totally covered by family subscriptions and user charges set at levels approved by parish governments.

Despite the expanding set of new approaches to EMS financing, it is apparent that reimbursement practices are generally disorganized and fragmented. From a financing perspective, EMS is still operated not as a system, but rather as a collection of unrelated elements. This is especially evident when current third-party financing provisions are considered.

On the average, 80 per cent of EMS patients are covered under one or more health insurance plans through such third-party carriers as Blue Cross/Blue Shield, Medicare/Medicaid, commercial insurance companies, and private programs. Those in rural areas are twice as likely to be covered as those in urban areas. Passage of a national health insurance program would be likely to increase this percentage still further.

At present, many insurance policies do

not provide coverage for out-of-hospital emergency medical services; policies that do include out-of-hospital benefits are typically limited in nature and extent of coverage. Few health insurance plans specify any coverage for either communications or system management costs where these are not included in transportation charges.

Common insurance restrictions limit coverage to selected patient conditions, set maximum allowable costs for defined services, and/or restrict benefits to hospital-based services. For example, 20 per cent of the total population insured through Blue Cross plans across the nation are not covered for emergency transportation; and one-third of all those covered by Blue Cross plans are limited to reimbursement for accident-related injuries only (i.e., sudden illness is excluded form emergency coverage). Some commercial policies provide benefits for EMS transportation services only if a patient is hospitalized following transportation. In some instances, treatment services rendered by emergency medical technicians and paramedics are also not covered.

As reflected in current third-party benefit structures, therefore, insurance benefits have not generally kept pace with changing concepts and developments in emergency medical services delivery. Coverage for the full range of emergent patient conditions requiring emergency medical care is often incomplete, and benefit limits are frequently restricted for expenses associated with necessary and appropriate out-of-hospital activities. Until third-party coverage is updated to reflect actual and necessary costs, their effect on out-of-hospital emergency services will continue to be far less than on in-hospital services.

ISSUES FOR THE FUTURE

While developing EMS systems have provided important insights into the costs and financing of emergency services, they have also raised important economic questions. These are difficult to answer but will have important implications for the future development of EMS systems.

1. *Who should pay the bill?* Whatever the cost of an EMS system in a particular community, someone must pay for it. This is an important question that must be faced in all communities. The underlying issue can be phrased in the language of the economist as follows: Is EMS a private or a public good? That is, should it be treated as a private service like most other medical care services or as a public service like fire and police protection? If the answer to this question is "private," it follows that the user(s) should pay for EMS through service charges, subscriptions, or other direct means. If the answer to the question is "public," it follows that the cost should be borne by all for whom services are available—i.e., in practice, by the taxpayers.

Whatever philosophical position is taken on this question, it is essential to recognize that citizens will end up paying one way or another for EMS system development and operation. This is an important corollary of one of the most famous theorems in the field of economics: "There is no such thing as a free lunch."

In struggling with this question, it is often useful to consider the various components of the EMS system—transportation, communications, management, and hospital services—in terms of their fundamental nature and current sources of support for these services. In most communities, because hospital-based services generally are relatively well supported through health insurance, it is convenient to consider these services as private. On the other hand, to the extent that out-of-hospital services are inadequately supported through private sources, there are significant pressures to consider them as public services and, hence, as eligible for support through governmental sources.

2. *What are the effects on EMS system structure?* How EMS systems are financed may significantly influence their development and evolution over time. This is perhaps most evident in the case of developmental financing programs, both federal and foundation-supported, which have substantially influenced the nature of EMS systems through extensive specifications of system structure and resource requirements. For example, the federal EMS program requires grantees to focus explicit attention on selected aspects of emergency system structure and operation as a condition for developmental funding.

In the operational realm, there is additional evidence from both EMS and other health care delivery contexts that system structure will tend to follow the sources and nature of funding. It is no coincidence, for example, that the best-financed component of the emergency medical services system—the hospital emergency room—is generally also the most well developed. Because there are few traditional funding sources for management and communications activities beyond the developmental funding stage, there is an apparent danger that the lack of future operational financing will selectively retard development of these important components of EMS systems in the future. In general, one can expect out-of-hospital activities to suffer most as developmental funding dwindles.

In addition, it is not only the amount of money available for selected activities that determines the patterns of development. Designation of those who receive the funding and therefore control the funds can also significantly influence development. This reflects the reality that true power in community programs often derives from financial control, and EMS is no exception to this general rule.

3. *Are there economies of scale in "regional" EMS systems?* An underlying rationale for the design and development of regional EMS systems is the improvement in efficiency that is expected to result from more appropriate use of resources and services on a regional basis. The organization of health resources and services on a regional basis is one of the dominant themes of this decade in health care delivery. This is reflected most clearly in the recent National Health Planning and Resources Development Act (P. L. 93-641). However, despite substantial federal and private foundation investments in health services regionalization, including EMS system regionalization, there is little evidence to date that such organized regional systems actually result in increased efficiencies and improved effectiveness. Important issues relating to the appropriateness of designated regional boundaries for different emergency services (e.g., burns, trauma, poisons), and the implications of alternative regional sys-

tem structures must still be examined as EMS systems mature.

4. *What trade-offs exist between EMS costs and service levels?* In a time of limited resources, serious questions must be raised about the costs associated with the various levels of service which can be provided in an EMS system. While extensive advanced life support throughout the nation is a worthy objective, the cost of such services will often require that communities fall short of this level of service, at least in the foreseeable future. They will need to set priorities that will permit the greatest improvement in service for the funds available, and inevitably, some objectives will have to be sacrificed in favor of others. How costs vary with differing levels and qualities of service is essential information if these design and development decisions are to be made in the most responsible manner possible.

CONCLUDING COMMENTS

In summary, it seems clear that available developmental funds have significantly increased public expectations and aspirations for improved emergency medical services. They have also resulted in significant improvements in many communities. These improvements can involve substantial increases in EMS costs, which must be financed on a continuing basis if the momentum toward expanded EMS service levels is to be maintained. However, it appears likely that uncertainties with respect to EMS funding will continue for the foreseeable future as long as fragmented sources of funding must be depended upon for operational financing.

Views on the above issues and questions range widely among EMS professionals in the EMS field. There can be little debate, however, that these will require considerably more attention in the future than they have received in the past. This is essential if better information is to be made available to those planning and managing EMS systems as well as to those setting national EMS policy.

Chapter 63

PREVENTION, CONSUMER EDUCATION, AND COMMUNITY INVOLVEMENT

Thomas C. Kennedy

THE PUBLIC'S ROLE IN EMERGENCY MEDICAL SERVICES (EMS)

Introduction

The population served by an EMS system is not simply a body of potential consumers, but also is a crucial operating component of the system. The ability of the system to scan its environment and react to an emergency situation depends almost exclusively on a voluntary response by members of the public within its service area. In order for other more specialized and highly skilled actors within the system—ambulance personnel, communications dispatchers, hospital staff—to respond to an emergency, the public must know how, and be willing, to gain access to these other components. They must know where to call for help.

Further, in order for access procedures to be efficient, the public also must know when to engage the rest of the system. They must be able to identify correctly a medical emergency. If a citizen's threshold for the definition of an emergency is too low, resources will be wasted, and the system will over-respond relative to the severity of the problem. On the other hand, if a citizen's definition threshold is too high, he will underestimate emergencies, underutilize the system, and perhaps cause unnecessary

pain, disability, or even death as a result (Mogielnicki, et al., 1974). An EMS system will also be more effective in time-critical situations if citizens can react to stabilize patients until specially trained help arrives. Correct procedures by members of the public should result in reduced response time and more economic use of the system's resources. In short, a well informed and willing public is necessary for an effective and efficient EMS system.

Defining the Problem

Emergency medical services are peculiar in that there is a lack of clear role differentiation between consumers and providers. There is a role overlap between the set of actors who deliver the service and the public whom the system serves.

We should begin by examining more closely the sets of actors necessary for an effective EMS system, and the functions that these actors perform. The gross classification of actors as either providers or consumers is oversimplified to the point of constraining a clear view of the problems to be overcome.

An EMS system contains all the people within its spatial bounds at any given time, *all* functioning as both potential consumers and potential providers, but with different tasks, interests, motivations, and levels of knowledge. The total population consists of

1397

people with differing potentials for becoming providers or consumers once an emergency has occurred.

Actors who normally are considered as providers, such as ambulance attendants, dispatchers, and Emergency Department physicians, certainly are characterized by high levels of skill, knowledge, motivation, and interest and, of course, a high probability at any given time of being called upon to utilize these characteristics. It is commonly agreed that these specialized actors are necessary, but they are not sufficient for the development of an EMS system. As part of a system, a set of interrelated functions, they are dependent on other actors, a willing and informed general public. All people within the spatial bounds of the system must be recognized as potential providers of simple, but often critical, functions. It is both characteristic and problematic that most people within an EMS system are unlikely to be called upon to provide these functions.

Similarly, all persons are potential consumers. Strictly speaking, consumers are the victims of emergency illness and injury who are assisted by EMS. Potential consumers, like potential providers, have different probabilities of becoming active consumers. The likelihood of becoming a victim is relatively low for most people, and it is difficult to identify operationally the distribution of these probabilities.

In planning and developing an EMS system, we must somehow deal with these probabilities of potential, a major problem for all EMS systems, and the problem addressed in this chapter is how to activate low probability actors. (In the remainder of the chapter "the public" will be used as a shorthand for "low probability potential actors.")

A ROLE FOR LOW PROBABILITY ACTORS

It is now commonplace to define the human and material components that respond to health emergencies as a system. Churchman (1968) defines a system as "a set of parts coordinated to accomplish a set of goals." This simple model fits well with the concept of a set of actors and technology directed toward the purpose of reducing mortality and disability rates attendant on emergency illness and injury.

We should note, however, that useful system definition proceeds from normative statements of purpose. There are an almost infinite number of ways to define a set of systematic relationships, since ultimately everything is related to everything else. Purpose is the critical guide to restricting system definition.

Systems do not exist in a vacuum, but operate within environments that contain opportunities and constraints. A system's environment is made up of the entities that are fixed or given from the system's point of view, its objectives and resources. As we shall see, it is necessary to consider the points of view of different levels of decision-making within a complex organizational system like EMS. Of course, the concept of environment is useful only to the extent that we can differentiate the effects of the entities that make up the universe external to the system. As with system definition, this differentiation is guided by the purpose of the system.

As Churchman (1968) points out, we must ask, "Can I do anything about it, and does it matter relative to my purpose?" if the answer to both questions is "yes," then "it" is part of the system. Alternatively, if the answer to the first question is "no" and to the second is "yes," then "it" is in the system's operational environment. Implicit or explicit in these determinations is a judgment of *how much* it matters and *how much* it can be controlled.

Perhaps the major problem associated with the allocation of resources to improve the delivery of emergency medical services, as with most other public services, is that these quantitative parameters, answers to the "how much" questions, are as yet only vaguely perceived. This is true along almost all dimensions of the system. A recent Rand study summarizes the situation well.

A few progressive ambulance services have implemented advanced systems of emergency medical care. These have been proclaimed successful and serve as goals to be achieved in other regions. However, the "documentation" of these successes has not been convincing, due to the use of performance measures that can be interpreted in very different ways, and that may be substantially influenced by unmeasured conditions outside the EMS system ... The validity of current objectives in the area of emergency ambulance services still remains to be evaluated through empirical investigation ... Research is still needed to establish the costs and benefits of different organizational frameworks for emergency services, and to provide guidelines for values of relevant parameters that specify which framework is to be preferred in a given region (Chaiken and Gladstone, 1974).

Ideally, EMS system decision-making should be able to assess the impact of proposed combinations of actors, facilities, and equipment in terms of death, disability, and suffering reduction. The present state of every EMS system might be described at the conceptual level as a hypothesized but untested ideal model, based almost entirely on input criteria or intuitive standards, and at the operational level as various approximations of this model at various stages of development toward it.

Given this situation, it is impossible to design programs that test the impact of public information and action on disability and mortality outcomes. Since the detection, reporting, and on-site treatment of emergencies by the public are linked to system outcomes through other components of the system, the best results we can design for are process measures. That is, we can attempt to design and measure the impact of programs for information and skill transfer, and the effect of this knowledge on behavior. Behavioral change, in turn, can be related to temporal parameters and to patient condition at the interface with other components of the system.

Although we have some strong intuitive feelings about the value of improving certain EMS functions, we have virtually no objective criteria for measuring the comparative benefits to be gained from marginal investments in the various components of the system. Notwithstanding, decisions have been, and are being, made to commit resources to the improvement of EMS systems. A brief examination of this decision process helps explain why so few resources have been allocated toward improving the functions of low probability potential actors.

The primary management decision bodies for local systems are EMS councils mandated by the Federal legislation of 1973. This management component is made up of representatives from each of the various actor sets that function at the operation level of the system. Emergency medical services, therefore, cannot be understood completely as a system, but rather must be examined simultaneously as a coalition or consortium of systems.

This is another characteristic peculiar to EMS relative to other service delivery systems. Whereas all organizations have to deal with conflicting and competing goals of the individuals within them, this constraint is made particularly acute within EMS councils because its members are all representing other systems, only a part, and perhaps a small part, of whose concerns are with EMS. The objectives of hospitals, police, and fire departments, as well as those of the general public, override, compete, and sometimes conflict with the objectives of the EMS system.

Public statements of goals and priorities are of limited use in determining the operational objectives of such a complexly motivated system management. Perhaps the best indicator of the purposes and priorities of an EMS system is the distribution of resources within it.

When we look at the resources allocated to the public component of an EMS system, it is not even clear by this criterion that the public is indeed considered an operational component of the system. So few resources have been allocated to the public component, compared to those allocated to ambulances, electronic communications equipment, and professional staff, that we might conclude that the system's management has really defined the public as part of the system's environment, something that matters relative to the purpose of the system but not something about which anything can be done. For example, consider that a single hospital staff position for 24-hour Emergency Department coverage may cost $150,000 per year, and that the operation of a conventional ambulance round-the-clock costs upward of $90,000 per year (Hanlon, 1973). Not one EMS system has spent even one-half of the latter amount on developing the functions of the system's public component. An analysis by Cretin (1974) indicates that reductions in prehospital mortality among heart attack victims depend more on shortening the typically long delay until the patient seeks medical help than on further reducing ambulance response times. This also may be true for victims of other illnesses and trauma, but these possibilities have been all but ignored by most EMS councils.

The pervasive de facto relegation of the public's function to the system's environment is a decision often made on ill-informed intuitive grounds by system managers with a biased view of the significance of other system components to mortality and disability outcomes. Lacking knowledge of the impacts of alternative marginal investments, EMS councils are essentially organizations that negotiate resource allocation on the basis of the perceived needs of each of the interests represented. Since actors concerned primarily with public functions are represented only weakly, few resources are allocated to improving public functions.

If resources allocated to answering questions about the effectiveness of controlling public functions and beyond are to be diverted to broader efforts to improve these functions, it will first be necessary to provide a larger role in system management for the public whose interests these functions most directly serve. There are, however, certain dilemmas attendant on this prescription.

To date, EMS councils have been structured according to the *tried* and *untrue* model of "citizen participation" that has failed in virtually every collective decision-making situation to which it has been applied. Downs offers a partial, but compelling, explanation of why the "public interest" that consumer representatives are supposed to guard is almost inevitably shortchanged within this kind of decision structure.

Specialization demands expert knowledge and information especially if competition is keen, but most men cannot afford to become expert in many fields simultaneously . . . Naturally, the men who stand to gain from exerting influence in a policy area are the men who can best afford the expense of becoming expert about it . . . In almost every policy area, (there are) men who earn their incomes there. This is true because most men earn their incomes in one area but spend them in many . . . For all these reasons, producers are much more likely to become influencers than consumers (Downs, 1957).

Downs concludes that "the cost of acquiring information and communicating opinions to government determines the structure of political influence. Only those who can afford to bear this cost are in a position to be influential."

There is little doubt that the failure of public service agencies to engage necessary consumer participation has been due in part to the high cost of becoming informed about the relevant issues, but broader

motivations also are involved. Even if information and communication costs were zero for all citizens, some would be more motivated than others to influence aspects of collective policy formation.

Most consumer representatives are members of what Olson (1965) calls "latent groups." A characteristic of these is seen in the fact that no individual member's contribution to a particular decision or action makes a perceptible difference to other members of the group, or to his own benefit. In other words, any large group decision has public good characteristics. Public goods are such that, once they are produced, no one within the range of their effects can be excluded from their consumption. Also, the consumption of such goods by any individual does not result in diminishing its consumption by another. This analysis further explains the failure of traditional consumer participation strategies.

"Only a separate and selective incentive will stimulate a rational individual in a latent group to act in a group-oriented way. In such circumstances group action can be obtained only through an incentive that operates, not discriminately, like the collective good, upon the group as a whole, but rather *selectively* toward the individuals in the group" (Olson, 1965).

Olson's model of the illogicality of consumer participation strongly implies a basic principle that must be applied to the design of collective decision-making organizations such as EMS councils. Participation must be rewarded as a private good.

The most obvious and straightforward strategy both for reducing information costs and for rewarding decisions for the public good as decisions also for the private good is to pay the delegates. The most effective way for a group to reduce the time, effort, and bargaining costs of decision-making is to delegate authority to a single individual or a small set of individuals. As we noted above, this is already being done for representatives of all other major functional components of the EMS system. Representatives of hospitals or public safety departments not only are often being paid to attend group decision functions and for gathering relevant knowledge of the system, but also may be rewarded within the institution that employs them for negotiating resource allocation to that institution. The public component likewise should have a professional delegate or delegates who can aim to equalize its role in the system's decision and negotiation process.

Strategies

Having discussed the prerequisite of a larger role for public participation, it remains to explore more thoroughly strategies for improving the function of the public at the operational level of the EMS system.

As was pointed out earlier, the operation of the EMS system critically depends on a public informed as to where and when to gain access to other components of the system. A single access phone number must be available to the public. The 9-1-1 number has some advantages but the principal advantage, one number nation-wide, depends on its becoming ubiquitous. Nine-one-one may yet be technically or financially infeasible in many areas. The overriding consideration is to have a single point through which help can be dispatched, and a close second best alternative to 9-1-1 is a single seven-digit number.

Since the amount of critical information per message informing where and when to gain access is small, and since this information must be disseminated as broadly as possible among the service population, mass media channels would seem the most appropriate channels of dissemination. Part of the public education task is to develop an optimum range of emergency recognition threshold, and thus messages describing the telephone access procedure should be linked with illustrations of appropriate health emergency situations. Further, since many people may not be aware of the role of the public safety component, a brief explanation of this function also should be included. The functions of the public in detecting and reporting emergencies are strongly interdependent, and should be explicitly linked into one message during an information campaign.

A simple pretest/post-test sample survey will at least indicate grossly whether the media campaign has succeeded in transferring information. A well controlled evaluation design, however, would be extremely difficult and costly, owing to the characteristics of the mass media and the number of rival hypotheses generated by an attempt to use a different EMS service area from which to draw a control population.

Fear of a large number of inappropriate calls may be retarding the developing and publicizing of 9-1-1 or other single access numbers for medical emergencies. A report by the President's Office of Telecommunications Policy observed that whereas "most communities do experience an initial period in which their rate of false calls increases [this] is to be expected since many people will want to dial the number to make sure that it is really in operation. This 'testing' of the number usually continues for a week or two. After that the rate of prank and nuisance calls tends to subside to previous levels" (Washington, D.C., U.S. Government Printing Office, 1973). The report concludes: "there is no reason to suspect that the (long-run) volume of such calls will be any greater with 9-1-1 than with the previous system."

If fear of inappropriate calls is blocking development of an access number, the nuisance factor can be estimated by initially limiting the information campaign to segments of the mass media, and monitoring the calls that follow. This strategy, however, controls only those calls coming from individuals described above as having a low threshold for emergency reporting.

Mogielnicki, et al. (1974) have suggested that "one way to reduce the volume of non-emergency medical calls on a central emergency number would be to provide an alternative publicized number on which medical information could be given to people to assist them in making decisions in both emergencies and other situations." Such an information number also would give recourse to people whose emergency definition threshold is too high, and who would tend to delay or take inappropriate action.

To test the impact of the alternative number on low-threshold callers, emergency number calls could be monitored to detect the hypothesized decline of inappropriate calls. The information number could be monitored for referrals to the emergency number in order to test for the hypothesized effect on high threshold callers.

In the final analysis, the proper technique for dealing with inappropriate calls is to avoid their stressing the response system by training dispatchers to screen calls, not by withholding access potential from the public.

Once we have determined how effective a public education campaign is at the level of information transfer, it is important to find out whether higher public information levels actually result in a higher proportion of true emergency cases flowing through the system. This determination can be made by pre- and post-information campaign measures of the mode of transportation by which true emergencies arrive at hospitals.

One important result of a well-known telephone access system should be a reduction of delay time between an emergency incident and the report of that incident. Report lags might be sampled by designing an appropriate item into ambulance report forms. Further, this data could usefully be disaggregated by specific illness and injury, because delay times probably are different for various types of incidents, and an ability to group and rank these differences will allow for better corrective strategies. In order to measure program impact, of course, samples must be monitored before and after the public information campaign.

Finally, since there is a public good aspect involved in emergency detection and reporting, it might be interesting to test the effect of a reward structure for correctly detecting and reporting emergencies.

TRAINING

Having every citizen trained in basic first-aid and life support skills is an ideal that is a long way from realization. National estimates indicate that probably less than 5 per cent of all emergency victims receive initial treatment prior to intervention by trained ambulance personnel, or prior to their arrival at a hospital Emergency Department.

Improvement of first-aid training programs can be developed through strategies that deal with the constraints militating against proper response.

A necessary first step is to manipulate the unwieldy concept "general public" into more specifically defined publics or target groups. That is, we might begin by attempting to define a profile of persons most likely to become candidates for lay emergency care training, most likely from two points of view: (1) that of the goals and objectives of the EMS system; and (2) that of the individual trainees. The next step will be to identify or create groups or organizations that have members with coincident characteristics.

From the point of view of the system,

priority for training should be placed on programs with the highest probability of need. This is one way of insuring that resources expended on training will be utilized most productively.

There are two major categories of training candidates who fit this criteria: those having high rates of contact with at-risk populations, and those who simply have high rates of contact with large groups of people.

Even in training "high probability of need" groups, we must realize that skill utilization is not likely to be intensive enough in itself to serve as a sufficient practice and feedback mechanism. Training programs must provide for continuous follow-up training, reinforcement of awareness, and monitoring; in short, they must be institutionalized. The usual procedure of bringing into a group an instructor who administers training and then withdraws may not be sufficient to maintain a necessary state of trainee competence over a period of time. Emergency care training can be institutionalized — linked to an ongoing group process — by each group's developing and maintaining an autonomous capacity for training, reinforcement, and performance monitoring. Not only should instructors be developed within a given group, but a coordination role also should be identified.

High contact groups are fairly evident and straightforwardly defined. Examples of such groups are transportation workers, hotel staff, employees in large office buildings, institutions, and manufacturing firms. Identification of high risk related groups is perhaps rather more complex.

Although it is true that emergency situations can strike anyone, anywhere, it is not true that each individual in the population is equally likely to become a victim of sudden injury or illness. As Waller and Klein have argued (1974): "Epidemiology as a field is predicated on the non-random distribution of disease in populations. As has been convincingly documented, injury events are not randomly distributed over time, location or population. An important corollary to this fact is that the distribution of different *severities* of injury is not random either."

O'Connell (1971) similarly criticizes the concept of "accident" as a factor in automobile injuries. He points out that the term "accident" suggests a randomness that rational preventive interventions would not affect. It is argued that auto crashes are not "accidents" at all, but rather "perfectly predictable outcomes of a particular transportation system utilizing a specific technology." Similar arguments can be made for emergency illnesses such as heart attack and stroke.

We are far from having perfect information as to how injury and illness probabilities are distributed, but it should be possible to define generally a number of at-risk groups whose characteristics—age, life-style, income, sex, health history—are correlated with a much greater than even chance of becoming emergency victims. Once a better defined epidemiology of emergency injury and illness has been established, training programs can be designed to address the most probable health problems of sets of individuals within the general public.

Response training for specific situations should be directed in most cases not at the risk population itself—who in critical cases will not be able to administer self-treatment—but at family members, work associates, friends, teachers, or nurses who spend a substantial amount of time with high risk individuals, and who have a high personal interest in their welfare.

When the EMS system management attempts to recruit volunteers for training, productivity criteria must be matched with opportunities and constraints relative to the motivations of potential trainees. These opportunities and constraints can be conceptualized as costs and benefits associated with training and proper utilization of learned skills. Individuals are more likely to volunteer for training and act on this training as these costs are reduced.

The principal rationale for shifting costs away from the trainee rests on the public good characteristics intrinsic to the delivery of emergency services. For example, a knowledge of correct response to an emergency is not likely to result in direct benefits for the responder. Any one individual's benefit from EMS training depends on another's knowledge and skill. That is, EMS involvement is characterized by public good effects. To the degree that these generalizations hold, potential trainees will not be motivated to incur costs—either time costs or monetary costs—for training. The same constraints may operate when trained individuals are faced with situations requiring application of their skills.

An important countervailing process that militates against these cost calculations is the personal satisfaction or psychic reward that accrues to those who intervene to assist a victim. By focusing training programs on those who have a personal interest in the welfare of at-risk individuals, the public good aspect of lay care is reduced.

There are other kinds of rewards that might have a similar effect. Symbolic or social awards might be made, such as public presentations or recognition through the mass media. Consideration also might be given to monetary rewards for proper lay intervention in emergency situations.

The operational role of the public in EMS is clustered around their interface with the public safety component of the system, but users also, of course, interface with hospital Emergency Departments. This topic will be taken up in Chapter 69.

References

Chaiken, J. M., and Gladstone, R. J.: Some Trends in the Delivery of Ambulance Services. Santa Monica, Rand Corp., 1974, p. 32. (Information needs for resource allocation decision-making in EMS systems is summarized in detail by Geoffrey Gibson: "Emergency medical services: the research gaps." Health Services Research, Spring 1974, pp. 6–21.)

Cretin, S.: A Model of the Risk of Death from Myocardial Infarction. M.I.T. Technical Report, 1974.

Churchman, C. W.: The Systems Approach. New York, Dell, 1968, p. 29.

Downs, A.: An Economic Theory of Democracy. New York, Harper and Row, 1957, p. 254.

Hanlon, J.: Emergency medical care as a comprehensive system. Health Services Reports 88, No. 7:579–587, 1973.

Mogielnicki, R. P., et al.: Patient and Bystander Response to Medical Emergencies. Cambridge, Mass.: M.I.T., 1974.

O'Connell, J.: The Injury Industry. New York, Commerce Clearing House, 1971, p. ix.

Office of Telecommunications Policy: Nine-one-one, The Emergency Telephone Number: A Handbook for Community Planning. Washington, D.C.: U.S. Govt. Printing Office, 1973, p. 42.

Olson, M. Jr.: The Logic of Collective Action. Cambridge, Mass., Harvard University Press, 1965.

Waller, J. A., and Klein, D.: Society, emergency and injury: inevitable triad? Research Directions Toward the Reduction of Injury. Washington, D.C.: U.S. Dept. H.E.W., 1971, p. 4.

Chapter 64

MANPOWER AND TRAINING

Gerald L. Looney

During the first half of this century, most nongovernmental health services (with the obvious exception of sanitation and general public health measures) were oriented toward individual patients and solo practitioners, and were almost entirely dependent on local initiative in small geographic or political areas. Many medical requirements and regulations as well as medical services were viewed by state and federal authorities as local affairs, and such standards and services varied widely from one town to the next. In this setting, communities supported general emergency services readily through police, fire, and disaster agencies, but the out-of-hospital medical component of these services was largely unsupported by public funds and considered to be the responsibility of individual physicians and hospitals.

However, as health care became increasingly institutionalized and hospitals became subject to fiscal accountability and balanced budgets by the beginning of the second half of the century, this primary source of emergency medical care steadily diminished. The lack of interest and involvement by medical institutions in the largely nonreimbursable problems of emergency care produced a period of "benign neglect" in which a previously adequate emergency medical system began to develop profound but predictable deficiencies. As the magnitude of these inadequacies was finally documented, they were eventually described in 1972 by the Assistant Secretary of Health, Education, and Welfare as "the hidden crisis in health care." In all the deficiencies found in this hidden crisis, none were greater than those in manpower and training.

It became apparent that new programs and materials with more medical input and orientation were needed. Initial attempts were not well supported or adequately funded, but most programs managed to compensate for this poverty with a wealth of enthusiasm. The first efforts were geared to the training of basic ambulance personnel, who were identified by the new title of "Emergency Medical Technician-Ambulance." The programs ranged from a minimal week-end course of about 20 hours to an extensive and extended course of 80 or more hours. Significant changes became apparent in this new effort to train emergency manpower: the courses now were frequently taught by physicians; the programs were often supported and housed in hospitals and other medical institutions; for the first time, emergency medical personnel were being taught specific medical skills not previously available in disaster and rescue training programs. Fortunately, some of these skills, such as cardiopulmonary resuscitation (CPR), are now available to all branches of emergency personnel and, occasionally, even to the general public.

One of the most familiar programs for the basic Emergency Medical Technician (EMT-I) was developed by the Committee on Injuries of the American Academy of Orthopedic Surgeons. This consisted primarily of a text, along with a series of slides to accompany the material in the text, and this material was subsequently integrated into the basic training program developed by Dunlap and associates for the National Highway Traffic Administration. Other excellent teaching aids were soon developed, and a variety of resources is now available to any individual or institution attempting to develop and maintain basic training courses for Emergency Medical Technicians (EMT-A or EMT-I).

Soon thereafter, but on a much more limited scale and involving primarily the cities of Seattle, Miami, Jacksonville, Columbus, and Los Angeles, pioneering efforts were under way to develop a more advanced level of Emergency Medical Technician called the EMT-II, more popularly known as "paramedic." As in the case of the original efforts for EMT-I training programs, widely different recommendations were made, ranging from 280 hours up to more than 1000 hours for this new level of training. Except for limited instruction on splinting or extrications, this new course was taught almost exclusively by doctors and nurses or other medical personnel, and it added a significant array of additional therapeutic measures to prehospital emergency care. The simple station-wagon or van-type ambulance with little if any medical equipment and staffed by poorly trained personnel had now become a sophisticated medical vehicle with well trained personnel that could properly be labeled a "Mobile Intensive Care Unit." Most of this improvement was made possible by marked change in earlier attitudes: emergency care was now viewed as a community responsibility, and public funds were made available to support these newer and more comprehensive emergency medical services.

As more and more areas of the country are upgrading their vehicles and training their personnel to the level of EMT-I, there is increasing interest in continuing this advancement to the level of EMT-II. Once again, there are no iron-clad requirements or uniform national approaches, but a series of texts are available that deal with the more comprehensive approach to the evaluation and treatment of cardiac problems as well as the drugs available in the paramedic's armamentarium. Given the current state of flux and the rapid evolution of enabling state legislation, no unique or lasting recommendations can be applied to out-of-hospital personnel.

However, it seems reasonable to predict that several modifications of the ambulance mechanical and medical equipment as well as new combinations of staffing and personnel will be tried in the future and perhaps perfected in various parts of the nation. Helicopters and fixed-wing aircraft are likely to be used more as emergency services are coordinated on a large scale, particularly in rural and remote areas, and as regional centers are developed for a variety of medical services. The final make-up of the ambulance crew is far from settled, but forgotten are the ambulance teams in large cities during the 1930's and early 40's, when a hospital-based ambulance often carried a driver, two attendants, and an intern. (Also forgotten is the fact that the intern in those days was the lowest paid and most economical member of the ambulance team!) One of the nation's last physician-staffed ambulance services in Pasadena has recently changed to paramedic staffing, and it seems unlikely that the physician will ever be a fixed or consistent member of a primary response (home or highway) ambulance team (although of interest is that the Russian System expanded the role of the physician in the ambulance.)* For secondary response (interhospital transfer) ambulances, however, physician staffing may be essential in critical cases, while a new level of emergency medical manpower, the hospital-based paramedic, may provide the core staff for such transfer vehicles.

Combination staffing may become a popular pattern in the future. Surprisingly, many municipalities now operate ambulances staffed by either EMT-I or EMT-II personnel, but almost never by a combination of the two. Some of the people who insist on this all-or-none phenomenon apparently believe that the prefix in paramedic was derived from the word "pair," while overlooking the fact that mixed EMT-I and EMT-II ambulance teams would immediately double paramedic coverage in a city without delay or extra expense. Furthermore, this combination staffing would provide a logical and obvious incentive for the EMT-II to review and teach and for the EMT-I to learn and advance on a career ladder.

As prehospital emergency personnel learn more medical procedures and skills, it is essential that their initial training as well as continuing education programs be integrated as much as possible with the education of in-house personnel. This may be more feasible as improved educational techniques such as programmed patient or computer-operated manikins are made available. These modern techniques provide a uniform and consistent source of patient teaching

---

*See p. 1489.

material for all emergency medical personnel, whether they are based in the hospital Emergency Department or in a distant field station. Furthermore, this educational integration and common orientation will allow much more rapid and accurate assessment of quality of care in out-of-hospital problems. Such quality evaluation programs are not yet available or operational in emergency care, but appear inevitable in the near future as better records and more data become available.

The advances of modern pharmacology and the potentials of future technology are of little benefit unless utilized by well trained and highly skilled emergency medical personnel.

Chapter 65

EMERGENCY MEDICAL SERVICES COMMUNICATIONS

Arthur H. Griffiths

INTRODUCTION

The communications requirements for support of emergency medical services are similar whether there is a single incident of sudden illness or injury, or a disaster involving large numbers of victims. Only after the system has been defined in terms of what services are to be provided, who is responsible for providing them and how they are to be provided, can the functional communications system requirements be determined. Some of these requirements, of course, are determined by the nature of emergency services; the remainder are dictated by *how* the services are to be provided.

The normal EMS cycle includes the following elements:

(1) *Incident.* The occurrence that generates the need for EMS.

(2) *Detection.* The action that determines that the incident took place.

(3) *Notification.* The action that informs the emergency resource control agency where and when the incident took place, and its nature.

(4) *Response.* The action that orders and directs the required emergency resources to the scene of the incident.

(5) *Closure.* The transport of emergency resources to the scene of the incident.

(6) *Action.* Those necessary acts that correct or alleviate conditions generated by the incident, including immediate care, medical control, and transport to a medical facility.

(7) *Return to station.* The return of all emergency resources to a state of readiness for a new cycle.

Once the incident has been detected, communications become a vital element to activate, control, and coordinate the total response of the system. Without an efficient communications system, emergency services cannot be expected to function effectively.

Reduction in response time is an often stated objective to improve emergency systems. Response time can be defined in more than one way, but the most valid definition is that which includes time from the instant of perceived need. Using this definition, it is apparent that a considerable reduction in response time can be brought about by simplifying the process of reporting the need for emergency services—the *notification* portion of the emergency cycle.

THE 9-1-1 TELEPHONE SYSTEM

Most Americans are unaware of how difficult it can be to report a need for emergency service in some parts of the U.S. Most of us have not committed to memory the telephone number to use in our own home territory, let alone the one to use when we are not on familiar ground. Some telephone books list dozens of emergency telephone numbers on the inside cover, and it is necessary to know which political jurisdiction serves a specific area in order to make the correct number selection. Further, the telephone operator (who may be located many miles away) may not be able to provide needed answers readily. Ideally, the number used should be one we have known since earliest childhood, and one valid throughout the U.S.

The "Emergency Medical Services Systems Act of 1973 (P.L. 93–154)" authorizes the appropriation of funds for grants to support the development of EMS systems. The Act itself and the regulations governing the administration of the Act require that an EMS system shall "join the personnel, facilities, and equipment of the system by a central communications system so that requests for emergency health care services will be handled by a communications facility which utilizes emergency medical telephonic screening; utilizes (or, within such period as the Secretary may prescribe, will utilize) the universal emergency telephone number 911; and will have direct communication connections and interconnections with the personnel, facilities, and equipment of the system and with other appropriate emergency medical services systems."

In 1967, the President's Commission on Law Enforcement and Administration of Justice recognized the need for simplifying the notification process, and recommended that "a single number should be established" for reporting police emergencies. The concept of a single nationwide telephone number for reporting emergencies is not new. It was realized in Great Britain more than 30 years ago, when that country established "9-9-9" as its national emergency number. Other countries in Europe and elsewhere have since established nationally uniform emergency telephone numbers.

In 1968, the American Telephone and Telegraph Company announced that it was making the number "9-1-1" available as an emergency system access telephone number. Independent telephone organizations also have endorsed this number. There are now in the U.S. over 600 "9-1-1" systems operating in communities of all sizes and serving a population in excess of 44 million. It is erroneous to assume that, since the telephone number is the same, all "9-1-1" systems are identical. The systems are configured to satisfy the areas that they serve, which is a euphemistic way of saying that they satisfy the political realities and the telephone exchange boundaries existing at the time the system is implemented. As a first step in planning for a "9-1-1" system, the following primary issues must be addressed and decisions made.

(1) *The scope of the services to be included in the "9-1-1" system.* As a minimum the system should include police, fire, and emergency medical services.

(2) *The area to be served by the pro-*

posed "9-1-1" system. Decisions here involve consideration of telephone system boundaries and political jurisdiction boundaries.

(3) *The location of the "9-1-1" answering center.* Decisions here must take into account available resources and system recurring costs. The U.S., for example, has more than 3500 emergency operating centers, built with matching funds from the Defense Civil Preparedness Agency (DCPA), which can be used for this purpose.

(4) *The existing public safety agencies in the "9-1-1" service area and their available resources and jurisdictions.* How will these agencies and the "9-1-1" system be organized into an operating public safety system?

(5) *The service areas (telephone exchange boundaries) and their relationship to the political jurisdiction(s) to be included within the "9-1-1" system.* These two sets of boundaries rarely coincide, especially in urban areas, and consequently can generate some costly proposals as solutions to jurisdictional problems.

Close examination of these stated primary issues should make clear that "9-1-1" is not something that can be ordered tomorrow from the telephone company and installed the following week.

The "9-1-1" system requires careful planning, many compromises, and dedication on the part of those responsible for its implementation. To define the commitment required for "9-1-1" implementation, the following is excerpted from the booklet published in May 1973 by the Office of Telecommunications Policy, Executive Office of the President, entitled "9-1-1 – The Emergency Telephone Number – A Handbook for Community Planning." °

How Does a Community Initiate Planning for 9-1-1?

Usually one or two individuals in a community become interested in 9-1-1 and decide that they would like to find out more about it. This

---

°This Office of Telecommunications Policy Publication provides the best coverage of this subject now available. It can be purchased from the Superintendent of Documents, U.S. Government Printing Office, Washington, D.C., 20402. Price $1.35. Stock number 2205–0003. Copies on a limited basis also are available from the Division of Emergency Medical Services Clearinghouse, 6525 Belcrest Road, West Hyattsville, Maryland 20782.

initiative may come from a private citizen, citizens' group, the police or fire chief, an elected official, or anyone else in the community who is concerned with emergency communications. After it has been determined that a wider interest in 9-1-1 exists, work can begin on learning how it might serve that particular area.

Because 9-1-1 will affect so many different segments of the community, it is usually best to select a task force or committee which will be responsible for investigating the issues involved with the implementation of 9-1-1. Each community will have to decide which individuals will be most valuable on such a committee, but generally it is best to consider the following persons:

(1) *The mayor or other elected official.* Either the mayor, a councilman, or other elected official should be represented on the planning committee. This person will be in a position to represent the local government and to indicate what governmental resources can be made available for 9-1-1 planning and implementation. In many cases a resolution or ordinance must be passed by the local government in order to approve expenditures or other resources allocated to 9-1-1; a representative on the planning board may pave the way for such formal approval.

(2) *The Chief of Police.* The Chief of Police is in a position to let the committee know exactly what his communications requirements are and how any proposed changes in the communications process may alter his operating procedures. He will also be familiar with the emergency communications system which is currently in use.

(3) *The Fire Chief.* Fire departments also have an immediate need for information. A fire in progress can greatly change in character within minutes and an early response can literally mean the difference between life and death. The fire chief will be able to detail his needs for emergency reporting.

(4) *Representatives from local ambulance services.* In many communities ambulances or rescue squads are dispatched directly from police or fire stations when an injury is reported. In those communities which are served by private ambulance companies or by hospital-operated emergency vehicles, representatives from these organizations should also be included in discussions of emergency reporting capabilities.

(5) *The local Civil Defense representative.* Communities usually have an appointed Civil Defense representative who is knowledgeable in procedures to follow in emergency situations. His experience in planning and setting up a local emergency operations center may be quite helpful in planning a 9-1-1 system.

(6) *Representatives from citizens' organizations.* Because 9-1-1 is first and foremost a system to benefit the citizen, local residents should be asked to indicate their current problems in obtaining emergency assistance and to respond to the suggestions made by the communications and public safety experts.

(7) *A communications consultant from the telephone company which serves the community.* The configuration of telephone equipment which serves a community is, in all likelihood, unique to that community. Only a telephone company representative will be able to suggest the alternatives available with present equipment and to explain his company's ability to respond to a request for 9-1-1 service.

If the planning committee is sufficiently broad-based in its composition, each issue which arises can be considered from a variety of viewpoints, and resolution of problem areas can be achieved early in the planning stages.

The "9-1-1" systems that develop as a result of these planning activities will take on various configurations and methods of operation. The compromises agreed upon will be those dictated by the combination of political jurisdiction boundaries, telephone switching system (exchange) boundaries, and the "people problems" faced and solved during the process of arriving at an acceptable plan.

The plan that finally evolves will probably result in a "9-1-1" system configuration resembling one of these three general patterns.

(1) *Centralized "9-1-1" call reception. Decentralized Emergency Service Dispatch (Relay).* All "9-1-1" calls are directed to a single answering center. The answering operator obtains all necessary and pertinent data from the caller, and then *relays* this information to the appropriate response agency(ies).

(2) *Centralized "9-1-1" call reception. Decentralized Emergency Service Dispatch (Transfer).* Incoming "9-1-1" calls are directed to a single answering center. The answering operator determines the nature of the emergency, and then *transfers* the call to the appropriate emergency service agency to obtain the necessary and pertinent data prior to dispatch.

(3) *Centralized "9-1-1" call reception. Centralized Emergency Service Dispatch.* All incoming "9-1-1" calls are received at a single centralized communications center that has the authority to control and coordinate the emergency services resources of the system.

Of the three configurations, the last probably is the most cost-effective and the most efficient. However, it is also the configuration most difficult to achieve because of "people problems."

THE RESOURCE CONTROL CENTER

The Emergency Medical Services Systems Act (EMS Systems Act) requires that the system "join the personnel, facilities, and equipment by a central communications system." The regulations define this to include "a system command and control center which is responsible for establishing those communications channels and providing those public resources essential to the most effective and efficient emergency medical services management of the immediate problem, and which has the necessary equipment and facilities to permit immediate interchange of information essential for the system's resource management and control." Thus, both the ACT and its regulations recognize the need for a Resource Control Center (RCC).

The RCC is the nerve center for the entire system. It is the center to which the *notification* action is directed. It receives all requests for system response. System resources are controlled and all necessary system liaison with other public safety and emergency response systems is coordinated, from this center.

A separate RCC for EMS exclusive of other emergency services, which lend support required on a day-to-day basis as well as during major emergencies or disasters, is not economically sound for most communities. Also, separate control centers for the various public safety and other service agencies makes coordination between agencies difficult. Good management principles require effective utilization of existing resources. Applying these principles to EMS communications systems requires interagency cooperation and multi-agency use of facilities, manpower, and all other resources.

Coordination between agencies can be improved by establishing their resource control functions in a common center. As mentioned in the "9-1-1" discussion, 3500 or more emergency operating centers exist and are available to be used as RCCs. By placing day-to-day resource control functions for police, fire, rescue, EMS, and other public safety-oriented services together in one center, it is possible to overcome most of the coordination problems that arise during a major emergency or disaster. The importance cannot be overemphasized for embedding the normal day-to-day EMS system within the organization and center which is planned for use during disaster conditions. This approach assures a functioning system that needs only to be augmented as necessary or possible to provide disaster response to the limit of its capabilities.

THE MEDICAL CONTROL FUNCTION

EMS communications systems, in addition to requiring resource coordination and control, also must provide for medical control of the system. Emergency Medical Services Systems Program Guidelines for the EMS Systems Act define medical control as "directions and advice provided from a centrally designated medical facility staffed by appropriate EMS personnel, operating under medical supervision, supplying professional support through radio or telephonic communication for on-site and in-transit, basic and advanced life support services given by field and satellite facility personnel." Medical control communications satisfy the communications requirements of the *action* element of the EMS cycle.

Federal Communications Commission (FCC) Rules and Regulations governing Emergency Medical Services Radio Communications have allocated a block of Ultra High Frequency (UHF) radio frequencies for use to satisfy the medical control function. The FCC licenses the use of any or all of this block of UHF frequencies when authorizing an EMS system's operation on the UHF band. This places a very heavy burden of responsibility upon those charged with the operation of the EMS system, which is authorized to use the block of frequencies almost as it sees fit. However, it must be remembered that every other EMS system also has the same set of frequencies authorized for its use. The potential is present for utter chaos if the managers of adjacent EMS systems fail to work out mutual noninterference frequency plans for real-time frequency usage management plans. An adequate number of discrete frequencies are available for adjacent systems to operate simultaneously without causing interference to each other, but this can be accomplished only by mutual agreement and strict adherence to those agreements. If left to chance, Murphy's law dictates that interference will occur, probably at a time when the most damage can ensue.

The problem of intersystem and intrasystem interference is most severe in the large metropolitan areas. The high population density areas will generate the greater amount of EMS activity, with a resulting need for more rigid control of the system if interference between elements of the system is to be avoided. This greater activity also increases the probability of interference with surrounding area systems. Consequently, great care must be exercised in the design of the communications facilities in these areas.

Other public safety communications systems are not affected by interference problems in the same manner as are EMS communications systems. First, they are not allocated a block of frequencies as are the medical services. Second, their normal channel usage time generally is quite short, whereas in the medical services a communications channel may be in use during the medical control phase for 30 minutes or more, denying use of that channel to any other potential user. For this reason, it is strongly recommended that the system's mode of operation be so arranged that the RCC is responsible for establishing the required communications channel for each incident. Thus, when an ambulance is dispatched, the RCC operator can assign a channel to be used by that ambulance for all of its communications with its medical control facility for the duration of that particular incident. In addition, the RCC should alert the medical control facility and assure that the assigned channel is established and usable. Some EMS systems have been configured so that these medical control channels are switched through the RCC to the medical control facility. This approach can be very cost-effective in eliminating costly duplication of equipment. It has the advantage of placing responsibility for system operation with a single organization, the RCC. Finally, by making the RCC responsible for communications system operation, it relieves the medical control facility (hospital) of responsibility for a portion of the EMS system's communications. Medical control *must* be provided with clear communications channels, but control and responsibility for the efficient operation of the EMS communications system should be left to professional communicators. It is a serious mistake to try to make communicators of medical professionals.

OPERATION AND MANAGEMENT

The establishment of a RCC implies the need for an organization responsible for the operation and management of the EMS systems communications. Such an organization is essential to any communications systems. Without some means of daily monitoring the operations of the system, its efficiency and effectiveness will decline. Radio communications in particular require almost military discipline to avoid becoming ineffective. An example will help defend this position. The FCC in its regulations states: "The Commission expects each licensee to take reasonable precautions to prevent unnecessary interference. If harmful interference develops, the commission may require any or all stations to monitor the transmitting frequency prior to transmission." Carelessness or disregard of the manner in which radio communications must be conducted, ignoring "circuit discipline," can totally destroy the usefulness of the circuit (channel). In telephone communications, if one tries to interrupt an "in use" circuit, a busy signal is received, and those using the circuit do not experience interference. With radio communications, such interruptions do interfere with the "in use" circuit and deny its use both to those using and to those attempting to use the channel. The need for an operating organization that can establish operating procedures, assure adherence to established procedures, and improve the over-all effectiveness of the system on a continuing basis is very real, if the communications system is to continue to satisfy the EMS system it was designed to support. An EMS communications system is *not* a collection of transmitters, receivers, towers, and antennas. Hardware does not make a system. It takes people functioning within the constraints of established procedures for use of that hardware to create an effective communications system.

As stated at the beginning of this discussion, communications requirements can be determined only after the EMS system has been defined. "Defined" in this sense implies that the system operational concepts are known, characterized, and established or agreed upon; that the EMS system's boundaries are established and its resources are known. "Defined" in this instance also means that bordering systems are known and that their impact or potential impact upon communications will be considered. The boundaries of an EMS system are described by existing natural patient care flow patterns. The EMS system must encompass a sufficient population base to be able to support and provide facilities for definitive care services to the majority of general, emergent, and critical patients. Where highly sophisticated critical care facilities are deficient within the system's boundaries, arrangements and procedures must be established to obtain these patient care services in adjoining systems. These elements all bear on the final configuration of the communications system that will best serve the EMS system.

Portions of the EMS communications requirements must be satisfied by radio, because its resources in part are mobile; therefore, Federal Communications Commission Rules and Regulations establish constraints on the communications system design. Present FCC regulations allocate both VHF and UHF frequencies to medical services. The VHF frequency allocations establish specific frequencies to be used for paging, low power portable (hand-held and not airborne) transmissions, and base and mobile station transmissions. The VHF frequencies *cannot* be used for the transmission of telemetry signals.

This prohibition limits the VHF freqency communication system to support of the Basic Life Support EMS system. Basic Life Support Services (BLS) provide the minimal acceptable level of care services available in an areawide EMS system. Advanced Life Support Services (ALS) provide the highest level of emergency care services, and do call for the use of telemetry. For EMS systems to have the maximum effect in

reducing death and disability, BLS Services must progress on to ALS Services. EMS system communications designs, therefore, should anticipate the ultimate transfer of EMS system communications to the UHF band. Neither EMS system communications planning nor equipment procurement is encouraged in other than the UHF band.

TELEMETRY

The term "telemetry" means measurement at a distance. At the present time, EMS systems use telemetry to transmit a patient's electrocardiogram from the patient's location to a medical control facility. The EKG provides a part of the data base necessary to establish a treatment protocol. The method employed to transmit the EKG is common to many telemetry and data transmissions. A reference audio tone (subcarrier) is made to change frequency in accordance with the data to be transmitted. If the potential generated by the heart goes positive, the subcarrier is made to increase in frequency, and conversely. This subcarrier tone is detected at the distant terminal and used to activate a recording device (strip chart). To assure compatibility between telemetry systems, the subcarrier frequencies used must be the same. The Federal Communications Commission has proposed that a Telemetry Standard published by the Office of Telecommunications Policy, Executive Office of the President be adopted as a required standard for the manufacture of these equipments.

Although telemetry now is used exclusively to transmit EKGs, it need not be limited to this one vital life sign, and neither should the use of telemetry necessarily be limited to use in dealing with the coronary patient. Telemetry is a new tool for EMS, and its full potential has yet to be established. There is no reason to assume that other, or new, sensors for vital life signs will not be adaptable for use in Emergency Medical Services.

Chapter 66

EMERGENCY MEDICAL SERVICES TRANSPORTATION

Robert L. Donald and Garry I. Briese

The "emergency medical transportation component" of an EMS system has often in the past been synonymous with the totality of emergency medical services. Although the transportation component certainly is the most visible and audible of the components, it must now be recognized as being only one of many. Here we will describe an emergency medical system as: "... a planned and functioning combination of personnel, equipment, and facilities related to the delivery of quality and effective emergency medical care (pre-hospital *and* in-hospital), and which is administered by public or private entities recognized by local authorities" (Briese, 1974).

Although such an integrated and functioning "system" may be lacking in a given community, every community has the essential building blocks for total system development. The manpower is generally available but often untrained. The communication and transportation elements may exist, but obsolescence often prevails. Too frequently, most basic plans for the development of an integrated system are lacking. Without proper organization, coordination, and evaluation, it is impossible to identify the system components needing alteration and/or improvement. We must remember that this emergency medical "system" is, in fact, another subsystem of the total health care delivery system. It must not be viewed as a separate and distinct entity.

Emergency medical services can be most effectively shown in relation to the passage of a patient through the patient-flow pattern of a "typical" incident. Figure 1 ac-

curately describes this passage and the total system's response. "The objective of the emergency medical transportation system is to provide, in the least possible time, safe and competent emergency medical treatment for the accident/sudden-illness victim. Sub-objectives, with their attendant measures of performance in parentheses, directed toward the accomplishment of this objective of the system include:

1. Least possible time required to respond to an accident/sudden-illness incident (total system response time)

2. Highest possible quality of treatment administered to the patient (patient condition, medical attendant proficiency, equipment types, and serviceability)

3. Least possible time required to transport the patient to the medical facility best able to administer to his needs (total system incident-to-hospital-treatment time)

4. Insurance of safe operations (accident rates, operator proficiency, vehicle serviceability)

5. The most effective use of resources (volume-to-capacity ratios, inventory levels-to-use ratios, benefit-cost ratios)

6. Continuous reporting of measures of performance relative to costs (cost-effectiveness).

The emergency medical transportation system is designed to perform in a ten-step mission cycle: (1) notification, (2) dispatch, (3) closure, (4) triage, (5) first-aid, (6) transport, (7) life support, (8) delivery, (9) disposition, and (10) recock, or return to the ready status which may involve logistical support. Each emergency call serviced involves sev-

EMERGENCY MEDICAL SERVICES FLOW CHART

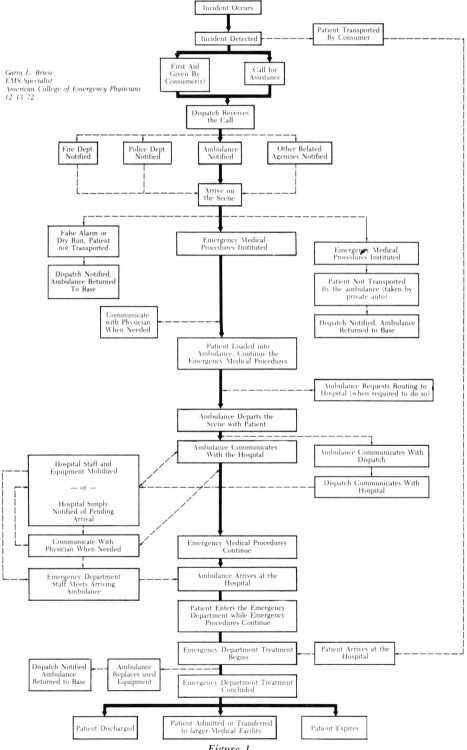

Figure 1

eral or all of these steps (a false alarm, for example, might include notification, dispatch, closure, no incident, recock). The process is initiated by the detection of the incident, but the emergency medical transportation system becomes involved only when notified. It is at this juncture that safeguards against false alarms may be inserted. Some missions may require only first-aid at the scene of the accident, but most calls will go full cycle" (Wyanf, 1971).

In the U.S., perhaps the most glaring discrepancy in the development of an integrated response system has been the inadequacy of the prehospital care administered to victims of accidents or sudden illness. The statistics and horror stories need not be repeated here. Let it suffice to say that great improvements have been instituted, and it is generally believed, although difficult to document, that a reduction in the mortality and morbidity of accident or sudden illness patients is under way.

This reduction, if actual, certainly cannot be attributed solely to improved prehospital emergency care. Other factors, such as increased usage of seat belts, decreased speed limits, citizen training in cardiopulmonary resuscitation, better automobile construction, and the increased home consumption of alcohol (as opposed to consumption in bars, etc.), certainly have had some effect in this mortality and morbidity reduction.

RESPONSIBILITY FOR THE PROVISION OF EMERGENCY AMBULANCE SERVICE

It is a citizen's right to have adequate prehospital emergency care guaranteed to him and his family, for, as Vogt said ". . . the greatest threat to the average citizen is not the fire in the home or the criminal in the street . . . but, it is the inability to get emergency medical care at a time when minutes mean life." A function of our government is to provide those services which the individual cannot better provide for himself. Emergency medical services, like fire control and law enforcement, should be considered one of those basic services and recognized as such. We are not stating that the government should operate the emergency medical service; rather it is the responsibility of our government to guarantee the adequate minimal level of care to all citizens. Government, in this usage, refers to all three levels, with emphasis being placed at the local level.

Whether this service can best be provided directly by the government, by private operators under contractual agreement, by a hospital-operated service, by volunteers, or by any other organizational option is immaterial. What is important is that a level of care be established in accordance with recognized national standards *and be insured by appropriate governmental level.*

For the development and maintenance of high quality emergency medical services programs, the government, whether local or state, seems to be the only institution of our society capable of insuring this level of care.

Not only must these high standards be initiated and implemented, they should also be enforceable by a local or state governmental agency. One should include such items as response times, staffing, training of personnel, billing procedures, and general outline of cost, as well as vehicles, with clearly documented standards and specifications.

Before concentrating on transportation as such, one more concept should be identified. A service area should have an emergency medical services system, *not* two or three or more. Integrated into this single system may be several ambulance companies or providers and multiple hospitals, but only *one* system. Tax support dollars should be diverted to the system, *not* divided, among the various components in some haphazard way. System control and responsibility should be clearly delegated to a usable responsible committee, council, or agency.

GROUND TRANSPORTATION

An "ambulance," according to Webster's Dictionary, "is a vehicle equipped for transporting the sick or injured." Although this is an adequate general definition, the National Academy of Sciences/National Research Council's Committee on Ambulance Design Criteria decided that a vehicle should not be termed an "ambulance" unless it has been designed, constructed, equipped, and staffed to handle trauma and medical emergencies outside the hospital Emergency Department. Specifically the Committee stated:

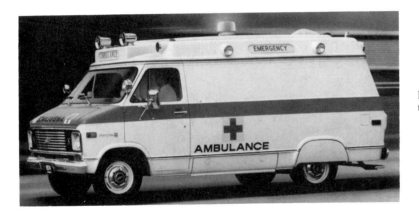

Figure 2. Van-style ambulance meeting federal specifications.

The ambulance is defined as a vehicle for emergency care which provides a driver compartment, and a patient compartment which can accommodate two emergency medical technicians and two litter patients so positioned that at least one patient can be given intensive life-support during transit; which carries equipment and supplies for optimal emergency care at the scene as well as during transport, for two-way radio communication, for safe-guarding personnel and patients under hazardous conditions, and for light rescue procedures; and which is designed and constructed to afford maximum safety and comfort, and to avoid aggravation of the patient's condition, exposure to complications, and threat to survival (Ambulance Design Criteria, 1973).

For many years, ambulance design depended on the amount of money the buyer wished to invest and the ingenuity of the builder in finding space to store the equipment the operator could afford. During this period, the public and the medical community accepted inadequate vehicles as ambulances, when in fact the vehicles were suit-able for nothing more than placing the victim in a recumbent position for a quick and often dangerous ride to the nearest hospital. These "ambulances" have been collectively referred to as "horizontal taxis." But, do not mistake ignorance for cognizant neglect. The public did not have any measurable performance criteria, and the medical community had not considered the provision of "emergency medical care" outside the hospital.

When, in 1957, the Trauma Committee of the American College of Surgeons, the American Association for the Surgery of Trauma, and the National Safety Council sponsored a nationwide survey of emergency services—and the results shocked those who read them—the committee developed a list of "Minimum Equipment for Ambulances." The publication of the "minimal" list of equipment in 1957 was the first dutiful recognition on the part of the national medical community of their responsibility in the insurance of adequate prehos-

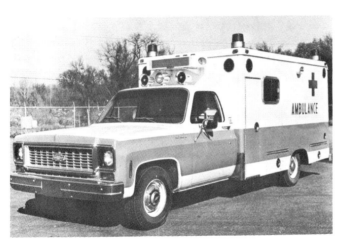

Figure 3. Modular-style ambulance meeting federal specifications.

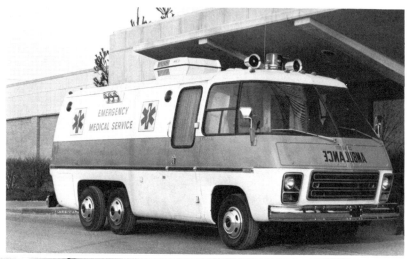

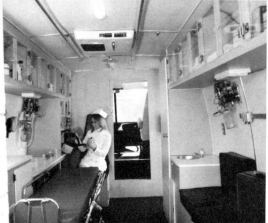
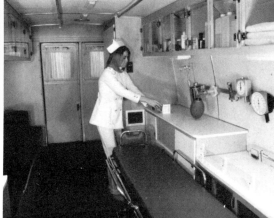

Figure 4. Regional life-support/critical transfer ambulance.

pital emergency care for their patients. Since that time, the medical community has participated in many different programs and stimulated many efforts to improve and upgrade community emergency medical care. The list was updated in 1969 as the "Essential Equipment for Ambulances" list, and is now the accepted standard nationally. However, with recent advances in prehospital emergency care, the "Essential Equipment" list should be reviewed and revised.

Two documents published by the Federal government perhaps have done more to stimulate improvement in the design of ambulances than anything else (Medical Requirements for Ambulance Design, 1969; Ambulance Design Criteria, 1971). Although more emergency ambulances meet these criteria today than met these "standards" in

1969, it is estimated that 70 per cent of the ambulances in use today still do not meet the "criteria." It is hoped that professional and provider awareness will reduce this percentage in the near future.

After nearly five years of increasing public and professional educational campaigns, great advances have been made, but these are at best limited when one views the over-all picture of the status of EMS in the U.S. Locally, perhaps, the prehospital emergency care problem has been solved in a few fortunate communities, but this is the exception rather than the rule. As long as a citizen cannot be assured of receiving an acceptable level of emergency medical care throughout the U.S., the job has not been completed.

Recently the federal government published another document that will have great impact on emergency ambulances. "Federal Emergency Medical Care Vehicle Specifications KKK-A-1822" was based on the earlier *Ambulance Design Criteria* and translated the Criteria's general concepts into specific engineering design sepcifications. This is a rather complicated document, and the potential user may well become confused while attempting to digest its facts. Special attention should be directed to Section 6, page 31, of the specifications. This section pertains to the correct ordering procedure for vehicles with these specifications. All federally funded programs will be required to use this specification for bidding procedures on ambulances.

Specific vehicle designs are especially suited to certain geographic and population density areas. These vehicles are in use in established systems throughout the country, and the potential buyer should study the performance results of any vehicle type before being committed to its purchase. System leaders in these communities will be glad to share their experiences with vehicle design in their particular area with other potential or established providers. A few inquiries before purchase may avoid many headaches afterward.

Ground transportation may well be the single most expensive component of a system and, therefore, should be given the time and thought it justly deserves.

HELICOPTERS IN EMERGENCY MEDICAL SERVICE

Owing to the unqualified success and the extensive "aeromedical evacuation" experience gained by the U.S. military during the Indochina War (Vietnam), various helicopter programs have been initiated throughout the United States.

"The three major benefits of helicopters vs. ground-based ambulances which are responsible for today's great interest in helicopters are:

1. faster response time (based on greater speed, straight-line travel and the elimination of the effects of traffic and deterring conditions)

2. service to inaccessible areas (where no road exists or where roads are impassable due to severe weather conditions)

3. smoother transport of the patient which is especially important for certain types of injuries such as cerebral hemorrhage or severe spinal injuries.

As a direct consequence of the speed and mobility of the helicopters, the benefits can also be stated in terms of increases in the size of the service area (or a reduction in the number of ambulance locations) for a given criterion response time" (Economics of Highway Ambulance Services, 1969).

The application and forte of the helicopter will obviously be in the rural, low population density areas of the country. The experiences of the Military Assistance to Safety and Traffic program has shown reasonable successes in rural service areas. The MAST program was begun in August 1969 as a pilot program to explore the feasibility of utilizing military helicopters and personnel to respond to civilian medical emergencies, particularly to highway accidents. "MAST was essentially an operational test, where military resources of known capability were meshed with local emergency medical services systems with a minimum of delay and administrative difficulty, and with no additional men, money, or equipment provided."

After the preliminary trial period, several conclusions were reached by the MAST experience which are of interest here:

"1. The degree of utilization of the military helicopters, once a responsive service was established, was not a function of any factors within the military, but was related to factors in the community which were not precisely identified.

2. The local community's emergency medical system must be highly organized and well-developed to fully integrate and make the most effective use of military air ambulances. An adequate emergency medical communication system is vital for making responsive and effective use of military air ambulances. It insures prompt notification, proper coordination, and direct communication between the military and various elements of the emergency medical system" (MAST — Report of Test Program, 1970).

The helicopter, therefore, except in very special instances, should be an adjunct to an existing operational emergency medical services system and should be utilized only as special situations dictate.

Recently Public Law 93–155 was signed, authorizing military units to assist civilian communities by providing emergency helicopter transportation. This law will, in effect, expand the pilot MAST program across the nation.

Of special note in the sucess of civilian helicopter operations should be the Maryland State Police helicopter operation as well as the Southeast Mississippi Air Ambulance Service District (Hattiesburg, Mississippi). The Maryland State Police operation began in 1969 and has transported over 2500 patients. Operating as an adjunct to the existing fire-rescue and ambulance services in the state has allowed the service to claim a survival rate of approximately 83 per cent. The primary reason attributed to this high survival rate has been getting the patients to properly staffed and equipped treatment centers in the shortest possible time. The Mississippi helicopter is the first such operation created and financed by a special taxing district. This program is the result of a federally sponsored and funded project in Mississippi to test the feasibility of helicopter operations (Project CARE-SOM: Coordinated Accident Rescue Endeavor—State of Mississippi). The project places a special tax on property holders in the district of $1.67 per year. (See the March-April 1974 issue of *Emergency Product News* for a complete story.)

The U.S. Department of Transportation has produced a document summarizing the "Helicopters in Emergency Medical Service NHTSA Experience to Date" (December 1972). This is available from the National Technical Information Service, 5285 Port Royal Road, Springfield, Virginia 22151.

Helicopter services are extremely expensive both to initiate and to maintain. Although in certain areas and in specific circumstances helicopter usefulness is unquestioned, many potential use locations must be eliminated because of the high cost-use ratio. There are, however, areas where the helicopter can be assigned multiple uses, and good experiences have been documented. These are generally the areas where its use for emergency medical services has been coupled with those of air search, police control, special personnel transport, fire control (both in communities and over forest areas), etc.

SPECIALIZED TRANSPORTATION

"In certain cases where definitive care is beyond the scope of the primary institu-

tion to which a critically ill or injured patient is delivered, secondary transfer must be arranged" (Boyd, 1972). Often these transfers are extremely risky to the patient. They are also quite necessary if the patient is going to survive. Although the physical facilities for transporting such critical patients have improved along with the generalized improvement in emergency medical services, the organization of statewide and regional networks for providing uniformly excellent critical care transfer is not available at the present time.

Several states, such as Indiana, Maine, Illinois, and Nebraska, have begun to implement programs to fill this significant void in the emergency medical services system. "The biggest problem, and the one on which we should concentrate our efforts and resources, is the EMS systems of rural areas, small communities, and isolated cities. Rather than continuing to spend funds and effort in metropolitan areas with already established or rapidly developing EMS systems, it is time we pay attention to the areas with the greater need" (Farrington, 1973). Even with the decrease in the death rate per million miles traveled to the lowest record ever (4.5 per million miles traveled), still 70 per cent of the automobile deaths occurred in rural areas.

Some areas have begun to utilize life-support units capable of providing specialized care to the patient. Further advances in development are manifested in the development of a vehicle capable of rendering multiple facets of specialized care. These are larger than the frequently utilized van or modular ambulance and have the advantages of more treatment space and more storage space. These are ideal for longer distance transport with continuing in-vehicle patient care. These are indeed regional life support units.

These regional life support units can provide the ultimate in specialized treatment for patients while they are being transferred to facilities capable of administering the required definitive care. The units eliminate the need for disease-specific units (coronary care, neonatal care, etc.). They will have the capability of rapidly converting from one function to another by an uncomplicated process of changing disease-specific equipment and personnel.

Perhaps the most difficult problem in the establishment of such regional life support units is physician and public education in the proper utilization of the unit. The awareness level of physicians must be increased in the area of early detection of potential patient disasters and in the area of the early transportation of the critical patient to specialized centers by these life support units. The general public must be made aware not only of the functions of these units, but also of the relatively high cost of the units, because the funding ultimately comes from the public, in one form or another.

SPECIAL SOLUTIONS TO SPECIAL PROBLEMS

Winter presents special problems for many of our nation's emergency medical services. The usual cold weather adaptations such as snow tires, low viscosity lubricants, anti-freeze and snow chains will adequately convert the "standard" ambulance for winter duty. However, freezing weather complicates all problems. For example, an initial patient survey is rather easily performed on a patient wearing "normal" street clothes. However, when the patient and the emergency medical technician are encased in snowmobile suits, immersed in a snow drift two miles from the closest road, and the wind chill index is −40° F., the survey becomes a major effort. Emergency care procedures are complicated and equipment becomes inoperable.

Many ambulance services have made special use of the snowmobile as a rescue device in transporting emergency medical technicians and equipment to the scene of an incident and in transporting the patient to the ambulance. Frostbite and hypothermia are as major concerns as hemorrhage control and airway maintenance. Plastic inflatable splints cannot be used because they crack and split in the cold. Esophageal airways must be warmed before insertion. Metal backboards cannot be used, or flesh will freeze to them. Special experience is needed to drive the ambulances on the winter roads if the ambulance is to arrive at the hospital intact. Special heaters are required to warm the patient compartment. Water cannot be applied to burns outside the ambulance because of rapid freezing. The problems are many and varied in the saga of winter vs. EMS.

Water is another problem. In areas where the population lives on islands or on boats (the Thousand Islands in the St. Lawrence Seaway, the Florida Keys, or a large marina), the emergency medical service system must be prepared to be able to gain access to these citizens as well as remove them. We are not aware of any specialized "marine" ambulance in use today in this country other than the U.S. Coast Guard Lifesaving boats. In any case, a water vehicle utilized for the transport of critically injured or ill patients should have the minimum life support equipment on board.

Some communities along the Florida Gulf Coast have utilized specially converted jeeps or other light-weight four-wheel drive vehicles capable of responding to drowning accidents on beaches inaccessible to conventional ambulances because of the low trafficability of the sand. These vehicles carry the essential life support equipment along with trained personnel. However, because of their specialized use, they are not available for the current federal ambulance funding. The rescue vehicles of the Honolulu Fire Department each carry a surfboard for water rescue; the Miami Fire-Rescue units carry Scuba equipment.

Other special problems such as farming accidents do not require specialized vehicles as much as they require knowledge of the specialized problems and the integration of solutions into the training of the emergency medical technician. Careful examination of the problems of a particular geographic area and the addition of these unique needs to the EMT training program will begin to make the training fully responsive to the need.

The transportation medium is only as good as the personnel who staff it. A well trained emergency medical technician can do an adequate job with only the barest of equipment. However, the converse is not true. Transportation is sub-system of the emergency medical care system and cannot stand independently. Transportation is dependent on training, communications, and equipment. Equipment is dependent on training and transportation. The interrelations are complex and varied.

CONCLUSION

The past five years have seen constantly increasing activities in the development of emergency transportation mechanisms, of the equipment carried, and of the personnel who man them. The next five years will certainly see developments far exceeding our current expectations. Projects are currently under way for the transmitting of pictures and sound from the scene of an accident or illness into the emergency department. Emergency medical technicians, emergency physicians assistants, and emergency nurses are being trained to higher and higher levels of patient care. Vehicle improvement has reached the point where ambulances are being *designed*, not converted from trucks and hearses. The past five years have brought EMS further than the entire preceding 25. Technical designs, equipment improvements, and advanced training, along with physician and public recognition, will convert this neglected disease of modern society, as stated by the National Research Council, into simply another problem eventually to be controlled by scientific technology, public interest, and man's love for mankind.

References

Boyd, D. R.: A total emergency medical services system for Illinois. Illinois Med. J. November, 1972.

Briese, R. J.: Economic Considerations for the Provision of Pre-Hospital Emergency Medical Services. *In* Emergency Medical Services Implementation Manual. Michigan Association of Regional Medical Programs, 1974.

Economics of Highway Ambulance Services. U.S. Department of Transportation, 1969.

Farrington, J. D.: The seven years' war. Bull. Am. Coll. Surg. November, 1973.

MAST—Report of Test Program. Interagency Study Group, 1970.

Wyanf, W. D.: A discussion of the emergency medical transportation problem—with a view towards a systematic planning process. Appalachia Med. September, 1971.

Chapter 67   DISASTER PREPAREDNESS

William F. Bouzarth and John P. Mariano

The purpose of this chapter is to stress methods for disaster preparedness, not only in individual hospitals but in such geographic areas as a Standard Metropolitan Statistical Area, a Comprehensive Health Planning Region, a state, and/or groups of adjacent states.

Details for preparing hospital disaster plans have been documented adequately by The American College of Surgeons, American Hospital Association, and the National Fire Protection Association. Special attention should be given to flexibility in planning, so that each hospital can quickly adapt to whatever casualties may result, whether from a relatively minor disaster or a major holocaust. For the latter, such as a train accident, tornado, or even a nuclear explosion, it is necessary that each hospital relate fully to a community-wide, region-wide, or state-wide medical disaster plan, as literally no hospital is so isolated that it need not be involved.

With few exceptions, community emergency medical service councils have emerged generally as the central body for coordinating plans for disasters. Such councils have included representatives from the professional and paraprofessional medical community to work with nonmedical and government agencies, and conceptually successful plans have been developed in this manner by the State of Illinois, the Hospital Council of Southern California, and the Philadelphia County Medical Society (Bouzarth and Mariano, 1969). The essential ingredient is cooperation by groups of responsible individuals to develop a comprehensive disaster plan for the community.

The key element in any plan is coordination of appropriate agencies whose personnel are accustomed or trained to perform disaster duties. Local catastrophes that result in multiple casualties occur frequently and characteristically without sufficient warning. Supportive activity, particularly in the early stages of the response, is usually quick but uncoordinated. Generally, coordination problems appear early, because the basic operational forces, usually municipal police and fire services, respond first to the emergency and then discover that the disaster situation requires extensive medical expertise. At this point it is necessary to summon professional medical decision-making personnel who have the ability to mobilize the medical community. It is therefore imperative that a comprehensive medical disaster plan have a sophisticated command, communications, and alert system capable of dispatching responsible medical and paramedical personnel promptly to the scene so that triage, treatment, and coordinated hospital transportation can be effected almost instantly. The triage medical command officer must assume the responsibility for activating the community-wide disaster plan.

AUTHORITY AND COMMUNICATIONS

The plan should delineate an alert phase for notifying key medical personnel when any emergency situation suggests potential mass casualty problems. For example, whenever three or more alarms are sounded in the Philadelphia Emergency Communications Center, the Chief Police/Fire Surgeon and other key personnel are notified immediately of the incident; he or the Police/Fire Surgeon on duty then proceeds to the scene to assume medical command, including triage and patient hospital transport. Simultaneously, the municipal main disaster control center contacts all hospitals in the affected sector, declaring a disaster alert. The hospitals respond with a report of their immediate capabilities to treat casualties. If the Philadelphia area medical disaster plan is activated, all hospitals communicate with their emergency operating center rather than with each other. The emergency operating center is in direct contact with the senior medical officer at the scene through a field disaster center. In the early stages, the field disaster center can be simply a police vehicle with walkie-talkie capability, or later, as sophisticated as a field-control trailer with emergency telephone and two-way radio service, loud-speaker equipment, and other such facilities, depending on the magnitude of the situation. In a practical sense, command of the emergency situation is assumed by the senior officer to arrive, usually a police supervisor or fire chief. This officer maintains control at the scene while requesting additional emergency aid in accordance with the local plan. Appropriate response should include the arrival of the plan's designated over-all commanding medical officer, who may be a surgeon in private practice.

The field disaster center—however simple or elaborate—must be utilized as the field control center through which all key personnel should report and coordinate disaster operations.

Not every community possesses the capability to install centralized command communications, nor may it be appropriate to a given community's medical disaster planning concept. In such cases, interhospital communications may present a weak link in the plan. After the Los Angeles earthquake, 67 per cent of hospitals had difficulty with interhospital communications despite the fact that Southern California had an organized hospital radio communication network! Hence, it appears that interhospital communications with sophisticated equipment are not entirely satisfactory, but if such radio equipment can be afforded, proper planning for its utilization can be a step in the right direction. Commercial systems with a medical band are also available, but are expensive.

Communications between hospitals pose a problem only when normal day-to-day channels are not functioning. This can occur even without a disaster or major medical problem. For example, hospital switchboards may become overloaded at inconvenient times. A random check made in Philadelphia indicated that most hospitals are very slow to answer from 6 to 8 P.M.

One hospital in particular had an overloaded switchboard during that time, and busy signals were received repeatedly. It was found that the nursing students received their calls through that switchboard, and it was during these hours that they were permitted to make and receive telephone calls. Hospital switchboards also can become overloaded when something happens in the community that slows traffic. When relatives become concerned because a member of the family has not returned home, they look first to the hospital Emergency Department. Telephone communications also can be disrupted by broken lines during bad weather. For instance, it is interesting to note that a recent ice storm in Philadelphia overloaded the city's circuits because of calls to employers to explain absences from work and idle chatter concerning the weather. It was impossible to contact hospitals for at least two hours. An electric power failure may close down hospital switchboards unless auxiliary power is available to illuminate lights on the board for incoming calls. Accidents can damage major trunk lines, or sabotage may destroy an entire communication network. In disaster situations, as the 1971 earthquake in California demonstrated, the Bell System can become overloaded with calls coming from a distance. During that time it was impossible to make a long distance call to that state. Thus, no area is immune to situations that could make interhospital communications impossible by the Bell Telephone System.

Interhospital communication may be necessitated by shortages of supplies such as blood or I.V. solutions; certain equipment such as incubators or surgical instruments may be required; there may be a need for extra nurses, x-ray technicians, or doctors. An overloaded hospital may wish to transfer patients, or in civil disorders patients who are prisoners may be transferred to selected hospitals to save guards. Another need for good interhospital communication is that the medical community may be the first to perceive a disaster situation, and hospitals must be able to warn other hospitals of the problem. Finally, in a major disaster it may become the responsibility of medical experts to delineate the "expectant group," that is, those patients whose prospects are so poor that they must be denied essential life-support such as blood and I.V. fluids in the interests of conserving such support for persons who may be salvaged. This is a difficult decision. With good interhospital communications, the senior physicians in various hospitals can make this decision jointly.

There are a few alternative ways in which interhospital communications can be maintained with somewhat greater dependability. First, a "hospital hot-line" whose number is known only to key personnel may be set up, and the telephone company asked to supply "essential service" for that line, which means that one has a much greater chance of making outgoing calls when regular circuits are busy. Of course, the hot-line should have an extension in the administrator's office as well as in the Emergency Department, should be painted red, and used only for medical emergencies. However, this procedure is more expensive than it sounds, and it may be difficult to convince the administrator of the need for the extra expenditure. Another suggestion is to reserve a phone number for patients' inquiries, separate from the hospital switchboard, and publish this number in the telephone directory. It will help prevent overloading when people are calling to find out about relatives. It has been suggested that hospitals purchase their own interhospital hot-lines, but this is extremely expensive unless hospitals are fairly close to each other.

A major disaster may well result, then, in disruption of telephone service and resort to the difficult, if not impossible, procedure of transporatation by messenger. If one is warned that a medical disaster has occurred, it may be sensible to set up a conference call among hospitals. The lines would thus be kept open, but this technique is expensive during the time it is in operation. If this fails, one would have to resort to other means.

Short-wave radio communication would solve the problem, but such arrangements are expensive, and large city hospitals may not be able to afford them. Also, it is difficult to obtain a short-wave band, and during disasters it may be difficult to get a priority call. If there is no area-wide hospital radio network, substitute methods for emergency communications can be prearranged and included in the plan as contingencies. For example, planners may contact "ham" operators' associations, such as R.A.C.E.S., to organize several mobile units for each hospital. These operators may park their cars outside the administrator's office or the Emergency Department to send and receive messages. Or, perhaps a nonemergency system may already exist, as in Philadelphia, where the Department of Public Property trucks equipped with two-way radios have no major emergency assignments. They can be assigned to hospitals to maintain mobile interhospital communications, but are sufficiently flexible to expand the service even beyond interhospital communications. Also,

---

TABLE 1   *List of Professional Medical Agencies*

County Medical Society
Trauma Committee/(American College of Surgeons;
    American College of Emergency Physicians;
    American Trauma Society)

Hospital Council
Nursing Association
Dental Association
Podiatry Association
Pharmaceutical Association
Veterinarian Association
Industrial Medical Associations

    Organizations such as these should be looked upon to provide the professional medical insight to the disaster plan and/or operations. Among services which they may provide are:

Medical support for on-site triage, treatment, and medical supervision.
Emergency staffing for stressed hospitals or improvised medical facilities.
Observers for test exercises.
Training faculty for emergency medical care courses.
Facilities and personnel to conduct forums and symposia.
Emergency Department operations for casualty treatment around-the-clock.
Medical supplies and emergency blood requirements.
Medical stockpiling.
Emergency drug supplies and other medical equipment and material.

a large tire company in Philadelphia has agreed to deploy their ten radio-equipped vehicles for the same purpose in any emergency.

Although it is difficult to use police and fire shortwave bands directly during a disaster, as a last resort messages can be sent between hospitals by means of this equipment. These emergency vehicles frequently stand parked outside the Emergency Department, having just delivered disaster victims. Another method to consider is the use of insurance teletype systems. In Philadelphia, the Blue Cross teletype system which has terminals in the majority of Philadelphia area hospitals, is used as an auxiliary communications network. Blue Cross has agreed to keep it operational 24 hours a day in event of disaster. Hospitals with central computer systems for business purposes can arrange to have them programmed for auxiliary communications from one hospital to another.

Another way to communicate is by helicopter. If helicopters cannot land in your area, obtain megaphones in advance so as to transmit voice messages to the pilot, who then could relay the messages to the desired hospital. AM-FM radio can also be utilized by prior agreement with Emergency Broadcast Stations (EBS) to announce medical emergency messages.

In brief, a short-wave radio band hospital network would be the best investment for disaster situations; otherwise, makeshift techniques prepared in advance may permit hospitals to communicate for mutual support.

RECOGNITION AND UTILIZATION OF RESOURCES

In order to identify the disaster resources of an area, pre-planning requires

TABLE 2 Government Agencies

Health Department
Fire Department
Police Department
Public Property Department
Welfare Department
School Department
Information Offices
Civil Defense
Sanitation Department
Armed Forces and Reserves
Rumor Services

Operational aspects of disaster planning cannot be accomplished without the complete cooperation of governmental agencies, particularly utilizing the services of the local government. Services available from these agencies are almost unlimited and include:

Professional civil defense personnel for readiness planning; coordination of operations and exercises; training; mutual aid of coordination; volunteer action.
Special services such as alert and warning systems, communications, emergency operating centers, emergency power and water supply.
Traffic control; transportation in concert with ambulance services; law and order; security and handling of prisoner patients.
Fire-fighting; land and water rescue operations; paramedic services.
Sanitation and temporary morgue operations; control of medical supply allocations or rationing.
Preparation of situation reports and dissemination to the mass media of emergency medical information.
Emergency shelter and housing provisions in conjunction with functions of national organizations.
Military hospitals for emergency room services and field triage teams.
Administrative guidance and on-site assistance for rehabilitation in major catastrophies.
Financial assistance for planning activities.
Military services for land, water, and air transport.
Packaged Disaster Hospitals (PDH) which serve best to expand the local existing hospital facilities to which they are assigned and stored, or can be set up in school gymnasiums, for example, or other facilities with such expansive floor space. PDH's can be "cannibalized" to use certain of the supplies in stressed hospitals or improvised medical facilities which may be set up on the disaster site.
Observers for test exercises.
Administrative guidance and funding source for council and planning activities.
Medical stockpile equipment and supplies such as first-aid material and stations; Hospital Reserve Disaster Inventory (HRDI) stockpiles.
Mass training programs.

TABLE 3   Private Agencies

Red Cross
Salvation Army
Voluntary and Private Ambulance and Rescue Companies
Scouts and Explorers
Civil Air Patrol
Radio and T.V.
Civil Rights Groups
Medical Insurance Groups
Amateur Radio Groups

One or more of the organizations in this category will be required for duty assignment for almost any disaster, regardless of its magnitude. Their services are essential and include:

On-site disaster and welfare services; volunteer disaster personnel for first aid service and transportation.
Litter bearers; "casualties" for test exercises; participation in first aid training programs.
Fixed wing and helicopter transport.
Comfort stations and mass feedings for rescue workers and victims.
On-site first aid/emergency care treatment, hospital transport and rescue operations. (These services from ambulance and rescue companies may overlap with similar municipal services. For example, in Philadelphia a sick or injured person could call upon (1) the City Fire Department; (2) Police Department; (3) one of many voluntary, or (4) fee-for-service ambulance organizations. A search of the telephone Yellow Pages is suggested.)

TABLE 4   Public Utilities and Transportation Agencies

Gas
Electric
Water and Sewage Plants
Telephone
Transportation Authorities
Turnpike Authorities
Harbor or Port Authorities
Tunnel and Bridge Operators

This category usually is looked upon for input to operations when the disaster situation is prolonged and exhaustive. Nevertheless, representatives from these organizations should be involved in all aspects of disaster planning. Some long-range services which they provide are:

Emergency heat, light, power, water, and sanitation provisions; transportation of personnel and supplies; evacuation services; mutual aid for essential services.
Emergency telephone installations and essential service listings in the Bell System.
Bus, trolley, taxi, subway, trains, and airport services.

TABLE 5   Other Organizations

Church Council
Trucking Companies
Armored Cars
Funeral Directors
Industrial Centers
Nuclear Plants
Colleges
Lions, Rotary, and other social/charitable clubs

Operationally, these organizations parallel those which are required during the prolonged disaster situation. However, planning and program promotion should not proceed without such services as:

Clergy, social, and miscellaneous voluntary services.
Industrial plant facilities for temporary shelter and/or clinical services.
Reserve for emergency heat, light, power, and transportation of personnel and supplies.
Security transportation.
Facilities and personnel for temporary morgue service.
Public relations and training programs.

recruitment from various agencies and groups. Indeed, compiling such a list is a task in itself. Many agencies appear on the surface to be local but in reality are part of state or national organizations. Occasionally, state or national organizations without local connections may rush in to help in a disaster. These well-meaning intrusions may add to the confusion. Tables 1 to 5 show agencies with some role to play in disasters. This list is not exhaustive, and changing times may make it inaccurate. Representatives of each of the agencies listed should be on call for at least telephone consultation or, if required, report to the main disaster headquarters or field control center to aid in the assessment of the disaster situation. Each representative should have the necessary expertise in his speciality to make final, on-the-scene decisions, and should have the authority to commit to immediate use his agency's resources.

TESTING THE PLAN

The most extensive and sophisticated plan is worthless unless it is periodically reviewed, seriously tested, and updated. Although no exercise can really simulate the genuine disaster situation, basic principles may be tested with a view toward timing mobilization, measuring the effectiveness of emergency communication systems and space allocations, etc. It is difficult to carry out satisfactory tests of a plan without some disruption of normal working-day activities, but hospital patients and staff usually are most understanding when the needs are explained adequately.

Occasionally a surprise odd-hour communications exercise will serve to point up basic gaps in the plan, such as deficiencies in fan-out and after-hour contacts of key disaster personnel. Once again, communications are the major weakness in disaster planning. This type of test can be performed with minimal effort at almost any time without any significant inconvenience to participants. Large-scale exercises are best accomplished on a regular basis through an area-wide effort.

SUMMARY

(1) Begin planning at once, preferably well before any emergency situation arises. It is infinitely better to modify an existing plan in the face of emergency than to have to create one. Work in concert with a total, area-wide effort.

(2) Assess the capabilities of the local and area-wide communications system with a view toward upgrading this aspect of the plan to satisfy appropriate operational requirements.

(3) Recognize the available medical and related resources that can be included in your plan. Although the duties performed by disaster personnel must be expanded as required during disaster situations, people do best when performing duties similar to those to which they are accustomed and for which they have been trained.

(4) Test, review, and update the plan periodically. No drill or exercise can ever approximate the real disaster situation, but any test is better than none at all. Short, frequent tests of portions of the plan are desirable. Occasional but regular large-scale exercises are equally desirable if performed with area-wide planning. Critique the drills as quickly as possible following the exercise, with a view toward recognizing deficiencies and improving the plan accordingly. It appears that the best plans develop in areas that have had major disasters; however, even so there are exceptions (Bouzarth, 1974).

References

Bouzarth, W. F., and Mariano, J. P.: Philadelphia regional emergency medical disaster operations plan (PREMDOP). Arch. Environ. Health 18:203, 1969.

Bouzarth, W. F.: Lessons "unlearned" from Hurricane Agnes. Penna. Med. 77:61, 1974.

Chapter 68

SPECIAL SERVICES

A. Poison Control Centers
B. Crisis Intervention Services

A. POISON CONTROL CENTERS

Sylvia Micik

Each year in the United States an estimated 5 million poisonings occur, a number that is steadily increasing. Poisonings are the fourth most frequent cause of accidental death, with only motor vehicle accidents, drownings, and burns more frequent. They result in over 5,000 deaths per year and a significant morbidity and disability at great cost to the nation.

Ninety per cent of the total cases involve children, making poisoning the most common pediatric medical emergency; the remaining 10 per cent mostly represent suicide attempts, industrial poisonings, and drug abuse in adults.

These poisonings place a very large demand on our emergency medical resources. They occur as a result of exposure to toxic substances, the number and variety of which seem to be almost limitless. With the increasing proliferation of new chemicals, new household products, and new drugs, the physician must have an easily accessible central information resource that will enable him to identify toxic substances and their contents, and will advise him of the expected clinical problems and appropriate therapeutic procedures.

With most poisoning incidents recognized in the asymptomatic stage, the public must also have prompt access to home management to prevent symptoms from appearing and to avoid Emergency Department visits. Treatment in the home can significantly reduce morbidity and can be initiated in 88 per cent of all incidents (Table 1).

It is in response to these clinical management needs that poison information or control centers have proliferated through the United States. The first was established by the Illinois Chapter of the Academy of Pediatrics in 1953, and now over 600 are in existence. They have become an essential component in the management of any poisoning.

When properly organized, funded, staffed, and integrated into a regional system of care for the victim of poisoning, these centers can effectively reduce the mortality and morbidity of this emergency condition. As part of this system, a poison control center provides the following services:

(1) A complete information resource on toxic substances for physicians, emergency medical service personnel, and the public.

(2) Telephone management of cases asymptomatic at discovery.

(3) Referral of symptomatic cases to designated facilities with poisoning care capabilities. (These designations should be determined by emergency medical area-wide planning.)

(4) Up-to-date management expertise to physicians treating symptomatic cases at these facilities and bedside consultation for critically ill patients.

(5) Coordination of transfer to specialized units for the critically ill.

(6) Education of EMS professionals (dispatchers, public safety personnel, emergency medical technicians, Emergency Department nurses, Emergency Department physicians).

(7) Education of the public concerning the need to act, how to obtain help and first aid measures.

(8) Establishment of effective prevention programs.

(9) Collection of data for clinical and epidemiologic studies and evaluation.

(10) Research and evaluation.

INFORMATION RESOURCE FILE

A complete data file with product and drug information and specific, detailed treatment procedures is crucial to the operation of the center and is most difficult to establish and maintain. It is necessary to utilize multiple sources of information for data entry (manufacturers, chemists, pharmacists, clinical toxicologists, the National Clearing-

TABLE 1   Calls to San Diego Poison Information Center, 1974

Total calls	18,802
Information calls	4,952
Poisoning incidents	13,850
Treated by telephone	11,924–88%
Directed to specialized facilities	1,926–12%

house for Poison Control Centers, literature reviews, and the Center's own clinical and epidemiologic experience). This data must be updated on a continuous (daily) basis. Access time to data for specific treatment must be less than 30 seconds. The presently available resource files consisting of card file (mechanical or electronic), computer, and computer generated microfiche (Poisindex System), all leave something to be desired. Our experience at the San Diego Poison Information Center has shown that both the card file and computer generated microfiche are necessary to achieve rapid access and continuous data entry. Some private corporations have been initiated which will update the information on a regular basis to hospitals who pay for the service.

TELEPHONE MANAGEMENT

Patients with poisoning can be clinically identified and separated according to the severity of their condition. Those patients who are asymptomatic at the time of discovery constitute the first category and represent approximately 85 per cent of all poisoning incidents. Typically they are children between the age of 18 months and three years who have been diagnosed by their mothers within five minutes of the time of poisoning. They need rapid access through a regional telephone number to a poison center staffed with personnel trained to assess the case and then provide treatment instructions over the telephone if the exposure has been toxic. Treatment consists primarily of removal of the poison to prevent symptoms. At the San Diego Poison Information Center, syrup of ipecac in doses of 15 cc. in patients under 30 pounds, 30 cc. in patients over 30 pounds, 60 cc. in adolescents and adults taken with eight ounces of ginger ale, is used to induce emesis. In the 5,000 cases in which these doses were used, no toxicity occurred. There were only five failures to induce emesis, a success rate of 99.9 per cent. A follow-up call is necessary to insure that emesis has occurred and that no symptoms have appeared.

After three years experience, the San Diego Poison Information Center has been able to report that 88 per cent of all incoming calls on poisoning incidents were treated effectively at home by telephone instructions (Table 1). Follow-up of these patients verified that they did not subsequently seek treatment at Emergency Departments.

TABLE 2 *San Diego Poison Information Center: Hospital Admissions Due to Poisoning in Children Aged 10 Years or Less*

HOSPITAL	1970°	1974	DECREASE(%)
A	44	33	−25
B	18	14	−22
C	11	6	−45
D	55	26	−53
E	30	14	−53
F	158	93	−41
TOTAL	316	186	−41

°Poison Information Center began operation in December 1971.

Since the initiation of this system of management in San Diego in 1971, there has been an average 40 per cent drop in hospital admissions for poisonings in the age group 0–10 years in a representative sample of hospitals (Table 2).

REFERRAL OF SYMPTOMATIC CASES

The second identifiable category of patient consists of those who are symptomatic at the time of discovery or who are not amenable to home management even though asymptomatic. (Cases involved ingestion of caustics (lye), two ounces or more of petroleum distillates, narcotics (Lomotil, Darvon, Methadone) and exposure to organic phosphate insecticides.) These patients need immediate first aid instructions, initiation of the emergency medical services transport system and/or referral to emergency facilities that have been designated by area-wide planning as having poisoning care capabilities. If such designations have not been made, the poison center itself must initiate the planning. Without the capability of referral to the appropriate facility, the poison center cannot affect the eventual outcome of these patients. Upon referral, the poison center notifies the emergency facility of the impending arrival and provides the physician with the necessary product information and detailed specific treatment procedures.

The third identifiable category of patient consists of the 3 to 5 per cent of victims who are critically ill when discovered (usually adult suicide attempts). In general, they enter the emergency medical services system directly without calling the center and require skilled medical treatment at the scene and en route to the hospital. In this situation the poison center is called upon to provide information to the physician directing the treatment in the field, and, later, for the physician treating the patient at the designated facility.

CLINICAL MANAGEMENT PROCEDURES AND CONSULTATION

Up-to-date emergency treatment protocols must be developed as part of the data file and must be available within a matter of seconds to the physician requesting information. In order for these protocols to reflect the latest medical knowledge and experience, a poison center needs a physician clinical toxicologist to be responsible for their development and for the over-all direction of the center. This specialist also acts as a consultant at the bedside of patients who are critically ill or have unique problems. A radio communication system can ensure his availability at all times.

Each center should also have a subspecialist consultant panel to provide additional expertise (e.g., snake venoms, plants, sea animals, etc.) and access to a laboratory to provide screening and quantitative toxicologic studies.

COORDINATION OF TRANSFER

Patients requiring unique services may need transfer to regional centers providing them. Although the transfer is a physician-to-physician referral, the poison center should coordinate the communications, the transfer of the patients, and the transfer of information.

EDUCATION OF EMERGENCY MEDICAL SERVICE PERSONNEL

Poison centers have the responsibility of creating the necessary educational programs to train all emergency medical service personnel in assessment and clinical management of poisoning. Their staff must participate in the education of public safety personnel, dispatchers, EMT-I's, EMT-II's (paramedics), Emergency Department nurses, and Emergency Department physicians. They must see to it that each rescue unit and Emergency Department has the appropriate supplies and medication to treat these patients.

The education of medical students and house staff who rotate through the center is an added responsibility. Fellowships in clinical toxicology should be offered in conjunction with the medical schools of that region.

PUBLIC EDUCATION

An integral part of a poison center's activities is the education of the public in recognizing poisoning, the need for immediate action, and where to call for help. We have found that this can be effectively accomplished through universal mailings of telephone stickers with the regional telephone number (in gas and electric bills, water bills, mailings to new residents, etc.), distribution of stickers and flyers through schools, clubs, military organizations, pharmacies, physicians' offices, clinics, and Emergency Departments. Use of the media—newspapers, radio, television, billboards, etc.—and use of the first aid and self-help courses available to the public through the EMS system also provide for wide dissemination of information. Contests, quizzes, coloring books, and drug hunts are used to gain active public participation.

PREVENTION PROGRAMS

The ultimate outcome of an effective poison control center should be a decrease in the incidence of poisonings, with eventual eradication of the disease itself. This can only come about by carrying out aggressive, innovative prevention programs. These programs must bring about changes in behavior of parents and children. They must result in the incorporation of preventive practices as part of an individual's life style.

Epidemiologic studies will identify high risk groups, and programs can be geared especially for them.

No matter how complete any education preventive program may be there is still a need to back it up with federal and state legislation. A poison control center can greatly influence the passage of legislation, requiring proper labeling of products and drugs, safety packaging, and control of marketing of hazardous substances.

DATA COLLECTION AND EVALUATION

Data must be collected on each poisoning incident, not only to assist in the day to

TABLE 3   San Diego Poison Information Center Data Collection Form

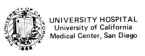

UNIVERSITY HOSPITAL
University of California
Medical Center, San Diego

| SHEET NO. |
| PRODUCT CODE |

POISON CENTER REGISTRATION DATA

DATE	TIME OF CALL		TIME OF POISONING		INTERVIEWER
		AM PM		AM PM	

NAME OF PRODUCT	SAFETY CLOSURE
	☐ YES ☐ NOT USED ☐ NO ☐ SPRAY

METHOD

INGESTION	☐ ml	INHALATION	SKIN	BITES/STINGS
Amount:	☐ mg	Duration, minutes:	% covered:	Number:

WOUNDS/PUNCTURES	EYE	OTHER
Number:	☐ Lg. Amt. ☐ Sm. Amt.	

SIGNS AND SYMPTOMS (CHECK ONE OR MORE)

☐ NONE	☐ ABDOMINAL PAINS	☐ DIFFICULTY SWALLOWING	☐ BURNS
☐ NAUSEA/VOMITING	☐ COUGHING, WHEEZING	☐ RASH	☐ RESP. DISTRESS
☐ DIARRHEA	☐ DROWSINESS	☐ UNCONSCIOUS	☐ FEVER
☐ HEADACHE	☐ ATAXIA	☐ SALIVATION	☐ RESP. DEPRESSION
☐ BURNING	☐ SWELLING	☐ PAIN	☐ CONVULSIONS
☐ TACHYCARDIA	☐ BLURRED VISION	☐ HYPOTENSION	☐ OTHER:

PATIENT	PHONE

WT.	SEX	AGE	Other Children Involved	☐ Human	PREVIOUS POISON
	☐ M ☐ F	Yrs. Mos.	☐ YES ☐ NO	☐ Animal ☐ Other:	☐ YES ☐ NO

WHY?
☐ ACCIDENT   ☐ INFO   ☐ SUICIDE   ☐ KICKS   ☐ AS PRESCRIBED   ☐ INTENTIONAL   ☐ OTHER:

CALL FROM

☐ DOCTOR	☐ PHARMACY	☐ PUBLIC	☐ ER OR HOSPITAL	☐ PUBLIC SAFETY	☐ AMBULANCE
☐ MILITARY	☐ SCHOOL	☐ VET	☐ AMBULATORY CLINICS	☐ OTHER AGENCIES:	

PHYSICIAN OR HOSPITAL REFERRED	NAME OF CALLER	PHONE
☐ YES ☐ NO		

INFORMATION REGARDING INGESTED PRODUCT
☐ BOOKS   ☐ CARDS   ☐ LABEL   ☐ MANUFACTURER   ☐ PREVIOUS KNOWLEDGE   ☐ POISINDEX   ☐ OTHER:

DISPOSITION

☐ IPECAC	☐ PRIVATE M.D.	☐ DILUTE	☐ CATHARTIC
☐ ER FACILITY CODE _____	☐ AMBULANCE	☐ OBSERVE	☐ IRRIGATE
☐ ACTIVATED CHARCOAL	☐ LAVAGE	☐ WASH	☐ NO Rx
☐ Treatment info to M.D. from references	☐ REFUSED ADVICE	☐ LIFE SUPPORT	☐ D.V.M.
☐ LOCAL COMPRESSES OR SOAKS	☐ FRESH AIR	☐ OTHER:	

HISTORY AND RX

FOLLOW-UP

☐ VOMITED FOLLOWING IPECAC
☐ HOSPITALIZED   NO. OF DAYS_____
☐ EXPIRED
☐ OTHER:

151-753 (Rev. 4-75) SIC 600

day management of the center and the public information and prevention programs, but also to delineate the epidemiology of the disease and its clinical manifestations. The data collection form of the San Diego Poison Information Center illustrates the nature of the information to be collected (Table 3). Review of the data also assists in the day-to-day update of the resource-treatment file and permits the addition of individual experiences and case reports. Trends can be easily identified and the appropriate information and prevention programs initiated.

Collection of data to document the cost effectiveness of the poison control center is necessary to justify continued financial support.

Most important of all, data must be collected to evaluate patient outcomes in terms of mortality and morbidity.

REGIONAL PLANNING – FUTURE DIRECTION FOR POISON CENTERS

Of the more than 600 poison centers in the United States most have developed haphazardly, each community attempting to establish one of its own, without regional planning. As a result, most are small without any independent existence from the Emergency Department and without specialized staff or budget. Information calls are answered by an Emergency Department clerk or available nurse or physician, many of whom are simply rotating through the Emergency Department and know little more than the caller. They rely on cards sent to them by the National Clearinghouse and a few texts for their information file (Lovejoy and Alpert, 1970). These sources alone are incomplete and cannot provide up-to-date product information and clinical management. Most have no access to a clinical laboratory for toxicologic studies. The number of calls handled by these centers is usually too small to justify a financial investment and too small to maintain expertise or benefit from clinical experience.

In 1970, Dr. Frederick Lovejoy of the Boston Poison Information Center surveyed 590 poison centers. He received replies from 404. Over 50 per cent of the centers received one or less calls per day. Fourteen per cent had no knowledge of how many calls they received. Seventy-two per cent had no telephone listing. Table 4 is a tabulation of this

TABLE 4   Survey of United States Poison Centers, 1970

1. Questionnaires sent, 590; replies received, 404
2. Center provides
   Information only   46
   Treatment only   2
   Both   356
3. Poison call information is usually given by (multiple answer):
   M.D.   185
   Nurse   250
   Pharmacist   81
   House staff   55
   Secretary   12
4. Center is open:
   24 hours per day and 7 days per week   380
   Less than 24 hours per day and 7 days per week   20
   No answer   4
5. Center provides information to:
   Health professionals only   61
   Public only   28
   Both   315
6. Number of calls received in 1965:
   Less than 400   224
   400 to 1000   65
   1000 to 2000   21
   2000 to 3000   14
   3000 to 4000   7
   More than 4000   17
   No answer   56
7. Does Center telephone have special listing in local telephone directory?
   Yes   110
   No   291
   No answer   3
8. Do you have access to clinical laboratories for necessary toxicologic analysis?
   Yes   358
   No   45
   No answer   1
9. Does your Center participate in prevention programs?
   Yes   281
   No   119
   No answer   4

(From Lovejoy, F. H., Jr., and Alpert, J. J.: Pediatr. Clin. North Am., 17:747, 1970.)

survey. Obviously, at this level of activity, neither the needs of the physician nor the needs of the public are being met.

Poison centers must be reorganized and consolidated into regional centers serving large populations with a national center responsible for standards of operation, a central information bank, and clinical and epidemiologic data analysis. They must be fully funded from federal, state and local sources and appropriately staffed. They must be part of a system of care for poison victims in a total emergency medical services system that has planned an organized stepwise management of the poisoning victim from initial discovery through recovery. Where this has

TABLE 5   San Diego Poison Information Center

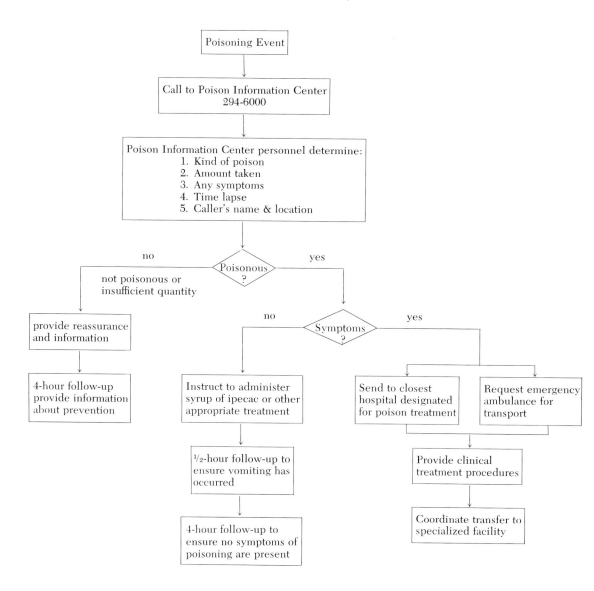

been done in other countries (Sweden), the mortality rate of patients with poisoning has dropped to 1 per cent. In the U.S. the mortality rate is 8 per cent. (Table 5 illustrates a system we have found effective in San Diego.) The impetus for planning and implementation of such a system must come from physicians. They must agree to arrange themselves and their facilities in such a way as to bring the benefits of the available clinical knowledge to each patient. Poison centers as part of this system can then make a significant contribution toward the reduction of the mortality and morbidity of this important medical emergency.

References

Adams, W. C.: Poison control centers: their purpose and operation. Clin. Pharmacol. Therap., *4*:293, 1963.

Arena, J. M.: Poisoning: Toxicology, Symptoms, Treatments. 3d ed. Springfield, Illinois, Charles C Thomas, 1975.

Crotty, J. J., and Verhulst, H. L. Organization and delivery of poison information in U.S. Pediatr. Clin. North Am. *17*:741, 1970.

Gleason, M. N., et al.: Clinical Toxicology of Commercial Products. 3d ed. Baltimore, Williams and Wilkins Co., 1969.

Govaerts, M.: Poison control in Europe. Pediatr. Clin. North Am. *17*:729–739, 1970.

Lovejoy, F. H., and Alpert, J. J.: A Future Direction for Poison Centers. Pediatric Clinics of North America, *17*:747, 1970.

Poisindex System. Micromedex, Inc., Denver, Colorado.

Robertson, W., and Ambuel, J. P.: Incorporating a poison control center into a pediatric teaching program. J. Med. Educ., *37*:217–219, 1962.

Teitelbaum, D.: New directions in poison control. Clin. Toxicol. *1*(1):3–13, March 1968.

Temple, A. R., and Done, A. K.: Organization of Emergency Treatment Facilities for Management of Acute Poisonings. pp. 107–115.

B. CRISIS INTERVENTION SERVICES

Robert L. Leopold

Sudden catastrophic illness, acute trauma, and life-threatening surgical emergencies represent true individual and family crises, yet little systematic thought has been given to means of providing useful crises intervention. Personal crisis is characterized by the inability of an individual or a small social system, such as a family, to control and to deal with an overwhelming situation. Some components of crisis may develop slowly, but the crisis itself usually erupts suddenly, and this very abruptness of onset contributes to a sense of helplessness, which is particularly strong in emergency medical and surgical situations.

The nature of most emergency situations, particularly trauma, allows the individual involved no warning of impending catastrophe. Thus, he is psychologically, as well as physically, unprepared for the dramatic alterations in his status from that of an individual adult to that of a bewildered, hurting, and dependent child. It is probable that the prognosis for sudden injury may be altered favorably if the victim has any advance warning, no matter how brief (Leopold and Dillon, 1960).

For the caretaking system to be able to intervene in a systematic way, the following components of crisis must be recognized.

(1) In crises, a person or small social system is thrown into disequilibrium by events that may be external or internal.

(2) At the time the crisis occurs, and until it is resolved, the individual and those around him (the "significant others") have heightened emotional vulnerability.

(3) With this heightened vulnerability, there is enhanced capacity for change, either in the direction of maturation or regression. Gerald Caplan* likens the person in crisis to an individual standing on one foot. Pushing him one way causes him to fall; nudging him the other way helps him to land solidly on both feet. This image seems apt, not only for the patient, but also for the significant others

---

*Personal communication.

in his life, since these others must deal with the realistic problems created and with their own feelings of concern or grief, often tinged with guilt.

(4) The resolution of crisis can be aided by skilled intervention at one or several appropriate levels. These include both the individual and the family system to which he belongs on the one hand, and the time sequences following the emergency on the other. Thus, intervention at the scene of an accident may take the form of realistic reassurance of the victim, and, at a later point in the course of the emergency illness, crisis intervention may need to deal with the mobilization of community resources.

(5) The period of relatively acute anxiety is moderately brief. The crisis may be resolved satisfactorily with the learning of new coping patterns; it may be resolved unsatisfactorily with the development of inadequate and partial solutions; or it may continue to exist as chronic immobilization, but without great anxiety.

Caretakers obviously have dealt with crises on an intuitive basis for many years. Recognition of crisis intervention as a technique had its origin following a catastrophic emergency situation, the Coconut Grove fire in Boston. Cobb and Lindemann (1944), noting the difficulty that fire victims and their families had in dealing emotionally with this catastrophe and its sequelae, recognized the crisis and the nature of the disabilities, and began to devise strategies for intervention. Caplan (1959) carried this work further in his approach to mental health consultation and its particular relationship to crisis intervention among Peace Corps volunteers. Leopold and Duhl (1963) stress the practical application of crisis intervention theory in medical and psychiatric emergencies among overseas personnel. Disaster as personal or family crisis has been well described by Barton (1969). However, strategies for crisis intervention following natural disaster have been minimal.

In the emergency care field, crisis intervention must be viewed both temporarily and in terms of the individual and the significant others whom the emergency of the individual involves. Intervention with the patient and his family must be viewed as a continuum. The concept of the case manager, which is gaining credence in the area of health care, has not developed to any significant extent in emergency services. Indeed, the very nature of emergency care tends to be episodic, with frequent changes in those giving care to the individual and with only sporadic and discontinuous attempts to deal with those others close to the patient. It seems appropriate that the model of the case manager will be adapted to the area of emergency care. The perspective of such a manager is useful as a way of viewing the interlocking systems of intervention needed for the individual and his family, particularly because of the mutual feedback between these systems.

The nature of the immediate crisis of the patient during a medical or surgical emergency is apparent. The specific configuration of the crisis will be determined by the type of illness or injury, the state of consciousness, the state of relative preparedness or unpreparedness for the occurrence, and its psychologic impact. It is understandable that physical care must take precedence over immediate crisis intervention. However, almost simultaneously with physical care, the nature of the crisis should be recognized and realistic reassurance given. Despite the shock of injury or the acute occurrence of myocardial infarction, the patient is likely to have urgent questions about his immediate and long term future. Failure to recognize the intensity of these questions and to respond to them deepens and fixes the psychologic components of crisis. During transport to a hospital, the patient is likely to be bewildered and confused by the sudden change from independence to regressive, painful dependency. Many patients will use the defense of denial, but bewilderment is never far from the surface of awareness. Simple and honest explanations can do much to allay these feelings. The patient also is quick to recognize the impact of his personal catastrophe on those around him, and to feel the need for their involvement.

The two systems of intervention—patient and family—are likely to meet in the hospital Emergency Department or after admission to the hospital. The patient's family can be expected to be stunned psychologically by the impact of the emergency. Their feelings may be expressed in a variety of ways, many of which are unpalatable to those whose primary concern is with the patient. The family may be querulous, demanding, hostile, dependent, or commonly will express a mixture of these emotions. Certain members of the family are most in crisis, and accordingly most vulnerable at the onset of the crisis situation, when their own world is thrown into disorder. Systematic intervention at the level of first contact, usually in the Emergency Department or the hospital, seems mandatory. The professional discipline of the intervenor is far less important than his capacity for compassion and ability to identify with the family in crisis. Commonly, the first intervenor with the family will be an overburdened nurse, an harassed house officer (in a teaching hospital), or not infrequently a volunteer worker. It is rare that social workers with special training in this area are involved at this level. By reason of the fact that Emergency Department personnel are likely to be the first intervenors, the care they can give is episodic. It is likely that the family will not see the primary intervenor after the initial contact, and that the next level of intervention will occur with another individual. If one could apply the case manager model to emergency situations, one could establish a continuity within both systems that would be sustained over a period of time.

After the resolution of the acute emergency situation, the crisis continues in altered form. As the first shocks wear off, both the patient and his family face the inevitable disruption of their lives, and not unexpectedly have difficulty in formulating a plan of action. Family difficulties will vary from financial concern to the arrangement of child care. In our current method of health care, we expect the family to deal with these realities at the time when they are most vulnerable and least able to cope. The family's anxiety is transmitted to the patient, who now must deal not only with the problems created by his own sudden illness or injury, but with the problems of those close to him. Despite this, the health care system today mobilizes its resources very slowly, if at all. Referral to the social service department a week after the crisis has begun is unlikely to speed immediate crisis resolution. It seems essential that a system of care be provided that can respond quickly, yet on a continuous basis.

For some patients and their families, the crisis will begin to resolve within the first week or ten days. This is particularly true if knowledgeable help has been provided and the potential for growth and maturity, coping with the situation mentioned earlier, has been aided. For those patients and their families requiring and able to obtain continuing intervention, existing resources again would entail a change of personnel, which is undesirable. Unfortunately, current crisis interventions tend to be delayed until the crisis is far advanced and often unmanageable; that is, a week or ten days after the incident itself. Help may be feasible at this point, but is far more difficult than at an earlier time when positions are less fixed and the potential for responding favorably is far greater.

Crisis intervention as a technique consists of far more than explanation and reassurance. Successful intervention aids the individual and the family to resolve the crisis in an efficient and acceptable way; it also helps those in crisis to improve their general ability to cope with difficult situations. Thus, crisis intervention not only represents an opportunity for speedy resolution from a current problem, but also allows the individual or family to gain strength for future use (Leopold, 1968).

In summary, there is adequate knowledge concerning crisis intervention to enable such intervention, applied in a systematic way, to stabilize the health of an emergency victim and the coping responses of those around him. Many of the facets of such a network are available, either directly or potentially. The task ahead is the organization of these component parts into a functioning and unified system.

References

Barton, A. H.: Communities in Disaster: A Sociological Analysis of Collective Stress Situations. New York, Anchor Books, 1969.

Caplan, G.: Concepts of Mental Health and Consultation. Children's Bureau Publication No. 373. Washington, D.C., U. S. Dept. of Health, Education and Welfare, 1959.

Caplan, G.: Manual for Psychiatrists Participating in the Peace Corps. Available from J. T. English, M.D., Chief Psychiatric Consultant, Peace Corps, Washington, D.C.

Cobb, S., and Lindemann, E.: Neuropsychiatric observations. From Symposium on the Management of the Coconut Grove Burns at the Massachusetts General Hospital. Ann. Surg. 117:814, 1943.

Leopold, R. L.: Some Notes on Theory and Practice. In Einstein, G. (ed.): Learning to Apply New Concepts to Casework Practice. New York, Family Service Association of America, 1968, pp. 9–33.

Leopold, R. L., and Dillon, H.: Psychiatric considerations in whiplash injuries of the neck. Pa. Med. J. 63:385, 1960.

Leopold, R. L., and Duhl, L. J.: The Peace Corps: a historical note on a new challenge to psychiatry. J. Nerv. Ment. Dis. 137:1, 1963.

Lindemann, E.: Symptomatology and management of acute grief. Am. J. Psychiatr. 101:141, 1944.

Chapter 69   # THE EMERGENCY DEPARTMENT

A. Organization and Staffing
B. Financing the Emergency Department
C. Evaluation
D. Categorization of Emergency Facilities
E. Education in the Emergency Department

A. ORGANIZATION AND STAFFING

James D. Mills

The modern Emergency Department necessarily performs a service oriented to the consumer. The primary rule of its operation is that each patient presenting himself will be seen courteously and be treated competently. Such a service represents a distinct expansion and improvement over the "accident wards" of an earlier period, which were concerned mostly with life-threatening, usually traumatic conditions.

The public has told us in the most emphatic way it can that this is what is desired. Case loads have increased beyond all expectations, and we are rewarded (or plagued) for having met a demonstrated need. When other medical resources in a community, and even within the hospital, "wind down" for evenings, weekends and holidays, the Emergency Department and its supporting services attempt to fill the gap.

The mission of the Emergency Department is to treat everyone with as much humanity as can be mustered, with special skill for the most acutely ill or injured patients. It is glaringly obvious when we fail to fulfill this mission, for the work of the Emergency Department is open for all to see. Achieving the goal is complex and requires a cohesive and ongoing relationship between professional staff, paramedical staff, and hospital administration.

The Emergency Department is the site of 5 per cent of physician visits in the United States (Gibson, 1973). As a major clinical department it interfaces with all the other departments in an ongoing working relationship to provide patient care.

Formerly the responsibility of an emergency room committee and staffed by house staff who had other responsibilities within the hospital, the Emergency Department is now more frequently being staffed with full-time emergency physician specialists whose primary responsibility is the evaluation, treatment, and disposition of patients presenting themselves to the Emergency Department. Some 10 per cent of these patients are admitted to the hospital, and this group tends to be sicker and to account for more

inpatient days than those admitted electively from other sources (Gibson, 1973).

The organizational response to this change in case load and in mode of operation, together with the need to interact with other departments, has been to create Emergency Departments within the medical staff hierarchy. As departments they assume the traditional responsibilities of departmental organization, with regularly scheduled meetings for patient care audit, death conferences, and related activites for improving patient care.

As the need for a more organized and effective emergency service became apparent, the official organ of the Joint Committee for Accreditation of Hospitals made appropriate findings and recommendations. When justified by the complexity of the service the JCAH recommends establishment of an Emergency Department within an existing medical staff to be headed by a chief who is a member of the active medical staff and who implements the policies and supervises the professional medical services. Developing within the AMA and also the AHA are sections on emergency medical care which will include the medical management of disasters.

Establishment of an Emergency Department recognizes its function as a major clinical service from the standpoint of direct responsibility for patients. As a department, its chief sits on the medical staff's executive committee and its interests are represented by a spokesman whose knowledge is reinforced by first-hand involvement in the work of the department. His position on the executive committee allows him continuous communication with other department heads and facilitates the resolution of differences before problems arise.

Medical staffs are aware that the Emergency Department, like the other services, must be a cooperative endeavor of the entire staff. Physicians and surgeons in other departments must stand ready to support the Emergency Department by accepting referrals and requests for consultations. To obviate misunderstanding, these responsibilities must be clearly spelled out in staff rules and regulations. In addition, referral lists should be published to assure definite referral lines on any given day.

Staff confrères usually are quite willing to discharge their responsibilities within their own areas of competence. They are entitled to know their obligations and to be assured of fair treatment. It is a fact that individual practices are busier than most physicians ever anticipated. Referrals from the Emergency Department impose an additional burden, necessary as it is. Emergency physicians can ease the load by accepting requests for stand-by practice coverage for outpatients, by arranging admission and writing initial orders at odd hours when this is desired (although there are increased malpractice risks in this service which the emergency physician should realize), and by smoothing the way when other physicians are seeing their patients within the often crowded Emergency Department.

The emergency physician augments the individual private practice of medicine. He knows that ongoing care of the individual patient within the Emergency Department is expensive and episodic and is rewarding for neither the physician nor the patient. In the attempt to create continuing doctor-patient relationships, he makes suitable referrals to primary physicians. For the other specialties, referrals are usually made according to a published monthly roster prepared from lists made by the various departments, although geographical referral has been used for patient convenience.

Disaster planning is a responsibility of the entire medical staff in harmony with other community resources. Since its impact on the Emergency Department is profound, due consideration should be given to the department's responsibility and response. As a fully staffed 24-hour facility likely to have early awareness of any catastrophe, it is the responsibility of the physician in charge of the ED to implement the disaster plan when needed. It is equally important to withhold this implementation when a maximum response will be counterproductive. Disasters may be large or small. An active Emergency Department should have the organizational capability of dealing with a predetermined number of seriously injured patients effectively by calling on its usual staff support. It needs to anticipate a situation when it will be overwhelmed and the maximum response disaster plan will be necessary.

PHYSICIAN STAFF

A basic physician staff is needed (and economically feasible) to be on the premises every hour of every day with case loads of 20,000 per year or more. In some areas, particularly when the conditions presenting tend to be more serious (such as high trauma regions) full staffing is justified with a lesser patient load. Four full-time physicians are the minimum required for this service (or four full-time equivalents if help by part-time physicians is used.) As the case load increases it is realistic to plan on one full-time emergency physician for each 7000 cases seen annually. Their work-hours are scheduled to cope with anticipated peak load hours. These numbers can be modified to meet the special needs of a given area and further altered as the use of paramedical help is increased, or if there are special features of the physical plant to be considered.

Since the early 1960s, Emergency Departments staffed full-time have relied for the most part on general practitioners and other physicians who have augmented their training and experience with specialized instructions in the crises they might expect to treat. This system was a giant step ahead of previous staffing with house physicians or rotating members of the attending staff. It represented the first generation of "on-line" emergency physicians. These physicians necessarily have had to deal with all the problems that present themselves on a daily basis.

Maintenance of professional performance is encouraged by the openness of the emergency facility together with departmental audits and review of records. Emergency physicians do their work in a hospital setting exposed to the counsel and also the criticism of their medical confrères. They are not encouraged to repeat their mistakes in the harsh light of this sort of exposure, nor is the physician whose personal needs make him avoid this exposure attracted to emergency medicine as a career.

There is no pretense that the ultimate in emergency care has been reached, even in departments with full-time staffs. There is evidence, however, to show that diastrous mismanagement of individual cases has not resulted in the huge malpractice judgments associated with other methods of staffing. Also, there is, not surprisingly, a trend to assume a consulting role in the areas in which the emergency physician has developed a special competence.

As the need for around-the-clock skilled professional care was demonstrated and warmly received by the consuming public and the lay press, and then by the medical establishment, the next stage in its evolution became obvious. It was the specialized graduate training of physicians whose career choice was Emergency Medicine. Within a five-year span, 30 university programs began to offer formalized residency training in Emergency Medicine. The graduates of these programs are just beginning to enter the active practice of Emergency Medicine and are greatly in demand to upgrade the quality of service. At the same time, the American College of Emergency Physicians has exerted leadership in the development of specialty certification, which will designate those men and women having demonstrated by training and examination that they qualify as certified emergency physician specialists.

NURSING STAFF

Within the department, patients are served by nurses, orderlies, and technicians from the laboratory, x-ray department, and the heart station. Nurses are a critical part of the team in a real sense, and are relied on to keep the work flowing, even to the point of goading the physician who is not keeping pace. They oversee the work of the orderlies; keep open a clear track for life-threatening emergencies; assist the clerical staff with triage; anticipate orders in crisis situations; deal with family; order supplies, drugs and equipment; spur on the laboratory; draw blood; start infusions; record vital signs serially; mind the monitors; and perform other duties for which they are qualified by their special training and experience.

From their point of view, the Emergency Department is an ideal place for a nurse to work. It is attractive to bright, young, energetic men and women who wish to keep their skills sharpened, and who enjoy working directly with physicians.

They are confident of their own worth and recognize that they are highly valued by

their medical colleagues. Esprit de corps derives from this mutual respect and enhances the work of the department. It helps in the recruitment of nurses which happily has not been a problem to the degree it is in other areas of the hospital. Maximum return from Emergency Department nurses is obtained by scheduling them entirely within the department rather than rotating them throughout the hospital.

Schedules for nurses are designed to use their hours most efficiently. This means that the traditional shifts are modified to suit the times of maximal patient load. In addition to the traditional shifts (7–3, 3–11, and 11–7) they may work 10 AM to 6 PM, 6 PM to 2 AM, and 2 AM to 10 AM. One or more nurses may be compensated to be on stand-by call at home to respond if needed.

When nursing work shifts are tailored to peak load hours, 7 to 9 nurses are required per day for each 100 patients seen.

Nurses are encouraged to participate in specialized training in their area of special competence. For this they should be assisted with subsidies offered by their employers. Their national organization, Emergency Department Nurses Association, has made significant progress in upgrading standards and offering postgraduate training opportunities.

Emergency Department nurses are employees of the hospital and organizationally are under the nursing service. The medical chief of the Emergency Department retains the responsibility for the technical supervision of the Emergency Department nurses. If in his view their work is technically unsatisfactory, there must be a mechanism for discharges or transfers from the department.

TECHNICIAN STAFFING

The title Emergency Medical Technicians is an earned one and implies that the technician has undergone basic and then more advanced EMT training. In the past decade we have observed and encouraged the evolution of the Emergency Department orderly to EMT status as he qualified first with the Red Cross first aid course, then with the basic EMT course designed by the Highway Safety Division of the Department of Transportation, and finally, with the advanced EMT courses offered by many of the community colleges. Important as a training resource have been the early and ongoing efforts of the American Academy of Orthopaedic Surgeons and the American College of Surgeons, who set standards and offer many organized training opportunities throughout the United States. The National Registry of Emergency Medical Technicians examines graduates and qualifies them as registered EMT's. Many young men enter this work because they have health career objectives. Some bring experience in paramedical work from the armed services.

EMT's prepare and dress wounds. They assist with resuscitation, inhalation therapy, cardiovascular monitoring, chest tubes, nasal packs, orthopedic procedures, and infusions. They do limited laboratory work within the department, prepare smears for bacteriology, take electrocardiograms, record laboratory data, and transport patients within the hospital. Four to five EMT's, working eight-hour shifts, are required for each 100 patients treated in a day. Heaviest EMT coverage is scheduled for the busiest hours.

One of the EMT's may take responsibility for scheduling and for quality of work performance. EMT's are employees of the hospital and, like nurses, are technically responsible to the Emergency Department chief. In a tightly knit department there is no practical problem in assuring that high standards are expected and required.

References

Gibson, G.: The Social System of Emergency Care in Emergency Medical Services. New York, Behavioral Publications, 1973.

Accreditation Manual for Hospitals. Joint Commission for Accreditation of Hospitals, Chicago, 1973.

Which E. R. coverage arrangement is best? Med. Economics. November 6, 1972, pp. 112–116.

B. FINANCING THE EMERGENCY DEPARTMENT

Karl G. Mangold

The financial aspects of emergency medical services represent a broad and complex topic that spans the entire emergency medical services system. This chapter, however, will be restricted to the financial realities of *the department* of emergency medicine within a hospital and how the economics of the department relate to the hospital, the consumer, and the physician.

It is essential for physicians involved in the entire spectrum of emergency medicine to have a working knowledge of the language of business and finance. It is beyond the scope of this chapter to provide a glossary of terms for the fundamentals of medical finance and accounting. However, listed below are examples of some terms that should be understood by all who desire to improve the quality of emergency medical services.

Terms

accounting systems
accounting, tax
accounts payable
accounts receivable
assets
audit procedure
auditing, governmental
auditing, internal
bad debt
balance sheet
billing
bond
bookkeeping, double entry
budget and budgeting
budget analysis
capital
cash flow
collateral
collection
contracts
contractual allowances
controller
corporation, nonprofit
cost accounting
cost accounting, departmental
cost center
cost leasing
cost per unit
costs, administrative (direct and indirect)
costs, controllable
costs, fixed
costs, noncontrollable
credit
debit
demography
depreciation expense
expense, medical liability
factoring
financing, debt
financing, equity
financing, long term
financing, short term
income
inventory
leverage
liability
lien
overhead
profit and loss statement
return on investment
revenue
write off

FINANCIAL IMPACT OF THE EMERGENCY DEPARTMENT ON THE HOSPITALS – DIRECT AND INDIRECT

The traditional attitude regarding Emergency Departments has been that they are an economic drain upon the hospital – that emergency services were "loss leaders." Prior to 10 years ago, most hospitals had quite high occupancy rates. Hospital administrators were convinced that "an open door emergency policy" would result in the hospital being overwhelmed by patients unable to handle their resultant financial obligation. The problem was that traditional cost accounting methods credited the Emergency Department "fees" as the sole departmental source of revenue. Most Emergency Departments were, and still are, cost accounted on a departmental basis. With such a method of departmental cost accounting, large amounts of revenue initiated by a functioning Emergency Department were not reflected as part of Emergency Department (ED) revenue. On the other hand, the costs applied *against* the ED were the accumulation of high personnel salaries, personnel fringe benefits, and other direct and indirect expenses, including general administrative costs.

The department method of cost accounting has obscured the real issue, i.e., the financial impact of the department of Emergency Medicine on the hospital. The easiest way to illustrate this impact is figuratively to close the Emergency Department and remove fiscally from the hospital's income statement and balance sheet all the cash flow generated by the ED. That is, remove all direct gross revenue generated by patients who entered the hospital via the Emergency Department and/or revenue generated by those patients who utilized the ancillary services while in the Emergency Department. Such a calculation reveals that frequently, in the average community hospital, 30 to 40 per cent of the entire hospital revenue is generated by patients who were seen exclusively or initially in the ED. In some county hospitals, and even in some university associated hospitals, this figure may reach as high as 70 to 80 per cent of the cash flow of the entire medical institution.

It has also been shown that the ancillary services of a hospital, such as pharmacy, laboratory, radiology, operating room, central supply, and inhalation therapy, generate 50 per cent of the gross revenue, which is 80 per cent of the hospital's profit. The remaining 50 per cent of the gross revenue is generated by bed utilization. However, this 50 per cent of gross revenue accounts for only 20 per cent of the hospital's profit. It is also well to understand that the so-called "nonprofit" hospital is, in reality, a nontaxable hospital. All hospitals, in order to survive, expand, replace equipment, purchase new equipment, etc., must have profits. An analysis of the use of ancillary services by emergency patients in a number of community hospitals reveals the following: 49 per cent of the patients had pharmacy charges; 18 per cent of the patients had laboratory charges; 35 per cent of the patients had radiology charges; 6 per cent of the patients had electrocardiographic charges; 2 per cent of the patients had inhalation therapy charges; and 28 per cent of the patients had central supply charges.

Further analysis of the same hospitals revealed that patients admitted to the hospital via the Emergency Department (as compared to elective admissions) stayed longer as inpatients and generated larger amounts of gross revenue because of much heavier utilization of ancillary services. Patients admitted through the Emergency Department usually are sicker and require more aggressive diagnostic and therapeutic modalities.

The financial impact of the department of Emergency Medicine is a complex one that must be viewed on a broad hospital fiscal impact basis rather than on a restricted departmental cost accounting basis. Admission rates and ancillary service utilization may have a profoundly positive impact on the hospital financial structure. Well organized, competent, ethical groups of emergency physicians who effectively manage and administrate a hospital Emergency Department may literally change patterns of hospital utilization by members of the medical community as well as patterns of hospital preferences by the lay community.

PLANNING AN EMERGENCY DEPARTMENT

Certain utilization factors are important in planning. The Emergency Department records for at least the last two years should be reviewed, noting the following:

(1) Percentage of primary care.

(2) Percentage of urgent care.

(3) Percentage of emergency care.

(4) Percentage of convenience usage, e.g., telephone orders, injections, laboratory work.

(5) Percentage of utilization for preoperative preparation for outpatient surgery and elective intradepartmental procedures.

(6) Percentage of patients seen within the department by their private doctors, the house staff, and the emergency physicians.

An estimate of potential patient utilization may be made by assuming 250 to 300 Emergency Department patient visits per year per thousand population in the hospital service area. (Be careful not to overstate the hospital service population.)

Consideration of the demographic distribution of physicians in the hospital and the hospital service area is essential. An area that is high in specialists and underserved in primary care physicians generally produces a greater Emergency Department volume.

Demographic studies of the population in a hospital service area are extremely important. Such studies will help determine whether patients who will utilize the hospital Emergency Department will be able to provide an adequate cash flow to sustain the emergency physician group. If there is a large indigent and welfare population, collections will be significantly lower. In California, for example, if all third-party carriers remunerated emergency physicians for their services in exactly the same manner utilized by the Department of Health under its Medi-Cal Program, the vast majority of emergency physician groups would not be able to survive economically.

The importance of a well-studied third-party demographic distribution for a specific service population cannot be overemphasized. A detailed study of the basic eight categories of their party carriers can generally project, with a fair degree of accuracy, the percentage of collection. An example of a typical third-party distribution in patients utilizing some California hospital Emergency Departments follows:

(1) Blue Cross—15 per cent.

(2) Blue Shield—15 per cent.

(3) Industrial—10 per cent.

(4) Medicare—6 per cent.

(5) Welfare—40 per cent.

(6) Champus—1 per cent.

(7) Other private insurance—10 per cent.

(8) No insurance—3 per cent.

By multiplying the above percentages by the expected rates of return from each of the third parties, it is easy to estimate the percentage of noncollection or bad debt expense.

The so-called "break-even point" for the hospital when calculated on the basis of the over-all financial impact that the Emergency Department has on the hospital, and assuming an admission rate of 10 per cent, can be as low as 600 patients per month. Depending on the fiscal relationship between the emergency physician group, the hospital, and the patient, the break-even point for a group of emergency physicians may be as low as 1,000 or 1,100 patients per month.

The financial "break-even point" for a group of emergency physicians depends on what they are prepared to accept as an irreducible minimum for their professional services. They must take into consideration their overhead expenses and the degree of autonomy they wish to retain or surrender. The greatest degree of autonomy or professional independence is achieved when there is absolutely no financial relationship with the hospital. However, total financial independence is directly related to a patient volume of at least 35,000 to 40,000 patients per year, plus a reasonably randomized distribution of third-party carriers. More concretely stated, a reasonable minimum break-even point would be approximately 1,200 patients per month, or 14,000 patients per year, assuming an average emergency physician charge per patient of $20.00, with the gross professional accounts receivable being purchased by the hospital at 85 per cent of the gross billing. This is predicated on the hospital's sharing the burden of the traditional bad debt expense. In return, the hospital generates inpatient revenue and utilization of existing ancillary services with little or no additional capital expenditure.

HOSPITAL GUARANTEES

Many hospital Emergency Departments do not have an adequate patient volume to sustain financially or attract full-time emergency physician groups, and yet have valid reasons for existing. Some departments have an adequate patient volume but, owing to the inequitable reimbursement methods by some of the third parties, cannot generate enough cash flow to be financially independent of the hospital. In these cases, a financial relationship between the emergency physician group and the hospital is usually the rule, at least for the period while the service is initially developed.

The so-called "guaranteed minimum" included in many contracts serves a multiplicity of purposes and exists for many reasons. In hospitals where the fees generated will not produce an adequate income to sustain the emergency physician group, the guaranteed minimum insures a sufficient income to continue Emergency Department coverage. It is hoped that, in time, an adequate cash flow will be generated so that the physicians are able to support themselves entirely by gross monies billed and received from their direct patient services.

The "guaranteed minimum" has taken many forms. Some contracts state that monies paid to the group are for its departmental administrative and management functions. Other guaranteed minimums are simply a dollar amount per month versus a percentage of gross professional billings, whichever is higher. At the present time, a fairly typical minimum guarantee for a physician group in an Emergency Department with 25,000 or fewer patient visits per year is approximately $17,000.00 per month versus 85 per cent of the gross professional charges, whichever is higher. Calculations are done on a monthly basis and a check is issued by the hospital to ther emergency physician group in the month following performance of professional services. Essentially, the hospital acts as the emergency physicians' billing and collection agent, with the emergency physician group paying the hospital 5 per cent of the gross for its billing and collection expense and sharing the bad debt to the extent of 10 per cent of gross. A total of 15 per cent of the gross professional charges is paid back to the hospital. In essence, the hospital purchases the emergency physician group's accounts receivable.

One of the simplest forms of guaranteed minimum is a sliding scale in which the dollar value of remuneration to the group changes as the patient volume changes. In this instance, the emergency physician group arranges to do its own billing. It is important to recognize this difference. The emergency physician group is now in the billing and collection business, which represents a heavy commitment of time and energy. If the sliding scale is used, it simply means that, as the patient volume increases, the dollar amount per patient which the hospital reimburses the physician group decreases. At a mutually agreed upon patient volume, the hospital reimburses the emergency physician group zero dollars per patient, and any financial relationship for that month is nonexistent. All calculations are performed and monies are reimbursed monthly. The essential factor in this type of arrangement is simplicity, in that the group and the hospital can calculate the so-called minimum guarantee quickly by counting the number of patients seen during the month. The sliding scale method avoids cross-audit of books, which is necessary if the guarantee is tied specifically to dollars collected by the group.

It is important to keep dollars in perspective: $17,000.00 per month appears to be a substantial amount of money. However, this money has to be distributed among a minimum of four full-time emergency physicians. The physician's net income is substantially reduced by professional expenses, including malpractice insurance and business overhead.

The route of choice for the emergency physician group is to attain complete autonomy from the hospital. Because of inadequate patient volume and other factors, this may initially be unobtainable in approximately 90 per cent of emergency physician group/hospital relationships. It is, however, becoming increasingly common, and certainly is beneficial to the development of the specialty of Emergency Medicine.

FEE SCHEDULES

The emergency physician uses the same relative value scale and fee schedule as any other physician in the community. For example, in California the usual relative value studies schedule is published by the California Medical Association. In other areas, the local Blue Shield relative value schedule or the relative value study produced by the American Medical Association entitled "CPT" (Current Procedural Terminology) may be utilized.

Regardless of the fee schedule used, it

is important that individual members of the physician group charge roughly the same fees for similar services. The group should agree on the fees for various procedures and produce a fee schedule all will follow. The relative value studies are a helpful guideline, but they must not be construed as an *absolute* fee schedule. The conversion factors that are utilized to derive a dollar figure on the traditional fee schedule should fall within the median of conversion factors that the community physicians use in their practices.

BILLING AND COLLECTION

The most widely utilized contractual system for billing emergency physician fees is for the group to pay the hospital 5 per cent of one's gross professional billings to act as a billing and collection agent and to pay the hospital 10 per cent of the gross billings as the physician's share of the bad debt expense. A combined bill of the emergency fees plus all hospital charges for that patient visit may then be produced by the hospital. Receiving one or simultaneous bills is a real service to third-party carriers and to the patient. A disadvantage in such a relationship is the close fiscal interrelationship between the emergency physician group and the hospital.

An increasing number of groups are using the mechanism of independent billing because it provides autonomy and independence. It is important to recognize that independent billing and its associated expenses may be costly. There is inherent in the practice of Emergency Medicine a much higher bad debt or noncollectable percentage of gross billings than in an office practice or in an inpatient hospital practice. If the emergency physician group decides that the economies are such that separate billing is financially viable, the group must hire expert help to manage the billing, collections, and personnel office.

An alternative is to contract out the billing and collection to a billing service, a financial management company, or to another emergency physician group already doing its own billing.

CONTRACT NEGOTIATION

It is beyond the scope of this short chapter to discuss the multiple parameters of an equitable hospital contract. Instead, some concepts and items which should be covered in an emergency physician contract will be listed, and detailed information should be sought in other references.

(1) Parties to the agreement (by name, corporate or DBA).
(2) Formalities: "Whereas," "Recitals," and "heretofores."
(3) Exclusivity.
(4) Clear description of duties of and coverage by emergency physicians.
(4a) Clear description of duties of medical staff.
(4b) Clear description of duties of the hospital.
(5) Term of agreement (beginning, end, continuance).
(6) Facilities (ED space).
(7) Relationship of parties involved.
(8) A clear statement as to whether the emergency physicians are independent contractors; that is: (a) not employees of the hospital; (b) not a joint venture between hospital and physician.
(9) Equipment and supplies (who is responsible for ordering, purchasing, etc.).
(10) Maintenance of facilities and equipment.
(11) Staff membership, staff privileges, delineation of Chief of the department and a departmental status statement.
(12) Statement of responsibility for other employees.
(13) Licensing: hospital/physician state licenses.
(14) Physician administrative responsibilities and compensation thereof; due process in medico-administrative matters — heard under whose jurisdiction.
(15) Number and competence of RNs and ancillary personnel staffing.
(16) Referral methods for continued care of patients.
(17) Financial arrangements:
(17a) Professional fees — mechanism of billing and collection — combined or separate billing.
(17b) Hospital fiscal guarantees; if applicable (how much and for what period of time?)
(18) Medical and financial records.
(19) Ethics and standards.
(20) Liability insurance, both professional and public.
(21) Amendments.
(22) Disagreements: mechanism for resolution, e.g., arbitration.
(23) Termination through loss of staff privileges.
(24) Scope of agreement succession: assignability and nonassignability.
(25) Physician group remuneration for development of the department over a period of years.

Here are some other parameters which sometimes are included in hospital/emergency physician contracts:

(1) Voluntary and involuntary retirement provisions.
(2) Treatment of hospital employees, visitors injured on premises, employee physicals, in-house responsibilities.
(3) Emergency treatment description.
(4) Limitation of services (e.g., no circular casts applied).
(5) Outside practice statement, "permissibility"?
(6) Teaching responsibilities.
(7) Professional courtesy policy.
(8) Policies and procedures of any kind.
(9) Rendering to physician group "the appropriate corporate resolution indicating that the Board of Directors authorize the various entities (administrator, executive, vice-president) to enter into this agreement."

Such a list incorporates just some of the parameters to be considered. Local needs, experiences, and expectations will influence such considerations.

EMERGENCY DEPARTMENT BUDGET

The physician director should make input into the budget during its preparation and certainly prior to its final approval by the board of trustees. Examples of financial management input which should be included are the following:

(1) Reports of departmental operation showing actual and budgeted income expenses.
(2) Patient statistics.
(3) Man hours worked by nonphysician personnel.
(4) Man hours cost per unit of service.
(5) Cost of supplies.
(6) Supply cost per unit service.
(7) Payroll expense.
(8) Comparative budget information.
(9) A record of past expendituress.
(10) Anticipation of future work loads considering identifiable trends.

Anyone may easily calculate the cost of operating a department of Emergency Medicine, since approximately 50 per cent of the costs go to payroll expenses.

C. EVALUATION

C. Gene Cayten

As Emergency Department visits have mushroomed from 18 million in 1958 to 60.1 million visits in 1972, a number of hospitals have taken different approaches to this increased demand. Evaluation of medical care in Emergency Departments must be appropriate to the role served by the hospital within the medical community, and to the particular goals of the department within the hospital and the community. For example, goals would be expected to differ for departments functioning within: (1) a rural or suburban community hospital (providing primary care for the patient's chief complaint and referral back to a family physician); (2) an urban university hospital functioning as a regional trauma center; (3) a hospital functioning as part of a comprehensive health care plan (e.g., Kaiser-Permanente); (4) a city general hospital. Despite the different goals necessitated by these diverse settings, most

Emergency Departments have at least the following common explicit objectives.

(1) Diagnosis, treatment, and/or stabilization of emergent medical conditions.
(2) Diagnosis and treatment of urgent medical conditions.
(3) Referral of patients with urgent conditions for follow-up.
(4) Symptomatic treatment of patients with non-urgent conditions.
(5) Referral of patients with non-urgent conditions for definitive diagnosis, treatment, and comprehensive care.

In addition to fulfilling these basic objectives, hospitals may want to develop further goals, depending on the type of patients seen and the general accessibility of health care. For example, an Emergency Department in an urban setting, where few patients have their own primary practitioners, might want to develop a program for early diagnosis of conditions for which early treatment would be important. Such a program would screen patients who came to the Department, regardless of their chief complaint, for the specific conditions to which they are at greatest risk according to age, sex, race, etc. For instance, women older than 35 years would be given pap smears while waiting; all patients would have blood pressure taken; and women over 35 would have a breast examination and be taught to do a self-examination.

GENERAL TYPES OF MEDICAL CARE APPRAISAL

The American Public Health Association defines evaluation as "the value or amount of success in achieving predetermined objectives." The evaluation of Emergency Department care measures how well the objectives of the department are fulfilled, i.e., the quality of care provided in fulfilling each objective. Evaluation methodology can be thought of most easily in terms of Donabedian's schema (1969): structure, process, and outcome. Structural evaluation measures the credentials and level of training of the personnel, and the facilities, equipment, and organization of the system. Structure is relatively easy to measure, but has not been shown to correlate consistently with outcome. Process assessment consists of measuring what is included in the actual performance of medical care, such as laboratory studies done, physician performance, etc. Such assessment assumes that good medical care results in a good outcome, and that bad medical care results in a bad outcome. Unfortunately, it often is an evaluation of record keeping. Outcome assessment measures variables such as mortality, morbidity, length of stay, and degree of disability, and assumes that patient outcomes are a reflection of the quality of care provided.

Outcomes that are collected most easily, such as mortality, frequently are quite insensitive measures of the quality of care, whereas the more sensitive outcome measures, such as long-term disability, frequently may not reflect validly the quality of the emergent phase of the patient's care. One major problem involved in the use of any long-term outcome measure, such as length of hospital stay or degree of disability, is the great difficulty of separating the effects of the care given in the Emergency Department from the effects of prehospital and in-hospital care.

Because structure, process, and outcome types of appraisal all have their limitations, a program of emergency medical services evaluation should include all three. They must be used selectively in such a way as to complement each other.

APPLICABILITY OF MEDICAL CARE APPRAISAL METHODS TO THE EMERGENCY DEPARTMENT

Present methods of appraisal of medical care are not uniformly applicable to the care rendered in an Emergency Department. It is helpful to think in terms of evaluating the care in the following patient categories.

(1) *Emergent.* Requires immediate medical attention. Any delay is definitely harmful to patient. Disorder is acute and severe and threatens life or function of patient.

(2) *Urgent.* Requires medical attention within a few hours. Patient is in actual or potential danger if not attended. Disorder is not immediately life-threatening or severe.

(3) *Non-urgent.* Does not necessarily require the services and resources of the Emergency Department. Disorder is not severe or life-threatening. Patient is not endangered by delay of 24 hours.

Table 1 lists a subjective estimate of the applicability of present techniques that fall under structure, process, and outcome as they relate to the care of patients' emergent, urgent, and non-urgent problems. Applicability as used here includes consideration of validity, reliability, and ease and cost of use.

TABLE 1   Adequacy of Type of Appraisal for Types of Problems Encountered in Emergency Department

	STRUCTURE	PROCESS	OUTCOME
Emergent	++	+++	++
Urgent	+	++	+
Non-Urgent	++	+	+ (+++)°

°Health status outcomes are not very useful, but medical system outcomes measures are.

Emergent Patient Care

In evaluating the care of the most seriously ill (emergent) patients, structure, process, and outcome measures are all quite useful. Structural evaluation in the form of surveys has been used in many different ways to appraise the ability of an Emergency Department to deal with life-threatening injuries. Surveys of the level of training of the physicians working in the Emergency Department and of the in-house availability of specialists would be expected to correlate well with the outcomes of emergent patients. Physicians who have completed an emergency physician residency would be expected to provide better care than those with less specific medical training.

In treating very severely ill patients, one also would expect both process and outcome appraisal to be useful, since good process should result in good survival and poor care should result in poor survival. If a patient in hemorrhagic shock has his intravascular volume replaced and his loss of blood stopped, he should live. If a patient with ventricular fibrillation is not defibrillated, he should die. In these patients, the severity of the presenting condition makes process criteria fairly sensitive measures of the quality of care, since they tend to relate directly with outcome. However, as an improved prehospital EMS system delivers patients to the Emergency Department, who previously were DOAs (Dead on Arrival), good care may not correlate with improved Emergency Department survival. When selecting outcome measures, it must be remembered that the outcomes of emergency care are dependent on all the following factors: (1) the nature and severity of victim's condition; (2) the victim's constitution (previous health conditions); (3) the nature and quality of care and treatment; and (4) the time elapsed from the occurrence of the incident to care and treatment.

Urgent Patient Care

In urgent cases, structural analysis or survey would be quite insensitive measures of quality of care, since the correlations with usual outcomes are imprecise. Urgent procedures like suturing a laceration, casting a fracture, and treating urinary tract infections might well be performed with equally satisfactory results by personnel ranging from physician specialists to medical corpsmen or nurse practitioners. Likewise, the facility and equipment are less likely to affect urgent care very favorably or unfavorably. Although some very well-established protocols have been developed for the type of care to be provided, very few of these regimens have been shown to have a strong correlation with the patient's health status.

Patients with urgent conditions are much less likely to die if their medical problems are not properly taken care of than are those with emergent conditions; therefore, mortality rates will not reflect adequately the quality of urgent care. Morbidity or complication rates are more likely to reflect the quality of care provided in the Emergency Department, but such rates are difficult to obtain because follow-up care data usually are not readily available.

Non-Urgent Patient Care

The statements made about the poor applicability of the usual forms of structure, process, and outcome measures to urgent patient care are even more true about non-urgent patients. It is unfortunate that the care provided to this group, which includes many patients seen in the Emergency Department, is the most difficult to measure. These non-urgent patients include those with chronic or acute minor conditions, and the "worried well." It is hard to see how the care provided in one visit to the Emergency Department can have much effect on the long-term health status of these individuals. Recently, health status indices have been developed to measure the effectiveness of emergency medical care. Work by Bush and Katz measuring degrees of disability and providing a scale of activities of daily living was originally designed for chronic diseases, and therefore might be considered applicable to non-urgent emergency care appraisal (Bush, et al., 1971; Katz, et al., 1970). There are two major drawbacks to the use of these indices to appraise emergency care:

(1) They require follow-up several months after the episode.

(2) At that point of measurement, it is very difficult to attribute differences in status to differences in the care provided in the prehospital and/or hospital Emergency Department and in followup phases of care. With

chronic medical problems, it would be very difficult to control for the care given before and after the emergency care.

EMERGENCY DEPARTMENT EVALUATION

In developing an Emergency Department evaluation program, the following general considerations should be kept in mind.

(1) Start simply and use existing data sources first. Existing data will point to areas in which further data is needed.

(2) Involve those being evaluated in setting up the specific methods and standards.

(3) Wherever possible, use methods that do not require hours of physician time.

(4) Develop a feedback mechanism so that those being evaluated get the results in an educational form, not a punitive one.

(5) Get acquainted with existing methods to avoid "reinventing the wheel."

(6) Get enough cases to control variables.

Structural Evaluation

The main instruments of structural evaluation of the Emergency Departments are (1) the surveys by the Joint Commission on Accreditation of Hospitals (JCAH); and (2) a categorization survey. Both of these instruments survey the organization, equipment, staffing, ancillary service, etc., of the Emergency Department.

The JCAH survey should be used as an opportunity to look critically at the various parameters beyond the minimum requirements. Ongoing methods of monitoring adherence to accepted standards could be useful. Such monitoring might involve a monthly check-sheet to be filled out by the nurse or physician in charge, and/or as one of the functions of the E.D. committee. Also, structural evaluation can be useful for interhospital comparisons.

Process Evaluation

Process evaluation methods in Emergency Departments have been fairly rudimentary. The two main methods used are direct observation and/or record audit. Direct observation is fraught with great expense, lack of reliability, and frequently lack of objectivity. Record audits are hindered by exaggerations of the usual drawbacks of in-house record audits: poor legibility, incompleteness, poor reflection of actual care provided, etc. Recently, some Emergency Departments have developed precoded records that can be computer-analyzed for some data. Developing a common data base to be computer-processed and used on a regional basis, as Boyd has done in Illinois for trauma, is an important long-term objective for Emergency Department evaluation (Boyd, et al., 1973).

As mentioned earlier, process evaluation should be geared toward emergent and urgent conditions. Some direct observation by the chief Emergency Department physician undoubtedly will reveal some examples of situations in which care could be improved.

Methods of conducting medical record audits should be designed according to the size of the Emergency Department and the availability of physician time. The following options should be considered in the program.

(1) Auditing all records vs. sampling.

(2) Use of physician vs. non-physician auditors.

(3) Use of implicit vs. explicit criteria.

(4) Use of nondiagnostic specific criteria (e.g., were vital signs, diagnosis, disposition, etc., recorded?).

(5) Use of diagnostic specific criteria (e.g., was urinalysis done for patients with the diagnosis of appendicitis?).

(6) Use of symptoms/sign-specific criteria (e.g., has an EKG been taken on patients whose chief complaint is crushing chest pain?).

Larger Emergency Department patient loads should incline an audit program toward record sampling, nonphysician auditors, and the use of explicit nondiagnostic, diagnostic, and symptom/sign-specific criteria.

Criteria should be developed with the following considerations: (1) Are they readily abstractable from the record? (2) Do they reflect care where a clear consensus has been established? (3) Are they sensitive to Emergency Department intervention? and (4) Do they correlate with outcomes?

Those records that do not fulfill the criteria should be screened out for further review by physicians. Nonphysicians should not be expected to make final judgments on the quality of care, even with the use of predetermined criteria. The development of diagnostic-specific and/or symptom/sign-specific criteria for the record audit of non-emergency problems would be be very complex and very difficult to prove valid.

Outcome Evaluation

Few Emergency Departments now use any outcome measures to evaluate the quality of care given, for the simple reason that there are few good outcome measures specific to the Department. A very small percentage of patients seen in the Emergency Department die there, and those few who do die usually do so more because of the state in which they arrived than because of any care that was or was not given. Nevertheless, careful clinicopathologic review of any deaths occurring in the Emergency Department or within 24 hours of admission regarding whether the death could have been prevented should be part of any Emergency Department audit program.

Likewise, the development of complications attributable to the care given in the Department would be very difficult to assess. Information regarding the occurrence of such complications after the patients were admitted, discharged, and/or referred elsewhere would be virtually impossible to compile on an ongoing basis. If complications developed during the entire hospitalization or an index of health status based on activity level, etc., is reviewed several months later, it usually is very difficult to attribute differences in results to differences in the quality of emergency care. It is too difficult to control for the care given before and after the emergency care.

Even if diagnostic-specific indices of severity could be developed to quantify the patient's condition on entering and leaving the Emergency Department, it is questionable that the difference in his condition over that period would be a valid measurement of the quality of care provided. Here again, the severity of the patient's condition on leaving the Department would be very heavily (and perhaps uncontrollably) influenced by his underlying injuries, illness, and general state of health.

Possibly, diagnostic- and/or problem-specific scales based on duration of time in the Emergency Department could be developed, and could be regarded as medical systems outcomes. For example, the time from entrance to the Emergency Department to that of entrance to the operating room for a patient with blunt trauma to the abdomen who is in shock could reflect the quality (efficiency) of the medical care system the patient has entered. This also would reflect the efficiency of ancillary services, radiology, blood bank, hematology, etc. Mean patient problem and/or diagnostic-specific Emergency Department times could be developed and used as a screening tool to select for evaluation cases in which time in the Emergency Department greatly exceeded the mean.

The quality of medical care provided to non-emergent conditions in the emergency room is impossible to measure in terms of existing medical outcome measures. Death, disability, and complications would be much too insensitive indices to reflect good or bad care. For non-urgent patients, the most important function of the Emergency Department visit is to gain access to the health care system; what actually is done in the Department during any single episode is of much less importance. Brook and Stevenson (1970) found that, of 141 non-urgent Emergency Department patients requiring x-rays for gastrointestinal problems, only 94 completed their x-ray studies, and only 37 of these knew whether the study was normal or abnormal. Thus, for non-urgent patients, it appears more appropriate to use medical system outcome measures such as patient satisfaction, efficiency of patient care, patient compliance with prescription and appointments, etc. Although these medical system outcome measures do not measure actual patient health status, there is general agreement that they are important in attaining good health status.

Evaluative data collected using structural, process, and outcome modes can be used in several ways: (1) it can be compared to data taken at some subsequent point in time to denote the extent of progress; (2) it can be compared to data taken from other Emergency Departments in similar settings and with similar types of patients; (3) it can be compared to existing standards of care as set forth by experts and professional organizations.

References

American Hospital Association. Hospital Statistics, 1972, p. 34.

Boyd, D. R., Lowe, R. J., and Nyhus, L. M.: Trauma registry, a new computer method for multifactorial evaluation of a major health problem. J.A.M.A., 223(4):422, 1973.

Brook, R. H., and Stevenson, B. S.: Effectiveness of pa-

tient care in an emergency room. N. Engl. J. Med. 283:904, 1970.

Bush, J. W., Chen, M. N., and Donald, L.: Social Indicators for Health Based on Function Status and Prognosis. University of California, San Diego, Health Index Project, Department of Community Medicine, La Jolla, California, p. 40.

Donabedian, A.: A Guide to Medical Care Administration. Vol. 2, Medical Care Appraisal—Quality and Utilization. New York, American Public Health Association, 1969.

Katz, S., et al.: Progress in the development of the index of ADL. Gerontology 10:20, 1970.

Schulberg, H. C., Sheldon, A., and Baker, F.: Program Evaluation in the Health Fields. New York Behaviorial Publication, Inc., 1969, p. 6.

D. CATEGORIZATION OF EMERGENCY FACILITIES

Richard A. Brose

The *why* and *how* of categorization of hospital emergency services are perhaps two of the more controversial aspects of emergency care systems. The history of such categorization is brief and has been confused to some extent by differing systems of classification recommended by professional organizations. Regardless of the system applied, the principle behind such actions is to identify sources of immediate definitive care for the life-threatened emergency patient. The "why" might simply be stated to be the best utilization of existing resources, yet such a statement deserves at least a brief discussion.

The expanding utilization of Emergency Departments over the past two decades includes a major workload of non-emergency patients who use the Emergency Department as their private physician substitute. Although this workload cannot be overlooked, categorization of facilities must concentrate on the identification of the hospital's ability to care effectively for the life-threatened patient at any time. This places emphasis on major medical and surgical cases, which generally comprise less than 10 per cent of the total workload of the Emergency Department.

Few Emergency Departments are sufficiently staffed or equipped to provide total patient care within the department without relying on support from other hospital departments. Categorization, therefore, reflects the ability and willingness of the total hospital to divert major resources to a limited number of patients requiring immediate definitive care.

Although Emergency Medicine and Emergency Nursing are becoming popular specialty areas, there still exists a chronic shortage of well-trained and experienced emergency service personnel. With this shortage, it appears desirable to concentrate the available personnel at specific facilities which have the capability to provide 24-hour definitive immediate care for the life-threatened patient rather than to expect every hospital to provide such services at all times.

Not every hospital that can provide 24-hour emergency service can also provide definitive specialized care immediately at any time. As one studies the utilization of emergency services, it does not appear that every hospital need attempt to provide such complex emergency services. Furthermore, groups of hospitals, operating under a categorization system, also can permit some of their members to provide only limited services for nonemergency patients without reducing the community's response capability.

In a multi-hospital service area, the keys to effective utilization of Emergency Departments lie in the prehospital emergency care and transportation system and in the education of the general public regarding the purposes of such categorization activities.

If life-threatened patients are routed to

comprehensive care centers, definitive care can realistically be expected within minutes or seconds. Other emergency patients, who are not life-threatened, may receive adequate and more rapid care at less definitive care centers without the interruption caused by the arrival of more critical patients. Finally, the nonemergency patients who want to be seen by a physician may find more rapid care at hospitals operating nonemergency outpatient clinics, which may replace previous emergency services.

The public response to categorized emergency services is more complex than it may first appear. Most patients, following even minor injuries, consider themselves to be an "emergency," and may seek care at comprehensive care centers. The problem of proper service selection by patients is compounded by the onset of pain, which may reflect major or minor medical problems. It is, therefore, unrealistic to believe that total patient distribution between categorized emergency services will be based on correct evaluation, especially by the patients themselves, and we must expect that nonemergency patients will continue to seek care at facilities prepared to deal with the life-threatened patient. It is more important to identify specific capabilities of each hospital so that the professional community and public safety personnel (police, fire, and ambulance services) can determine the appropriate facility for the life-threatened patient.

Emergency service categorization is considered by some to be valid only in urban multihospital service areas and not applicable to rural areas, where several counties may be served by only one hospital and several physicians. If the purpose of categorization is to identify the capabilities of the total hospital to care for the life-threatened patient as previously stated, the principle is as valid for rural hospitals as for their urban counterparts.

As space here is too limited to debate such issues, we will assume that the reader agrees with the "why" of categorization and begin the discussion of "how" to categorize.

A categorization system generally is based on numerous factors within the hospital which include personnel staffing, training programs and preparation of available personnel, equipment and supplies, physical characteristics of the hospital, specialty services available, administrative structure of the Emergency Department, communications systems, and patient workload.

External factors such as geographic location, classification of other hospitals, patient flow patterns, and others should also be considered in the development of the total system.

With this information in hand, it is recommended that each facility be rated at its lowest possible response capability rather than at its maximum response capability. In other words, the ability of most hospitals to provide immediate definitive care at 2 A.M. on a Sunday morning is quite different from the ability at 10 A.M. on a weekday morning, when most of the attending staff are at the hospital. As we have no control over the occurrence of life-threatening emergencies, the facility should be rated on its ability at 2 A.M., not 10 A.M.

HOW MANY CATEGORIES AND WHAT TO CALL THEM?

The recommendations of professional organizations vary considerably in the number of categories and the names for each. Some areas have simply designated which of their hospitals provide emergency service, thus placing each in a "Go" or "No Go" position, which may be too simplified a categorization to be meaningful. Other recommendations encourage five or six categories of emergency services. This, however, may be confusing to the general public and even to practicing health professionals. In an attempt to reach a happy medium, three categories seem appropriate for discussion here, as some major distinctions may be made between them.

Recommended names or titles for each category also vary considerably. Terms such as "comprehensive," "major," "general," "basic," "emergency," "first aid," "limited," etc., commonly are found in health service publications. The terms we shall use are: Major Emergency Service, Emergency Service, and Limited Emergency Service (Table 1).

In any event, whatever the number and names chosen for local use, they should be selected so that they will be meaningful to the general public, to public safety services, and to health professionals.

TABLE 1 Categorization of Emergency Facilities Guidelines

	MAJOR EMERGENCY	EMERGENCY	LIMITED EMERGENCY
Types of Patients	Life-threatened Emergency Routine	Emergency Routine	Routine
Emergency Department Staffing	Emer. Physicians, Nurses, Paramedical, Clerical & Admin.	Emer. Physicians, Nurses, Paramedical, Clerical	Specially trained non-physician staff. Phys. — on call
Specialty Staffing	Anes., Gen. Surg., Int. Med., Peds., Ob.-Gyn., Psych. *WITHIN THE HOSPITAL AT ALL TIMES Others on call within 30-min. time*	As required *On Call Within 30-min. time*	Call-list recommended
Other Hospital Departments (For support)	Staffed non-phys. at all times: X-ray, Lab., Blood Bank, IT, EKG, EEG, Pharm., other as req.	Staffed non-phys. at all times: X-ray, Lab., Blood Bank, IT, EKG, other as req.	Cardiopulmonary resuscitation services
Other Hospital Departments (For transfer)	Operating room, ICUs, Delivery & Newborn Nursery, Psych. Rec., other as required *Staffed — 24 hr.*	ICUs, Delivery & Newborn, Psych., other as req. *Staffed — 24 hr.* Operating Room, Other as req. *On Call*	No requirement
Facilities	Large — capable of multi-critical patient care in E.D.	Large to med. Capable of at least 1 crit pt. care in E.D.	No requirement
Equipment & Supplies	Major commitment, life-support & definitive care	Major commitment, life-support & delayed definitive care	Cardiopulmonary resuscitation
Communications	Telemetry two-way radio intercom system	Telemetry two-way radio intercom system (optional)	No requirement
Administration	Dept. status Policy & proced. manuals	Dept. status or Committee — policy & proc manuals	Policy & proced. manuals
Training Program	Active — Interdiscip.	Active — Interdiscip.	CPR Team

Major Emergency Service

This category of service represents the most immediate and definitive care available within the hospital grouping and requires the most complex staffing, equipment, and facilities. To meet the needs of critical patients immediately, the emergency department must be staffed at *all* times with highly trained emergency physicians, nurses, and other appropriate paramedical staff in sufficient numbers to deal with expected workloads.

Such facilities generally are large, can accommodate multiple critical patients at the same time within the Emergency Department and should be equipped and supplied to facilitate high quality care by the Emergency Department staff and those of the specialty staff who may be called to provide more definitive care within the Department. Complete cardiopulmonary resuscitation capability must *always* be available, as well as other life support measures.

The Major Emergency Service is distinguished by its ability to transfer immediately the responsibility of critical patients to specialty staff who are on call from *within* the hospital at all times. Most recommendations list Anesthesia, General Surgery, Internal Medicine, Pediatrics, and Obstetrics-Gynecology as the specialty areas to be available constantly from within the hospital. Some systems, desiring to meet the total needs of all emergency patients, have added Psychiatry to the required in-house availability of specialties. Other specialties are on call as required. Obviously, most hospitals, even major teaching hospitals, will not have boarded specialists available within the hospital at all times; therefore, residents in their second year of specialty training, or beyond, are given in-house responsibility for support of the Emergency Department. It appears that only major teaching hospitals will have this capability for the foreseeable future.

Immediate in-hospital support from other departments is also required for the Major Emergency classification in order to provide complete diagnostic and treatment procedures. Such services as radiology, medical laboratory, blood bank, pharmacy, electrocardiography, and inhalation therapy must be able to provide immediate support to the Emergency Department. Still other hospital services (e.g., operating room, delivery room, intensive care units, newborn nursery, and psychiatric receiving) should be ready to accept patients from the Emergency Department without delay, and therefore require constant staffing by qualified personnel.

With the expanded role of the Emergency Department into the community via telemetry-equipped ambulances and paramedical personnel, the capability of telemetric monitoring and two-way radio supervision of paramedics is the logical function of the Major Emergency Service. As critical patients will be directed to these facilities for definitive care, this additional responsibility may improve the care of the patient even before his arrival at the Emergency Department door. Adequate communications in terms of intradepartmental and interdepartmental messages should also be considered. Such systems should not rely on normal telephone usage, but rather on intercom systems.

Finally, the administrative structure of the Emergency Department should have equal status with that of any other hospital department. Included with administrative procedures should be written policies and procedures concerning all types of emergency patients, their treatment and processing within the department.

Emergency Service

This category of service represents immediate life-supporting care within the Emergency Department and, thus, requires around-the-clock staffing by experienced emergency physicians, nurses, and other paramedical personnel. Equipment and supplies must also be adequate for any procedure performed within the department.

The major difference between this category and the Major Emergency Service is that specialty physician support is *not* required around-the-clock from within the hospital, but is on call during normal slack times of hospital operation. Anesthesia, General Surgery, Internal Medicine, Pediatrics, and Obstetrics and Gynecology should be available within 30 minutes to support the emergency patient.

Hospital departments that support procedures normally carried out by emergency physicians (e.g., radiology, laboratory, blood bank) must be staffed at all times by qualified nonphysician personnel. Other hospital departments which receive emergency patients (e.g., intensive care units, delivery rooms) must also be staffed constantly by qualified personnel to assure continued life-support care. Some relief from staffing costs is available within this category, as some services (e.g., operating room teams) may be on call, corresponding to those specialty physicians also on call.

External two-way radio communications systems with ambulances are recommended, but telemetry monitoring is generally considered optional. Inter- and intradepartment communications should not rely on phone lines, but on intercom systems.

Administrative structure of the department may have equal status with other hospital departments or may be governed by a multidiscipline committee of which the emergency physician is Chairman. Policy and procedure manuals covering all phases of treatment and administrative management of emergency patients should be considered vital.

Limited Emergency Service

Unlike the two categories previously discussed, the Limited Emergency Service does *not* require a physician to be present at all times. Most limited services do maintain call lists of physicians in general or Family Practice, Internal Medicine, and General Surgery, who agree to see patients within the department within 30 minutes after notification. This type of response obviously does not attempt to provide immediate definitive care for the life-threatened emergency patient and such patients should be routed to other hospitals with more definitive care available.

Even though ambulance transported cases will not bring life-threatened patients to a Limited Emergency Service, there remains the likelihood that such patients will arrive from time to time by private auto or some other noncontrolled conveyance. Therefore, it is necessary to maintain specially trained, nonphysician personnel within the hospital capable of basic cardiopulmonary resuscitation and other patient stabilization measures. It is also necessary that procedures be established to facilitate the rapid and safe transport of these patients to hospitals equipped to provide more definitive care.

If specialty services are available within the hospital (e.g., intensive care units), the requirements of staffing by qualified personnel is equivalent to other hospitals with such services. Otherwise, staffing of other hospital departments to support the emergency service may be on call as necessary.

Communication systems requirements are minimal and usually are determined by intrahospital policies.

Administrative structures, especially dealing with policy and procedure manuals for nonphysician personnel in the treatment and administrative management of emergency patients, are vital to the adequate support of patients. Delegation of responsibilities to nonphysician personnel and the limits of those responsibilities must be carefully delineated in writing to avoid confusion, patient mismanagement, and possible legal action.

CATEGORIZATION EXTENDED TO INPATIENT CARE

Do all hospitals with the same emergency service category have the identical inpatient care capability? To the contrary, it is unlikely that any two hospitals will be identical in the quality of care they can provide for various types of critical patients. Few hospitals, nationally, can provide the best possible care for every type of patient. Some hospitals, by choice, have specialized in some types of critical inpatient care. Others, by circumstance, provide less than desirable quality of care for certain types of patients.

It is obvious that critical patients brought to any level of emergency service require prompt transfer to some type of inpatient service where life-support and definitive care may be continued for days, weeks, or months, as necessary. In 1975, the evaluation of critical inpatient care capability became part of some categorization systems, and recommendations from the federal government suggested rating the care capabilities relating to specified kinds of critical patients. These patient types included trauma; burns; acute coronary, poisons, drug overdoses and alcohol detoxification; high-risk neonates; and critical psychiatric patients. Some systems have expanded that listing to include other acute medical problems and acute obstetric crises.

How does one quantify the quality of care available at any hospital? There are no quick, easy, and readily acceptable criteria at present; yet, such evaluation must again focus on the professional and support services available to the critically ill patient.

It has been recommended that, for each of the types of patients described above, inpatient care be graded into three levels that describe the clinical sophistication necessary to meet patient needs adequately.

A Level 3 for any of the above patients would indicate that prompt and continuous definitive care is available to deal with any complication associated with the primary diagnosis. This would provide the highest possible quality care for critical patients.

A Level 2 for any of the above patients would indicate a lesser degree of sophistication in providing continuous definitive care, and perhaps would suggest that some patients with particularly complex problems should be transferred to a Level 3 service at another hospital.

A Level 1 for any of the above patients would indicate that continuous definitive care was not available and that patients with more than routine needs would best be transferred to a higher level service.

Level 0 simply indicates that inpatient care for the specified type of patient is not available within the hospital.

Although specific criteria to measure such levels of care have not yet been established nationally, such measures must include the professional manpower available to the patient, the sophistication of that manpower, the equipment and supplies available for diagnostic and therapeutic procedures, and the physical facilities of the hospital. As a rule of thumb, the higher the level of inpatient care, the greater the demand for professional staff sophistication and complex diagnostic and therapeutic procedures.

Thus every hospital within the system would have a specified level of emergency service and specified levels of inpatient care for the types of patients previously described. Not all levels need be the same for different types of patients, and a hospital with an Emergency Service categorization rating may have inpatient care services at Levels 3, 2, 1 or 0 for specified types of patients. With this type of categorization, the system can identify which hospital is best prepared to deal with a specific type of critical patient.

SUMMARY

The categorization of emergency facilities should be an integral part of any emergency services system. The effects of categorization are maximized if prehospital patient transport is controlled to assure patient distribution to appropriate facilities. The basis of categorization is an appraisal of the total hospital capability to provide immediate and long term definitive care to the life-threatened patient at any time. Differentiation between emergency service categories is largely dependent on physician availability within the Emergency Department. Inpatient critical care is also largely dependent on the sophistication of physician staff. However, both the Emergency Department categorization and the level of inpatient care for specified types of critical patients also depends on: (1) nonphysician staffing; (2) specialty services available for diagnosis and therapy; (3) equipment and supplies; (4) physical facilities; (5) communications; and (6) administrative structure.

Although multihospital urban areas appear to benefit more from categorization of services, rural hospital categorization is recommended to identify resources for the rural patient. Guidelines for emergency service categorization are available from a number of professional organizations now, and guidelines for Inpatient Care Level evaluation should soon be available.

References

American Medical Association: Categorization of Hospital Emergency Capabilities. Chicago, 1971.

Committee on Acute Medicine, American Society of Anesthesiology: Community-wide emergency medical services. J.A.M.A., *204*:595, 1968.

Emergency Medical Services. Proceedings of the Airlie Conference, American College of Surgeons and American College of Orthopaedic Surgeons, 1969.

Forkosh, D. S.: A plan for the organization of emergency medical services on Chicago's north side. Ill. Med. J. *142*:209–212, 1972.

Illinois Department of Health: The Critically Injured Patient. Chapter 3: Regionalization and Categorization. Springfield, 1971.

Joint Committee of Accreditation of Hospitals: Accreditation Manual for Hospitals. Chicago, 1970.

Kansas City Area Hospital Association: Categorization of Emergency Services. Kansas City, 1973, 1974.

National Academy of Sciences, National Research Council, Division of Medical Services: Accidental Death and Disability: The Neglected Disease of Modern Society. Washington, 1966.

Youmans, R., and Brose, R.: A basis for classifying hospital emergency services. J.A.M.A., *213*:1647, 1970.

E. EDUCATION IN THE EMERGENCY DEPARTMENT

Gerald L. Looney

Following the Second World War, the American health system began to change rapidly and started exploration of new areas of service such as basic and clinical research. At the same time, it neglected earlier areas of public service such as emergency care, particularly if these earlier services were unacknowledged and unfunded by new-found Federal money. Emergency medical care was left virtually unattended and unsupervised, and the most crucial aspect of health care began to be regarded as separate and remote from hospitals and the developing health system.

Unfortunately, this neglect of emergency care problems did not stop at the Emergency Department door. As physicians left ambulance runs to assume increasing obligations in research laboratories and on patient wards, the problems of emergency care also left the concern of physicians and the curricula of medical schools and postgraduate training programs. The medical management of trauma and other emergency problems had always been difficult to teach, and as medicine began to be carved into smaller and smaller areas of physician specialties, emergency care had no single base and no consistent advocacy and attention. It is not surprising that subsequent health personnel were trained with virtually no exposure to the problems of emergency care, and no ability even to recognize or diagnose the deficiencies in emergency medical services, much less the skill to treat them.

The current local and national interest in the problems of EMS is long overdue, and it has rapidly become evident that one of the greatest deficiencies is a lack of adequately trained personnel at all levels, even in the hospital Emergency Department. Unfortunately, as attempts are made to upgrade both the quality and quantity of emergency medical manpower, an immediate dilemma arises: because of the urgency and time limitations inherent in the definition of an emergency, the classic patient presentation and discussion can rarely be used in this new medical specialty. Unlike training in most other physician specialties, it obviously is impossible to schedule real emergency patients for a certain clinic or classroom at certain hours, and it is unjustifiable to delay the prompt evaluation and immediate treatment of emergency patients so that they can be used as teaching material at a later time or in a different location. One of the best solutions to this dilemma may be the use of medical simulation. In other areas of medical education, simulation serves as a valuable adjunct to live patient teaching, but for emergency medicine simulation may become a primary teaching mode, with live case presentations assuming a secondary role.

Simulation in emergency training has already been proved and widely accepted for demonstrating the management of a variety of specific emergency problems, particularly through the use of manikins to teach cardiopulmonary resuscitation. A wide range of manikins and simulators have been developed to teach a number of emergency techniques, such as endotracheal intubation, emergency childbirth, insertion of intravenous fluids, etc. These simple simulators generally are limited to a single technique or procedure, and there have been other attempts to develop a live "simulator" through the use of the programmed patient. These highly trained and sophisticated "patients" can teach a variety of single or mixed emergency medical problems, but so far have had limited use. These programmed patients are not readily trained except in comprehensive centers; they cannot be mass-produced; they cannot be used repeatedly for injections or practicing other medical procedures; they are too fragile for easy packaging or shipment; and their maintenance and upkeep is considerable, since they cannot be stored between teaching sessions. Some of these problems have been overcome by the development of a synthetic, but most realistic, manikin controlled by a computer. This life-like manikin, called Sim I, was designed to teach medical personnel the skills required in the administration of anesthesia, and then in turn to test the effectiveness of the teaching and the effectiveness of the student's skills.

Certain desirable educational benefits were immediately obvious after using the simulator: (1) it allowed for planned and gradual increase in the difficulty of the skill to be taught; (2) it permitted the student an almost unlimited repetition of any phase of the procedure being taught; (3) it reinforced the student's learning opportunity by providing him with an immediate feedback of his own performance; and (4) it made it possible for each student to proceed at his own pace.

Controlled experiments with Sim I also showed unequivocally that the use of simulators provides a twofold advantage over conventional methods. The first is that residents in anesthesiology trained on the simulator reach an acceptable professional level of performance in fewer elapsed days, thus saving time in personnel training. Second, residents trained on the simulator require fewer trials in the operating room to reach the required level of skill, thus posing significantly less threat to patient safety. It also was observed in the operating room that residents trained on the simulator were better organized, exhibited more confidence, and were less error-prone. Subsequent training was applied to different levels of medical personnel, ranging all the way down to ward attendants learning to measure vital signs. Even personnel of lesser skill trained on the computer-controlled manikin showed marked improvement and net saving of training time, with significant improvements in student performance.

The positive result noted in the training of anesthesiology personnel could be even more profound in the training of emergency medical personnel, since the anesthesiologists already had two significant advantages: (1) they were able to schedule and collect their clinical material and responsibilities at a given time in a given location; and (2) there was already a large cadre of fully trained and qualified instructors available to supervise trainees in this clinical setting. These two advantages do not exist, and perhaps may never exist, in emergency medicine, and the possible adaptation of Sim I for emergency medical training may be very important for future efforts to standardize teaching and certification of emergency personnel.

Sophisticated educational technology, whether with programmed patients or lifelike simulated patients, will not be the total answer to education problems in the Emergency Department. As in the case of prehospital emergency medical personnel, the best initial approach in this new area of medical education may be a variety of approaches. Then, as the specialty itself becomes more discrete and defined and as different approaches demonstrate their inherent advantages and disadvantages, a more uniform methodology can be developed.

No matter what the eventual course content or educational philosophy involved, all educational programs in the Emergency Department must face one inescapable deficiency: of all the inadequate records generated in the health care system, particularly in terms of the developing peer review efforts and quality of care evaluation attempts, the most inadequate records of all and the greatest medical data deficiencies emanate from the hospital Emergency Department.

A major step toward solving some of these inadequacies may be the adaptation of a limited version of the Problem Oriented Medical Record system advocated by Weed. Much of this system is designed to organize and maintain data on repeated progress notes and long term follow-up care, conditions that are not present in the setting of the Emergency Department. However, the separation of data obtained from history and physical examination into subjective and objective categories, and the organization of a data base, may be beneficial for the treating physician as well as subsequent reviewers. Likewise, the development of a distinct and comprehensive problem list for each patient, or at least for complicated medical and traumatic problems, may keep to a minimum deficiencies in data and in treatment. The goal of "zero defects" is appropriate for the entire health system, and is particularly appropriate in the Emergency Department; this area is geared only for acute and episodic care, and there is little or no opportunity for follow-up and a minimal chance to review decisions or correct mistakes.

Chapter 70

OTHER HOSPITAL RESOURCES

A. Specialized Patient Care Units
B. Operating Rooms

A. SPECIALIZED PATIENT CARE UNITS

R Adams Cowley

INTRODUCTION

The immediate medical needs of many critically ill or injured persons cannot be met by the limited resources of the Emergency Department or the general wards of the community hospital. Intensive, specialized care, therefore, is required for the trauma emergency, the coronary emergency, critical neonatal problems, severe burn cases, and others. To meet these special needs, specialized patient care units have been created, first in the metropolitan teaching hospitals where support is feasible, and then extending throughout the community as their value is proved. Now, many highly sophisticated care centers receive the patient either directly from the scene, or after he has been stabilized for the moment at another facility or in the Emergency Department of the same hospital.

The specialized intensive care units (ICUs) are an important element in the continuity of the patient's treatment from the recognition of the disease or injury, initial treatment, surgery, and intensive care, through rehabilitation. As such, these units are a part of the over-all Emergency Medical System.

In this section we will first examine the principles applicable to all ICUs, and then highlight unique aspects of specialized units.

PHILOSOPHY AND DEVELOPMENT

The philosophy for developing an intensive care unit is best described by Collins, who states: "it is impossible to conceive that bringing the sickest patients, the best personnel, and proper equipment together in the same place at the same time will not give patients the best possible chance for survival. Failure to survive in this unit undoubtedly indicates failure to survive in any other portion of the hospital" (Collins and Ballinger, 1969).

The widespread development of anes-thesia recovery rooms after World War II was the beginning of a trend toward a variety of intensive care units, although in 1863 Florence Nightingale described the recovery room in small country hospitals (Nightingale, 1863). One of the rationales for expanding the function of the recovery room to a more sophisticated unit was to provide not only immediate life support but also efficient and economical extended care. The nursing personnel shortage and the unavailability of medical staff when needed, together with the inability to locate and utilize life-saving equipment scattered throughout the hospital, made it mandatory that patients with life-threatening problems should be congregated in one area. The new philosophy of grouping patients according to the severity of illness rather than the disease entity provided economy in nursing and medical care and demonstrated an improvement in survival and lessening of morbidity.

However, the development and refinement of special equipment to monitor and assist in providing respiratory, cardiac, and metabolic care was yet to come; it awaited the modification for clinical use of physiologic and biochemical techniques developed in the laboratory. As this technology has advanced, so has the ability of the physician to support and control patient management. Physiologic response measurements and biochemical microtechniques have made available a wealth of pertinent information to aid in patient management and in understanding disease processes. Although great strides have been made, further improvement in technical procedure is needed. For example, the use of noninvasive monitoring and telemetering of patient data with immediate retrieval and analysis will both decrease charting and sifting of information by the physician and nurse and reduce infection related to invasive procedures.

The concept of "physician-in-charge" in intensive care units is now generally accepted over the more conventional physician-patient relationship. As a result of having over-all management authority, the physician-in-charge can institute uniform patient management protocols necessary for maximum utilization of personnel and resources and assessment of results achieved. Today, physicians are being trained specifically to assume management responsibility for the ICU.

The establishment of ICUs also has resulted in the development of the team concept of patient care, allowing protocols to be established for effective patient management. For example, resuscitation demands a team effort following a pre-planned step-by-step protocol.

With the advent of ICUs, young physicians were given the opportunity to apply the principles of physiology and biochemistry taught in medical school and to see how these tools are used in patient management. Medical research was enhanced by concentrating medical problems of mutual interest to the clinician and basic scientist in a single area, creating a kind of clinical laboratory.

Proved successful management of patients in ICUs has fostered further specialization, e.g., medical, surgical, respiratory, coronary, stroke, trauma, burn, spinal cord injury, neonatal, and shock units. Focusing on the particular needs of the patient they serve, these units demonstrate improved patient care, cost effectiveness, increased opportunities for education and research, and the development of innovative techniques. Undoubtedly, other special units will be added to the list as the future confirms the trend toward increasing specialization.

AREAS FOR FURTHER STUDY

INFECTION

As with many excellent forms of therapy, the ICU has its undesired side-effects. One of the most stubborn problems encountered as a result of congregating critically ill patients in one area is the control of both exogeneous and endogenous infections. As a consequence of total body response to the initiating illness or accident, many patients seem to lose their host defense mechanism and become more susceptible to environmental bacteria and iatrogenic infection. Even though the physician and nurse are trained in preventing transmission of infection, laziness and carelessness continue to be major problems.

Technologic advances in unit design, air circulation, and noninvasive procedures, along with improved antibiotic regimens and ways of establishing total cleanliness, will each contribute to the development of a safer environment for the ICU patient. However, the key to infection control is staff training and cooperation in adhering to high cleanliness standards.

LOSS OF CONTINUITY

Another area of concern is the potential loss of patient care continuity through isolation in the ICU. The ICU physician sees the patient in an isolated phase of his total care program, which makes it difficult to relate personally with each patient. Without special efforts, care provided in the ICU by both the nursing and physician staff can become impersonal.

PSYCHIATRIC PROBLEMS

Finally, psychiatric problems,* which have received much attention, can be of serious consequence for both the patient and the staff. The patient undergoes emotional stress due to his isolation, lack of sleep caused by hourly therapy and procedures, disorientation as to the passage of time, and bombardment with auditory and visual stimuli. The patient may have the feeling of impending disaster while listening to the constant monotony of respirators, monitors beeping, and alarms sounding, all the time wondering when his alarm will sound. With this orientation, the patient may misinterpret overheard conversations regarding therapy as being detrimental to his condition. Generally, the nurse has a close working relationship with the medical staff and is able to provide total patient care. These should be ideal; however, the intensity of the ICU environment and the responsibility for life and death decisions eventually cause many nurses to seek positions in a less stressful environment.

Of necessity, access to the ICU by visitors and spectators must be restricted, not only for the patient's welfare but also to shield family members from possibly disturbing sights. Infection control and uninterrupted patient care require limits on visi-

---

*See also Chapter 76.

tation privileges. Although it is difficult for the family, this policy generally is accepted once it is explained properly.

Many investigations into these problem areas are under way, with the goal of maximizing the benefits of the ICU while developing new ways of controlling the problems.

GENERAL CONSIDERATIONS IN ALL INTENSIVE CARE UNITS

All specialized ICUs adhere to the basic principle of congregating in one service area those patients who require ever-present, highly skilled personnel and supportive equipment until their medical crisis is resolved. Thus, "an intensive care unit can most simply be defined as a special place in a hospital for taking care of the sickest patients" (Collins and Ballinger, 1969).

LOCATION

The criteria for selecting the location of an ICU are its proposed purpose, size, and function.

The general ICU should be a geographic extension of the operation room/recovery room complex. It should be readily accessible to the Emergency and Radiology Departments and the clinical laboratory. Ideally, these facilities should be on the same floor in order to minimize movement of the patient, supplies, and equipment. Subspecialty units should be in close proximity to the main ICU to facilitate sharing of special equipment and highly skilled personnel, although in practice most are located within their respective departments.

SIZE AND PLAN

The size of any ICU depends on the number of hospital beds (Wiklund, 1969). Generally, units larger than 15 beds are unwieldy. Units with 10 to 15 beds should contain an elevated central nursing station permitting observation of all patients. Separate cubicles for patients demand more floor space and make visual contact and accessibility more complicated, but offer the advantages of privacy, sound proofing, and better infection control.

CUBICLES

The traditional open ward beds separated by curtains offer advantages in observation, conservation of floor space, and cleanliness, but detract from privacy, quiet, and infection control. The three-wall, open-end cubicles, which allow adequate observation, have proved the best of suggested space configurations. Large pieces of equipment, e.g., x-ray machines, respirators, hypothermia units, etc., can be moved in and out with ease. Staff have ready access to the patient's side and more room in which to maneuver; in a cardiac arrest situation this is essential. The upper one-third of the wall partition between cubicles should contain large glass windows that allow observation of the patient and yet assure him of some degree of privacy. Provision should be made for a few closed cubicles for infection control and for isolation of the dying patient.

In general, it is preferable for all equipment, such as spotlights, intravenous poles, etc., to be suspended from the ceiling or wall of the cubicle, rather than on the floor. Monitors and other items for continuous patient care also should be installed on the wall, out of the way but easily observed and readily accessible. This allows more floor space around the bed and makes for easier cleaning.

There can never be too many service outlets in the cubicle. Adequate outlets are need for electrical equipment, gases, suction, air, and water, and should be mounted on the wall or suspended overhead. During the design phase, planning for large empty conduits interconnecting all areas and cubicles can save expensive renovations at a later date when additional equipment is obtained.

LIGHTING

Proper lighting in an ICU is critical for good patient care. Separate lighting for halls, cubicles, and nursing station does much to prevent interruption of sleep. Adjustable spotlights suspended from the ceiling facilitate the performance of venous and arterial "cut-downs," dressing changes, and close examinations of local areas. Simulation of night and day by varying light intensities gives the patient a feeling of time progression and helps to alleviate his disorientation.

OTHER SPACE NEEDS

Planning for adequate floor space for various needs such as storage area, offices, staff rest areas, medical preparation room, and so on prevents costly renovations at a later date. Insufficient storage space can be a daily irritation and hazard in the ICU. Medical carts, beds, hypothermia units, respirators, and other items of patient care not in use must be conveniently stored nearby, but not underfoot. Immediate life-saving equipment such as defibrillators, spare monitoring equipment, resuscitation boards, medication carts, and sets all must have space near the patient area for ready availability. It generally is thought desirable to have a utility room area where equipment can be cleaned and washed and soiled linens and gowns collected, and a place where sterile supplies can be stored. The nurses' medical preparation room should be located in a quiet area off the busy thoroughfare. It should be well-lit, designed with adequate shelf and bench space for preparing medications, and should contain a refrigerator for storing certain medications at the proper temperature. There should be a physician and nurse lounge, with nearby toilet, shower, and locker space. A comfortable and attractive family waiting and visiting area with toilet and telephone facilities is desirable. Other space needs include offices for the medical and nursing supervisors, charting areas, an x-ray viewing room, and a conference room large enough for classroom teaching. If the ICU is located far from the general hospital clinical laboratory, a small clinical laboratory adjacent to the unit is of great value for doing those clinical studies needed immediately for patient care and research. Intercom and telephone communication links are essential.

ELECTRICAL HAZARDS

A poorly conceived electrical system, or one without proper safeguards, is hazardous to the patient's welfare in an intensive care environment. Fibrillations can be produced by small leakages of current passing through a saline-filled catheter fixed into the patient's bloodstream, also a good conductor of electricity. Without proper grounding of all electrical equipment in the unit, those life-saving lines can provide excellent electrical conduction when electrical devices are attached to the patient.

The patient's survival often depends on electrical life-support equipment, and therefore an automatically engaged emergency power supply is mandatory and must be tested periodically. Throughout any unit, there must be adequately spaced 220-volt lines for apparatus requiring this source of power, such as portable x-ray equipment and housekeeping cleaning devices. These outlets should be designed with special sockets to prevent inadvertent plugging in of 110-volt equipment, with dire consequences.

MONITORING

Monitoring in an ICU depends on the unit's purpose. Generally, there should be three types: physiologic, biochemical, and infection surveillance. The physiologic monitoring includes measurement of the temperature, heart and respiratory rate, electrocardiogram, central venous pressure, arterial pressure, wedge pulmonary pressure, and urine output. Biochemical monitoring includes routine sampling of blood for gases and electrolytes, as well as measuring respiratory gas values. All physiologic monitoring systems, whenever possible, should contain adjustable controls for setting upper and lower ranges of each parameter, so that unacceptable measurements will trigger visual and auditory alarms. Results of biochemical investigations (e.g., electrolytes, hemoglobin and hematocrit, arterial blood gases, respiratory gas values, etc.) must be immediately available. Infection surveillance includes regular culturing of floors, walls, equipment, tracheostomies, catheters, wounds, and dressings. Infection control is discussed more fully below.

CARTS

Specially designed carts vastly improve the unit's ability to give both emergency and routine care. A variety of carts (CPR carts, monitoring carts, medication carts) are available on the market. They should have adequate-sized wheels for steady rolling and should be constructed of easily cleaned materials. Sealing a properly stocked cart can provide security to the user in the event of an emergency. A broken seal indicates that something has been removed from the cart and that it should be restocked and sealed. Stretchers for patient transportation are standard, but new carts are appearing on the market that will move the patient on and off the carts without lifting by attendants or nurses.

X-RAY

All routine procedures, including peripheral arteriography or venography, can be performed adequately by the available portable x-ray models. The mobile x-ray unit can be moved to the patient's side and turned rapidly, and is time-saving compared to the fixed overhead x-ray installation, which also is more costly. With current Federal regulations, fixed overhead installations would require that patients be separated by lead walls. Two-way tracking, overhead cables, and additional construction costs are prohibitive, and accumulation of dust and foreign particles on the equipment is undesirable. For these reasons, portable apparatus is currently recommended for all but special procedures which are best done in the x-ray facility.

INFECTION CONTROL

Cleanliness is the key word in infection control. Cleanliness of the cubicles, the equipment, and the staff are of vital importance. Improper catheterization and intravenous line penetrations, and dust and droplet nuclei from coughing, sneezing, draining intestinal contents, and wounds, are sources of infection. However, the main source of contamination is cross-infection secondary to sloppy technique by both physicians and nurses. Although cleanliness is the primary means of prevention, environmental factors can inhibit the spread of bacteria. For example, cubicles with barriers between the patients impede convectional circulation of bacteria-laden dust and droplet nuclei. Air conditioning systems can either contribute to or help alleviate infection problems. Commercial units that recirculate air can recirculate bacteria as well if the filters are not cleaned and disinfected regularly. Studies demonstrate that air conditioning units that introduce fresh filtered air into the unit are best. Recirculation units with proper filters and care, providing ten changes of air per hour, can effectively remove most dust and suspended droplets from the air. Recently developed laminar air flow systems are of limited value in a general ICU because of the cost and the necessity of keeping the cubicle closed. Ultraviolet irradiation as a means of sterilizing environmental air has been disappointing because the intensity needed is detrimental to patients and staff.

Strictly enforced dress codes, handwashing procedures, and guidelines for the conduct of invasive procedures will reduce the spread of infection. Constant bacteriologic surveillance and re-evaluation of the antibiotic policy are necessary components of infection control.

The gravity of infection control in the ICU cannot be stressed too often. Critically ill or injured patients are especially susceptible to infection, especially trauma and burn patients with open wounds. It is an indictment and a challenge to modern medicine that we frequently pull the patient through the initial emergency, whether it be multiple injuries sustained in an auto accident or severe burns, only to have him succumb to infection.

NURSING CARE

Undoubtedly, the backbone of the ICU is the nursing staff. It is the nurse who provides most patient care, spends the most time with the patient, and interacts with the family. In addition to the special technical training required, workshops, seminars, and discussion groups must provide the nurse with an understanding of the psychologic problems of the patient and his family. The nurse also must be given an outlet for the expression of emotions related to the stress of the ICU environment, and must have sufficient training in the appropriate specialty area in order to feel secure in dispensing care. Depending on the type of ICU, nurse patient ratio could be as low as 1:1 or as high as 4:1. All ICUs must have 24-hour nurse coverage, of course, and one nurse-in-charge who has over-all responsibility for nursing care, nurse training, and continuing education.

OTHER SPECIALIZED PERSONNEL

A complete program requires the expertise of numerous professionals representing various disciplines. In addition to the regular nursing and physician staffs, specialists in various technologies contribute to the program. The inhalation therapist adjusts and sets respiratory equipment and usually assumes responsibility for cleaning and repair. In smaller ICUs this person is responsible for all respiratory care, including the collection and analysis of blood gases. Physical therapists assist in preventing and treating pulmonary complications. They also teach patients (and nurses) the correct way to cough, turn, and sit up, and assist the patient in achieving these goals before discharge from the unit. Specially trained technicians in larger ICUs perform special studies such as cardiac output, ventilatory studies, etc. Finally, the cardiologist, radiologist, nephrologist, psychiatrist, infectious disease consultant, and neurologist all fulfill their roles as consultants by providing further expertise when needed.

TYPES OF INTENSIVE CARE UNITS

ANESTHESIA RECOVERY ROOM

The purpose of the anesthesia recovery room is to care for and observe postsurgical patients as they recover from anesthesia by making certain that airway obstruction does not occur, and that shock does not develop from medication or bleeding. The patient usually stays for only a short time, generally four to eight hours. If complications develop requiring further care, the patient is transferred to the general ICU. The anesthesia recovery room is located adjacent to the operation room and ideally near the ICU for continuity of patient care.

SURGICAL INTENSIVE CARE UNIT

Historically, the surgical ICU was a part of the postanesthesia recovery room. Today, the surgical ICU, a separate entity, is a continuation of the postanesthesia recovery unit; it provides pulmonary and circulatory support by specially trained medical and nursing personnel, and special equipment to surgical patients requiring intensive, long term care (generally two to five days). The unit must have a separate room for isolating patients with infection and, as with many speciality units, must contain a

room for the dying patient where he can be visited by the family in privacy without interfering with the function of the rest of the unit.

CARDIAC SURGICAL UNIT

Even more specialized than the surgical ICU unit, the cardiac surgical unit serves cardiac surgery patients, many of whom have had heart failure or are in some phase of congestive failure prior to surgery. In addition, they often have reduced pulmonary and hepatic function from long-standing chronic passive congestion, and most need careful monitoring and ventilatory support over extended periods (usually two to seven days). In such a unit there generally is found a cardiologist on the team as a consultant, in addition to the surgical and anesthesia staffs. Psychiatric consultation can become necessary, as these patients frequently develop unique emotional problems.

Since most cardiac surgical operation rooms contain the capability for special equipment such as pump oxygenators, counterpulsation equipment, hypothermia, and special monitoring techniques, the cardiac surgical unit should be close to this operation room to allow direct patient transfer, bypass of the anesthesia recovery room, and continuation of many of the therapeutic functions already established.

CORONARY CARE UNIT

In contrast to the cardiac surgical unit, the coronary care unit provides constant intensive observation and immediate emergency treatment for persons suffering acute coronary attacks. Patients may remain for as long as three weeks, depending on the availability of "step-down" observation units. Generally, the CCU is situated in the vicinity of the cardiology or medical service, although it is not dependent on any special location. As with most specialty units, it should contain a room for physician consultation, a sleeping room, a lounge for nursing personnel, and a comfortable family waiting room.

TRAUMA UNIT

A trauma unit is equipped for the management of severe multiple trauma that requires the presence or immediate availability on a 24-hour basis of multidisciplinary trauma teams and consultants capable of resuscitating and stabilizing, on short notice, victims of severe multiple injuries. Since many patients can exsanguinate rapidly, an operation room must be available at all times for emergency surgery. If operation rooms are on other floors and the unit is located in a large trauma population area, the unit should have its own operation room. Ideally, it should be near the Emergency Department also. The length of stay in the trauma unit generally is three to seven days. After recovery and stabilization patients are transferred to a less intensive care area; they seldom are transferred to a general hospital bed or home.

RESPIRATORY CARE UNIT

An outgrowth of medical interest in acute respiratory problems, these units provide intensive respiratory assistance, therapy, and monitoring for patients with chronic lung disase such as emphysema, chronic bronchitis, drug overdose, and neurologic paralysis, and occasionally for those with chest and head injuries. It usually is located near the medical or pulmonary service of the hospital, but can be anywhere. The length of stay is two to 21 days.

BURN UNIT

The burn unit is designed to manage the very special problems, surgical, medical, and psychologic, of the severe burn victim who requires long term care, rehabilitation, and counseling. Since infection is always a life-threatening problem, methods in management using special techniques are mandatory. It is the burn unit that new designs and techniques in isolation are being sought for improved infection control. Provision for physical therapy is especially important in this unit to help reduce deformity and disability in these patients.

NEONATAL NURSERY INTENSIVE CARE UNIT

These units are geared to manage premature newborns, many with congenital defects or other critical illness who could not survive in many hospital environments because of the lack of proper equipment (incubators, infant respirators, etc.). These units are most logically organized on a regional basis for economy and improved survival. The problems encountered in these infants require special nursing and physician care that utilizes equipment of the proper size and provides the proper environment for survival. It must be located near the pediatric service so that pediatricians can be readily available for assistance and consultation. Infants may stay for days or weeks, until care can be provided at a local hospital or at home.

DRUG AND ALCOHOL ABUSE CENTERS

Patients with drug or alcohol problems usually are seen in the Emergency Department, but this may not have the facilities for their management, and the other patients may be greatly disturbed by them. Persons with alcoholic or drug emergencies can be transferred immediately to this special center, which can provide appropriate care and help them with their crisis. Centers can be located outside the general hospital environment or as a separate receiving area within the hospital. The patient usually stays in this acute environment for 24 to 48 hours, after which he is either admitted for long term care or discharged home.

CONCLUSION

Other types of special care units are already in operation or will become part of the Emergency Medical System in the future. These include neurologic ICUs, stroke units, spinal cord injury centers, pediatric trauma units, and poison control centers. These facilities, and those discussed above, each contribute to the total scheme of Emergency Medical Services. Some are better utilized on a regional basis, whereas others may serve local needs, depending on patient populations, cost, medical resources, and other factors.

The future will reinforce this trend toward specialization and maximum use of special units, as part of the total emergency medical system. This trend can only improve patient care, enhance medical research and technology, and provide educational opportunities, at the same time making best use of financial and human resources.

References

Baue, A. E., et al.: Organization of a cardiac surgical unit. Angiology 25:43, 1974.

Baxter, S.: Psychological problems of intensive care. Nurs. Times 71(1):22, 1975.

Bergen, R.: Intensive care in hospitals. J.A.M.A. 206:1393, 1968.

Carroll, W. W.: Joint Commission Accreditation Standards for Anesthesia Services and Intensive Care Units. Clin. Anesthesiol. 10(3):49, 1974.

Collins, J. A., and Ballinger, W. F., II.: The surgical intensive care unit. Surgery 66:614, 1969.

Dornette, W. H.: An electrically safe surgical environment. Arch. Surg. 107:567, 1973.

Dornette, W., and Durbin, R.: Design and construction of an intensive care facility. Hosp. Manage. 91(2):35, 1961, and 91(3):51, 1961.

Haldeman, J. C.: Elements of progressive patient care. U.S. Department of Health, Education and Welfare, USPHS Report of February 1959.

Hay, D., and Oken, D.: The psychological stresses of intensive care unit nursing. Psychosom. Med. 34:109, 1972.

Holmdahl, M. H.: The respiratory care unit. Anesthesiology 23:559, 1962.

Hudak, C. M., Gallo, B. M., and Lohr, T.: Critical Care Nursing. Philadelphia, J. B. Lippincott, Co., 1973.

Jacobs, T. T.: Organizing and operating an intensive care unit. Hospitals 39:69, 1965.

Kornfeld, D. S., Zimberg, S., and Malm, J. R.: Psychiatric complications of open-heart surgery. N. Engl. J. Med. 273:287, 1965.

Kinney, J. M.: Problems in design of intensive care units. Anesthesiology 25:204, 1964.

Kinney, J. M.: The intensive care unit. Bull. Am. Coll. Surg. 51:201, 1966.

Langhorne, W. H.: The coronary care unit: a year's experience in a community hospital. J.A.M.A. 201:662, 1967.

Lockward, H. J., Giddings, L., and Thoms, E. J.: Progressive patient care. J.A.M.A. 172:112, 1960.

National Academy of Sciences—National Research Council. Workshop on intensive care units (Hamilton, W. K., chairman). Anesthesiology 25:192, 1964.

Nightingale, F.: Notes on Hospitals, 3d ed. London, Longman, Green, Longman, Roberts, & Green, 1863, p. 89.

Noehren, T., and Friedman, I.: A ventilation unit for special intensive care of patients with respiratory failure. J.A.M.A. 203:641, 1968.

Petty, T. L., et al.: Essentials of an intensive respiratory care unit. Chest 59:554, 1971.

Petty, T. L., et al.: Intensive respiratory care unit; review of ten years experience. J.A.M.A. 233:34, 1975.

Public Health Service Publication No. 1250: Coronary care units: specialized intensive care units for acute myocardial infarction patients. October, 1964.

Safar, P.: Respiratory Therapy. Philadelphia, F. A., Davis Co., 1965.

Sanford, J. P.: Infection control in critical care units. Crit. Care Med. 2:211, 1974.

Tanser , A. R., and Wetten, B. G.: Multipurpose intensive care unit in a district general hospital. Br. Med. J. 3:227, 1973.

Travis, K., et al.: Report on the first year's activities of a multidisciplinary respiratory intensive care unit. Crit. Care Med. 1:235, 1973.

Wiklund, P. E.: Intensive care units: design, location, staffing, ancillary areas, equipment. Anesthesiology 31:122, 1969.

B.   OPERATING ROOMS

R Adams Cowley

Critically ill and injured patients requiring immediate and extensive surgery are commonly admitted to community hospitals as well as large general hospitals associated with medical schools. The operating room is an integral part of the life-saving procedure and is a necessary hospital resource to provide immediate appropriate care for the emergency critically ill and injured. However, unlike those hospitalized with acute or chronic disease, the individual with a life-threatening problem is usually an unwelcome patient because the hospital often is neither prepared nor geared to handle his emergency (Cowley, 1967).

In this section, we will examine the need for a dedicated operating room and highlight design and location criteria as well as equipment and staffing requirements.

BACKGROUND: THE NEED

With trauma patients, "for every 30 minutes that elapse before definitive care, the mortality rate can be expected to increase threefold" (Foster, 1969). An analysis of military casualities, as well as the patient population of the Maryland Institute for Emergency Medicine (MIEM), has revealed that the mortality varies inversely with the length of time intervening between injury and definitive care (Cole, 1970).

To combat this time limitation, total preparedness for treatment of any life-threatening injury or illness must be the basic philosophy of any emergency health care delivery system. *The fight for survival begins at admission.* All severely traumatized patients can be assumed to be dying and therefore cannot wait for extensive evaluation. Rapid assessment, endotracheal intubation, continuous positive pressure ventilation, and circulatory support often become mandatory. And often, early, aggressive surgery must be a part of resuscitation efforts (Cowley, 1976).

Therefore, in the hospital that has assumed responsibility for trauma care, the need becomes apparent for an available, dedicated operating room. Any system of emergency health care delivery designed to provide immediate care without waiting is bound to fail if an operating room and anesthesiology and nursing staff are not available on a moment's notice. Many multiple trauma victims cannot survive their injuries without immediate surgery. The delay of even minutes can be fatal. Therefore, immediate access to a fully staffed, fully equipped operating room is necessary if the life is to be saved.

It is often impossible to meet this demand by using the general hospital's operating rooms where elective procedures are scheduled. The patient must wait while the room is vacated; the schedules of the room and the surgeons are disrupted; the room is not always staffed during periods of increased trauma incidence—nights, weekends, and holidays. The general OR nursing staff may not have the expertise required for the complex, intraoperative care of the trauma victim. Therefore, general operating rooms are inadequate, and if the hospital is committed to care of trauma victims, an operating room must be available for emergency surgery.

AVAILABILITY

To provide multiple trauma care capability, at least two operating rooms are necessary in the trauma operating suite. Multiple emergency admissions are common and may require more than one operating room. Also, patients often require follow-up procedures, sometimes soon after the original operations. One room should be available for incoming emergencies and the other for back-up for multiple admissions and for scheduled and emergency follow-up procedures.

LOCATION AND DESIGN

The trauma operating rooms should be adjacent to the accident receiving area in the Emergency Department. If possible, they should be near the radiology department. The time lost waiting for elevators or transport to another part of the hospital can cost lives.

The rooms should be large enough for several surgeons to carry out a number of procedures simultaneously. Essentially, the rooms should be of the size and design to accommodate a thoracic or cardiovascular procedure. The latest environmental nosocomial infection control system should be incorporated.

Necessary equipment includes multisystem monitoring devices, radiologic support (either fixed or portable), resuscitative equipment such as defibrillators, and surgical instruments for all types of surgery, including neurosurgical, orthopedic, thoracic, vascular, and abdominal surgery. Emergency drugs and fluids for resuscitation and volume replacement should be on hand. Items for providing anesthesia are those found in any standard major operating room. Specific fixed equipment, such as oxygen, suction, anesthetic gas outlets, is also standard.

Storage for supplies is generally inadequate in most operating room designs. The trauma operating room needs greater storage space because of the equipment and supplies required for managing multiple surgical procedures simultaneously under one anesthetic.

It is somewhat expensive to have a full complement of equipment and instruments to care for all types of injuries in each operating room, but dying patients cannot wait for supplies and equipment that should have been on hand.

STAFFING

A competent staff should be available at all times to handle any emergency. Staffing must be provided 24 hours a day, seven days a week. Weekends, holidays, and summers are high trauma periods; therefore, increased staff is maintained during these periods.

An all-RN staff is necessary to provide the high quality, high priority type of nursing care needed for trauma patients with their complex metabolic, respiratory, and physiologic problems. The nursing staff must give intraoperative care to the multiple system injured patients. This requires ingenuity in positioning, draping, and instrumentation. The staff must also be skilled in all types of monitoring and have working knowledge of all instruments used in multisystem surgery.

The operating room staff must work as a team. There must be specific suture and instrument routines—there is no place for an individual surgeon's idiosyncrasies in trauma surgical care. The staff should have a thorough knowledge of the capabilities of each team member. Pre-planning is important.

TRAINING

Intensive in-service education must be available for all operating staff members treating the emergency victim. Pre-planning for emergency surgery should include knowledge of (1) instrumentation, (2) emergency drugs, (3) emergency equipment such as electrocardiogram with defibrillator and the cardiac pacer, (4) fluid replacement, and (5) resource people throughout the hospital.

There is no room for panic. Emergency is the rule rather than the exception. But with a little bit of time, planning, foresight, and knowledge of the capabilities of the OR staff, those capabilities can be used to the fullest to provide successful surgical management.

CONCLUSION

For a trauma facility to successfully save lives, it must include operating rooms adjacent to the trauma receiving area. The rooms must be fully equipped, fully staffed, and immediately available.

To equip and staff operating rooms to receive trauma patients is expensive. Therefore, it should not be the responsibility of every hospital. Rather, selected hospitals with the capability and the commitment for this type of care should develop the specialized facilities necessary if lives are to be saved.

References

Cole, W. H.:The need for improved first aid care in motor vehicle accidents. J. Trauma 10:184, 1970.

Cowley, R A.: A study of shock and trauma in man utilizing the resources of a clinical shock trauma unit. Maryland State Med. J. 16:63, 1967.

Cowley, R A.: The resuscitation and stabilization of major multiple trauma patients in a trauma center environment. Clin. Med. 83:14, 1976.

Foster, J.: Helicopters make sense in medical care. Mod. Hosp. 112(2):79, 1969.

Chapter 71

FOREIGN MODELS OF ORGANIZATION OF EMERGENCY MEDICAL SERVICES

A. INTRODUCTION

Patrick B. Storey

The characteristics of an effective emergency care system described in the preceding chapters are expressed organizationally in different ways in the many differing communities of the U.S. Ultimately, one might envision a national system so arranged that in our highly mobile society any citizen anywhere would know exactly what to expect and precisely how to gain rapid access into the system.

There are many determinants of how such a system would develop, including such major ones as the geographic area involved, the degree of urbanization, the state of development of the general health care system, and the nature of the social contract that is reflected in the governmental mechanism.

These and other issues will determine how a system is put together, but certain common elements must be used to create such a system. Certainly, there is a uniform basic goal — to get help to a victim as quickly as possible and to transport him safely to where he needs to go. And certainly there are basic ingredients of such a system: manpower must be trained and deployed wisely; there must be good communications; facilities and equipment must be adequate and accessible; the public must be educated to use the system effectively; and there has to be effective review and evaluation, with a capability to change as the advancing competence of medicine dictates such change.

The following chapters depict to some extent how other nations have tried to put their emergency care systems together, conditioned by the particular constraints of their territories and social contracts. A consideration of these systems may yield mutually useful information.

The vast territories of Australia and the Soviet Union force upon responsible authorities the consideration of distance and time. The need to integrate the private and public sectors is shown in Sweden and Israel. The possibility of a single responsible nongovernmental agency as the coordinating mechanism is described in Israel's Magen David Adom (Red Shield of David), an organization similar to the Red Cross and Red Crescent. The potential of central direction and fixed responsibility is illustrated in the Hungarian and Soviet models . The problems inherent in delivering services in the super-city under different social and economic conditions are shown in Moscow and in Tokyo.

These are some of the issues discussed by our colleagues from other countries in the following pages.

B. EMERGENCY MEDICAL SERVICES IN AUSTRALIA

G. Anthony Ryan

Australia is roughly the same size as the continental U.S., with its population of 13 million concentrated in the Southern and Eastern coastal areas. Eighty per cent of the population live in urban areas, with 60 per cent living in the capital cities of the six states. Historically, each state developed as a separate colony, and even though federation occurred in 1901 there are still marked differences in approach to the provision of health services between states. However, throughout Australia, first aid in emergencies is supplied by ambulance services, with definitive medical care being provided by the Casualty (Emergency) Departments of public, i.e., government-subsidized, hospitals.

ORGANIZATION

Ambulance services of each state are under the direction of a central, nonprofit organization, with locally organized operating units. In the four Eastern states of Queensland, New South Wales, Victoria, and Tasmania, the central authority is set up under an Act of Parliament. The power of these authorities to regulate the services provided lies in their control of the distribution of the subsidies provided by each state government. There is a strong tradition of local autonomy in the operating centers, and persuasion, rather than regulation, is used to effect changes.

There is no Act of Parliament in South Australia or Western Australia, services there being provided by the St. John Ambulance Association, a voluntary organization, with the aid of government subsidies. In the territories controlled by the Federal government, the Australian Capital Territory, and the Northern Territory, there is no legislation governing ambulance services, which are provided by the government hospitals and departments concerned.

The size of the operating units varies considerably between states. Victoria has 16 ambulance regions, each region with a headquarters and several substations, administered as a single service. In the other states the size of the units tends to be much smaller, except in the largest cities. The range is from a one-vehicle, volunteer service in a small rural town to one, such as that serving Melbourne, with over 1300 officers and 100 vehicles for a population of over 2 million.

STAFFING

In the larger cities ambulance officers are full-time; in the smaller, rural areas volunteers are used. Victoria, New South Wales, and Western Australia have central, residential, training schools in which training courses are held for all grades of ambulance officer. Within each service there is a career structure through several grades of ambulance officer to superintendent, who

has charge of a service. Successful completion of the appropriate training courses is a prerequisite for promotion. The level of pay for ambulance officers is about the same as that of the police and fire services.

COMMUNICATIONS

Throughout Australia there is a universal emergency telephone number — '000' — which is called for either the police, fire, or ambulance services. These emergency calls are directed to the ambulance service switchboard, from whence an ambulance is dispatched to the site of the emergency by telephone or two-way radio as appropriate. Communication with hospitals for urgent cases is by direct telephone line to the Casualty Department. There is central coordination of each service for emergency and routine transport cases, using radio control in all but the smallest services.

TRANSPORT AND EQUIPMENT

A variety of ambulance types are used, based on car or light truck conversions. Victoria has developed a standard ambulance based on a light truck with modified suspension to achieve a better ride, and this is slowly being accepted throughout the state. It has two regular berths, with two emergency stretchers, air-conditioning, and generous stowage space for standard equipment, including bag and mask oxygen equipment and suction apparatus. Most services carry an analgesic inhaler using Trilene or nitrous oxide for use of patients in considerable pain.

Fixed-wing aircraft are used as ambulances on a regular basis in Victoria, New South Wales, and Queensland, commonly for transport of patients between rural areas and treatment centers in the principal cities. Emergency flights are made as required. A helicopter service is provided for emergencies by an ambulance service in a semi-rural area near Melbourne, with a considerable subsidy.

FINANCE

Financial support for the services comes from government subsidies, donations, fees charged for transport on a minimum charge plus mileage basis, and subscribers' fees. The latter are derived from members of insurance plans whereby, on payment of an annual fee, the member and his family are carried free for up to certain substantial limits of mileage. Reciprocal arrangements are made with other services for reimbursements for services provided in other states.

In New South Wales and Queensland a considerable proportion of income is derived from fund-raising social activities organized by the local units. The exact proportions of income derived from each source vary considerably from state to state, and from service to service, so no over-all figure can be given.

UTILIZATION

The bulk of the workload of Australian ambulance services consists of non-emergency transport of patients between hospitals and homes. A committee of the Australian Medical Association, with support from the National Health and Medical Research Council, has completed a detailed study of the workload operations of Australia's ambulance services. Preliminary data from this survey give a national figure of 98 ambulance trips per 1000 population, of which about 15 per cent are emergencies, and one-third of these are due to road crashes. Needless to say, there is considerable variation between states in these proportions, depending on the policy regarding the number of routine transport cases of the "taxi" type. Research directed at the operations of emergency medical services in Melbourne revealed that, although the ambulance service was operating at a satisfactory level, there was a breakdown of communication at the interface between ambulance service and hospital, and also some defects in the operations of the hospitals concerned.

In summary, Australia has developed an organized system of ambulance services having a considerable degree of local autonomy, but with central direction and coordination. The ambulance services are run as nonprofit public organizations with government subsidy. Standards of training, equipment, and organization generally are good. The few evaluations of the service performance confirm this judgment of quality.

There are recognized deficiencies in standardization of equipment within and between services, and in co-ordination with hospitals and treatment centers; moves are being made to correct these.

References

Bain, C. J., et al.: Australian Ambulance Services. Sydney, Australian Medical Association. 1975.

Ryan, G. A.: Casualty care in car crashes. Int. J. Epidemiol. 3:31, 1973.

Ryan, G. A., and Clark, P. D.: The emergency care of traffic injury: care before hospital. Med. J. Aust. 1:1173, 1972.

Stuckey, E. S.: The Australian Medical Association Ambulance Survey. National Road Safety Symposium. Canberra, Commonwealth Department of Shipping and Transport, 1972.

C. THE EMERGENCY MEDICAL SYSTEM IN HUNGARY

Béla Bencze and Aurel A. Gábor

In Hungary, the recorded history of emergency care started two centuries ago when Queen Maria Theresia edited a law on first aid and life-saving. A century later, the Sanitary Enabling Bill designated these as governmental tasks. Before long, in 1887, the Budapest Voluntary Life-Saving Society was founded, followed by numerous smaller services over the country.

After World War II, the entire network of ambulance stations and vehicles had to be reconstructed. In 1948, all life-saving and ambulance societies were unified and nationalized within a modern state organization: The Hungarian National Emergency and Ambulance Service (NEAS), and recent legislation states that "in the context of emergency and ambulance matters, NEAS is the curative and preventive, organizatory and methodological, educational and scientific, institution of, and adviser to, the Ministry of Health; its range of function reaches out to the whole territory of the country."

Not all prehospital care is provided by NEAS. Emergencies occurring in the patients' home are dealt with, as a rule, by the Area General Practitioner, or by one duty officer on holidays, Sundays, and at night. If hospitalization appears necessary, NEAS performs simple ambulance transport. In emergency cases not seen by a doctor, however, an emergency crew would ride in the ambulance. In case of accident, intoxication, grave hemorrhage, suicide, childbirth, or life-threatening condition, the public is entitled to call for NEAS help by dialing its free call number "0–4." Sometimes the GP himself will ask for a medical officer to accompany the patient during transport if his condition is critical or he is in need of the facilities of a medically-manned ambulance.

In the vast majority of cases, emergency prehospital care is given predominantly by NEAS. We distinguish clearly between "emergency" and "critical condition." For example, a bout of glaucoma certainly represents a real emergency, although it is not at all life-threatening—"only" the sight is at stake. A postoperative stage may represent a most critical condition, without generally having anything in common with an unforeseen emergency. The characteristics of an emergency are that: (1) it usually occurs suddenly, with no, or hardly any, warning, in the midst of complete health, or in the uneventful course of some disease; (2) it is, or seems to be, a "grave" condition as judged by those present; (3) it displays a high time factor as a main hallmark.

Time factor, again, reflects the actual biologic meaning of the elapsing "absolute" time in the context of a given pathologic process; the term "five minutes" alone does not make sense. In complete airway obstruction, it means eternity; in severe arterial bleeding, a halfway point to irreversibility; in shock, a noticeable delay; in chronic diseases, hardly anything at all.

In everyday practice, emergency situations are classified as follows.

(1) Immediate danger to life, with a necessarily lethal outcome unless properly treated, e.g., severe arterial bleeding.

(2) Severe condition, not necessarily lethal but potentially life-threatening at any moment, e.g., myocardial infarction.

(3) Danger not to life but to organs, or provoking severe pain and suffering, e.g., renal colic.

(4) No real danger to the patient but disturbing normal activities around him, e.g., hysterical fit.

The paramount aim of emergency medical care on the spot is to achieve a more favorable time factor, and to reduce the danger of transport trauma by stabilizing the patient's altered physiologic equilibrium. Of course, one tries also to alleviate pain and other complaints. Not infrequently, emergency care for less severe cases becomes definitive making hospitalization unnecessary.

In order to cope with all the duties as enacted, by law, a precisely designed organization is absolutely essential. NEAS represents a comprehensive, unique unified, nationwide governmental organization, dependent directly on the Ministry of Health. The Headquarters comprise the Directory General with its ten departments and groups. Under the immediate leadership of the Directory General, there are 20 so-called Emergency and Ambulance Organizations, plus its own hospital and a Flight Group. It will be recalled that Hungary has a territory of about 34,000 square miles, and approximately 10 million inhabitants, 2 million of whom live in the capital, Budapest.

An Emergency Ambulance Organization consists of five to 14 stations. The leading station controls all emergency and transport activities over the territory of the given Organization. Substations only perform operative work as instructed. The Head of Organization is a senior physician in charge, aided by his staff. They work permanently under the control of the Directory General, and are responsible for all activities performed by the leading station and its subordinates. There are 160 stations in all in Hungary.

The Budapest E.-A. Organization also controls the Central Dispatching Group, which is responsible for coordinating activities of the individual Organizations all over the country, in addition controlling deployments immediately within the capital. This

Group is headed by a Senior Physician-On-Duty round the clock, who is a kind of deputy of the Director General in urgent operative affairs.

Apart from the uniform free call number of NEAS "0-4," there are several other separate special telephone lines within the Service that connect with cooperating institutions and corporations such as Fire Brigade, Police, Traffic Police, and Public Transport. Furthermore, VHF systems with several channels provide for connecting the Central Dispatching Group with all leading stations, for connecting these with their respective substations, and for emergency and transport deployment control en route.

In larger cities, emergency care through NEAS is supplied by a medical officer, an attendant, and a driver; in smaller cities and villages, by a qualified attendant. Medically manned ambulances are outfitted with the most important drugs, fluids, and instruments for life-saving and other emergency intervention. Even those not medically manned carry equipment such as Ruben's bellows, Ambu suction pump, vacuum mattress, and a standard outfit of bandage material and medicaments.

In the capital and in county centers, Ambulances for Special Emergencies (ASE) also are established to deal with major accidents and other very severe conditions, resuscitation cases, and extraordinary situations such as a major catastrophe. The ASE carries more equipment, including EKG, defibrillator, pacemaker, respirator (Bird—Mark 8), etc. Its driver's medical competence equals that of a skilled attendant; its attendant is a qualified one with particular ASE training. Its leader is always an M.D., generally a senior specialist, accompanied sometimes by a second medical officer.

Teaching and training of personnel is done within the NEAS. A new ambulance attendant undergoes first, two weeks of elementary training, followed by an examination; second, supervised practical work; and third, a qualification course that takes half a year, ending in a State examination. Much later, and subject to extremely exacting stipulations, some can be admitted to another two-year course at the academy (college)

level, in order to become Junior Emergency Medical Officers (JEMO); definitely a higher degree than EMT! Along with these candidates, medical students in the tenth semester are allowed to attend a special course in oxyology (emergency and ambulance medicine), delivered at the University but by the NEAS' own teaching staff, in order to become JEMOs during the last year of studies.

Both full-time and part-time ambulance doctors have various medical specializations, but they are deployed in all kinds of emergencies. Since emergency and ambulance medicine represents a self-contained discipline, further specialization within the specialty of "oxyology" cannot be justified.

In Budapest, there is one hospital of the NEAS. It actually was the first to realize the concept of what today is called an Emergency Department. In spite of its very modest number of beds as compared to the over-all number in Budapest (85 beds vs. some 30,000), it takes about 15 to 20 per cent of cases brought in as emergencies. This is made possible by the existence of a Transitory Ward where mild cases can have a short stay under qualified supervision; here, all necessary examinations are done, the diagnosis established, and the patients can then return home for further treatment by the Area G.P.

The Flight Group operates two medium range aircraft of the Morava type (two-engine prop), and two STOL machines, type Pilatus Turbo Porter (single-engine prop-jet). All these serve only for transport. The purchase of helicopters for emergency deployments is being considered at present.

The experience of several decades has shown that the matter of emergency medical care has been settled satisfactorily by the territorial health care system, on the one hand, and by the special structure and function of NEAS on the other hand. Regular medical deployment, and the trend of providing highly qualified medical care at the site of the emergency, have led to the development of a new medical specialty, oxyology, or emergency and ambulance medicine.

D. EMERGENCY MEDICAL CARE SYSTEM IN TEL-AVIV

Yehezkiel Kishon

Tel-Aviv is the largest city in Israel in terms of population, which has tripled, particularly within the past three decades, to about 400,000 inhabitants. This city now is not only the administrative, financial, commercial, and cultural center of the central area of Israel, but also the home of its "light industries." Finally, because of its beach, hotels, and recreation areas, it has become a center of attraction for thousands of tourists and local visitors. This population growth, within an area of about 50 thousand dunams (12,500 acres), explains in part the serious problems that arise in handling the municipal services. It is estimated that, during a typical day, about 800,000 people (almost one quarter of the population of Israel) live, work, or pass through Tel-Aviv, which has an area of less than 1 per cent of the size of Israel. This growth of population of the city, with its resulting crowding, plays a major role in the consideration of the organization of emergency medical care.

TRAINING AND KNOWLEDGE OF EMERGENCY CARE AMONG THE POPULATION

Because of the pattern of life led by the people living in Israel, most of whom have been affected directly by military and hostile activities for the past 50 years, the population is well aware of the importance of emergency care; many have taken one or more courses in this field at some time in their lives. Starting in the youth movement or in the elementary and high schools, and later in the regular army or during active reserve service, many courses in emergency care are given, either at beginners' or at a more advanced level. Promotion in the police and in the army, as well as licenses for some jobs such as bus-drivers and cab-drivers, involve special examinations—both theoretical and practical—in emergency care, including resuscitation. In addition, special courses for citizens are held by the Train-

ing Department of Magen David Adom, on a voluntary basis. During the year 1973 almost 3000 residents took these courses in the area of Tel-Aviv alone.

MAGEN DAVID ADOM (RED SHIELD OF DAVID)

This is a society whose aims and activities are similar to those of the Red Cross. Among other functions, this organization maintains Emergeny Care Services that can be further divided into the following branches: (1) emergency care stations and posts; (2) ambulance service; (3) voluntary blood transfusion service; (4) physicians' service; and (5) emergency care beach stations during bathing seasons. The means for carrying out these activities are provided by municipal and local councils, by contributions of members all over the country, and by the government of Israel. The society also receives financial support from its centers in other countries.

Emergency Care Stations

Within the area of the city of Tel-Aviv five emergency stations are now functioning, and all citizens know that they can call for emergency help by using the telephone number 1-0-1. One of the stations works on a 24-hour basis; the others operate during the daytime only. Two additional new and well-equipped stations are planned in the near future, one with underground rooms. The main station (located near the Headquarters of Magen David Adom) is staffed by a physician on a 24-hour basis; another station, in the Jaffa section of Tel-Aviv, is staffed by a physician during daytime only. In all there are five physicians in this work, all experienced in traumatology and with a sound knowledge of general medicine.

All stations are staffed with attendants who have had the basic course in emergency care given by the Training Department of the Magen David Adom. This basic evening course, of three months' duration, includes a study of cardiopulmonary resuscitation, application of splints and bandages, and control of bleeding. Following an additional advanced course, the attendant is capable of parenteral administration of drugs and infusions under a physician's order and supervision. The Central Station is staffed by ten attendants during the day time, and two during the night. The station provides, in addition to routine facilities for first aid treatment, the following services: artificial ventilation; tracheal intubation; tracheostomy; defibrillation; treatment of shock; and respiratory care.

Ambulance Service

Ambulances are being operated within the area of Tel-Aviv by Magen David Adom, both for primary transportation (from the scene of accident to either the nearest hospital or the emergency care station) and for secondary transportation (from station to the hospital). Five ambulances are ready for calls during daytime, and two at night. They are staffed by a medical driver and an attendant, both having received the same training as the attendants working in a station. The methods and rules of transporting injured patients are particularly emphasized in the course for these drivers. Complete cardiopulmonary resuscitation cannot be given by the staff of this ambulance, but basic initial steps such as control of hemorrhage, mouth-to-mouth resuscitation, and closed cardiac massage are being taught, and may be applied by them.

Voluntary Blood Transfusion Service

This service includes the Blood Transfusion Bank in Tel-Aviv, which provides blood to all the hospitals in Tel-Aviv and its vicinity. This service also is responsible for a predetermined level of reserve of blood in Israel during an emergency. Recently, a Blood Insurance program has been initiated, whereby donation of a pint of blood during one year entitles the members of the donor's family to receive blood whenever necessary.

Physician's Night Service

In order to secure satisfactory emergency medical care for acutely ill patients in the city of Tel-Aviv, a new system of medical service has been developed and has been in operation for some time. Physicians with experience in internal and general medicine, most of them from the staff of the hospitals in Tel-Aviv and its vicinity, are available for ambulance calls between 7:00 P.M. and 8:00 A.M. Two such units operate every night in the area of Tel-Aviv. When these receive a call through the communication system, they visit the patient at his house and, following medical examination, determine whether he requires hospitalization. If so, another ambulance is sent for this purpose. If hospitalization is not needed, the patient is directed by the physician to the appropriate clinic. A regular fee for this night call has been set with Medical Insurance, which returns 75 per cent of the charge. The average number of night calls in the area of Tel-Aviv is about 80 per night.

Beach Emergency Care Stations

Thousands of residents and tourists use the beach of Tel-Aviv during the bathing season (May to September). Near-drowning, heatstroke, bone fractures (because of rocks in the sea), laceration, and abrasions are examples of accidents seen at the beach. The casualties are taken care of by the personnel of seven emergency care beach stations distributed along the coast, each staffed by two daytime attendants during the season. In 1973, 16,500 people received service at these beach stations; more than 4,000 were treated during each of the months of July and August.

Other Emergency Services

Magen David Adom in Tel-Aviv provides Emergency Care Units for public and social affairs in which large numbers of people are gathered, e.g., concerts, theater performances, football matches, carnivals, and similar events. These units each consist of two attendants, with first aid kits and stretchers (with ambulances and additional stretchers where needed).

In order to meet the special demand of mass casualties, larger ambulances are stored and ready for such emergencies. These are equipped with standard first-aid kits, stretchers, communication systems, and a power generator. In addition, volunteers all over the city, who have taken the basic courses in first-aid, are organized and divided into small working teams according to their residential area. When needed, these can be reached and rushed to the scene of an accident.

OTHER FACILITIES FOR EMERGENCY MEDICAL CARE

Magen David Adom is the main body concerned with daily accidents and other emergency events occurring within the area of Tel-Aviv, but other institutions also are involved in this field. There are public and private organizations in Israel that provide medical care to their members through their general clinics. Many of these clinics are located in Tel-Aviv, and nearby accident casualties or acutely ill patients occasionally are brought there for emergency treatment. All the clinics are equipped with first aid kits and trained medical personnel who offer some help during working hours (from 8:00 AM. until 4:00 P.M.). Transportation to hospitals, if necessary, is accomplished either by Magen David Adom or by their own ambulances. Finally, schools and other public institutions frequently have their own first aid stations, usually with a registered nurse, where medical treatment can be initiated. Teachers and students also are encouraged to take special courses in first-aid and resuscitation. Recently, private ambulance companies have begun to operate well-equipped, staffed vehicles for transportation of acutely ill patients to hospitals. The phone numbers of these ambulances are published in all newspapers. Similarly, private practitioners in Tel-Aviv have started a night service similar to that operated by Magen David Adom.

EMERGENCY SERVICE UNITS IN HOSPITALS

Three municipal hospitals are located within the area of Tel-Aviv (Ichilov, Hadassah, and Donolo) and provide emergency medical services in the city. In addition, two other hospitals just outside Tel-Aviv (Sheba Medical Center in Tel-Hashomer and Beilinson Hospital in Petach-Tikva) can be linked to the system in case of need (e.g., mass casualties or accidents). A special medical committee appointed two years ago by the Minister of Health outlined the optimal set-up in the Admitting Ward of the hospitals to meet the requirements of everyday casualties as well as mass ones. Special attention has been given to emergency facilities for artificial ventilation, tracheal intubation, tracheostomy, defibrillation, treatment of shock, and other life-saving procedures. Minimal criteria for manpower, training standards, and equipment have been outlined and adopted by the authorities. Intensive Coronary Care Units are functioning in three of the five above-mentioned hospitals (Ichilov, Sheba Medical Center, and Beilinson), with six beds each. In addition, an Intermediate Coronary Care Unit with 14 monitored beds operates at the Sheba Medical Center, and a similar unit has been built in Beilinson Hospital. A special traumatologic center has been planned at the Sheba Medical Center. Much effort has been spent to provide the necessary emergency services in the hospitals in and around the largest city in Israel, and all possible contingencies have been considered.

FIRE BRIGADE RESCUE TEAM

A new emergency medical system began early in 1977 in one of the suburbs of the greater Tel-Aviv area. Should this pilot project succeed, the system will be extended over the whole municipal area.

All those who volunteer for this duty from the Fire Brigade will receive a comprehensive course of instruction of about 50 hours' duration. The instructors will be physicians of the Intensive Coronary Care Unit, Sheba Medical Center. The volunteers will receive instruction on recognition of emergency symptoms and signs and how to deal with them on a provisional basis.

The team will consist of two men (on a 24-hour basis), and they will respond to any call for help involving a person who is unconscious or in shock. The team, appropriately equipped for cardiac monitoring and resuscitation, will be able to ventilate the patient either manually or by automatic respirator. Closed-chest massage will be instituted manually when necessary.

The central dispatching system operating for the Fire Brigade vehicles will be used to communicate with the physician-on-call in the Intensive Coronary Care Unit. There are plans for the electrocardiogram of the patient being transmitted through radio communication to the physician-on-call, who will advise the rescue team regarding medical treatment en route. Once the patient is in a relatively stable condition, he will then be transported to the related medical center.

SUMMARY

The population of about 800,000 inhabitants within Tel-Aviv is taken care of by various medical care systems, the main one dealing with emergency cases being Magen David Adom. This service is maintained through five emergency care stations, seven small beach stations, and ambulances operated by five physicians assisted by attendants and auxiliary personnel. Occasionally, military medical units and helicopters may be called to the scene of an accident or a catastrophe if it is too big to be handled by the local emergency services.

E. TOKYO EMERGENCY MEDICAL SERVICES

Arthur E. Rikli

Tokyo is the world's largest city and also one of the most thriving. Metropolitan Tokyo has a population of approximately 12 million people living in an area of 800 square miles, a population concentration of 15,000/square mile. Japan's population — about one-half that of the U.S. — is squeezed into an area slightly less than that of California. The net result is a very heavy demand on emergency services.[*]

The responsibility for providing emergency medical services is not specified by Japanese law. Accidents made up 6.2 per cent of total deaths in 1972, an increase from 3.6 per cent in 1950, and they follow stroke, cancer, and heart disease as the fourth leading cause of death in Japan.

ORGANIZATION

Metropolitan Tokyo, like other major cities, has its central city and its surburban area. The organization of public and private services has followed the development of population concentrations and political subdivisions. Although there are many variations in the composition, source, and financing of EMS in different geographic areas, some dominant characteristics are common to most.

Emergency medical service is not an administrative entity, nor is it considered to be a major health problem either at the national or local level of public or private health agencies. Most emergency services are provided by private clinics, with or without beds, which usually are owned and operated by one or two doctors. Second to private clinics in providing EMS are private hospitals, which by Japanese law are any medical facilities with more than 20 beds. National hospitals and university hospitals in recent years have been called on more frequently to take emergency medical cases, especially at night, weekends, and holidays, when the physicians operating private clinics are not readily available.

The organization and availability of emergency services is influenced by the nine forms of Japan's national compulsory health insurance program. Insurance fees paid for services to accident victims are substantially higher than those for other medical services. This fee schedule serves as an in-

---

[*]Credits to:
Tokyo Fire Department, Ambulance Division.
  1st Assistant Chief Yukuyo Honda, Chief of Ambulance Division; Fire Captain Isao Igoshi, Assistant Chief of Planning Section.
W. J. Stephens, M.B. ChB. M.R.C.G.P. D.R.C.O.G.
  A Study of the Health Service in Japan with Particular Reference to Primary Medical Care.
  Report to the Nuffield Foundation.
Dr. Atsuaki Gunji, Assistant Professor, The Heart Institute of Japan, Tokyo Women's Medical College.

centive for the private sector to provide these services, thus reducing the necessity for the public sector to supply them.

Since Tokyo has experienced the ravages of earthquakes, floods, and fires, it has a well organized Fire Department that plays a very prominent role in bringing together the person and the emergency services he requires. The Department's ten major administrative units include the Ambulance Division, which is divided into the Ambulance Section, Ambulance Medical Section, and Ambulance Control Center. Seven Fire Districts serve central Tokyo, and the eighth Fire District co-ordinates services to suburban Tokyo. The Department's fiscal 1974 budget was Y58,184,480,000 ($1 = Y285), equal to 3.24 per cent of the total Tokyo government budget. Y197,465,000 was allocated to the Ambulance Division.

TRANSPORTATION

Persons requiring emergency services usually are transported to health facilities providing the services, rather than having the services brought to them. Some services necessary to sustain life or stabilize the clinical condition of the patient are provided before the person is taken to second level medical services. Although both public and private carriers provide emergency service transportation, and a few hospitals have their own ambulances, the major source of ambulance service is the Tokyo Fire Department.

The Tokyo Fire Department has 148 ambulances. Also available are one large helicopter with 20 seats, and four helicopters with seven seats, which are used primarily in rescue operations. These units are manned by firemen specially trained in rescue operations and first aid, and are ready to provide service at all times. Their goal is to provide service within three minutes to all areas, and they claim that this service is now provided to 70 per cent of the metropolitan Tokyo area.

The number of trips made by ambulance increased from 178,828 in 1969 to 247,559 in 1974, and the number of patients transported increased from 171,937 in 1969 to 228,893 in 1974 (Table 1). This extra demand for ambulance services has not been accompanied by an equal increase in medical facilities or manpower to take care of the

TABLE 1   Statistics

The Tokyo Fire Department reports the following statistics:

1. Ambulance Runs by Cause (1974)

Acute illness	139,690
Injuries	39,002
Traffic accidents	36,653
Transport hospital to hospital	7812
Crimes	7775
Labor accidents	5107
Suicides	4184
Others	7336
	247,559

2. Need for Transportation of Patients (1974)

Slight	116,234
Moderate	93,114
Serious	16,361
Dangerous	2396
Died	788
	228,893

3. Type of Patients by Age (1973)

Type of Patient	Total	Adults	Children
Traffic accidents	45,456	38,621	6835
Injury	38,459	29,713	8746
Accident	3723	3086	637
Suicides and crime	10,684	10,188	496
Acute illness	130,534	104,051	26,483
	228,856	185,659	43,197

additional cases. The same period has seen a decrease in the number of traffic accident cases, possibly the result of increased penalties associated with traffic accidents.

The Tokyo Fire Department's assessment of need for transporting 228,893 patients in 1974 was as shown in Table 1. The high number of patients with slight need suggests that there should be a change in the policy of providing ambulance service to all that request it, or that a public education program and/or penalties should be instituted in order to prevent misuse of the ambulance service.

The demand for ambulance services is greatest during the period from 4:00 P.M. until 12:00 A.M. Acutely ill patients account for 66 per cent of cases during the period between midnight and 8:00 A.M.; during the remainder of the day they account for less than 50 per cent.

COMMUNICATIONS

When a person requires EMS, he may rely on his traditional source of medical service—his family physician, a private hospital or clinic—or he may dial 119, using the telephone or the special emergency dialing red box found in many public telephone booths. The red box requires no coins, and also can be used for calling the police department number, 110.

When 119 is dialed (the same number used for reporting fires), the call will be answered in the central city by the Control Center in the Headquarters Office. Calls from the suburban area are answered by the eighth District Headquarters Office. The dispatcher then, by direct telephone line, requests the nearest fire station to send an ambulance. The Ambulance Control Center maintains close contact with the ambulance personnel by two-way radio, providing information regarding first aid measures to be taken, and the availability of beds and doctors in hospitals that have been approved for EMS. Twenty-four ambulances have been equipped recently with electrocardiographic telephone attachments so that they may obtain services from Tokyo Women's Medical College to assist them in determining the disposition of cardiovascular patients and related problems. The Nippon Medical School and Hospital is expanding its EMS and also will participate in providing this service to the Tokyo Fire Department, along with six other hospitals.

The Ambulance Control Center maintains a perpetual inventory of emergency facilities, equipment, supplies, and physician services that are available. In addition to answering information needs of the ambulance personnel, the Control Center also provides information services to individuals, hospital personnel, or physicians. This service was computerized in 1976, when the Tokyo Fire Department moved into its new Headquarters Building.

A Medical Information Center is operated by the Medical Society in the Shibuya district in central Tokyo, and a computerized service is operated by the Kanagawa District Medical Society in the political subdivision located south of Metropolitan Tokyo.

Local medical associations have started bringing pressure on the government and on their colleagues to improve the organization of medical care by providing emergency centers for Sundays, public holidays, and perhaps ultimately for night work.

FACILITIES

In Tokyo, acute emergencies are accepted by 507 hospitals or clinics. Of these, 476 are priviately owned. As previously noted, national and university hospitals are now accepting some emergency cases, and are expanding their EMS.

There are a total of 282 fire stations: 218 in the city and 64 in the suburban area. Each of the 72 main fire stations has associated with it one to six branch stations, a total of 210. There are 148 ambulances with first aid equipment, but no drugs or intravenous fluids, stationed with the fire engines at these stations. One ambulance is equipped with a hyperbaric chamber and an accompanying car for a physician. This is used to transport serious cases of burns or poisoning while oxygen is administered. Another specialized ambulance is available for use in time of earthquakes.

In 1973, 3114 cases were refused admission by hospitals or clinics certified to accept emergency cases: 1316 because all emergency beds were occupied, 1173 because the patient required medical skills beyond those of the physician at that facility, and 552 for other reasons. The Tokyo Department of Health as yet has been unsuccessful in its efforts to classify hospitals into primary, secondary, and tertiary emergency care facilities for the purpose of expediting emergency admissions.

MANPOWER

All hospitals and clinics certified to accept emergency cases are required to maintain 24-hour services of a physician, and to reserve a specified number of beds for emergency cases. There are no requirements covering the ambulance or the qualifications of its staff.

The Tokyo Fire Department has 1273 firemen responsible for ambulance duty, each of whom has received a minimum of 228 hours of training for ambulance duty. Seventy ambulances are manned with a driver and three attendants, and 70 have only two attendants. The training includes (emergency) life survival measures; the management of bleeding, fracture, or burn cases; problems associated with pregnancy and poisoning; and other traditional first aid measures. When more sophisticated medical care is required, either a physician is called for assistance or the care is deferred until the patient arrives at the clinic or hospital.

PUBLIC EDUCATION

Public and private industrial agencies such as the Tokyo Fire Department, railroad workers, postal employees, utility employees, as well as private industries, have organized safety programs that include training in accident prevention and some first aid. There is a Japanese Red Cross Agency that operates some hospitals, has played a role in disaster relief, has assisted with collection and distribution of blood and blood products, and has distributed first aid training materials.

There appears to be no active public education program to emphasize the need for EMS or the role that individuals might play in the alleviation of human suffering and sustaining life through first aid and accident prevention measures. Also, there is no concerted effort to develop the arrangement of personnel, facilities, and equipment for effective co-ordination and delivery of emergency health services to appropriate geographic areas.

The lack of public demand to improve EMS for Tokyo raises questions. Are the present services satisfactory, or is there an unrecognized need for improving them? The absence of an active public education program denies the public the information required to answer such questions intelligently.

F. THE STOCKHOLM EMERGENCY MEDICAL CARE SYSTEM

Thorsten Thor

ORGANIZATION IN BROAD OUTLINE

In Stockholm, the responsibility for seeing that an emergency medical care system operates within every medical care district rests with the highest local authority—the County Council and those communes that are independent of County Council jurisdiction.

A medical care system with doctors on call is maintained at most somatic and psychiatric hospitals and also at medical centers in the various subdistricts of the medical care area.

In the general medical care system operating at present, most contacts take place when doctors call at the patients' homes. In some of the subdistricts, patients living outside the actual "Stockholm area" are treated at the central medical units of the district or at surgeries when they have been specially advised to go there by a doctor. From the point of view of examination and treatment, the system of personal visits to the patient's home means that the doctor can

obtain a good impression of the home environment on which to base his medical opinion. The advantages gained thereby, however, do not compensate for the fact that it often is difficult to carry out a safisfactory examination and provide the treatment required in the home of the patient, owing to inadequate lighting, for example, and other circumstances. A considerable part of the visiting doctor's time also is taken up in traveling to and from patients. From both the medical and the organizational standpoint, therefore, it would seem desirable to increase the number of visits by patients to medical centers and to the surgeries of district medical officers. Cases reported in which the condition of the patient is so serious that he neither could, nor should, be examined or treated by a doctor at home are taken in at the hospital Emergency Departments. Patients travel to hospital by taxi, in their own car, or by ambulance in more serious cases. Great efforts are made to see that only those patients in need of the qualified resources of the hospital are referred to the Emergency Departments. It is unavoidable, however, that patients who on their own initiative seek the advice of a hospital doctor sometimes believe themselves to be in a worse condition than they really are. This means that Emergency Departments not infrequently have to take in patients who could have been better treated by the doctor on duty at the central emergency medical unit of the district, or even in their own homes.

Organization in the Inner Stockholm Area

This medical care area covers the communes of Stockholm, Solna, Sundbyberg, and Lidingö, and also the parish of Nacka in Nacka Commune, and has a population of 900,000. The district medical officers in this area are not obliged to be available for emergency medical service within the area at present. The responsibility for this service is in the hands of the Stockholm Medical Association, which by agreement makes doctors available for on-call duty within the area. Approximately 175 doctors serve in this organization.

The 24-hour day is divided into four six-hour spells of duty, and normally four doctors are on call during each spell between 7:00 A.M. and 1:00 A.M., and two during the night. In summertime, when the standard of health usually improves, the number of doctors is reduced to three and one respectively. At times when there is an increase in the number of sick persons in the area, during influenza epidemics, for instance, extra doctors can be added to the staff. In order to serve in the Inner Stockholm Medical Service, the doctor must be fully qualified and have had at least three years' hospital experience.

A transport company is under contract to the County Council to provide cars to be used by doctors called out. The contract stipulates that the cars shall be equipped as emergency vehicles, fitted with communication radio and car telephone, oxygen apparatus, mucus-suction unit, and first aid kit. The transport company is paid for each journey made.

Telephone calls for the doctor on duty are received by the Medical Information Unit, which is manned 24 hours per day by State-registered nurses with long experience of their profession. They must be able to make a preliminary judgment based on the information given over the telephone, and decide whether the patient needs immediate hospital attention, and if so whether an ambulance will be required; whether the doctor on duty should go to the patient's home; or whether the symptoms are not sufficiently serious to justify this, so that the patient without inconvenience could himself attend the surgery of the regular district medical officer during usual surgery hours. When a visit to the patient's home is necessary, the call for the doctor is transmitted to the cars by radio or by radio telephone; by means of the latter, the doctor also can contact the patient in order to obtain any further information required.

During 1973, the calls for the doctor on duty totaled more than 80,000, and the number of visits made to patients was about 74,700. The difference in the figures is due to the fact that a number of calls for a doctor were later found to be unnecessary as the patient's condition had improved so much that no doctor was required, or else had deteriorated to such an extent that immediate hospital treatment was essential.

Organization in the Outer Areas of the Stockholm County Council Region

The area covered includes the whole of the County Council Region with the exception of the communes of Stockholm, Solna, Sunbyberg, Lidingö, and the parish of Nacka in Nacka Commune. The medical care district is divided into 13 smaller subdistricts. The total population of these districts amounts to approximately 500,000.

The emergency medical care system in each district is operated in principle by the district medical officers. In practice, however, most emergency cases are attended to by medical officers temporarily appointed to the service. Doctors holding these appointments are recruited mainly from a group of about 200 doctors and advanced medical students. In order to reduce the workload of district medical officers and their deputies and to utilize doctors' working hours more effectively, medical centers have been established in some of the outer districts, where in principle the patients themselves must attend for examination and treatment. In addition, home visits are undertaken to a limited extent.

Calls for the doctor on duty—as in the

Inner Stockholm Area—are received at the same Medical Information Unit at which nurses make the initial appraisal as to whether the case needs a doctor's attention. The calls are forwarded by telephone to the different doctors on duty, there being no "doctors' cars" at their disposal. As a rule, doctors in the outer districts use taxis or their own cars to reach patients. Since incoming calls for doctors within the whole of the County Council Region are channeled through the Medical Information Unit, there is great advantage in the fact that a centralized opinion can be reached on the various requirements in respect of medical care. Minor changes in the organization of the County Council medical care system can also be heeded more easily when all incoming calls are connected through one channel only.

In 1973, 54,500 calls were received and 45,300 visits were made to patients' homes. The relatively large divergence in the figures is due not only to the same factors as those applying in the Inner Stockholm Area, but also to the fact that, to a considerable extent, the doctors themselves telephone the patient before the visit and thereby are able to decide whether there is a real need to visit his home.

ROUND-THE-CLOCK EMERGENCY SERVICES AT HOSPITALS

Each hospital has a casualty ward for the reception of acute medical and surgical cases of illness and injury. This unit, manned by doctors and nursing personnel 24 hours per day, has special emergency rooms equipped with the machinery required for immediate treatment, such as EKG apparatus, defibrillator, etc. When the patient requires more examination or treatment than is available in the casualty ward, the hospital X-ray Department and Laboratory (working 24 hours per day) and other facilities can be utilized.

Parallel with the continuous emergency preparedness at hospitals and in the open care system, there is also an emergency organization ready to come into immediate operation in the event of a disaster in which local resources would be inadequate to save lives or limit the effects of injury. This organization, planned to function at the scene of an accident, consists of groups ap-

pointed for the purpose: doctors and nurses available to be sent from hospitals to assign priority to victims needing hospital treatment, and also to take immediate steps to save life and give first aid to the injured. In order to meet the needs of hospital care in the event of major accidents with far-reaching consequences, it is possible at short notice to raise the level of preparedness of personnel at hospital casualty reception wards. Special disaster plans have been drawn up for this purpose. It is estimated that the normal reception capacity could be doubled within about one hour, and, within about three hours after the sounding of the alarm, doubled once again to deal with approximately 400 injured persons at all the County Council hospitals. In this way, a high standard of operational readiness can be maintained.

MEDICAL TRANSPORT

The medical transport organization of the County Council consists of 79 ambulances, of which 29 are available 24 hours per day, the others being "day" ambulances undertaking primarily the transport of sick persons during daytime. All ambulances are similarly equipped with oxygen apparatus, aspirator, and medical supplies, and therefore can be utilized during the transport of urgent cases of illness and accident without the need for outside assistance. Since the ambulances are directed wholly by radio, a very high level of readiness can be maintained for urgent medical transport.

Each ambulance is manned by two drivers specially trained for service with their particular vehicle. Training consists of three weeks' theory at a medical training school, followed by four weeks' practical work at a hospital, primarily in wards dealing with cases of acute illness. Personnel receive further training each year, and have the opportunity of working at a hospital to gain information and learn about new developments in medicine. The County Council at present has no ambulances specially equipped for a particular purpose, such as myocardial infarction. As a rule, doctors and nurses do not travel with the ambulance sent out in response to an urgent call. When a patient is being moved between different hospitals, special medical personnel—as the exception rather than the rule—may accompany him if special care and attention are required during transport.

In urgent cases, a caller obtains an ambulance by dialing the telephone number 90 000. In less urgent cases when an ambulance is required, calls can be made to specified direct telephone numbers. The call is connected to a special Central Alarm Unit, manned round the clock, where on the basis of information received it is decided whether the transport should be carried out by ambulance and if so the degree of urgency, or whether some other vehicle could be used without inconvenience. When any doubts arise in assessing a case, the personnel of the Central Alarm Unit have facilities for consulting the nurses of the Medical Care Information Unit via a direct telephone connection, or by transferring the caller directly to the Information Unit.

The Central Alarm Unit is responsible for giving directions to all ambulances, and it is the duty of the Unit, when there are temporary reductions in the number of ambulances available in any part of the County Council region, to ensure that they are shared equally so that a high level of readiness for acute medical transport can be maintained. Since the Central Alarm Unit has to assess transport requirements, in addition to directing medical transport, it is essential that its staff are well experienced in ambulance work and acute medical care, and moreover can judge the degree of medical care required on the basis of information given by the caller.

FEES

Every patient seeking medical care must pay a small fee at a hospital or when the doctor visits his home. The charge is 12 Kr. per hospital visit and 20 Kr. per home visit. The doctors on duty serving in an outer district under the medical care system, as well as those on call in the Inner Stockholm Area, receive a special payment in addition to that made by the patient.

As the highest authority responsible for medical care, the County Council meets the full cost of transport.

No charge is made to the patient carried by ambulance within the Stockholm County Council Region. The entire cost is met by the County Council, but a small refund is obtained from the Regional Social Insurance

Office for each journey undertaken. The annual gross cost of medical transport is Kr:20.6 million, and refunds received amount to approximately Kr:7.5 million.

EXPERIENCE GAINED

It has been found that only about 50 per cent of calls received by the doctor on duty via telephone no. 90 000 lead to action being taken by him. In some cases the condition of the patient is so serious that there can be no question of waiting for the doctor to arrive, and the patient instead should be taken immediately to hospital; in other cases, the symptoms of illness are so mild that the patient without risk can wait and see the doctor during normal surgery hours the following day. The reason for the unusually high percentage of patients who are given other directions, instead of being visited by the doctor on duty, would appear to be that the regular medical centers at present are too understaffed to deal with emergency cases during normal surgery hours, and turn away far too high a proportion of patients who then are forced to call the doctor on duty. One prerequisite if overloading of the emergency medical system is to be avoided, therefore, is for adequate reception resources to be made available at the regular medical centers.

Another feature of the experience gained is that, to an exceptionally high extent, the doctors on duty are called out to new housing estates where newly-built blocks of flats are let at high rents. A large proportion of the residents in these areas are young low-income families in which the parents lack knowledge and experience in the care of children. Much of the work of the doctor on call in these areas, therefore, consists of attention to sick children. As the same experience has gradually become evident in respect of newly-built housing estates in the inner Stockholm area, it seems that the high number of emergency calls for doctors in such districts reflects a feeling of social insecurity, which in turn appears to be due to pressure of financial circumstances and the birth rate in the newly-formed families.

With regard to medical transport, it has been found that about 20 per cent of the ambulance journeys—approximately 140,000 annually—are for urgent medical or accident cases. Since ambulance transport within the County Council region is free of charge, a certain amount of abuse occurs, and patients not infrequently call for an ambulance to take them to hospital when they could very well travel by taxi. The excuse usually given is that the patient has no money to pay for a taxi.

G.   EMERGENCY MEDICAL SERVICES IN THE U.S.S.R.

Patrick B. Storey

INTRODUCTION

Emergency medical care in the Soviet Union is a discrete component of the universal system of comprehensive health services guaranteed to the Soviet people as a constitutional right.

Emergency care is viewed in two separate phases: (1) provision of 24-hour coverage by the neighborhood primary care system to its enrollees; and (2) the ability at the larger community level to move highly qualified help rapidly to the victim of trauma or sudden serious illness.

The two phases are administered separately. The first, the Neotlozhnaya, is administered by the local polyclinic, the medical staff of which are obliged to arrange their work schedules to provide seven-day 24-hour availability. Patients are instructed to use this system for problems that are not threatening to life or limb. The second, the Skoraya, is organized on a community-wide basis such as a city or a region; the public is instructed to dial 03 to connect directly with it in case of sudden emergency need. In small communities the two phases are combined, and in the city of Tbilisi, capital of the Republic of Georgia, with a population of 900,000, the Neotlozhnaya and Skoraya functions have been combined on an experimental basis for the past five years.*

Another way of viewing the difference between the Neotlozhnaya and the Skoraya is to remember that the former represents the continuing every-day care system for a given segment of the community, whereas the latter represents a separate discrete organizational effort to deal with the larger community problem of sudden onset of disaster, and is not to be used in place of the Neotlozhnaya. This separation produces a certain amount of confusion, but its absence is what gluts American emergency care facilities with about 70 per cent of patients who do not represent true emergencies.

The remainder of this discussion will concern only the Skoraya. A detailed description, based on the experience of the Leningrad Skoraya, has been published by M. A. Messel (1975), and has just been translated into English. More limited treatises also are available in English (Fry, 1969; Storey, 1972; Storey and Ross, 1971).

ORGANIZATION

The basic principle of the Skoraya is to bring highly qualified service to the patient as quickly as possible. The Skoraya has two main functions: to bring help and to provide transportation. Organization, manpower, and communications are built around this principle and these two functions.

The city of Moscow must provide emergency services to 7 million inhabitants and 2 million additional daily transients into the city. The principal station and nerve-center of the Skoraya is located in central Moscow, with 22 substations distributed throughout the city. Special telephone lines connect these stations, and general ambulances and crews are stationed at them.

All ambulances sent out to provide medical care are staffed by a physician and a team, usually including a feldsher (physician-assistant) and an attendant. Both the

*The Russian word Neotlozhnaya (Nye-ot-lozh'-na-ya) means "urgent." The word Skoraya (Skor'-a-ya) means "rapid." The full title of the Skoraya is "Skoraya Meditsinskaya Pomosch," which means "rapid medical service."

physician and the feldsher are specially trained in emergency medicine and in the function of the Skoraya (Storey, 1972). The ambulances may be general duty or specialized, i.e., specially equipped to handle myocardial infarction, stroke, poisoning, shock, and pediatric emergencies. The physician staff may be full-time or half-time, spending a full shift at their basic hospital. This is particularly true for the specialized ambulance staff. The feldshers are full-time.

TRANSPORTATION

The Skoraya maintains the bed inventory of all hospitals in Moscow. It also has its own hospital base at the Sklifosovsky Institute for Research in Emergency Care, which is used especially for trauma victims. The ambulance team decide whether to keep the patient or leave him at home. If they decide to hospitalize him they select the hospital nearest his home, i.e., the one with which his own polyclinic is connected; if his condition demands immediate and/or special attention, however, they take him to the most appropriate hosipial. The Skoraya is responsible for knowing the bed status of every hospital, but it also has final authority on admissions. A hospital must accept a patient brought in by the Skoraya.

Ambulances used for secondary transportation, e.g., for scheduled transport of patients from home to hospital, or hospital to hospital, etc., are staffed only with driver and attendant, except in the case of maternity patients, for whom the ambulance team includes a feldsher-midwife.

COMMUNICATIONS

Throughout the Soviet Union the telephone number 03 is reserved for emergency medical care. All pay-phones are equipped with a button that obviates the need for a coin in order to dial 01 for fire; 02 for police; and 03 for the Skoraya.

All calls go directly in to a central dispatching office, and none to any of the substations. This principle is rigorously enforced. The dispatching center switchboards are staffed by feldshers or nurses experienced in the Skoraya, and supervised on a 24-hour basis by a Skoraya

physician. The center is divided into incoming and outgoing components. When the call comes in, a card is made up containing name, address, and nature of emergency. Information is secured from the caller and a decision made about disposition, with or without consultation from the physician, depending on the nature of the call. The card then is transferred by conveyor belt to the outgoing section where contact is made either with the central Skoraya teams, or with a peripheral substation close to the site of call, or by radiophone with a vehicle known to be in the area. An ambulance out on call may have its mission upgraded by radiophone.

One minute is allowed for assignment of the call, and two more minutes for the ambulance team to indicate that it is on the way. The first 3 minutes are a function of organization, staffing, and communication, which can be tightly controlled. The next four minutes are subject to external variables such as distance, traffic flow, weather, and geographic terrain. Since Kiev is a river-port city with many residents along the shore and on the islands, two of the ambulances are speedboats. "Chronometric" studies are used to revise Skoraya procedures in order to increase speed and efficiency of service.

Telemetry is not developed. The need for it is not so urgent since the Skoraya teams are headed by specially trained physicians.

FEATURES

Some characteristics of the Skoraya, although perhaps not transferable to other social environments, are of considerable heuristic interest to all concerned with emergency care.

(1) The Skoraya is an essential, major integrated component of the Soviet health care system that provides emergency care under medical lines of control. Such a complex medical service is not a function of the Fire Department, the Police Department, or any voluntary or proprietary agency.

(2) Its basic principle is to bring the best in modern medical care to the victims of disaster, rather than to bring patients to the source of care. The system thus is designed to move the medical service forward and to diminish that critical period of transportation

that separates the victim of serious mishap from expert medical help.

(3) Since the system is a medical responsibility, all ambulances sent out on emergency calls are staffed by physicians and physician-assistants (feldshers) who are specially trained in emergency care. This assures faster physician attention and direct medical control of life-threatening situations. This is considered important because much of modern medical care is technologically sophisticated, and complex aspects of diagnosis and management of serious illness or injury require the competence of specially trained physicians.

(4) With physicians available on every ambulance, assistants can be trained to play a supportive rather than a substitutional role. This allows for development of an efficient team approach to emergency care.

(5) Physicians are available to decide whether to leave the patient home, remanding him to his own physician, or to hospitalize him. It is useful and significant to note that the former happens in about 70 per cent of cases.

(6) Since the emergency care subsystem is integrated into the general care system, patients can be brought to appropriate health facilities without delay and with minimal error.

(7) Central co-ordination of the emergency system allows for the support of regular ambulance teams with specialized ambulances and teams when necessary.

(8) The Skoraya, as a discrete subsystem of the general system of health care, actively stimulates and co-ordinates service and research with other medical disciplines. Two striking examples are in the areas of traumatology and resuscitation. Many problems of orthopedics, cardiology, thromboembolic disease, etc., must involve shared management between the hospital subsystem and the Skoraya.

(9) The Skoraya exists as an organized entity, and other subsystems can be developed in relation to it. For example, medical stations staffed by physician-assistants can be maintained at every subway station or other point of convergence of great numbers of people, because the Skoraya is almost instantly available to cover emergency cases.

(10) The Skoraya, because it is part of the medical care system, has become a medical specialty with its own: (a) scientific research base; (b) educational requirements and opportunities; (c) organizational set-up for personnel, facilities, and equipment; (d) system of conferences and national and international assemblies; and (e) medical literature.

References

Fry, J.: Medicine in Three Societies. M.T.P. Chiltern House, 1969.

Messel, M. A.: Urban Emergency Medical Service of the City of Leningrad. Published by the Fogarty International Center for Advanced Study in the Health Sciences, Department of Health, Education and Welfare Publication No. (NIH) 75–671, 1975.

Storey, P. B.: Medical Care in the U.S.S.R. Report of the U.S. Delegation on Health Care Services and Planning. Published by the Fogarty International Center for Advanced Study in the Health Sciences, Department of Health, Education and Welfare Publication No. 72–60, 1972.

Storey, P. B.: The Soviet Feldsher as a Physician's Assistant. Published by the Fogarty International Center for Advanced Study in the Health Sciences, Department of Health, Education and Welfare Publication No. 72–58, 1972.

Storey, P. B., and Ross, R. B.: Emergency medical care in the Soviet Union. A study of the Skoraya. J.A.M.A. 217:588, 1971.

Part V

LEGAL AND LEGISLATIVE ASPECTS OF EMERGENCY CARE

Chapter 72

MEDICOLEGAL PROBLEMS OF EMERGENCY MEDICINE

James E. George

BACKGROUND

Medical malpractice ranks as one of the major headaches of modern health practitioners and health care institutions. Most physicians, nurses, and health care administrators have a constant, free-floating awareness of medicolegal problems, but few fully appreciate the unstructured complexity of the collision between law and medicine until they have been intimately involved themselves. After such an encounter, the memory lingers, and one is more attuned to medicolegal prophylaxis. It is hoped that this chapter will serve to crystallize some of the medicolegal problem areas in the Emergency Department and offer some approaches to these problems.

Is there a medical malpractice crisis? The answer is both "no" and "yes." There is no solid evidence to indicate that more negligent medical care is provided today than in the past, but on the other hand there *is* a growing atmosphere of crisis in the minds of health care providers and insurers. This crisis mentality has been encouraged by sensational news-reporting of some negligence cases, increasing health consumerism, and, above all, ever-rising professional liability insurance premiums and even a paucity of insurance companies who are willing to underwrite professional medical liability.

With the air so filled with "crisis," there is no doubt that the facts have been blurred. The President's Commission on Medical Malpractice produced a study of the malpractice problem, which resulted in a number of dissenting opinions from both physicians and attorneys, as well as questions about insurance industry data that had been gathered to support past premium hikes. The Medical and Chirurgical Faculty of the State of Maryland conducted a study of Maryland malpractice in 1971 that eroded two malpractice myths. First, no evidence was found to sustain the assumption that hospital Emergency Departments were high-risk areas; on the contrary, more malpractice emanated from in-patient hospital areas and the physician's office than from Emergency Departments. Second, foreign-trained physicians practicing in Maryland did not contribute a larger percentage of claims than physicians trained in the U.S.

Regardless of the magnitude of the malpractice problem, the practical fact remains that most physicians, especially those in Emergency Departments, have consciously or unconsciously modified their practice habits to make some provision for the practice of "defensive medicine." The high pressure environment of the practice of modern emergency medicine affords inadequate time for leisurely diagnosis and consultation when in doubt. An unceasing flow of patients in search of immediate treatment, attended by various emotionally strained family members and friends, serves to keep Emergency Department staff in a state of constant tension. This environment contains many pitfalls of which the professional should be aware.

Space requires that this chapter be succinct, but it is intended to provide the practitioner with an overview of many relevant medicolegal considerations in the practice of emergency medicine. The reader should bear in mind constantly that the outcome of a legal case depends on the particular facts of the case in question, and that changing one peculiar item can result in an entirely different legal outcome. Since statutory law and case law vary from state to state, the reader should exercise caution in strictly applying this legal information to his own personal or professional legal problems. Although the following pages acknowledge basic legal concepts that can be applied broadly for general guidance, the appropriate state statute books and local counsel should be consulted for specific legal advice when necessary.

NEGLIGENCE

Medical malpractice is synonymous with professional medical negligence, a specific tort action within the broad area of law known as civil law. Law in the U.S. generally is divided into the criminal law and the civil law. Criminal law involves a legal action filed by a state or by the U.S. against a particular offending individual or individuals, and deals with the definition of crimes and their punishments. Civil law is the other broad category of U.S. law, and concerns itself with legal actions brought by one individual against other individuals. Contracts, domestic relations, torts, etc., are some examples of the subdivisions that comprise the broad category of civil law. Civil wrongs committed by an individual against another individual are called *torts*. A particular tort or civil wrong can also constitute a criminal wrong, such as assault and battery. This subjects the offending individual to both civil and criminal liability for the act committed. The tort of *negligence* is the particular tort with which physicians usually are concerned, for herein lies malpractice.

Black's Law Dictionary (West Publishing Co., 4th ed., 1951) defines negligence as "the omission to do something which a reasonable man, guided by those ordinary considerations which ordinarily regulate human affairs, would do, or the doing of something which a reasonable and prudent man would not do." Conduct that fails to meet a standard of care recognized in the law for the protection of others against unreasonable risks of harm generally can be said to constitute negligence. The law expects all citizens

to conduct their personal and business affairs in a reasonable safe manner so as to protect others from unnecessary harm. This rule of conduct applies to all activities, from driving an automobile to performing professional tasks. A physician may be liable for professional negligence when his conduct fails to meet an accepted standard of care in his profession and a patient is damaged as a result.

Four particular elements must be alleged and proved in a court of law in order to sustain a lawsuit for negligence brought by a complaining party (the plaintiff) against the offending party (the defendant). These elements of negligence include pre-existing duty, breach of duty, damages, and proximate cause. If the plaintiff fails to prove any one of these four elements, his suit for negligence will not be sustained.

DUTY AND ITS BREACH

The plaintiff in a negligence action must prove that the defendant owed the plaintiff a duty to use due care. The court usually looks to the relationship between the parties to determine whether there is a duty of due care owed the plaintiff by the defendant. The health practitioner's duty (whether he is physician, nurse, technician, or whatever) arises from his voluntary entrance into a health care relationship with the patient.

From this health practitioner-patient relationship evolves the duty to conduct oneself according to the standard of care expected of a reasonably trained, prudent health practitioner confronting the same or similar circumstances. The duty of due care of the "reasonable man" was at one time confined by the courts to the particular locality in which the individual practiced, and was known as the "locality rule." Therefore, if one practiced in a university setting, one was held to the standard of care of the university medical center, and one practicing in a rural area was held to the standard of care of the rural practitioner in that locality. However, the development of mass transportation and communications, along with recent advances in modern medicine, have gradually prompted the courts to discard the locality rule and to hold that the U.S. comprises one medical community from New York to California. There is an ever-increasing trend to impose textbook standards of care on the health practitioner.

Breach of duty, whereby an individual's conduct does not comply with the anticipated, reasonable standard of care, can occur by way of *malfeasance* when an *affirmative act* does not comport with the acceptable standard of care. Breach of duty also can occur by *nonfeasance* when *failure to act* results in damages to a patient that could have been avoided by taking appropriate action in compliance with acceptable medical practice under the circumstances. Failure to resuscitate a patient in cardiopulmonary arrest, when good medical practice would have dictated that he *should* be resuscitated, is an example of breach of duty and negligence by nonfeasance.

DAMAGES

The third element the plaintiff must prove is that he sustained damages by virtue of the alleged negligence. If an individual has not been damaged in some discernible fashion, he will not be successful in a suit for negligence. Monetary damages are an integral part of a suit for negligence, since the purpose of such civil redress is to obtain some financial award from the court for the damages suffered. A patient would not have a viable suit for negligence, for example, if he unknowingly received an erroneous medication that caused him absolutely no ill-effects whatever. If there have been no damages, the court will not entertain an action for negligence.

CAUSATION

The last necessary element of negligence is *proximate cause*. Black's Law Dictionary defines proximate cause as "that which, in a natural and continuous sequence, unbroken by any efficient intervening cause, produces the injury, and without which the result would not have occurred." The following is a clinical example of proximate cause. If a patient trips in the Emergency Department, bruises his knee, and sues for his myocardial infarction three months later, he would be hard pressed to prove proximate cause in a suit for negligence. If, however, the patient's myocardial infarction occurred moments after his

fall in the Emergency Department, he would have a much better basis for proving proximate cause. The latter requires that there be some reasonable cause-and-effect relationship between the act complained of and the damages sustained by the patient.

OTHER GENERAL LEGAL PRINCIPLES

Res Ipsa Loquitur

One of many legal principles which has been a cause of growing concern for the medical profession has been the doctrine of *res ipsa loquitur*, a Latin phrase that means "the thing speaks for itself." This legal doctrine evolved through time as a mechanism to assist a plaintiff in recovering damages in the face of circumstances in which it would be almost impossible for him to prove all of the elements of negligence. An example in which *res ipsa loquitur* applies in a clinical situation would be the patient who enters the surgical suite for a routine appendectomy, and later awakens in the recovery room paralyzed from the waist down. It would be almost impossible for the patient to prove negligence, because he was asleep during the time the unexpected paralysis occurred.

For the plaintiff to raise *res ipsa loquitur* on his behalf, he must prove that his damages would not have occurred in the absence of somebody's negligence, that the instruments which caused the damage must have been under the defendant's control at all times, and that the patient himself must not have done anything that could have contributed to his own injury. When the plaintiff accomplishes this task, the legal effect is to shift the burden of proof from the plaintiff to the defendant, who must now prove that he was not negligent. In recent years some courts have applied and misapplied this doctrine broadly, resulting in an injudicious expansion of the doctrine of *res ipsa loquitur*. This has caused great apprehension on the part of the medical profession and the defense bar.

Statute of Limitations

How long may a patient wait to file a complaint for negligence? The answer depends on each state's peculiar Statute of Limitations, which is a law formulated on the thesis that it is against public policy to let the threat of a lawsuit linger forever. The time limit thus placed upon the period during which a complaint may be filed in court depends on the type of complaint filed, such as a contract action or a tort action. Statutes of Limitations for negligence actions usually are two to three years. If a plaintiff fails to file his action within the period allowed by the Statute of Limitations, the court will prevent him from doing so thereafter. A key factor here is to know when the limiting time period actually begins to run. Some states permit it to start when the negligent act occurred, whereas other states regard it as beginning when the patient actually discovers that a negligent act has been committed against him. In the case of minors, the Statute of Limitations does not begin to run until they are emancipated or reach the age of majority, which is 18 years of age in some states and 21 in others. A court may consider a minor legally emancipated if he marries or is economically independent from his family.

Agency Law

The law of agency is a last area of interest to emergency medicine. The hospital Emergency Department cast of characters includes physicians, nurses, the hospital administration, and a variety of hospital employees. Relationships often found among these individuals include employer-employee and independent contractor relationships. The exact nature of the relationship among the above persons is important in order that the legal liabilities of the parties involved may be determined.

In some cases the liability will fall entirely upon one party, whereas in others the liability may be shared to different degrees among the parties involved. The Emergency Department staff should be aware of the legal rule that each individual is responsible for his own torts, regardless of whether he is an independent contractor, employee, etc. Also, an employee's torts committed within the scope of his employment can render his employer vicariously liable. However, the torts of an independent contractor generally are not imputed to the employer if the latter has no significant con-

trol over the actions of the independent contractor.

The above legal maxims are subject to as many variables as can be created by the unique facts of each case. Whenever a lawsuit is brought against the hospital and its professional staff, the attorneys for both the hospital and the physicians or nurses inevitably begin analyzing the facts to show that responsibility rests exclusively with the other party. Also, in this day of increasingly inaccessible malpractice insurance, attorneys for the insurance company frequently attempt to deny liability for damages.

The only conclusion that can be safely drawn is that the plaintiff will attempt to join all possible defendants in a negligence suit so as to assure recovery from somebody. If the plaintiff wins, the court may instruct the defendants and their attorneys to decide among themselves who will pay for what portion of the damages.

DUTY TO PROVIDE EMERGENCY CARE

Under the common law, neither the physician nor the private hospital had an affirmative duty to render medical treatment. As a result it was possible for private hospitals and some public hospitals to refuse to admit a patient for emergency treatment. Today, as a result of a series of important legal decisions that were the outgrowth of abuses in Emergency Department treatment policies, this situation has been reversed completely. The right of a hospital to refuse emergency service to a patient has become substantially curtailed.

An important case leading to this change was *Wilmington General Hospital v. Manlove*, 184 A.2d. 135 (S. Ct., Delaware, 1961). In Manlove, the parents of a four-month-old infant with a recent history of fever and diarrhea brought the child to the hospital Emergency Department. Since the child had been under the care of private pediatricians, no physician or nurse examined or treated the child. The child was sent home by the nurse, who explained to the parents that the hospital's policy was to decline emergency treatment to persons already under the care of a private physician. Shortly thereafter, the child died of bronchopneumonia.

The key issue before the court was whether the hospital had a duty to provide emergency treatment in the face of an unmistakable emergency. The Court held that it did. The hospital's liability was based primarily upon the parents' reliance on the hospital's capacity to render emergency care, and the fact that this was a case that could be held to involve an unmistakable emergency. This decision, and others of its kind, have fostered an "open door" hospital emergency department policy. If a hospital holds itself out to the public as having the capability to render emergency treatment, it cannot deny such treatment to persons who have reasonably relied on such representations. In the *Manlove* case this duty outweighed the hospital's internal policies.

Federal legislation, such as the Hill-Burton Act, has also limited significantly a hospital's ability to refuse to render emergency care. A hospital that has received a Hill-Burton grant from the Federal government has the responsibility to provide a certain amount of "free" medical care for indigent patients.

State laws and regulations also have recognized the duty of hospitals to provide emergency medical care. For example, New York has adopted the following law (Chapter 712, June 11, 1973): "...In cities with a population of one million or more, a general hospital must provide emergency medical care and treatment to all persons in need of such care and treatment and applying to such hospital therefore. . . ." In addition, the Joint Commission on Accreditation of Hospitals, which determines the standards for the accreditation of hospitals, has stated that adequate advice or initial treatment shall be given to any ill or injured person who presents himself to the hospital.

Therefore, it is clear that hospital Emergency Departments and emergency practitioners have a positive duty to render treatment to persons in need of it. Hospitals have found that one of the best means of assuming these increased responsibilities is to staff Emergency Departments with practitioners who specialize in emergency medicine. In fact, the responsibilities are so great that any hospital that does not have a qualified emergency physician on duty in the Emergency Department might conceivably find that it is unable to discharge its full legal duty to the public.

PROBLEM AREAS

It is important to apply these general legal principles to specific problem areas that arise in the practice of emergency medicine. These include: (1) consent to treatment; (2) medical records; (3) the reporting of certain events; (4) blood alcohol requests by police on arrested motorists; (5) abandonment of patients; (6) difficulties encountered through interaction between Emergency Department physicians and the rest of the medical staff; and (7) problems relating generally to the proper and efficient use of space, equipment, and personnel.

Consent to Treatment

ASSAULT AND BATTERY

This broad problem area comprises legal theories relating to assault and battery as well as consent. A single assault and battery incident can result in two lawsuits—a criminal action by the state against the individual, and a civil action for money damages brought by the person claiming injury from assault and battery. Assault and battery are two separate causes of action that can be tried individually or jointly, depending on the facts. Assault is defined as the unlawful placing of an individual in apprehension of immediate bodily harm without his consent. Battery is defined as the unlawful touching of another individual without his consent. If it were not for the patient's consent, health practitioners would be routinely accused of assault and battery.

EXPRESS AND IMPLIED CONSENT

There are two major types of consent—express and implied. A patient gives his express consent to treatment when he gives the health practitioner his explicit permission to treat him. On the other hand, implied consent does not involve such a direct expression of permission. The actions of the patient are deemed sufficient to imply to a reasonable person that the patient has consented to treatment. An example of implied consent is a case in which a person rolls up his sleeve to receive an injection, but does not expressly authorize the injection. Implied consent also exists if a patient is not mentally competent because of psychosis, drugs, alcohol, organic disease, or unconsciousness. These conditions of mental incompetence may present the practitioner with an emergency condition that, according to public policy, should be treated as promptly as possible to save life. In addition, courts have held that implied consent exists in such situations because it is believed that the patient, if mentally competent, would have given his consent to treatment necessary to save his life.

INFORMED CONSENT

The doctrine of informed consent has been developed recently to describe further the quality of the patient's consent. According to this doctrine, which is somewhat vague and differs from jurisdiction to jurisdiction, the patient must be competent to give his consent and must understand all the reasonable risks and benefits inherent in the proposed procedure. In obtaining the patient's informed consent, the physician is held to the standard of care of the reasonably trained, prudent physician confronting a similar patient under similar circumstances. If damages result from a procedure performed by the physician and no informed consent is obtained, the physician can be liable for a technical battery upon the patient and therefore be responsible for all resulting damages. Under these circumstances, the plaintiff would not be required to prove the necessary elements of negligence.

REFUSAL OF TREATMENT

In general, consent must be obtained from the patient in order to treat him. A mentally competent adult patient cannot be forced to receive treatment, even in the face of a life-threatening emergency. Thus, Jehovah's Witnesses have presented a continuous problem in the consent area. Some states have permitted courts to issue orders requiring patients to consent to life-saving treatment. Other states have refused to issue orders and have reaffirmed a competent individual's right to refuse treatment if he so wishes. The result often depends on the peculiar clinical facts.

MINORS

Consent for treatment of minors must be obtained from parents, kinfolk, or legal guardian, whichever, is appropriate under the circumstances. Parental consent is not necessary for treatment of minors who have been emancipated by virtue of maririage, statute, or economic independence. In addition, if emergency conditions require immediate treatment, minors can obtain such treatment without parental consent. A reasonable effort must always be made to obtain parental consent. In cases of borderline emergency, such as slight lacerations, the treatment should be given to minors even if appropriate consent cannot be secured. It is better to err on the side of treatment than on that of nontreatment. Nontreatment carries with it the threat of a neligence suit, whereas treatment may occasion possible nonpayment of the bill for services rendered. Some states have passed legislation that provides for treatment of minors without parental consent in suspected cases of venereal disease or drug abuse.

INTOXICATED PATIENTS

Persons who are intoxicated or extremely belligerent often cause problems in regard to consent. Emergency Department personnel including physicians and nurses, often react with hostility toward such patients, and in many cases are inclined to avoid treating them unless they are cooperative. It must be recognized by Emergency Department staff that, in some instances, intoxicated people have a diminished capacity either to grant or withhold their consent for treatment. To avoid possible liability for failure to treat an intoxicated patient, the physician should make every reasonable effort to quiet the patient and to insure his understanding of the seriousness of the injury in order, to obtain his knowing consent to treatment.

Emergency Departments often deal with persons recently arrested or previously incarcerated. Since these individuals retain their constitutional rights despite their arrest, their consent to examination and treatment must be obtained prior to their receiving treatment in the Emergency Department. Deviation from this procedure could result in civil liability for assault and battery.

Medical Records

It is essential that every hospital should accurately prepare and properly store medical records, which are the subject of constant review by the hospital's administrative and medical staff and by professional reviewing agencies. They also are potentially critical documents in legal proceedings brought against the hospital and staff.

The Joint Commission on Accreditation of Hospitals has formulated Standard V, dealing with record keeping and emergency services, which states: "A medical record shall be kept for every patient receiving emergency services; it shall become an official hospital record." The Joint Commission further delineates the particulars that must be present in the Emergency Department medical record. These include the following: (1) adequate patient identification and consent; (2) information about the time of the patient's arrival, means of arrival, and by whom transported; (3) pertinent history of the injury or illness, including details relative to first aid or emergency care given to the patient prior to his arrival at the hospital; (4) vital signs; (5) names of attending physicians and nurses; (6) diagnosis and treatment given; and (7) final disposition, including instruction given to the patient and/or his family relative to necessary follow-up. These essentials should be present to one degree or another within the bounds of the Emergency Department medical record; probably the greatest sin committed by Emergency Department staffs everywhere is to neglect to record all this vital information.

A patient's medical record is a confidential document, and hospital personnel are precluded from divulging privileged information contained therein. However, a court of law can order the release of confidential information, and failure to comply with this order can result in a contempt of court decree. As a protective measure, it is recommended that the patient's written consent be obtained before any information contained in a medical record is released other than pursuant to a court order. This will eliminate the danger of a subsequent lawsuit for breach of the patient's right to confidentiality.

Reportable Events

All states, either by statute or administrative regulation, require the reporting by health care personnel of certain events. These include, but are not limited to, rape, child abuse, gunshot or stab wounds, venereal disease, drug addiction, and patients who are dead upon arrival at the hospital.

RAPE

In view of the frequency with which Emergency Departments are confronted with alleged rape situations, a brief discussion of this subject is in order. Rape is defined generally as unlawful carnal knowledge of a woman by a man, not her husband, forcibly against her will and with penetration, however slight, of the male genitalia into those of the female. A second category of rape is statutory rape, which is defined generally as sexual intercourse by a male with a female under statutory age, either with or without the female's consent. The Emergency Department physician's medicolegal task is not to diagnose rape, but to conduct a thoroughly documented history and physical examination of the alleged victim.

Although the Emergency Department setting does not usually permit the staff to conduct the totally comprehensive, compassionate type of examination envisioned by many feminist groups, there is room for much improvement in the conduct of most rape examinations. Important considerations in the staff's approach to the alleged rape victim should include obtaining the patient's consent, history, physical examination, and laboratory studies. Clothing should be saved and the proper authorities should be notified. Appropriate consent should be written and witnessed, and should permit examination, collection of specimens, photographs (if necessary), and release of information to proper authorities. History should reveal time, person(s), place, and circumstances. It is necessrary to ask whether the patient was under the influence of drugs or alcohol at the time, and whether she has bathed since the assault. Vaginal specimens should be tested for motile sperm, acid phosphatase, and blood group antigens of semen. A specimen should be cultured for possible *Neisseria gonorrhoeae*, and a VDRL should be obtained. A urine pregnancy test should be conducted to determine if the patient was pregnant at the time of the alleged assault.

The above specimens should be taken in the presence of a witness, documented in writing, and handed directly to the examining pathologist or laboratory technician, if possible. In the absence of the above procedure, these specimens should be labeled and placed in a locked receptacle to which only the examining pathologist has access. If the police wish to conduct these studies, the specimens should be handed directly to the police, and a witnessed receipt should be executed to document this transfer. These procedures are necessary to insure that no gaps appear in the evidentiary chain. Any undocumented handling of these specimens might be sufficient to destroy their value as evidence in a court of law. The results of these tests may be given to the adult patient, to her parents or legal guardian if she is a minor, or to the police, provided that the latter are in possession of proper authorization from the court.

Finally, the treating physician should counsel the patient about the prevention of pregnancy, venereal disease, and psychic trauma, and also arrange for the follow-up care of the patient in whatever way is clinically indicated. Failure to attend to the above necessities may result in civil suit for negligence if damages occur from such oversight.

CHILD ABUSE

The Emergency Department inevitably encounters the manifold problems of the battered child syndrome. Battered children are defined as those who have received serious physical injuries at the hands of their parents or other caretakers. Willful starvation or other deprivation of the child by the caretaker also is classified as child abuse, although it may not involve the physical contact of a battering.

Most abused children are under the age of four. Generally speaking, the younger the abused child, the greater is the danger, because the incidence of death from battering is much higher in younger than in older children.

All states have statutes or regulations providing for some degree of reporting of suspected cases of child abuse. Some of these reporting laws are permissive and allow the reporter to use his discretion in deciding whether or not to report. Others are mandatory reporting laws that require reporting under penalty of fine and/or imprisonment. There traditionally has been a paucity of battered child reports, due in part to a variety of circumstances including reporter reluctance, but recently these reports have been increasing.

Some states provide immunity from civil or criminal liability for those who report suspected battered children. The approved reporting party varies among states, but the trend is toward broadened reporting requirements authorizing *any person* who reasonably suspects an abused child to report that suspicion.

The recent California case of Thomas Robinson and the Arroyo Grande Hospital was settled before trial for damages in excess of $600,000. This case involved the issue of whether failure to report a suspected battered child would be grounds for a civil suit for negligence. The unreported battered child in this case sustained irreparable brain damage, for which the natural father filed suit. The defendant physician, who failed to report, was sufficiently impressed with the possibility of civil liability for negligence that he settled the matter rather than go to trial.

There is a reported instance, currently in litigation, of a physician sued by the mother for slander in reporting her child as a suspected case of child abuse. This occurred in a state with immunity legislation, and can easily happen if one is less than discreet in the presence of other people.

Thus, it is apparent that one can incur legal entanglements whether or not one reports suspected battered children. However, health care personnel have a high social responsibility to report suspected cases of child abuse, and should do so in compliance with the letter as well as the spirit of the law.

D.O.A.

The patient who is brought to the hospital dead on arrival (D.O.A.) presents still another reportable event for the Emergency Department. The case is routinely reported to the medical examiner for investigation as to possible foul play and as to whether any benefit could be derived from a postmortem examination.

The emergency physician's professional responsibility in the case of the D.O.A. is to pronounce the patient dead. All tissue and body fluid specimens should be drawn only by the medical examiner. Nothing should be done by Emergency Department staff that might serve to alter the appearance of the corpse; this only complicates the evidence-gathering function of the medical examiner. All clothing and other appurtenances attached to the corpse should be preserved for the medical examiner with as little handling as possible.

OTHER REPORTABLE EVENTS

Acts of social violence often are legally required to be reported. These include gun-shot wounds and stab wounds, as well as assault and battery with a variety of other potentially deadly weapons.

Venereal diseases often have found ready treatment access to the Emergency Department, and suspected cases increasingly present for treatment as the venereal epidemic spreads. Many states require reporting of V.D. to the Department of Health. The Emergency Department should adopt a method of complying with such requirements where they exist.

A similar epidemic development in the U.S. is drug addiction. It is a constant amazement to learn of the increasing variety of drugs to which addicts can become habituated. The Emergency Department should be aware of Health Department Requirements for reporting cases of drug addiction.

Blood Alcohol Request and the Police

Drunk drivers invariably find themselves in the hospital Emergency Department. They arrive in a variety of conditions, ranging from dead to severely injured to unharmed but "under the influence." Police often accompany these motorists to the Emergency Department and request or demand the staff to draw blood specimens for alcohol analysis by the police.

The case of *Schmerber v. California*, 384 U.S. 757, decided by the U.S. Supreme Court in 1966, dealt with the problem of blood alcohol in a typical situation. Schmerber was arrested for driving under the influence of intoxicating liquor. He was taken to the Emergency Department by police, who ordered a physician to draw a blood sample. Schmerber refused to comply but offered no physical resistance. The U.S. Supreme Court commented at length about the constitutional issues of the case, and held that there was no violation of Schmerber's Fourth Amendment right to be free from unreasonable search and seizure. It also held that there was no violation of the Fifth Amendment's prohibition against self-incriminating testimony.

The Court, however, did not say anything about the possible civil liability of the Emergency Department staff for assault and battery in performing a venipuncture without the consent of the patient. An emergency physician, nurse, or technician can be liable for assault and battery for touching a patient without the patient's consent. Therefore, staff should exercise caution when attempting to cooperate with police and confronting a patient unwilling to submit to a blood alcohol test.

The police sometimes attempt to mislead the staff into believing that the motorist's arrest warrant is a legal document capable of forcing them to draw the blood specimen against their will. Staff should be aware that only a court order is capable of forcing an individual to do something against his will. This force stems from the fact that one can be imprisoned for failing to obey a court order.

If the staff decide to draw the blood alcohol specimen, all contents should be properly recorded on hospital forms and appropriately witnessed. The patient's skin should be prepared with non-alcohol-containing substances, and the blood should be injected into clearly identified test tubes. If the police take the specimen, have them sign to that effect. Above all, staff should refrain from drawing the patient's blood specimen without his documented consent.

Abandonment

No matter what the scope of his practice, the emergency physician must be concerned with the problem of legal abandonment. This is the unilateral termination of the physician-patient relationship by the physician without the patient's consent, and without giving the patient sufficient opportunity to secure the services of another competent physician. Since the emergency physician's responsibility may extend beyond initial care, he should inform the patient of the necessary follow-up steps in his treatment. One means of proof that such information was provided would be an instruction sheet for a particular injury signed by the patient and ideally witnessed by a third party other than the treating physician or nurse. Such a document, however, does not provide ironclad protection, since it would still be open to attack on the grounds that the patient did not fully understand the nature of the document he was signing or the medical procedures outlined thereon. All patients should be instructed that, if complications arise, they should seek further medical attention from their family physician or from the treating Emergency Department itself.

Abandonment can occur during the transfer of a patient between different hospital Emergency Departments. It generally is the responsibility of the initial department to stabilize the patient's condition, determine whether he is physically capable of withstanding a transfer, clear his admission with the second hospital, and insure the patient's well-being until he is received by the latter. If it fulfills its responsibilities in these areas, the transferring hospital will minimize its own exposure to a potential lawsuit for negligence and abandonment.

A patient can suffer abandonment over the telephone. A typical example is a situation in which a patient returns home after receiving treatment in an Emergency Department, experiences a recurrence of symptoms, calls the Department, and is told not to worry about it until the morning. If that patient becomes ill during the night, the department is potentially liable for both negligence and abandonment. It is essential, therefore, that Emergency Department personnel should never engage in telephone diagnosis or treatment. Each patient in the above factual situation, night or day, should be instructed to return for immediate treatment.

Medical Staff Relationships

One of the most important relationships in the Emergency Department is between the emergency physicians and the remainder of the hospital medical staff. If this relationship is strained owing to personal, professional, or other reasons, it inevitably causes a diminished level of patient care, and obviously enhances a climate of confusion in which lawsuits more easily arise.

Emergency physicians should become members of the medical staff by the same procedure to which other physicians seeking hospital privileges are subjected. They also should be exposed to interdepartmental peer review of their work and, in turn, should participate in peer review of other members of the medical staff where appropriate.

The Emergency Department should be positioned in the hospital bureaucracy in such a fashion as to assure administrative competitiveness with other segments of the hospital. This allows the department to acqiuire its fair share of personnel and equipment that is indispensable for providing high quality emergency medical care. It also permits the department to protect itself agiainst possible abuse of its facilities and personnel for practices that are not appropriately conducted in the modern Emergency Department (e.g., elective outpatient blood transfusions, etc.).

The medical stafff member who instructs his patient to meet him in the Emergency Department for treatment, and then fails to appear or call to treat the patient, is a constant source of confusion for Emergency Department staff. The prime question for the Department is whether it should exercise control over this patient and institute diagnosis and treatment. If the patient's problem is nonemergent and he wishes only to see his family physician, there is little problem for the staff. However, the situation can become more troublesome when the patient's condition is potentially harmful, such as a complaint of chest pain.

Good patient care under these conditions dictates that the Emergency Department staff intervene to institute diagnosis and treatment of potential problem patients when the patient's private physician is unavailable. Obviously, some effort should be made to contact the patient's physician, but administrative considerations should never interfere with patient care. When there is any element of doubt, it is usually more prudent to err on the side of treating the patient than to withhold treatment. This course of action naturally presupposes that the patient has consented to treatment.

The Emergency Department physician also encounters the occasional difficulty of being asked to write admission orders for patients admitted through the Emergency Department to other members of the medical staff. He should be aware that he is extending his potential liability out of the Emergency Department and into the special care unit or ward to which the patient has been admitted.

Once the patient's status has been converted from outpatient to inpatient, the responsibility for his care passes through a gray zone from the Emergency Department physician to the attending physician. The first formal event witnessing this transfer is the writing of temporary orders pending the attending physician's arrival to examine the patient. This responsibility should be exercised by the attending physican after being informed of the patient's initial diagnosis and status by the emergency physician. If the emergency physician is a full-time practitioner who has contracted away his own admission privileges at the hospital, it is even more imperative that initial admission orders be written by the physician to whom the patient has been admitted.

The obvious question raised by the admission order issue is how soon after admission should the patient be seen by the attending physician. The answer obviously depends on the clinical facts. If the patient's condition is serious, he should be seen immediately upon admission. With decreasing severity of the patient's condition, the attending physician can be afforded a slightly longer time before he sees the patient. Certainly, all admitted patients should be seen within an hour or so. These guidelines are subject to some variation depending on how long the patient has been retained for "observation" in the Emergency Department. In practice, more observation occurs during the night hours. However, under no conditions should the attending physician attempt to "observe" the patient in the Emergency Department when good medicine dictates that the patient be admitted forthwith. Some of the juiciest malpractice cases have arisen from bastardized Emergency Departments that have been converted by the medical staff into wholesale holding areas. This is poor emergency medicine that probably borders on administrative negligence on the part of the hospital administration.

Manpower, Space, and Equipment

Other Emergency Department problems center around manpower, space, and equipment. Insufficient personnel (e.g., nurses, aides, technicians, etc.) and inadequately trained personnel are a constant source of legal hazard for the Emergency Department. Also, hospitals without adequate, trained emergency physician coverage of their Emergency Department are fast falling below the standard of care expected of such departments. The university hospital Emergency Department is not immune from this fault.

The Emergency Department should have enough space and equipment in which to handle initial diagnosis and treatment of emergency and nonemergency conditions. Laryngoscopes, defibrillators, ventilation bags and masks, etc., must be readily available and in satisfactory working order. The hospital should be aware that deficiencies in Emergency Department manpower, space, and equipment can result in state revocation of the hospital's license, Federal withholding of Medicare payments, and liability for negligence. It is the responsibility of the medical staff and the hospital to see to it that such deficiencies are remedied where they exist.

CONCLUSION

This chapter has been intended to present the reader with an overview of some of the medicolegal problems of the practice of emergency medicine. Certain recommendations and conclusions can be stated. First, the ever-present threat of a malpractice suit dictates that all emergency physicians and nurses should carry adequate amounts of professional liability insurance. Second, emergency physicians and nurses should be qualified to practice modern emergency medicine and should maintain those qualifications. And third, the Emergency Department must be granted appropriate recognition within the hospital bureaucracy as the "doorway" to the hospital.

Chapter 73   LEGISLATIVE ASPECTS

Alan S. Kaplan

This chapter is directed toward the non-lawyer health planner/provider who is faced with the problem and the challenge of designing and implementing an emergency medical services system. It will first describe the various kinds of "legislation," and then discuss each system component in terms of its current legislation.

It is not a legal guide, for that is within the province of the lawyer. Detailed legal questions and advice should be sought from the appropriate source as needed. This chapter will draw attention to the existing legislation with the broadest of definitions.

Traditionally, we regard legislation as the act or process of law-making; laws are viewed as rules of conduct established and enforced by an authority, i.e., government. However, for the purposes of this chapter we need a broader view of the process and the authority, as there are at least 12 possible combinations of "laws" . . . three in general terms and four in more specific language. The three general terms include national, state, and local. The four specific terms are laws, regulations/license, executive order, and court rulings.

In addition to these seven categories, one must consider resolutions and promulgated standards by organized groups and appropriations acts.

The Federal laws of principal interest in the emergency care field are the Emergency Medical Services Act (P.L. 93–154); the National Highway Safety Act (P.L. 89–564); and the Federal Communications Commission Law. It also is well to be aware of the general contract authority that the Federal Government has, as well as the type of research carried out by the National Institutes of Health. Included also should be some of the general authorities under the Defense Department and through the Executive Office of the President; for example, the Office of Telecommunications Policy.

State and local laws vary greatly. Actually, there are few laws that currently affect emergency services systems. (State Statutes on Emergency Medical Services. DHEW Pub. 72–2017.)

The question of whether legislation is really needed is an important one. Legislation that is too rigid or too premature may be a hindrance to system development. Legislation that is too detailed may become an impediment. For example, in some of the early work done with physician extenders and nurse practitioners, the advocates were so effective and caused passage of legislation so complex that the law became impossible to administer, almost destroying the programs and their concepts. It therefore is wise to use the "lowest" level of legislative authority, where the administration usually is more flexible and errors can be corrected more easily.

At the "lowest level" are the standard, resolution, guideline, policy, etc., established by local organizations. An appropriate example is a medical society calling for an ambulance to bring a patient to the nearest hospital. If that patient dies as a result of not having been taken to the nearest facility, what happens? The authorties cannot ticket the ambulance attendant nor confine him to jail. But a lawsuit can be instituted that probably will result in the strict enforcement of such a resolution by the people involved, and even the threat of this will very often bring compliance. This type of resolution often is more effective because it involves local people in their own situations. Interested individuals and organizations sometimes emerge from such circumstances. This often is very effective in precipitating the second level of activity, the court ruling.

Interpretation of the law or regulation by the judge and/or jury established precedent and leads to the same situation as if a law were passed. This in essence is the second level of legislative activity. The separate but equal doctrine, in contrast to the 1954 Supreme Court ruling, is a distinct example. There have been cases in the past in which specific laws and judicial interpretations were precipitated in order to force such a ruling, but this usually is a time-consuming and costly process that is not a feasible step toward the implementation and development of an EMS system.

The executive order is a still higher level of "legislative" activity. Issued under the general laws covering an executive, the order carries the force of law and can even command appropriations. It is important to remember this latter point, for although the prestige of an organization issuing a standard or resolution carries weight, it often is not sufficient to command appropriations except, of course, by the organization itself. Examples of executive orders affecting EMS are seen in the states of Maryland and Illinois. At the national level, the Emergency Medical Services Demonstration Special Projects emanated essentially from the executive action of the President.

This is a very effective tool simply because, more often than not, it can be used with relative ease once the executive has agreed to issue such an order. Here again, the dangers of being too precise must be stressed. The mechanism for achieving this executive order depends primarily on one's ability to meet with the executive or his key aids and to present them with sound facts, thereby convincing them that such an order would be beneficial to the development of an EMS system in the jurisdiction over which the executive has responsibility.

The law—or legislative act—is the highest level of legislative action. The Emergency Medical Services (EMS) Act of 1974 (P.L. 93–154) is an example of a national act. By itself it authorizes and generally frames the emergency medical system and the methods that the branch can use to achieve the purposes of the Act. However, it is not so self-contained that it can be effective. It needs regulations. Passage of a legislative act is not as simple to achieve as that of the executive order, and it is far more complex than a simple resolution adopted by a local organization. Before embarking on a legislative course, it is wise to read one of the outstanding texts currently available on the process of achieving legislation. *The Dance of Legislation* by Eric Redman (Simon and Schuster, 1973) is quite useful for anyone interested in achieving EMS legislation at the State or local level. This publication involves a health program of social significance readily envisioned by anyone desiring to implement an EMS system.

Despite the previous warning about too precise legislation, we now must caution just the opposite. The success of any enacted legislation is its careful and thoughtful administration. The "regulations" are the tools to accomplish this. In the EMS Act, for example, if care had not been used to adopt the GSA specifications for ambulance purchases the Federal Government would have promulgated a double standard for civilian ambulances. At the same time, because the issue of categorization was not yet clarified, guidance and criteria had to be established in the regulations that would be precise but not absolute. It is important for those who are writing or suggesting content for regulations to observe these guidelines. Regulations usually are written in draft by professionals most familiar with the subject matter. The lawyers then convert these concepts into the proper legal language. It is precisely at this point in the legislative dance that the nonlawyer can have his greatest impact, if he has not been involved with the legislation itself.

A closely related legislative action is licensing. On a par with regulations, it is a direct consequence of a regulatory act. It is a controlling mechanism and can be a double-edged sword. In some cases it can be used to deter progress; in others it is an impetus. Again, it must be implemented and utilized carefully.

A final legislative action is appropriations. There usually are sufficient laws with powers broad enough to allow a broad connotation, e.g., "demonstration project" authority. In such a case, appropriation of funds for specific action under such legislative act will, in fact, be implementing or enabling legislation. Although this probably is the least satisfactory method of achieving enactment or implementatinon of an EMS system, this legislative action may be one of the better mechanisms in a case in which money is the major problem.

In summary, there are laws, regulations and licensing activities that result from legislative actions and require executive follow-through; there are orders that stem directly from the general powers embodied in the executive; and there are court rulings that are manifestations of actions through the judicial system. On a nonlegal basis, but often with as much legal force, there are resolutions, policies, standards, and actions promulgated by professional or lay groups, which by weight of those organizations' prestige can be considered standards of social and/or moral actions—implying law. Each of the above can occur on the nationwide (Federal) and State or local levels, and can be conflicting if not carefully and thoughtfully administered.

LEGISLATION AS IT SPECIFICALLY RELATES TO EMERGENCY MEDICAL SERVICES SYSTEMS COMPONENTS

Communications

"Communications" basically refers to radio communications and telemetry, and in both instances is covered by strict Federal communications laws and regulations. These legal aspects of the EMS Communications are extremely technical in nature and should be properly handled by an experienced and knowledgeable person. Two useful guides are the Office of Telecommunications Policy Book on 9-1-1 and the American Hospital Association's booklet on EMS Communications, *A Guide For Hospital Participation In An Emergency Medical Services System.* This is an instance in which there is a nationwide law followed by regulations that affect Federal, State, and local activities. In certain cases, State and local guidelines for communications systems and procedures are promulgated; e.g., state of Illinois MERCI Communications Manual, or local communications procedures as established by fire rescue services and local medical societies, such as in Montgomery County, Maryland.

Ambulances

Laws covering ambulances vary from state to state, most of which have antiquated laws. A model ambulance ordinance has been developed in cooperation with the National Safety Council, the American Medical Commission on EMS, and other organizations. In addition, there are the previously mentioned Federal standards that are an outgrowth of the U.S. Department of Transportation regulations as established by the National Highway Safety Act. Some medical societies and fire rescue services have been much more specific in their designs for equipment and the number and level of training of attendants.

Facilities

Reference here is made primarily to hospital Emergency Departments. At the present time they are not covered under any specific law, although generally accredited hospitals must follow the rules and regulations of the Joint Commission on Hospital Accreditation. Here is an example of a nationwide private organization issuing regulations and standards covering operation of an emergency facility. The American Medical Association's standards on categorization also should be reviewed. Several useful guides include *Guidelines for Design and Function of a Hospital Emergency Department* (American College of Surgeons) and *Emergency Services: The Hospital Emergency Department in an Emergency Care System* (American Hospital Association).

The EMS Act of 1974 strongly recommends categorization, and the regulations indicate that the facilities must be systematized in accordance with a formulated method of classifying hospital emergency capabilities, but they do not specifically spell out which method should be used. The categorization guidelines established by the American Medical Association are suggested as one course of action, but it also is noted that certain states have other categorization procedures. Dr. Oscar P. Hampton's article in *Prism* (July 1974, Volume 2, Number 7), *A Rating System for Emergency Departments,* reviews some of the pros and cons of the AMA system and suggests possible alternative courses of action. This is still a controversial area that needs to be considered carefully in the development of an EMS system. The question of hospital categorization from a public point of view, and the need for understanding the hospital capability from the ambulance attendant's standpoint, also should be taken into account.

Manpower

There is general agreement that ambulance attendants must be relatively well trained individuals, but the level of training has not been fully decided. The Department of Transportation 81-Hour Course, which upon completion leads to registration as an Emergency Medical Technician (EMT), is considered basic at present.

Careful planning in the use of legislation can be effective in this area. For example, the passage of the Cardio-Rescue Technician (CRT) legislation in the State of Maryland resulted in the development of such technicians and the ability of the fire rescue services actually to perform cardiopulmonary resuscitation. Until that time the Medical Practices Act in that State had precluded such treatment. In this particular instance the law was not extremely precise, but left it to the regulatory and licensing boards to establish the appropriate criteria. The appropriate professional personnel were then able to assist those boards in establishing the licensing, examinations, and training criteria.

Consumer Education

At the present time there is very little in the way of legislation for consumer education. This reflects the general weakness of health education and the general failure of accident prevention programs. Attention is called to the National Occupation and Safety Health Act, especially as it relates to mine safety, but the present effect on EMS development is practically nil.

Organization

The structuring of the EMS system is primarily the responsibility of local and State organizations. Very often, however, one group will run the ambulances, another will administer the hospitals, and a third will attempt to exert influence on the physicians. Basically it can be said that there is no existing organizational framework or legislative base to provide a unifying, single, controlling force on the EMS System, but there is a model EMS Act (DHEW Pub. #72-2016) that might serve as such. Currently the organization may be identified as a confederation of providers, consumers, and patients, all cognizant of the fact that any given time there could be a great deal of interchangeability.

The establishment of local "EMS councils" has contributed favorably toward influencing the development of community EMS systems. A council affords an opportunity for the consumer, the provider, the fire rescue personnel, and others to convene on common ground to discuss problems and to assist mutually in the development of the EMS system. Guidelines for establishing an EMS Council have been developed by the AMA Commission on Emergency Medical Services (*A Kit: Emergency Medical Services Rx Emergency Care for Yourself, Your Family, Your Community*). In our own experience in establishing an EMS Council, it is important to have a set of agreed bylaws that spell out in detail the functions of the Council and its organization and procedure.

Since the strength of the Council lies in its recognition by the basic health planning bodies and the local government, it is important to have a resolution of endorsement passed by local government. The power invested in the EMS Council is advisory, but action cannot be taken without their guidance.

To achieve success in developing an EMS system, the people involved must be committed to an honest, common-bond relationship. These qualities, aided by laws, resolutions, and regulations, will bring about the successful implementation of such a system.

Part VI

SOCIOECONOMICS OF EMERGENCY MEDICINE

Chapter 74

PATTERNS AND TRENDS OF UTILIZATION OF EMERGENCY MEDICAL SERVICES

Geoffrey Gibson

In 1972 there were over 60 million visits to hospital Emergency Departments in this country, and this figure is increasing by well over 5 million each year. If we exclude visits to federal and long term hospitals, Table 1 shows that Emergency Department visits went up from 9 million to 56 million between 1954 and 1972. This increase of 495 per cent is larger than any other measure of hospital use. In 1954, there were 17 Emergency Department visits per hospital bed: by 1972 there were 63; in 1954, there were 1807 Emergency Department visits at the average hospital: by 1972 there were 9585. Indeed, if one includes only those 4726 hospitals with an Emergency Department (and this number significantly is declining by over 100 each year), there are an average of 11,851 visits for each hospital with an Emergency Department. Even within the context of growing hospital outpatient activity, Emergency Department visits in 1954 accounted for less than one-fifth of all outpatient visits, whereas by 1972 they accounted for over one-third. This rise is particularly marked when it is expressed as rates per thousand population to standardize for population growth. Thus, in 1954 there were 58 visits per thousand population, and by 1972 this had gone up to 272 visits per thousand population per year.

UTILIZATION TRENDS FOR EMERGENCY DEPARTMENTS

Not only has there been a fivefold increase in the rate of use over the past two

TABLE 1   Utilization Data for Nonfederal, General Short Term U.S. Hospitals, 1954–1972

	1954	1972	PERCENTAGE CHANGE
Number of Hospitals	5212	5843	12
Number of Inpatient Beds	553,068	883,681	60
Number of Inpatient Admissions	18,391,657	30,776,923	67
Number of Inpatient Days	143,455,065	242,845,009	69
Total Outpatient Department			
Visits:	50,408,617	166,983,161	231
Referred	10,850,922	54,284,669	400
Clinic	26,405,125	56,690,545	115
Emergency Department	9,418,755	56,007,947	495
Emergency Department Visits:			
per bed	17	63	
per hospital	1807	9585	
per 1000 population	58	272	

Sources: American Hospital Association, *J.A.H.A., Guide Issue*, Volume 29, Number 8 (1955) and *Hospital Statistics* (1973).

TABLE 2   Hospital Emergency Department
Utilization in the Ten Largest U.S. Cities, 1972

	VISITS	VISITS PER 1000 POPULATION
New York	3,364,045	426
Chicago	1,125,329	335
Los Angeles	725,930	267
Philadelphia	841,832	431
Detroit	655,920	434
Houston	320,498	260
Baltimore	674,426	744
Dallas	288,536	342
Washington	472,781	625
Cleveland	380,710	507

Source: American Hospital Association, *Hospital Statistics*, 1973.

decades, but the 1972 rate, being a nation-wide average, varies greatly by location and patient characteristics. Table 2 shows that the utilization rate varies from 260 visits per thousand population in Houston to 754 in Baltimore, and in New York City alone there were 3.4 million visits in 1972. This variation of utilization rates is clearly not only a function of the availability of Emergency Departments and health care, but also of the differing demographic mix of the populations. Indeed, Emergency Department use varies markedly by patient characteristics as shown in Table 3, which reports previously unpublished data from the National Center for Health Statistics' Health Interview Survey. Thus, for every 100 people in 1967 there were 430 physician visits in total (for all treatment sites), and of these, ten took place in a hospital Emergency Department; in 1969 there were also 430 total visits per 100 population, but 11 of these took place in an Emergency Department. Utilization rates in Emergency Departments are higher for males than for females; they decrease with age, and are much lower for whites than for nonwhites. Between 1967 and 1969, these rates increased for females (but not for males), for nonwhites (but not for whites), for children (but not for adults). The trend data for income and education groups are not clear.

The data in Table 3, of course, are utilization rates that indicate an increase in the absolute number of Emergency Department visits. By itself this information does not present the proportion of all physician

TABLE 3   Total Physician Visits (all sites) and Emergency Department Physician Visits
Per Annum Per 100 Population, 1967 and 1969.

	1967 PHYSICIAN VISITS PER 100 POPULATION		1969 PHYSICIAN VISITS PER 100 POPULATION	
	ALL SITES	E.D.	ALL SITES	E.D.
All persons	430	10	430	11
Sex: Males	380	12	370	12
Females	480	9	470	10
Age: Under 5	570	17	570	20
5–14	270	11	280	12
15–24	400	12	370	12
25–34	440	12	440	13
35–44	430	11	410	9
45–54	430	7	430	7
55–64	510	4	510	8
65–74	600	6	610	6
75 and over	600	8	620	5
Race: White	450	10	440	10
Nonwhite	310	13	350	18
Years of Education				
Under 5	370	12	410	12
5–8	400	10	400	10
9–12	430	11	415	12
13	500	9	470	10
Family Income:				
Less than $3000	460	10	480	12
$3000–4999	410	11	450	14
$5000–6999	420	13	390	10
$7000–9999	430	11	410	11
$10,000–and over	450	8	435	10

TABLE 4 Emergency Department Physician Visits as Percentage of Total Physician Visits, 1967 and 1969.

| | E. D. VISITS AS PERCENTAGE OF TOTAL PHYSICIAN VISITS: | |
	1967	1969
All persons	2.3	2.5
Sex: Males	3.1	3.2
Females	1.8	2.1
Age: Under 5	2.9	3.5
5–14	4.0	4.3
15–24	3.0	3.2
25–34	2.7	2.9
35–44	2.5	2.2
45–54	1.6	1.6
55–64	0.9	1.6
65–74	1.0	1.0
75 and over	2.7	0.8
Race: White	2.2	2.3
Nonwhite	4.2	5.1
Years of Education:		
Under 5	3.2	2.9
5–8	2.5	2.5
9–12	2.5	2.9
13	1.8	2.1
Family Income:		
Less than $3000	2.2	2.5
$3000–4999	2.9	3.1
$5000–6999	3.1	2.5
$7000–9999	1.8	2.3
$10,000–and over	1.8	2.3

visits that take place in an Emergency Department. This is set out in Table 4, which shows that there has been an increase not only in absolute utilization rates, but also in the proportion of all physician visits accounted for by hospital Emergency Departments. It also indicates differences by demographic characteristics of patients. For example, a higher proportion of all physician visits take place in an Emergency Department for nonwhites than for whites; this also is true of males compared to females, of younger to older, of low-educated to high-educated, and low income persons to high income persons.

Up to this point several conclusions may be drawn about trends and patterns of utilization of Emergency Departments, and we summarize them here before explaining why they have occurred.

(1) Hospital Emergency Department visits have increased from 9 million in 1954 to 56 million in 1972.

(2) The average hospital Emergency Department had 1807 visits in 1954 and 11,851 in 1972.

(3) There were 58 Emergency Department visits per thousand population in 1954 compared to 272 in 1972.

(4) Among the ten largest U.S. cities, Baltimore and Washington have the highest utilization rates (754 and 625, respectively, Emergency Department visits per year per thousand population).

(5) In 1969, for every 100 persons there were 430 physician visits in total, and 11 of these visits took place in an Emergency Department.

(6) Over the last decade there has been an absolute increase in Emergency Department visits, and also a relative increase in Emergency Department use compared to all other treatment sites. This increase in the proportion of all health care that is received through an Emergency Department has been particularly marked for nonwhites, males, those under 25 years of age, and those who are poor and undereducated.

(7) Less than one-third of Emergency Department visits represent clinical emergencies, and between one-half and two-thirds are for routine primary health care.

REASONS FOR INCREASED EMERGENCY DEPARTMENT USE

It is clear that these trends cannot be accounted for by an increase in the incidence of clinical emergencies. Instead, they represent the consequences of hospital Emergency Departments assuming, or rather being forced to assume, a primary health care function for patients who are unwilling or unable to secure health care in alternative ways. For this reason, the following list of causes of increased Emergency Department use also constitutes a catalog of the decreasing ability of the health care system outside the Emergency Department to provide primary health care to substantial portions of the population.

(1) In most inner city areas, private physicians who relocate or die are not being replaced, and thus contribute to the situation in which large concentrations of low income groups have neither physical nor financial access to a private ambulatory health care system.

(2) High levels of geographic mobility have left substantial numbers of patients without a regular family physician.

(3) Physicians increasingly are unavailable at night or at weekends, and are reluctant to make house calls.

(4) There has been a decrease in the number of general practitioners who function as primary care physicians of first contact.

(5) Increasing physician specialization also has resulted in the patient not knowing which specialist to call, in the arrangement of office hours by appointment only, and in physician unwillingness to accept responsibility for a patient's problem outside his field of interest.

(6) The independent capacity of the physician to treat emergency conditions optimally in his private office has decreased with the increase in medical science and technology.

(7) The needed technical and human resources increasingly are concentrated in hospitals where they are available (through the Emergency Department) on a 24 hour basis and are geographically accessible to urban populations lacking alternative ambulatory delivery sites.

(8) Patients increasingly accept and have confidence in the Emergency Department as a facility for acute and non-acute conditions, and prefer to be treated there rather than by a private physician.

(9) The reimbursement policies of health insurance plans cover treatment in Emergency Departments, but not if it is rendered on office visit or house calls.

The most important aspect of this list of reasons for increased Emergency Department use is that the reasons lie outside the EMS system itself. Because of this, it is extremely unlikely that the Emergency Department will be able to influence the demand for its services. Its use is now a function of wider trends in the entire health care system, and will continue to be determined primarily by these exogenous trends of health care access. Emergency Departments are the one entry point and treatment site in the health care arena that can neither deny or delay access. Hospitals can delay access to inpatients, and private physicians can refuse to take on new patients, but the hospital Emergency Department does not have this option. It must for legal and ethical reasons accept all comers. It can "triage" incoming patients in the sense of treating the clinically emergent first, and after initial examination may even refer the non-urgent

to other treatment sites, but it may not refuse or turn away patients without placing itself in severe legal jeopardy and violating the "Hospital Licensing Code" in most states.

Thus, as I have indicated in greater detail elsewhere (Gibson, 1973) the present activities of the hospital Emergency Department, as well as its future role, will be determined mainly by the nature of the wider health care system, rather than by the EMS subsystem. In an era of (1) rising health expectations; (2) the certainty of reduced financial barriers to utilization (with National Health Insurance); and (3) a lack of any concomitant increase in the capacity to meet this growing demand, the hospital Emergency Department stands alone as the only entry point to health care without an ability to control its own intake in either quality or quantity. Because of this, it is forced into a role of the 24-hour "rainbarrel" of ambulatory health care to collect the "leaks" from the rest of the system. One important consequence of this is that substantial numbers of patients regard the Emergency Department as their regular source of health care. Thus, in a recent study in Buffalo, New York, where 888 patients were interviewed in 22 hospital Emergency Departments, 23 per cent said they received all of their health care from the Emergency Department. All these patients were asked about their health care utilization over the previous 30 days, and Table 5 shows this previously unpublished information. For these patients the Emergency Department is not only the single most important source of health care, but it accounts for more health care than all other treatment sites put together. In terms of Emergency Department visits as a proportion of all doctor visits, nonwhites are much more likely (69 per cent) to receive their medical care at the Emergency Department than are whites (47 per cent). This also is true of poor compared to rich patients, and low-educated compared to high-educated ones. In general, the fewer contacts patients have with physicians, the more likely it is that contact will be made in an Emergency Department. Table 5 also gives comparative data for the entire U.S. population, and indicates much greater use by this population (both relatively and absolutely) of Emergency Departments for general medical care. However, these figures relate to visits and not to severity of complaint.

TABLE 5 *Mean Number of Physician Visits in Past 30 Days by Site and Patient Characteristics in 888 Emergency Department Patients in Buffalo, New York.*

CHARACTERISTICS:	SITES				TOTAL		E.D. VISITS AS % OF ALL VISITS
	E.D.	O.P.D.	DOCTOR'S OFFICE	NONHOSP. CLINIC	PER MONTH°	PER ANNUM°°	
Age:							
0–4 years	0.6	0.9	0.9	0.7	3.1	49.2	39
5–18 years	0.4	0.3	0.4	0.3	1.4	28.8	58
19–39 years	0.4	0.3	0.6	0.2	1.5	30.0	56
40–64 years	1.0	0.1	0.9	0.4	2.4	40.8	59
56+ years	0.5	0.2	1.8	0.0	2.5	42.0	43
Sex:							
Male	0.5	0.3	0.6	0.6	2.0	36.0	50
Female	0.6	0.3	0.9	0.1	1.9	34.8	55
Race:							
White	0.4	0.3	0.9	0.4	2.0	36.0	47
Nonwhite	1.0	0.4	0.3	0.2	1.9	34.8	69
Annual Family Income:							
$0–2999	1.1	0.6	1.0	0.6	3.3	39.6	49
$3000–4999	0.4	0.2	0.7	0.1	1.4	28.8	58
$5000–6999	0.4	0.3	0.5	0.2	1.4	28.8	58
$7000–9999	0.4	0.2	0.7	0.1	1.4	28.8	58
$10,000–14,999	0.3	0.1	0.5	0.1	1.0	24.0	65
$15,000+	0.3	0.2	0.8	0.0	1.3	27.6	56
Education (grades completed):							
0–4	0.2	0.1	1.7	0.1	2.1	37.2	39
5–9	0.4	0.4	0.7	0.1	1.6	31.2	54
9–12	0.7	0.3	0.6	0.1	1.7	32.4	63
13+	0.4	0.1	0.6	0.1	1.2	26.4	64
U.S. Population	0.0	0.0	0.3	0.0	0.5	5.6	3

°Excluding current E.D. visit.
°°Including current E.D. visit, which is added to monthly total and multiplied by 12 to give annual totals.

It is quite clear, then, that hospital Emergency Departments already have a substantial role in providing ambulatory health care, and one that is almost certain to increase. If any of the current versions of national health insurance is passed to raise demand by lowering financial barriers without simultaneously increasing health services supply, it is inevitable that a substantial part of the increased utilization will be concentrated in already overcrowded Emergency Departments.

SUMMARY AND CONCLUSIONS

Hospital Emergency Department visits have increased from 9 million in 1954 to 56 million in 1972, the largest single increase of any aspect of health care utilization. Ex-pressed as a utilization rate, there were 58 Emergency Department visits per thousand population in 1954, compared to 272 in 1972. A substantial part of this increased utilization is not attributable to any increase in emergencies, but instead to a growing reliance by significant proportions of the population on the Emergency Department as the regular source of primary health care. This, in turn, has resulted from general trends in the wider health care system that adversely affect access to care through traditional non-Emergency Department sites. Thus the Emergency Department has been forced to assume a role of 24-hour "rain-barrel" for ambulatory health care to collect the "leaks" of unmet demand from all other sectors. Significantly, the Emergency Department is particularly vulnerable to this function, since it is the one entry point or treatment site in health care that lacks the option of denying or delaying access. Because of this, hospital Emergency Departments now have a substantial role in providing primary health care to segments of the population, many of whom look to them as their regular or even sole source of care. With national health insurance, this role will expand even further.

References

Gibson, G.: Emergency medical services: a facet of ambulatory care. Hospitals *47*:59, 1973.

Gibson, G.: The Social System of Emergency Medical Care. *In* Noble, J. (ed.): Emergency Medical Services: Behavioral and Planning Perspectives. New York, Behavioral Publications, Inc., 1974.

Gibson, G., et al.: Emergency Medical Services in the Chicago Area. Center for Health Administration Studies, University of Chicago, 1970.

Chapter 75

EPIDEMIOLOGIC FACTORS IN EMERGENCY CARE

Julian A. Waller

Epidemiology is the study of the distribution and determinants of disease and other health-related phenomena within the community, and several epidemiologic concepts are relevant to an assessment of emergency health services, and to planning, implementation, and evaluation of changes. One of these concepts is the basic and well-documented assumption that the distribution of the frequency of injury and illness among the population is not random; neither is the distribution of the severity of injury or illness. Even if disease cannot be prevented, if the nature of the nonrandom frequencies can be identified, it is possible to ensure that services will be most available when and where disease, and especially serious disease, most often is found.

If identification can be made *when* and *where* disease is most likely to be serious—as measured by death, disability, and discomfort—it often is possible also to determine *why* it is more serious under certain circumstances, and to bring about appropriate countermeasures. There is increasing evidence, for example, that one reason why highway crashes in suburban and rural areas are more likely to be fatal than in urban areas is because the necessary emergency care often is not available when and where it is needed (Waller, J. A., et al., 1964).

A second relevant epidemiologic concept is that a single cause may have several effects, and a single effect may be the result of multiple causes. For example, excessive use of alcohol as a causal agent may contribute: (1) to the initiation of a highway crash; (2) to the severity of the crash (as measured by extent of damage to the vehicle); (3) perhaps to greater sensitivity of tissues to injury; (4) to biases against compassionate treatment; (5) to problems in evaluation of the nature and extent of injury; and (6) to the frequency of complications of therapy.

Conversely, permanent brain damage or even death as outcomes may be the result not only of the kinetic forces of the crash, but also of: (1) how they are imparted to the head; (2) the presence of cerebral edema secondary to alcohol; (3) reduced consciousness because of the alcohol; and (4) problems in clearing an airway because discovery of the crash is delayed, the design of the vehicle or other aspects of the environment do not permit easy access to the patient or extrication, personnel are inadequately trained or have insufficient experience, or necessary equipment is not available.

The uses of epidemiologic concepts and techniques to assess and improve emergency care will be considered in the examination of three types of situations: (1) distribution and determinants of emergencies and their outcomes; (2) distribution and determinants of emergency services; and (3) evaluation of the effects of any changes within the emergency care system.

DISTRIBUTION AND DETERMINANTS OF EMERGENCIES AND THEIR OUTCOMES

Perhaps the most important introductory comment that must be made about the distribution of emergencies is that they are not predominantly related to injuries. Since the major recent thrust in the improvement of emergency care began with the emergency care standard in 1967 of the U.S. Department of Transportation, many people have assumed that trauma, and highway trauma in particular, is the most common problem. The pattern, of course, varies from one community to another. However, although injury events do comprise a substantial proportion of emergencies, and especially more serious emergencies, they commonly represent only a minority of all problems seen in Emergency Departments (although they are a modest majority of those seen in ambulances) (King and Sox, 1967).

The concept of an emergency is that it is an acute situation for which the time or place cannot be anticipated. This may be true for an individual event, but it does not apply when over-all distributions are examined. It is quite possible to predict when, where, and among which groups emergencies of specific types are most and least likely to occur, and even to predict the approximate proportions of the distributions.

In illustration, Youmans' data from the University of Kansas Medical Center (1970) show that the proportion of true emergencies (conditions requiring care within one half-hour to avoid harmful outcome) increases from 28 per cent of all Emergency Department patients during the day shift to 49 per cent in the evening and 64 per cent at night. Over-all, however, 50 per cent of all patients (emergency and non-emergency) were seen during the day, 39 per cent in the evening, and 11 per cent at night, and emergencies during these shifts comprised respectively 14 per cent, 19 per cent, and 7 per cent of all patients in the 24 hours. These figures, of course, would vary somewhat from one community to another depending on the local pattern of use of the emergency department for nonurgent conditions.

It also is apparent from Youmans' study that the Emergency Department now serves more as an outpatient facility than as a place for treating real emergencies. Over a three- or four-year period, there was a 42 per cent increase in visits for real emergencies, but a 345 per cent increase in other visits, a pattern that has been documented in many other hospitals as well.

Certain factors associated with injury or illness itself bring about a true increase in more serious events during evening and night-time hours. The most prominent of these factors is excessive consumption of alcohol — largely a night-time and weekend activity. Alcohol is much more highly correlated with serious injury than with minor trauma, although it plays an appreciable role there too. About one-half of all serious injuries to adults involve consumption of alcohol, whether the trauma is attempted homicide, suicide, highway crashes, falls, drownings, or fire-related injuries (Waller, 1970). Alcohol is probably a factor in about 15 per cent of less serious injury events. Because of circadian rhythms of the human body, there is a suggestion that heart attacks and other health problems might be more serious at night than during the day, thus placing greater demands on the emergency care system at a time when staff capabilities may be minimal.

Identifiable variations in the distribution of injury or illness over time may occur not only within a period of a day or a week, but from one season to another. Trends in type and severity of injury or illness also may be found over a period of years because of changes in life-style and technology.

Injuries to arms, for example, are no longer seen as a result of cranking starters on automobiles, and are seldom seen from wringer-type washing machines except among welfare recipients who, under regulations of some social service agencies, are permitted to buy only washing machines of this outmoded and dangerous type. (Not surprisingly, these injuries substantially increase the costs to the agency.) Except in rural areas, burns from wood and kerosene stoves are less common than in the past.

These types of trauma have largely been replaced by crushing injuries to the chest from impacts with automobile steering columns, serious head injury from windshields and from motorcycle crashes, and other injuries from power lawnmowers, workshop equipment, snowmobiles, snowblowers, and various other accouterments of an affluent society. Illness too has reflected these changes, as the frequency of acute myocardial infarction has increased over the years, presumably because of the alterations in diet, work, and leisure patterns.

However, technology and legislation

also can produce other changes that reduce the frequency and severity of injury or illness events over time. Injury is the result of man's failure to maintain complete control over sources of physical energy (kinetic, chemical, thermal, electric, radiation) in his environment. Such control exists as long as the capability of the person exceeds the demands of the task involved in exposure to or use of the energy source. If the task exceeds the performance, the energy becomes available to injure, and the nature and extent of the resulting injury depend on how the energy is transferred to the body. As Hippocrates noted, impact to the head with a hard, sharp object causes more brain damage than does impact with a soft, blunt one. The higher the transfer rate of energy per unit of time and body space, the greater the resulting injury.

Traditionally, we have been concerned with making people more capable to perform tasks, and legislation such as that requiring drivers to show at least minimal competence and to be licensed undoubtedly has contributed to some reduction in the frequency of highway injury over the years. But so have design improvements to reduce task demands, such as better highway geometry and signs that have high visibility and legibility. The technology for better highways and for the promotion of product safety far exceeds current application, and recent emphasis on these areas should mean further reduction in the frequency of potential injury events over the next several years.

Other important changes involve reducing the energy transfer even if the task demand is greater than performance. Successful examples of this strategy include: (1) the use of fuses and circuit breakers in buildings; (2) energy-absorbing steering columns; (3) high penetration-resistant windshields; (4) lap and shoulder restraints in automobiles; (5) breakaway signposts and properly designed and placed guard rails on highways; (6) helmets for motorcyclists; and (7) flame-retarding fabrics and building components. Again, the recent surge of interest in product safety, and the establishment of the National Highway Safety Bureau (now the National Highway Traffic Safety Administration) and of the Consumer Product Safety Commission, should result in continued progress in reducing the frequency and severity of actual injury.

The introduction of penetration-resistant windshields, for example, has markedly changed the character of emergency and definitive care for facial injuries, and the passage of legislation in Australia making wearing of passenger restraints compulsory has brought about startling reductions in the need for neurosurgical staffs at night and weekends and for personnel to supervise long term rehabilitation. In the prevention of disease, such technologic changes as improved canning techniques, better refrigeration, and public water and sewerage systems have greatly altered the patterns of use of emergency care facilities. Haddon (1970) has described the various strategies for injury and illness control in several seminal papers that should be required reading for all who wish to understand and deal with this field.

The distribution of the frequency and severity of emergencies varies not only according to time but also according to place and person. Rural areas appear to have more serious crashes because of poorer roads, somewhat higher speeds, severe single vehicle collisions with trees and rocks, etc., and problems of emergency care. Slum areas have more serious fires, recreational areas more drownings, nonwhite urban neighborhoods more assaults, and white neighborhoods more suicides. The older the population, the greater the frequency of heart attacks and serious falls. The younger the population, the greater the number of calls about possible toxic ingestion. Where high hazard industries exist, such as lumbering and mining, the frequency of severe trauma is greater. Conversely, there are fewer fractures among the elderly in communities with high fluoride content (three or more parts per million) in the drinking water, because bone is denser and apparently sturdier. Periodic high levels of air pollution over several days because of local industrial, traffic, and climatic patterns may bring about epidemics of acute respiratory and circulatory failure that can stretch the health care system to its limits.

The important point is that planning of emergency services for a community must involve assessment of basic demographic characteristics of the population, both resident and transient, and of environmental characteristics. This assessment should be repeated at least every five years, because the character and needs of communities and neighborhoods are constantly changing over time.

DISTRIBUTION AND DETERMINANTS OF EMERGENCY SERVICES

Distinction must be made between the distribution of the availability of services and of the services actually sought and provided. The former is much easier to determine than is the latter, although such questions as whether those services available are below or beyond what a particular community actually needs are only now beginning to be considered with any degree of sophistication. The reader is referred to two papers by Gibson (1973, 1974) that deal with some of the relevant conceptual questions and problems.

Let us examine first the distribution and determinants of availability of services. In an examination of ambulance services in 25 American cities, Gibson (1973) reports that availability of ambulances per 100,000 population varied from 1.78 to 13.52, and total use per 1000 persons ranged from 13.3 to 90.4. Some estimates from rural areas suggest availability of about two ambulances per 100,000 and utilization rates of about 30 to 40 per 1000.

Use of ambulance and other emergency services, of course, will depend not only on the numbers and types of emergencies that occur, but also on the cost and availability of other means of transportation and emergency service. If the cost of ambulance service to the consumer is minimal, an increase in "abuse" can be expected, that is, in the proportion of runs for conditions that are not true emergencies. If physicians are not readily available to substantial segments of the community, either because of problems in scheduling or because of cost, it can be anticipated that hospital Emergency Departments will be used increasingly for outpatient care. Both types of unanticipated (but not unforeseeable) use of emergency facilities have increased markedly in recent years, especially in urban slums.

Beginning in the 1950s, studies indicated that ambulance services available, whether adequate in numbers or not, tended to be quite inadequate in the probable quality of service that could be provided (Hampton, 1960). These assessments were based on such criteria as personnel training that often did not reach even the level of the Red Cross standard or advanced first aid courses, absence of equipment for ambulance-to-hospital communication, management of airway and respiration, splinting, utilization in some cases of one-man ambulance crews, and absence of regional coordination of services. As more methodical assessments of problems and resources began to be made during the latter half of the 1960s and the early 1970s, these deficits were found to be distributed quite uniformly throughout the nation, both urban and rural.

Only anecdotal data are available about the causes of these inadequacies, but three factors appear to predominate.

(1) A general failure by the medical community to consider ambulance service or other aspects of the prehospital phase as a relevant part of the health care system, and a consequent lack of interest in promoting adequate training, equipment, or coordination.

(2) Insufficient funding of ambulance services because neither government nor health insurers were willing to support legitimate costs.

(3) The predominant role of morticians in the field as the only group with anything approaching a suitable vehicle with, in some instances, a substantial conflict of interest between their ambulance and mortuary services.

Each of these factors appeared to reinforce the others, poor quality leading to inadequate funding and unwillingness of others either to help or to replace the morticians, and vice versa.

Data about the training of police officers to provide emergency care, and about the adequacy of hospital Emergency Departments, also indicate a rather uniform absence of quality until the early 1970s. Although some university-affiliated hospitals and large urban medical centers have had many and diverse specialists, with well organized services and house staff on duty 24 hours a day, most hospitals in urban, suburban, and especially rural areas have lacked nurses and physicians trained and experienced in emergency care who are available around the clock, and have further lacked ongoing supervision and monitoring by an Emergency Department director or committee (Owens, 1965; Kanwit and Gettinger, 1971). Furthermore, even the best of hospitals usually had inadequate signs in the community or around the hospital to ensure that the Emergency Department could be found easily. Thus, the best Emergency Departments usually, but not invariably, have been in large facilities in urban centers, and the least adequate ones have been in small suburban or rural hospitals.

All this is in the process of changing, and to date the changes appear to be distributed fairly uniformly. The major determinants of change, based on anecdotal data only, are as follows.

(1) The emphasis placed upon the emergency care system *as a system* by the Department of Transportation emergency care standard of 1967. This provided both positive incentives for change (money, new research, systems guidance, and a new 81-hour emergency medical technician training curriculum) and negative incentives (threatened loss of federal highway funds) if change did not take place.

(2) Pressures because of greater public use of Emergency Departments for ambulatory care, so that physicians became motivated to take more interest in emergency care, to upgrade services, and in some cases to specialize in this field.

(3) Growing willingness by state and local governments and insurers to support emergency services, but often only if those services met minimal standards.

But what about the distribution and determinants of services actually sought and provided? Are there gaps between what is now available (or becoming available) and what is being used? The answer is "yes," for a variety of reasons. First, there is evidence that, even with rather serious injury or illness, there may be substantial delays before help is sought. With myocardial infarction, this delay is often six hours or longer after the development of signs or symptoms. A recent study by G. Keller (1973) attributes some of this delay to prolonged decision-making by the sick or injured person and by friends or relatives called for advice, but some also is the result of incomplete advice by doctors and nurses about

how to call an ambulance or get to the hospital. Other data show that, in some cases, physicians may refuse to help at all. At night or in rural areas there may be serious problems in getting assistance, even though theoretically it is available.

Through ignorance or poor advice many people who need an ambulance arrive at the hospital by other means, and some who should use other transportation take an ambulance instead. As noted earlier, this is sometimes because it is the least expensive mode. Gibson's data (1974) for 181 persons with emergent conditions in Chicago revealed that 44 per cent used an ambulance, 34 per cent drove themselves, 17 per cent were driven by someone else or took a taxi, and 5 per cent walked or used public transportation. These data also are supported by other studies in rural areas. Conversely, about 15 per cent of all ambulance runs in Gibson's study were for nonemergencies.

Recent work by Frazier and colleagues at New Haven (1973) shows that misdiagnosis, or wrong action after correct diagnosis, is much more common among highly trained ambulance personnel than had been hoped, and experience in Vermont and suburban areas of Baltimore suggests that one reason why this may occur among emergency care personnel of all types is that some kinds of emergencies are seen so seldom that staffs are unable to retain either knowledge or skills.

Finally, there appear to be biases that militate against equal treatment for certain types of patients. Gibson (1973) notes that in Chicago "whites are much more likely than non-whites to use a private ambulance while non-whites are much more likely to be taken by police paddy-wagons. Given the inferiority of police vehicles, it seems that while blacks receive the same quantity of ambulance services as whites the quality of service received is substantially lower than that for whites." Also documented is the fact that care for young persons who have acute life-threatening illness is likely to be much more heroic than for individuals aged 30 or older who are incapacitated (Waller, 1973). Persons who attempt suicide, become sick or injured after drinking heavily, or are injured in ways not to the liking of the hospital staff (e.g., on snowmobiles or motorcycles) are sometimes the recipients of substantial insult to add to their injury.

EVALUATION OF EFFECTS OF CHANGES IN EMERGENCY SERVICES

There has been an absolute paucity of studies examining the contribution of problems in emergency care to the frequency of unnecessary death and disability, and no adequate studies have been completed of the effects of change in the system on patient outcome. The few reports that have been completed suggest that perhaps one in every four or five persons who die of highway trauma on the North American continent might have survived if care were different (Perrine, M. W., et al., 1971; Gertner, H. R., et al., 1972; Frey, C. F., et al., 1969).

These studies have come from areas with different population densities and services, and have used different criteria of survivability. For example, a person who would be deemed beyond hope despite the best care and facilities that might reasonably be expected in a small rural community might be considered salvageable if he were injured near a major trauma center. Apparently no study has yet applied both criteria comparatively to the same series of patients.

One study in a rural area found that about half of the problems that were associated with death from survivable injury occurred during the prehospital phase of care, and the other half occurred during the hospital phase (Perrine, M. W., et al., 1971). In that report it was estimated that almost all persons who died at the crash site died of nonsurvivable injuries, whereas this was true for only about one-half of those who died after being moved.

Another study in an urban area of persons who died of abdominal injury after arrival at the hospital also reported that about one-half died of survivable injury, and further identified that those hospitals in which such deaths were most likely to occur were ones in which the staff had only occasional exposure to persons with this type of trauma (Gertner, H. R., et al., 1972). In each of these few reports, emphasis appears to have been placed on examination of fatalities because such studies are easier and less costly, and on highway deaths because autopsy data are much more likely to be available.

The purpose of evaluation is to identify to what extent, under what circumstances, and for what reason attempts to change the system have brought about desired effects, and to what extent, where, and why they

have been ineffective or even counterproductive. The institution of the "911" central dispatch system in New York City, for example, has been reported by New York newspapers to have resulted at least for a short time in clogging of the telephone lines with calls for minor emergencies or even nonemergencies, so that in some cases disasters have occurred because persons with real emergencies have been unable to get through to obtain help.

In order to observe change and its effects, it is first necessary to have baseline information systematically gathered over a sufficient period, both about the independent variables (such as numbers and types of trained persons) to be changed and about the dependent variables (such as death or disability) to be affected by these changes. Such data should be collected not only for the area in which the changes will be introduced, but also in a comparison area that presumably will not undergo similar alteration during the same period.

The reason for this is that the fact that anticipated changes occur in the program area does not necessarily mean that they would not have occurred even if no effort were made (and consequently money were saved). This can only be determined by comparison before and after with an area in which effort is not made. To date, no such evaluation appears to have been carried out of attempts to improve emergency services. Instead evaluation, where it has been attempted, is limited to examination of conditions before and after in the program area only.

Three types of before-after evaluation are possible (either with or without use of a comparison area). These are assessment of changes: (1) in "input" measures such as improvements in training or equipment; (2) in "process" such as the application of that training; and (3) in "outcome" such as reduced morbidity or mortality. It generally is assumed—although it is not necessarily true, as will be shown—that changes in input will invariably lead to changes in process, and that this in turn will affect outcome.

Most of the recent improvements in emergency care noted earlier have in fact been changes in input—better training and equipment, improved communications, changes in staffing patterns, better regional cooperation, etc. Only rarely are attempts being made to determine whether these result in actual changes in behavior, or if not, why not.

Frazier and colleagues (1973), for example, found that emergency medical technicians quite often do not make correct diagnoses in the presence of cardinal signs or symptoms, and sometimes, as in the case of persons with strokes, do not carry out mandated procedures such as giving oxygen, even if the correct diagnosis is made. This seems to occur because the EMTs fail to understand the underlying physiologic mechanisms, thus indicating the need for more basic training.

On the other hand, critique sessions held for ambulance and nursing personnel in Vermont suggest that appropriate procedures may not be carried out in some cases because in rural areas there is only limited opportunity to obtain sufficient experience to maintain knowledge and skills. In other cases, these individuals may not apply splints or perform other procedures because some physicians still believe ambulance and nursing personnel are incapable, and consequently forbid such activities with their patients. Sometimes police officers will not permit ambulance crews the time to do effective extrication or splinting at the scene even if traffic is not backed up. Such data can be obtained—and corrective actions taken—only if a specific attempt is made to determine what is happening and why.

Finally, there is the knotty problem of evaluation of outcome, which to date has never been attempted successfully. Because of the normal biologic gradient of disease, it can be anticipated that a large proportion of patients will improve no matter how inadequate services are; that some will not improve or will even get worse no matter how good the care; and that in only a small proportion of cases will there be an actual relationship between care provided and outcome. Although there is general agreement that satisfaction with care is an insensitive outcome measure, there is some controversy over whether the most appropriate criterion should be reduction in disability, decrease in case fatality ratio, avoidance of unnecessary deaths (and how is this to be assessed?), or some other measure or combination of measures.

Ideally, these measures as dependent variables should be examined in the presence of various combinations of system components. For example, case fatality ratios could be compared for patients with similar problems who are taken by "poor" ambulances to "poor" hospitals (as measured by input or process criteria), by "good" ambulances to "poor" hospitals, by "poor" ambulances to "good" hospitals, or by "good" ambulances to "good" hospitals. In the light of the apparent current trend toward increasingly sophisticated examination and improvement of the emergency care system, it is anticipated that appropriate outcome evaluation will be possible not too far in the future.

References

Frazier, W. H., Lally, P. P., and Cannon, J. F.: EMT performance evaluation: a clinical trial. Proceedings of 17th Conference of American Association For Automotive Medicine, Oklahoma City, Oklahoma, November 14–17, 1973, p. 279.

Frey, C. F., Huelke, D. F., and Gikas, P. W.: Resuscitation and survival in motor vehicle accidents. J. Trauma 9:292, 1969.

Gertner, H. R., Baker, S. P., Rutherford, R. B., and Spitz, W. U.: Evaluation of the management of vehicular fatalities secondary to abdominal injury. J. Trauma 12:425, 1972.

Gibson, G.: Evaluative criteria for emergency ambulance systems. Soc. Sci. Med. 7:425, 1973.

Gibson, G.: Guidelines for research and evaluation of emergency health services. Health Serv. Res. 89:99, 1974.

Haddon, W., Jr.: On the escape of tigers: an ecologic note. Am. J. Public Health 60:2229, 1970.

Hampton, O. P., Jr.: Transportation of the Injured. Bull. Amer. Coll. Surg. 45:55, 1960.

Hippocrates: On Injuries of the Head. In The Genuine Works of Hippocrates. Translated by Adams, F. Baltimore, Williams & Wilkins Co., 1939.

Kanwit, J. H., and Gettinger, C. E.: Hospital emergency services in Vermont. Burlington, Vermont, Vermont Department of Health, 1971.

Keller, G. D.: A study of bystander communications behavior in medical emergencies: report of a pilot study. Presented at American Public Health Association meeting in San Francisco, 1973.

King, B. G., and Sox, E. D.: An emergency medical services system: analysis of workload. Public Health Rep. 82:995, 1967.

Owens, C.: Colorado Study of Emergency Treatment Facilities. In Bi-Regional Emergency Medical Services Seminar Report. University of Nevada, Reno, 1965.

Perrine, M. W., Waller, J. A., and Harris, L. S.: Alcohol and highway safety: behavioral and medical aspects. Burlington, Vermont, Psychology Department, University of Vermont, 1971.

Waller, J. A.: Alcohol, Other Drugs, and Injury—Implications for Interagency Approaches. In Stoller, A., and Luby, B. (eds.): Interdisciplinary Seminars on Medical and Psychiatric Aspects of Alcohol and Drug Dependence. Australia, University of Melbourne, 1970.

Waller, J. A.: Emergency care for fatalities from injury and illness in the nonhighway setting. J. Trauma, 12:54, 1973.

Waller, J. A., Curran, R., and Noyes, F.: Traffic deaths: a preliminary study of urban and rural fatalities in California. Calif. Med. 101:272, 1964.

Youmans, R. L.: Emergency service experience. J. Kans. Med. Soc. 71:90, 1970.

Chapter 76   THE WORK ENVIRONMENT

George R. Schwartz

Whenever a word or phrase gets used consistently it is likely to have some validity. For years, physicians and nurses have spoken of the Emergency Department as "The Pit." This implies a seething, dangerous place set in some dank subterraneous chamber. Many Emergency Departments have been situated in badly lighted basement areas, poorly maintained, and often administratively forgotten. As medical sophistication has increased and respect for Emergency Departments and their function within a hospital has grown, newer facilities have evolved. Nonetheless, certain unpleasant elements often remain. As physicians, nurses, and paramedical personnel devote their careers to emergency medicine, it is important to isolate some of the less desirable aspects and to attempt to lessen their impact upon those working within such an environment.

The amount of sensory stimuli present often is enormous, with people moving in every direction, telephones ringing, monitors beeping, and everywhere a feeling of "what will come next?"—all in a framework of time pressure. These stimuli not only affect the nervous system but cause measurable physiologic effects, including peripheral vasoconstriction, hypertension, changes in bowel mobility, gastric acid and intestinal secretion, hormonal changes, and many others.

In addition, there are sights, sounds, and smells of human suffering and disease. In the Emergency Department the staff frequently is exposed to the results of violence, mangled bodies, and death in the young. Although hospital staffs have become hardened to seeing elderly people dying, it is always difficult to avoid the severe emotional effect of seeing young people dead in the prime of their lives—or even before that, in the innocence of childhood.

Certain degrees of stress and sensory input are important for function, but high continued stress leads to performance decrement, particularly when associated with sleep and circadian cycle alteration. Moreover, the 24-hour shifts at some Emergency Departments surpass the ability of most individuals to maintain efficiency. Such long shifts should be interdicted, since performance decrement reflects directly on quality of patient care. With 24-hour work periods, there is a pattern of performance deterioration. The performance peak occurs after six to ten hours, and then drops off to a low point at 22 hours. Thus, shift durations should not be longer than 12 hours in busy settings.

Patients come to Emergency Departments unprepared, frequently upset, in crisis, worried, or desperately afraid. Frequently they act out their emotional turmoil by hostility or anger directed at nurses or physicians.

Added to the potential turmoil is the need for 24-hour coverage and consequent shift changes. A situation easily manageable emotionally in the afternoon may require tremendous control at 4:00 A.M., especially during the first few nights before personal patterns have readjusted at least partially. The effects of circadian cycle shifts in hospital personnel have not been explored in depth. The greatest experience comes from the military and the space program in which studies were made of psychologic reactivity and performance at various hours. Those who change shifts frequently are in constant dysrhythmia and experience sleep disturbances,

1526

irritability, and decreased performance. Of particular importance is the decrease in frustration tolerance found in such people. In addition, with sleep alterations, the myriad diurnal or circadian rhythms of which more than 100 are known cannot readjust rapidly, and never do in some cases, even with prolonged night work. The effects of sleep deprivation and fatigue may be severe.

RESPONSES TO THE ENVIRONMENT

For some personnel the environment proves to be overwhelming, and after a brief period they choose other types of medical work.

However, a phenomenon has been observed in some of those who stay that, although milder, is similar to that in survivors of Hiroshima and soldiers from Vietnam. Robert Jan Lifton called it "Psychic Numbing." This phenomenon allows for survival in a stressful environment, but with less compassion toward others.

Medical education involves a great deal of desensitization. In order to work effectively, the physician and nurse must not respond too emotionally to a situation if a high level of functioning is to be preserved. A balance must be kept. The depersonalization and distance is necessary on some occasions, but the ability to shift gears psychically must be maintained.

As "psychic numbing" proceeds, there is more concentration on technical tasks, and less concern with the patient and his feelings. There is more intellectualization, and human concerns become expressed in technical jargon. In the early stages of this numbing, tempers are raw and people irritable, but if it is allowed to proceed to a more advanced stage there is increased apathy and acceptance.

The staff members in such units often experience changes in their lives including less general empathy, poor sleep, more rapid automobile driving, and a feeling of hypervigilance. Although this may permit adequate function with emotional protection, the end-result can be decreased morale and dehumanization of the Emergency or Critical Care Department, along with behavioral changes in some staff members.

How can improvements be made? How can the environment be engineered to reduce the need for emotional protection? Certain aspects cannot change. People in crisis will continue to respond to their inner turmoil. Death is a reality that will not go away. The Emergency Department staff must function and, to some extent, protect itself against excessive emotional response.

However, Emergency Departments can be designed to reduce sensory stimuli. For example, sound-proofing and newer types of carpeting can change sound levels significantly. Analysis of staff movements can allow development of a facility in which there is less walking and less confusion. Orderly procedures can help. Telephones need not ring (they can light, or can be designed to make modest sounds). Pages are rarely needed. The environment should be "bioengineered" for staff and patient comfort and privacy to the extent possible.

Those responsible for scheduling can do so with awareness of circadian cycles and can attempt to minimize transitions. Special rooms for the staff can be provided offering some "escape" for mealtimes. An important element is to allow expression of feelings and concerns. Staff meetings that offer an opportunity to discuss difficult problems, unexpected deaths, the management of grief, etc., can reduce the need to block out such emotions. Certainly, limitation of shift duration in busy Departments is important.

An actively involved social service department can assist, as can conferences with religious leaders. Conferences with psychiatrists, unless they are actively involved on a daily basis in the Department, are rarely necessary. In some instances they may have negative effects upon the staff.

THE PATIENT AND FAMILY—PEOPLE IN CRISIS

When people make an appointment with their physician, they have time to prepare, even if it is a frightening experience. However, when an acute medical situation arises—be it sudden accident or illness—they arrive unprepared at an Emergency Department. Faced by sudden forces outside their control, there often is a feeling of helplessness and frustration. Waiting increases the level of tension, as does uncertainty. If death comes, it is unexpected and catastrophic for the family.

The physician's traditional established

relationship with the patient and family allows him to be a comforting person, but when the physician is someone the family doesn't know, it adds to their uncertainty. This places an additional burden on the emergency physician—the need to establish trust and rapport quickly.

A great source of concern for the family is lack of knowledge about a patient's condition. When a loved one is behind closed doors, with no word from the nurse or physician, people think of the worst situation they can imagine. Similarly, patients upon whom procedures such as blood tests, x-rays, etc., are being performed become fearful from not knowing.

Medical staff should have a deep personal commitment to the skilled technology of medicine, but also should understand its broader humanistic caring function.

The Emergency Department staff must communicate to the greatest extent possible with the patient and his family. Long, elaborate technical explanations are not called for, but instead simple, easy-to-understand words. The patient should be reassured, even if it seems likely that death is imminent. If the patient's condition is deteriorating rapidly, the family should be told at frequent intervals that the staff is doing its best but that the situation is very grave. This allows some time for emotional preparation.

It is important that the physician should not delegate this task to others unless he cannot spare the few seconds required. If the clinical situation demands constant physician presence, a nurse should inform the family. It is a mistake to send someone with the least medical knowledge to do this.

In the waiting area, families should be provided with comfortable chairs. Simple things like the availability of warm drinks offer some comfort and a feeling of being in a caring environment. Human comfort should be the overriding concern in the design of waiting areas.

Recent developments have introduced ombudsmen, neighborhood health workers, and others who provide a conduit for information and who can decrease tension in the waiting areas. These workers should be employed when available, but not as a replacement for the physician's or nurse's involvement with the family. Too frequently, such people are used as messengers when the nurses and physicians find it difficult to meet the families.

The truth is sometimes hard to confront that death is an inevitable part of life, and that a patient dying despite the maximum concern and treatment by the physician and other staff does not represent failure. Part of the art of medicine, which must be employed frequently in an Emergency Department, is the knowledge of how to provide comfort to the survivors. They may have great guilt if there was a delay in bringing the patient, or may regret some small conflict they had with the person now dead and beyond apologies. The physician can do much at this time to reduce needless guilt, and to offer support if their world seems to have crashed.

Social workers can provide a good deal of assistance, but should not supplant the physician and nurse. Religious leaders may be of great help, and suitable telephone numbers should be available so that they may be summoned.

A very real danger, however, is the delegation of the caring functions to nonmedical personnel, leaving a cadre of dehumanized technicians. Henry Ford originally began with one man seeing an automobile through all its stages. Then, for efficiency, he developed a highly specialized group of workers—but he knew the dangers and predicted that the development of specialization would lead to technicians concerned with their part, but not the whole.

There is a parallel here with some aspects of medicine: although perhaps not to such an extreme extent, similar tendencies are obvious, e.g., an increased concentration on small specialty areas. In the Emergency Department there is a continual need to look at the whole patient in the context of his family or friends. Whether the emergency is minor or major, they come seeking relief. The emergency staff is in a unique and privileged position to offer them relief and, if need be, to refer them into an appropriate system of continuing care. But "care" means just that. No organic disease exists apart from a person in distress. Patients don't consult physicians because certain organs are affected, but because they feel ill.

Because of the variety of demands presently imposed on the emergency physician, we must await future developments that should reduce the number of patients presenting at Emergency Departments, but will increase the percentage of those with more serious conditions. This will allow more time for each patient, and will permit the flowering of the art of the emergency physician.

References

Adams, O. S., and Chiles, W. D.: Prolonged human performance as a function of the work-rest cycle. Aerosp. Med. *34*:132, 1963.

Aschoff, J.: Circadian rhythms in man. Science *148*:1247, 1965.

Bartter, F., Delea, C. S., and Halberg, F.: A map of blood and urinary changes related to circadian variations in adrenal cortical functions and normal subjects. Ann. N.Y. Acad. Sci. 98:969, 1962.

Beranek, L. L.: Noise Reduction. New York, McGraw-Hill Book Co., 1960.

Bernard, V. W., Ottenberg, P., and Redl, F.: Dehumanization: A Composite Psychological Defense in Relation to Modern War. *In* Schwebel, M. (ed.): Behavioral Science and Human Survival. Palo Alto, Calif., Stanford University Press, 1965.

Brantigan, J. W.: Physician fatigue – some lessions from the cockpit. Hosp. Physician, Sept., 1973, p. 13.

Broadbent, D. C.: Effects of Noise on Behavior. *In* Harris, C. M. (ed.): Handbook of Noise Control. New York, McGraw-Hill Book Co., 1957, pp. 1–34.

Cooper, G. D., Adams, H. B., and Cohen, L. D.: Personality changes after sensory deprivation. J. Nerv. Ment. Dis. *140(2)*:103, 1965.

Corcoran, D. W. J.: Influence of task complexity and practice on performance after loss of sleep. J. Appl. Psychol. *48*:339, 1964.

Falk, S. A., and Woods, N. F.: Hospital noise levels and potential health hazards. N. Engl. J. Med. 289:15, 774, 1974.

Hale, H. B.: Adrenal cortical activity associated with exposure to low frequency sounds. Am. J. Physiol. *171*:732, 1952.

Harrison, T. R.: The most distressing symptom. J.A.M.A. *198*:1, 52, 1966.

Jerison, H. J.: Effects of noise on human performance. J. Appl. Physiol. *43(2)*:96, 1959.

Kales, A.: Psychophysiological studies of insomnia. Ann. Intern. Med. *71*:625, 1969.

Kleitman, N.: Sleep and Wakefulness. Chicago, University of Chicago Press, 1965.

Levi, L.: Emotional Stress. New York, American Elsevier Publishing Co., 1967.

Lifton, R. J.: Home from the war, the psychology of survival. Atlantic, Nov., 1972, pp. 56–73.

Luby, E. D.: Biochemical, psychological and behavioral responses to sleep deprivation. Ann. N.Y. Acad. Sci. 96:71, 1962.

Luce, T. S.: Vigilance as a function of stimulus variety and response complexity. Hum. Factors 6:101, 1964.

Rogers, D.: The doctor himself must become the treatment. Pharos, Oct., 1974, pp. 124–129.

Schwartz, G. R.: Psychological and behavioral responses of hospital staff involved in the care of the critically ill. Crit. Care Med. 2:1, 48, 1974.

Schwartz, G. R.: Psychic numbing in the Emergency Department. Emergency Medical Services 4:1, 31, 1975.

Selye, H.: Stress and Disease. Science *122*:625, 1955.

Smith, E. L., and Laird, D. A.: The loudness of auditory stimuli which affects stomach contractions in human beings. J. Acoust. Soc. Am. 2:94, 1930.

Von Gierke, H. E.: On noise and vibration exposure critera. Arch. Environ. Health *11*:327, 1965.

Wilkins, W. L.: Group Behavior in Long-Term Isolation. *In* Appley, M. H., and Trumbull, R. (eds.): Psychological Stress, New York, Appleton-Century-Crofts, 1966.

Wilkinson, R. J.: The effect of lack of sleep on visual watch-keeping. Q. J. Exp. Psychol. *12(1)*:36, 1960.

Chapter 77

EMERGENCY CARE, HEALTH MAINTENANCE ORGANIZATIONS, AND NATIONAL HEALTH INSURANCE

A. The Health Maintenance Organization
B. National Health Insurance

A. THE HEALTH MAINTENANCE ORGANIZATION

Thomas N. Perloff

The Health Maintenance Organization (HMO) as an organized health care delivery system has a great potential for the introduction of innovations into the provision of emergency care services. Because HMOs are contractually responsible for providing "total" health care, they must emphasize the accessibility of primary care, which in turn reduces the need for "improper" utilization of emergency care resources. Revenues are fixed yearly by the prepaid premium, so that HMOs must budget expenditures carefully and must scrutinize closely all expensive modalities such as emergency care. Also, because they are organized delivery systems, HMOs have the medical management structure to make changes in areas such as manpower utilization, medical record-keeping, and quality assurance that are integral to the delivery of effective and efficient emergency medical care.

PROVISION OF EMERGENCY CARE

The HMO is structured to receive prepaid payments from subscribers and to provide the medically determined number of specified services. Payment to the provider is made on a capitation basis and includes both the benefits of hospital care and provision of all professional medical services. Financial incentives are derived from maintaining health, thereby minimizing the utilization of hospital services, which are the most costly mode of care. The prototypal HMOs are organized on a closed panel group practice basis, but a number of open panel "independent practice associations" have been organized recently.

HMOs provide emergency care in a variety of ways. Those with large enrollments are able to provide emergency care by utilizing their own delivery systems. For example, the Kaiser Health Plan operates its own hospitals and Emergency Departments, and the Health Insurance Plan of Greater New York operates a centralized off-hour emergency physician service. Moderate-sized HMOs are able to provide some emergency care directly and contract with existing emergency care systems for the remainder. Some of these HMOs maintain separate emergency or triage units, keep skeletal staffs in their centers for off-hour emergencies, or have detailed communications systems for arranging for emergency care. Small and new HMOs utilize existing community emergency care resources, concentrating on improving access for their enrollees and providing competent follow-up care. In all cases, HMOs provide indemnity insurance coverage for out-of-area emergencies.

EMPHASIS ON PRIMARY CARE

The first innovative aspect of the Health Maintenance Organization's delivery of emergency care follows from its emphasis on primary care. A defining characteristic of the HMO is its emphasis on the provision of comprehensive and accessible primary care. It is contractually bound to provide first access care, to provide care over a specified time period, and to integrate information about the utilization of specialty resources for the enrollee. The emphasis on health maintenance and preventive medicine implies a commitment to primary preventive action and to the early detection of disease. This emphasis is expressed in financial terms through the HMO's "first dollar" coverage of professional medical services.

HMOs, accordingly, are organized around the provision of primary care. The most common form of organization is the multi-specialty group practice. The hospital phase of care is still critical in an individual case, but its organizational significance is secondary. New enrollees are encouraged to make contact with the HMO before an acute episode develops in order to establish a data base, select a personal physician, and educate the individual in the workings of the system. A continuing emphasis is placed on utilizing the primary care provider as the entry point into the rest of the health care delivery system.

This HMO emphasis on primary care has important implications for the delivery of emergency medical care. First, the enrollee has a guaranteed source of primary care and therefore does not need to use the Emergency Department as his "family physician;" emergency resources can then be used properly for the delivery of emergency care. Second, every enrollee has access to a well organized medical data base to facilitate timely treatment. Third, the enrollee has an explicitly identified personal physician who can be consulted for further information and who can continue the management of a prolonged treatment plan. Lastly, the HMO has accepted the responsibility for organizing a specialty and "extraordinary" care service system to supplement the emergency care system.

BUDGETING OF RESOURCES

The HMO's budget is substantially set by its premium rate. Unlike traditional fee-for-service practices, the HMO receives no additional revenues for providing additional services. Indeed, there is some fear that the HMO will withhold some medically necessary services as a means of containing expenditures, but against this can be set: (1) the possibility that failure to treat may lead to the need for more expensive treatments in the future; (2) the development of quality assurance programs; and (3) the existence of other legal and contractual checks. The fact remains that the HMO has a strong legal and financial incentive to economize on the use of expensive modalities of care.

The HMO can address this by negotiating as a sophisticated and large purchaser of community emergency resources. In addition to its market position, the HMO can point to other factors that can lower cost, such as the existence and accessibility of a data base and of clear lines of referral for follow-up. Furthermore, the HMO has a strong incentive to organize patient health education programs about the judicious use of emergency resources. It must balance the desire to deny payment for improper Emergency Department visits against the need to keep its enrollees satisfied with their membership. Lastly, because the HMO is a closed system, it must have detailed data

on which to make business decisions about alternative methods of delivering emergency care. It should be able to determine how much its enrollees are spending for emergency care outside the system and to balance this against the cost of setting up more sophisticated internal emergency care facilities.

ORGANIZATION OF THE DELIVERY SYSTEM

The last innovative way in which the HMO delivers emergency care relates to the fact that it is an organized health care delivery system. This implies that organizational and management insights have been applied to the way in which care is delivered. The HMO, thus, has both the capability to disseminate new technologies and the financial incentive to economize on the use of health care resources.

One example of this capability is the use of health manpower. The HMO can employ new health manpower such as "middle level" practitioners (e.g., nurse clinicians, physician's assistants) because it has the medical management structure to use and supervise them properly. As a group practice, the HMO has multiple professional resources to develop treatment protocols, to supervise the laying-on-of-hands, and to audit the activity of the nurse practitioner or physician's assistant. Because of its financing mechanism it has the ability to substitute resources so that the most expensive factor of production, the physician's time, can be utilized optimally. Lastly, the prepaid group practice structure allows the practitioner to schedule educational time systematically and to evaluate different treatment approaches. HMOs accordingly have utilized emergency medical technicians, developed the role of the nurse practitioner as a triage agent, and worked out roles for other "paraprofessionals" in the delivery of emergency care.

Another example of the advantage of the HMO as an organized delivery system involves the medical record and flow of medical information. Most HMOs use the problem-oriented medical system that includes development of a data base, charting in a problem-oriented manner, use of treatment protocols, and the ability to audit treatment. This medical practice system is consistent with preventive medicine emphasis on primary prevention and early detection of disease. Because the HMO is a closed health care delivery system, comprehensive patient medical information can easily be made accessible to the myriad of health care providers who might need it. As noted above, this can be crucial in the delivery of emergency medical care, since it implies that consistent data is readily available.

A final example of the advantages of an organized delivery system such as an HMO in the delivery of emergency care involves quality assurance. Beside the structural factors such as group practice, a total medical record system, and the use of multiple professionals, the HMO has financial and contractual incentives to develop a well-articulated quality assurance program. The HMO must be able to demonstrate to its subscribers that it is not scrimping on the delivery of care as a cost-containing measure. Quality assurance programs are important in the area of emergency care because emergency treatment has significant impact, is a field prone to errors, and is extremely visible.

In summary, evolution of the HMO concept is in its early phase, as is maturation of the emergency medical care system in the U.S. Certain attributes of the HMO system will greatly influence the development of emergency services. The degree to which planned linkages occur will be a critical issue in determining the structure and function of a total community system of health care.

References

Gumbiner, R.: HMO. Putting It All Together. St. Louis, C. V. Mosby Co., 1975.

Kress, J. R., and Singer, J.: HMO Handbook: A Guide for Development of Prepaid Group Practice Health Maintenance Oorganizations. Rockville, Md., Aspen Systems Corp., 1975.

MacColl, W. A.: Group Practice and Prepayment of Medical Care. Washington, D.C., Public Affairs Press, 1966.

Solomon, M. A., and Batt, T.: Analysis of the Emergency Medical Services in Health Maintenance Organizations. Washington, D.C., Group Health Association of America, Inc., 1975.

Somers, A. R.: The Kaiser-Permanente Medical Care Program. A symposium. New York, The Commonwealth Fund, 1971.

B. NATIONAL HEALTH INSURANCE

Thomas N. Perloff

National Health insurance represents a nation-wide approach to restructuring the financing of health care on a more equitable basis. It can be combined with a reshaping of the delivery system, as in the case of the British National Health System, or can be simply a financing mechanism, as in the case of the prototypal German "mandated health insurance" approach. There can be significant variation in the degree to which income or purchasing ability is redistributed, in the definition of covered health services, and in the universality of individuals covered.

Major national health insurance initiatives have been proposed periodically in the U.S. In this century, major proposals have been made during the Progressive Era in the 1910s, during the New Deal era in the 1930s, immediately after the second World War, and in the late 1960s and 1970s. The most recent thrusts have been spurred by the catastrophic financial consequences of major illness, and by the significant over-all rise in health care cost. All the parties most intimately involved in the delivery of health care—including organized health professionals, health insurers, organized consumers, legislators, and governmental health and welfare administrators—seem to agree on the need for national health insurance, but a political consensus on the exact nature of the program has not yet coalesced.

Even though a national health insurance program has not yet been passed into law, a number of consequences and questions for the delivery of emergency care can be discerned.

MORE UNIVERSAL COVERAGE OF EMERGENCY CARE

There is apparent general agreement that the financing of emergency care should be universally assured, permitting the development and operation of an effective system of care for all potential consumers. Other problems will remain.

(a) No assurance of availability. National health insurance might assure the financing of emergency medical care, but not the availability of that care. Financing is just one of the constraints that limit the availability of emergency care in geographic locales such as the inner city, rural areas, and other underserved communities. Other constraints, such as improvement of facilities, personal insecurity, and the amenities of practice, will have to be addressed directly before emergency care is universally available.

(b) Uncertainty as to the breadth of coverage. Although the need for universal coverage of emergency care is recognized generally, the question of the breadth of services to be covered is still open. Some open questions are: (1) what constitutes emergency ill health?; (2) will covered services be defined by the content of the service or by the provider who performs the service?; (3) how will extraordinary care services be covered?; and (4) how extensive will be the definition of first contact care to be covered?

MORE GOVERNMENTAL ACCOUNTABILITY

As the proportion of public funds supporting emergency care increases, the amount of governmental supervision of these services also will increase. The public will need to be assured that its tax dollars are being expended properly and effectively. The technology of such supervision is in its infancy, but government will be forced to refine this capability as the amounts of public expenditure grow. Accountability will demand the following.

(a) Improved information systems. One of the first requirements for increased public accountability will be the need for improved and standardized information systems. A consensus will have to be reached on (1) the stage in the care process at which this information is needed; (2) what nomenclature will be utilized; (3) how the information will be transmitted; and (4) how patient confidentiality will be protected.

(b) More concentration of outcomes. As the evaluation process becomes more sophisticated, a greater emphasis will be placed on the outcomes of care. In less sophisticated stages of evaluation of technology, the focus has been on the structure and process of providing emergency care. Variables in these areas are easier to measure so that meaningful results can be educed at relatively low cost. As the technology advances, it will become increasingly possible to analyze the outcomes of alternative approaches to providing care.

MORE APPROPRIATE UTILIZATION OF EMERGENCY CARE RESOURCES

As noted above, the main driving forces behind current interest in national health insurance are the catastrophic costs of prolonged illness and the general rise in the cost of all care. The existence of these problems suggests that there are structural imbalances in the American health care delivery system. Correcting these will necessitate more changes than simply adjusting the financing schemes. Emergency care resources will need to be utilized more appropriately.

(a) Increased planning. Government will undoubtedly place a greater emphasis on health planning as it picks up more of the emergency care tab. Many issues still need to be resolved, such as the responsibilities of different levels of government and the roles of the different parties in the planning process. Emergency care will be an early focus of these increased activities because it is highly visible, expensive, and not well organized today. Thus, there will be an even greater emphasis on categorization and regionalization of care as the role of government increases.

(b) Improved interface with primary care. If emergency care resources are to be utilized more appropriately, greater emphasis will need to be placed on the interface with primary health care. There will be an increased concern with medical information exchange between subsystems, with patient education concerning the proper utilization of facilities, and with the fixing of professional responsibility for continuity of care. This will change the nature and tempo of most Emergency Departments so that they can focus more directly on emergency care.

(c) Increased unit cost of emergency care. One of the corollaries of these activities is that the cost of a unit of emergency care service will increase, since Emergency Departments will no longer be expected to handle as many routine first access problems, but instead true emergencies. This will reduce the number of visits and shrink the activity base over which overhead costs are spread. Those emergency facilities that continue to exist will be more specialized, and thus more expensive resources will be utilized to a much fuller extent. Society should benefit from this, however, not only because emergencies will be treated more effectively, but also because primary care will be provided in a more appropriate setting.

In summary, a clear political consensus is emerging on the need to make the financing of health care more equitable through national health insurance. Whatever the final form of this financing program, there will be profound implications for the delivery of emergency care. There will be more universal coverage of emergency care, but no assurances of availability or comprehensiveness. Government will increasingly demand accountability over the quality of service, necessitating improved information systems and concentration on the outcomes of care. Lastly, there will be explicit public pressure to improve the utilization of emergency care resources through planning and better articulated interfaces with primary health care systems. Thus, national health insurance should provide a significant impetus toward rationalizing the financing and organization of emergency care.

References

Davis, K.: National Health Insurance. Washington, D.C., Bookings Institution, 1975.

Eilers, R. D., and Moyerman, S. S.: National Health Insurance. Homewood, Ill., Richard D. Irwin, Inc., 1971.

Hirshfield, D. S.: The Lost Reform. The Campaign For Compulsory Health Insurance in the United States from 1932 to 1943. Cambridge, Mass., Harvard University Press, 1970.

INDEX

INDEX

Numbers in *italics* refer to illustrations; those followed by (t) refer to tables.

i